BRIEF CONTENTS

T0198251

Evolve®

YOU'VE JUST PURCHASED
MORE THAN
A TEXTBOOK!

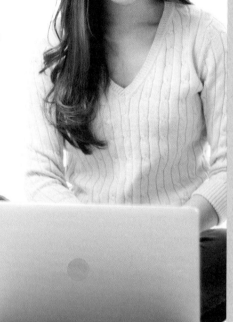

Enhance your learning with Evolve Student Resources.

These online study tools and exercises can help deepen your understanding of textbook content so you can be more prepared for class, perform better on exams, and succeed in your course.

Activate the complete learning experience that comes with each NEW textbook purchase by registering with your scratch-off access code at

http://evolve.elsevier.com/kostelnick/longterm/

If your school uses its own Learning Management System, your resources may be delivered on that platform. Consult with your instructor.

If you rented or purchased a used book and the scratch-off code at right has already been revealed, the code may have been used and cannot be re-used for registration. To purchase a new code to access these valuable study resources, simply follow the link above.

KOSTELNICK
Scratch Gently
to Reveal Code

REGISTER TODAY!

ELSEVIER

You can now purchase Elsevier products on Evolve!
Go to evolve.elsevier.com/shop to search and browse for products.

2019v1.0

NINTH EDITION

MOSBY'S TEXTBOOK FOR
LONG-TERM CARE
NURSING ASSISTANTS

Clare Kostelnick, RN, BSN
Professor Emeritus and Nurse Assistant Instructor
Des Moines Area Community College
Ames, Iowa

ELSEVIER

Elsevier
3251 Riverport Lane
St. Louis, Missouri 63043

MOSBY'S TEXTBOOK FOR LONG-TERM CARE NURSING
ASSISTANTS, NINTH EDITION

ISBN: 978-0-323-87488-5

Copyright © 2024 by Elsevier, Inc. All rights reserved.

No part of this publication may be reproduced or transmitted in any form or by any means, electronic or mechanical, including photocopying, recording, or any information storage and retrieval system, without permission in writing from the publisher. Details on how to seek permission, further information about the Publisher's permissions policies and our arrangements with organizations such as the Copyright Clearance Center and the Copyright Licensing Agency, can be found at our website: www.elsevier.com/permissions.

This book and the individual contributions contained in it are protected under copyright by the Publisher (other than as may be noted herein).

Notice

Practitioners and researchers must always rely on their own experience and knowledge in evaluating and using any information, methods, compounds or experiments described herein. Because of rapid advances in the medical sciences, in particular, independent verification of diagnoses and drug dosages should be made. To the fullest extent of the law, no responsibility is assumed by Elsevier, authors, editors or contributors for any injury and/or damage to persons or property as a matter of products liability, negligence or otherwise, or from any use or operation of any methods, products, instructions, or ideas contained in the material herein.

Previous editions copyrighted 2020, 2015, 2011, 2007, 2003, 1999, 1994, and 1988

Executive Content Strategist: Sonya Seigafuse
Content Development Manager: Danielle Frazier
Senior Content Development Specialist: Maria Broeker
Publishing Services Manager: Deepthi Unni
Project Manager: Sindhuraj Thulasingam
Design Direction: Ryan Cook

Printed in Canada

Last digit is the print number: 9 8 7 6 5 4 3 2 1

Working together
to grow libraries in
developing countries

www.elsevier.com • www.bookaid.org

To my husband, Charlie, for his love and support for over 50 years.

And to my children and grandchildren who bless me every day with their inspiration, love, and devotion.

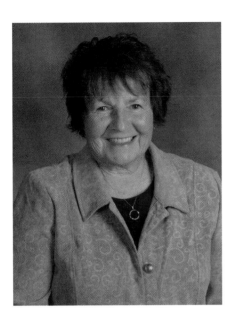

Clare Kostelnick is professor emeritus at Des Moines Area Community College, where she continues to teach nursing assistant courses. She received her BSN from the Brokaw School of Nursing of Illinois Wesleyan University, Bloomington, Illinois. She began her career as a registered nurse serving in the US Army Nurse Corps. Her assignments included Ft. Sam Houston, Texas; Ft. Ord, California; and Ft. Leonard Wood, Missouri. Having achieved the rank of captain, she spent most of her military career working in emergency care.

Clare's 49 years of nursing experience also includes working in critical care as a staff nurse, a home care and hospice staff nurse, a long-term care staff nurse and consultant, and a coordinator of an assisted living facility. While at Des Moines Area Community College, she taught health occupations, medical terminology, emergency care, and CPR. She has taught nursing assistant classes for over 25 years.

Having worked as a nursing assistant herself during high school and college, Clare identifies with students as they begin their rewarding careers caring for others. She loves the profession of nursing and enjoys passing on to students the enormous possibilities that this career offers. She feels honored to play a role in the formation of future health care professionals. Clare is active in volunteer work with her parish and veterans' groups. She and her husband, Charlie, reside on their acreage, Timberlea Farm, near the Des Moines River Valley, where they grow Aronia berries. They enjoy traveling and camping but especially look forward to family gatherings when their five grown children, their spouses, and ten grandchildren return to the farm.

REVIEWERS

Mary Barr, RN
Instructor (retired)
Patient Care Technician
Lancaster County Career and Technology Center
Willow Street, Pennsylvania

Kathy R. House, BSN, MSN-Edu, RN
Dean of Health Sciences
J Renee College
Elgin, Illinois

Suzanne Pinos, MSN
Adjunct Instructor, Nursing
Palm Beach State College
Lake Worth, Florida

Cherie R. Rebar, PhD, MBA, RN, CNE, CNEcl, COI, FAADN
Professor of Nursing
Galen College of Nursing
Louisville, Kentucky

Fatima D. Reyes, RN, MS, CCRN
Program Coordinator
Avid CNA School
Streamwood, Illinois

Katianna Yoakum, BSN(c)
University of Kentucky
Lexington, Kentucky

ACKNOWLEDGMENTS

The contributions of many individuals and agencies have made this ninth edition of *Mosby's Textbook for Long-Term Care Nursing Assistants* possible. I would especially like to express my appreciation to the following:

- My colleagues at Des Moines Area Community College, especially Pam Vandenberg, RN, MSN, and my daughter, Christine Sorensen, RN, BSN, for their ongoing support and excellent nursing advice.
- Connie Booth, RN, MSN, for providing contact information that opened up this writing opportunity for me.
- Cathy Wetzeler, RN, BSN, CWOCN, for her expert consultation on wound care.
- Mary Madison, RN, RAC-CT, CDP, for her contribution to electronic records and MDS content, and to PointClickCare for screen shots.
- The staff of the Eastern Star Masonic Home (Boone, IA), especially Mona Lerdal, RN, DON, for advice and help with photo shoots.
- The staff of Northcrest Community (Ames, IA), especially Amy Van Landen, RN, DON, for advice and help with photoshoots and for welcoming students to their facility for valuable clinical experience.
- Steve Lochray, RN (Director of Clinical Services), of Green Hills Retirement Center (Ames, IA) for assistance with photographs and clinical experiences.
- Elizabeth Hummer, MA, CCC-SLP, for her contribution to dysphagia content and corresponding photography. Special thanks to model Patricia Bennett.
- Tony Mack and Brian O'Toole, physical therapists from Boone County Hospital Rehabilitation Services, for their advice and photo assistance.
- Karen Vanbuskirk, RN, for her expert advice on low-vision concepts.
- Father Tim Johnson for his spiritual guidance, concern, and attention to residents of local care centers and for agreeing to a photo.
- Those individuals who served as reviewers for this ninth edition: Mary Barr, Fatima Demonteverde Reyes, Kathy R. House, Suzanne Pinos, Cherie Rebar, and Katianna Yoakum.
- The artists at Graphic World Illustration Studios in St. Louis, MO, for their excellent artwork.
- The talented and dedicated Elsevier/Mosby staff, especially:
  - Sonya Seigafuse (Executive Content Strategist, Education Content) for overseeing this edition.
  - Maria Broeker (Senior Content Development Specialist), whom I have been extremely fortunate to work with over the years. Maria quickly found a solution to any problem, question, or obstacle. She is extremely efficient, thorough, patient, and kind. Her experience and professionalism contributed greatly to the success of this edition.
  - Sindhuraj Thulasingam (Project Manager) for providing advice in a timely manner and keeping the project on track.
- My husband, Charles Kostelnick, whose writing experience and talent far outweigh mine. While working fervently to meet his own publication deadlines, he would always stop to help me with my current dilemma. He has been there by my side for 48 years to offer expert English language advice. Thanks, Charlie, for all your support!
- I would also like to express sincere appreciation to those individuals residing in long-term care centers. Often, I would sit with them in their rooms and listen to their stories—filled with wisdom, sacrifice, loss, and love. They have much to teach the younger generations. They candidly shared with me their feelings, ideas, and suggestions about topics that would improve their stay in care centers. These heartfelt conversations echo in my mind as I try my best to enable students to offer competent and compassionate care to seniors.

And finally, I am grateful for the input and inspiration received from students who use these resources. I so admire your fresh, energetic, and altruistic view on life. Your work as a nursing assistant will be one of the most rewarding careers you will ever experience!

Clare Kostelnick

As with previous editions of *Mosby's Textbook for Long-Term Care Nursing Assistants,* the ninth edition serves to prepare students to function as nursing assistants in nursing centers. This textbook serves the needs of students and instructors in community colleges, technical schools, high schools, nursing centers, and other agencies. As students complete their education, the book is a valuable resource for the competency test review. As part of one's personal library, the book is a reference for the nursing assistant who seeks to review or learn additional information for safe care.

Residents are presented as *persons* with dignity and value who have a past, a present, and a future. Caring—understanding, protecting, and respecting the person's rights—and respecting residents as persons with dignity and value are attitudes conveyed throughout the book.

Nursing assistants of today and tomorrow must have a firm understanding of the legal principles affecting their role. Both federal and state laws directly and indirectly define their roles, range of functions, and limitations. Nursing assistant roles and functions also vary among states and nursing centers. Therefore, emphasis is given to nursing assistant responsibilities, limitations, and professional boundaries that focus on the legal and ethical aspects of the role. This includes reporting abuse.

Nursing assistant functions and role limits also depend on effective delegation. Building on the delegation principles presented in Chapter 1, *Delegation Guidelines* boxes are presented as they relate to procedures. They empower the student to seek information from the nurse and the care plan about critical aspects of the procedure and the observations to report and record. Step 1 of most procedures refers the student to the appropriate *Delegation Guidelines* boxes.

Since the first edition, safety and comfort have been core values of *Mosby's Textbook for Long-Term Care Nursing Assistants.* Therefore *Promoting Safety and Comfort* boxes focus the student's attention on the need to be safe and cautious and to promote comfort when giving care. Step 1 of most procedures refers the student to the appropriate *Promoting Safety and Comfort* boxes.

Besides legal aspects, delegation, and safety and comfort, work ethics also affect how nursing assistants function. To foster a positive work ethic, Chapter 3 focuses on workplace behaviors and practices. The goal is for the nursing assistant to be a proud, professional member of the nursing and health teams.

Being a productive and efficient member of the nursing team requires teamwork, time management, and communication skills. Good communication skills are needed when interacting with residents. Two features address these issues:

- *Teamwork and Time Management* boxes suggest ways to efficiently work with and help other nursing team members.
- *Focus on Communication* boxes suggest what to say and questions to ask when interacting with residents, visitors, and the nursing team.

- Persons with dementia present other challenges. *Residents With Dementia* boxes provide insights and care measures to promote the quality of life for persons with dementia.

ORGANIZATIONAL STRATEGIES

These concepts and principles—the resident as a person, ethical and legal aspects, delegation, safety and comfort, and work ethics—serve as the guiding framework for this book. Other organizational strategies and values include:

- Understanding the work setting and the individuals in that setting
- Respecting residents as physical, social, psychologic, and spiritual beings with basic needs and protected rights
- Respecting personal choice and the person's dignity
- Appreciating the role of cultural heritage and religion in health and illness practices
- Understanding that knowledge about body structure and function is needed to give safe care and to safely perform nursing skills
- Following the principle that learning proceeds from the simple to the complex
- Recognizing that certain concepts and functions are foundational—safety, body mechanics, and preventing infection are central to other procedures
- Embracing the nursing process as the basis for planning and delivering nursing care and the role that nursing assistants play in assisting with the process

CONTENT ISSUES

With every edition, revision and content decisions are made. When changes are made in laws or in guidelines and standards issued by government agencies, accrediting agencies, or associations, the decisions are easy. Content and new figure decisions also are based on state curricula and competency testing services. Reviews from instructors in various regions of the country and from those practicing in long-term care settings played an important contribution to the revisions of this edition. Every attempt is made to make the book as up to date as possible, with changes sometimes made right before publication. With such issues in mind, new content includes:

- COVID-19 infection control concepts
- New Centers for Disease Control and Prevention (CDC) illustrations of donning and removing PPE
- Detailed description of masks and other PPE
- Stop the Bleed concepts and illustrations
- New information from International Diet Dysphagia Standardisation Initiative (IDDSI) concerning dysphagia and dietary intake

- Pressure injury classifications
- Eye wash station
- External female catheter
- Ceiling-mounted lift systems
- Shredding bin for confidential documents
- Blanket warmer
- Gown with shoulder snaps
- Infrared thermometers
- Wrist manometers for blood pressure
- Emergency cart
- Evacuation plans
- Expanded content on depression
- Expanded content on autism spectrum disorder
- New information from the National Institute of Health (NIH) on helping someone in emotional pain and newly instituted 988 emergency number

FEATURES AND DESIGN

Besides content issues, attention is given to improving the book's features and designs (see Student Preface). It has been my experience while teaching nursing assistant courses that most students begin this training very enthusiastically and motivated. It is our job, as instructors, to kindle that flame and to help students develop the skills and competence they will need to be successful. The features previously described are designed to take learning to the next level. When students readily understand how the material can be applied, they gain ownership of that knowledge. It is my most sincere wish that this book will be a valuable resource as you help train the students that will be caring for our loved ones in long-term care centers. May they treasure the value of offering care that is competent, respectful, dignified, and compassionate.

Clare Kostelnick

This book was designed for you. It was designed to help you learn. The book is a useful resource as you gain experience and expand your knowledge.

This preface gives some study guidelines and helps you use the book. When given a reading assignment, do you read from the first page to the last page without stopping? How much do you remember? You will learn more if you use a study system. A useful study system has these steps:

- Survey or preview
- Question
- Read and record
- Recite and review

PREVIEW

Before you start a reading assignment, preview or survey the assignment. This gives you an idea of what the assignment covers. It also helps you recall what you already know about the subject. Carefully look over the assignment. Preview the chapter title, headings, subheadings, and terms or ideas in bold print or italics. Also survey the objectives, key terms, key abbreviations, boxes, and review questions at the end of the chapter. Previewing only takes a few minutes. Remember, previewing helps you become familiar with the material.

QUESTION

After previewing, you need to form questions to answer while you read. Questions should relate to what might be asked on a test or how the information applies to giving care. Use the title, headings, and subheadings to form questions. Avoid questions that have one-word answers. Questions that begin with what, how, or why are helpful. While reading, you may find that a question does not help you study. If so, just change the question. Remember, questioning sets a purpose for reading, so changing a question only makes this step more useful.

READ AND RECORD

Reading is the next step. Reading is more productive after determining what you already know and what you need to learn. Read to find answers to your questions. The purpose of reading is to:

- Gain new information
- Connect new information to what you already know

Break the assignment into smaller parts. Then answer your questions as you read each part. Also mark important information—underline, highlight, or make notes. Underlining and highlighting remind you of what you need to learn. Go back and review the marked parts later. Making notes results in more immediate learning. To make notes, write down important information in the margins or in a notebook. Use words and statements to jog your memory about the material. At times, you may have further questions about the material you have read. Write these questions in your notes and bring them to your next class session. It may help to have the instructor explain the concept further.

You need to remember what you read. To do so, work with the information. Organize information into a study guide. Study guides have many forms. Diagrams or charts show relationships or steps in a process. Creating simple flash cards is an easy method to memorize definitions for abbreviations. Notetaking in outline format is also very useful. The following is a sample outline.

1. Main heading
   a. Second level
   b. Second level
      i. Third level
      ii. Third level
2. Main heading

RECITE AND REVIEW

Finally, recite and review. Use your notes and study guides. Answer the questions you formed earlier. Also answer other questions that came up when reading and answering the Review Questions at the end of a chapter. Answer all questions aloud (recite).

Reviewing is more about *when* to study rather than what to study. You already determined what to study during the preview, question, and reading steps. The best times to review are right after the first study session, 1 week later, and before a quiz or test.

This book was also designed to help you study. Special design features are described on the next pages.

I hope you enjoy learning and your work. You and your work are important. You and the care you give make a difference in the person's life!

Objectives tell what is presented in the chapter.

Key Terms are the important words and phrases in the chapter. Definitions are given for each term. The key terms introduce you to the chapter content. They are also a useful study guide.

Key Abbreviations are a quick reference of the abbreviations used in the chapter. They are listed after Key Terms.

Focus on Rehabilitation boxes alert you to considerations and insights about rehabilitation and restorative care.

Blue, bolded type is used to highlight the key terms in the text. You again see the key term and read its definition. This helps reinforce your learning.

Boxes and tables contain important rules, principles, guidelines, signs and symptoms, nursing measures, and other information in a list format. They identify important information and are useful study guides.

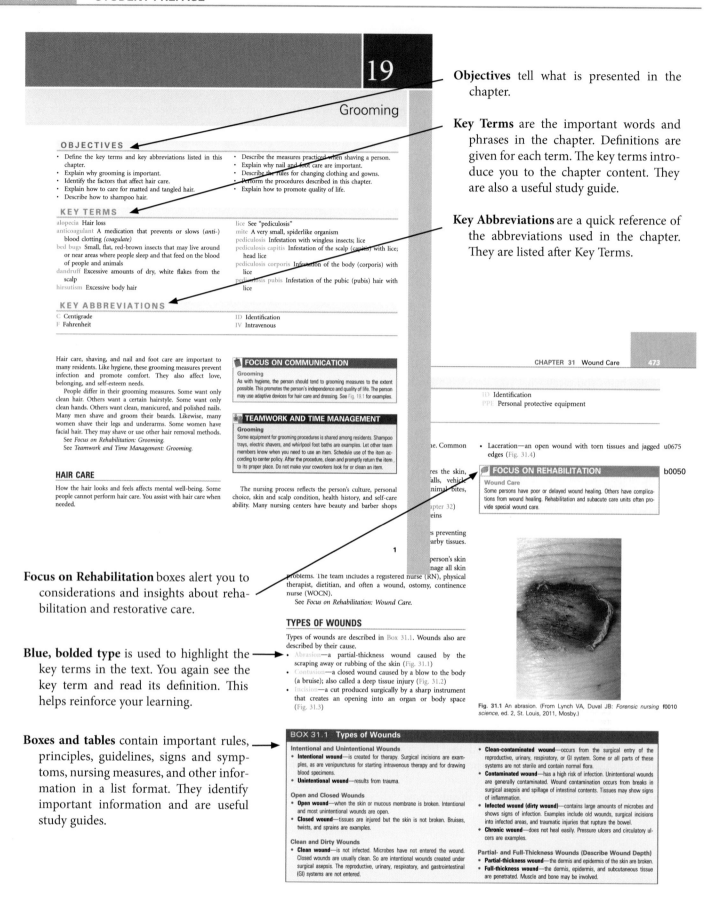

19
Grooming

OBJECTIVES

- Define the key terms and key abbreviations listed in this chapter.
- Explain why grooming is important.
- Identify the factors that affect hair care.
- Explain how to care for matted and tangled hair.
- Describe how to shampoo hair.
- Describe the measures practiced when shaving a person.
- Explain why nail and foot care are important.
- Describe the rules for changing clothing and gowns.
- Perform the procedures described in this chapter.
- Explain how to promote quality of life.

KEY TERMS

alopecia Hair loss
anticoagulant A medication that prevents or slows (*anti-*) blood clotting (*coagulate*)
bed bugs Small, flat, red-brown insects that may live around or near areas where people sleep and that feed on the blood of people and animals
dandruff Excessive amounts of dry, white flakes from the scalp
hirsutism Excessive body hair

lice See "pediculosis"
mite A very small, spiderlike organism
pediculosis Infestation with wingless insects; lice
pediculosis capitis Infestation of the scalp (*capitis*) with lice; head lice
pediculosis corporis Infestation of the body (corporis) with lice
pediculosis pubis Infestation of the pubic (pubis) hair with lice

KEY ABBREVIATIONS

C Centigrade
F Fahrenheit

ID Identification
IV Intravenous

Hair care, shaving, and nail and foot care are important to many residents. Like hygiene, these grooming measures prevent infection and promote comfort. They also affect love, belonging, and self-esteem needs.

People differ in their grooming measures. Some want only clean hair. Others want a certain hairstyle. Some want only clean hands. Others want clean, manicured, and polished nails. Many men shave and groom their beards. Likewise, many women shave their legs and underarms. Some women have facial hair. They may shave or use other hair removal methods.

See *Focus on Rehabilitation: Grooming.*
See *Teamwork and Time Management: Grooming.*

HAIR CARE

How the hair looks and feels affects mental well-being. Some people cannot perform hair care. You assist with hair care when needed.

FOCUS ON COMMUNICATION

Grooming
As with hygiene, the person should tend to grooming measures to the extent possible. This promotes the person's independence and quality of life. The person may use adaptive devices for hair care and dressing. See Fig. 19.1 for examples.

TEAMWORK AND TIME MANAGEMENT

Grooming
Some equipment for grooming procedures is shared among residents. Shampoo trays, electric shavers, and whirlpool foot baths are examples. Let other team members know when you need to use an item. Schedule use of the item according to center policy. After the procedure, clean and promptly return the item to its proper place. Do not make your coworkers look for or clean an item.

The nursing process reflects the person's culture, personal choice, skin and scalp condition, health history, and self-care ability. Many nursing centers have beauty and barber shops

---

ID Identification
PPE Personal protective equipment

...e. Common
...res the skin,
...alls, vehicle
...nimal bites,

...apter 32)
...eins

...es preventing
...arby tissues.

...person's skin
...nage all skin
problems. The team includes a registered nurse (RN), physical therapist, dietitian, and often a wound, ostomy, continence nurse (WOCN).

See *Focus on Rehabilitation: Wound Care.*

TYPES OF WOUNDS

Types of wounds are described in Box 31.1. Wounds also are described by their cause.

- **Abrasion**—a partial-thickness wound caused by the scraping away or rubbing of the skin (Fig. 31.1)
- **Contusion**—a closed wound caused by a blow to the body (a bruise); also called a deep tissue injury (Fig. 31.2)
- **Incision**—a cut produced surgically by a sharp instrument that creates an opening into an organ or body space (Fig. 31.3)
- **Laceration**—an open wound with torn tissues and jagged u0675 edges (Fig. 31.4)

FOCUS ON REHABILITATION   b0050

Wound Care
Some persons have poor or delayed wound healing. Others have complications from wound healing. Rehabilitation and subacute care units often provide special wound care.

Fig. 31.1 An abrasion. (From Lynch VA, Duval JB: *Forensic nursing* f0010 *science*, ed. 2, St. Louis, 2011, Mosby.)

BOX 31.1   Types of Wounds

Intentional and Unintentional Wounds
- **Intentional wound**—is created for therapy. Surgical incisions are examples, as are venipunctures for starting intravenous therapy and for drawing blood specimens.
- **Unintentional wound**—results from trauma.

Open and Closed Wounds
- **Open wound**—when the skin or mucous membrane is broken. Intentional and most unintentional wounds are open.
- **Closed wound**—tissues are injured but the skin is not broken. Bruises, twists, and sprains are examples.

Clean and Dirty Wounds
- **Clean wound**—is not infected. Microbes have not entered the wound. Closed wounds are usually clean. So are intentional wounds created under surgical asepsis. The reproductive, urinary, respiratory, and gastrointestinal (GI) systems are not entered.

- **Clean-contaminated wound**—occurs from the surgical entry of the reproductive, urinary, respiratory, or GI system. Some or all parts of these systems are not sterile and contain normal flora.
- **Contaminated wound**—has a high risk of infection. Unintentional wounds are generally contaminated. Wound contamination occurs from breaks in surgical asepsis and spillage of intestinal contents. Tissues may show signs of inflammation.
- **Infected wound (dirty wound)**—contains large amounts of microbes and shows signs of infection. Examples include old wounds, surgical incisions into infected areas, and traumatic injuries that rupture the bowel.
- **Chronic wound**—does not heal easily. Pressure ulcers and circulatory ulcers are examples.

Partial- and Full-Thickness Wounds (Describe Wound Depth)
- **Partial-thickness wound**—the dermis and epidermis of the skin are broken.
- **Full-thickness wound**—the dermis, epidermis, and subcutaneous tissue are penetrated. Muscle and bone may be involved.

✳ SHAVING

Many men shave for comfort and mental well-being. Many women shave their legs and underarms. Women with coarse facial hair may shave or they may use other hair removal methods. See Box 19.1 for shaving rules.

Safety razors or electric shavers are used (Fig. 19.12). Usually residents are required to have their own electric shavers. If the center's shaver is used, clean it after every use. Follow the manufacturer instructions for brushing out whiskers. Also follow center policy for cleaning electric shavers.

Safety razors (blade razors) involve razor blades. They can cause nicks and cuts. Older persons with wrinkled skin are at risk for nicks and cuts. Therefore, safety razors are not used on persons who have healing problems or for those who take anticoagulants. An anticoagulant is a medication that prevents or slows down *(anti-)* blood clotting *(coagulate)*. Bleeding occurs easily and is hard to stop. A nick or cut can cause serious bleeding. Electric shavers are used.

Soften the beard before using an electric shaver or safety razor. Do so by applying a moist, warm washcloth or towel for a few minutes. Then pat dry the face and apply talcum powder if using an electric shaver. If using a safety razor, lather the face with soap and water or shaving cream.

See *Residents with Dementia: Shaving.*
See *Delegation Guidelines: Shaving.*
See *Promoting Safety and Comfort: Shaving.*

Caring for Mustaches and Beards

Mustaches and beards need daily care. Food can collect in the whiskers. So can mouth and nose drainage. Daily washing and combing are needed. Ask the person how to groom the mustache or beard. *Never trim a mustache or beard without the person's consent.*

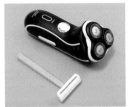

Fig. 19.12 Electric shaver *(top)* and safety razor *(bottom)*.

▣ RESIDENTS WITH DEMENTIA

Shaving
Safety razors are not used to shave persons with dementia. They may not understand what you are doing. They may resist care and move suddenly. Serious nicks and cuts can occur. Use electric shavers for these persons.

▣ DELEGATION GUIDELINES

Shaving
Before shaving a person, you need this information from the nurse and the care plan:
- What shaver to use—electric or safety
- If the person takes anticoagulants
- When to shave the person
- What facial hair to shave
- The location of tender or sensitive areas on the person's face
- What observations to report and record:
  - Nicks (report at once)
  - Cuts (report at once)
  - Bleeding (report at once)
  - Irritation
- When to report observations
- What specific resident concerns to report at once

Residents With Dementia boxes focus on information and care measures needed for persons with dementia.

Delegation Guidelines describe what information you need from the nurse and care plan before performing a procedure. They also tell you what information to report and record.

---

488   CHAPTER 31 Wound Care

✳ Applying Warm and Cold

Protect the person from injury during heat and cold applications. Follow the rules listed in Box 31.8.
See *Focus on Communication: Applying Warm and Cold.*
See *Teamwork and Time Management: Applying Warm and Cold.*
See *Delegation Guidelines: Applying Warm and Cold.*
See *Promoting Safety and Comfort: Applying Warm and Cold.*

▣ TEAMWORK AND TIME MANAGEMENT

Applying Warm and Cold
After applying warm or cold, check the person and the application every 5 minutes. Plan your work so that you can stay in or near the person's room. For example, during the application:
- Make the bed and straighten the person's unit.
- Provide care to the roommate if you are assigned to this person.
- Help the person complete a daily or weekly menu.
- Read cards and letters to the person, with consent.
- Address envelopes and other correspondence for the person.
- Take time to visit with the person.

▣ DELEGATION GUIDELINES

Applying Warm and Cold
Before applying warm or cold, you need this information from the nurse and the care plan:
- The type of application—warm compress or pack, commercial compress, warm soak, sitz bath, aquathermia pad; ice bag, ice collar, ice glove, cold pack, or cold compress
- How to cover the application
- What temperature to use
- The application site
- How long to leave the application in place
- What observations to report and record:
  - Complaints of pain or discomfort, numbness, or burning
  - Excessive redness
  - Blisters
  - Pale, white, or gray skin
  - *Cyanosis* (bluish color)
  - Shivering
  - Rapid pulse, weakness, faintness, and drowsiness (sitz bath)
  - Time, site, and length of application
- When to report observations
- What specific resident concerns to report at once

▣ FOCUS ON COMMUNICATION

Applying Warm and Cold
The person may not tell you about pain or discomfort. The person may not know what symptoms to report. For heat and cold applications, you need to ask:
- "Does the application feel too hot or too cold?"
- "Do you feel any pain, numbness, or burning?"
- "Are you warm enough?"
- "Do you feel weak, faint, or drowsy?" If yes: "Tell me how you feel."

▣ PROMOTING SAFETY AND COMFORT

Applying Warm and Cold
Safety
Check the person every 5 minutes. Also follow these safety measures:
- *Sitz bath.* Blood flow increases to the perineum and rectum. Therefore, less blood flows to other body parts. The person may become weak or feel faint. Drowsiness can occur from the bath's relaxing effect. Observe for signs of weakness, fainting, or fatigue. Also protect the person from injury. Keep the call light within reach and prevent chills and burns.
- *Commercial hot and cold packs.* Read warning labels and follow the manufacturer instructions.
- *Aquathermia pad:*
  - Follow electrical safety precautions (Chapter 11).
  - Check the device for damage or flaws.
  - Follow the manufacturer instructions.
  - Place the heating unit on an even, uncluttered surface. This prevents it from being knocked over or knocked off the surface.
  - Make sure the hoses do not have kinks or bubbles.
  - Use a flannel cover to insulate the pad. It absorbs perspiration at the application site. (Some centers use towels or pillowcases.)
  - Secure the pad in place with ties, tape, or rolled gauze. Do not use pins. They can puncture the pad and cause leaks.
  - Do not place the pad under the person or under a body part. This prevents the escape of heat. Burns can result if heat cannot escape.
  - Give the key used to set the temperature to the nurse. This prevents anyone from changing the temperature.

Some persons have medicated patches or ointments applied to the skin. Do not apply heat over such areas.

Comfort
Cold applications can cause chills and shivering. Provide for warmth. Use bath blankets or other blankets as needed.

Heading icons alert you to associated procedures. Procedure boxes contain the same icon.

Focus on Communication boxes suggest what to say and questions to ask when interacting with residents, visitors, and the nursing team.

Promoting Safety and Comfort boxes focus your attention on the need to be safe and cautious and promote comfort when giving care. "Safety" and "Comfort" subtitles are used.

Teamwork and Time Management boxes suggest ways to efficiently work with and help nursing team members.

BOX 31.8 Rules for Applying Warm and Cold

- Know how to use the equipment. Follow the manufacturer instructions for commercial devices.
- Measure the temperature of moist applications. Use a bath thermometer or follow center policy for measuring temperature.
- Follow center policies for safe temperature ranges.
- Do not apply *very hot* (above 106°F [46.1°C]) applications. Tissue damage can occur.
- Ask the nurse what the temperature should be.
  - Warm—cooler temperatures are needed for persons at risk.
  - Cold—warmer temperatures are needed for persons at risk.
- Know the exact site of the application. Ask the nurse to show you the site.
- Cover dry warm or cold applications before applying them. Use a flannel cover, towel, or other cover as directed by the nurse.
- Provide for privacy. Properly screen and drape the person. Expose only the body part involved. Avoid unnecessary exposure.
- Maintain comfort and body alignment during the procedure.
- Observe the skin every 5 minutes for signs of complications. See *Delegation Guidelines: Applying Warm and Cold.*
- Do not let the person change the temperature of the application.
- Know how long to leave the application in place. See *Delegation Guidelines: Applying Warm and Cold.* Carefully watch the time. Warm and cold are applied no longer than 15 to 20 minutes.
- Follow the rules of electrical safety when using electrical appliances to apply heat.
- Place the call light within the person's reach.
- Complete a safety check before leaving the room. (See the inside of the front cover.)

NATCEP® in the procedure title bar alerts you to those skills that are part of competency evaluations. Ask your instructor for a list of the skills tested in your state.

Procedure icons in the title bar alert you to associated content areas. Heading icons and procedure icons are the same.

Play icons in the procedures alert you to related video clips available online on *Evolve Student Learning Resources.*

Color illustrations and photographs visually present key ideas, concepts, or procedure steps. They help you apply and remember the written material.

Procedure boxes are written in a step-by-step format. They are divided into "Quality of Life," "Preprocedure," "Procedure," and "Postprocedure" sections for easy studying. The "Quality of Life" section lists six simple courtesies that show respect for the resident as a person.

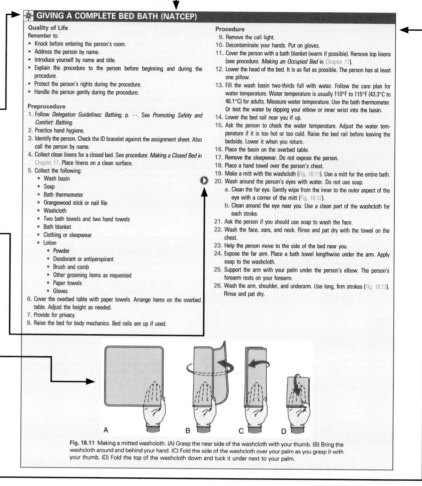

✳ GIVING A COMPLETE BED BATH (NATCEP)

Quality of Life
Remember to:
- Knock before entering the person's room.
- Address the person by name.
- Introduce yourself by name and title.
- Explain the procedure to the person before beginning and during the procedure.
- Protect the person's rights during the procedure.
- Handle the person gently during the procedure.

Preprocedure
1. Follow *Delegation Guidelines: Bathing*, p. ··. See *Promoting Safety and Comfort: Bathing.*
2. Practice hand hygiene.
3. Identify the person. Check the ID bracelet against the assignment sheet. Also call the person by name.
4. Collect clean linens for a closed bed. See procedure: *Making a Closed Bed* in Chapter 17. Place linens on a clean surface.
5. Collect the following:
   - Wash basin
   - Soap
   - Bath thermometer
   - Orangewood stick or nail file
   - Washcloth
   - Two bath towels and two hand towels
   - Bath blanket
   - Clothing or sleepwear
   - Lotion
     - Powder
     - Deodorant or antiperspirant
     - Brush and comb
     - Other grooming items as requested
     - Paper towels
     - Gloves
6. Cover the overbed table with paper towels. Arrange items on the overbed table. Adjust the height as needed.
7. Provide for privacy.
8. Raise the bed for body mechanics. Bed rails are up if used.

Procedure
9. Remove the call light.
10. Decontaminate your hands. Put on gloves.
11. Cover the person with a bath blanket (warm if possible). Remove top linens (see procedure: *Making an Occupied Bed* in Chapter 17).
12. Lower the head of the bed. It is as flat as possible. The person has at least one pillow.
13. Fill the wash basin two-thirds full with water. Follow the care plan for water temperature. Water temperature is usually 110°F to 115°F (43.3°C to 46.1°C) for adults. Measure water temperature. Use the bath thermometer. Or test the water by dipping your elbow or inner wrist into the basin.
14. Lower the bed rail near you if up.
15. Ask the person to check the water temperature. Adjust the water temperature if it is too hot or too cold. Raise the bed rail before leaving the bedside. Lower it when you return.
16. Place the basin on the overbed table.
17. Remove the sleepwear. Do not expose the person.
18. Place a hand towel over the person's chest.
19. Make a mitt with the washcloth (Fig. 18.11). Use a mitt for the entire bath.
20. Wash around the person's eyes with water. Do not use soap.
    a. Clean the far eye. Gently wipe from the inner to the outer aspect of the eye with a corner of the mitt (Fig. 18.12).
    b. Clean around the eye near you. Use a clean part of the washcloth for each stroke.
21. Ask the person if you should use soap to wash the face.
22. Wash the face, ears, and neck. Rinse and pat dry with the towel on the chest.
23. Help the person move to the side of the bed near you.
24. Expose the far arm. Place a bath towel lengthwise under the arm. Apply soap to the washcloth.
25. Support the arm with your palm under the person's elbow. The person's forearm rests on your forearm.
26. Wash the arm, shoulder, and underarm. Use long, firm strokes (Fig. 18.13). Rinse and pat dry.

Fig. 18.11 Making a mitted washcloth. (A) Grasp the near side of the washcloth with your thumb. (B) Bring the washcloth around and behind your hand. (C) Fold the side of the washcloth over your palm as you grasp it with your thumb. (D) Fold the top of the washcloth down and tuck it under next to your palm.

OBRA and CMS highlights inform you of requirements by the Omnibus Budget Reconciliation Act of 1987 (OBRA) and the Centers for Medicare and Medicaid Services (CMS).

❖ Abuse in Nursing Centers

OBRA requires these actions if abuse is suspected within the center:
- The incident is reported at once to the administrator. It also is reported at once to other officials as required by federal and state laws.
- All claims of abuse are thoroughly investigated.
- The center must prevent further potential for abuse while the investigation is in progress.
- Investigation results are reported to the center administrator within 5 days of the incident. They also are reported to other officials as required by federal and state laws.
- Corrective actions are taken if the claim of abuse is found to be true.

Box 2.8 lists some severe cases of elder abuse. The abusers were convicted of crimes.

The examples of abuse that follow are more common. However, such abuse is still wrong. It will be investigated. If the abuse allegation is substantiated, you can lose your job. In addition, the state nursing assistant registry will be notified. Nursing assistants have lost their certification (registration) because of elder abuse.
- A person constantly crying out for help is taken to his room. He is left alone with the door closed.
- A person is told to be nice, otherwise care will not be given.
- A person cannot control her bowels. She is called "dirty" and "disgusting."

- The nurse uses the person's phone to call a friend.
- A person lies in a wet and soiled bed all night.
- Money is taken from a person's wallet.
- A person uses the call light a lot. It is taken away from the person.
- A person's mouth is forced open. Food is forced into the person's mouth.
- A person is told that her son does not visit because she is so mean.

Domestic Abuse

Domestic abuse—also called domestic violence, intimate partner abuse, partner abuse, and spousal abuse—occurs in relationships. One partner has power and control over the other through abuse. Fear and harm occur. Usually more than one of the following is present:
- *Physical abuse*—unwanted punching, slapping, grabbing, choking, poking, biting, pulling hair, twisting arms, or kicking. It may involve burns and weapons. Physical injuries occur. Death is a constant threat.
- *Sexual abuse*—unwanted sexual contact.
- *Verbal abuse*—unkind and hurtful remarks. They make the person feel unwhole, unattractive, and without value.
- *Economic abuse*—controlling money. Having or not having a job is controlled by the abuser. So are paychecks, money gifts from family and friends, and money for household expenses (food, clothing).

Activities-of-Daily-Living Flow Sheet

ORDER/INSTRUCTION	TIME	JAN 1	FEB 2	MAR 3	4	APR 5	MAY 6	7	JUN 8	9	JUL 10	11	AUG 12	13	SEP 14	15	16	OCT 17	18	NOV 19	20	DEC 21	22	23	24	25	26	27	28	29	30	31
Dressing I=Independent S=Set up A=Assist T=Total Care	11-7																																
	7-3																																
	3-11																																
Grooming, Combing Hair I=Independent S=Set up A=Assist T=Total Care	11-7																																
	7-3																																
	3-11																																
Shave Men Daily	11-7																																
Shave Women every ___ days	7-3																																
	3-11																																
Trim Fingernails Weekly	11-7																																
	7-3																																
	3-11																																

Fig. 19.29 Charting sample.

QUALITY OF LIFE

Grooming measures promote comfort. They also help the person's body image and self-esteem needs. Clean hair, nails, and garments all help mental well-being. So does a clean-shaven face or a well-groomed beard or mustache. A person's pride may be boosted by a visit to the hair salon. It may be your responsibility to transport the person by wheelchair if the salon is a distance.

The person may not have energy for some procedures. The nurse tells you what care to give and when to give it. Encourage and allow personal choice when possible. Grooming practices vary from person to person. Always assist as needed.

Carefully handle the person's grooming products, shaver, hair dryer, brush and comb, perfumes, and other personal care items. Garments also need your attention. Do not break zippers, tear clothing, lose buttons, or cause other damage. Treat the person's property with care and respect.

Respect the person's privacy by helping with putting on a robe over a hospital gown when walking in hallways. This prevents the person from exposing the backside inadvertently.

Sometimes family members want to help with grooming. For example, they want to help style the person's hair. Or they want to apply lotion to the person's hands and feet. With the person's permission, allow family members to assist with grooming measures as much as safely possible. This promotes social interaction. It also involves the family in the person's care.

Report your observations to the nurse. Also record your observations and the care given according to center policy (Fig. 19.29). This information is needed to meet the person's needs.

Quality of Life boxes at the end of each chapter bridge the chapter's focus with how to promote the resident's rights and enhance quality of life when giving care.

TIME TO REFLECT

Mrs. Martin is a retired beautician who resides at the nursing center. She has recently suffered a stroke and has right-sided weakness. She always takes pride in her personal appearance. You are working the day shift and have many residents to help with morning care and transport to the dining room before breakfast is served. Mrs. Martin refuses to let you transport her by wheelchair to the dining room table until her hair is fixed and her makeup is applied. How could you approach this situation?

Time to Reflect boxes give you the chance to review a scenario that might really happen to you at the workplace. Think about how you would react in the described setting. These stories are designed to help you apply the information you have learned in the current chapter.

REVIEW QUESTIONS

Circle the BEST answer.

1. A person has alopecia. This is
   a. Excessive body hair
   b. Dry, white flakes from the scalp
   c. An infestation with lice
   d. Hair loss
2. Which prevents hair from matting and tangling?
   a. Bedrest
   b. Daily brushing and combing
   c. Daily shampooing
   d. Cutting hair
3. A person's hair is not matted or tangled. When brushing hair, start at the
   a. Forehead and brush backward
   b. Hair ends
   c. Scalp
   d. Back of the neck and brush forward
4. Brushing keeps the hair
   a. Soft and shiny
   b. Clean
   c. Free of lice
   d. Long

Review Questions are useful study guides. They help you to review what you have learned. They can also be used when studying for a test or the competency evaluation. Answers are given at the back of the book, beginning on p. 298.

CONTENTS

The Nursing Assistant Working in Long-Term Care

OBJECTIVES

- Define the key terms and key abbreviations listed in this chapter.
- Describe the types, purposes, and organization of long-term care centers.
- Describe members of the nursing team.
- Describe the interdisciplinary team.
- Describe the programs that pay for health care.
- Explain why standards are met.
- Explain the history and current trends affecting nursing assistants.
- Explain the laws that affect nursing assistants.
- List the reasons for denying, suspending, or revoking a nursing assistant's certification, license, or registration.
- Describe the training and competency evaluation requirements for nursing assistants.
- Identify the information in the nursing assistant registry.
- Explain how to obtain certification, a license, or registration in another state.
- Describe what nursing assistants can do and their role limits.
- Describe the standards for nursing assistants developed by the National Council of State Boards of Nursing.
- Explain why a job description is important.
- Describe the delegation process.
- Explain your role in the delegation process.
- Explain how to accept or refuse a delegated task.
- Explain how to promote quality of life.

KEY TERMS

accountable Being responsible for one's actions and the actions of others who performed delegated tasks; answering questions about and explaining one's actions and the actions of others

acute illness A sudden illness from which a person is expected to recover

Alzheimer disease (AD) A disease that affects brain tissue; memory loss and confusion increase until the person cannot tend to simple personal needs

assisted living residence (ALR) Provides housing, personal care, support services, health care, and activities in a homelike setting

board and care home Provides rooms, meals, laundry, and supervision to independent residents in a homelike setting; group home

case management A nursing care pattern; a case manager (an RN) coordinates a person's care from admission through discharge and into the home setting

chronic illness An ongoing illness, slow or gradual in onset; it has no cure; the illness can be controlled and complications prevented with proper treatment

delegate To authorize another person to perform a nursing task in a certain situation

group home See "board and care home"

health care provider A medical doctor, doctor of osteopathy, nurse practitioner, or physician assistant

hospice A health care agency or program for persons who are terminally ill

independence Not relying on or requiring care from others

interdisciplinary team The many health care workers whose skills and knowledge focus on the person's total care; health team

job description A document that describes what the center expects you to do

licensed practical nurse (LPN) A nurse who has completed a 1-year nursing program and has passed a licensing test; called licensed vocational nurse (LVN) in some states

licensed vocational nurse (LVN) See "licensed practical nurse"

Medicaid A health care payment program sponsored by the federal government and operated by the states

Medicare A federal health insurance program for persons 65 years of age or older and younger people with certain disabilities

nurse practitioner (NP) A registered nurse (RN) who has completed graduate education at the master's or doctoral level and has obtained national board certification

nursing assistant A person who gives basic nursing care under the supervision of a licensed nurse; nurse aide, nursing attendant, orderly, unlicensed assistive personnel, and health care assistant are some other titles

nursing center Provides health care and nursing care to persons who need regular or continuous care; licensed nurses are required; nursing facility or nursing home

nursing facility (NF) See "nursing center"

nursing home See "nursing center"

nursing task Nursing care or a nursing function, procedure, activity, or work that can be delegated to nursing assistants when it does not require an RN's professional knowledge or judgment

nursing team Those who provide nursing care—RNs, LPNs/LVNs, and nursing assistants

physician assistant (PA) A medical professional who may diagnose, treat, and prescribe medication for patients. They often work together with other health care providers.

registered nurse (RN) A nurse who has completed a 2-, 3-, or 4-year nursing program and has passed a licensing test

responsibility The duty or obligation to perform some act or function

skilled nursing facility (SNF) Provides health care and nursing care for residents who have many or severe health problems or who need rehabilitation; may be part of a nursing center or a hospital

KEY ABBREVIATIONS

AD Alzheimer disease
ALR Assisted living residence
ARNP Advanced registered nurse practitioner
CNA Certified nursing assistant, certified nurse aide
DON Director of nursing
HMO Health maintenance organization
LNA Licensed nursing assistant
LPN Licensed practical nurse
LVN Licensed vocational nurse
NATCEP Nursing assistant training and competency evaluation program

NCSBN National Council of State Boards of Nursing
NP Nurse practitioner
OBRA Omnibus Budget Reconciliation Act of 1987
PA Physician assistant
PPO Preferred provider organization
RN Registered nurse
RNA Registered nurse aide
SNF Skilled nursing facility
STNA State-tested nursing assistant
UAP Unlicensed assistive personnel

Working in long-term care offers many new and rewarding experiences. Your focus is the resident—the person needing care. You must provide quality care and promote the person's quality of life. This includes promoting the person's independence. Independence means not relying on or requiring care from others.

LONG-TERM CARE CENTERS

Long-term care centers provide health care to persons who cannot care for themselves at home. They do not need hospital care. Care needs range from simple to complex. Medical, nursing, dietary, recreational, rehabilitative, and social services are provided. So are housekeeping and laundry services.

Persons in long-term care centers are often referred to as *residents*. They usually are not called *patients*. This is because the center is their temporary or permanent home. Some centers may choose a different title for the people they care for. *Clients* and *persons served* are other titles. In assisted living units, the term *tenant* is often used for the people who receive care. Your facility policy will tell you which term is preferred. In this textbook, the term *resident* will be used when referring to the people cared for in long-term care centers.

Residents may be older or disabled. Some are recovering from illness, injury, or surgery. Long-term care centers are designed to meet their needs. Some people return home when well enough. Others need nursing care until death.

Purposes and Goals

Long-term care serves to *promote physical and mental health*. Most residents have one or more health problems. They are helped and encouraged to:

- Understand and accept the limits of their health problems.
- Understand and accept physical and mental changes.
- Function within those limits.
- Focus on abilities, not disabilities.
- Do as much for themselves as possible.
- Change habits that make health problems worse.
- Eat properly and exercise.

The goal of comprehensive care is to help the person maintain the highest possible level of function with all members of the health care team, including the resident and family, involved in the process.

Board and Care Homes

Board and care homes (group homes) provide rooms, meals, laundry, and supervision to independent residents in a homelike setting. Care is given that meets the person's basic needs. A safe setting and supervision are provided. So are housekeeping and transportation services. There is an emergency call system and a 24-hour caregiver. This person may be a nursing assistant.

Residents usually can dress themselves. They usually tend to grooming and bathroom needs with little help. They may receive help with personal care and medication reminders as needed.

Assisted Living Residences

Assisted living residences (ALRs) provide housing, personal care, support services, health care, and activities in a homelike setting (Chapter 43). Many residences look like apartment buildings. Some are part of retirement communities or nursing centers.

The person has a room or an apartment. Help is given as needed with personal care, meals, or taking medications. Two or three meals a day are provided. Housekeeping, laundry, transportation services, and social and recreational activities are provided. There is access to health and medical care.

Nursing Centers

A nursing center provides health care and nursing care to persons who need regular or continuous care. Nursing facility (NF) and nursing home are other names. Licensed nurses are required.

Residents have more complex health problems than do board and care or ALR residents. These services are provided:

- Medical care
- Nursing care (Fig. 1.1)
- Dietary services
- Rehabilitation
- Recreation
- Social services
- Laundry
- Housekeeping
- Maintenance

Skilled nursing facilities (SNFs) provide health care and nursing care for residents who have many or severe health problems or who need rehabilitation. The SNF may be part of a nursing center or a hospital.

SNFs provide more complex care than nursing centers. Many persons are admitted from hospitals. They need to recover or have rehabilitation after an illness, injury, or surgery. Some return home; others do not.

Long-term care also serves to *treat chronic illness*. A chronic illness is an ongoing illness, slow or gradual in onset. It has no cure. The illness can be controlled and complications prevented with proper treatment. An acute illness is a sudden illness from which the person is expected to recover. An acute illness may require hospital care.

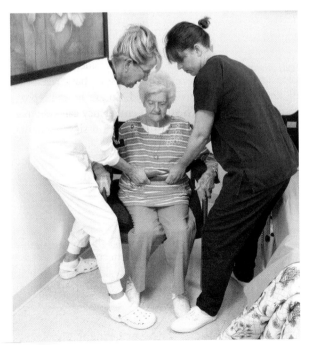

Fig. 1.1 A nursing assistant is helping a nurse with a resident's care.

Communicable diseases are prevented. A communicable disease can be spread from one person to another (Chapter 14). The common cold, influenza (flu), and corona viruses are examples. They can cause major health problems for older and disabled persons. Often you are the first person to detect signs and symptoms of a communicable disease.

Rehabilitation or restorative care helps persons return to their highest possible level of physical and mental function (Chapter 42). They are helped to become or remain as independent as possible. This includes persons who need nursing center care until death.

Rehabilitation starts when a person is admitted to the center. Weakness after an acute illness is common. *Deconditioning* is the process of becoming weak from illness or lack of exercise (Chapter 24). Strokes, fractures, and surgery are common causes. All staff members follow the rehabilitation plan.

Other Services

Some nursing centers offer learning experiences for students. They study to become nurses, nursing assistants, doctors, or other health team members. All students focus on the center's purposes and goals.

Many nursing centers have special care units. Hospice and memory care units are common.

- *Hospices.* A hospice is a health care agency or program for persons who are terminally ill. Such persons no longer respond to treatments aimed at cures. Usually they have less than 6 months to live. The physical, emotional, social, and spiritual needs of the person and family are met. The focus is on comfort, not cure. Children and pets can visit. Family and friends can assist with care. Hospice care is provided by hospitals, nursing centers, and home care agencies. Hospice services can also take place in the person's home.
- *Memory Care Units (Dementia Care Units).* These units are for persons with Alzheimer disease and other dementias (Chapter 40). The building may be a self-contained, free-standing facility or connected to a long-term care center. Alzheimer disease (AD) affects brain tissue (Chapter 40). Memory loss and confusion increase until the person cannot tend to simple personal needs. Over time, the person forgets names of self and others. The person may wander and become agitated and combative. The unit is usually closed off from the rest of the center. The doorways may be secured and passcodes necessary to enter or exit. This provides a safe setting for residents to wander freely. AD worsens over time. When wandering is no longer a problem, a closed unit may no longer be needed. The person may be transferred to another unit in the center.
- *Rehabilitation and Subacute Care.* Some nursing centers and hospitals provide rehabilitation and subacute care. Subacute care requires intensive, skilled nursing care. It is more complex and requires a higher ratio of licensed nurses. Often the stay is for a few weeks or months. Persons on these units may be called *patients* or *clients*. If problems occur, the person may need long-term care.

Nursing Center Organization

Nursing centers are usually owned by an individual or a corporation. Some are owned by government agencies. Some are nonprofit facilities, and others may be operated by a faith-based organization. The owners control policies to ensure that safe care is provided. Local, state, and federal rules must be followed.

Each center has an administrator. The administrator plans, directs, and oversees the delivery of health care. Department directors report to the administrator (Fig. 1.2). Most nursing centers have nursing, therapy, and food service departments. They also have housekeeping, maintenance, and laundry departments. A human resources director handles personnel matters such as hiring staff. A finance director handles resident billing. A social services director meets the social needs of residents and families. An activity director plans resident activities.

By law, nursing centers must have a medical director. This person is a doctor. This doctor consults with the staff about medical problems not handled by a resident's doctor. Guidance is given about resident care policies and programs. Nurse practitioners (NPs) and physician assistants (PAs) may also provide valuable services to residents in long-term care settings. Different states have different regulations concerning the degree of independence of their practice. Some work closely with a physician. The term health care provider will be used in this textbook to refer to a medical doctor, osteopathic doctor, physician assistant, nurse practitioner, or advanced registered nurse practitioner (ARNP).

Nursing Service

Nursing service is a large department. The director of nursing (DON) is a registered nurse (RN). The DON is responsible for the entire nursing staff. This includes giving safe care.

Nurse managers (usually RNs) assist the DON. They manage and carry out nursing department functions. Shift managers coordinate resident care for a certain shift. Other managers are responsible for a nursing area or a certain function. Staff development, restorative nursing, infection control, and continuous quality improvement are examples.

Each nursing unit usually has a charge nurse. This may be titled as a charge nurse, unit manager, or nurse supervisor. Charge nurses are usually RNs. In some states, licensed practical nurses/licensed vocational nurses (LPNs/LVNs) are charge nurses. The charge nurse is responsible for all resident care and for the actions of nursing staff on a unit. Staff RNs report to the charge nurse. LPNs/LVNs report to staff RNs or to the charge nurse. You report to the nurse supervising your work.

Nursing education (staff development) is part of nursing service. Nursing education staff:
- Plan and present educational programs (inservice programs).
- Provide the nursing team with new and changing information.
- Teach the nursing team how to use new equipment and supplies.
- Review key policies and procedures on a regular basis.
- Educate and train nursing assistants.
- Conduct new employee orientation programs.
- Provide programs that meet federal and state educational requirements.

Organizational chart

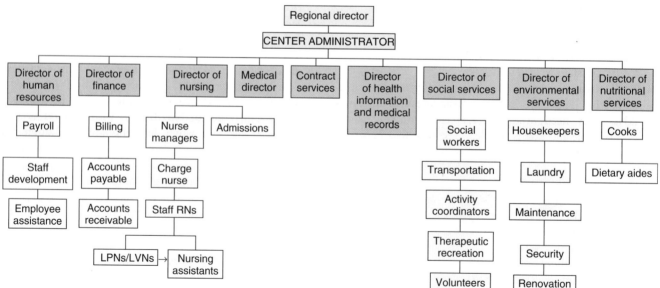

Fig. 1.2 Organization of a nursing center.

THE NURSING TEAM

The nursing team involves those who provide nursing care—RNs, LPNs/LVNs, and nursing assistants. Their roles and responsibilities differ. All focus on the needs of residents and families.

Registered Nurses

A registered nurse (RN) has completed a 2-, 3-, or 4-year nursing program and has passed a licensing test.

- Community college programs—2 years
- Hospital-based diploma programs—2 or 3 years
- College or university programs—4 years

RNs assess, make nursing diagnoses, plan, implement, and evaluate nursing care (Chapter 5). They develop care plans for each person and provide care. They also delegate nursing care and tasks to the nursing team. They evaluate how the care plans and nursing care affect each person. RNs teach persons how to improve health and independence. They also teach the family.

RNs carry out the health care provider's orders. They may delegate them to LPNs/LVNs or nursing assistants. RNs do not prescribe treatments or medications. However, RNs can study to become *clinical nurse specialists* or *nurse practitioners*. These RNs have limited diagnosing and prescribing functions.

Licensed Practical Nurses and Licensed Vocational Nurses

A licensed practical nurse (LPN) has completed a 1-year nursing program and has passed a licensing test. Hospitals, community colleges, vocational schools, and technical schools offer programs. Some programs are 10 months long; others take 18 months. Some high schools offer 2-year programs.

Graduates take a licensing test for practical nursing. After passing the test, the person receives a license to practice and the title of *licensed practical nurse.* Licensed vocational nurse (LVN) is used in some states. LPNs/LVNs must have a license required by the state in which they work.

LPNs/LVNs are supervised by RNs, licensed doctors, and licensed dentists. They have fewer responsibilities and functions than RNs. They need little supervision when the person's condition is stable and care is simple. They assist RNs in caring for acutely ill persons and with complex procedures.

Nursing Assistants

Nursing assistants give basic nursing care under the supervision of a licensed nurse. *Nurse aide, nursing attendant, orderly, health care assistant,* and *unlicensed assistive personnel (UAP)* are some other titles. For consistency, the term *nursing assistant* will be used in this textbook.

Nursing assistants give much of the care provided in nursing centers. To work in a nursing center, they must have formal training and pass a competency test.

See *Focus on Rehabilitation: Nursing Care Patterns.*

 FOCUS ON REHABILITATION

Nursing Care Patterns

Case management is often used in rehabilitation and subacute care. In case management, a case manager (an RN) coordinates a person's care from admission through discharge and into the home setting. The case manager communicates with the person's doctor and the health team. There also is communication with the insurance company and community agencies as needed. The case manager also helps the health team work together.

THE INTERDISCIPLINARY TEAM

The interdisciplinary team *(health team)* involves the many health care workers whose skills and knowledge focus on the person's total care (Table 1.1). The team provides supportive services for the overall goal of quality resident care (Fig. 1.3). They work together to meet each person's needs. Many health care workers are involved in the care of each person. Coordinated care is needed. An RN leads this team.

See *Focus on Communication: The Interdisciplinary Team.*

 FOCUS ON COMMUNICATION

The Interdisciplinary Team

Many staff members work together to provide a person's care. Each member has a different role. Health team members must communicate often. You may have questions or concerns about a person and the respective care. Tell the team leader. The leader will communicate with other health team members.

PAYING FOR HEALTH CARE

Health care is a major focus in society. The goals are to provide health care to everyone and to reduce the high cost of care. Hospital and nursing center care is costly. So are doctor visits, drugs, medical supplies, and home care. Most people cannot afford these costs. Some avoid medical care because they cannot pay. Others pay doctor bills but go without food or drugs. Health care bills cause worry, fear, and emotional upset. If the person has insurance, some care costs are covered. Rarely is the total cost of care covered.

These programs help pay for health care:

- *Private insurance* is bought by individuals and families. The insurance company pays for some or all health care costs.
- *Group insurance* is bought by groups or organizations for individuals. This is often an employee benefit.
- Medicare is a federal health insurance program for persons 65 years of age or older. Some younger people with certain disabilities are covered. Part A pays for some hospital, SNF, hospice, and home care costs. Part B helps pay for

TABLE 1.1 Health Team Members

Title	Description	Credentials
Activities director	Assesses, plans, and implements recreational needs	Varies with state and/or employer; ranges from no training to bachelor's degree
Audiologist	Tests hearing; prescribes hearing aids; works with persons who are hard of hearing	Master's degree or higher; state license
Cleric (clergyman; clergywoman)	Assists with spiritual needs	Priest, minister, rabbi, sister (nun), deacon, or other pastoral training
Clinical laboratory technologist	Performs complicated laboratory tests on blood, urine, and other body fluids, secretions, and excretions; organizes, supervises, and performs diagnostic analyses	Bachelor's degree; national certification test; license in some states
Clinical nurse specialist	Provides nursing care and consults in a nursing specialty—geriatrics, critical care, diabetes, rehabilitation, and wound care are examples	Registered nurse (RN) with master's degree or doctorate as a clinical nurse specialist
Dental hygienist	Focuses on preventing dental disorders; supervised by a licensed dentist	Completion of a dental hygiene program; state license
Dentist	Prevents and treats disorders and diseases of the teeth, gums, and oral structures	Doctor of dental science (DDS) or doctor of dental medicine (DMD); state license
Dietitian and nutritionist	Assesses and plans for nutritional needs; teaches good nutrition, food selection, and preparation	Bachelor's degree; registered dietitian (RD) must pass a national registration test; license or certification in some states
Licensed practical/vocational nurse (LPN/LVN)	Provides direct nursing care, including giving drugs, under the direction of an RN	State-approved program (usually 1 year in length); state license
Medical or clinical laboratory technician	Collects samples and performs laboratory tests on blood, urine, and other body fluids, secretions, and excretions	Associate's degree; national certifying test; license in some states
Medical records and health information technician	Maintains medical records; transcribes medical reports; files records; completes required reports	Associate's degree; credentialing test
Medication assistant-certified (MA-C)	Gives medications as allowed by state law under the supervision of an RN or LPN/LVN	Certified nursing assistant with additional education and training as required by state law; state certification
Nurse practitioner	Plans and provides care with the health team; does physical exams, health assessments, and health education	RN with master's degree or higher and clinical experience in an area of nursing; certification test may be required
Nursing assistant	Assists nurses and gives nursing care; supervised by an RN or LPN/LVN	Completion of a state-approved training and competency evaluation program to work in long-term care or home care agencies receiving Medicare funds; state registry; state certification or license
Occupational therapist (OT)	Assists persons to learn or retain skills needed to perform daily activities; designs adaptive equipment for daily living	Master's degree or higher; national certification; state license
Occupational therapy assistant	Performs tasks and services supervised by an OT	Associate's degree; national certification; license in some states
Pharmacist	Fills medication orders written by doctors; monitors and evaluates medication interactions; consults with doctors and nurses about medication actions and interactions	Pharm.D. degree; state license
Physical therapist (PT)	Assists persons with musculoskeletal problems to restore function and prevent disability	Master's degree or higher; state license
Physical therapy assistant	Performs tasks and services supervised by a PT	Associate's degree; national certification or license in some states
Physician (doctor)	Diagnoses and treats diseases and injuries	Medical school graduation (MD), residency, and national board certification; state license
Physician's assistant (PA)	Assists in diagnosis and treatment; performs medical tasks, often working closely with a doctor	Master's degree or higher; national certification exam; license in some states
Podiatrist	Prevents, diagnoses, and treats foot disorders	Doctor of podiatric medicine (DPM); state license
Radiographer/radiologic technologist	Takes x-rays and processes film for viewing	Associate's degree or higher; license in some states
Registered nurse (RN)	Assesses, makes nursing diagnoses, plans, implements, and evaluates nursing care; supervises LPNs/LVNs and nursing assistants	Associate's degree, diploma, bachelor's, or master's degree; state license
Respiratory therapist (RT)	Assists in treating lung and heart disorders; gives respiratory treatments and therapies	Associate's degree; national certification test; license in most states
Social worker	Deals with social, emotional, and environmental issues affecting illness and recovery; coordinates community agencies to assist patients, residents, and families	Bachelor's degree or higher; 2 years supervised work experience for clinical social workers; license, certification, or registration
Speech-language pathologist	Evaluates speech and language and treats persons with speech, voice, hearing, communication, and swallowing disorders	Master's degree; supervised work experience and national test for licensure in most states

Modified from Bureau of Labor Statistics, US Department of Labor. *Occupational outlook handbook,* 2021 edition. Available at: https://www.bls.gov/ooh/healthcare/home.htm.

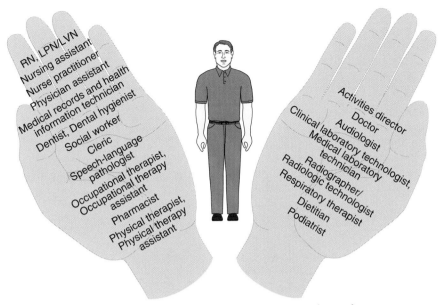

Fig. 1.3 Members of the health team. The person is the focus of care.

doctors' services, outpatient hospital care, physical and occupational therapists, some home care, among other services. Part B is voluntary. The person pays a monthly premium.

- Medicaid is a health care payment program. It is sponsored by the federal government and operated by the states. People with low incomes usually qualify. So do some older, blind, and disabled persons. There is no insurance premium. The amount paid for covered services is limited. Medicaid may also pay for care once a person's resources have run out. See *Promoting Safety and Comfort: Paying for Health Care.*

👤 PROMOTING SAFETY AND COMFORT

Paying for Health Care
Safety
Some conditions can be prevented with proper care. Medicare will pay a lower rate for such conditions if they are acquired during a hospital stay. Pressure injuries (Chapter 32) and certain types of falls, trauma, and infections are examples. You must assist the nursing and health teams in preventing such conditions.

Prospective Payment Systems

Prospective payment systems limit the amount paid by insurers, Medicare, and Medicaid. Prospective means *"before"* care.

- *Medicare severity-adjusted diagnosis-related groups (MS-DRGs)* are for hospital costs.
- *Resource utilization groups (RUGs)* are for SNF payments.
- *Case mix groups (CMGs)* are used for rehabilitation centers.

Length of stay and treatment costs are determined for each group. If the treatment costs are less than the amount paid, the agency keeps the extra money. If costs are greater, the agency takes the loss.

MANAGED CARE

Managed care deals with health care delivery and payment (Box 1.1). Insurers contract with doctors and hospitals for reduced rates or discounts. The insured person uses doctors and agencies providing the lower rates. If others are used, care is covered in part or not at all. The person pays for costs not covered by insurance.

Managed care limits the choice of where to go for health care. It also limits the care that doctors provide. Managed care is common for Medicaid and Medicare coverage.

Managed Care as Preapproval for Services

Many insurers must approve the need for health care services. If the need is approved, the insurer pays for the services. If the need is not approved, the person pays for the costs. The preapproval process depends on the insurer.

BOX 1.1 Types of Managed Care

Health Maintenance Organization (HMO)—provides health care services for a prepaid fee. For the fee, persons receive needed services offered by the HMO. Some have an annual physical exam. Others need hospital care. Whatever services are used, the cost is covered by the prepaid fee. HMOs focus on preventing disease and maintaining health. Keeping someone healthy costs far less than treating illness.

Preferred Provider Organization (PPO)—is a group of doctors and hospitals. They provide health care at reduced rates. Usually the agreement is between the PPO and an employer or an insurance company. Employees or those insured receive reduced rates for the services used. The person can choose any doctor or hospital in the PPO.

This preapproval process is also called *managed care*. It includes monitoring care. The purpose is to reduce unneeded services and procedures. The insurer decides what to pay. With health maintenance organizations (HMOs) and preferred provider organizations (PPOs), the insurer may decide where the person goes for services.

MEETING STANDARDS

Nursing centers must meet certain standards. Standards are set by the federal and state governments. They also are set by accrediting agencies. Standards relate to center policies and procedures, budget and finances, and quality of care. A center must meet standards for:

- *Licensure.* A license is issued by the state. A center must have a license to operate and provide care.
- *Certification.* This is required to receive Medicare and Medicaid funds.
- *Accreditation.* This is voluntary. It signals quality and excellence.

The Survey Process

Surveys are done to see if the center meets set standards. A survey team will:

- Review policies and procedures.
- Review medical records.
- Interview staff, residents, and families.
- Observe how care is given.
- Observe if dignity and privacy are promoted.
- Check for cleanliness and safety.
- Review budgets and finances.
- Make sure the staff meets state requirements. (Are doctors, nurses, and other health care providers licensed? Are nursing assistants on the state registry?)

The survey team decides if the center meets the standards. If standards are met, the center receives a license, certification, or accreditation.

Sometimes problems are found. A problem is called a *deficiency* (Box 1.2). The center is given time to correct it, usually 60 days. Sometimes less time is given. The agency can be fined for uncorrected or serious deficiencies. It can lose its license, certification, or accreditation. The center may not be allowed to have nursing assistant students learn at their facility.

Your Role

You have an important role in meeting standards and in the survey process. You must:

- Provide quality care.
- Protect the person's rights.
- Provide for the person's and your own safety.
- Help keep the center clean and safe.
- Conduct yourself in a professional manner.
- Have good work ethics.
- Follow center policies and procedures.
- Answer questions honestly and completely.

BOX 1.2   Common Nursing Center Deficiencies

Surveyors cited nursing homes because they failed to:

- Watch each resident carefully and provide assistive devices to prevent accidents.
- Provide the care and services needed to attain or maintain the highest quality of life possible.
- Protect residents from abuse, mistreatment, neglect, and/or theft of personal property.
- Keep each resident free from unneeded physical restraints.
- Provide activities to meet each person's needs.
- Listen to resident or family groups or act on their complaints or suggestions.
- Hire only people with no legal history of abusing, neglecting, or mistreating residents.
- Report or investigate any acts of abuse, neglect, or mistreatment.
- Keep the nursing home area free of dangers that cause accidents.

From www.medicare.gov.

THE NURSING ASSISTANT IN LONG-TERM CARE

Federal and state laws and nursing center policies combine to define the roles and functions of each health team member. Everyone must protect residents from harm. To do so, you need to know:

- What you can and cannot do.
- Your legal limits.

Laws, job descriptions, and the person's condition shape your work. So does the amount of supervision you need.

History and Current Trends

For decades, nursing assistants have helped nurses with basic nursing care. Often called *nurse's aides*, they gave baths and made beds. They helped with grooming, elimination, and other needs. Their work was similar in hospitals and nursing centers. Until the 1980s, training was not required by law. Nurses gave on-the-job training. Some hospitals, nursing centers, and schools offered nursing assistant courses.

Before the 1980s, team nursing was common. An RN was the team leader. The RN assigned care to nurses and nursing assistants. Care was assigned according to each person's needs and condition. It also depended on the staff member's education and experiences.

Primary nursing was common in the 1980s. RNs planned and gave care. Many hospitals only hired RNs. Meanwhile, nursing centers relied on nursing assistants for resident care.

Home care increased during the 1980s. Prospective payment systems limit health care payments. To reduce care costs, hospital stays also are limited. Therefore patients are discharged earlier than in the past. Often they are still quite ill and need home care.

Efforts to reduce health care costs include:

- *Hospital closings.* Many do not make enough money to stay open.

- *Hospital mergers.* Hospitals merge to share resources and to avoid the same costly services. For example, one hospital offers heart surgery; the other serves women and children.
- *Health care systems.* Agencies join together as one provider of care. A system often has hospitals, nursing centers, and home care agencies. It also has hospice settings, ambulance services, and doctors. For example, a hospital patient needs long-term care. The person transfers from the hospital to a system nursing center. The person is transported by the system-owned ambulance service. After rehabilitation, the person returns home. The system-owned home care agency provides needed services in the home setting. The person's care stays within the system from the hospital to the home setting.
- *Managed care.* Insurers have contracts with doctors, hospitals, and health care systems for reduced rates.
- *Staffing mix.* Hospitals hire RNs, LPNs/LVNs, and nursing assistants. Most hospitals require a state-approved nursing assistant training and competency evaluation for employment. More training is given for tasks not in the training program.

Federal and State Laws

The US Congress makes federal laws that all 50 states must follow. State legislatures make state laws. For example, the New York legislature makes state laws for New York. The Texas legislature makes state laws for Texas. You must know the federal and state laws that affect your work. They provide direction for what you can do.

See Chapter 2 for other laws affecting your work.

Nurse Practice Acts

Each state has a nurse practice act. It protects the public's welfare and safety by regulating nursing practice in that state. A nurse practice act:
- Defines RN and LPN/LVN.
- Describes the scope of practice for RNs and LPNs/LVNs.
- Describes education and licensing requirements for RNs and LPNs/LVNs.
- Protects the public from persons practicing nursing without a license. Persons who do not meet the state's requirements cannot perform nursing functions.

Nursing assistants. A state's nurse practice act is used to decide what nursing assistants can do. Some nurse practice acts also regulate nursing assistant roles, functions, education, and certification requirements. Other states have separate laws for nursing assistants.

Legal and advisory opinions about nursing assistants are based on the state's nurse practice act. So are any state laws about their roles and functions. If you do something beyond the legal limits of your role, you could be practicing nursing without a license. This creates serious legal problems for you and the nurse supervising your work.

Nursing assistants must be able to function with skill and safety. Like nurses, nursing assistants can have their certification (p. ··) denied, revoked, or suspended. The National Council of State Boards of Nursing (NCSBN) lists these reasons for doing so:
- Substance abuse or dependency
- Abandoning, abusing, or neglecting a resident
- Fraud or deceit. Examples include the following:
  - Filing false personal information
  - Providing false information when applying for initial certification or to have it reinstated
- Violating professional boundaries (Chapter 2)
- Giving unsafe care
- Performing acts beyond the nursing assistant role
- Misappropriation (stealing, theft) or misusing property
- Obtaining money or property from a resident (e.g., through fraud, falsely representing oneself, use of force)
- Having been convicted of a crime (e.g., murder, assault, kidnapping, rape or sexual assault, robbery, sexual crimes involving children, criminal mistreatment of children or a vulnerable adult [Chapter 2], drug trafficking, embezzlement [to take a person's property for one's own use], theft, and arson [starting fires])
- Failing to conform to the standards of nursing assistants (p. ··)
- Putting residents at risk for harm
- Violating a resident's privacy
- Failing to maintain the confidentiality of resident information

The Omnibus Budget Reconciliation Act of 1987 ❖

The Omnibus Budget Reconciliation Act of 1987 (OBRA) is a federal law. Its purpose is to improve the quality of life of nursing center residents.

OBRA sets minimum training and competency evaluation requirements for nursing assistants. Each state must have a nursing assistant training and competency evaluation program (NATCEP). A nursing assistant must successfully complete a NATCEP to work in a nursing center, hospital long-term care unit, or home care agency receiving Medicare funds.

The training program. OBRA requires at least 75 hours of instruction. Some states require more hours. At least 16 hours of supervised practical training are required. Such training occurs in a laboratory or clinical setting (Fig. 1.4). Students perform nursing care and tasks on another person. A nurse supervises this practical training (clinical practicum or clinical experience).

The training program includes the knowledge and skills needed to give basic nursing care. Areas of study include the following:
- Communication
- Infection control
- Safety and emergency procedures
- Residents' rights
- Basic nursing skills
- Personal care skills
- Feeding methods

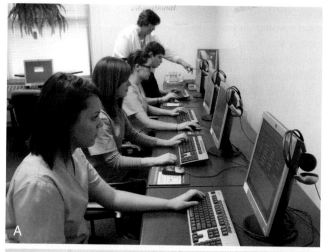

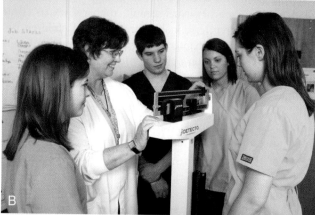

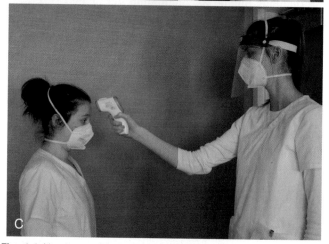

Fig. 1.4 Nursing assistant training program. (A) Students study in a classroom setting. (B) An instructor demonstrates a skill in a laboratory setting. (C) Students practice skills in a clinical setting.

- Elimination procedures
- Skin care
- Transferring, positioning, and turning methods
- Dressing
- Helping the person walk
- Range-of-motion exercises
- Signs and symptoms of common diseases

- How to care for cognitively impaired persons (those who have problems with thinking and memory)

Competency evaluation. The competency evaluation has a written test and a skills test (Appendix A). The written test has multiple-choice questions. Each has four choices. Only one answer is correct. The number of questions varies from state to state.

The skills test involves performing nursing skills. You will perform certain skills learned in your training program.

You take the competency evaluation after your training program. Your instructor tells you when and where the tests are given and may help you complete the application. There is a fee for the evaluation. If working in a nursing center, the employer pays this fee. You are told the place and time of the tests after your application is processed. Some states give a choice of test dates and sites.

Your training prepares you for the competency evaluation. If you listen, study hard, and practice safe care, you should do well. If the first attempt was not successful, you can retest. OBRA allows at least three attempts to successfully complete the evaluation. Some states require repeating a nurse assistant training course if the student fails the competency evaluation three times.

Nursing assistant registry. OBRA requires a nursing assistant registry in each state. It is an official record or listing of persons who have successfully completed that state's approved NATCEP. The registry has information about each nursing assistant:

- Full name, including maiden name and any married names
- Last known home address
- Registry number and the date it expires
- Date of birth
- Last known employer, date hired, and date employment ended
- Date the competency evaluation was passed
- Information about findings of abuse, neglect, or dishonest use of property. It includes the nature of the offense and supporting evidence. If a hearing was held, the date and its outcome are included. The person has the right to include a statement disputing the finding. All information stays in the registry for at least 5 years.

Any agency (hospital, nursing center, home care agency) can access registry information. You also receive a copy of your registry information. The copy is provided when the first entry is made and when information is changed or added. You can correct wrong information.

Other OBRA requirements. Retraining and a new competency evaluation program are required for nursing assistants who have not worked for 24 months. It does not matter how long you worked as a nursing assistant. What matters is how long you did *not* work. States can require:

- A new competency evaluation.
- Both retraining and a new competency evaluation.

Nursing centers must provide 12 hours of educational programs to nursing assistants every year. Performance reviews also are required. That is, your work is evaluated. These requirements help ensure that you have the current knowledge and skills to give safe, effective care.

◆ See *Teamwork and Time Management: Other OBRA Requirements.*

▶▶ TEAMWORK AND TIME MANAGEMENT

Other OBRA Requirements

Educational programs in nursing centers are commonly called *inservice programs* or *inservice training.* Some are required; others are optional. Program announcements and schedules are posted on bulletin boards on nursing units, in staff locker rooms and lounges, and by the time clock. Some notices may be included with your paycheck or sent through email. Know how your agency posts inservice information. Check those areas often.

Such training is scheduled before your shift begins, during your shift, or after your shift. If scheduled before work, plan to arrive early. If scheduled after work, plan to stay late. Arrange for transportation and child care as needed (Chapter 3). Some inservice training may be exercises done on a computer or watching video recordings online.

If the program is during your shift, plan with your coworkers. Some staff stay on the unit while others attend the program. Staff on the unit tend to all residents. A person may have special care needs while you are off the unit. Share this information with the staff who will provide such care. When you return to the unit, thank your coworkers for helping you. Help your coworkers when they leave the unit to attend inservice programs.

Certification

Each state's NATCEP must meet OBRA requirements. Some states require more training hours. Each state has its own competency evaluation program. After successfully completing your state's NATCEP, you have the title used in your state:

- Certified nursing assistant (CNA) or certified nurse aide (CNA), which is used in most states
- Licensed nursing assistant (LNA)
- Registered nurse aide (RNA)
- State-tested nursing assistant (STNA)

   Working in another state. To work in another state, you must meet that state's registry requirements. First, contact the state agency responsible for NATCEPs and the nursing assistant registry. To find that agency, do one of the following:

- Contact your current nursing assistant registry.
- Go to the NCSBN website. Find the link to the state agency.

Then apply to the state agency to be a CNA (LNA, RNA, STNA). The state uses one of these terms: *endorsement, reciprocity,* or *equivalency.* The terms mean that:

- Your application for CNA (LNA, RNA, STNA) is reviewed to see if you meet the state's requirements:
- Your certification (license, registration) is current and in good standing.
- You meet that state's education, work, and legal requirements.
- Certification (a license, registration) is granted if the requirements are met.
- Follow the application instructions. Expect to:
- Complete the required forms.

- Provide proof of successfully completing a NATCEP. You may need to send a copy of the certificate of completion from your NATCEP. Do not send the original.
- Request written registry verification from the state in which you are currently certified (licensed, registered). Pay the required fee.
- Provide fingerprints.
- Pay the required application fee.

   A criminal background check is done. Registry information is checked. Expect an investigation if the check shows a criminal history or if the check shows findings of abuse, neglect, dishonest use of property, or other action against you.

   You must be truthful. False or misleading information may result in:

- Denial of certification (a license, registration).
- Disciplinary action.
- A fine.

   The review results in one or more of the following:

- Being granted or denied certification (a license, registration)
- Having to take a competency test, which may be the written test, the skills test, or both
- Having to take an NATCEP in that state

ROLES AND RESPONSIBILITIES

Nurse practice acts, OBRA, state laws, and legal and advisory opinions direct what you can do. To protect persons from harm, you must understand what you can do, what you cannot do, and the legal limits of your role. In some states, this is called *scope of practice.* The NCSBN calls it *range of functions.*

   Licensed nurses supervise your work. You assist them in giving care. You also perform nursing tasks related to the person's care. A nursing task is the nursing care or a nursing function, procedure, activity, or work that can be delegated to nursing assistants when it does not require an RN's professional knowledge or judgment. Often you function without a nurse in the room. At other times you help nurses give care. In some centers, you assist doctors with procedures. The rules in Box 1.3 will help you understand your role.

BOX 1.3 Rules for Nursing Assistants

- You are an assistant to the nurse.
- A nurse assigns and supervises your work.
- You report observations about the person's physical and mental status to the nurse (Chapter 5). Report changes in the person's condition or behavior at once.
- The nurse decides what should be done for a person. The nurse decides what should not be done for a person. You do not make these decisions.
- Review directions and the care plan with the nurse before going to the person.
- Perform only those tasks for which you are trained.
- Ask a nurse to supervise you if you are not comfortable performing a nursing task.
- Perform only the nursing tasks that your state and job description allow.

The range of functions for nursing assistants varies among states and centers. Before you perform a nursing task ensure that:

- Your state allows nursing assistants to do so.
- It is in your job description.
- You have the necessary education and training.
- A nurse is available to answer questions and to supervise you.

You perform nursing tasks to meet the person's hygiene, safety, comfort, nutrition, exercise, and elimination needs. You also handle and move persons, make observations, and collect specimens. You help admit and discharge residents. You also measure temperatures, pulses, respirations, and blood pressures. And you help promote the person's mental comfort.

Box 1.4 describes the limits of your role—the nursing tasks that you should never do. State laws differ. You must know what you can do in the state in which you are working. For example, you move from Vermont to Maine. You must learn the laws and rules in Maine. Or you might work in two states. For example, you work in centers in Illinois and Iowa. You must know the laws and rules of both states.

State laws and rules limit nursing assistant functions. Your job description reflects those laws and rules. A center can further limit what you can do, and so can a nurse based on the person's needs. However, no center or nurse can expand your range of functions beyond what your state's laws and rules allow.

Nursing Assistant Standards

OBRA defines the basic range of functions for nursing assistants. All NATCEPs include those functions (p. ··). Some states allow other functions. NATCEPs also prepare nursing assistants to meet the standards listed in Box 1.5.

Job Description

The job description is a document that describes what the center expects you to do (Fig. 1.5). It also states educational requirements.

Always obtain a written job description when you apply for a job. Ask questions about it during your job interview. Before accepting a job, tell the employer about:

- Functions you did not learn.
- Functions you cannot do for moral or religious reasons.

BOX 1.4 Role Limits for Nursing Assistants

- ***Never give medications (drugs, medicines).*** This includes medications given orally, rectally, vaginally, and by injection. It also includes medications given by application to the skin, eyes, ears, and nose. Nor do you give medications directly into the bloodstream or through an intravenous (IV) line. Nurses give medications. Many states allow nursing assistants to give medications after completing a state-approved medication assistant training program. The function must be in your job description and you must have the necessary supervision.

- ***Never insert tubes or objects into body openings. Do not remove them from the body.*** You must not insert tubes into a person's bladder, esophagus, trachea, nose, ears, bloodstream, or surgically created body openings. Exceptions to this rule are the procedures you will study during your training. Giving enemas is an example. To perform them, they must be in your job description and you must have the necessary supervision.

- ***Never take oral or phone orders from doctors.*** Politely give your name and title and ask the doctor to wait for a nurse. Promptly find a nurse to speak with the doctor.

- ***Never perform procedures that require sterile technique.*** With sterile technique, all objects in contact with the person are free of microorganisms (Chapter 14). Sterile technique and procedures require skills, knowledge, and judgment beyond your training. You can *assist* a nurse with a sterile procedure. However, you will not perform the procedure yourself.

- ***Never tell the person or family the person's diagnosis or medical or surgical treatment plans.*** This is the doctor's responsibility. Nurses may clarify what the doctor has said.

- ***Never diagnose or prescribe treatments or medications for anyone.*** Doctors diagnose and prescribe.

- ***Never supervise others, including other nursing assistants.*** This is a nurse's legal responsibility. You will not be trained to supervise others. Supervising others can have serious legal problems.

- ***Never ignore an order or request to do something. This includes nursing tasks that you can do, those you cannot do, and those that are beyond your legal limits.*** Promptly and politely explain to the nurse why you cannot carry out the order or request. The nurse assumes you are doing what you were told to do unless you explain otherwise. You cannot neglect the person's care.

BOX 1.5 Nursing Assistant Standards

The nursing assistant:

- Performs nursing tasks within the range of functions allowed by the state's nurse practice act and its rules.
- Is honest and shows integrity in performing nursing tasks. (*Integrity* involves following a code of ethics [Chapter 2].)
- Bases nursing tasks on education and training. Also bases them on the nurse's directions.
- Is accountable for behavior and actions while assisting the nurse and helping residents.
- Performs delegated aspects of the person's nursing care.
- Assists the nurse in observing residents. Also assists in identifying their needs.
- Communicates:
  - Progress toward completing delegated nursing tasks.
  - Problems in completing delegated nursing tasks.
  - Changes in the person's status.
- Asks the nurse to clarify what is expected when unsure.
- Uses educational and training opportunities as available.
- Practices safety measures to protect the person, others, and self.
- Respects the person's rights, concerns, decisions, and dignity.
- Functions as a member of the health team. Helps implement the care plan (Chapter 5).
- Respects the person's property and the property of others.
- Protects confidential information unless required by law to share the information.

Modified from National Council of State Boards of Nursing, Inc. *Model nursing practice act and model nursing administrative rules.* Chicago: Author; 2021.

POSITION DESCRIPTION/PERFORMANCE EVALUATION

Job Title: Certified Nursing Assistant (CNA), Skilled Nursing Facility   Supervised by: Licensed Nurse

Prepared by: _____ Date: _____ Approved by: _____ Date: _____

Job Summary: Provides direct and indirect resident care activities under the direction of an RN or LPN. Assists residents with activities of daily living, provides for personal care and comfort, and assists in the maintenance of a safe and clean environment for an assigned group of residents.

DUTIES AND RESPONSIBILITIES:

E=Exceeds the Standard   M=Meets the Standard   NI=Needs Improvement

Demonstrates Competency in the Following Areas:	E	M	NI
Assists in the preparation for admission of residents.	2	1	0
Assists in and accompanies residents in the admission, transfer, and discharge procedures.	2	1	0
Provides morning care, which may include bed bath, shower or whirlpool, oral hygiene, combing hair, back massage, dressing resident, changing bed linen, cleaning overbed table and bedside stand, straightening room, and other general care as necessary throughout the day.	2	1	0
Provides evening care, which includes hand/face washing as needed, oral hygiene, back massage, pericare, freshening linen, cleaning overbed table, straightening room, and other general care as needed.	2	1	0
Notifies RN/LPN when resident complains of pain.	2	1	0
Assists with post-mortem care.	2	1	2
Assists nurses in treatment procedures.	2	1	0
Provides general nursing care such as positioning residents, lifting and turning residents, applying/utilizing special equipment, assisting in use of bedpan or commode, and ambulating the residents.	2	1	0
Performs all aspects of resident care in an environment that optimizes resident safety and reduces the likelihood of medical/health care errors.	2	1	0
Measures and records temperature, pulse, respiration, weight, blood pressure, and intake-output.	2	1	0
Makes rounds with outgoing shift. Knows whereabouts of assigned residents.	2	1	0
Makes rounds with oncoming shift to ensure the unit is left in good condition.	2	1	0
Adheres to policies and procedures of the center and the Department of Nursing.	2	1	0
Participates in socialization activities on the unit.	2	1	0
Turns and positions residents as ordered and/or as needed, making sure no rough surfaces are in direct contact with the body. Moves and turns with proper and safe body mechanics and with available resources.	2	1	0
Checks for reddened areas or skin breakdown and reports to RN or LPN.	2	1	0
Ensures residents are dressed properly and assists, as necessary. Ensures that clothing is properly stored in bedside stand or on hangers in closet. Ensures that all residents are clean and dry at all times.	2	1	0
Checks unit for adequate linen. Cleans linen cart. Provides clean linen and clothing. Makes beds.	2	1	0
Treats residents and their families with respect and dignity.	2	1	0
Follows center policies and procedures when caring for persons who are restrained.	2	1	0
Prepares residents for meals. Serves and removes food trays. Assists with meals or feeds residents, if necessary.	2	1	0
Distributes drinking water and other nourishments to residents.	2	1	0
Performs general care activities for residents on Isolation Precautions.	2	1	0
Answers residents' signal lights promptly. Anticipates residents' needs and makes rounds to assigned residents.	2	1	0
Assists residents with handling and care of clothing and other personal property (including dentures, eyeglasses, contact lenses, hearing aids, and prosthetic devices).	2	1	0
Transports residents to and from various departments, as requested.	2	1	0
Reports and, when appropriate, records any changes observed in condition or behavior of residents and unusual incidents.	2	1	0
Participates in and contributes to Resident Care Conferences.	2	1	0
Follows directions, both oral and written, and works cooperatively with other staff members.	2	1	0

Fig. 1.5 Nursing assistant job description. Note that the job description is also a performance evaluation tool. (Modified from Medical Consultants Network, Inc., Englewood, CO.)

POSITION DESCRIPTION/PERFORMANCE EVALUATION—cont'd

	E	M	NI
Establishes and maintains interpersonal relationships with residents, family members, and other center personnel while ensuring confidentiality of resident information.	2	1	0
Has the ability to acquire knowledge of and develop skills in basic nursing procedures and simple charting.	2	1	0
Attends in-service education programs, as assigned, to learn new treatments, procedures, skills, etc.	2	1	0
Maintains personal health in order to prevent absence from work due to health problems.	2	1	0

Professional Requirements:

	E	M	NI
Meets dress code standards. Appearance is neat and clean.	2	1	0
Completes annual education requirements.	2	1	0
Maintains regulatory requirements.	2	1	0
Meets center's standards for attendance.	2	1	0
Consistently completes and maintains assigned duties.	2	1	0
Wears identification while on duty.	2	1	0
Practices careful, efficient, and non-wasteful use of supplies and linen. Follows established charge procedure for resident charge items.	2	1	0
Attends annual review and department in-services, as scheduled.	2	1	0
Attends at least 75% of staff meetings. Reads and returns all monthly staff meeting minutes.	2	1	0
Represents the center in a positive and professional manner.	2	1	0
Actively participates in the Continuous Quality Improvement (CQI) activities.	2	1	0
Complies with all center policies regarding ethical business practices.	2	1	0
Communicates the mission, ethics, and goals of the center, as well as the focus statement of the department.	2	1	0
Possesses a genuine interest and concern for older and disabled persons.	2	1	0

TOTAL POINTS _____ _____ _____

Regulatory Requirements:

• High school graduate or equivalent

• Current Certified Nursing Assistant (CNA) certification

• Current Basic Life Support for Healthcare Providers certification within three (3) months of hire date

Language Skills:

• Ability to read and communicate effectively in English

• Additional languages preferred

Skills:

• Basic computer knowledge

Physical Demands:

• See "Physical Demands" policy.

I have received, read, and understand the Position Description/Performance Evaluation above.

_____   _____
Name/Signature   Date Signed

Fig. 1.5, cont'd

Clearly understand what is expected before taking a job. Do not take a job that requires you to:

- Act beyond the legal limits of your role.
- Function beyond your training limits.
- Perform acts that are against your morals or religion.

No one can force you to do something beyond the legal limits of your role. Sometimes jobs are threatened for refusing to follow a nurse's orders. Often staff obey out of fear. That is why you must understand:

- Your roles and responsibilities.
- What you can safely do.
- The things you should never do.
- Your job description.
- The ethical and legal aspects of your role (Chapter 2).

See *Focus on Communication: Job Description*.

FOCUS ON COMMUNICATION

Job Description

Your training prepares you to perform certain nursing tasks. The center may not let you do everything you learned. Other centers may want you to do things that you did not learn. Use your job description if you need to discuss these issues with the nurse.

For example, Mr. Wey is in the bathroom when the nurse brings a medication to him. The nurse tells you to give him the pill when he comes out of the bathroom. If you give the medication, you are performing a task and responsibility beyond the limits of your role. With respect, you must firmly refuse to follow the nurse's direction. You can say: "I'm sorry, but I cannot give Mr. Wey that pill. I was not trained to give medications, and that task is not in my job description. I'll let you know when Mr. Wey comes out of the bathroom."

DELEGATION

Nurse practice acts give nurses certain responsibilities. They also give them the legal authority to perform nursing actions. A responsibility is the duty or obligation to perform some act or function. For example, RNs are responsible for supervising LPNs/LVNs and nursing assistants. Only RNs can carry out this responsibility.

Delegate means to authorize another person to perform a nursing task in a certain situation. The person must be competent to perform a task in a given situation. For example, you know how to give a bed bath. However, Mr. Jones is a new resident. The RN wants to spend time with him and assess his nursing needs. You do not assess. Therefore the RN gives the bath.

Who Can Delegate

RNs can delegate nursing tasks to LPNs/LVNs and nursing assistants. In some states, LPNs/LVNs can delegate tasks to nursing assistants. RNs and LPNs/LVNs can delegate only tasks within their scope of practice. And they can delegate only the tasks in your job description.

Delegation decisions must protect the person's health and safety. The delegating nurse is legally accountable for the nursing task. Accountable means to be responsible for one's actions and the actions of others who performed the delegated tasks. It also involves answering questions about and explaining one's actions and the actions of others.

The delegating nurse must make sure that the task was completed safely and correctly. If the RN delegates, the RN is responsible for the delegated task. If the LPN/LVN delegates, they are responsible for the delegated task. The RN also supervises LPNs/LVNs. Therefore the RN is legally accountable for the tasks that LPNs/LVNs delegate to nursing assistants. The RN is accountable for all nursing care.

Nursing assistants cannot delegate. You cannot delegate any task to other nursing assistants or to any other worker. You can ask someone to help you, but you cannot ask or tell someone to do your work.

Delegation Process

To make delegation decisions, the nurse follows a process. The person's needs, the nursing task, and the staff member doing the task must fit. The nurse decides whether to delegate the task to you. The person's needs and the task may require a nurse's knowledge, judgment, and skill. You may be asked to assist.

Do not get offended or angry if you cannot perform a task usually delegated to you. The nurse decides what is best for the person at the time. That decision is also best for you at that time. You must not do something that requires a nurse's judgment. For example, you always care for Mrs. Mills. Now she is weak and not eating well. The nurse wants to observe and evaluate the changes in her condition. The nurse gives needed care. At this time Mrs. Mills needs the nurse's judgment and knowledge.

The person's circumstances are central factors in delegation decisions. Delegation decisions must result in the best care for the person. Otherwise the person's health and safety are at risk. Also, the nurse may face serious legal problems. If you perform a task that places the person at risk, you may face serious legal problems.

The NCSBN describes the delegation process in four steps.

Step 1—Assess and Plan

Step 1 is done by the nurse. To safely delegate, the nurse needs to understand the person's needs. And the nurse needs to know your knowledge, skills, and job description. The nurse then decides if it is safe to delegate the nursing task. It must be safe for the person and safe for you. If unsafe, the nurse stops the delegation process. If it is safe for the person and you, the nurse moves to step 2.

Step 2—Communication

Step 2 involves the nurse and you. The nurse must provide clear and complete directions. The nurse must ensure that you understand the directions. The nurse asks you questions to ensure you understand. The nurse may ask you to explain what you are going to do. Do not be insulted by such questions. The nurse must ensure that you give safe care. This protects the person and you.

Before performing a delegated nursing task, you must have the opportunity to discuss the task with the nurse. Make sure that you:

- Ask questions about the delegated task.
- Ask questions about what you are expected to do.
- Tell the nurse if you have not done the task before. Also tell the nurse if you have not done it often.
- Ask for needed training or supervision.
- Restate what specific resident concerns to report to the nurse.
- Explain how and when you will report your progress in completing the task.
- Know how to contact the nurse for an emergency.
- Know what the nurse wants you to do during an emergency.

After completing a delegated task, you report and record the care given. You also report and record your observations. See "Reporting and Recording" in Chapter 4.

Step 3—Surveillance and Supervision

Surveillance means to keep a close watch over someone or something. *Supervise* means to oversee, direct, or manage. In this step, the nurse observes the care you give. The nurse ensures that you complete the task correctly. The nurse also observes the person's condition and response to your care. The nurse is alert for signs and symptoms that signal a possible change in the person's condition. This way the nurse, with your help, can act before the person's condition changes in a major way.

Sometimes problems arise in completing a nursing task. By supervising you, the nurse can detect and solve problems early. This helps you complete the task safely and on time.

After you complete the task, the nurse may review and discuss what happened with you. This helps you learn. If a similar situation happens in the future, you have ideas about how to adjust.

Step 4—Evaluation and Feedback

This final step is done by the nurse. *Evaluate* means to judge. The nurse decides if the delegation was successful. *Feedback* means to respond. The nurse tells you what you did correctly. If you did something wrong, the nurse tells you that, too. Feedback is another way for you to learn and improve the care you give.

The Five Rights of Delegation

The NCSBN's *Five Rights of Delegation* is another way to view the delegation process. To use the "five rights," the nurse answers the questions listed in the four steps described earlier. The five rights are:

- *The right task.* Can the task be delegated? Is the nurse allowed to delegate the task? Is the task in your job description?
- *The right circumstances.* What are the person's physical, mental, emotional, and spiritual needs at this time?
- *The right person.* Do you have the training and experience to safely perform the task for this person?

- *The right directions and communication.* The nurse must give clear directions. The nurse tells you what to do and when to do it. The nurse tells you what observations to make and when to report back. The nurse allows questions and helps you set priorities.
- *The right supervision.* In this step, the nurse:
  - Guides, directs, and evaluates the care you give.
  - Demonstrates tasks as necessary and is available to answer questions. The less experience you have with a task, the more supervision you need. Complex tasks require more supervision than basic tasks. Also, the person's circumstances affect how much supervision you need.
  - Assesses how the task affected the person and how well you performed the task.
  - Tells you what you did well and how to improve your work. This helps you learn and give better care.

Your Role in Delegation

You perform delegated nursing tasks for or on a *person*. You must protect the person from harm. You have two choices when a task is delegated to you. You either *agree* or *refuse* to do the task. Use the *Five Rights of Delegation* in Box 1.6.

BOX 1.6 The *Five Rights of Delegation* for Nursing Assistants

The Right Task
- Does your state allow you to perform the task?
- Were you trained to do the task?
- Do you have experience performing the task?
- Is the task in your job description?

The Right Circumstances
- Do you have experience performing the task given the person's condition and needs?
- Do you understand the purposes of the task for the person?
- Can you perform the task safely under the current circumstances?
- Do you have the equipment and supplies to safely complete the task?
- Do you know how to use the equipment and supplies?
- Is this the correct time to perform the task?

The Right Person
- Are you comfortable performing the task?
- Do you have concerns about performing the task?
- Have you received the correct training to perform the task?

The Right Directions and Communication
- Did the nurse give clear directions and instructions?
- Did you review the task with the nurse?
- Do you understand what the nurse expects?

The Right Supervision and Evaluation
- Is a nurse available to answer questions?
- Is a nurse available if the person's condition changes or if problems occur?

Modified from National Council of State Boards of Nursing, Inc. *The five rights of delegation.* Chicago: Author; 2019. Available at: https://www.ncsbn.org/NGND-PosPaper_06.pdf

Accepting a Task

When you agree to perform a task, you are responsible for your own actions. What you do or fail to do can harm the person. *You must complete the task safely.* Ask for help when you are unsure or have questions about a task. Report to the nurse what you did and the observations you made.

Refusing a Task

You have the right to say no. Sometimes refusing to follow the nurse's directions is your right and duty. You should refuse to perform a task when:

- The task is beyond the legal limits of your role.
- The task is not in your job description.
- You were not prepared to perform the task.
- The task could harm the person.
- The person's condition has changed.
- You do not know how to use the supplies or equipment.
- Directions are not ethical or legal.
- Directions are against center policies.
- Directions are not clear or not complete.
- A nurse is not available for supervision.

Use common sense. This protects you and the person. Ask yourself if what you are doing is safe for the person.

Never ignore an order or a request to do something. Tell the nurse about your concerns. If the task is within the legal limits of your role and in your job description, the nurse can help increase your comfort with the task. The nurse can:

- Answer your questions.
- Demonstrate the task.
- Show you how to use supplies and equipment.
- Help you as needed.
- Observe you performing the task.
- Check on you often.
- Arrange for needed training.

Do not refuse a task because you do not like it or do not want to do it. You must have sound reasons. Otherwise, you place the person at risk for harm. You also could lose your job.

See *Focus on Communication: Refusing a Task.*

 FOCUS ON COMMUNICATION

Refusing a Task

A nurse may delegate a task that you did not learn in your training program. The task is in your job description. You can say, "I know this task is in my job description but I did not learn it in school. Can you show me what to do and then observe me doing it? That would really help me."

A nurse may ask you to do something that is not in your job description. With respect, you must firmly refuse the nurse's request. You can say, "I'm sorry. I am not trained to do that. That task is not in my job description. Can I help you with something else?"

QUALITY OF LIFE

Nursing center care is always focused on the resident. The interdisciplinary team helps all residents to become or remain as independent as possible. This promotes their quality of life. Always remember to let residents do as much for themselves as safely possible. This helps their feelings of independence. Do not do or take over tasks that residents can do themselves.

The work you do has value. By continuing to learn, you increase your skills and knowledge. It adds to your value. It offers you more opportunities. Your current training is just the start of a lifetime of learning and possibilities.

Some states have higher levels of nursing assistants. Medication assistant-certified (MA-C) or certified medication aide (CMA) are examples. These are nursing assistants with extra training. Supervised by a licensed nurse, they give medications as allowed by state law.

You can continue to learn in many ways. Find out the options available in your state and center. Take advantage of them. Be proud of your training. And never stop learning!

TIME TO REFLECT

You have been caring for Mrs. Clark for several weeks. She resides in the care center due to a stroke. You have developed a good relationship with Mrs. Clark and with her daughter, Janet, who visits daily. Janet tells you she is concerned about how much her mother's care is costing. She is afraid her mother's resources will soon be depleted. Janet tells you she wants to take her mother home to live with her. She asks if you would consider leaving your job at the nursing center and come work for them in their home. How would you respond to this offer from Janet?

▌ R E V I E W   Q U E S T I O N S

Circle the BEST answer.

1. Helping persons return to their highest physical and mental function is called
   - **a.** Maintaining independence
   - **b.** Promoting health
   - **c.** Preventing disease
   - **d.** Rehabilitation
2. Which provides 24-hour nursing care?
   - **a.** Board and care homes
   - **b.** Assisted living residences
   - **c.** Nursing centers
   - **d.** Residential care facilities
3. Who controls policy in a nursing center?
   - **a.** The director of nursing
   - **b.** The owner
   - **c.** The health team
   - **d.** Medicare and Medicaid
4. A health care program for terminally ill persons is a
   - **a.** Hospice
   - **b.** Board and care home
   - **c.** Skilled nursing facility
   - **d.** Home care agency

5. The nursing team does *not* include
   a. Doctors
   b. LPNs/LVNs
   c. Nursing assistants
   d. RNs
6. Who is responsible for the entire nursing staff?
   a. The case manager
   b. The RN
   c. The director of nursing
   d. The medical director
7. Nursing assistants are supervised by
   a. RNs and LPNs/LVNs
   b. Other nursing assistants
   c. The health team
   d. The medical director
8. The nursing assistant's role is to
   a. Meet Medicare and Medicaid standards
   b. Assist nurses in giving care
   c. Carry out the doctor's orders
   d. Manage care
9. Medicare is for persons who
   a. Are 65 years of age and older
   b. Are part of a PPO
   c. Have group insurance
   d. Have low incomes
10. A survey team is at your center. A team member asks you some questions. You should
    a. Refer all questions to the nurse
    b. Answer as the DON tells you to
    c. Give as little information as possible
    d. Give honest and complete answers
11. What state law affects what nursing assistants can do?
    a. Standards for nursing assistants
    b. OBRA
    c. Nurse practice act
    d. Medicaid
12. Your nursing assistant certification can be revoked for
    a. Refusing a nursing task
    b. Asking the nurse questions
    c. Performing acts beyond your role
    d. Keeping the person's information confidential
13. Which requires a training and competency evaluation program for nursing assistants?
    a. Medicare
    b. Medicaid

c. NCSBN
d. OBRA
14. As a nursing assistant, you
    a. Must perform all nursing tasks as directed by the nurse
    b. Make decisions about a person's care
    c. Need a written job description before employment
    d. Give a medication when a nurse tells you to
15. As a nursing assistant, you
    a. Can take verbal or phone orders from doctors
    b. Are responsible for your own actions
    c. Can remove tubes from the person's body
    d. Can ignore a nursing task if it is not in your job description
16. Who assigns and supervises your work?
    a. Other nursing assistants
    b. The health team
    c. Nurses
    d. Doctors
17. You are responsible for
    a. Supervising other nursing assistants
    b. Delegation decisions
    c. Completing delegated tasks safely
    d. Deciding what treatments are needed
18. A task is in your job description. Which is *false*?
    a. The nurse must delegate the task to you.
    b. The nurse can delegate the task if the person's circumstances are right.
    c. You must have the necessary education and training to complete the task.
    d. You must have clear directions before you perform the task.
19. You can refuse to perform a task for these reasons *except*
    a. The task is beyond the legal limits of your role
    b. The task is not in your job description
    c. You do not like the task
    d. A nurse is not available to supervise you
20. You decide to refuse a task. What should you do?
    a. Delegate the task to a nursing assistant
    b. Communicate your concerns to the nurse
    c. Ignore the request
    d. Talk to the director of nursing

See Appendix A for answers to these questions.

2

Resident Rights, Ethics, and Laws

OBJECTIVES

- Define the key terms and key abbreviations listed in this chapter.
- Describe the purpose and requirements of the Omnibus Budget Reconciliation Act of 1987 (OBRA).
- Identify the person's rights under OBRA.
- Explain how to protect the person's rights.
- Explain the ombudsman role.
- Describe ethical conduct.
- Describe the rules of conduct for nursing assistants.
- Explain how to maintain professional boundaries.

- Explain how to prevent negligent acts.
- Give examples of false imprisonment, defamation, assault, battery, and fraud.
- Describe how to protect the right to privacy.
- Explain the purpose of informed consent.
- Explain your role in relation to wills.
- Describe elder and domestic abuse.
- Explain how to promote quality of life.

KEY TERMS

abuse The willful infliction of injury, unreasonable confinement, intimidation (to threaten, to hurt or punish), or punishment that results in physical harm, pain, or mental anguish; depriving the person (or the person's caretaker) of the goods or services needed to attain or maintain well-being

assault Intentionally attempting or threatening to touch a person's body without the person's consent

battery Touching a person's body without the person's consent

boundary crossing A brief act or behavior outside the helpful zone

boundary sign An act, behavior, or thought that warns of a boundary crossing or violation

boundary violation An act or behavior that meets your needs, not the person's needs

civil law Laws concerned with relationships between people

crime An act that violates a criminal law

criminal law Laws concerned with offenses against the public and society in general

defamation Injuring a person's name and reputation by making false statements to a third person

ethics Knowledge of what is right conduct and wrong conduct

false imprisonment Unlawful restraint or restriction of a person's freedom of movement

fraud Saying or doing something to trick, fool, or deceive a person

invasion of privacy Violating a person's right not to have own name, photo, or private affairs exposed or made public without giving consent

involuntary seclusion Separating a person from others against the person's will, keeping the person confined to a certain area, or keeping the person away from own room without consent

law A rule of conduct made by a government body

libel Making false statements in print, writing, or through pictures or drawings

malpractice Negligence by a professional person

neglect Failure to provide the person with the goods or services needed to avoid physical harm, mental anguish, or mental illness

negligence An unintentional wrong in which a person did not act in a reasonable and careful manner and a person or the person's property was harmed

ombudsman Someone who supports or promotes the needs and interests of another person

professional boundary That which separates helpful behaviors from behaviors that are not helpful

professional sexual misconduct An act, behavior, or comment that is sexual in nature

protected health information Identifying information and information about the person's health care that is maintained or sent in any form (paper, electronic, oral)

representative Any person who has the legal right to act on the resident's behalf when the resident does not have the ability

self-neglect A person's behaviors that self-threaten health and safety

slander Making false statements orally

standard of care The skills, care, and judgments required by a health team member under similar conditions

tort A wrong committed against a person or the person's property

treatment The care provided to maintain or restore health, improve function, or relieve symptoms

vulnerable adult A person 18 years old or older who has a disability or condition that presents the risk to be wounded, attacked, or damaged

will A legal document of how a person wants property distributed after death

KEY ABBREVIATIONS

DON Director of nursing

HIPAA Health Insurance Portability and Accountability Act of 1996

OBRA Omnibus Budget Reconciliation Act of 1987

In 1987, the US Congress passed the Omnibus Budget Reconciliation Act (OBRA). This federal law applies to all 50 states. OBRA requires that nursing centers provide care in a manner and in a setting that maintains or improves each person's quality of life, health, and safety. It also requires nursing assistant training and competency evaluation (Chapter 1). Resident rights are a major part of OBRA.

❖ Resident Rights

Residents have rights as US citizens. For example, they have the right to vote. They also have rights relating to their everyday lives and care in a nursing center. These rights are protected by federal and state laws. Nursing centers must protect and promote such rights. The center cannot interfere with a resident's rights.

Some residents are incompetent (not able). They cannot exercise their rights. A representative (partner, adult child, court-appointed guardian) does so for them. A representative is any person who has the legal right to act on the resident's behalf when the resident cannot do so for oneself.

Nursing centers must inform residents of their rights. Centers must also inform residents of all rules about resident conduct and responsibilities in the center. This is done orally and in writing. Such information is given before or during admission to the center, as needed during the person's stay, and when laws (state or federal) or center rules change. It is given in the language the person uses and understands.

- Medical terms are avoided to the extent possible.
- An interpreter is used if the person speaks and understands a foreign language or communicates by sign language.
- Written translations are provided in the foreign languages common in the center's geographic area.
- Sign language and other communication aids are used as necessary.
- Large-print texts are available for persons with impaired vision.

Resident rights (Box 2.1) are posted throughout the center (Fig. 2.1). Those that affect your role are described in this chapter.

Information

The *right to information* means access to all records about the person. They include the medical record, contracts, incident reports, and financial records. The request can be oral or written.

The person has the right to be fully informed of one's own health condition. Information is given in a language and in words the person can understand. Interpreters are used as needed. Sign language or other aids are used for those with hearing losses.

The person must also have information about one's own health care provider. This includes the name, specialty, and how to contact the health care provider.

Report any request for information to the nurse. *Do not give the information just described to the person or family.*

Refusing Treatment

The person has the *right to refuse treatment*. Treatment means the care provided to maintain or restore health, improve function, or relieve symptoms. A person who does not give consent or refuses treatment cannot be treated against one's own wishes. The center must find out what the person is refusing and why. For example, a person learned to walk after a hip fracture. However, the person refuses to walk. The center must:

- Find out the reason for the refusal.
- Educate the person about the problems that can result from not walking.
- Offer other treatment options.
- Continue to provide all other services.

Advance directives are part of the right to refuse treatment (Chapter 45). They include living wills and instructions about life support. *Advance directives* are written instructions about health care when the person is not able to make such decisions.

Report any treatment refusal to the nurse. The nurse may change the person's care plan.

Privacy and Confidentiality

Residents have the *right to personal privacy*. Staff must provide care in a manner that maintains privacy of the person's body. The person's body is exposed only as necessary. Only staff directly involved in care and treatments are present. The person must give consent for others to be present. For example, a student wants to observe a treatment. The person's consent is needed for the student to observe.

A person has the right to use the bathroom in private. Privacy is maintained for all personal care measures such as bathing and dressing. Protect privacy by:

- Closing privacy curtains, doors, and window coverings.
- Removing residents from public view.
- Providing clothes or draping the person to prevent unnecessary exposure of body parts.

Leaving the person without a gown or bed covers violates the person's right to privacy. So does leaving the room door open when the person uses the bathroom or bedpan.

Residents have the right to visit with others in private—in areas where others cannot see or hear them. If requested, the

BOX 2.1 Resident Rights

- To be treated with dignity and respect and to receive quality care.
- To exercise one's rights as a center resident and as a US citizen.
- To be informed orally and in writing of one's rights and center rules. This is done in a language the person understands.
- To access all records about oneself, including current clinical records.
- To obtain copies of one's records. This is at the resident's expense.
- To refuse treatment.
- To refuse to take part in experimental research. This is the development and testing of new treatments and medications.
- To make advance directives (Chapter 45).
- To be informed of Medicare benefits and services. This includes costs and charges covered and not covered.
- To file complaints with the appropriate state agency about abuse, neglect, and the misuse of one's property.
- To be informed of center services and of the charges for those services.
- To choose one's health care provider.
- To know the name, specialty, and contact information of the health care provider responsible for one's care.
- To be fully informed of one's total health status, including medical condition.
- To be informed of:
  - Any accident or injury that may need medical attention.
  - A change in one's physical, mental, or psychosocial status.
  - The need to stop, change, or add a treatment.
  - A decision to transfer or discharge the person.
  - A change in the person's room or roommate.
  - A change in the person's rights under federal or state law.
- To manage one's personal and financial affairs.
- To be fully informed in advance about one's care and treatment. This includes changes in care and treatment.
- To privacy and confidentiality:
  - Of personal and medical records
  - Of treatment and personal care
  - Of written and phone communications
  - During visits with family and friends
- When meeting with resident groups
- To voice grievances and have them solved promptly.
- To see the results of federal and state surveys. The person also has the right to see the plans to correct problems or areas of weakness.
- To perform services for the center or to refuse to perform services.
- To send and receive mail that is not open. To buy supplies to send mail.
- To receive information from one's health care provider and community and state agencies responsible for protecting developmentally disabled and mentally ill persons.
- To have and use personal items and clothing.
- To share a room with one's spouse (husband, wife) when married residents live in the same center (Chapter 10).
- To take one's medications without help if able.
- To receive notice before one's room or roommate is changed.
- To refuse to change to a different room.
- To have reasonable notice about a transfer or discharge (Chapter 30).
- To be free from physical and chemical restraints (Chapter 13).
- To be free from abuse (verbal, sexual, physical), bodily punishment, and involuntary seclusion.
- To be cared for in a manner and in a setting that maintains or enhances quality of life.
- To choose activities, schedules, and health care that meet one's interest.
- To interact with community members inside and outside the center.
- To make choices about one's life in the center.
- To organize and take part in resident groups.
- To take part in social, religious, and community activities.
- To a setting and services that consider one's needs and choices.
- To be informed of one's health and medical condition in a language that is understandable. That language is used when the person takes part in care planning.
- To a clean, comfortable, and homelike setting. This includes temperature, lighting, and sound levels.
- To closet space.
- To visit with one's spouse, family, and friends at any reasonable hour.

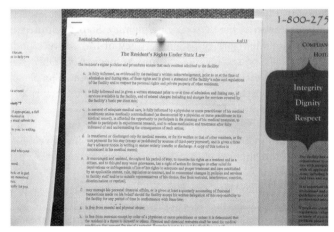

Fig. 2.1 Resident rights are posted in the nursing center.

center must provide private space. Offices, chapels, dining rooms, meeting rooms, and outdoor spaces are used as needed.

Residents have the right to make phone calls in private (Fig. 2.2). The calls must not be where they can be overheard.

Therefore phones are not used in offices or at the nurses' station. Centers provide cordless phones or phone jacks in resident rooms. Phones are at the correct height for use by persons in wheelchairs. Phones for persons who are hearing impaired are also available. Some residents have their own cell phones, electronic tablets, or laptop computers for communication.

The right to privacy also involves mail. The person has the right to send and receive mail without others interfering. No one can open mail the person sends or receives without the person's consent. Unopened mail is given to the person within 24 hours of delivery to the center. Mail the person sends is delivered to the postal service within 24 hours when there is regular delivery or pickup service.

Information about the person's care, treatment, and condition is kept confidential. So are medical and financial records. Consent is needed to release them to other agencies or persons.

You must provide privacy and protect confidentiality. Staff do not have the right to look at a resident's medical record if it does not pertain to the care they are giving. Sometimes it is necessary to have written notes about the care you have offered.

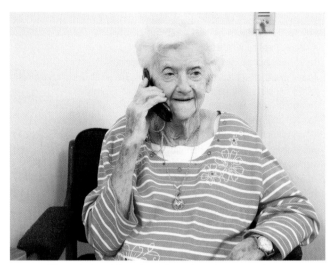

Fig. 2.2 A resident is talking privately on the phone.

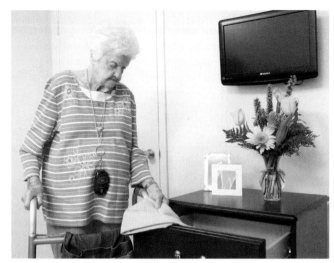

Fig. 2.4 A resident is choosing what clothing to wear.

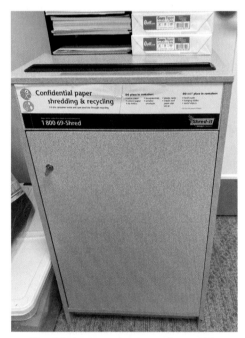

Fig. 2.3 A secure document disposal bin

Once the information has been entered or conveyed, the paper should be placed in a secure document disposal bin (Fig 2.3) or shredded. It is common to have flow sheets or records to document vital signs or weights. These should not be left in public view. Keeping this information private shows respect for the person. It also protects the person's dignity.

Personal Choice

Residents have the *right to make their own choices*. They can choose their own doctors. They also have the right to take part in planning and deciding about their care and treatment. They can choose activities, schedules, and care based on their preferences. They can choose when to get up and go to bed, what to wear, how to spend time, and what to eat (Fig. 2.4). They can choose friends and visitors inside and outside the center.

Personal choice promotes quality of life, dignity, and self-respect. You must allow personal choice when safely possible.

Grievances

Residents have the *right to voice concerns, questions, and complaints about treatment or care*. The problem may involve another person. It may be about care that was given or not given. The center must promptly try to correct the matter. No one can punish the person in any way for voicing the grievance.

Work

The person does not work for care, care items, or other things or privileges. The person is not required to perform services for the center.

However, the person has the *right to work or perform services if desired*. Some people like to garden, repair or build things, clean, sew, mend, fold laundry, or cook. Other persons need work for rehabilitation or activity reasons. The desire or need for work is part of the person's care plan. Residents volunteer or are paid for their services.

Taking Part in Resident Groups

The person has the *right to form and take part in resident groups*. Some centers have resident councils that meet on a regular basis. Families have the right to meet with other families. These groups can discuss concerns and suggest center improvements. They also can support each other, plan activities, and take part in educational activities.

Residents have the right to take part in social, cultural, religious, spiritual, and community events. They have the right to request help in getting to and from events of their choice.

Personal Items

Residents have the *right to keep and use personal items*. This includes clothing and some furnishings. The type and amount of personal items allowed depend on space needs and the health and safety of others.

Treat the person's property with care and respect. These items have great value to the resident just as your possessions have value to you. They also relate to personal choice, dignity, a homelike setting, and quality of life.

The person's property is protected. Items are labeled with the person's name. The center must investigate reports of lost, stolen, or damaged items. Police help is sometimes needed. The person and family are advised not to keep jewelry and other costly items in the center.

Protect yourself and the center from being accused of stealing a person's property. Do not go through a person's closet, drawers, purse or wallet, or other space without the person's knowledge and consent. A nurse may ask you to inspect closets and drawers. Center policy should require that a coworker and the person or legal representative be present. The coworker is a witness to your activities. Follow center policy for reporting and recording the inspection.

Freedom From Abuse, Mistreatment, and Neglect

Residents have the right to be free from verbal, sexual, physical, and mental abuse. *Abuse* means:

- The willful infliction of injury, unreasonable confinement, intimidation (to threaten to hurt or punish), or punishment that results in physical harm, pain, or mental anguish.
- Depriving the person (or the person's caretaker) of the goods or services needed to attain or maintain well-being.

They also have the right to be free from *involuntary seclusion*:

- Separating a person from others against the person's will
- Keeping the person confined to a certain area
- Keeping the person away from one's own room without consent

No one can abuse, neglect, or mistreat a resident. This includes center staff, volunteers, and staff from other agencies or groups. It also includes other residents, family members, friends, visitors, and legal representatives. Nursing centers must investigate suspected or reported cases of abuse. They cannot employ persons who:

- Were found guilty of abusing, neglecting, or mistreating others by a court of law.
- Have a finding entered into the state's nursing assistant registry (Chapter 1) about abuse, neglect, mistreatment, or wrongful acts involving the person's money or property. A *finding* means that a state has determined that the employee abused, neglected, mistreated, or wrongfully used the person's money or property.

Freedom from Restraint

Residents have the *right not to have body movements restricted*. Restraints and certain medications can restrict body movements. Some medications can restrain the person because they affect mood, behavior, and mental function. Sometimes residents are restrained to protect them from harming themselves or others. A doctor's order is needed for restraint use. Restraints are not used for staff convenience or to discipline a person.

They are used only if required to treat the person's medical symptoms. Restraints are discussed in Chapter 13.

Quality of Life

Residents have the *right to quality of life*. Nursing centers must care for residents in a manner and in a setting that promotes dignity and respect for self. This means that staff provide care in a manner that maintains or enhances the person's self-esteem and feelings of self-worth. Staff must promote physical, mental, and psychosocial well-being. Protecting resident rights promotes quality of life. It shows respect for the person.

The person is spoken to in a polite and courteous manner. Good, honest, and thoughtful care enhances the person's quality of life. Box 2.2 lists OBRA-required actions that promote dignity and privacy.

Activities

Residents have the *right to activities that enhance each person's physical, mental, and psycho-social well-being*. The intent is to promote self-esteem, pleasure, comfort, education, creativity, success, and independence. They must have a purpose and relate to the person's needs, interests, culture, and background. Centers also provide religious services for spiritual health. Activities must have meaning for the person. They are meaningful when they:

- Reflect the person's interests and lifestyle.
- Are enjoyed by the person.
- Help the person feel useful or produce something useful.
- Provide a sense of belonging.

Activities may involve large or small groups. A concert is a large group activity. A card game is a small group activity. Other activities involve two people, or the person does something alone such as writing a letter or playing a computer game.

You assist residents to and from activity programs. You may need to help them with activities.

See *Teamwork and Time Management: Activities.*

See *Focus on Communication: Activities.*

TEAMWORK AND TIME MANAGEMENT

Activities

Residents may need help getting to and from activity programs. Know when an activity begins and ends. Do the following before assisting residents to activity areas.

- Assist with elimination needs and hand washing.
- Assist with grooming measures such as brushing and combing hair. A person may want to apply some aftershave or perfume and/or makeup.
- Make sure the person wears the correct clothing and footwear for the activity.
- Make sure the person has needed assist devices (e.g., eyeglasses, hearing aids, cane, walker).

Allow 15 to 20 minutes to assist residents to and from the activity area. Help your coworkers as needed.

You may have to help residents with activities (Fig. 2.5). If not, use the activity time wisely. Provide needed care and visit residents who cannot leave their rooms. You can also clean and straighten rooms, bathrooms, shower rooms, and utility rooms.

BOX 2.2   OBRA-Required Actions That Promote Dignity and Privacy

Courteous and Dignified Interactions
- Use the right tone of voice.
- Use good eye contact.
- Stand or sit close enough as needed.
- Use the person's proper name and title (e.g., "Mrs. Crane").
- Gain the person's attention before interacting with the person.
- Use touch if the person approves.
- Respect the person's social status.
- Listen with interest to what the person is saying.
- Do not yell at, scold, or embarrass the person.

Privacy and Self-Determination
- Drape properly during care and procedures to avoid exposure and embarrassment.
- Drape properly in chair.
- Use privacy curtains or screens during care and procedures.
- Close the room door during care and procedures as the person desires; also close window coverings.
- Knock on the door before entering; wait to be asked inside.
- Close the bathroom door when the person uses the bathroom.

Maintain Personal Choice and Independence
- Person smokes in allowed areas.
- Person takes part in activities according to own interests.
- Person takes part in scheduling activities and care.
- Person gives input into the care plan about preferences and independence.
- Person is involved in room or roommate change.
- The person's items are moved or inspected only with the person's consent.

Courteous and Dignified Care
- Groom hair, beards, and nails as the person wishes.
- Assist with dressing in the right clothing for time of day, season, and personal choice.
- Promote independence and dignity in dining.
- Respect private space and property (e.g., change radio or TV stations only with the person's consent).
- Assist with walking and transfers. Do not interfere with independence.
- Assist with bathing and hygiene preferences. Do not interfere with independence.
    - Appearance is neat and clean.
    - The person is clean shaven or has a groomed beard and mustache.
    - Nails are trimmed and clean.
    - Dentures, hearing aids, eyeglasses, and other devices are used correctly.
    - Clothing is clean.
    - Clothing is properly fitted and fastened.
    - Shoes, hose, and socks are properly applied and fastened.
    - Extra clothing is worn for warmth as needed (e.g., sweaters and lap blankets).

📋 FOCUS ON COMMUNICATION

Activities
You may need help assisting residents to and from activity programs. Politely ask a coworker to help you. Share this information with your coworker:
- What time you need the help
- How much of the coworker's time you need
- The residents you need help with
- If the person walks or uses a wheelchair
- What assist devices are used (e.g., eyeglasses, hearing aids, cane, walker)

Be sure to say "please" when asking for help and thank the person for helping you. For example: "Jane, can you please help me assist two residents to the concert? It starts at 1:00 so I'll need your help at 12:45. Mr. Harris needs his glasses and hearing aid. He'll use a walker. Mrs. Juarez uses a wheelchair. She needs her glasses and a blanket for her lap. The blanket is in her wheelchair. The concert is over at 2:00. Please help me then, too. Thank you so much for helping me."

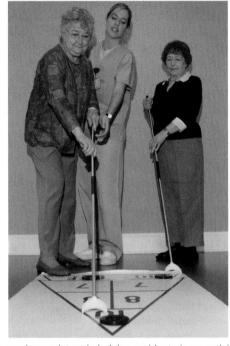

Fig. 2.5 A nursing assistant is helping residents in an activity program.

❖ Environment

Residents have the *right to a safe, clean, comfortable, and homelike setting.* The person is allowed to have and use personal items to the extent possible.

The center must provide a setting and services that meet the person's needs and preferences. The setting and staff must promote the person's independence, dignity, and well-being. The center must try to change schedules, call systems, and room arrangements to meet the person's desires and needs.

For example, the center must make changes when a person:
- Refuses a bath but prefers a shower.
- Prefers to have a shower at a different time or on a different day.
- Refuses a shower because of the fear of falling.
- Is uneasy about the staff assigned to help.
- Is worried about falling.
- Cannot reach or use the call light.
- Cannot reach personal items.
- Does not like the food served.

OMBUDSMAN PROGRAM

The Older Americans Act is a federal law. It requires a long-term care ombudsman program in every state. An ombudsman is someone who supports or promotes the needs and interests of another person. Long-term care ombudsmen are employed by a state agency. Some are volunteers. They are not nursing center employees. They act on behalf of nursing center and assisted-living residents.

Ombudsmen protect the health, safety, welfare, and rights of residents. They:

- Investigate and resolve complaints.
- Provide services to assist residents.
- Provide information about long-term care services.
- Monitor nursing center care.
- Monitor nursing center conditions.
- Provide support to resident and family groups.
- Help the resident and family resolve conflicts within the family.
- Help the center manage difficult problems.
- Educate residents, families, and the public about long-term care issues and concerns.
- Represent residents' interests before local, state, and federal governments.

Residents have the right to voice grievances and disputes. They also have the right to communicate privately with anyone of their choice. They can share concerns with anyone outside the center.

❖ *OBRA requires that nursing centers post the names, addresses, and phone numbers of local and state ombudsmen. This information must be posted where residents can easily see it.*

A resident or family may share a concern with you. You must know state and center policies and procedures for contacting an ombudsman. Ombudsman services are useful when:

- There is concern about a person's care or treatment.
- Someone interferes with a person's rights, health, safety, or welfare.

ETHICAL ASPECTS

Ethics is knowledge of what is right conduct and wrong conduct. Morals are involved. It also deals with choices or judgments about what should or should not be done. An ethical person behaves and acts in the right way and does not cause anyone harm.

Ethical behavior also involves not being *prejudiced* or *biased*. To be prejudiced or biased means to make judgments and have views before knowing the facts. Judgments and views usually are based on one's values and standards. They are based on the person's culture, religion, education, and experiences. The person's situation may be very different from your own. For example:

- Children want their mother to have nursing home care. In your culture, children care for older parents at home.
- A person has many tattoos and body piercings. You do not like tattoos or body piercings.

BOX 2.3 Code of Conduct for Nursing Assistants

- Respect each person as an individual.
- Know the limits of your role and knowledge.
- Perform only those tasks that are within the legal limits of your role.
- Perform only those tasks that you have been prepared to do.
- Perform no act that will cause the person harm.
- Take medications only if prescribed and supervised by a doctor.
- Carry out the directions and instructions of the nurse to your best possible ability.
- Follow the center's policies and procedures.
- Complete each task safely.
- Be loyal to your employer and coworkers.
- Act as a responsible citizen at all times.
- Keep the person's information confidential.
- Protect the person's privacy.
- Protect the person's property.
- Consider the person's needs to be more important than your own.
- Report errors and incidents at once.
- Be accountable for your actions.

- An 83-year-old man does not want life-saving measures. You believe that everything must be done to save a life.

Do not judge the person by your values and standards. Do not avoid persons whose standards and values differ from your own.

Ethical problems involve making choices. You must decide what is the right thing to do. For example:

- You find a coworker in an empty room drinking from a cup. You smell alcohol on her breath. She asks you not to tell anyone.
- A resident has bruises all over her body. She told the nurse that she fell. She tells you that her son is very mean to her. She asks you not to tell the nurse.

Professional groups have codes of ethics. The code has rules, or standards of conduct, for group members to follow. The American Nurses Association (ANA) has a code of ethics for registered nurses (RNs). The National Federation of Licensed Practical Nurses (NFLPN) has one for licensed practical nurses/licensed vocational nurses (LPNs/LVNs). The rules of conduct in Box 2.3 can guide your thinking and behavior. See Chapter 3 for ethics in the workplace.

Boundaries

A *boundary* limits or separates something. For example, a fence forms a boundary. You stay inside or outside the fenced area. As a nursing assistant, you help residents and families. Therefore you enter into a helping relationship with them. The helping relationship has professional boundaries.

Professional boundaries separate helpful behaviors from behaviors that are not helpful (Fig. 2.6). The boundaries create a helpful zone. If your behaviors are outside the helpful zone, you are overinvolved with the person or underinvolved. The following can occur:

- **Boundary crossing.** This is a brief act or behavior outside the helpful zone. The act or behavior may be thoughtless or something you did not mean to do. Or it could be on purpose if it meets the person's needs. For example, you give a

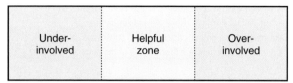

| Under-involved | Helpful zone | Over-involved |

Fig. 2.6 Professional boundaries. (Modified from National Council of State Boards of Nursing, Inc.: *Professional boundaries: a nurse's guide to the importance of appropriate professional boundaries*, Chicago, https://www.ncsbn.org/ProfessionalBoundaries_Complete.pdf)

crying patient a hug. The hug meets the person's needs at that time. If giving a hug meets your needs, the act is wrong. Also, it is wrong to hug the person every time you see each other.

- **Boundary violation.** This is an act or behavior that meets your needs, not the person's. The act or behavior is not ethical. It violates the code of conduct in Box 2.3. The person could be harmed. Boundary violations include:
- Abuse (p. 25).
- Giving a lot of information about yourself. You tell a person about your personal relationships or problems.
- Keeping secrets with the person.
- **Professional sexual misconduct.** This is an act, behavior, or comment that is sexual in nature. It is sexual misconduct even if the person consents or makes the first move.

Some boundary violations and some types of professional sexual misconduct also are crimes. To maintain professional boundaries, follow the rules in Box 2.4. Be alert to boundary signs. Boundary signs are acts, behaviors, or thoughts that warn of a boundary crossing or violation (Box 2.5).

BOX 2.4 Rules for Maintaining Professional Boundaries

- Follow the code of conduct listed in Box 2.3.
- Talk to the nurse if you sense a boundary sign, crossing, or violation.
- Avoid caring for family, friends, and people with whom you do business. This may be hard to do in a small community. Always tell the nurse if you know the person. The nurse may change your assignment.
- Do not date, flirt with, kiss, or have a sexual relationship with current residents. The same applies to family members of current residents.
- Do not make sexual comments or jokes.
- Do not use offensive language.
- Do not discuss your sexual relationships with residents or their families.
- Do not say or write things that could suggest a romantic or sexual relationship with a resident or family member.
- Use touch correctly. Only touch or handle sexual and genital areas when necessary to give care. Such areas include the breasts, nipples, perineum, buttocks, and anus of both males and females.
- Do not accept gifts, loans, money, credit cards, or other valuables from a resident or family member.
- Do not give gifts, loans, money, credit cards, or other valuables to a resident or family member.
- Do not borrow from a resident or family member. This includes money, personal items, and transportation.
- Maintain a professional relationship at all times. Do not develop any personal relationship or friendship with the resident or family member.
- Do not visit or spend extra time with a resident who is not part of your assignment.
- Do not share personal or financial information with a resident or family member.
- Do not help a resident or family member with finances.
- Do not take a resident home with you. This includes for holidays or other events.
- Ask these questions before you date or marry a person whom you cared for. Be aware of the risk for sexual misconduct.
- How long ago did you assist with the person's care?
- Was the person's care short term or long term?
- What kind and how much information do you have about the person? How will that information affect your relationship with the person?
- Will the person need more care in the future?
- Does dating or marrying the person place the person at risk for harm?

BOX 2.5 Boundary Signs

- You think about the person when you are not at work.
- You organize your work and provide other care around the person's needs.
- You spend free time with the person. You visit with the person during breaks, meal times, when off duty, and so on.
- You trade assignments with other staff so you can provide the person's care.
- You give more care or attention to the person at the expense of other residents.
- You believe that you are the only one who understands the person and the person's needs.
- The person gives you gifts or money.
- You give the person gifts or money.
- You share information about yourself with the person.
- You talk about your work situation with the person.
- You flirt with the person.
- You make comments that have a sexual message.
- You tell the person "off-color" jokes.
- You notice more touch between you and the person.
- You use foul, vulgar, or offensive language when talking to the person.
- You and the person have secrets.
- You choose the person's side when there is disagreement with other staff or the family.
- You select what you report and record. You do not give complete information.
- You do not like questions about the care you give or your relationship with the person.
- You change how you dress or your appearance when you will work with the person.
- You receive gifts from the person after the person leaves the center.
- You have contact with the person after the person leaves the center.

See *Focus on Communication: Professional Boundaries.*

📋 FOCUS ON COMMUNICATION

Professional Boundaries

Some residents and families want to thank the staff for the care given. Some send thank-you cards and letters. Some offer gifts—candy, cookies, money, gift certificates, flowers, and so on. Accepting gifts is a boundary violation. When offered a gift, you can say:

- "Thank you so much for thinking of me. It's very kind of you. However, it is against center policy to accept gifts of any kind. I do appreciate your offer."
- "Thank you for wanting me to have the flowers your friend sent. They are lovely. However, it is against center policy to receive gifts. Let me help you find a way to take them home."

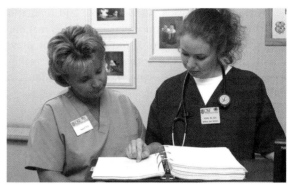

Fig. 2.7 A nurse and nursing assistant review the policy and procedure manual. It is kept at the nurses' station.

LEGAL ASPECTS

Ethics is about what you *should or should not do.* Laws tell you what you *can and cannot do.* A law is a rule of conduct made by a government body. The US Congress and state legislatures make laws. Enforced by the government, laws protect the public welfare.

Criminal laws are concerned with offenses against the public and society in general. An act that violates a criminal law is called a crime. If found guilty of a crime, the person is fined or sent to prison. Murder, robbery, rape, kidnapping, and abuse (p. ··) are crimes.

Civil laws are concerned with relationships between people. Examples of civil laws are those that involve contracts and nursing practice. A person found guilty of breaking a civil law usually has to pay a sum of money to the injured person.

Torts

Tort comes from the French word meaning "wrong." Torts are part of civil law. A tort is a wrong committed against a person or the person's property. Some torts are *unintentional,* meaning harm was not intended. Some torts are *intentional,* however, meaning harm was intended.

Unintentional Torts

Negligence is an unintentional wrong. The negligent person did not act in a reasonable and careful manner. As a result, a person or the person's property was harmed. The person causing the harm did not intend or mean to cause harm. The person failed to do what a reasonable and careful person *would have done.* Or the person did what a reasonable and careful person *would not have done.* The negligent person may have to pay damages (a sum of money) to the one injured.

Malpractice is negligence by a professional person. A person has professional status because of training and the service provided. Nurses, doctors, dentists, and pharmacists are examples.

What you do or do not do can lead to a lawsuit if harm results to the person or property of another. Standard of care refers to skills, care, and judgments required by a health team member under similar conditions. Standards of care come from:

- Laws, including nurse practice acts.
- Textbooks.
- Center policy and procedure manuals (Fig. 2.7). These explain how to perform certain procedures.
- Manufacturer instructions for equipment and supplies.
- Job descriptions.
- Approval and accrediting agency standards.
- Standards and guidelines issued by government agencies. The following actions could lead to charges of negligence:
- A nurse asks you to apply a hot soak. You fail to test water temperature. The water is too hot. The person is burned.
- Mrs. Fong needs help getting to the bathroom. You do not answer her call light promptly. She gets up without help. She falls and breaks an arm.
- You use a mechanical lift to transfer Mr. Rossi from bed to a chair. You do not follow the manufacturer instructions for using the lift. Mr. Rossi slips out of the lift and falls to the floor. He fractures a hip.
- Mrs. Clark complains of chest pain. You do not tell the nurse. Mrs. Clark has a heart attack and dies.
- The door to the assisted living residence is supposed to be locked at night. Mr. Augustine goes outside and slips on the ice. He is not discovered for several hours. He later dies of hypothermia.
- Two residents have the same last name. You do not identify the person before a procedure. You perform the procedure on the wrong person. Both residents are harmed. One had a procedure that was not ordered. The other did not have a needed procedure.

You are legally responsible *(liable)* for your own actions. The nurse is liable as your supervisor. However, you still have personal liability. Remember, sometimes refusing to follow the nurse's directions is your right and duty (Chapter 1).

Intentional Torts

Intentional torts are acts meant to be harmful. The act is done on purpose.

Defamation is injuring a person's name and reputation by making false statements to a third person. Libel is making false statements in print, writing, or through pictures or drawings. Slander is making false statements orally. Never make false statements about a resident, coworker, or any other person. Examples of defamation include:

- Implying or suggesting that a person uses drugs.
- Saying that a person is insane or mentally ill.
- Implying or suggesting that a person steals money from the staff.

False imprisonment is the unlawful restraint or restriction of a person's freedom of movement. It involves:

- Threatening to restrain a person.
- Restraining a person.
- Preventing a person from leaving the agency.

Invasion of privacy is violating a person's right not to have one's own name, photo, or private affairs exposed or made public without giving consent. You must treat the person with respect and ensure privacy. Only staff involved in the person's care should see, handle, or examine the person's body. Box 2.6 provides measures to protect privacy.

The Health Insurance Portability and Accountability Act of 1996 (HIPAA) protects the privacy and security of a person's health information. Protected health information refers to identifying information and information about the person's health care that is maintained or sent in any form (paper, electronic, oral). Failure to follow HIPAA rules can result in fines, penalties, and criminal action, including jail time. Always follow center policies and procedures. Some centers have specific policies that staff must sign regarding the use of personal cell phones and social media. Direct any questions about the person or the person's care to the nurse. Also follow the rules for using computers and other electronic devices (Chapter 4).

Fraud is saying or doing something to trick, fool, or deceive a person. The act is fraud if it does or could harm a person or the person's property. Telling a person or family that you are a nurse is fraud. So is giving wrong or incomplete information on a job application.

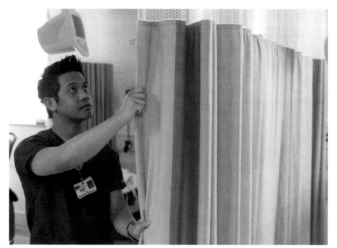

Fig. 2.8 Pulling the privacy curtain around the bed helps protect the person's privacy.

Assault and battery may result in both civil and criminal charges. Assault is intentionally attempting or threatening to touch a person's body without the person's consent. The person fears bodily harm. Threatening to "tie down" a person is an example of assault. Battery is touching a person's body without the person's consent. Consent is the important factor in assault and battery. The person must consent to any procedure, treatment, or other act that involves touching the body. The person has the right to withdraw consent at any time.

Protect yourself from being accused of assault and battery. Explain to the person what you are going to do and get the person's consent. Consent may be verbal—"yes" or "okay." Or it can be a gesture—a nod, turning over for a back rub, or holding out an arm for you to take a pulse.

Informed Consent

Persons have the right to decide what will be done to their body and who can touch their body. The doctor is responsible for informing each person about all aspects of treatment. Consent is informed when the person clearly understands:

- The reason for a treatment, procedure, or care measure.
- What will be done.
- How it will be done.
- Who will do it.
- The expected outcomes.
- Other treatment, procedure, or care options.
- The effects of not having the treatment, procedure, or care measure.

Persons under legal age (usually 18 years) cannot give consent, nor can persons with mental incompetence. Such persons may be unconscious, sedated, or confused. Or they have certain mental health disorders. Informed consent is given by a responsible party—a wife, husband, daughter, son, or legal representative.

Consent is given when the person enters the center. A form is signed giving general consent to treatment. Special consent forms are required before admission to a secured memory care

---

BOX 2.6   Protecting the Right to Privacy

- Keep all information about the person confidential.
- Provide covering when the person is being moved in hallways.
- Screen the person. Close the privacy curtain as in Fig. 2.8. Close the door when giving care; also close window coverings.
- Expose only the body part involved in care or a procedure.
- Do not discuss the person or the person's treatment with anyone except the nurse supervising your work. "Shop talk" is a common cause of invasion of privacy.
- Ask visitors to leave the room when care is given.
- Do not open the person's mail.
- Never share information about a resident on social media sites.
- Never post pictures of residents on social media sites.
- Allow the person to visit with others in private.
- Allow the person to use the phone in private.
- Follow center policies and procedures required to protect privacy.

unit (Chapter 40). Certain procedures performed by the health care provider require special consents. The health care provider informs the person about all aspects of the procedure. The nurse may be given this responsibility.

You are never responsible for obtaining written consent. In some centers, you can witness the signing of a consent. When a witness, you are present when the person signs the consent.

See *Focus on Communication: Informed Consent.*

📋 FOCUS ON COMMUNICATION

Informed Consent

There are different ways to give consent:

- *Written consent.* The person signs a form agreeing to a treatment or procedure. You are not responsible for obtaining written consent.
- *Verbal consent.* The person says aloud the consent (e.g., says "yes" or "okay").
- *Implied consent.* For example, you ask Mr. Ahmad if you can check his blood pressure. He extends his arm. His movement implies consent.

Before any procedure, explain the steps to the person. This is how you obtain verbal or implied consent. Also explain each step during a procedure. This allows the person the chance to refuse at any time.

Wills

A will is a legal document of how a person wants property distributed after death. You can ethically and legally witness a will signing. Or you can refuse to do so without fear of legal action.

A person may ask you to prepare a will. You must politely refuse. Explain that you do not have the legal knowledge or ability to prepare a will. Report the request to the nurse. The nurse will speak to the person or a family member about contacting a lawyer.

Do not witness a will signing if you are named in the will. Doing so prevents you from getting what was left to you. As a witness, be prepared to testify that:

- The person was of sound mind when the will was signed.
- The person stated that the document was the last will.

Many centers do not let nursing assistants witness wills. There may be administrative staff members specifically trained to do this. Know your center's policy before you agree to witness a will. If you have questions, ask the nurse. If you witness a will, tell the nurse.

REPORTING ABUSE

Some persons are mistreated or harmed on purpose. This is abuse, defined as:

- The willful infliction of injury, unreasonable confinement, intimidation, or punishment that results in physical harm, pain, or mental anguish. *Intimidation* means to make afraid with threats of force or violence.
- Depriving the person (or the person's caregiver) of the goods or services needed to attain or maintain well-being.

Abuse also includes involuntary seclusion. Abuse is a crime. All persons must be protected from abuse. This includes persons in a coma.

The abuser is usually a family member or caregiver—spouse, partner, adult child, and others. The abuser can be a friend, neighbor, landlord, or other person. Both men and women are abusers. Both men and women are abused.

State laws, accrediting agencies, and OBRA do not allow centers to employ persons who were convicted of abuse, neglect, or mistreatment. Before hiring, the center must thoroughly check the applicant's work history. All references are checked. Efforts must be made to find out about any criminal records.

Most states require employees of long-term care facilities to receive training regarding elder abuse. This training is repeated periodically. All employees should be familiar with how to report abuse. The center also checks the nursing assistant registry for findings of abuse, neglect, or mistreatment. It also is checked for misusing or stealing a person's property.

Vulnerable Adults

Vulnerable comes from the Latin word *vulnerare,* which means "to wound." Vulnerable adults are persons 18 years old or older who have disabilities or conditions that put them at risk to be wounded, attacked, or damaged. They have problems caring for or protecting themselves due to:

- A mental, emotional, physical, or developmental disability. See Chapter 41 for a discussion about "developmental disabilities."
- Brain damage.
- Changes from aging.

All residents, regardless of age, are vulnerable. Older persons and children are at risk for abuse.

See *Residents with Dementia: Vulnerable Adults.*

👤 RESIDENTS WITH DEMENTIA

Vulnerable Adults

Some persons have behaviors that threaten their own health and safety. This is called self-neglect. Causes include declining health and chronic disease. Other causes are disorders that impair judgment or memory. Alzheimer disease and dementia are examples. The warning signs of self-neglect are:

- Hoarding. The person saves, hides, or stores things. Newspapers, magazines, food containers, and shopping bags are examples.
- Not having food, water, heat, and other necessities.
- Not taking needed medications.
- Refusing medical treatment for serious illnesses.
- Dehydration—poor urinary output, dry skin, dry mouth, confusion.
- Poor hygiene.
- Wearing the wrong clothing for the weather.
- Confusion.

Elder Abuse

Elder abuse is any knowing, intentional, or negligent act by a caregiver or any other person to an older adult. The act causes harm or serious risk of harm. Elder abuse can take these forms:

- *Physical abuse.* This involves inflicting, or threatening to inflict, physical pain or injury. Grabbing, hitting, slapping, kicking, pinching, hair-pulling, or beating are examples. It also includes *corporal punishment*—punishment inflicted directly on the body. Beatings, lashings, and whippings are examples. Depriving the person of a basic need also is physical abuse.

- *Neglect.* Failure to provide the person with the goods or services needed to avoid physical harm, mental anguish, or mental illness is called neglect. This includes failure to provide health care or treatment, food, clothing, hygiene, shelter, or other needs. In health care, neglect includes but is not limited to:
- Leaving persons lying or sitting in urine or feces.
- Keeping persons alone in their rooms or other areas.
- Failing to answer signal lights.
- *Verbal abuse.* Using oral or written words or statements that speak badly of, sneer at, criticize, or condemn the person. It includes unkind gestures, threats of harm, or saying things to frighten the person. For example, Mr. Garcia is told he will never see family members again.
- *Involuntary seclusion.* Confining the person to a certain area. People have been locked in closets, basements, attics, bathrooms, and other spaces.
- *Financial exploitation or misappropriation.* To *exploit* means to use unjustly. *Misappropriate* means to dishonestly, unfairly, or wrongly take for one's own use. The older person's resources (money, property, assets) are misused by another person. Or the resources are used for the other person's profit or benefit. The person's money is stolen or used by another person. Or a person's property is misused. For example, a son sells his mother's house without her consent.
- *Emotional or mental abuse.* This involves inflicting mental pain, anguish, or distress through verbal or nonverbal acts. Humiliation, harassment, ridicule, and threats of punishment are examples. It includes being deprived of needs such as food, clothing, care, a home, or a place to sleep.
- *Sexual abuse.* The person is harassed about sex or is attacked sexually. The person may be forced to perform sexual acts out of fear of punishment or physical harm.
- *Abandonment.* *Abandon* means to leave or desert someone. The person is deserted by someone who is supposed to provide care.

There are many signs of elder abuse. The abused person may show only some of the signs in Box 2.7.

Federal and state laws require the reporting of elder abuse. The Elder Justice Act became law in 2010. This law outlines how suspected abuse should be reported. It states that centers that receive federal funding must report abuse immediately or they will be fined. It also states that an employee who reports suspected abuse cannot be punished by that center. If abuse is suspected, it must be reported.

You may suspect abuse. If so, discuss the matter and your observations with the nurse. Give as many details as possible. The nurse contacts community agencies that investigate elder abuse and law enforcement. They act at once if the problem is life threatening. The nurse may contact health team members as needed.

Follow the center's policy for reporting abuse. Many centers post the phone numbers for reporting abuse. Any employee

---

BOX 2.7 Signs of Elder Abuse

- Living conditions are unsafe, unclean, or inadequate.
- Personal hygiene is lacking. The person is not clean. Clothes are dirty.
- Weight loss—there are signs of poor nutrition and poor fluid intake.
- Assist devices are missing or broken (e.g., eyeglasses, hearing aids, dentures, cane, walker).
- Medical needs are not met.
- Frequent injuries—conditions behind the injuries are strange or seem impossible.
- Old and new injuries (e.g., bruises, pressure marks, welts, scars, fractures, punctures) occur.
- Complaints of pain or itching in the genital area occur.
- Bleeding and bruising around the breasts or in the genital area occur.
- Burns appear on the feet, hands, buttocks, or other parts of the body. Cigarettes and cigars cause small circlelike burns.
- Pressure injuries (Chapter 32) or contractures (Chapter 23) occur.
- The person seems very quiet or withdrawn.
- The person shows unexplained withdrawal from normal activities.
- The person seems fearful, anxious, or agitated.
- Sudden change in alertness occur.
- Depression is evident.
- Sudden changes in finances are reported.
- The person does not seem to want to talk or answer questions.
- The person is restrained. Or the person is locked in a certain area for long periods.
- The person cannot reach toilet facilities, food, water, and other needed items.
- Private conversations are not allowed. The caregiver is present during all conversations.
- Strained or tense relationships with a caregiver occur.
- Frequent arguments with a caregiver occur.
- The person seems anxious to please the caregiver.
- Medications are not taken properly. Medications are not bought or too much or too little of the medication is taken.
- Emergency room visits may be frequent.
- The person may change doctors often. Some people do not have a doctor.

---

working in a long-term care setting must first stop an abusive action. Next, the employee must report it to the supervisor. Remember, you cannot be punished for reporting suspected abuse.

Helping abused older persons is not always easy or possible. Some abuse is not reported or recognized. The investigating agency may not have access to the person. Sometimes older persons are abused by a spouse or adult child. A victim may want to protect the spouse or child. Some victims are embarrassed or believe the abuse is deserved. A victim may fear what will happen. The victim may think that the present situation is better than no care at all. Some people fear not being believed if they report the abuse themselves.

❖ Abuse in Nursing Centers

OBRA requires these actions if abuse is suspected within the center:

- The incident is reported at once to the administrator. It also is reported at once to other officials as required by federal and state laws.
- All claims of abuse are thoroughly investigated.
- The center must prevent further potential for abuse while the investigation is in progress.
- Investigation results are reported to the center administrator within 5 days of the incident. They also are reported to other officials as required by federal and state laws.
- Corrective actions are taken if the claim of abuse is found to be true.

Box 2.8 lists some severe cases of elder abuse. The abusers were convicted of crimes.

The examples of abuse that follow are more common. However, such abuse is still wrong. It will be investigated. If the abuse allegation is substantiated, you can lose your job. In addition, the state nursing assistant registry will be notified. Nursing assistants have lost their certification (registration) because of elder abuse.

- A person constantly crying out for help is taken to his room. He is left alone with the door closed.
- A person is told to be nice, otherwise care will not be given.
- A person cannot control her bowels. She is called "dirty" and "disgusting."
- A person is turned in a rough and hurried manner.

- The nurse uses the person's phone to call a friend.
- A person lies in a wet and soiled bed all night.
- Money is taken from a person's wallet.
- A person uses the call light a lot. It is taken away from the person.
- A person's mouth is forced open. Food is forced into the person's mouth.
- A person is told that her son does not visit because she is so mean.

Domestic Abuse

Domestic abuse—also called domestic violence, intimate partner abuse, partner abuse, and spousal abuse—occurs in relationships. One partner has power and control over the other through abuse. Fear and harm occur. Usually more than one of the following is present:

- *Physical abuse*—unwanted punching, slapping, grabbing, choking, poking, biting, pulling hair, twisting arms, or kicking. It may involve burns and weapons. Physical injuries occur. Death is a constant threat.
- *Sexual abuse*—unwanted sexual contact.
- *Verbal abuse*—unkind and hurtful remarks. They make the person feel unwhole, unattractive, and without value.
- *Economic abuse*—controlling money. Having or not having a job is controlled by the abuser. So are paychecks, money gifts from family and friends, and money for household expenses (food, clothing).
- *Social abuse*—controlling friendships and other relationships. The abuser controls phone calls, car use, leaving the home, and visits with family and friends.

Residents can suffer from domestic abuse. For example, a husband slaps his wife during a visit. Or a wife uses her husband's money for herself rather than buying her husband's medications.

Domestic abuse is a safety issue. Like child and elder abuse, domestic abuse is complex. The victim often hides the abuse. The victim may protect the abusive partner. State laws vary about reporting domestic abuse. However, the health team has an ethical duty to give information about safety and community resources. If you suspect domestic abuse, share your concerns with the nurse. The nurse gathers information to help the person.

Under OBRA, the resident has the right to be free from abuse, mistreatment, or neglect. If a resident is abused by anyone, the abuse must be reported. This includes abuse by a partner.

BOX 2.8 Prosecuted Cases of Elder Abuse

- A resident was complaining of pain while being cleaned. To stop him from complaining, a nursing assistant stuck a rag down his throat.
- A patient was screaming. To stop the patient from screaming, a nurse poured water down her throat.
- A nursing assistant beat and kicked a 92-year-old man who was lying on the floor.
- A nursing assistant stepped on a resident's face.
- A person was visiting his grandmother. While there, he sexually abused a patient with head injuries.
- A female patient in a wheelchair was dragged into a room by a nursing assistant. The nursing assistant forced the patient to have sex with him.
- A nursing assistant teased and taunted a resident with dementia.
- A health care worker repeatedly insulted an older woman because her son was gay.
- A nursing assistant forced a person to urinate in bed. Then the nursing assistant made fun of the person.
- Two older women lived in a board and care home. Both had Alzheimer disease. They were left in a room with blood splattered on the walls. The carpet was caked with feces, vomitus, and urine. The women were partially dressed. One woman was tied to the bed with a sheet.
- A nursing assistant failed to feed a resident who could not feed herself. A video camera caught the nursing assistant dumping the person's food into trash cans.
- A resident could not talk. She totally depended on the staff for care. She did not have a bowel movement for 26 days. She was given a laxative every 3 days. No other treatment was given for her constipation.
- Caregivers willfully neglected to give medications to residents.

From American Society on Aging: *Elder abuse and neglect: prosecution and prevention*, San Francisco, Author.

QUALITY OF LIFE

Residents have the right to a comfortable and safe setting. To protect them from harm, you must understand your roles and responsibilities. What you do and how you do it affects their quality of life.

OBRA's purpose is to improve the quality of life of nursing center residents. The law requires training and competency evaluation programs for nursing assistants working in long-term care. These programs provide nursing assistants with the knowledge and skills needed to give basic nursing care. You must always practice within the legal limits of your role.

Residents have the right to be free from abuse, mistreatment, and neglect. Nursing centers have procedures for investigating all cases of suspected abuse. Be alert for signs and symptoms of abuse. If you suspect that a person is being abused, report the matter to the nurse. Share your observations with the nurse. Everything you do must maintain or improve each person's quality of life, health, and safety. If you remember this, your job will be rewarding and enjoyable.

⚡ TIME TO REFLECT

Mr. Leeds has dementia. He does not want to take the pills that the nurse is trying to give him. As you walk by the room, you overhear the nurse shout: "Open your mouth and take these pills now! If you don't, you'll be spending the rest of the day locked in this room!" You are troubled by what you heard and later decide to talk privately with the director of nursing (DON) about the conversation. The DON listens to your account and then says: "Mr. Leeds has been a big challenge lately. I believe the nurse was just trying her best to get him to take his pills. Let's not make a big deal over this." What would you do from here?

▌ REVIEW QUESTIONS

Circle the BEST answer.

1. OBRA is a
   a. State law
   b. Federal law
   c. State agency
   d. Federal agency
2. A son has the legal right to act on his mother's behalf. The son is his mother's legal
   a. Ombudsman
   b. Representative
   c. Caregiver
   d. Health care provider
3. A daughter wants to read her father's medical record. What should you do?
   a. Give her the medical record
   b. Ask the resident if you can give the daughter the medical record
   c. Tell the nurse
   d. Tell her that she cannot do so
4. A resident refuses to have a shower. What should you do?
   a. Tell her that she cannot refuse a shower
   b. Tell her daughter
   c. Give her a bath instead
   d. Tell the nurse
5. A resident has a phone in his room. He wants to make a phone call. What should you do?
   a. Leave the room
   b. Tell the nurse
   c. Ask him to use the phone at the nurses' station
   d. Close the privacy curtain so you can stay in the room to finish your tasks
6. Who decides how to style a person's hair?
   a. The person
   b. The nurse
   c. You
   d. The ombudsman

7. Residents do *not* have a right to
   a. A private room
   b. Refuse treatment
   c. Contact an ombudsman
   d. Make personal choices
8. Residents have the right to be free from the following *except*
   a. Disease
   b. Abuse
   c. Involuntary seclusion
   d. Neglect
9. Who selects activities for a resident?
   a. The nurse
   b. You
   c. The person's representative
   d. The person
10. A long-term care ombudsman
    a. Is employed by the nursing center
    b. Investigates resident complaints
    c. Grants a nursing center a license or certification
    d. Can prevent a resident from leaving the center
11. Which action does *not* promote a person's dignity?
    a. Restraining the person
    b. Providing privacy during personal care
    c. Making sure the person has needed assist devices
    d. Listening to the person
12. Which is the correct way to address a person?
    a. "Hello, sweetie"
    b. "Hello, Mr. Garcia"
    c. "Hello, Jim"
    d. "Hello, Grandpa"
13. Which does *not* promote dignity or privacy?
    a. Knocking before entering the person's room
    b. Closing the bathroom door when the person uses the bathroom
    c. Assisting with bathing and hygiene preferences
    d. Moving the person's items as you prefer

14. Ethics is
    a. Making judgments before you have the facts
    b. Knowledge of what is right conduct and wrong conduct
    c. A behavior that meets your needs, not the person's
    d. Skills, care, and judgments required of a health team member
15. Which is ethical behavior?
    a. Sharing information about a resident with your family
    b. Accepting gifts from a resident's family
    c. Reporting errors
    d. Calling your family before answering a call light
16. To maintain professional boundaries, your behaviors must
    a. Help the person
    b. Meet your needs
    c. Be biased
    d. Show that you care
17. Which is *not* a crime?
    a. Abuse
    b. Murder
    c. Negligence
    d. Robbery
18. Threatening to touch the person's body without the person's consent is
    a. Assault
    b. Battery
    c. Defamation
    d. False imprisonment
19. Restraining a person's freedom of movement is
    a. Assault
    b. Battery
    c. Defamation
    d. False imprisonment
20. Photos of Mr. Bose are shown to others without his consent. This is
    a. Battery
    b. Fraud
    c. Invasion of privacy
    d. Malpractice
21. A person asks if you are a nurse. You answer "yes." This is
    a. Negligence
    b. Fraud
    c. Libel
    d. Slander
22. Informed consent is when the person
    a. Fully understands all aspects of one's own treatment
    b. Signs a consent form
    c. Is admitted to the center
    d. Decides how to distribute property after death
23. Which is *not* a sign of elder abuse?
    a. Stiff joints and joint pain
    b. Old and new bruises
    c. Poor personal hygiene
    d. Frequent injuries
24. These statements are about domestic abuse. Which is *true*?
    a. It always involves physical harm
    b. It always involves violence
    c. One partner has control over the other partner
    d. Only one type of abuse is usually present
25. You suspect a person was abused. What should you do?
    a. Tell the family
    b. Call the police
    c. Tell the nurse
    d. Ask the person about the abuse

See Appendix A for answers to these questions.

3

Work Ethics

KEY TERMS

confidentiality Trusting others with personal and private information

courtesy A polite, considerate, or helpful comment or act

gossip To spread rumors or talk about the private matters of others

harassment To trouble, torment, offend, or worry a person by one's behavior or comments

priority The most important thing at the time

professionalism Following laws, being ethical, having good work ethics, and having the skills to do your work

stress The response or change in the body caused by any emotional, physical, social, or economic factor

stressor The event or factor that causes stress

work ethics Behavior in the workplace

KEY ABBREVIATIONS

OBRA Omnibus Budget Reconciliation Act of 1987

TB Tuberculosis

As a nursing assistant, you must act and function in a professional manner. Professionalism involves following laws, being ethical, having good work ethics, and having the skills to do your work. Laws and ethics are discussed in Chapter 2. Laws are rules of conduct made by government bodies. Ethics deals with right and wrong conduct. It involves choices and judgments about what to do or what not to do. An ethical person does the right thing. In the workplace, certain behaviors (conduct), choices, and judgments are expected. Work ethics deals with behavior in the workplace. Your conduct reflects your choices and judgments. Work ethics involves:

- How you look.
- What you say.
- How you behave.
- How you treat others.
- How you work with others.

To get and keep a job, you must conduct yourself in the right manner.

HEALTH, HYGIENE, AND APPEARANCE

Residents, families, and visitors expect the health team to look and act healthy. For example, a person is told to stop smoking, yet sees health team members smoking. If you are not clean, people wonder if you give good care. You are part of the health team. Your health, hygiene, and appearance need careful attention.

Your Health

You must give safe and effective care. To do so, you must be physically and mentally healthy. Otherwise you cannot function at your best.

- *Diet.* You need a balanced diet (Chapter 20). Start your day with a good breakfast. To maintain your weight, balance the calories you take in with your energy needs. To lose weight, take in fewer calories than your energy needs. Avoid foods high in fat, oil, and sugar. Also avoid salty foods and crash diets.

- *Sleep and rest.* Sleep and rest are needed for health and to do your job well. Most adults need about 7 hours of sleep daily. Fatigue, lack of energy, and irritability mean you need more rest and sleep.
- *Immunizations, tests, and physical exams. Your facility may have requirements that ensure that you are healthy enough to perform tasks. A physical exam may be required prior to being hired. Preventing the spread of infectious diseases (Chapter 14) to residents is another concern. You may be required to undergo **TB** (tuberculosis) testing on a regular basis. Proof of immunization or immunity against childhood illness is often required. Periodic vaccines for influenza and coronal viruses may be required. The facility will let you know if these are provided at no cost to you.*
- *Body mechanics.* You will bend; carry heavy objects; and handle, move, and turn persons. These tasks place stress and strain on your body. You need to use your muscles correctly (Chapter 15).
- *Exercise.* Exercise is needed for muscle tone, circulation, and weight loss. Walking, running, swimming, and biking are good forms of exercise. Regular exercise helps you feel better physically and mentally. Consult your health care provider before starting a vigorous exercise program.
- *Your eyes.* You will read instructions and take measurements. Wrong readings can cause the person harm. Have your eyes checked. Wear needed eyeglasses or contact lenses. Provide enough light for reading and fine work.
- *Smoking.* Smoking causes lung, heart, and circulatory disorders. Smoke odors stay on your breath, hands, clothing, and hair. Hand washing and good personal hygiene are needed.
- *Drugs.* Some drugs affect thinking, feeling, behavior, and function. Working under the influence of drugs affects the person's safety. Take only medications ordered by a health care provider. Take them in the prescribed way.
- *Alcohol.* Alcohol is a drug that depresses the brain. It affects thinking, balance, coordination, and mental alertness. Never report to work under the influence of alcohol. Do not drink alcohol while working. Like other drugs, alcohol affects the person's safety.

Your Hygiene

Personal hygiene needs careful attention. Bathe daily. Use a deodorant or antiperspirant to prevent body odors. Brush your teeth often—upon awakening, before and after meals, and at bedtime. Use a mouthwash to prevent breath odors. Shampoo your hair often. Style your hair in a simple, attractive way. Keep your fingernails clean, short, and neatly shaped.

Foot care prevents odors and infection. Wash your feet daily. Dry thoroughly between the toes. Cut toenails straight across after bathing or soaking them.

Your Appearance

Good health and hygiene practices help you look and feel well. Follow the practices in Box 3.1. They help you look clean, neat, and professional (Fig. 3.1). Always follow the dress code policy at the center where you are employed.

BOX 3.1 Practices for a Professional Appearance

- Practice good hygiene.
- Wear uniforms that fit well. They are modest in length and style. Follow the center's dress code.
- Keep uniforms clean, pressed, and mended. Sew on buttons. Repair zippers, tears, and hems. Pant legs should not drag on the floor.
- Wear a clean uniform daily.
- Wear your name badge or photo identification (ID) at all times when on duty. Make sure it can be seen. Wear it according to center policy.
- Wear undergarments that are clean and fit properly. Change them daily.
- Wear undergarments in the correct color for your skin tone. Do not wear colored (e.g., red, pink, blue) ones that can be seen through white and light-colored uniforms.
- Cover tattoos (body art). They may offend others.
- Follow the center's dress code for jewelry. Wedding and engagement rings may be allowed. Rings and bracelets can scratch a person. Confused or combative persons can easily pull on jewelry (necklaces, dangling earrings), as can young children.
- Do not wear jewelry in pierced eyebrows, nose, lips, or tongue while on duty.
- Follow the center's dress code for earrings. Usually small, simple earrings are allowed. For multiple ear piercings, usually only one set of earrings is allowed.
- Wear a wristwatch with a second (sweep) hand.
- Wear clean stockings or socks that fit well. Change them daily.
- Wear shoes that fit properly, are comfortable, give needed support, and have nonskid soles. Do not wear sandals or open-toed shoes.
- Clean and polish shoes often. Wash and replace laces as needed.
- Keep fingernails clean, short, and neatly shaped. Long nails can scratch a person and can puncture gloves that are worn for protection. Nails must be natural.
- Do not wear nail polish or fake nails. Chipped nail polish and acrylic nails may provide a place for microbes to grow.
- Have a simple, attractive hairstyle. Hair is off your collar and away from your face. Use simple pins, combs, barrettes, and bands to keep long hair up and in place. When serving food, some centers require hair coverings to be worn.
- Keep beards and mustaches clean and trimmed.
- Use makeup that is modest in amount and moderate in color. Avoid a painted and severe look.
- Do not wear perfume, cologne, or aftershave lotion. Cigarette smoke may linger on clothing. These scents may offend, nauseate, or cause breathing problems in residents.

Good work ethics involves the qualities and traits described in Box 3.2. They are necessary for you to function well (Fig. 3.2).

Being dependable is important. You must be at work on time and when scheduled. Undependable people cause everyone problems. Other staff must take on extra work to compensate. Fewer people give care. Quality of care suffers. You want coworkers to work when scheduled. Otherwise, you have extra work. You have less time to spend with residents. Likewise, coworkers also expect you to work when scheduled.

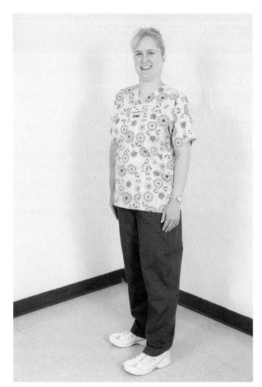

Fig. 3.1 This nursing assistant is well groomed. Her uniform and shoes are clean. Her hair has a simple style. It is away from her face and off her collar. She does not wear jewelry.

PREPARING FOR WORK

Information on job-seeking skills is covered in Chapter 46. To keep your job, you must function well and work well with others. You must:

- Work when scheduled.
- Get to work on time.
- Stay the entire shift.

Absences and tardiness (being late) are common reasons for losing a job. Child care and transportation issues often interfere with getting to work. Plan for them in advance by having a backup plan to cover unexpected circumstances.

Child Care

Someone needs to care for your children when you leave for work, while you are at work, and before you get home from work. Also plan for emergencies:

- Your child care provider is ill or cannot care for your children that day.
- A child becomes ill while you are at work.
- You will be late getting home from work.

Transportation

Plan for how you get to and from work. If you drive, keep your car in good working order. Keep enough gas in the car, or leave early to get gas.

Carpooling is an option. Carpool members depend on each other. If the driver is late leaving, everyone is late for work. If

---

BOX 3.2 Qualities and Traits for Good Work Ethics

- **Caring.** Have concern for the person. Help make the person's life happier, easier, or less painful.
- **Dependable.** Report to work on time and when scheduled. Perform delegated tasks. Keep obligations and promises.
- **Considerate.** Respect the person's physical and emotional feelings. Be gentle and kind toward residents, families, and coworkers.
- **Cheerful.** Greet and talk to people in a pleasant manner. Do not be moody, bad tempered, or unhappy while at work.
- **Empathetic.** Empathy is seeing things from the person's point of view—putting yourself in the person's place. How would you feel if you had the person's problems?
- **Trustworthy.** Residents and staff have confidence in you. They believe you will keep information confidential. They trust you not to gossip about residents or the health team.
- **Respectful.** Residents have rights, values, beliefs, and feelings. These may differ from yours. Do not judge or condemn the person. Treat the person with respect and dignity at all times. Also show respect for the health team.
- **Courteous.** Be polite and courteous to residents, families, visitors, and coworkers. See p. ·· for common courtesies in the workplace.
- **Conscientious.** Be careful, alert, and exact in following instructions. Give thorough care. Do not lose or damage the person's property. Follow facility policies.
- **Honest.** Accurately report the care given, your observations, and any errors.
- **Cooperative.** Willingly help and work with others. Also take that "extra step" during busy and stressful times.
- **Enthusiastic.** Be eager, interested, and excited about your work. Your work is important.
- **Self-aware.** Know your feelings, strengths, and weaknesses. You need to understand yourself before you can understand the residents.

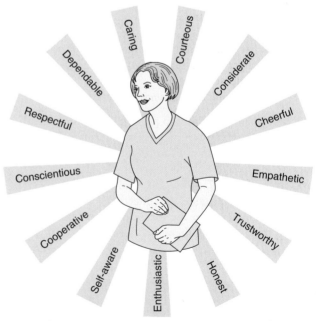

Fig. 3.2 Good work ethics involves these qualities and traits.

one person is not ready when the driver arrives, everyone is late for work. Carpool with persons you trust to be ready and on time. When you drive, leave and pick up others on time. As a passenger, be ready to be picked up on time.

Know your bus or train schedule. Know what other bus or train to take if delays occur. Always carry enough money for fares to and from work.

Always have a backup plan for getting to work. Your car may not start, the carpool driver may not go to work, or public transportation may not operate.

TEAMWORK

How you look, how you behave, and what you say affects everyone in the center. Practice good work ethics.
- Work when scheduled.
- Be cheerful and friendly.
- Perform delegated tasks.
- Be available to help others. Help willingly.
- Be kind to others.

You are an important member of the health team. Quality of care is affected by how you work with others and how you feel about your job.

Attendance

Report to work when scheduled and on time. The entire unit is affected when just one person is late. Call the center if you will be late or cannot go to work. Follow the center's attendance policy in your employee handbook. Poor attendance can cause you to lose your job.

Be *ready to work* when your shift starts. Store your coat, purse, backpack, and other items before your shift starts. Use the restroom when you arrive at the center. Arrive on your nursing unit a few minutes early. This gives you time to greet others and settle yourself.

Attendance also means staying the entire shift. Prepare for child care emergencies. Watching the clock for when your shift ends gives a bad image. You may need to work overtime. Prepare to stay longer if necessary. When it is time to leave, report off duty to the nurse.

See *Teamwork and Time Management: Attendance.*

TEAMWORK AND TIME MANAGEMENT

Attendance

Sometimes a staff member is late for work or does not show up for work. Until a replacement arrives, you and other staff members have extra work. Resident care cannot suffer.

To promote teamwork and manage your time:
- Ask the nurse how you can help.
- Do not complain about not having enough staff.
- Ask the nurse to list the most important tasks and care measures.

Your Attitude

You need a good attitude (see Box 3.2). Show that you enjoy your work. Listen to others. Be willing to learn. Stay busy and use your time well.

Your work is very important. Nurses, residents, and families rely on you to give good care. They expect you to be pleasant and respectful. You must believe that you and your work have value.

Always think before you speak. These statements signal a bad attitude:
- "That's not my resident."
- "I can't. I'm too busy."
- "I didn't do it."
- "I don't feel like it."
- "It's not my fault."
- "Don't blame me."
- "It's not my turn. I did it yesterday."
- "Nobody told me."
- "That's not my job."
- "You didn't say that you needed it right away."
- "I work harder than anyone else."
- "No one appreciates what I do."
- "I'm tired of this place."
- "Is it time to leave yet?"
- "Good luck. I had a horrible day."

Gossip

To gossip means to spread rumors or talk about the private matters of others. Gossiping is unprofessional and hurtful. To avoid being a part of gossip:
- Remove yourself from a group or setting where people are gossiping.
- Do not make or repeat any comment that can hurt a person, family member, visitor, coworker, or the center.
- Do not make or repeat any comment that you do not know is true. Making or writing false statements about another person is defamation (Chapter 2).
- Do not talk about residents, family members, visitors, co-workers, or the center at home or in social settings.

Confidentiality

The person's information is private and personal. Confidentiality means trusting others with personal and private information. The person's information is shared only among health team members involved in the person's care. Privacy and confidentiality are rights protected by OBRA. Center, family, and coworker information also is confidential.

Avoid talking about residents, families, the center, or co-workers when others are present. Share information only with the nurse. Do not talk about residents, families, the center, or coworkers in hallways, elevators, dining areas, or outside the center. Others may overhear you. Residents and visitors are very alert to comments. They think you are talking about them or their loved ones. This leads to wrong information and wrong impressions about the person's condition. You can easily upset the person or family. Be very careful about what, how, when, and where you say things.

Do not eavesdrop. To eavesdrop means to listen in or overhear what others are saying. It invades a person's privacy.

Many centers have intercom systems. They allow for communication between the bedside and the nurses' station (Chapter 16). The person uses the intercom to signal when help is needed. Someone at the nurses' station answers the intercom. The nursing team also uses the intercom to communicate with each other. Be careful what you say over the intercom. It is like a loudspeaker. Others nearby can hear what you are saying.

See *Focus on Communication: Confidentiality.*

 FOCUS ON COMMUNICATION

Confidentiality

Your family members and friends may ask you about people they know in the center. They may ask about residents, their families, or employees. For example, your mother says: "Mrs. Drew goes to our church. I heard that she's in your nursing home. What's wrong with her?"

Do not share any information with your family and friends. Doing so violates the person's right to privacy and confidentiality (Chapter 2). You can say: "I'm sorry, but I can't tell you about anyone in the center. It is unprofessional and against center policies. And it violates the person's right to privacy and confidentiality. Please don't ask me about anyone in the center."

Hygiene and Appearance

How you look affects the way people think about you and the center. If the staff are clean and neat, people think the center is clean and neat. They think the center is unclean if the staff are messy and not tidy. People also wonder about the quality of care given.

Home and social attire is often improper at work. You cannot wear jeans, halter tops, tank tops, or short skirts. Clothing must not be tight, revealing, or sexual. Females cannot show cleavage, the tops of breasts, or upper thighs. Males must avoid tight pants and exposing their chests. Only the top shirt button is open. Follow the practices in Box 3.1.

Speech and Language

Your speech and language must be professional. Speech and language used in home and social settings may be improper at work. Words used with family and friends may offend residents, families, visitors, and coworkers. Remember the following:

- Do not swear or use foul, vulgar, or abusive language.
- Do not use slang.
- Control the volume and tone of your voice. Speak softly and gently.
- Speak clearly. The person may have a hearing impairment (Chapter 33).
- Do not shout or yell.
- Do not fight or argue with a person, family member, visitor, or coworker.

Courtesies

A courtesy is a polite, considerate, or helpful comment or act. Courtesies are easy. They take little time or energy; and they mean so much to people. Even the smallest kind act can brighten someone's day.

- Address others by their correct title (e.g., Miss, Mrs., Ms., Mr., Doctor). Use a first name only if the person asks you to do so.
- Say "please." Begin or end each request with "please."

- Say "thank you" when someone does something for you.
- Apologize. Say "I'm sorry" when you make a mistake or hurt someone. Even little things—like bumping someone in the hallway—need an apology.
- Be thoughtful. Compliment others. Wish others a happy birthday, a happy day or weekend off, or a happy holiday.
- Wish the person and family well when they leave the center: "Stay well" or "stay healthy" are good phrases to use.
- Hold doors open for others. If you are at the door first, open the door and let others pass through.
- Hold elevator doors open for others coming down the hallway.
- Let residents, families, and visitors enter elevators first.
- Stand to greet visitors and families.
- Help others willingly when asked.
- Give praise. If you see a coworker do or say something that impresses you, tell that person. Also tell your coworkers.
- Do not take credit for another person's deeds. Give the person credit for the action.

Personal Matters

You were hired to do a job. Personal matters cannot interfere with the job, otherwise care is neglected. You could lose your job for tending to personal matters while at work. To keep personal matters out of the workplace:

- Make personal phone calls or text messages during meals and breaks. Using a personal phone while providing care for a resident is unacceptable. Many employee handbooks have a policy concerning personal cell phone usage while at work.
- Do not let family and friends visit you on the unit. If they must see you, have them meet you during a meal or break.
- Make appointments (doctor, dentist, lawyer, and others) for your days off.
- Do not use the center's computers, printers, fax machines, copiers, or other equipment for your personal use.
- Do not take center supplies (pens, paper, and others) for your personal use.
- Do not discuss personal problems.
- Control your emotions. If you need to cry or express anger, do so in a private place. Get yourself together quickly and return to your work.
- Do not borrow money from or lend it to coworkers. This includes meal money and bus or train fares. Borrowing and lending can lead to problems with coworkers.
- Do not sell things or engage in fundraising. For example, do not sell your child's candy or raffle tickets to coworkers.
- Turn off personal pagers and cell phones.
- Do not send or check text messages while on duty. Do this on your break.

Meals and Breaks

Meal breaks are usually 30 minutes. Other breaks are usually 15 minutes. Meals and breaks are scheduled so that some staff are always on the unit. Staff remaining on the unit cover for the staff on break.

Staff members depend on each other. Leave for and return from breaks on time. That way other staff can have their turn. Do not take longer than allowed. Tell the nurse when you leave and return to the unit.

Job Safety

You must protect residents, families, visitors, coworkers, and yourself from harm. Everyone is responsible for safety. Negligent behavior affects the safety of others (Chapter 2). Safety practices are presented throughout this book. These guidelines apply to everything you do:

- Understand the roles, functions, and responsibilities in your job description.
- Know the contents and policies in the employee handbook and policy and procedure manuals.
- Know what to do in emergency situations. Take fire drills and other training sessions seriously.
- Know what is right and wrong.
- Know what you can and cannot do.
- Develop the desired qualities and traits of nursing assistants.
- Follow the nurse's directions and instructions.
- Question unclear directions and things you do not understand.
- Help others willingly when asked.
- Follow center rules.
- Attend required training sessions and ask for any training that you might need.
- Report measurements, observations, the care given, the person's complaints, and any errors accurately (Chapter 4).
- Accept responsibility for your actions. Admit when you are wrong or make mistakes. Do not blame others. Do not make excuses for your actions. Learn what you did wrong and why. Always try to learn from your mistakes.
- Handle the person's property carefully and prevent damage.

Planning Your Work

You will give care and perform routine tasks on the nursing unit. Some tasks are done at certain times. Others are done by the end of the shift.

The nurse, the Kardex, the care plan, and your assignment sheet help you decide what to do and when (Chapters 4 and 5). This is called *priority setting*. A *priority* is the most important thing at the time. Setting priorities involves deciding:

- Which person has the greatest or most life-threatening needs.
- What tasks the nurse or person needs done first.
- What tasks need to be done at a set time.
- What tasks need to be done when your shift starts.
- What tasks need to be done at the end of your shift.
- How much time it takes to complete a task.
- How much help you need to complete a task.
- Who can help you and when.

Priorities change as the person's needs change. A person's condition can improve or worsen. New residents are admitted.

BOX 3.3 Planning Your Work

- Discuss priorities with the nurse.
- Know the routine of your shift and nursing unit.
- Follow unit policies for shift reports.
- List tasks that are on a schedule (e.g., some persons are turned or offered the bedpan every 2 hours).
- Judge how much time you need for each person and task.
- Identify the tasks to do while residents are eating, visiting, or involved with activities or therapies.
- Plan care around meal times, visiting hours, rest periods, and therapies. Also consider recreation and social activities.
- Identify when you will need help from a coworker. Ask a coworker to help you. Give the time when you will need help and for how long.
- Schedule equipment or rooms for the person's use (e.g., the shower room).
- Review delegated tasks. Gather needed supplies beforehand.
- Do not waste time. Stay focused on your work.
- Leave a clean work area. Make sure rooms and utility areas are neat, clean, and orderly.
- Be a self-starter. Have initiative. Ask others if they need help. Follow unit routines, stock supply areas, and clean utility rooms. Stay busy.

Others are transferred to other nursing units or discharged. These and many other factors can cause priorities to change.

Setting priorities is hard at first. It becomes easier as you gain experience. You can ask the nurse to help you set priorities. Plan your work to give safe, thorough care and to make good use of your time (Box 3.3).

MANAGING STRESS

Stress is the response or change in the body caused by any emotional, physical, social, or economic factor. Stress is normal. It occurs every minute of every day. It occurs in everything you do.

A *stressor* is the event or factor that causes stress. Many stressors are pleasant—watching a child play, planning a party, laughing with family and friends, enjoying a nice day. Some are not pleasant—illness, injury, family problems, death of loved ones, divorce, money concerns. Many parts of your job are stressful.

No matter the cause, stress affects the whole person.

- *Physically*—sweating, increased heart rate, faster and deeper breathing, increased blood pressure, dry mouth, and so on
- *Mentally*—anxiety, fear, anger, dread, depression, and using defense mechanisms (Chapter 39)
- *Socially*—changes in relationships, avoiding others, needing others, blaming others, and so on
- *Spiritually*—changes in beliefs and values and strengthening or questioning one's belief in God or a higher power

Prolonged or frequent stress can threaten your health. Physical and mental health problems can occur. Some problems are minor (e.g., headaches, stomach upset, sleep problems, muscle tension). Others are life threatening (e.g., high blood pressure, heart attack, stroke, ulcers).

Dealing with stress is important. If your job causes stress, it affects your family and friends. If you have stress in your personal life, it affects your work. Stress affects you, the care you give, the person's quality of life, and how you relate to co-workers. These guidelines can help you reduce or cope with stress:

- Exercise regularly. It has physical and mental benefits—cardiovascular health, weight control, tension release, emotional well-being, and relaxation.
- Get enough rest and sleep.
- Eat healthily.
- Plan personal and quiet time for you. Read, take a hot bath, go for a walk, meditate, or listen to music. Do what makes you feel good.
- Use common sense about what you can do. Do not try to do everything that family and friends ask you to do. Consider the amount of time and energy that you have.
- Do one thing at a time. The demands on you may seem overwhelming. List each thing that you have to do. Set priorities.
- Do not judge yourself harshly. Do not try to be perfect or expect too much from yourself.
- Give yourself praise. You do good and wonderful things every day.
- Have a sense of humor. Laugh at yourself. Laugh with others. Spend time with those who make you laugh.
- Talk to the nurse if your work or a person is causing too much stress. The nurse may be able to help you deal with the matter.
- Do not be afraid to seek professional help if you feel stress and anxiety are overcoming your daily life. Counseling and support groups can be very helpful.

HARASSMENT

Harassment means to trouble, torment, offend, or worry a person by one's behavior or comments. Harassment can be sexual; or it can involve age, race, ethnic background, religion, or disability. You must respect others. Do not offend others by your gestures, remarks, or use of touch. Do not offend others with jokes, photos, or other pictures (e.g., drawings, cartoons). Harassment is not legal in the workplace. Bullying can be a form of harassment.

See *Focus on Communication: Harassment.*

📋 FOCUS ON COMMUNICATION

Harassment

You have the right to feel safe and unthreatened. If someone's comments make you uncomfortable, you can say: "Please don't say things like that. It's unprofessional." If someone's actions make you uneasy, you can say: "Please don't do that. It's unprofessional." Leave the area. Report the person's statements or actions to the nurse.

Sexual Harassment

Sexual harassment involves unwanted sexual behaviors by another. The behavior may be a sexual advance or it may be a request for a sexual favor. Some remarks, comments, and touching are sexual. The behavior affects the person's work and comfort. In extreme cases, the person's job is threatened if sexual favors are not granted.

Victims of sexual harassment may be men or women. Men harass women or men. Women harass men or women. You might feel that you are being harassed. If so, report the matter to the nurse and the human resources officer.

Be careful about what you say or do. Even innocent remarks and behaviors can be viewed as harassment. Employee orientation programs address harassment. You might not be sure about your own or another person's remarks or behaviors. Postings on social media can be unkind and hurtful. Do not offend a coworker with disrespectful remarks on social media sites. Do not share any personal information about residents or coworkers on social media. Do not express negative views about your facility or administration. You cannot be too careful.

DRUG TESTING

Drug and alcohol use affect resident and staff safety. Quality of care suffers. Those who use drugs or alcohol are late to work or absent more often than staff who do not use such substances. Therefore drug testing policies are common. Review your center's policy for when and how you might be tested.

👥 QUALITY OF LIFE

Your job as a nursing assistant is important. Residents, families, and visitors believe you will give safe and effective care. They trust that you will:

- Work when scheduled.
- Arrive at work on time.
- Stay the entire shift.
- Complete your assignments.
- Be well groomed.
- Be pleasant and courteous.

Your work ethic affects quality of life. Good work ethic helps people feel safe, secure, loved, and cared for. If you want to make their lives happier, easier, and less painful, you will practice a good work ethic.

❓ TIME TO REFLECT

Two nursing assistants are finishing their shifts and enter the elevator to leave the building. One mentions how tired and stressed she feels after taking care of Mrs. Thornton today: "I must have changed her pants five times in 2 hours and it wasn't pretty." The other agrees: "It was the same way yesterday for me." Suddenly a young woman in the back of the elevator says: "Excuse me, but Helen Thornton is my grandmother and I don't appreciate hearing you talk about her like that!" What do you think should happen to these nursing assistants?

REVIEW QUESTIONS

Circle the BEST answer.

1. Which will *not* help you do your job well?
   a. Enough rest and sleep
   b. Regular exercise
   c. Using drugs and alcohol
   d. Good nutrition

2. Which is *not* a good hygiene practice?
   a. Bathing daily
   b. Using a deodorant
   c. Brushing teeth after meals
   d. Having long and polished fingernails

3. You are getting ready for work. Which is *not* a good practice?
   a. Wearing jewelry
   b. Ironing your uniform
   c. Wearing your name badge
   d. Styling hair up and off your collar

4. Empathy is
   a. Feeling sorry for a person
   b. Seeing things from the other person's point of view
   c. Being polite to others
   d. Saying kind things

5. Which statement reflects a good work attitude?
   a. "It's not my fault."
   b. "I'm sorry. I didn't know."
   c. "That's not my job."
   d. "I did it yesterday. It's your turn."

6. A coworker says that a doctor and nurse are dating. This is
   a. Gossip
   b. Eavesdropping
   c. Confidential information
   d. Sexual harassment

7. Which is professional speech and language?
   a. Speaking clearly
   b. Using vulgar words
   c. Shouting
   d. Arguing

8. Which is *not* a courteous act?
   a. Saying "please" and "thank you"
   b. Wanting others to open doors for you
   c. Saying "I'm sorry"
   d. Complimenting others

9. You are on a meal break. Which is *false*?
   a. You can make personal phone calls
   b. Family members can meet you
   c. You can take a few extra minutes if needed
   d. The nurse needs to know that you are off the unit

10. You are planning your work. You should do the following *except*
    a. Discuss priorities with the nurse
    b. Ask others if they need help
    c. Stay busy
    d. Plan care so that you can watch the person's TV

11. These statements are about stress. Which is *false*?
    a. Stress affects the whole person
    b. A stressor is an event that causes stress
    c. All stress is unpleasant
    d. Stress is normal

12. Which does *not* help reduce stress?
    a. Exercise, rest, and sleep
    b. Blaming yourself for things you did not do
    c. Planning quiet time
    d. Having a sense of humor

13. Which is *not* harassment?
    a. Using touch to comfort a person
    b. Joking about a person's religion
    c. Asking for a sexual favor
    d. Acting like a disabled person

14. Which is *not* an example of good teamwork?
    a. Completing tasks promptly
    b. Offering to help a coworker
    c. Complaining about not enough staff
    d. Asking the nurse if you can help

15. Which is *not* an example of a cheerful worker?
    a. Greeting people in a pleasant manner
    b. Being moody
    c. Smiling at residents
    d. Enjoying a conversation

16. Being eager, interested, and excited about your work shows
    a. Empathy
    b. Enthusiasm
    c. Cooperation
    d. Respect

17. Perfume, cologne, or aftershave lotion used by staff
    a. Is acceptable and can be worn freely
    b. Should be used to cover up cigarette odors
    c. May cause nausea or breathing problems for some residents
    d. Shows a well-groomed employee

18. Personal cell phone usage while at work
    a. Should be limited to break times when off the unit
    b. Is acceptable while caring for a resident
    c. Is acceptable if the resident does not mind
    d. Has no restrictions

19. You accidently knock a resident's picture frame to the floor and the glass breaks. What should you do?
    a. Say nothing and pretend it did not happen
    b. Hide it in the trash receptacle
    c. Admit what happened to the nurse and resident
    d. Say nothing but try to buy a new one that is similar

20. A coworker was just notified that her father died. She is scheduled to work the next day. What would be a solution for the situation?
    a. The unit would have to work short staffed
    b. Understanding coworkers might offer to work her shift
    c. The workers on the previous shift will work overtime
    d. The residents will have to do without certain care

See Appendix A for answers to these questions.

4

Communicating With the Health Team

OBJECTIVES

- Define the key terms and key abbreviations listed in this chapter.
- Explain why health team members need to communicate.
- Describe the rules for good communication.
- Explain the purpose, parts, and information found in the medical record.
- Describe the legal and ethical aspects of medical records.
- Describe the purpose of the Kardex.
- Describe the purpose of the care plan.
- List the information you need to report to the nurse.
- List the rules for recording information in a medical record.
- Use the 24-hour clock, medical terminology, and abbreviations.
- Explain how computers and other electronic devices are used in health care.
- Explain how to protect the right to privacy when using computers and other electronic devices.
- Describe the rules for answering phones.
- Explain how to problem solve and deal with conflict.
- Explain how to promote quality of life.

KEY TERMS

abbreviation A shortened form of a word or phrase

care plan A record of the measures to be offered to best care for the resident

chart See "medical record"

communication The exchange of information—a message sent is received and correctly interpreted by the intended person

conflict A clash between opposing interests or ideas

diagnosis The term used when symptoms, signs, or reasons for a problem are identified

Kardex A type of card file that summarizes information found in the medical record—medications, treatments, diagnoses, routine care measures, equipment, and special needs

medical record A written or electronic document of a person's condition and response to treatment and care; often referred to as a chart, clinical record, or health record

prefix A word element placed before a root; it changes the meaning of the word

progress note A written description of the care given and the person's response and progress

recording The written account of care and observations; charting

reporting The oral account of care and observations

root A word element that contains the basic meaning of the word

suffix A word element placed after a root; it changes the meaning of the word

word element A part of a word

KEY ABBREVIATIONS

ADL Activities of daily living
EHR Electronic health record
EMR Electronic medical record
EPHI Electronic protected health information
HIPAA Health Insurance Portability and Accountability Act

MDS Minimum data set
OBRA Omnibus Budget Reconciliation Act of 1987
PHI Protected health information
POC Point of care

Health team members must communicate with each other to give coordinated and effective care. They share information about:
- What was done for the person.
- What needs to be done for the person.
- The person's response to treatment.

For example, the doctor ordered a blood test for Mrs. Carter. Food and fluids affect the test results. Mrs. Carter must fast for 10 hours before the blood is drawn. A nurse tells the dietary department that Mrs. Carter will have breakfast later. She explains the breakfast delay to you and Mrs. Carter. A technician tells the nurse the blood sample was drawn. The nurse orders the meal. A dietary worker brings the tray to the nursing unit. You serve Mrs. Carter's tray. After she is done eating, you remove the tray and observe what she ate. You report your observations to the nurse. The nurse records your observations in Mrs. Carter's medical record.

Team members communicated with each other and Mrs. Carter. Her care was coordinated and effective. She knew that she was not neglected or forgotten.

You need to understand the basic aspects and rules of communication. Then you can learn how to communicate information to the nursing and health teams.

COMMUNICATION

Communication is the exchange of information—a message sent is received and correctly interpreted by the intended person. For good communication:

- Use words that mean the same thing to you and the receiver of the message. Avoid words with more than one meaning. What does "far" mean—10 feet, 50 feet, or 100 feet?
- Use familiar words. You will learn medical terms. If someone uses a term that you do not understand, ask what it means. You must understand the message. Otherwise communication does not occur. Likewise, avoid terms that the person and family do not understand.
- Be brief and concise. Do not add unrelated or unnecessary information. Stay on the subject. Do not wander in thought or get wordy.
- Give information in a logical and orderly manner. Organize your thoughts. Present them step by step.
- Give facts and be specific. Give the receiver a clear picture of what you are saying. You report a pulse rate of 110. It is more specific and factual than saying the "pulse is fast."
- Look at the person you are communicating with. Eye contact is an important part of good communication.
- Speak clearly in a normal tone of voice. Be sure you have the person's attention before beginning to speak. Provide your undivided attention to the speaker.
- Ask questions if you do not understand what is said. Asking questions shows that you are listening and willing to learn.

THE MEDICAL RECORD

The medical record (chart) is a written or an electronic account of a person's condition and response to treatment and care.

❖ *The Omnibus Budget Reconciliation Act of 1987 (OBRA) calls it the clinical record.*

The health team uses it to share information about the person. The record is permanent. Sometimes it is used months or years later if the person's health history is needed. The record is also a legal document. It can be used in court as legal evidence of the person's problems, treatment, and care.

The record has many forms. Each page has the person's name, room and bed number, and other identifying information. This helps prevent errors and improper placement of records. The record includes the person's:

- Admission sheet (also referred to as a face sheet).
- Health history.
- Physical examination results.
- Doctor's orders.
- Doctor's progress notes.

- Progress notes (nursing team and health team).
- Graphic sheet (vital signs, weights, etc.).
- Flow sheets.
- Immunization/vaccination records.
- Care plan.
- Minimum data set (MDS).
- Records and assessments.
- Laboratory results.
- X-ray reports.
- Intravenous (IV) therapy record or tube feeding record.
- Respiratory therapy record.
- Consultation reports.
- Assessments from nursing, social services, dietary services, and recreational therapy.
- Special consents.

Health team members record on the forms for their departments. Other team members read the information. It tells the care provided and the person's response (Fig. 4.1). An example of an electronic chart is seen in Fig. 4.2.

Nursing centers have policies about medical records and who can see them. Policies address:

- Who records.
- When to record.
- Abbreviations.
- Correcting errors.
- Ink color.
- Signing entries.

Some centers allow nursing assistants to record observations and care. Others do not. You must know your center's policies. Many centers are using electronic health records/electronic medical records (EHRs/EMRs). As with paper charting, you will need to know the center's policies on electronic charting.

Professional staff involved in a person's care can review charts. Cooks, laundry, housekeeping, and office staff do not need to read charts. Some centers let nursing assistants read charts. If not, the nurse shares needed information.

You have an ethical and legal duty to keep the person's information confidential. You may know someone in the center. If you are not involved in the person's care, you have no right to review the person's chart. To do so is an invasion of privacy because you did not have a need to know this information.

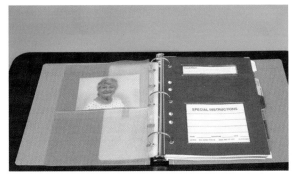

Fig. 4.1 A medical record.

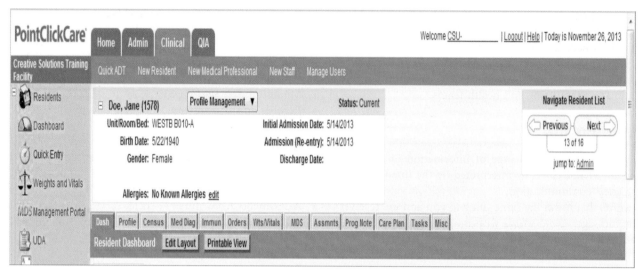

Fig. 4.2 Sample of an electronic resident chart. (Courtesy PointClickCare®.)

❖ *Under OBRA, residents have the right to know the information in their medical records.* A resident or a legal representative may ask you for the chart. Report the request to the nurse. The nurse deals with this request.

The following parts of the medical record relate to your work.

The Admission Sheet

The admission sheet (also known as the face sheet) is completed when the person is admitted to the center. It has the person's identifying information—legal name, birth date, age, gender (male or female), address, and marital status. It also has the person's Medicare, social security number, and insurance information. The names and contact information of the person's legal representative, guardian, and family members are included. Other information includes known allergies, diagnoses, date and time of admission, doctor's name, religion, and church or place of worship.

Each person receives an identification (ID) number. It is on the admission sheet. Information about advance directives is also recorded here. An advance directive is a document stating a person's wishes about life support measures (Chapter 45).

Use the admission sheet to fill out other forms that require the same information. That way the person does not have to answer the same question many times.

Progress Notes

The progress note is a written description of the care given and the person's response and progress (Fig. 4.3). The nurse records:

• Signs and symptoms.

Date	Time	Nursing Margin	Other Depts Margin
3-19	1700	Out with family for dinner. Jane Doe, LPN	
	1930	Returned from outing accompanied by her son. States she had a pleasant time Mary Smith, CNA	
3-20	0900	IN BED. COMPLAINS OF HEADACHE. T 98.4 ORALLY, RADIAL PULSE 72 AND REGULAR, RESPIRATIONS 18 AND UNLABORED. BP 134/84 LEFT ARM LYING DOWN. ALICE JONES, RN NOTIFIED OF RESIDENT COMPLAINT AND VITAL SIGNS. ANN ADAMS, CNA	
	0910	In bed resting. States she has had a headache for about 1/2 hour. Denies nausea and dizziness. No other complaints. PRN Tylenol given. Instructed resident to use signal light if headache worsens or other symptoms occur. Alice Jones, RN	
	0945	Resting quietly. Denies headache at this time. T 98.4 orally, radial pulse 70 and regular, respirations 18 and unlabored. BP 132/84 left arm lying down. Alice Jones, RN	

Fig. 4.3 Progress notes. Note that other members of the health team also can record on this form. *BP,* Blood pressure; *PRN,* as needed; *T,* temperature.

Activities of Daily Living Flow Sheet

ORDER/INSTRUCTION	TIME	JAN 1	2	FEB 3	4	5	(MAR) 6	7	8	APR 9
Bowel Movements L = Large M = Medium S = Small IC = Incontinent	11-7	M								
	7-3			L						
	3-11									
Bladder Elimination I = Independent IC = Incontinent FC = Foley catheter	11-7	/	/	/	/					
	7-3	/	/	/	/					
	3-11	/	IC	/	/					
Weight Bearing Status TT = Toe touch AT = As tol. P = Partial F = Full NWB = No weight bearing	11-7	AT	AT	AT	AT					
	7-3	AT	AT	AT	AT					
	3-11	AT	AT	AT						
Transfer Status ML = Mech lift SBA = Stand by assist; Assist of 1 or 2	11-7	SBA	SBA	SBA	SBA					
	7-3	SBA	SBA	SBA	SBA					
	3-11	SBA	SBA	SBA	A-1					
Activity A = Ambulate GC = Gerichair T = Turn every 2 hrs. W/C = Wheelchair	11-7	T	T	T	T					
	7-3	A	A	A	A					
	3-11	A	A	A	A					
Safety LT = Lap tray BR = Bed rails BA = Bed alarm SB = Seat belt	11-7									
	7-3									
	3-11									
Feeding Status I = Independent S = Set up F = Staff feed SP = Swallow precautions TL = Thickened liquids	Breakfast	S	S	S	S					
	Lunch	S	S	S	S					
	Supper	S	S	S	S					
Amount of food taken in %	Breakfast	75	100	100	75					
	Lunch	75	75	100	75					
	Supper	50	50	50	75					
Bath and Shampoo every Monday & Thursday on 7-3 shift T = Tub S = Shower B = Bed bath	11-7									
	7-3		T							
	3-11									
Oral Care Own/Dentures/No teeth I = Independent S = Set up A = Assist	11-7	S	S	S	S					
	7-3	S	S	S	S					
	3-11	S	S	S	S					
Dressing I = Independent S = Set up A = Assist T = Total care	11-7	A	A	S	S					
	7-3									
	3-11	A	A	A	A					
Grooming: Washing Face and Hands Combing Hair I = Independent S = Set up A = Assist T = Total care	11-7	A	A	A	A					
	7-3	A	A	A	A					
	3-11	A	A	A	A					
Trim Fingernails weekly Thursday	11-7									
	7-3		✓							
	3-11									
Lotion Arms and Legs twice daily	11-7									
	7-3	✓	✓	✓	✓					
	3-11	✓	✓	✓	✓					
Shave Men daily Shave Women every Monday & Thursday on 7-3 shift	11-7									
	7-3		✓							
	3-11									
Amount Between-Meal Nourishment taken in %	AM	100	75	100	50					
	PM	100	100	75	75					
	HS	50	75	75	75					
Intake and Output	11-7									
	7-3									
	3-11									
Vital Signs Every Thursday	11-7									
	7-3		✓							
	3-11									
Weight Every Thursday	11-7		✓							
	7-3									
	3-11									

Fig. 4.4 Some items on an activities of daily living (ADL) flow sheet.

- Information about treatments and medications.
- Information about teaching and counseling.
- Procedures performed by the health care provider.
- Visits by other health team members.

Progress notes are recorded when there is an unusual event, a problem, or a change in the person's condition. ❖ *OBRA requires that summaries of care be written at least every 3 months.* They reflect the person's progress toward the goals set in the care plan (Chapter 5). They also reflect the person's response to care. Some centers require summaries more often.

Flow Sheets

The activities of daily living (ADL) flow sheet is used to record a person's ability to perform ADL (Fig. 4.4). This flow sheet addresses hygiene, food and fluids, elimination, rest and sleep, activities, walking, vital signs, behaviors exhibited, and social interactions.

Many centers use electronic flow sheets where assistants record resident care. These flow sheets are part of a point of care (POC) module within an EHR. The nursing assistant records all care and interactions with the resident on small computer terminals called kiosks (Fig. 4.5). The information is recorded soon after the care is given. Entering data on a computer is often easier and faster than paper charting. Electronic charting eliminates the need for paper flow sheets. The nursing assistant's entries are used to gather information for completion of the MDS. Recorded information can also be used to help determine staffing needs.

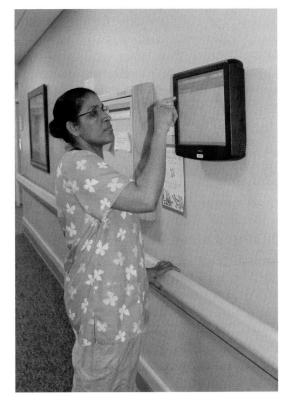

Fig. 4.5 A nursing assistant enters information at a touch-screen kiosk.

Other flow sheets are used to record frequent measurements and observations. Vital sign measurements (Chapter 27) and fluid intake and output records (Chapter 20) are examples.

THE KARDEX

The Kardex is a type of card file. It summarizes information found in the medical record—medications, treatments, diagnoses, routine care measures, equipment, and special needs. The Kardex is a quick, easy source of information about the person (Fig. 4.6).

THE CARE PLAN

Many facilities use a major portion of the care plan (Fig. 4.7) to convey measures that need to be taken to meet the resident's needs. Care plans need to be accurate and readily available to the nursing assistant. Some centers print a copy of the current care plan and post it in the resident's room or bathroom (for example, inside the medicine cabinet door). Other facilities may have this information printed on cards that the nursing assistant carries in a pocket. Still other facilities have this information stored in electronic devices that the nursing assistant has easy access to. You will be trained to the method that your facility uses. This information is updated regularly by the nurse.

RESIDENT CARE CONFERENCES

❖ OBRA requires two types of resident care conferences:
- *Interdisciplinary care planning conference.* This is held regularly to review and update care plans. It also is held to develop care plans for new residents. The nurse, health care provider, and other health team members may attend.
- *Problem-focused conference.* This is held when one problem affects a resident's care. Only staff directly involved with the problem attend.

The resident has the right to take part in these planning conferences. Often the family is involved. The resident may refuse actions suggested by the health team.

Many centers are now including nursing assistants in the resident's care conference. You often know a resident well because of your daily and frequent contact with the resident. You may be asked to attend these conferences. Always share your ideas and observations. You also play a key role in helping ◆ the resident meet personal goals.

REPORTING AND RECORDING

The health team communicates by reporting and recording (Fig. 4.8). Reporting is the oral account of care and observations. Recording *(charting)* is the written account of care and observations.

See *Focus on Communication: Reporting and Recording.*

Reporting

You report care and observations to the nurse. Report to the nurse at these times:
- Whenever there is a change from normal or a change in the person's condition—report these changes at once
- When the nurse asks you to do so
- When you leave the unit for meals, breaks, or other reasons
- Before the end-of-shift report
  When reporting, follow the rules in Box 4.1.

End-of-Shift Report

The nurse gives a report at the end of the shift. This is called the *end-of-shift report.* It is given to the nursing team of the oncoming shift. The nurse reports about:
- The care given.

> **📋 FOCUS ON COMMUNICATION**
>
> **Reporting and Recording**
> The terms "small," "moderate," and "large" mean different things to different people. Is small the size of a dime? Or is it the size of a quarter? In health care, different meanings can cause serious problems. Give accurate descriptions and measurements. If you have a question, ask the nurse to look at what you are trying to describe.

- The care to give during other shifts.
- The person's current condition.
- Changes in the person's condition.

In some centers, the entire nursing team hears the end-of-shift report as it comes on duty. In other centers, only nurses hear the report. After the report, information is shared with nursing assistants.

Many centers use "walking rounds" to provide end-of-shift reports. These walking rounds usually include the nurse going off duty and the nurse coming on duty. In some centers, the nursing assistants are also included in walking rounds. This team moves from room to room to see each resident. A brief report about the resident is shared with the members of the oncoming shift. If only the nurses participate in the walking rounds, information is passed on to the assistants and other team members.

See *Teamwork and Time Management: End-of-Shift Report.*

See *Promoting Safety and Comfort: End-of-Shift Report.*

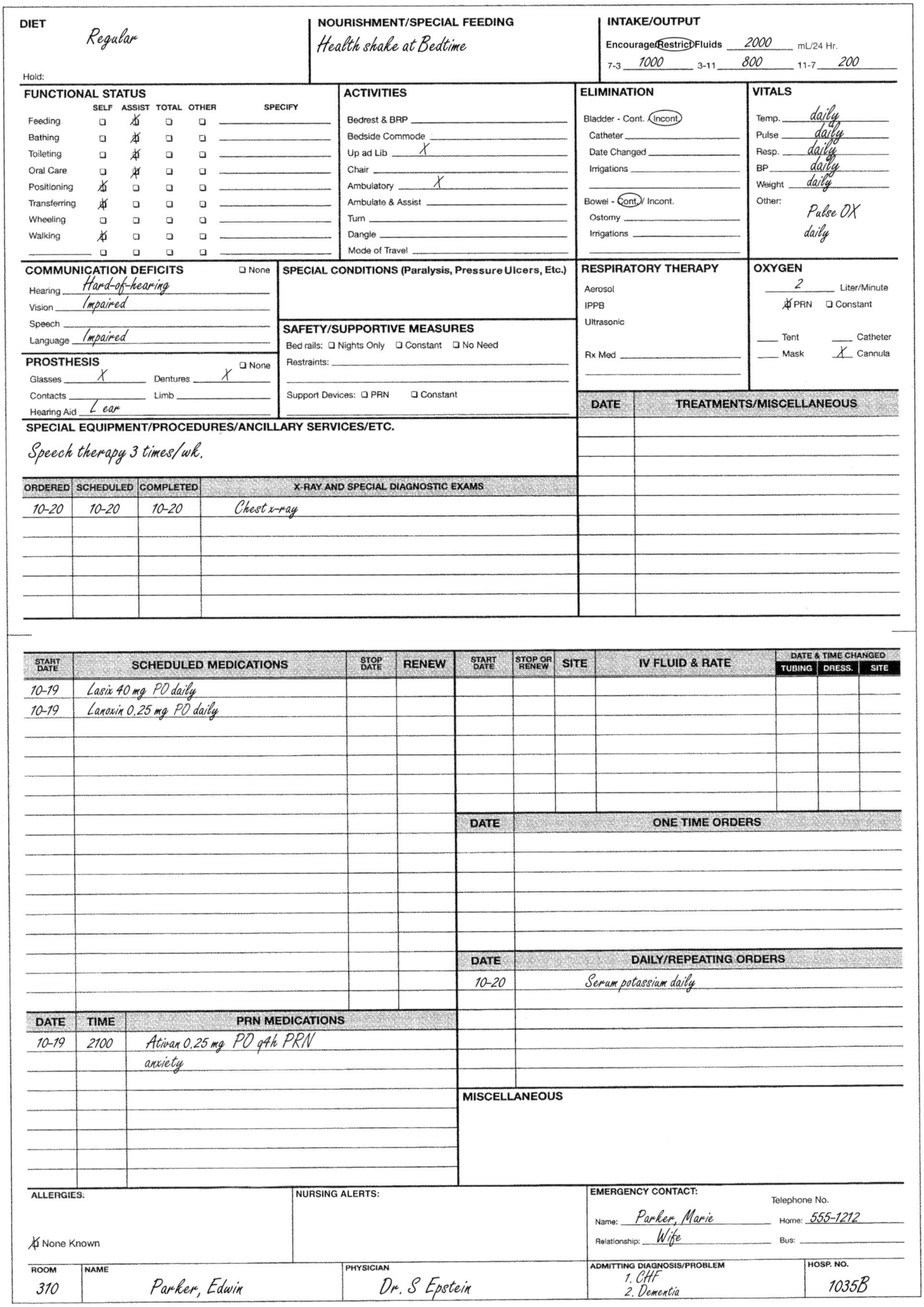

DIET: Regular
Hold:

NOURISHMENT/SPECIAL FEEDING: Health shake at Bedtime

INTAKE/OUTPUT
Encourage/(Restrict) Fluids 2000 mL/24 Hr.
7-3 1000 3-11 800 11-7 200

FUNCTIONAL STATUS

	SELF	ASSIST	TOTAL	OTHER	SPECIFY
Feeding	☐	X	☐	☐	
Bathing	☐	X	☐	☐	
Toileting	☐	X	☐	☐	
Oral Care	☐	X	☐	☐	
Positioning	X	☐	☐	☐	
Transferring	X	☐	☐	☐	
Wheeling	☐	☐	☐	☐	
Walking	X	☐	☐	☐	
	☐	☐	☐	☐	

ACTIVITIES
Bedrest & BRP
Bedside Commode
Up ad Lib X
Chair
Ambulatory X
Ambulate & Assist
Turn
Dangle
Mode of Travel

ELIMINATION
Bladder - Cont. (Incont)
Catheter
Date Changed
Irrigations
Bowel - (Cont) / Incont.
Ostomy
Irrigations

VITALS
Temp. daily
Pulse daily
Resp. daily
BP daily
Weight daily
Other: Pulse OX daily

COMMUNICATION DEFICITS ☐ None
Hearing Hard-of-hearing
Vision Impaired
Speech
Language Impaired

SPECIAL CONDITIONS (Paralysis, Pressure Ulcers, Etc.)

SAFETY/SUPPORTIVE MEASURES
Bed rails: ☐ Nights Only ☐ Constant ☐ No Need
Restraints:
Support Devices: ☐ PRN ☐ Constant

PROSTHESIS ☐ None
Glasses X Dentures X
Contacts Limb
Hearing Aid L ear

RESPIRATORY THERAPY
Aerosol
IPPB
Ultrasonic
Rx Med

OXYGEN
2 Liter/Minute
X PRN ☐ Constant
Tent Catheter
Mask X Cannula

SPECIAL EQUIPMENT/PROCEDURES/ANCILLARY SERVICES/ETC.
Speech therapy 3 times/wk.

ORDERED	SCHEDULED	COMPLETED	X-RAY AND SPECIAL DIAGNOSTIC EXAMS
10-20	10-20	10-20	Chest x-ray

DATE	TREATMENTS/MISCELLANEOUS

START DATE	SCHEDULED MEDICATIONS	STOP DATE	RENEW
10-19	Lasix 40 mg PO daily		
10-19	Lanoxin 0.25 mg PO daily		

START DATE	STOP OR RENEW	SITE	IV FLUID & RATE	DATE & TIME CHANGED: TUBING	DRESS.	SITE

DATE	ONE TIME ORDERS

DATE	DAILY/REPEATING ORDERS
10-20	Serum potassium daily

DATE	TIME	PRN MEDICATIONS
10-19	2100	Ativan 0.25 mg PO q4h PRN anxiety

MISCELLANEOUS

ALLERGIES: X None Known

NURSING ALERTS:

EMERGENCY CONTACT:
Name: Parker, Marie Telephone No. Home: 555-1212
Relationship: Wife Bus:

ROOM: 310
NAME: Parker, Edwin
PHYSICIAN: Dr. S Epstein
ADMITTING DIAGNOSIS/PROBLEM: 1. CHF 2. Dementia
HOSP. NO.: 1035B

Fig. 4.6 A sample Kardex. *BP*, Blood pressure; *BRP*, bathroom privileges; *CHF*, congestive heart failure; *IPPB*, intermittent positive pressure breathing; *IV*, intravenous; *OX*, oxygen; *PO*, orally; *PRN*, as needed. (Modified from Briggs Corporation, Des Moines, IA.)

QUICK PLAN OF CARE – This document is a quick reference for caregivers and serves as the major piece of the resident care plan; see back for focused goals and additional approaches.

CODE STATUS: ☐ CPR ☐ No CPR
HIGH RISK: ☐ Fall ☐ Skin ☐ Elopement

Resident name:_____ Prefers to be called:_____

COGNITION/SENSORY/COMMUNICATION ☐ See goal
Alert ☐ No ☐ Yes
Short term memory loss ☐ No ☐ Yes
Verbal ☐ No ☐ Yes ☐ Occasional
Hearing aids ☐ Night ☐ Left ☐ To nurse at night
Glasses ☐ No ☐ Yes ☐ Yes, but doesn't always wear
*Special notes*_____

MOOD/BEHAVIOR ☐ See goal
Insomnia ☐ No ☐ Yes
Combative ☐ No ☐ Yes
Wanders ☐ No ☐ Yes
Other _____

NUTRITION/DIETARY ☐ See goal
Diabetic ☐ No ☐ Yes
Dining area ☐ Main dining ☐ Prefers own room ☐ HWH
Texture modification ☐ No ☐ Yes, _____
Liquids ☐ Regular ☐ Thickened, _____
_____ **Straws:** ☐ No ☐ Yes
Other _____
Perfers MEDs: ☐ In room ☐ In dining room ☐ Either

CONTINENCE AND HYGIENE ☐ See goal
Toileting ☐ Alone ☐ SBA ☐ Assist of one or two
Per ☐ BR ☐ Urinal ☐ Commode
Urinary ☐ Continent ☐ Incontinent ☐ Catheter
Bowel ☐ Continent ☐ Incontinent ☐ Ostomy
Product used ☐ No ☐ Yes, **Size** _____
Bathing ☐ Whirlpool ☐ Shower ☐ Bed bath
Oral care ☐ Alone ☐ Set up ☐ Assist ☐ Dependent
Dentures ☐ Yes ☐ No–**Assist needed** ☐ Yes ☐ No
Partials ☐ Upper ☐ Lower–**Assist needed** ☐ Yes ☐ No
Special notes _____

MISCELLANEOUS
TED hose/support stockings ☐ No ☐ Yes
Report to nurse ☐ Intake ☐ Output
Braces/splints ☐ No ☐ Yes, _____
Oxygen ☐ No ☐ Yes_____ Liters/ via _____
Dominant hand ☐ Left hand ☐ Right hand
Other _____

PHYSICAL FUNTIONING ☐ See goal
Bed mobility ☐ Alone ☐ SBA ☐ Assist of one ☐ Assist of two ☐ Slide sheet
Transferring ☐ Alone ☐ SBA ☐ Assist of one ☐ Assist of two
Per ☐ Standing lift ☐ Floor/ceiling lift ☐ Gait belt
Ambulation ☐ Alone ☐ SBA ☐ Assist of one ☐ Assist of two
Assistive devices used ☐ Walker ☐ Wheelchair ☐ Gait belt
Dressing ☐ Alone ☐ SBA ☐ Assist of one ☐ Assist of two
Special notes _____
_____
_____
_____
B/P check only ☐ L arm OR only ☐ R arm _____

PAIN/COMFORT ☐ See goal ** Always report non-verbal symptoms to nurse
Chronic pain issues ☐ No ☐ Yes, related to _____
Routine pain meds ☐ No ☐ Yes *PRN pain meds* ☐ No ☐ Yes
Non-med pain interventions ☐ No ☐ Specifically, _____
_____
_____

SKIN ☐ See goal ☐ See TAR for ordered treatments
Intact ☐ No ☐ Yes If no, describe _____
Preventive interventions ☐ Geri sleeves ☐ Fleece sleeves ☐ Gel pad
☐ Booties/heel protectors ☐ Foot cradle in bed ☐ Other cushion, _____
Other _____
** Always observe skin during assist w/ bathing/ ADLs and report redness, open areas, changes, etc.**

ACTIVITIES/INTERESTS ☐ See goal

MISCELLANEOUS CARE TIPS/INFO
_____
_____
_____
_____
_____
_____
_____
_____
_____
_____
_____
_____

FAMILY and/or PERSONAL INFO

SAFETY INTERVENTIONS ☐ See goal
Side rails ☐ Top half ☐ Bottom half ☐ Mobility rails ☐ Padded railings ☐ No side rails *Geri chair* ☐ No ☐ Yes
Bed lowered to floor (while in bed) ☐ No ☐ Yes *Floor mat beside bed (while in bed)* ☐ No ☐ Yes
WanderGuard ☐ No ☐ Yes If yes, describe purpose: _____
*Other*_____
_____
_____
_____
_____
_____

Nurse/s signature: _____ Date: _____

Fig. 4.7 A sample care plan.

Recording

When recording on the person's chart, you must communicate clearly and thoroughly. Follow the rules in Box 4.1.

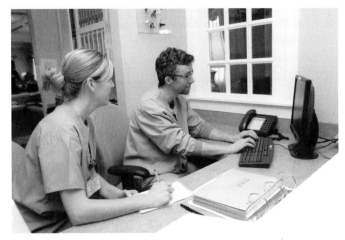

Fig. 4.8 The nursing assistant uses notes to report to the nurse.

TEAMWORK AND TIME MANAGEMENT

End-of-Shift Report

Two staff members are present at the end of a shift—the staff going off duty and the staff coming on duty. The entire oncoming shift may attend the end-of-shift report. If so, staff members going off duty answer all call lights, provide care, and tend to routine tasks. If only nurses attend the end-of-shift report, nursing assistants of the oncoming shift also answer call lights, provide care, and tend to routine tasks.

The end of shift is a time for good teamwork. Continue to do your job. Your attitude is important. If going off duty, avoid saying or thinking the following:

- "I'm ready to go home. Let them do it."
- "It's their turn. I've been here all day (evening or night)."
- "No one helped us when we came on duty."

Some centers have clear duties for the two shifts. For example, those going off duty continue to answer call lights. They know about changes in the person's condition and care plan and about new orders. They also know about the care needs of new residents. The oncoming shift has yet to learn this information. The oncoming shift uses this time to perform routine tasks for the shift and to collect needed supplies and equipment.

BOX 4.1 Rules for Reporting and Recording

Reporting

- Be prompt, thorough, and accurate.
- Give the person's name and room and bed number.
- Give the time your observations were made or the care was given.
- Report only what you observed or did yourself.
- Report care measures that you expect the person to need. For example, you expect that the person will need the bedpan during your meal break.
- Report expected changes in the person's condition. For example, you expect that the person may be tired after physical therapy.
- Give reports as often as the person's condition requires. Or give them when the nurse asks you to.
- Report any changes from normal or changes in the person's condition. Report these changes at once.
- Use your written notes to give a specific, concise, and clear report (see Fig. 4.8).

Recording
General Rules

- Follow center policies and procedures for recording. Ask for needed training.
- Include the date and time for every recording. Use conventional time (AM or PM) or 24-hour clock time according to center policy (p. ··).
- Use only center-approved abbreviations (p. ··).
- Use correct spelling, grammar, and punctuation.
- Do not use ditto marks.
- Sign all entries with your name and title as required by center policy.
- Make sure each form has the person's name and other identifying information.
- Record only what you observed and did yourself. Do not record for another person.
- Never chart a procedure, treatment, or care measure until after it is completed.
- Be accurate, concise, and factual. Do not record judgments or interpretations.
- Record in a logical and sequential manner.

- Be descriptive. Avoid terms with more than one meaning.
- Use the person's exact words when possible. Use quotation marks to show that the statement is a direct quote.
- Chart any changes from normal or changes in the person's condition. Also chart that you informed the nurse (include the nurse's name), what you told the nurse, and the time you made the report.
- Do not omit information.
- Record safety measures. Examples include placing the call light within reach, assisting a person when up, or reminding a person not to get out of bed.

Paper Charting

- Always use ink. Use the ink color required by the center.
- Make sure writing is readable and neat.
- Never erase or use correction fluid. Draw a line through the incorrect part. Date and initial the line. Write "mistaken entry" over it if this is center policy. Then rewrite the part. Follow center policy for correcting errors.
- Do not skip lines. Draw a line through the blank space of a partially completed line or to the end of the page. This prevents others from recording in a space with your signature.

Electronic Charting

- Log in using your username and password. Do not chart using another person's username.
- Check the time your entry is made. Make sure it is the intended time.
- Check for accuracy. Review your entry before saving.
- Save your entries. Unsaved data will be lost.
- Follow the vendor's instructions for changing or striking-out a mistaken entry. Most electronic charting systems keep a record of what was entered before a change was made. This works in the same manner as drawing a line through a mistaken entry in paper charting. The first entry is still visible.
- Log off after you are done charting. This prevents others from charting with your username.
- Remember to follow the center's policy on privacy while charting.

👤 PROMOTING SAFETY AND COMFORT

End-of-Shift Report

Safety

You may not hear the end-of-shift report as you come on duty. Yet you need to answer call lights and give care before the nurse shares new information with you. To give safe care:

- Check the care plan or Kardex before granting a request. The person's condition or care plan may have changed. There may be new orders from the doctor.
- Ask a nurse about the care needs of new residents. If necessary, politely interrupt the end-of-shift report to ask your questions.
- Do not take directions or orders from another nursing assistant. Remember, nursing assistants cannot supervise or delegate to other nursing assistants.

The charting sample in Fig. 4.9 shows how the rules apply. Anyone who reads your charting should know:

- What you observed.
- What you did.
- The person's response.

Reporting and Recording Time

The 24-hour clock (military time or international time) has four digits (Fig. 4.10). The first two digits are for the hours: 0100 = 1:00 AM; 1300 = 1:00 PM. The last two digits are for minutes: 0110 = 1:10 AM. The AM and PM abbreviations are not used.

As Box 4.2 shows, the hour is the same for morning times, but AM is not used. For PM times, add 12 to the clock time. If it is 2:00 PM, add 12 + 2 for 1400. For 8:35 PM, add 12 + 835 for 2035.

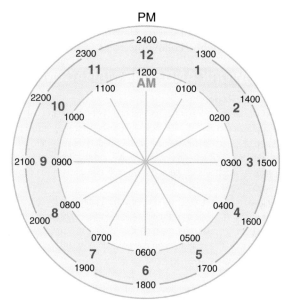

Fig. 4.10 The 24-hour clock.

Some centers use 0000 for midnight. Others use 2400. Follow center policy.

MEDICAL TERMS AND ABBREVIATIONS

Medical terms and abbreviations are used in health care. Someone may use a word or phrase that you do not understand. If so, ask a nurse to explain its meaning. Otherwise, communication does not occur. A medical dictionary is also useful for learning new words.

Date	Time	Nursing Margin / Other Depts Margin
4/10	1045	Requested assistance to lie down. States. "I don't feel well. I have a little upset stomach."
		Denies pain. VS taken. T-99(O). P-76 regular rate and rhythm. R-18 unlabored.
		BP 134/84 L arm lying down. Signal light within reach. Paula Jones, RN notified at 1040
		of resident's complaint and VS. Mary Jensen, CNA ────────
	1100	Asleep in bed. Appears to be resting comfortably. Color good. No signs of
		discomfort or distress noted at this time. Paula Jones, RN ────────
	1145	Refused to go to the dining room for lunch. Complains of nausea. Denies
		abdominal pain. Has not had an emesis. Abdomen soft to palpation. Good bowel
		sounds. VS taken. T-98.2̶ 99.2. P-76 regular rate and rhythm. R-18 unlabored. *(Mistaken entry 4-10, PJ)*
		BP-134/184. States she will try to eat something. Full liquid room tray ordered.
		Paula Jones, RN ────────

Fig. 4.9 Charting sample. *BP*, Blood pressure; *P*, pulse; *R*, respirations; *T*, temperature; *VS*, vital signs.

BOX 4.2   24-Hour Clock

AM Conventional Time	24-Hour Time
12:00 MIDNIGHT	0000 or 2400
1:00 AM	0100
2:00 AM	0200
3:00 AM	0300
4:00 AM	0400
5:00 AM	0500
6:00 AM	0600
7:00 AM	0700
8:00 AM	0800
9:00 AM	0900
10:00 AM	1000
11:00 AM	1100

PM Conventional Time	24-Hour Time
12:00 NOON	1200
1:00 PM	1300
2:00 PM	1400
3:00 PM	1500
4:00 PM	1600
5:00 PM	1700
6:00 PM	1800
7:00 PM	1900
8:00 PM	2000
9:00 PM	2100
10:00 PM	2200
11:00 PM	2300

Like all words, medical terms are made up of parts of words or word elements—prefixes, roots, and suffixes (Box 4.3). Most are from Greek or Latin. They are combined to form medical terms. To translate a term, the word is separated into its elements.

Prefixes, Roots, and Suffixes

A prefix is a word element placed before a root. It changes the meaning of the word. The prefix *olig-* ("scant, small amount") is placed before the root *uria* ("urine") to make *oliguria*. It means "a scant amount of urine." Prefixes are always combined with other word elements. They are never used alone.

The root is the word element that contains the basic meaning of the word. It is combined with another root, with prefixes, and with suffixes. A vowel (an *o* or an *i*) is added when two roots are combined or when a suffix is added to a root. The vowel makes the word easier to pronounce.

A suffix is a word element placed after a root. It changes the meaning of the word. Suffixes are not used alone. When translating medical terms, begin with the suffix. For example, *nephritis* means "inflammation of the kidney." It was formed by combining *nephron-* ("kidney") and *-itis* ("inflammation").

Medical terms are formed by combining word elements. Remember, prefixes always come before roots. Suffixes always come after roots. A root can be combined with prefixes, roots, and suffixes. The prefix *dys-* ("difficult") is combined with the root *pnea* ("breathing"). This forms *dyspnea*, which means "difficulty breathing."

Roots can be combined with suffixes. The root *mast* ("breast") combined with the suffix *-ectomy* ("excision or removal") forms *mastectomy*, which means "the removal of a breast."

BOX 4.3   Medical Terminology

Prefix	Meaning
a-, an-	without, not, lack of
ab-	away from
ad-	to, toward, near
ante-	before, forward, in front of
anti-	against
auto-	Self
bi-	double, two, twice
brady-	slow
circum-	around
contra-	against, opposite
de-	down, from
dia-	across, through, apart
dis-	apart, free from
dys-	bad, difficult, abnormal
ecto-	outer, outside
en-	in, into, within
endo-	inner, inside
epi-	over, on, upon
eryth-	Red
eu-	normal, good, well, healthy
ex-	out, out of, from, away from
hemi-	half
hyper-	excessive, too much, high
hypo-	under, decreased, less than normal
in-	in, into, within, not
inter-	between
intra-	within
intro-	into, within
leuk-	white
macro-	large
mal-	bad, illness, disease
meg-	large
micro-	small
mono-	one, single
neo-	New
non-	Not
olig-	small, scant
para-	beside, beyond, after
per-	by, through
peri-	around

BOX 4.3 Medical Terminology—cont'd

Prefix	Meaning
poly-	many, much
post-	after, behind
pre-	before, in front of, prior to
pro-	before, in front of
re-	again, backward
retro-	backward, behind
semi-	half
sub-	under, beneath
super-	above, over, excess
supra-	above, over
tachy-	fast, rapid
trans-	across
uni-	One

Root (Combining Vowel)	Meaning
abdomin (o)	abdomen
aden (o)	gland
adren (o)	adrenal gland
angi (o)	vessel
Arterio	artery
athr (o)	joint
Broncho	bronchus, bronchi
card, cardi (o)	heart
cephal (o)	head
chole, chol (o)	Bile
chondr (o)	cartilage
Colo	colon, large intestine
cost (o)	Rib
crani (o)	skull
cyan (o)	blue
cyst (o)	bladder, cyst
cyt (o)	Cell
dent (o)	tooth
Derma	skin
duoden (o)	duodenum
encephal (o)	brain
enter (o)	intestines
fibr (o)	fiber, fibrous
gastr (o)	stomach
gloss (o)	tongue
gluc (o)	sweetness, glucose
glyc (o)	sugar
gyn, gyne, gyneco	woman
hem, hema, hemo, hemat (o)	blood
hepat (o)	liver
hydr (o)	water
hyster (o)	uterus
ile (o), ili (o)	ileum
Laparo	abdomen, loin, flank
laryng (o)	larynx
lith (o)	stone
mamm (o)	breast, mammary gland
mast (o)	mammary gland, breast
Meno	menstruation
my (o)	muscle
myel (o)	spinal cord, bone marrow

Root (Combining Vowel)	Meaning
Necro	death
nephr (o)	kidney
neur (o)	nerve
ocul (o)	Eye
oophor (o)	ovary
ophthalm (o)	Eye
orth (o)	straight, normal, correct
oste (o)	bone
ot (o)	Ear
ped (o)	child, foot
pharyng (o)	pharynx
phleb (o)	vein
Pnea	breathing, respiration
pneum (o)	lung, air, gas
proct (o)	rectum
psych (o)	mind
Pulmo	lung
py (o)	Pus
rect (o)	rectum
rhin (o)	nose
salping (o)	eustachian tube, uterine tube
splen (o)	spleen
sten (o)	narrow, constriction
stern (o)	sternum
stomat (o)	mouth
therm (o)	heat
Thoraco	chest
thromb (o)	clot, thrombus
thyr (o)	thyroid
toxic (o)	poison, poisonous
Toxo	poison
trache (o)	trachea
urethr (o)	urethra
urin (o)	urine
Uro	urine, urinary tract, urination
uter (o)	uterus
vas (o)	blood vessel, vas deferens
ven (o)	vein
vertebr (o)	spine, vertebrae

Suffix	Meaning
-algia	pain
-asis	condition, usually abnormal
-cele	hernia, herniation, pouching
-centesis	puncture and aspiration of
-cyte	Cell
-ectasis	dilation, stretching
-ectomy	excision, removal of
-emia	blood condition
-genesis	development, production, creation
-genic	producing, causing
-gram	record
-graph	a diagram, a recording instrument
-graphy	making a recording
-iasis	condition of
-ism	a condition

BOX 4.3 Medical Terminology—cont'd

-itis	inflammation	-plegia	paralysis
-logy	the study of	-ptosis	falling, sagging, dropping down
-lysis	destruction of, decomposition	-rrhage, -rrhagia	excessive flow
-megaly	enlargement	-rrhaphy	stitching, suturing
-meter	measuring instrument	-rrhea	profuse flow, discharge
-oma	tumor	-scope	examination instrument
-osis	condition	-scopy	examination using a scope
-pathy	disease	-stasis	maintenance, maintaining a constant level
-penia	lack, deficiency		
-phagia	to eat or consume, swallowing	-stomy, -ostomy	creation of an opening
-phasia	speaking	-tomy, -otomy	incision, cutting into
-phobia	an exaggerated fear	-uria	condition of the urine
-plasty	surgical repair or reshaping		

Combining a prefix, root, and suffix is another way to form medical terms. *Endocarditis* has the prefix *endo-* ("inner"), the root *card* ("heart"), and the suffix *-itis* ("inflammation"); therefore, the term means "inflammation of the inner part of the heart."

Abdominal Regions

The abdomen is divided into regions (Fig. 4.11). They are used to describe the location of body structures, pain, or discomfort. The regions are:

- Right upper quadrant (RUQ).
- Left upper quadrant (LUQ).
- Right lower quadrant (RLQ).
- Left lower quadrant (LLQ).

Directional Terms

Certain terms describe the position of one body part in relation to another. These terms give the direction of the body part when a person is standing and facing forward (Fig. 4.12).

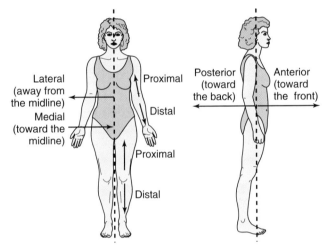

Fig. 4.12 Directional terms describe the position of one body part in relation to another.

- *Anterior (ventral)*—at or toward the front of the body or body part
- *Distal*—the part farthest from the center or from the point of attachment
- *Lateral*—away from the midline; at the side of the body or body part
- *Medial*—at or near the middle or midline of the body or body part
- *Posterior (dorsal)*—at or toward the back of the body or body part
- *Proximal*—the part nearest to the center or to the point of origin

Abbreviations

Abbreviations are shortened forms of words or phrases. They save time and space when recording. Each center has a list of accepted abbreviations. Obtain the list when you are hired. Use only those accepted by the center. If you are not sure that an abbreviation is acceptable, write the term out in full. This promotes accurate communication.

Common abbreviations are on the inside of the back cover for easy use.

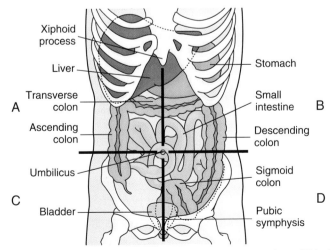

Fig. 4.11 The four abdominal regions. (A) Right upper quadrant. (B) Left upper quadrant. (C) Right lower quadrant. (D) Left lower quadrant.

Common Terms and Phrases

Some terms and phrases apply to basic care and safety. Because they are used throughout this book, they are presented in Box 4.4. Some are presented as key terms in other chapters.

COMPUTERS AND OTHER ELECTRONIC DEVICES

Computer software programs collect, send, record, and store information. Information is retrieved when needed.

The health team uses computers and faxes to send messages and reports to the nursing unit. This reduces clerical work and phone calls. Information is sent with greater speed and accuracy.

EHRs are used for everything found in a paper chart and more. The record includes weights and vital signs. Baseline and goal information is entered and then measured against information entered by the nursing assistant or other members of the health team. When an abnormal or beyond-limits measurement is entered, an alert is sent within the system. The nursing assistant may be asked to reweigh or retake the vital sign in question to ensure accuracy. If an abnormal measurement does exist, the nurse is notified.

Computers and other electronic devices save time. Quality care and safety are increased. Fewer errors are made in recording. Records are more complete. Staff are more efficient. Communication among team members is enhanced through the use of the EHR.

Computers store vast amounts of information. Therefore the right to privacy must be protected. Each staff member using computers and other electronic devices is issued a username and password. They are used to access, send, receive, or store protected health information (PHI).

You must follow the center's policies when using computers and other electronic devices. You must keep PHI and electronic protected health information (ePHI, EPHI) confidential. The Health Insurance Portability and Accountability Act (HIPAA) was passed to protect the privacy rights of persons. Follow the rules in Box 4.5 and the ethical and legal rules about privacy, confidentiality, and defamation (Chapter 2). Failure to comply with HIPAA regulations may result in a monetary fine of $10,000 for each violation. PHI should always be closely monitored by all team members.

TELEPHONE COMMUNICATION

You will answer phones at the nurses' station or in resident rooms. You need good communication skills. The caller cannot see you, but you give much information by your tone of voice, how clearly you speak, and your attitude. Behave as if you are speaking to someone face to face. Be professional and courteous. Also practice good work ethics. Follow the center's policy and the guidelines in Box 4.6.

Personal Cell Phone Use

Wireless (cell phone) use is widespread and commonly used by many individuals. Cell phones have many benefits to help people communicate with each other. However, cell phone use in the workplace has some negative aspects. Many nursing centers and other places of employment have policies to ensure that cell phone use is not abused. Some centers do not allow nursing assistants to carry their personal cell phones with them while they work. This policy

---

BOX 4.4 Common Health Care Terms and Phrases

Activities of daily living (ADL)	The activities usually done during a normal day in a persons life	**Dyspnea**	Difficult, labored, or painful (dys) breathing (pnea)
Assist device	Any item used by the person or staff to promote the persons function or safety (hand rails, grab bars, transfer lifts, canes, walkers, wheelchairs, eating devices, and so on)	**Feces**	The semisolid mass of waste products in the colon that are expelled through the anus
		Fever	Elevated body temperature
Atrophy	The decrease in size or the wasting away of tissue	**Fowler position**	A semi-sitting position; head of bed is raised between 45 and 60 degrees
Call light	Part of the call system that allows the person to signal the nurses station for help	**Incontinence**	Not being able to control urination (urinary incontinence) or defecation (fecal incontinence)
Care plan	A written guide about the persons care; provides staff with approaches to reach the residents goals	**Pressure injury**	A localized injury to the skin and/or underlying tissue, usually over a bony prominence
Cognitive function	Involves memory, thinking, reasoning, ability to understand, judgment, and behavior	**Prone**	Lying on the abdomen with the head turned to one side
Contracture	The lack of joint mobility caused by abnormal shortening of a muscle	**Semi-Fowler position**	Head of bed is raised 30 degrees; or head of bed is raised 30 degrees and knee portion is raised 15 degrees
Dementia	The loss of cognitive and social function caused by changes in the brain; the loss of cognitive function	**Supine**	The back-lying or dorsal recumbent position
		Vital signs	Temperature, pulse, respirations, and blood pressure
Dysphagia	Difficulty (dys) swallowing (phagia)	**Voiding**	Urinating

BOX 4.5 Using the Center's Computer and Other Electronic Devices

- Computers
- Never tell anyone your username or password. If someone has your information, that person can access, record, send, receive, or store protected health information (PHI) under your name. It will be hard to prove that someone else did so and not you.
- Do not write down, post, or expose your username or password in a manner that is not secure. For example, do not write them on a note pad or post them at your work station.
- Change your password often. Follow center policy.
- Do not use another person's username or password.
- Follow the rules for recording (see Box 4.1).
- Enter data carefully. Double-check your entries.
- Prevent others from seeing what is on the screen:
  - Position the monitor so the screen cannot be seen in the hallway or by others.
  - Be aware of anyone standing behind you.
  - Stand or sit with your back to the wall if recording on a mobile computer unit.
  - Do not leave the computer unattended.
- Log off after completing your entry. Log back in later if you are interrupted and need to leave the computer.
- Do not leave printouts where others can read them or pick them up.
- Shred or destroy computer-printed documents or worksheets (Chapter 2). Follow center policy.
- Send email and messages only to those needing the information.
- Do not use email for information or messages that require immediate reporting. Give the report in person. (The person may not read the email in a timely manner.)
- Do not use email or messages to report confidential information. This includes addresses, phone numbers, and social security numbers. The computer system may not be secure.
- Do not use the center's computer to:
  - Send personal email messages.
  - Send or receive email or messages that are offensive, not legal, or sexual.
  - Send or receive email or messages for illegal activities, jokes, politics, gambling (including football and other sports pools), chain letters, or other nonwork activities.
  - Post information, opinions, pictures, or comments on Internet message boards.
  - Take part in Internet discussion groups.
  - Upload, download, or send materials containing a copyright, trademark, or patent.
- Remember that any communication can be read or heard by someone other than the intended person.
- Remember that deleted communications can be retrieved by authorized staff.
- Remember that the center has the right to monitor your use of computers or other electronic devices. This includes Internet use.
- Do not open another person's email or messages.
- Follow center policy for misdirected emails.

Faxes
- Use the center's approved "cover sheet." The sheet has instructions about:
  - The confidentiality of PHI.
  - The receiver's responsibilities about PHI and if the fax is received in error (misdirected fax).
- Complete the "cover sheet" according to center policy:
  - Name of the person to receive the PHI
  - Receiver's fax number
  - Date
  - Number of pages being faxed
  - Department name
  - Name and phone number of the person sending the fax
- Follow center policy for a misdirected fax.
- Do not leave sent or received faxes unattended in the fax machine or lying around.

BOX 4.6 Guidelines for Answering Phones

- Answer the call after the first ring if possible. Be sure to answer by the fourth ring.
- Do not answer the phone in a rushed or hasty manner.
- Give a courteous greeting. Identify the nursing unit and give your name and title. For example: "Good morning. Three center. Mark Wills, nursing assistant."
- Write the following information when taking a message:
  - The caller's name and phone number (include area code and extension number)
  - The date and time
  - The message
- Repeat the message and phone number back to the caller.
- Ask the caller to "Please hold" if necessary. First find out who is calling. Then ask if the caller can hold. Do not put callers with an emergency on hold.
- Do not lay the phone down or cover the receiver with your hand when not speaking to the caller. The caller may overhear confidential conversations.
- Return to a caller on hold within 30 seconds. Ask if the caller can wait longer or if the call can be returned.
- Do not give confidential information to any caller. Resident and employee information is confidential. Refer such calls to a nurse.
- Transfer the call if appropriate.
  - Tell the caller that you are going to transfer the call.
  - Give the name of the department if appropriate.
  - Give the caller the phone number in case the call gets disconnected or the line is busy.
  - End the conversation politely. Thank the person for calling and say goodbye.
  - Give the message to the appropriate person.

ensures that nursing assistants are giving their undivided attention to the care of the residents. It also helps to protect the privacy of the resident. Pictures or audio recordings of residents should never be taken with a cell phone. This is a violation of the person's privacy. Some centers actually use cell phones or pagers for staff members to communicate with each other. Follow the center's policy regarding cell phone use at the workplace.

DEALING WITH CONFLICT

People bring their values, attitudes, opinions, experiences, and expectations to the work setting. Differences often lead to conflict. Conflict is a clash between opposing interests or ideas. People disagree and argue. There are misunderstandings and unrest.

Conflicts arise over issues or events. Work schedules, absences, and the amount and quality of work performed are examples. The problems must be worked out. Otherwise, unkind words or actions may occur. The work setting becomes unpleasant. Care is affected.

To resolve conflict, identify the real problem. This is part of *problem solving*. The problem-solving process involves these steps:

- Step 1: Define the problem. *A nurse ignores me.*
- Step 2: Collect information about the problem. Do not include unrelated information. *The nurse does not look at me. The nurse does not talk to me. The nurse does not respond when I ask for help. The nurse does not ask me to help with tasks that require two people. The nurse talks to other staff members.*
- Step 3: Identify possible solutions. *Ignore the nurse. Talk to my supervisor. Talk to coworkers about the problem. Change jobs.*
- Step 4: Select the best solution. *Talk to my supervisor.*
- Step 5: Carry out the solution. *See below.*
- Step 6: Evaluate the results. *See below.*

Communication and good work ethics help to prevent and resolve conflicts. Identify and solve problems before they become major issues. To deal with conflict:

- Ask your supervisor for some time to talk privately. Explain the problem. Give facts and specific examples. Ask for advice in solving the problem.
- Approach the person with whom you have the conflict. Ask to talk privately. Be polite and professional.
- Agree on a time and place to talk.
- Talk in a private setting. No one should hear you or the other person.
- Explain the problem and what is bothering you. Give facts and specific behaviors. Focus on the problem. Do not focus on the person.
- Listen to the person. Do not interrupt.

- Identify ways to solve the problem. Offer your thoughts. Ask for the coworker's ideas.
- Set a date and time to review the matter.
- Thank the person for meeting with you.
- Carry out the solution.
- Review the matter as scheduled.
  See *Focus on Communication: Dealing with Conflict.*

FOCUS ON COMMUNICATION

Dealing With Conflict

You may find it hard to talk to someone with whom you have a conflict. This is hard for many people. However, letting the problem or issue continue only makes the matter worse. The following may help you to start talking to the person:

- "You say 'no' when I ask you to help me. I help you when you ask me to. This really bothers me. Can we talk privately for a few minutes?"
- "I heard you tell John that you saw me sitting in Mrs. Gordon's room. You seemed angry when you said it. Can we talk privately? I want to explain why I was sitting and find out why that bothers you."
- "The new schedule shows me working every weekend this month. Please tell me why. The employee handbook says that we work every other weekend."

QUALITY OF LIFE

Health team members must communicate with each other for effective and co-ordinated care. Communication must be factual, concise, and understandable. It must be presented in a logical way. This helps the health team provide high-quality resident care. False or incomplete information can harm the person.

Resident information is personal and confidential. Always protect the right to privacy. Share information only with the health team members involved in the person's care. Never share it with the person's family or friends without the person's consent.

TIME TO REFLECT

Mrs. Freeman is being admitted to the nursing center for restorative care following a hip fracture. Melissa is a nursing assistant working today and she knows Mrs. Freeman because they attend the same church. After greeting Mrs. Freeman and helping her get settled, Melissa begins recording her care. Suddenly she thinks she should let her mother know that Mrs. Freeman has been admitted. She logs on to the computer and sends her mother and other relatives an email. She also posts a message on a social media site about Mrs. Freeman's arrival at the care center. What do you think of Melissa's actions? How should this situation be dealt with from here?

REVIEW QUESTIONS

Circle the BEST answer.

1. Information about the person's advance directives would be found in the
   a. Admission sheet (face sheet)
   b. Graphic sheet
   c. Lab results
   d. Flow sheet

2. Which of the following would not be found on the activities of daily living (ADL) flow sheet?
   a. Hygiene measures
   b. Food and fluid intake
   c. Lab results
   d. Elimination

3. Under OBRA residents have the right to
   a. Know the information in their medical record
   b. Record in their medical record
   c. Remove pages from their medical record
   d. View the records of other residents

4. OBRA requires that summaries of care (progress notes) be written at least
   a. Every month
   b. Every other month
   c. Every 3 months
   d. Every year

5. To communicate, you should do the following *except*
   a. Use terms with many meanings
   b. Be brief and concise
   c. Present information logically and in sequence
   d. Give facts and be specific

6. Mr. Yu is discharged from the center. His medical record is
   a. Destroyed
   b. Sent home with him
   c. Permanent
   d. Stored on a computer

7. These statements are about medical records. Which is *false?*
   a. They are used to communicate information about residents
   b. They are a written or electronic account of illness and response to treatment
   c. They can be used as evidence of the care given
   d. Anyone working in the center can read them

8. A person is weighed daily. The measurement is recorded on the
   a. Admission sheet
   b. Kardex
   c. Flow sheet
   d. Progress notes

9. Where does the nurse describe the nursing care given?
   a. Admission sheet
   b. Activities of daily living flow sheet
   c. Progress notes
   d. Kardex

10. When recording, you do the following *except*
    a. Use ink
    b. Include the date and time
    c. Erase errors
    d. Sign all entries with your name and title

11. These statements are about recording. Which is *false?*
    a. Use the person's exact words when possible
    b. Record only what you did and observed
    c. Sign your initials to a mistaken entry
    d. Chart a procedure before completing it

12. In the evening the clock shows 9:26. In 24-hour clock time this is
    a. 9:26 PM
    b. 1926
    c. 0926
    d. 2126

13. A suffix is
    a. Placed at the beginning of a word
    b. Placed after a root
    c. A shortened form of a word or phrase
    d. The main meaning of the word

14. Which term relates to the side of the body?
    a. Anterior
    b. Lateral
    c. Posterior
    d. Proximal

15. These statements are about computers in health care. Which is *false?*
    a. Computers are used to collect, send, record, and store information
    b. The person's privacy must be protected
    c. All employees have the same password
    d. Computers link one department to another

16. You have access to the center's computer. Which is *true?*
    a. Email and messages are sent only to those needing the information
    b. Email is used for reports the nurse needs at once
    c. You can open another person's email
    d. You can use the computer for your personal needs

17. Mrs. Parks asks you to answer her phone because she is unable to reach it. How should you answer?
    a. "Good morning. Mrs. Park's room."
    b. "Good morning. Third floor."
    c. "Hello."
    d. "Good morning. Tammy Brown, nursing assistant, speaking."

18. A coworker is often late for work. This means extra work for you. To resolve the conflict, you should do the following *except*
    a. Explain the problem to your supervisor
    b. Discuss the matter during the end-of-shift report
    c. Give facts and specific behaviors
    d. Suggest ways to solve the problem

See Appendix A for answers to these questions.

5

Assisting With the Nursing Process

OBJECTIVES

- Define the key terms and key abbreviations listed in this chapter.
- Explain the purpose of the nursing process.
- Describe the steps of the nursing process.
- Explain your role in each step of the nursing process.
- Explain the difference between objective data and subjective data.
- Identify the observations that you need to report to the nurse.
- Explain the purpose of care conferences.
- Explain how to promote quality of life.

KEY TERMS

assessment Collecting information about the person; a step in the nursing process

comprehensive care plan A written guide about the individual care a person should receive; developed by the interdisciplinary team (IDT); care plan

evaluation To determine if goals in the planning step were met; a step in the nursing process

goal That which is desired for or by a person as a result of nursing care

implementation To perform or carry out nursing measures in the care plan; a step in the nursing process

interdisciplinary team (IDT) Members of the departments found in a nursing center activities, dietary, nursing, social services, rehabilitation, etc.

medical diagnosis The identification of a disease or condition by a doctor

nursing diagnosis Describes a health problem that can be treated by nursing measures; a step in the nursing process

nursing intervention An action or measure taken by the nursing team to help the person reach a goal

nursing process The method nurses use to plan and deliver nursing care; its five steps are assessment, nursing diagnosis, planning, implementation, and evaluation

objective data Information that is seen, heard, felt, or smelled by an observer; signs

observation Using the senses of sight, hearing, touch, and smell to collect information

planning Setting priorities and goals; a step in the nursing process

Resident Assessment Instrument (RAI) Helps staff to gather information on a resident's strengths and needs, which must be addressed in an individualized care plan.

Resident Assessment Protocols (RAP) Identify social, medical, and psychological problems and form the basis for individualized care planning

signs See "objective data"

skilled care Daily services provided by an RN and/or therapist for rehabilitation or other complex services; provided in nursing centers for short periods of time

subjective data Things a person tells you about that you cannot observe through your senses; symptoms

symptoms See "subjective data"

triggers Information that is collected from the MDS for the care area assessments (CAAs)

utilization Putting planned care into action in an efficient manner

KEY ABBREVIATIONS

ADL Activities of daily living
CAA Care area assessment
CMS Centers for Medicare & Medicaid Services
IDT Interdisciplinary team
MDS Minimum Data Set

OBRA Omnibus Budget Reconciliation Act of 1987
POC Point of care
RAI Resident Assessment Instrument
RAP Resident Assessment Protocols
RN Registered nurse

Nurses communicate with each other about the person's strengths, problems, needs, and care. This information is shared through the nursing process. The nursing process is the method nurses use to plan and deliver nursing care. It has five steps:

- Assessment
- Nursing diagnosis
- Planning
- Implementation
- Evaluation

The nursing process focuses on the person's nursing needs. The person and nursing team need good communication.

Each step is important. If done in order with good communication, nursing care is organized and has purpose. All nursing team members do the same things for the person. They have the same goals. The person feels safe and secure with consistent care. Each resident has a unique path toward achieving the highest level of well-being.

The nursing process is used for all age groups. It is ongoing. New information is gathered and the person's needs may change. However, the steps are the same. You will see the continuous nature of the nursing process as each step is explained.

ASSESSMENT

Assessment involves collecting information about the person. Nurses use many sources. CMS recommends the use of a Resident Assessment Instrument (RAI). The RAI provides a structured approach for applying a problem identification process. The RAI consists of three basic components:

1. Minimum Data Set (MDS)
2. Resident Assessment Protocols (RAPs)
3. Utilization Guidelines

A health history is taken. This tells about current and past health problems. The family's health history is important. Many diseases are genetic. That is, the risk for certain diseases is inherited from parents. For example, a mother had breast cancer, so her daughters are at risk. Information from the doctor is reviewed, as are test results and past medical records.

A registered nurse (RN) assesses the person's body systems and mental status. You play a key role in assessment. You make many observations as you give care and talk to the person. Observation is using the senses of sight, hearing, touch, and smell to collect information.

- You *see* how the person lies, sits, or walks. You see flushed or pale skin. You see red and swollen body areas.
- You *listen* to the person breathe, talk, and cough. You use a stethoscope to listen to the heartbeat and to measure blood pressure.
- Through *touch*, you feel if the skin is hot or cold, or moist or dry. You use touch to take the person's pulse.
- *Smell* is used to detect body, wound, and breath odors. You also smell odors from urine and bowel movements.

Objective data (signs) are seen, heard, felt, or smelled by an observer. You can feel a pulse. You can see urine color. Subjective data (symptoms) are things a person tells you about that you cannot observe through your senses. You cannot feel or see the person's pain, fear, or nausea.

Box 5.1 lists the basic observations you need to make and report to the nurse. Box 5.2 lists the observations that you must report at once. Make notes of your observations. Use them to report and record observations. Carry a note pad and pen in your pocket. Note your observations as you make them. The

---

BOX 5.1   Basic Observations

Ability to Respond
- Is the person easy or hard to wake up?
- Can the person give own name, the time, and location when asked?
- Does the person identify others correctly?
- Does the person answer questions correctly?
- Does the person speak clearly?
- Are instructions followed correctly?
- Is the person calm, restless, or excited?
- Is the person conversing, quiet, or talking a lot?

Movement
- Can the person squeeze your fingers with each hand?
- Can the person move arms and legs?
- Are the person's movements shaky or jerky?
- Does the person complain of stiff or painful joints?

Pain or Discomfort
- Where is the pain located? (Ask the person to point to the pain.)
- Does the pain go anywhere else?
- How does the person rate the severity of the pain—mild, moderate, severe?
- How does the person rate the pain on a scale of 0 to 10 (Chapter 25)?
- When did the pain begin?
- What was the person doing when the pain began?
- How long does the pain last?
- How does the person describe the pain?
  - Sharp
  - Severe
  - Knifelike

- Dull
- Burning
- Aching
- Comes and goes
- Depends on position
- Was a pain-relief drug given?
- Did the pain-relief drug relieve the pain? Is the pain still present?
- Is the person able to sleep and rest?
- What is the position of comfort?

Skin
- Is the skin pale or flushed?
- Is the skin cool, warm, or hot?
- Is the skin moist or dry?
- What color are the lips and nail beds?
- Is the skin intact? Are there broken areas? If so, where?
- Are sores or reddened areas present? Is there a rash?
- Are bruises present? Where are they located?
- Does the person complain of itching? If yes, where?
- Is swelling present under the skin? If so, where?

Eyes, Ears, Nose, and Mouth
- Is there drainage from the eyes? What color is the drainage?
- Are the eyelids closed? Do they stay open?
- Are the eyes reddened?
- Does the person complain of spots, flashes, or blurring?
- Is the person sensitive to bright lights?
- Is there drainage from the ears? What color is the drainage?

BOX 5.1   Basic Observations—cont'd

- Can the person hear? Is repeating necessary? Are questions answered appropriately?
- Is there drainage from the nose? What color is the drainage?
- Can the person breathe through the nose?
- Is there breath odor?
- Does the person complain of a bad taste in the mouth?
- Does the person complain of painful gums or teeth?

Respirations
- Do both sides of the person's chest rise and fall with respirations?
- Is breathing noisy?
- Does the person complain of pain or difficulty breathing?
- What is the amount and color of sputum?
- What is the frequency of the person's cough? Is it dry or productive?

Bowels and Bladder
- Is the abdomen firm or soft?
- Does the person complain of gas?
- What are the amount, color, and consistency of bowel movements?
- What is the frequency of bowel movements?
- Can the person control bowel movements?
- Does the person have pain or difficulty urinating?
- What is the amount of urine?
- What is the color of urine?
- Is the urine clear? Are there particles in the urine?
- Does the urine have a foul smell?
- Can the person control the passage of urine?
- What is the frequency of urination?

Appetite
- Does the person like the food served?
- How much of the meal is eaten?
- What foods does the person like?
- Can the person chew food?
- What is the amount of fluid taken?
- What fluids does the person like?
- How often does the person drink fluids?
- Can the person swallow food and fluids?
- Does the person complain of nausea?
- What is the amount and color of material vomited?
- Does the person have hiccups?
- Is the person belching?
- Does the person cough when swallowing?

Activities of Daily Living
- Can the person perform personal care without help?
  - Bathing?
  - Brushing teeth?
  - Combing and brushing hair?
  - Shaving?
- Which does the person use: toilet, commode, bedpan, or urinal?
- Does the person feed oneself?
- Can the person walk?
- What amount and kind of help is needed?

Other
- Is the person bleeding from any body part? If yes, where and how much?

BOX 5.2   Observations to Report at Once

- A change in the person's ability to respond:
  - A responsive person is no longer responding
  - A nonresponsive person is now responding
- A change in the person's mobility:
  - The person cannot move a body part
  - The person is now able to move a body part
- Complaints of sudden, severe pain
- A sore or reddened area on the person's skin
- Complaints of a sudden change in vision
- Complaints of pain or difficulty breathing
- Abnormal respirations
- Complaints or signs of difficulty swallowing
- Vomiting
- Bleeding
- Vital signs outside their normal ranges

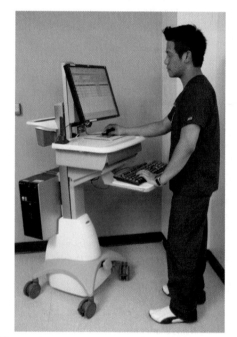

Fig. 5.1 The nursing assistant uses a computer to note observations.

center may provide electronic devices for this purpose (Fig. 5.1).

The assessment step never ends. New information is collected with every resident contact. New observations are made. The person shares more information, and often the family adds more information.

❖   The Omnibus Budget Reconciliation Act of 1987 (OBRA) requires completion of the Minimum Data Set (MDS) for nursing center residents. A sample of the first page of the MDS form can be seen in Fig. 5.2. The MDS is an assessment and screening tool. It provides extensive information about the

Resident _____ Identifier _____ Date _____

MINIMUM DATA SET (MDS) - Version 3.0
RESIDENT ASSESSMENT AND CARE SCREENING
Nursing Home Comprehensive (NC) Item Set

Section A	Identification Information

A0050. Type of Record

Enter Code [ ]
1. **Add new record** → Continue to A0100, Facility Provider Numbers
2. **Modify existing record** → Continue to A0100, Facility Provider Numbers
3. **Inactivate existing record** → Skip to X0150, Type of Provider

A0100. Facility Provider Numbers

A. **National Provider Identifier (NPI):**
[ ][ ][ ][ ][ ][ ][ ][ ][ ][ ]

B. **CMS Certification Number (CCN):**
[ ][ ][ ][ ][ ][ ][ ][ ][ ][ ][ ]

C. **State Provider Number:**
[ ][ ][ ][ ][ ][ ][ ][ ][ ][ ][ ][ ][ ][ ]

A0200. Type of Provider

Enter Code [ ]
Type of provider
1. **Nursing home (SNF/NF)**
2. **Swing Bed**

A0310. Type of Assessment

Enter Code [ ][ ]
A. **Federal OBRA Reason for Assessment**
01. **Admission** assessment (required by day 14)
02. **Quarterly** review assessment
03. **Annual** assessment
04. **Significant change in status** assessment
05. **Significant correction** to **prior comprehensive** assessment
06. **Significant correction** to **prior quarterly** assessment
99. **None of the above**

Enter Code [ ][ ]
B. **PPS Assessment**
PPS Scheduled Assessments for a Medicare Part A Stay
01. **5-day** scheduled assessment
02. **14-day** scheduled assessment
03. **30-day** scheduled assessment
04. **60-day** scheduled assessment
05. **90-day** scheduled assessment
PPS Unscheduled Assessments for a Medicare Part A Stay
07. **Unscheduled assessment used for PPS** (OMRA, significant or clinical change, or significant correction assessment)
Not PPS Assessment
99. **None of the above**

Enter Code [ ]
C. **PPS Other Medicare Required Assessment - OMRA**
0. **No**
1. **Start of therapy** assessment
2. **End of therapy** assessment
3. **Both Start and End of therapy** assessment
4. **Change of therapy** assessment

Enter Code [ ]
D. **Is this a Swing Bed clinical change assessment?** Complete only if A0200 = 2
0. **No**
1. **Yes**

Enter Code [ ]
E. **Is this assessment the first assessment** (OBRA, Scheduled PPS, or Discharge) **since the most recent admission/entry or reentry?**
0. **No**
1. **Yes**

Fig. 5.2 Sample slupage of Minimum Data Set. (From Centers for Medicare & Medicaid Services: MDS 3.0 nursing home comprehensive [NC] version 1.11.2, October 2021. https://www.cms.gov/Medicare/Quality-Initiatives-Patient-Assessment-Instruments/NursingHomeQualityInits/Downloads/Archive-Draft-of-the-MDS-30-Nursing-Home-Comprehensive-NC-Version-1140.pdf)

Resident _____ Identifier _____ Date _____

Section G	Functional Status

G0110. Activities of Daily Living (ADL) Assistance
Refer to the ADL flow chart in the RAI manual to facilitate accurate coding

Instructions for Rule of 3
- When an activity occurs three times at any one given level, code that level.
- When an activity occurs three times at multiple levels, code the most dependent, exceptions are total dependence (4), activity must require full assist every time, and activity did not occur (8), activity must not have occurred at all. Example, three times extensive assistance (3) and three times limited assistance (2), code extensive assistance (3).
- When an activity occurs at various levels, but not three times at any given level, apply the following:
  ○ When there is a combination of full staff performance, and extensive assistance, code extensive assistance.
  ○ When there is a combination of full staff performance, weight bearing assistance and/or non-weight bearing assistance code limited assistance (2).
If none of the above are met, code supervision.

1. ADL Self-Performance
Code for **resident's performance** over all shifts - not including setup. If the ADL activity occurred 3 or more times at various levels of assistance, code the most dependent - except for total dependence, which requires full staff performance every time

Coding:

Activity Occurred 3 or More Times
0. **Independent** - no help or staff oversight at any time
1. **Supervision** - oversight, encouragement or cueing
2. **Limited assistance** - resident highly involved in activity; staff provide guided maneuvering of limbs or other non-weight-bearing assistance
3. **Extensive assistance** - resident involved in activity, staff provide weight-bearing support
4. **Total dependence** - full staff performance every time during entire 7-day period

Activity Occurred 2 or Fewer Times
7. **Activity occurred only once or twice** - activity did occur but only once or twice
8. **Activity did not occur** - activity did not occur or family and/or non-facility staff provided care 100% of the time for that activity over the entire 7-day period

2. ADL Support Provided
Code for **most support provided** over all shifts; code regardless of resident's self-performance classification

Coding:
0. **No** setup or physical help from staff
1. **Setup** help only
2. **One** person physical assist
3. **Two**+ persons physical assist
8. ADL activity itself **did not occur** or family and/or non-facility staff provided care 100% of the time for that activity over the entire 7-day period

	1. Self-Performance	2. Support
	↓ Enter Codes in Boxes ↓	
A. Bed mobility - how resident moves to and from lying position, turns side to side, and positions body while in bed or alternate sleep furniture	☐	☐
B. Transfer - how resident moves between surfaces including to or from: bed, chair, wheelchair, standing position (**excludes** to/from bath/toilet)	☐	☐
C. Walk in room - how resident walks between locations in his/her room	☐	☐
D. Walk in corridor - how resident walks in corridor on unit	☐	☐
E. Locomotion on unit - how resident moves between locations in his/her room and adjacent corridor on same floor. If in wheelchair, self-sufficiency once in chair	☐	☐
F. Locomotion off unit - how resident moves to and returns from off-unit locations (e.g., areas set aside for dining, activities or treatments). **If facility has only one floor**, how resident moves to and from distant areas on the floor. If in wheelchair, self-sufficiency once in chair	☐	☐
G. Dressing - how resident puts on, fastens and takes off all items of clothing, including donning/removing a prosthesis or TED hose. Dressing includes putting on and changing pajamas and housedresses	☐	☐
H. Eating - how resident eats and drinks, regardless of skill. Do not include eating/drinking during medication pass. Includes intake of nourishment by other means (e.g., tube feeding, total parenteral nutrition, IV fluids administered for nutrition or hydration)	☐	☐
I. Toilet use - how resident uses the toilet room, commode, bedpan, or urinal; transfers on/off toilet; cleanses self after elimination; changes pad; manages ostomy or catheter; and adjusts clothes. Do not include emptying of bedpan, urinal, bedside commode, catheter bag or ostomy bag	☐	☐
J. Personal hygiene - how resident maintains personal hygiene, including combing hair, brushing teeth, shaving, applying makeup, washing/drying face and hands (**excludes** baths and showers)	☐	☐

MDS 3.0 Nursing Home Comprehensive (NC) Corrected Version 1.14.0 DRAFT

Fig. 5.2, Cont'd

person. Examples include memory, communication, hearing and vision, physical function, and activities.

The MDS has several hundred items that are answered by members of the interdisciplinary team (IDT). The IDT is composed of staff members from many departments in the center. MDS records are completed shortly after admission, each quarter, and annually. If the resident is receiving skilled care, the MDS is completed more frequently. Skilled care is daily care performed by the RN or therapist for complex procedures or during rehabilitation. The MDS is also completed when there is a change in the person's health status or if hospice (end-of-life) care is given at the center.

Completed MDS records are used to calculate payment to the facility for the care provided to each resident. The information you record in a paper chart or a point-of-care (POC) electronic record is a very important piece of the MDS process. An RN signs the MDS as complete when all members of the IDT have entered data for the sections of the MDS they are responsible for assessing.

Chapter 4 discussed the use of paper flow sheets and electronic charting using devices known as kiosks. Many electronic health records (EHRs) use POC modules. Assistants record the care provided to the residents as well as any observations. Fig. 5.3 shows an example of a POC chart for a resident. After information is entered on this screen, you can click on an icon to enter more specific information on another screen. Fig. 5.4 shows what you would see on a kiosk as you enter information about the percentage of the noon meal (lunch) consumed by the resident under your care.

Information that you and other members of the IDT record in the MDS is analyzed and used to create the resident's care plan. The care plan is reviewed quarterly after completion of another MDS record to see if changes to the plan are needed.

NURSING DIAGNOSIS

The RN uses assessment information to make a nursing diagnosis. A nursing diagnosis describes a health problem that can be treated by nursing measures. The problem may already exist or may develop.

Nursing diagnoses and medical diagnoses are not the same. A medical diagnosis is the identification of a disease or condition by a doctor. Cancer, stroke, heart attack, infection, and diabetes are examples. Doctors and other health care providers order medication, therapies, and surgery to cure or heal.

A person can have many nursing diagnoses. They deal with the total person—physical, emotional, social, and spiritual needs. They may change as assessment information changes. Or new nursing diagnoses are added (e.g., "Acute Pain" is added after surgery).

PLANNING

Planning involves setting priorities and goals for each resident. Nursing measures or actions are chosen to help the person meet the goals. The person, family, and health team help the RN plan the care.

Priorities relate to what is most important for the person. Maslow's theory of basic needs is useful for setting priorities (Chapter 6). The needs are arranged in order of importance. Some needs are required for life and survival (e.g., oxygen, water, food). They must be met before all other needs. They have priority and must be done first.

Goals are then set. A goal is that which is desired for or by a person as a result of nursing care. Goals are aimed at the person's highest level of well-being and function—physical, emotional, social, and spiritual. Goals promote health and

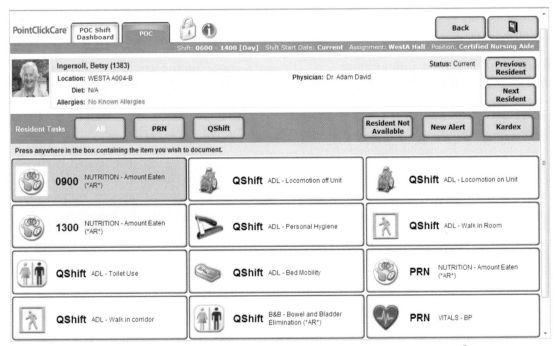

Fig. 5.3 Sample of point of care (POC) resident screen. (Courtesy PointClickCare®.)

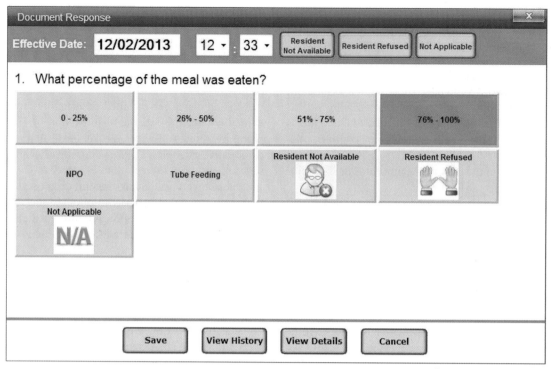

Fig. 5.4 Sample of resident data entry screen. (Courtesy PointClickCare®.)

prevent health problems. They also promote rehabilitation and comfort.

Nursing interventions are chosen after goals are set. An *intervention* is an action or measure. A nursing intervention is an action or measure taken by the nursing team to help the person reach a goal. *Nursing intervention, nursing action,* and *nursing measure* mean the same thing. A nursing intervention does not need a doctor's order. However, some nursing measures come from a health care provider's order. For example, a doctor orders that Mrs. Lange walk 50 yards two times a day. The nurse includes this order in the care plan.

Interdisciplinary Care Planning Conference

❖ OBRA requires regular interdisciplinary care planning conferences for each person. The comprehensive care plan (care plan) is a written guide about the care a person should receive. The interdisciplinary team develops it. The resident and family give input. The care plan includes nursing diagnoses and goals. It has the resident's problems, goals for care, and actions to take to help the person solve health problems. The care plan and goals belong to the resident but the approaches (also called interventions) belong to the staff caring for the resident.

The problems identified on the MDS give triggers (clues) for the care area assessments (CAAs). For example, Mr. Gomez is weak from illness and lack of exercise. The MDS shows that he can walk only a few steps. This triggers the CAAs. A care plan is developed to solve the problem. The goal is for Mr. Gomez to be able to walk to the dining room for meals each day. Staff from occupational therapy, physical therapy, and nursing work to solve the problem. The actions to help Mr. Gomez reach the goal are:

- Occupational therapy to work with Mr. Gomez on strengthening exercises daily.
- Physical therapy to work with Mr. Gomez on walking and strengthening exercises daily.
- Nursing staff member to walk Mr. Gomez 20 yards twice daily.

The care plan also states the person's strengths. For example, Mrs. Jacobson can walk without help. This strength increases her independence. The health team helps Mrs. Jacobson continue to walk on her own.

A comprehensive care plan is developed for each person. Care plan suggestions are welcomed from all team members, including nursing assistants. You use the care plan to give care. It is a communication tool. It tells what care to give and when. The nursing assistant plays an important role in having the resident ready for various therapy sessions. It is very important that residents have had their personal care needs tended to prior to a therapy session. It is also important that the resident's therapy sessions allow for periods of rest for the resident.

Care plan forms vary in each center. It may be in the person's chart, in a notebook, in a Kardex, posted in the resident's room, or on a computer. The plan must be carried out. The care plan is revised as the person's needs change. It is important that you review a resident's care plan often so you know the problems and goals of each person you care for.

See *Focus on Communication: Interdisciplinary Care Planning Conference.*

📋 **FOCUS ON COMMUNICATION**

Interdisciplinary Care Planning Conference

You spend a lot of time with the residents. You see what they like and do not like. You see what they can do and what they cannot do. Residents talk to you. They tell you about their families and interests. You make observations every time you are with them. Share this information during care conferences. Also share your ideas about the person's care. Your sharing can improve the person's quality of life. For example, you can say:

- "Mr. Antonio never eats his squash. He says that he misses the fresh green beans and broccoli from his garden. Can he have those more often?"
- "Mrs. Clark can use her feet to propel her wheelchair. Why do we have to push her wheelchair?"
- "Miss Walsh never talks when her family visits. She just sits there. Yet she talks to her roommate all the time."

IMPLEMENTATION

To *implement* means to perform or carry out. The implementation step is performing or carrying out nursing measures in the care plan. Sometimes the term **utilization** is used to determine if services are necessary and appropriate.

Nursing care ranges from simple to complex. The nurse delegates nursing tasks that are within your legal limits and job description. The nurse may ask you to assist with complex measures.

You report the care given to the nurse. In some centers, you record the care given. Report and record *after* giving care, not before. Also report and record your observations. Observing is part of assessment. New observations may change the nursing diagnoses. If so, care plan changes are made. To give correct care, you need to know about any changes in the care plan.

Assignment Sheets

The nurse communicates delegated tasks to you. An assignment sheet is used for this purpose (Fig. 5.5). The assignment sheet tells you about:

- Each person's care.
- What measures and tasks need to be done.
- Which nursing unit tasks to do. Cleaning kitchenettes and utility rooms and stocking shower rooms are examples. Cleaning equipment such as walkers and wheelchairs may be other tasks.

Talk to the nurse about any unclear assignment. You can also check the care plan and Kardex if you need more information. See *Teamwork and Time Management: Assignment Sheets.*

TEAMWORK AND TIME MANAGEMENT

Assignment Sheets

Use your assignment sheet to organize your work and to set priorities.

- What do you need to do first?
- What can be done while the person is having breakfast, lunch, or dinner?
- What can you do while the person is at therapy (physical, occupational, etc.) or an activity?

Assignment Sheet

Date: _9–10_
Shift: _Day_
Nursing assistant: _John Reed_
Supervisor: _Mary Adams, RN_

Breaks: _1000_ _1400_
Lunch: _1230_
Unit Tasks: _Pass ice water at 0900_
Clean utility room at 1430

Check the care plan for other care measures and information

	Functional status/other care measures and procedures
Room # _501A_ Name: _Mrs. Ann Lopez_ ID Number: _S1514491530_ Date of birth: _11/04/1925_ VS: _Daily at 0700_ T ____ P ____ R ____ BP ____ Wt: _Weekly (Monday at 0700)_ ____ Intake ____ BM ____ Bath: Portable tub Shampoo Bed rails	Total assist with ADL Stand-pivot transfers Uses w/c Incontinent of bowel and bladder – uses briefs Bilateral passive ROM exercises to extremities twice daily Turn and reposition q2h when in bed Wears eyeglasses and dentures Diet: High fiber (Total Assist)
Room # _510B_ Name: _Mr. Mark Monroe_ ID Number: _D4468947762_ Date of birth: _12/29/1926_ VS: _2 times daily, at 0700 and 1500_ 0700: T ____ P ____ R ____ BP ____ 1500: T ____ P ____ R ____ BP ____ Wt: _Daily at 0700_ ____ Intake ____ Output ____ BM ____ Bath: Shower	Independent with ADL Independent with ambulation Attends exercise group every morning Continent of bowel and bladder – q4h bathroom schedule to maintain continence Wears eyeglasses Coughing and deep breathing exercises q4h Diet: Sodium-controlled (Independent)

Fig. 5.5 Sample assignment sheet. Note: This assignment sheet is a computer printout. *ADL*, Activities of daily living; *q2h*, every 2 hours; *q4h*, every 4 hours; *ROM*, range of motion; *w/c*, wheelchair.

- Do you need to reserve a room (shower room, tub room) or equipment (portable tub, shower chair)?
- What do you need help with?
- How many coworkers are needed to complete tasks such as turning and transferring a person?
- Ask a coworker to help you. Tell the person what you need help with, when you need the help, and how long the task will take.
- Check off tasks as you complete them.
- Review the assignment sheet throughout the day and especially at the end of your work shift.

EVALUATION

Evaluation means to measure. The evaluation step involves determining if goals in the planning step were met. Progress is evaluated. Goals may be met totally, in part, or not at all. Assessment information is used for this step. Changes in nursing diagnoses, goals, and the care plan may result.

The nursing process never ends. Nurses constantly collect information about the person. Nursing diagnoses, goals, and the care plan may change as the person's needs change.

YOUR ROLE

You have a key role in the nursing process. The nurse uses your observations for nursing diagnoses and planning. If you are not sure whether to report an observation, it is better to report it to the nurse. Let the nurse decide if the information is important for the care of the resident. You may help develop the care plan. In the implementation step, you perform tasks in the care plan. Your assignment sheet tells you what to do. Your observations are used for the evaluation step. You are a very important member of the IDT.

QUALITY OF LIFE

Residents have the right to take part in their care planning. OBRA requires that each person be included in the process. The person may refuse actions suggested by the health team. Involving the person in the care planning process helps the team better meet the person's needs. You are a key member of the team. Share your observations and ideas. They can help the team provide better care.

TIME TO REFLECT

Mr. Carter has been a resident of the nursing center for over a year. You are very familiar with the help he needs with his activities of daily living (ADL). This morning when you arrive to help him get up and begin dressing, you notice that his speech is slurred and he is not able to move his right arm. Are these significant observations? What should you do next? You have six additional residents you need to help before breakfast is served.

REVIEW QUESTIONS

Circle the BEST answer.

1. Which is *not* a step in the nursing process?
   a. Observation
   b. Assessment
   c. Planning
   d. Implementation
2. The nursing process
   a. Involves guidelines for care plans
   b. Is a care conference
   c. Involves triggers
   d. Is the method nurses use to plan and deliver nursing care
3. What happens during assessment?
   a. Goals are set
   b. Information is collected
   c. Nursing measures are carried out
   d. Progress is evaluated
4. Which is a symptom?
   a. Redness
   b. Vomiting
   c. Pain
   d. Pulse rate of 78

5. Which is a sign?
   a. Nausea
   b. Headache
   c. Dizziness
   d. Dry skin
6. Which should you report at once?
   a. The person had a bowel movement
   b. The person complains of sudden, severe pain
   c. The person does not like the food served for lunch
   d. The person complains of stiff, painful joints
7. Which should you report at once?
   a. The person can no longer move a body part
   b. The person answers questions correctly
   c. The person has a breath odor
   d. The person walked to the dining room
8. Measures in the nursing care plan are carried out. This is
   a. A nursing diagnosis
   b. Planning
   c. Implementation
   d. Evaluation

9. Which statement about the nursing process is *true?*
   a. It is done without the person's input
   b. You are responsible for it
   c. It is used to communicate the person's care
   d. Steps can be done in any order
10. The comprehensive care plan is
    a. Written by the doctor
    b. The measures to help the person
    c. The same for all persons
    d. Also called the Kardex
11. What is used to communicate the nursing tasks delegated to you?
    a. The care plan
    b. The Kardex
    c. An assignment sheet
    d. Care conferences
12. Which is a nursing diagnosis?
    a. Cancer
    b. Heart attack
    c. Kidney failure
    d. Pain

See Appendix A for answers to these questions.

6

Understanding the Resident

OBJECTIVES

- Define the key terms listed in this chapter.
- Identify the parts that make up the whole person.
- Explain Abraham Maslow's theory of basic needs.
- Explain how culture and religion influence health and illness.
- Identify the emotional and social effects of illness.
- Describe persons cared for in nursing centers.
- Identify the elements needed for good communication.
- Describe how to use verbal and nonverbal communication.
- Explain the methods and barriers to good communication.
- Explain how to communicate with persons who have behavior problems.
- Explain how to communicate with persons who have disabilities or who are comatose.
- Explain why family and visitors are important to the person.
- Identify the courtesies given to the person, family, and friends.
- Explain how to promote quality of life.

KEY TERMS

body language Messages sent through facial expressions, gestures, posture, hand and body movements, gait, eye contact, and appearance

comatose The state of being unable to respond to stimuli

disability Any lost, absent, or impaired physical or mental function

esteem The worth, value, or opinion one has of a person

holism A concept that considers the whole person; the whole person has physical, social, psychologic, and spiritual parts that are woven together and cannot be separated

need Something necessary or desired for maintaining life and mental well-being

nonverbal communication Communication that does not use words

optimal level of function A person's highest potential for mental and physical performance

paraphrasing Restating the person's message in your own words

self-actualization Experiencing one's potential

self-esteem Thinking well of oneself and seeing oneself as useful and having value

verbal communication Communication that uses written or spoken words

---

The resident is the most important person in the nursing center. Age, religion, and nationality are several of numerous factors that make each person unique. So do culture, education, occupation, and lifestyle. Each person is important and special. Each has value. The person is treated as someone who thinks, acts, feels, and makes decisions.

You will care for many residents. Many are old; however, some younger people with disabilities may reside in care centers. Each person has fears, needs, and rights. Each has suffered losses—loss of home, family, friends, and body functions. Family and community roles have been lost, too.

CARING FOR THE PERSON

For effective care, you must consider the whole person. Holism means *whole*. Holism is a concept that considers the whole person. The whole person has physical, social, psychologic, and spiritual parts. These parts are woven together and cannot be separated (Fig. 6.1).

Each part relates to and depends on the others. As a social being, a person speaks and communicates with others. Physically, the brain, mouth, tongue, lips, and throat structures must function for speech. Communication is also psychologic. It involves thinking and reasoning.

To consider only the physical part is to ignore the person's ability to think, make decisions, and interact with others. It also ignores the person's experiences, lifestyle, culture, religion, joys, sorrows, spiritualities, and needs.

Disability and illness affect the whole person. For example, Mrs. Butler had a stroke. She requires help with her physical needs. She had to leave her home. Relationships with her husband and children are changed. She is angry with God for letting this happen to her. The health team plans care to help her deal with her problems.

Addressing the Person

You must know and respect the whole person to provide effective, quality care. Too often a person is referred to as a

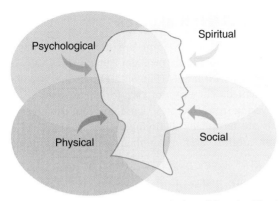

Fig. 6.1 A person is a physical, psychological, social, and spiritual being. The parts overlap and cannot be separated.

room number. For example: "12A needs the bedpan," rather than "Mrs. Brown in 12A needs the bedpan." This type of address strips the person of identity. It reduces the person to a thing.

Residents are not things. They are not your relatives or children. They are complex, adult human beings. Follow these rules to address them with dignity and respect:

- Call residents by their titles—"Mrs. Jones," "Mr. Nguyen," "Miss Turner," or "Dr. Gonzalez."
- Do not call residents by their first names unless they ask you to.
- Do not call residents by any other name unless they ask you to.
- Do not call residents "Grandma," "Papa," "Sweetheart," "Honey," or other names.

BASIC NEEDS

A need is something necessary or desired for maintaining life and mental well-being. According to Abraham Maslow, a famous psychologist, basic needs must be met for a person to survive and function. According to this theory, the needs are arranged in order of importance. Lower-level needs must be met before the higher-level needs. Basic needs, from the lowest level to the highest level, are:

- Physical needs
- Safety and security needs
- Love and belonging needs
- Self-esteem needs
- The need for self-actualization

People normally meet their own needs. When they cannot, it is usually because of disease, illness, injury, or advanced age. Those who are ill or injured usually seek health care.

Physical Needs

Oxygen, food, water, elimination, rest, and shelter are needed for life. They are needed to survive. A person dies within minutes without oxygen. Without food or water, a person feels weak and ill within a few hours. The kidneys and intestines must function. Otherwise, poisonous wastes build up in the

blood. This can cause death. Without enough rest and sleep, a person becomes very tired. Without shelter, the person is exposed to extremes of heat and cold.

You help the person meet physical needs. You need to truly understand their importance. When choking, how do you feel? How do you feel when you are thirsty or hungry? How do you react without enough sleep? What are your fears when you need to use the bathroom right away?

Safety and Security Needs

Safety and security needs relate to feeling safe from harm, danger, and fear. Many people are afraid of nursing centers. Some care involves strange equipment. Some care causes pain or discomfort. People feel safer and more secure if they know what will happen. For every task, even a simple bath, the person should know:

- Why it is needed.
- Who will do it.
- How it will be done.
- What sensations or feelings to expect.

Many persons do not feel safe and secure when admitted to a nursing center. They are not in their usual, secure home settings. They are in a strange place with strange routines. Strangers care for them. They may not have the comfort of their close friends or family. Some become scared and confused.

Be kind and understanding. Introduce yourself and other staff members. Show them the new setting. Introduce them to other residents. Listen to their concerns. Explain all routines and procedures. You may have to repeat information many times. Sometimes the information may need repeating for many days or weeks until the person feels safe and secure. Be patient.

Love and Belonging Needs

Love and belonging needs relate to love, closeness, and affection. They also involve meaningful relationships with others. There are many cases in which people became weaker or died because they lacked love and belonging. This is seen in older persons who have outlived family and friends.

Family, friends, and the health team can meet love and belonging needs. The center is the person's home. You must help the person feel loved and accepted. Remind the person that you are there to help.

Self-Esteem Needs

Esteem is the worth, value, or opinion one has of a person. Self-esteem means to think well of oneself and to see oneself as useful and having value. People often lack self-esteem when ill, injured, older, or disabled. For example:

- An older man once built his own home and worked a farm. He supported and raised a family. Now he cannot dress or feed himself.
- Cancer treatments caused a woman to lose her hair. She does not feel attractive or whole.
- A person has a slow, crippling disease.

- A woman had a leg amputated and wonders whether she will ever be mobile again.

You must treat all persons with respect. Although it takes more time, encourage them to do as much for themselves as possible. This helps increase self-esteem.

The Need for Self-Actualization

Self-actualization means experiencing one's potential. It involves learning, understanding, and creating to the limit of a person's capacity. This is the highest need. Rarely, if ever, is it totally met. Most people constantly try to learn and understand more. This need can be postponed and life will continue.

EFFECTS OF ILLNESS AND DISABILITY

People do not choose sickness or injury. When they occur, they have physical, psychologic, and social effects. Some result in disabilities. A disability is any lost, absent, or impaired physical or mental function. It may be temporary or permanent.

Normal activities—work, driving, fixing meals, yard work, hobbies—may be hard or impossible. Daily activities bring pleasure, worth, and contact with others. People often feel angry, upset, and useless when unable to perform them. These feelings may increase if others must help with routine functions.

Some people feel alone and isolated after outliving family and friends. Those who are disabled or have chronic illnesses may have many fears and concerns about nursing centers. They may feel lonely and abandoned by family and friends. They may fear depending on strangers. Many fear increasing loss of function. Some express their fears; others do not or cannot.

Anger is a common response to illness and disability. Persons who need nursing center care are often angry. The person may direct anger at you. However, the person is usually angry at the situation. You might have problems dealing with the person's anger. If so, ask the nurse for help.

You can help the person feel safe, secure, and loved. Take an extra minute to "visit," to hold a hand, or to give a hug. (Remember to maintain professional boundaries; see Chapter 2.) Show that you are willing to help with personal needs. Respond promptly. Treat each person with respect and dignity.

Optimal Level of Function

Sometimes the health team cannot prevent increasing loss of function. However, residents are helped to maintain their optimal level of function. This is the person's highest potential for mental and physical performance. Encourage the person to be as independent as possible. Always focus on the person's abilities, not on disabilities.

Hospital patients are often treated as sick, dependent people. Promoting this "sick role" in a nursing center reduces quality of life. The health team focuses on improving the person's quality of life. You must help each person regain or maintain as much physical and mental function as possible.

NURSING CENTER RESIDENTS

Most residents are older. Some are alert and oriented. Often they have chronic health problems that prevent them from living alone or with family (Fig. 6.2). Others are very confused and disoriented. They cannot care for themselves. Still others are recovering from fractures, acute illnesses, or surgery. Some residents are terminally ill (dying). They need special care to maintain comfort and make their last days as peaceful as possible.

Alert, Oriented Residents

Alert and oriented residents know who they are and where they are. They know the year and the time of day. These people need nursing center care because of physical problems. Some are paralyzed from a stroke, injury, or birth defect. Others are disabled from arthritis or multiple sclerosis. Still others have chronic heart, liver, kidney, or respiratory diseases.

The amount of care required depends on the degree of disability. Because these persons are alert and oriented, they may have problems adjusting to a nursing center. The care plan includes measures to help the person accept the nursing center as home.

Confused and Disoriented Residents

Many persons are mildly to severely confused and disoriented. Some cannot find the dining room. Others do not know the month or year. Others have more severe problems. For example, a man thinks he is waiting for a train. Or an older

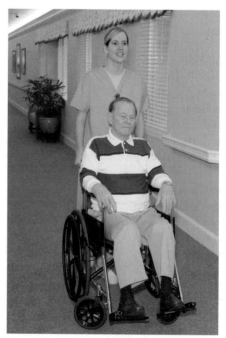

Fig. 6.2 This older person needs nursing center services.

woman wants to feed her baby. The most severely disoriented persons do not know who they are.

Sometimes confusion and disorientation are temporary. This is especially true for new residents. Some persons have Alzheimer disease and other dementias. Confusion and disorientation are permanent and become worse (Chapter 40).

Complete Care Residents

Some people are very disabled. They may also be confused and disoriented. They need total assistance with all activities. They cannot meet any of their own needs, nor can they say what they need or want. They may not be able to express that they are in pain. The nursing assistant must watch for clues that they may be in pain (Chapter 25). The health team must keep them clean, safe, and comfortable. You must treat them with respect and compassion. Touch, massage, and music may provide comfort and decrease loneliness.

Short-Term Residents

Some people need nursing center care to recover from fractures, acute illness, or surgery. Often they are younger than most residents. They may need tube feedings, wound care, rehabilitation, or other treatments. Others may need therapy programs: physical, occupational, speech and language, or respiratory. Some need restorative nursing care (Chapter 42). The goal is to help them regain their optimal level of function so they can return home.

Some people are cared for at home. They are admitted to nursing centers for short stays. This is *respite care.* Respite means rest or relief. The caregiver can take a vacation, tend to business, or simply rest. Respite care may last from a few days to several weeks.

Lifelong Residents

Birth defects and childhood injuries and diseases can cause disabilities. Intellectual disabilities and Down syndrome are common causes. A disability occurring before 22 years of age is called a *developmental disability* (Chapter 41). It may be a physical impairment, intellectual impairment, or both.

The person with a developmental disability has limited function in at least three of these areas:

- Self-care
- Understanding or expressing language
- Learning
- Mobility
- Self-direction
- Independent living
- Financial support for one's self

The person needs lifelong assistance, support, and special devices. Some nursing centers admit developmentally disabled children and adults.

Residents With Mental Health Disorders

Some people have problems coping or adjusting to stress (Chapter 39). Their behavior and function are affected. In severe cases, self-care and independent living are impaired. Some persons have physical and mental illnesses.

Terminally Ill Residents

Terminally ill persons are dying. They may have advanced cancer, liver, kidney, respiratory, or other diseases. Some are alert and oriented; others are comatose. Comatose means being unable to respond to stimuli (p. 77). The person may still feel pain. Often pain is shown by grimacing or groaning.

Some persons have severe pain. They need frequent care to maintain comfort. Promptly report any sign of discomfort to the nurse. Medications for pain relief are important, as is the care you provide. Turning and repositioning, giving gentle back rubs, careful touching, and holding a hand promote comfort and peace. Many centers work with hospice programs. The goal is to provide quality care to persons who are terminally ill (Chapters 1 and 45).

BEHAVIOR ISSUES

Many people accept illness and disability as part of aging. Others do not adjust well. They have some of the following behaviors. These behaviors are new for some people. For others, they are lifelong. They are part of one's personality.

- *Anger.* Anger is a common emotion caused by fear, pain, dying and death, among other things. Loss of function and loss of control over health and life are causes. Anger is a symptom of some diseases that affect thinking and behavior. Some people are generally angry. Anger is communicated verbally and nonverbally (p. 72). Verbal outbursts, shouting, raised voices, and rapid speech are common. Some people are silent. Others are uncooperative. They may refuse to answer questions. Nonverbal signs include rapid movements, pacing, clenched fists, and a red face. Glaring and getting close to you when speaking are other signs. Violent behaviors can occur.
- *Demanding behavior.* Nothing seems to please the person. The person is critical of others. The person wants care given at a certain time and in a certain way. Loss of independence, loss of health, and loss of control of life are causes, as are unmet needs.
- *Self-centered behavior.* The person cares only about own needs. The needs of others are ignored. The person demands the time and attention of others. The person becomes impatient if needs are not met.
- *Aggressive behavior.* The person may swear, bite, hit, pinch, scratch, or kick. Fear, anger, pain, and dementia (Chapter 40) are causes. Protect the person, others, and yourself from harm (Chapter 11).
- *Withdrawal.* The person has little or no contact with family, friends, and staff. The person spends time alone and does not take part in social or group events. This may signal physical illness or depression. Some people are generally not social, preferring to be alone.
- *Inappropriate sexual behavior.* Some people make inappropriate sexual remarks, or they touch others in the wrong

way (Chapter 10). Some disrobe or masturbate in public. These behaviors may be on purpose or be caused by disease, confusion, dementia, or side effects from medications.

Some behaviors are not pleasant. You cannot avoid the person or lose control. Good communication is needed. Behaviors are addressed in the care plan. The care plan may include some of the guidelines in Box 6.1.

See *Teamwork and Time Management: Behavior Issues.*

See *Focus on Communication: Behavior Issues.*

TEAMWORK AND TIME MANAGEMENT

Behavior Issues

Persons who are demanding can take a lot of time. A simple task such as filling a water pitcher can take several minutes. The pitcher may be too full or not full enough. The water may be too warm or too cold. Or the person may have a list of other care needs.

This may happen to you or to coworkers. Learn to recognize these situations. Offer to help coworkers with the person or other tasks. Hopefully they also will help you.

FOCUS ON COMMUNICATION

Behavior Issues

Anger is a common response to illness and disability. Residents may be angry with their situations. A person may direct anger at you. You might have difficulty dealing with the person's anger. You must continue to act in a professional manner. Remain calm. Do not yell at or insult the person. Listen to the person's concerns. Provide needed care. Try not to take the statements personally. If a resident says hurtful things, you can kindly say, "Please don't say those things. I'm trying to help you." Tell the nurse about the person's behavior.

Caring for demanding or angry persons can be hard. Ask the nurse or coworkers to help if needed.

COMMUNICATING WITH THE PERSON

You communicate with residents every time you give care. You give information to the person. The person gives information to you. Your body sends messages all the time—at the bedside, in hallways, at the nurses' station, in the dining room, and elsewhere. The person and family are aware of what you say and what you do. Good work ethics and understanding the person are needed for good communication. What you say and do also is important.

Effective Communication

For effective communication between you and the person, you must:

- Follow the rules of communication:
  - Use words that have the same meaning for you and the person.
  - Avoid medical terms and words not familiar to the person.

BOX 6.1   Dealing With Behavior Issues

- Recognize frustrating and frightening situations. Put yourself in the person's situation. How would you feel? How would you want to be treated?
- Treat the person with dignity and respect.
- Answer questions clearly and thoroughly. Ask the nurse to answer questions you cannot answer.
- Keep the person informed. Tell the person what you are going to do and when.
- Do not keep the person waiting. Answer call lights promptly. If you tell the person that you will do something, then do it promptly.
- Explain the reason for long waits. Ask if you can get or do something to increase the person's comfort.
- Stay calm and professional, especially if the person is angry or hostile. Often the person is not angry at you but at another person or situation.
- Do not argue with the person.
- Listen and use silence (p. 76). The person may feel better if able to express feelings.
- Protect yourself from violent behaviors (Chapter 11).
- Report the person's behavior to the nurse. Discuss how to deal with the person.

  - Communicate in a logical and orderly manner. Do not wander in thought.
  - Give facts and be specific.
  - Be brief and concise.
- Understand and respect the resident as a person.
- View the person as a physical, psychologic, social, and spiritual human being.
- Appreciate the person's problems and frustrations.
- Respect the person's rights.
- Respect the person's religion and culture.
- Give the person time to understand the information that you give.
- Repeat information as often as needed. Repeat what you said. Use the exact same words. Do not give the person a new message to process. If the person does not seem to understand after repeating, try rephrasing the message. This is very important for persons with hearing problems.
- Ask questions to see if the person understood you.
- Be patient. People with memory problems may ask the same question many times. Do not say that you are repeating information. Accept the memory loss as a disability.
- Include the person in conversations when others are present. This includes when a coworker is assisting you with care.
  See *Residents with Dementia: Effective Communication.*

Verbal Communication

Words are used in verbal communication. Words are spoken or written. You talk to the person. You find out how the person is feeling and share information. Most verbal communication involves the spoken word. Follow these rules:

- Face the person. Look directly at the person.

- Position yourself at the person's eye level. You may have to sit or squat by the person.
- Control the loudness and tone of your voice.
- Speak clearly, slowly, and distinctly.

🕐 RESIDENTS WITH DEMENTIA

Effective Communication

Communicating with persons who have dementia is often difficult. The Alzheimer's Disease Education and Referral Center (ADEAR) recommends the following:

- Gain the person's attention before speaking. Call the person by name.
- Choose simple words and short sentences.
- Use a gentle, calm voice.
- Do not talk to the person as you would a baby.
- Do not talk as if the person was not there.
- Keep distractions and noise to a minimum.
- Help the person focus on what you are saying.
- Allow the person time to respond. Do not interrupt.
- Try to provide the word the person is struggling to find.
- State questions and instructions in a positive way.

- Do not use slang or vulgar words.
- Repeat information as needed.

- Ask one question at a time. Wait for an answer.
- Do not shout, whisper, or mumble.
- Be kind, courteous, and friendly.

The written word is used when the person cannot speak or hear but can read. The nurse and care plan tell you how to communicate with the person. The devices shown in Fig. 6.3 are often used. The person also may have poor vision. When writing messages:

- Keep them brief and concise.
- Use a black felt pen on white paper or a dry erase board.
- Print in large letters.

Some persons cannot speak or read. Ask questions that require "yes" or "no" answers. The person can nod, blink, or use other gestures to respond accordingly. Follow the care plan. A picture board may be helpful (Fig. 6.4).

Persons who are deaf may use sign language (Fig. 6.5). See Chapter 33.

Nonverbal Communication

Nonverbal communication does not use words. Messages are sent with gestures, facial expressions, posture, body movements, touch, and smell. Nonverbal messages more accurately reflect a person's feelings than words do. They are usually involuntary and hard to control. A person may say one thing

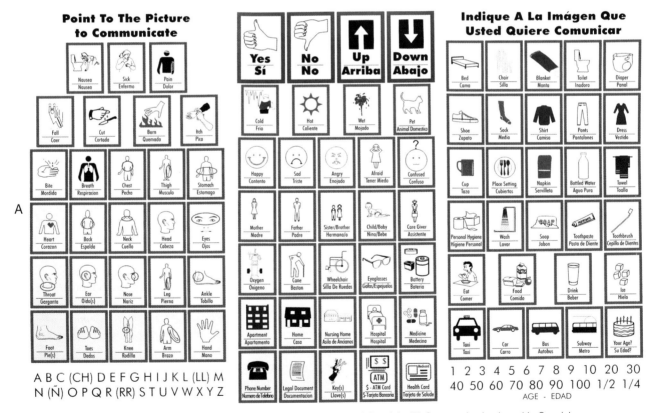

Fig. 6.3 Communication aids. (A) Picture board in English and Spanish. (B) Communication board in Spanish. (C) Magic slate.

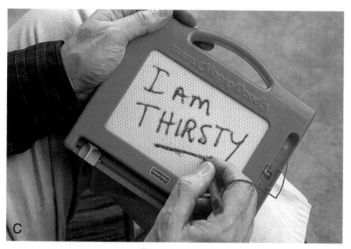

● ESTOY/TENGO
I AM

○ Dificultad para respirar
Short Of Breath
○ Frustrado/a
Frustrated
○ Náuseas
Nauseous
○ Ansiedad
Anxious
○ Decepcionado/a
Disappointed
○ Cansado/a
Tired
○ Somnoliento/a
Drowsy
○ Mejor
Better
○ Sed
Thirsty
○ Calor
Hot
○ Frío
Cold

○ Inseguro/a (con lo que está sucediendo)
Unsure Of What Is Happening)
○ Arcadas
Gagging
○ Dolor
In Pain
○ Mareado/a
Light Headed
○ Miedo
Afraid
○ Solo/a
Lonely
○ Enfadado/a
Angry
○ Mojado/a
Wet
○ Peor
Worse
○ Hambre
Hungry

● QUIERO
I WANT

○ Que me hagan una succión
Suctioned
○ Sentarme
To Sit Up
○ Agua
Water
○ Bañarme
Bath
○ Anteojos
Eyeglasses
○ Calcetines
Socks
○ Hacer una llamada
Make A Call
○ Darme vuelta a la derecha
To Turn Right
○ Que apaguen la luz
Lights Off
○ En silencio
It Quiet

○ Más control
More Control
○ Recostarme
To Lie Down
○ Hielo
Ice
○ Champú
Shampoo
○ Un cepillo para el pelo
Hairbrush
○ Un orinal
Urinal
○ Llamar a la enfermera, Ver TV
Call Lights,TV
○ Darme vuelta a la izquierda
To Turn Left
○ Que bajen las luces
Lights Dim
○ Dormir
To Sleep

○ Sentirme reconfortado/a
To Be Comforted
○ Orar
Prayer
○ Ejercicio físico
Exercise
○ Crema para el cuerpo
Lotion
○ Masaje
Massage
○ Chata para orinar
Bedpan
○ Almohada
Pillow
○ Enciendan la luz
Lights On
○ Cobija
Blanket
○ Descansar
To Rest

EZ BOARD DE VIDATAK
SISTEMA INNOVADOR DE COMUNICACIÓN PARA PACIENTES
EZ BOARD BY VIDATAK
AN INNOVATION IN PATIENT COMMUNICATION

● QUIERO VER A UN/A
I WANT TO SEE

○ Médico
Doctor
○ Terapeuta respiratorio
Respiratory Therapist
○ Enfermera
Nurse
○ Terapeuta físico
Physical Therapist
○ Capellán
Chaplain
○ Asistente
Assistant
○ Trabajador social
Social Worker
○ Mi familia
My Family

● QUIERO LIMPIARME
I WANT TO CLEAN

○ La boca
Mouth
○ Los dientes
Teeth
○ La cara
Face
○ La nariz
Nose
○ Las manos
Hands
○ El cabello
Hair

! 1 2 3 4 5 6 7 8 9 0 - + =   ¡Gracias! Thank You
Q W E R T Y U I O P [ ]   ¡Te quiero mucho! I Love You
A S D F G H J K L : '
Z X C V B N M , . ?
SPACE
VIDATAK EZ BOARD

Para prevenir infecciones, se ruega no usar esta pizarra con diferentes pacientes. For infection control purposes, please do not reuse this board between patients.

B

C

Fig. 6.3 cont'd

but act another way. Watch the person's eyes, hand movements, gestures, posture, and other actions. Sometimes these movements tell you more than words.

Touch

Touch is a very important form of nonverbal communication. It conveys comfort, caring, love, affection, interest, trust, concern, and reassurance. Touch means different things to different people. The meaning depends on age, gender, experiences, and culture.

Cultural groups have rules or practices about touch. They relate to who can touch, when it can occur, and where on the body it is appropriate (Chapter 7).

Some people do not like to be touched; respect the person's choice. For those who accept touch, remember that touch can show caring and warmth. Stroking or holding a hand can comfort a person. Touch should be gentle. It should not be

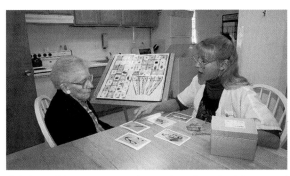

Fig. 6.4 A resident uses a picture board and picture cards to communicate.

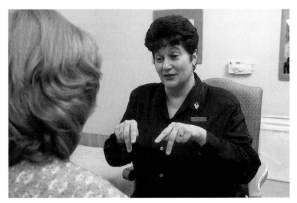

Fig. 6.5 Sign language is used to communicate.

hurried, rough, or sexual. To use touch, follow the person's care plan. Remember to maintain professional boundaries.

Body Language

People send messages through their body language. This can include any of the following:
- Facial expressions (see Chapter 7)
- Gestures
- Posture
- Hand and body movements
- Gait
- Eye contact

Slumped posture may mean the person is not happy or not feeling well. A person may deny pain but protect the affected body part by standing, lying, or sitting in a certain way. Many messages are sent through body language.

Your actions, movements, and facial expressions send messages. So do the ways you stand, sit, walk, and look at the person. Your body language should show interest and enthusiasm. It should show caring and respect for the person. Often you will need to control your body language. Control reactions to odors from body fluids, secretions, excretions, or the person's body. Many odors are beyond the person's

control. Embarrassment and humiliation increase if you react to odors.

Communication Methods

Certain methods help you communicate with others. They result in better relationships. More information is gained for the nursing process.

Listening

Listening means to focus on verbal and nonverbal communication. You use sight, hearing, touch (when appropriate and accepted), and smell. You focus on what the person is saying. You observe nonverbal clues. They can support what the person says, or they can show other feelings. For example, Mr. Ho says, "I want to stay here. That way my daughter won't have to care for me." You see tears, and he looks away from you. His verbal says "happy," but his nonverbal says "sadness."

Listening requires that you care and have interest. Follow these guidelines:
- Sit down if possible and face the person.
- Eliminate background noises. Ask permission to mute the person's television or turn down their radio.
- Be sure the person can see your face if eye contact is desired.
- Lean toward the person (Fig. 6.6). Do not sit back with your arms crossed.
- Respond to the person. Nod your head. Say "uh huh," "mmm," or "I see," then repeat what the person says. Ask questions.
- Avoid communication barriers.

Paraphrasing

Paraphrasing is restating the person's message in your own words. You use fewer words than the person did. Paraphrasing:
- Shows you are listening.
- Allows the person to see if you understand the message.
- Promotes further communication.

The person usually responds to your statement. For example:

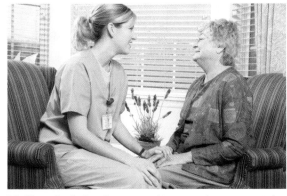

Fig. 6.6 Listen by facing the person. Have good eye contact. Lean toward the person.

Mr. Ho: My wife was crying after she spoke with the doctor. I don't know what they talked about.

You: You don't know why your wife was crying.

Mr. Ho: He must have told her that I have a tumor.

Direct Questions

Direct questions focus on certain information. You ask the person something you need to know. Some direct questions have "yes" or "no" answers. Others require more information. For example:

You: Mr. Ho, do you want to shave this morning?

Mr. Ho: Yes.

You: Mr. Ho, when would you like to do that?

Mr. Ho: Could we start in 15 minutes? I'd like to call my son first.

You: Yes, we can start in 15 minutes. Did you have a bowel movement today?

Mr. Ho: No.

You: You said you didn't eat well this morning. Can you tell me what you ate?

Mr. Hot: I only had toast and coffee. I just don't feel like eating this morning.

Open-Ended Questions

Open-ended questions lead or invite the person to share thoughts, feelings, or ideas. The person chooses what to talk about. The person controls the topic and the information given. Answers require more than a "yes" or "no" response. For example:

- "What do you like about living with your daughter?"
- "Tell me about your grandson."
- "What was your wife like?"
- "What do you like about being retired?"

The person chooses how to answer. Responses to open-ended questions are longer. They give more information than do responses to direct questions.

Clarifying

Clarifying lets you make sure that you understand the message. You can ask the person to repeat the message, say you do not understand, or restate the message. For example:

- "Could you say that again?"
- "I'm sorry, Mr. Ho. I don't understand what you mean."
- "Are you saying that you want to go home?"

Focusing

Focusing is dealing with a certain topic. It is useful when a person rambles or wanders in thought. For example, Mr. Ho talks at length about food and places to eat. You need to know why he did not eat much breakfast. To focus on breakfast you say, "Let's talk about breakfast. You said you don't feel like eating."

Silence

Silence is a very powerful way to communicate. Sometimes you do not need to say anything. This is true during sad times. Just being there shows you care. At other times, silence gives time to think, organize thoughts, or choose words. Silence is useful when making decisions. It also helps when the person is upset and needs to gain control. Silence on your part shows caring and respect for the person's situation and feelings.

Sometimes pauses or long silences are uncomfortable. You do not need to talk when the person is silent. The person may need silence. Dealing with silence gets easier as you gain experience in your role. See Chapter 7.

Communication Barriers

Communication barriers prevent the sending and receiving of messages, causing communication to fail. You must avoid these barriers:

- *Using unfamiliar language.* You and the person must use and understand the same language. If not, messages are not accurately interpreted. See the Spanish Vocabulary and Phrases Glossary on Evolve Student Learning Resources.
- *Cultural differences.* The person may attach different meanings to verbal and nonverbal communication. See Chapter 7.
- *Changing the subject.* Someone changes the subject when the topic is uncomfortable. Avoid changing the subject when possible.
- *Giving your opinion.* Opinions involve judging values, behaviors, or feelings. Let others express feelings and concerns without adding your opinion. Do not make judgments or jump to conclusions.
- *Talking a lot when others are silent.* Talking too much is usually because of nervousness and discomfort with silence. Silences have meaning. They show acceptance, rejection, and fear. They also show the need for quiet and time to think.
- *Failure to listen.* Do not pretend to listen. It shows lack of interest and caring. This causes poor responses. You miss reports of pain, discomfort, or other symptoms that you must report to the nurse.
- *Pat answers.* Avoid use of such responses as "Don't worry," "Everything will be okay," and "Your doctor knows best." These make the person feel that you do not care about such concerns, feelings, and fears.
- *Illness and disability.* Some illnesses, injuries, and birth defects affect speech, hearing, vision, cognitive function, and body movements. Verbal and nonverbal communication are affected.
- *Age.* Values and communication styles vary among age groups.

RESIDENTS WITH DISABILITIES

A person may acquire a disability any time from birth through old age. Disease and injury are common causes. For example, children can develop hearing problems from ear infections. Head injuries from accidents can impair cognitive function. Spinal cord injuries can affect movements. And loud noise (music, machines) is linked to hearing loss. The cause of disability or the age of onset does not matter. The person does not choose to have a disability.

The person has to adjust to the disability. For many people this can be long and hard (Chapter 42).

You will care for many people with disabilities. Your attitude is important for effective communication. People with disabilities have the same basic needs as you and everyone else. They feel joy, sorrow, happiness, sadness, and other emotions just like you and everyone else. They laugh, cry, have families, go to school, work, get married, and pay bills just like you and everyone else. And they certainly have the right to dignity and respect.

To communicate with persons who have certain disabilities, see persons:
- Who have speech impairments—Chapter 33.
- Who are hard of hearing—Chapter 33.
- Who are blind—Chapter 33.
- Who are confused—Chapter 40.
- With Alzheimer disease and other dementias—Chapter 40.

Common courtesies and manners (*etiquette*) apply to any person with a disability. See Box 6.2 for disability etiquette. The guidelines are from Easter Seals, an organization that helps persons with disabilities and their families.

The Person Who Is Comatose

Recall from earlier in this chapter, comatose means being unable to respond to stimuli. The person who is comatose is unconscious. The person cannot respond to others. Often the person can hear and can feel touch and pain. Pain may be shown by grimacing or groaning. Assume that the person hears and understands you. Use touch and give care gently. Practice these measures:

- Knock before entering the person's room.
- Tell the person your name, the time, and the place every time you enter the room.
- Give care on the same schedule every day.
- Explain what you are going to do. Explain care measures step by step as you do them.
- Tell the person when you are finishing care.
- Use touch to communicate care, concern, and comfort.
- Tell the person what time you will return.
- Tell the person when you are leaving the room.

FAMILY AND FRIENDS

Family and friends help meet safety and security, love and belonging, and self-esteem needs. They offer support and comfort. They lessen loneliness. Some also help with the person's care. This helps both the person and the family. The family knows they are doing something to help the person. And the person's physical and emotional needs are met. The presence or absence of family or friends affects the person's quality of life.

The person has the right to visit with family and friends in private and without unnecessary interruptions (Fig. 6.7). You may need to give care when visitors are there. Protect the right to privacy. Do not expose the person's body in front of visitors. Politely ask them to leave the room. Show them where to wait. Promptly tell them when they can return. A partner or family member may want to help you. If the resident consents, you may allow the person to stay.

Treat family and friends with courtesy and respect. They have concerns about the person's condition and care. They need support and understanding. However, do not discuss the person's condition with them. Refer their questions to the nurse. Visiting rules depend on center policy and the person's condition. Dying persons usually can have family members present all the time. This is policy for hospice units. Know your center's visiting policies and what is allowed for the person. During times of high incidence of infectious disease, visiting rules may need to be restricted. This can be very difficult for residents and for family members.

BOX 6.2 Disability Etiquette

- Ask if the person needs help before acting. If the person says "no," then respect those wishes. If the person wants help, ask what to do and how to do it.
- Extend the same courtesies to the person as you would to anyone else.
- Allow the person privacy.
- Treat adults as adults. Do not use the person's first name unless requested.
- Sit or squat to talk to a person in a wheelchair or chair. This puts you and the person at eye level.
- Think before giving directions to a person in a wheelchair. Think about distance, weather conditions, stairs, curbs, steep hills, and other obstacles.
- Do not hang on or lean on a person's wheelchair.
- Do not pat a person who is in a wheelchair on the head.
- Allow the person extra time to say or do things. Let the person set the pace in walking, talking, or other activities.
- Speak directly to the person. Do not address questions intended for the person to a companion.
- Do not be embarrassed if you use words that relate to a disability. For example, you say, "See you later" or "I've got to run."

Modified from Easter Seals, *Disability etiquette*, 2021, https://www.easterseals.com/explore-resources/facts-about-disability-etiquette.html.

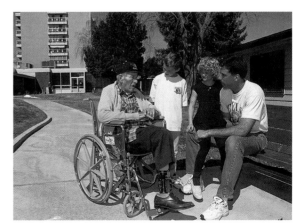

Fig. 6.7 A resident visits with family.

A visitor may upset or tire a person. Report your observations to the nurse. The nurse will speak with the visitor about the person's needs.

QUALITY OF LIFE

The resident is the most important person in the nursing center. Each person has physical, psychologic, social, and spiritual needs. You must know and respect the whole person to provide quality care. This includes promoting physical, mental, spiritual, and social well-being. Try to not focus on physical needs alone. Consider the person's thoughts and feelings. Small gestures make a difference. For example, give a person time to pray before eating if this is valued. While giving care, ask about the person's friends and family. Or simply say, "How are you feeling today?" Respect all of the person's needs. All interact and affect the person's well-being. Provide care that focuses on the person as a whole.

You will care for people from different cultures and religions (Chapter 7). Learn as much as you can about a person's religious, spiritual, and cultural beliefs and practices. This will help you understand the person and give better care.

Illness and disability affect quality of life. Normal tasks and activities that bring pleasure and contact with others may be hard or impossible. People often feel angry, frustrated, and useless. You can help by treating each person

with dignity and respect. You also help each person reach or maintain an optimal level of function. Always focus on the person's abilities, not on disabilities.

Family and visitors are important to the person. They can offer support and comfort, and enhance the person's quality of life. Always treat them with respect. If visiting needs to be restricted due to influenza or coronal virus outbreaks, try to assist the resident and family with other forms of communication. Using online programs such as Zoom or Facetime allows residents to visit virtually with their family members. Window visits may also be beneficial.

TIME TO REFLECT

Mrs. Thomas is a resident who is comatose. Today you are giving her a bed bath. You have been talking to her and telling her what you will be doing next. You request help from another assistant when it is time to turn her on her side. As you tell Mrs. Thomas that you will be turning her, the other assistant says, "Don't you know she is in a coma? She can't hear you. Save your breath." How would you react in this situation?

REVIEW QUESTIONS

Circle the BEST answer.

1. Which basic need is the *most* essential?
   a. Self-actualization
   b. Self-esteem
   c. Love and belonging
   d. Safety and security

2. Based on Maslow's theory of basic needs, which person's needs must be met *first*?
   a. The person who wants another blanket
   b. The person who wants mail opened
   c. The person who asks for more water
   d. The person who is crying

3. A person says, "What are they doing to me?" Which basic needs are *not* being met?
   a. Physical needs
   b. Safety and security needs
   c. Love and belonging needs
   d. Self-esteem needs

4. A person tends a garden behind the nursing center. This relates to
   a. Self-actualization
   b. Self-esteem
   c. Love and belonging
   d. Safety and security

5. These are statements about illness and disability. Which is *false*?
   a. They are matters of personal choice
   b. They affect normal activities
   c. Anger is a common response
   d. A goal is for the person to maintain optimal level of function

6. Alert and oriented residents need nursing center care because they
   a. Are very disabled and confused
   b. Have trouble remembering things
   c. Have physical problems
   d. Are dying

7. A person wants care given at a certain time and in a certain way. Nothing seems to please the person. The person is most likely demonstrating
   a. Angry behavior
   b. Demanding behavior
   c. Withdrawn behavior
   d. Aggressive behavior

8. A person is demonstrating problem behavior. You should do the following *except*
   a. Put yourself in the person's situation
   b. Tell the person what you are going to do and when
   c. Ask the person to be nicer
   d. Listen and use silence

9. Which is *false*?
   a. Verbal communication uses the written or spoken word
   b. Verbal communication is the truest reflection of a person's feelings
   c. Messages are sent by facial expressions, gestures, posture, and body movements
   d. Touch means different things to different people

10. To communicate with a person you should
    a. Use medical words and phrase
    b. Change the subject often
    c. Give your opinions
    d. Be quiet when the person is silent

11. Which might mean that you are *not* listening?
    a. You sit facing the person
    b. You have good eye contact with the person
    c. You sit with your arms crossed
    d. You ask questions
12. Which is a direct question?
    a. "Do you feel better now?"
    b. "What are your plans for home?"
    c. "What will you do at home?"
    d. "Why can't you sleep?"
13. A person wants to take a shower. You say, "You would like to take a shower." This is
    a. A communication barrier
    b. A direct question
    c. Paraphrasing
    d. An open-ended question
14. Focusing is useful when
    a. A person is rambling
    b. You want to make sure you understand the message
    c. You want the person to share thoughts and feelings
    d. You need certain information
15. Which reply promotes effective communication?
    a. "Don't worry"
    b. "Everything will be just fine"
    c. "This is a good nursing center"
    d. "You seem sad. Would you like to talk?"

16. Which is *not* a barrier to communication?
    a. Using silence
    b. Giving your opinions
    c. Changing the subject
    d. Illness
17. A person uses a wheelchair. For effective communication, you should
    a. Lean on the wheelchair
    b. Pat the person on the head
    c. Direct questions to the companion
    d. Sit or squat next to the person
18. A person is comatose. Which action is *not correct*?
    a. Assume that the person can hear and can feel touch
    b. Explain what you are going to do
    c. Perform care quickly and silently
    d. Tell the person when you are leaving the room
19. A person has many visitors. Which is *false*?
    a. They can help meet basic needs
    b. Privacy should be allowed
    c. The nurse answers their questions about the person's care
    d. Visitors can stay in the room when care is given
20. A visitor seems to tire a person. What should you do?
    a. Ask the person to leave
    b. Tell the nurse
    c. Stay in the room to observe the person and visitor
    d. Find out the visitor's relationship to the person

See Appendix A for answers to these questions.

7

Culture, Religion, and Spirituality

OBJECTIVES

- Define the key terms and key abbreviations listed in this chapter.
- Understand how culture can play a role in offering care to persons.
- Describe the basic characteristics of culture.
- List the health beliefs of select cultural groups.
- Understand how religion can play a role in offering care to persons.
- List the beliefs that correspond with some of the major religious faiths.

- Identify methods to understand and respect individuals of various cultures and faiths.
- Understand how gestures, personal space, use of touch, and eye contact can influence how care is received.
- Learn ways to help persons practice their beliefs while receiving care.
- Explain how to promote quality of life.

KEY TERMS

agnostic A person who believes it is impossible to know if a god exists

atheist A person who does not believe in the existence of a god or deity

bias To prefer something or someone, often without sound judgment

cleric A leader or representative from an organized religion (e.g., pastor, priest, rabbi)

culture The beliefs, practices, customs, and language of a group of people that is passed on between generations

ethnicity A classification of people based on national origin or culture

extended family A family composed of parents, their children, grandparents, aunts, uncles, and cousins

fast To refrain from consuming food (sometimes food and drink)

nuclear family A family consisting of parents and their children

personal space The distance that people require to comfortably communicate

prejudice Forming an opinion without having facts or information

race A classification of persons based on physical and biologic characteristics

religion Spiritual beliefs, needs, and practices

sensitivity The ability to appreciate the personal characteristics of others

spirituality A person's need to find meaning and purpose in life

stereotyping Believing that everyone in a group is the same

KEY ABBREVIATIONS

CMS Centers for Medicare & Medicaid Services

RN Registered nurse

Nursing assistants will care for people who come from many cultures, races, and nationalities. They may practice religions that are different from your own. It is important to respect these differences. Bias means to prefer something or someone, often without sound judgment. Prejudice is similar and involves forming an opinion without having facts. One way to avoid bias and prejudice is to understand the person's beliefs. Being sensitive to the beliefs of the residents you care for is very helpful. This enables trusting relationships.

CULTURE AND ETHNICITY

Culture is the characteristics of a group of people—language, values, beliefs, habits, likes, dislikes, and customs. They are passed from one generation to the next. The person's culture influences health beliefs and practices. Culture also affects thinking and behavior during illness and when in a nursing center.

Ethnicity is a classification of people based on national origin and shared culture. There are many ethnic groups that reside in the United States. Members of these groups often share language, customs, and beliefs. They usually come from the same geographic region. Examples are African Americans, Asian Americans, European Americans, Hispanic Americans, Middle Eastern Americans, and Native Americans. These groups may also have smaller groups within them.

While residing in a care center, members of various ethnic groups may wish to continue practicing their customs and beliefs. At times, this may not be easy. They may miss certain foods that they previously enjoyed. Perhaps they miss practicing a tradition related to a holiday. Some may wear clothing that is typical for their culture. There are ways the nursing assistant can help a resident observe cultural desires. Some cultures may have beliefs that influence their hygiene practices. Encouraging residents to share their customs helps the staff to understand. Take time to find out about the customs and beliefs of the residents you care for. Box 7.1 lists some guidelines for relating to persons from various cultures.

Some people have beliefs about what causes and cures illness. They may perform rituals to rid the body of disease. A person may believe that illness is caused by exposure to hot or cold. They believe that a "hot-cold" balance is necessary for health. If hot caused the illness, cold is used for the cure. Likewise, hot is used to cure illnesses caused by cold. Keep this in mind if someone refuses an ice pack that has been prescribed as treatment. The person may view it as a conflict instead of a remedy. Some cultures may include herbs and botanicals as methods of healing. Acupuncture, coin rubbing, cupping, or meditation may be important practices for other cultures. Many have beliefs and rituals about dying and death (Box 7.2). Some cultures require people of the same gender to provide care, especially if it requires exposure of the body. This would be important to remember, for example, when a female resident refuses to allow a male assistant to bathe her.

PERSONAL SPACE AND GESTURES

Personal space is the distance that people require to comfortably communicate or interact. Persons from some cultures stand very close to each other. They may even touch while communicating. Other cultures, however, stand farther away. This can also vary from one individual to another. In some cultures, it is acceptable to greet a person by shaking hands. In some cultures, only men may shake hands with men.

BOX 7.1 Guidelines for Relating to Persons from Various Cultures

- Review your own personal beliefs and experiences.
- Set aside any values, biases, and attitudes that are judgmental.
- Plan care according to the communicated needs and cultural background.
- Encourage the person to share.
- Be sensitive to the uniqueness of the person.
- Be attentive to signs of fear, anxiety, and confusion.
- Communicate respect by using a kind and attentive approach.
- Develop trust by listening and giving the person your full attention.
- Adopt special measures when the person speaks a different language.
- Use an appropriate language dictionary.
- Use an interpreter who is culturally sensitive.
- Use a caring tone of voice.
- Use gestures and pictures.
- Keep messages simple.

Modified from Giger JN. *Transcultural nursing: assessment and intervention*, ed 8, St. Louis, 2021, Mosby.

BOX 7.2 Religion and Dietary Practices

Church of Jesus Christ of Latter-Day Saints (Mormon)
- Alcohol, beverages containing caffeine (coffee and tea) are avoided.
- Fruits, vegetables, grains, and nuts take the place of meats.
- Meats, sugar, cheeses, and spices are limited.
- Fasting is practiced.

Greek Orthodox
- Fasting is required during the Great Lent and before other holy days.
- Meat, fish, and dairy products are not eaten during a fast.

Hinduism
- Pork, fowl, ducks, snails, and crabs are avoided.
- No beef is eaten. The cow is a sacred animal to Hindus.
- Products from cows—milk, yogurt, and butter—are allowed.
- Days of fast include Hindu holidays, Sundays, birthdays, and marriage and death anniversaries.

Islam (Muslim)
- All pork and pork products are forbidden.
- Tea and coffee are discouraged.
- Alcohol is not allowed.
- Fasting is practiced on Mondays and Thursdays, for 6 days during the Shawwal (the tenth month of the Islamic calendar), and during the entire month of Ramadan (the ninth month of the Islamic calendar). Fasting means no food or drink from sunrise to sunset.

Judaism (Jewish Faith)
- Foods must be kosher. (*Kosher* means "fit, proper, or correct.") Food must be prepared according to Jewish law. Fig. 7.6 shows some common symbols for kosher food packages.
- Meat of kosher animals can be eaten—cows, goats, and lambs.
- Chickens, ducks, and geese are kosher fowl.
- Kosher fish have scales and fins—tuna, sardines, carp, salmon, herring, whitefish, and so on. Lobster, shrimp, and clams are not allowed.
- Milk, milk products, and eggs from kosher animals and fowl are allowed.
- Meat and milk cannot be cooked together.
- Meat and milk products cannot be eaten at the same meal. They cannot be served on the same plate.
- Meat and milk products are not prepared or served with the same utensils and dishes. Two sets of utensils and dishes are needed. They are washed and stored separately.
- Fermented grain products are not consumed during Passover (e.g., cookies, noodles, alcohol).

Roman Catholic
- Abstaining from meat and fasting is required on Ash Wednesday and Good Friday. In addition, abstaining from meat is required on all Fridays during Lent. Fasting pertains to persons age 18–59. Some elderly people may still follow the custom of fasting.
- Not eating food is required for 1 hour before receiving Holy Communion, although the elderly and ill persons are exempt. Water and medications are allowed.

Seventh-Day Adventist
- Coffee, tea, and alcohol are avoided.
- Beverages with caffeine (colas) are avoided.
- Some groups have restrictions about meat, fish, and fowl.
- A vegetarian diet is encouraged.

In some cultures, it is unacceptable to touch the person on the top of the head. Gestures may also have different meanings to different cultures. In the United States we nod our head up and down for "yes." In another culture, this gesture may indicate a sign of respect rather than understanding. For some cultures, exposing the sole of the foot or pointing with the foot is an unkind gesture. It is very important to understand how the person you are caring for feels about personal space and the use of touch and gestures. If you do make a mistake, apologize to the person you may have offended.

EYE CONTACT

Eye contact is another factor that has different meanings. For many people, making direct eye contact shows that the person is interested in the conversation. Some cultures, however, may think that eye contact is showing disrespect or that the speaker is being challenged. Do not assume that a person is not being attentive when keeping the head down and avoiding eye contact with you. The person may be showing humility and respect.

The perception of time and time management may differ among cultures. Some persons in certain cultures may have a relaxed sense of time. They may feel it does not matter if they arrive late for an appointment. They may believe that personal relationships are more important than punctuality.

Families play an important role in different cultures. A nuclear family consists of parents and their children living in one setting. An extended family is composed of parents, their children, grandparents, aunts, uncles, and cousins. When a person resides in a care center there may be times when the extended family comes to visit. If possible, help them find a larger space where they can visit without disturbing others. In some cultures, it may be important for the family members to offer certain forms of care to the individual who is ill or dying. If you are not sure whether the family member should be giving the care, ask the nurse.

HYGIENE, GROOMING, AND DRESS PRACTICES

Some cultures have practices that affect their hygiene, grooming, and dress (Chapters 18 and 19). For example, some African Americans may wear their hair in tight braids. These are not routinely removed when the person's hair is shampooed. For some people a sponge bath is not acceptable. The person may have the need to have water poured over the body. Residents may have specific clothing items that reflect their religion, culture, or spirituality. Examples might include head coverings such as a bonnet, hijab, kippah, yarmulke, turban, cap, or scarf. Fig. 7.1 shows examples of various Muslim American head coverings. Always ask before removing such items. Some people of specific faiths may wear a special undergarment under their clothing. Some may wear jewelry such as a necklace, cross, or medal. Various types of tribal jewelry and bracelets may also hold significance to some people. Always treat these with respect and do not remove unless the person asks you to do so. When offering personal care or assisting the person with dressing, ask the person how to care for the items. Be mindful of where these objects are safely stored.

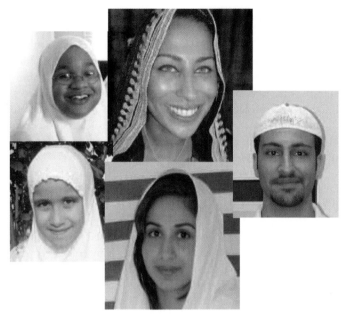

Fig. 7.1 Common Muslim-American head coverings. (From *Muslim Head Covering Poster*, Office for Civil Rights and Civil Liberties. From https://www.dhs.gov/office-civil-rights-and-civil-liberties)

RELIGION AND SPIRITUALITY

Religion relates to spiritual beliefs, needs, and practices. Often culture and religion are connected. Not all individuals practice a religion. An atheist is a person who does not believe in the existence of a god or deity. An agnostic is a person who believes it is impossible to know if a god exists. Spirituality describes a person's need to find meaning and purpose in life. A person could be spiritual without belonging to an organized religion. Those people who do believe in a supreme being or god may follow the beliefs of an organized religion. Tables 7.1 and 7.2 list some of the organized religions and denominations in the United States. A person's religion influences health and illness practices. Some individuals see illness as having not only physical causes but also spiritual causes. Religion and spiritual practices may have beliefs and practices about daily living, behaviors, relationships with others, diet (see Box 7.2), healing, days of worship, birth and birth control, medications, treatments, and death (Box 7.3).

Many people find comfort and strength from religion, especially during illness. Religion, faith, and spirituality can help improve physical and emotional health. The overall quality of life can be enhanced by faith and spirituality. Many people turn to their faith or spiritual beliefs when faced with a health care decision. Residents may want to pray and observe religious practices (Fig. 7.2).

According to the Nursing Home Abuse Center:

Spiritual care for the elderly is an important part of the aging process. Bereavement and depression can become a sad fact of life for seniors. Religion, faith, and spirituality can help improve physical and emotional health, as well as enhance the overall quality of life. Spirituality is often referred to as "the breath of life." It can describe a feeling people get from things

TABLE 7.1 Largest Denominational Families in the United States

Denomination	% US Population (2017)
Roman Catholic Church	20.8
Baptist	15.4
Methodist/Wesleyan	4.7
Lutheran	3.7
United Church of Christ	1.8
Church of Jesus Christ of Latter-Day Saints	1.6
Presbyterian	2.2
Assemblies of God	0.3
Episcopal	21.2
Congregational/United Church of Christ	0.4
Jehovah's Witnesses	0.8
Seventh-Day Adventist	0.6
Orthodox Church in America	0.5
Christian Churches (Unspecified)	7.4

Data reported via Pew Research Center. (2019). *Religion in America: U.S. religious data, demographics and statistics.* Retrieved from https://www.pewforum.org/religious-landscape-study/; Giger JN. *Transcultural nursing*, ed 8, St. Louis: Elsevier; 2021.

TABLE 7.2 Largest Organized Religions in the United States

Religion	% US Population (2008)	% US Population (2017)
Christianity	76.7	70.6
Judaism	1.2	1.9
Islam	0.6	0.9
Buddhism	0.5	0.7
Hinduism	0.4	0.7
Other faiths	0.3	1.5

Data reported via Pew Research Center. (2019). *Religion in America: U.S. religious data, demographics and statistics.* Retrieved from https://www.pewforum.org/religious-landscape-study/; Giger JN. *Transcultural nursing*, ed 8, St. Louis: Elsevier; 2021.

BOX 7.3 Examples of Death Rites

In *Israel* it is disrespectful to leave a dying person alone, so a relative remains to ensure that the soul does not leave the body. Rituals may start before a death has occurred. Jewish law requires burial within 24 hours unless the Sabbath intervenes. The eyes of the deceased are to be closed at death, and the body is left untouched until a family member or Jewish undertaker is contacted for ritual proceedings

In Vietnam, dying persons are helped to recall past good deeds and to achieve a fitting mental state. Death at home is preferred over death in the hospital. In some areas, a coin or jewels (a wealthy family) and rice (a poor family) are put in the dead person's mouth. This is from the belief that these items will help the soul go through encounters with gods and devils and the soul will be born rich in the next life.

The Chinese have an aversion to death and anything concerning death. Autopsy and disposal of the body are not prescribed by religion. Donating body parts is encouraged. The eldest son makes all arrangements. The body is buried in a coffin. After 7 years, the body is exhumed and cremated. The urn, containing the ashes, is buried in the family tomb. White, yellow, or black clothing is worn for mourning.

In India, Hindu persons are often accepting of God's will. The person's desire to be clear-headed as death nears must be assessed in planning treatment. A time and place for prayer are essential for the family and the person. Prayer helps them deal with anxiety and conflict. The Hindu priest reads from Holy Sanskrit books. Some priests tie strings (meaning a blessing) around the neck or wrist. After death, the son pours water into the mouth of the deceased. Blood transfusions, organ transplants, and autopsies are allowed. Cremation is preferred.

In *Saudi Arabia* it is believed that only Allah knows the true prognosis for a patient, so confronting a patient with a grave prognosis shatters hope and can create mistrust. Islamic regulations (fatwah) state that life support can be discontinued if certain conditions are met. After death, the body must be washed ceremonially (possibly by a family member) after which no non-Muslim is allowed to touch the body. Internment is usually carried out within a day and the body is buried in the ground wrapped in a shroud without a coffin. Cremation is not allowed.

Modified from D'Avanzo CE, *Pocket guide to cultural health assessment*, ed 4, St Louis, 2008, Mosby.

place on one day and a Catholic Mass may take place on a different day. Many times, nursing centers offer bible study programs for persons who are interested. Some residents may find interest in leading a bible study session or providing music for a religious service. Assist residents to participate as needed Some care centers will have videorecorded religious services. Many denominations have offered live-streamed versions of their service. Some residents may need assistance with logging onto the Internet site where these are available. Radio broadcasts of religious services are also offered.

Some residents may leave the center to worship. A family member or volunteer may offer them transportation. Your role may be to assist the resident with hygiene and dressing before leaving for a religious service. It may be necessary to transport the person by wheelchair to the entrance for pickup by a family member or friend.

that are enjoyable to them—a connected feeling that can be found in spending time with family, being in nature, painting or the arts, and anything that causes people to "light up."

This changes over time and spiritual activities for seniors may be different than for younger people. For example, walking in nature may no longer be possible as people age but connections might be made in different places, such as birdwatching, for example.

Nursing centers offer religious services. Some nursing centers have chapels or meditation areas for prayer or worship (Fig. 7.3). These services may vary according to the particular faith that is practiced. For example, a Jewish service may take

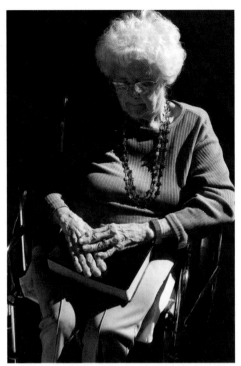

Fig. 7.2 A woman prays with hands on her prayer book. (From iStock.com/Lisa Thornberg)

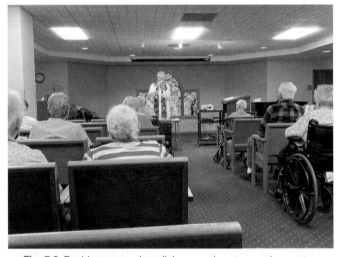

Fig. 7.3 Residents attend a religious service at a nursing center.

At times a person may request to see a spiritual leader or adviser. Report this to the nurse at once. There may be a chaplain that is associated with the care center. Some residents may request a visit from a specific cleric associated with their faith. Some people believe that a person should receive a special blessing or sacrament when they are seriously ill. Make sure the room is neat and orderly. Have a chair ready for the cleric. Provide privacy during the visit. Some people may receive Communion every Sunday. Some denominations may stress the benefit of receiving Communion before surgery or when the

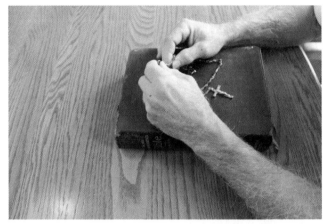

Fig. 7.4 A Holy Bible and rosary have special meaning for the person.

person is ill. They may need assistance with their personal cares before the cleric or church representative arrives for the visit.

Residents may have religious or spiritual objects in their rooms that hold special meaning to them. Examples include bibles, prayer books, crosses, rosaries, pictures, statues, and other objects (Fig. 7.4). Always treat these items with respect and do not move the items unless the resident gives permission. Never place an object on top of a Holy Bible, Koran, Torah, or any other sacred book.

> ### 👤 PROMOTING SAFETY AND COMFORT
>
> **Safety**
> **_Hazards of Candles_**
> Some religious customs and rituals involve lighting candles or votive lights. For example, in the Jewish faith, lighting a menorah has special meaning. Because of the risk of accidental fire, however, the **Centers for Medicare & Medicaid Services** (CMS) does not allow candles with flames to be burned in resident rooms. The resident or family member may not be aware of the danger of candles. For some religions small, battery-powered lights may be substituted.

It may be customary for some individuals to say a blessing before meals (Fig. 7.5) or to pray aloud before bedtime. In addition, some individuals may have religious dietary practices that they follow. They may fast or refrain from eating certain foods during religious holy days. Some religions require that individuals refrain from eating pork or beef. Some do not consume caffeine or alcohol. Still others may require a vegetarian diet. Box 7.2 lists some common dietary practices for select religions. Always be respectful of their religious practices. Offer a substitute item if they refuse a particular food on the menu due to a religious custom.

Some people practicing certain faiths may feel they must pray at certain times of the day. They may find it necessary to pray in a certain position or face a particular direction (Fig. 7.7). They may have a special rug that is placed on the floor. They may wish to be given time to pray privately or read

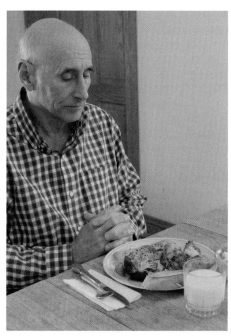

Fig. 7.5 This man prays a blessing before his meal.

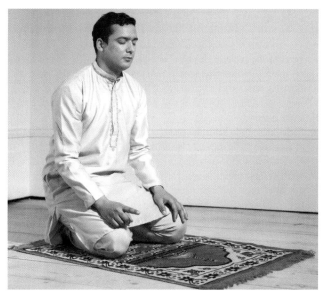

Fig. 7.7 Person kneeling during prayer on a prayer rug. (From iStock Photo.com/ImageSource)

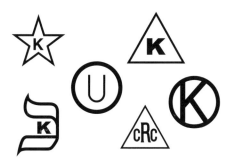

Fig. 7.6 Common kosher symbols on food packaging. (From Burks W, Eigenmann P, James J.M, *Food allergy*, ed. 1, Philadelphia, Elsevier, 2012.)

their holy book. Some faiths believe in special rituals of cleansing before praying.

The nursing process reflects the person's culture, spirituality, and religion. The care plan includes the person's cultural, spirituality, and religious practices. The person's wishes and needs are communicated to caregivers. Each person has unique needs and requires understanding. As the person's health declines, special considerations may take place. The person may request to see a spiritual advisor. Once death occurs, there may be special actions that take place (see Box 7.3).

Sensitivity is the ability to appreciate the personal characteristics of others. You must respect and accept the person's culture, religion, and spirituality. You do not have to agree or adopt the culture or religious beliefs of those in your care, but you must understand that they are important to those people.

Likewise, you do not try to force your religion, spirituality, or cultural beliefs on other people. An example of how a nursing assistant might be helpful would be to agree to read aloud passages from a person's holy book if the person requests this and the person's eyesight is poor. You will meet people from various cultures and religions. It is impossible to understand thoroughly *all* the beliefs of every religion, culture, religion, or spiritual practice, but try to show sensitivity to these issues. Learn about their beliefs and practices. Box 7.4 lists some characteristics of a few religions. Recognizing what is important to the person helps you understand and give better care.

A person may not follow all beliefs and practices of the preferred culture or religion. Some people do not practice a religion. Each person is unique. It is very important to know that not all members of a culture or religion will behave in the same way. Do not judge the person by your standards, and do not force your ideas on the person. Never ridicule or make fun of a person's beliefs or practices.

QUALITY OF LIFE

You will care for people from various cultures and religions. Learn as much as you can about a person's religious, spiritual, and cultural beliefs and practices. This will help you understand the person and give better care. Consider the person's thoughts and feelings. Small gestures make a difference. For example, give a person time to pray before eating if this is valued. Respect the person's customs and rituals. Enable the person to practice these as desired. When a person is ill or disabled, religious or spiritual beliefs can play an important role in recovery. Often, a sense of hope increases when spirituality and religion play a role. Always allow privacy for residents to visit with a cleric or member of their place of worship. Make sure you respect any religious items residents may have in their room.

BOX 7.4   Examples of Health Care Beliefs Related to Religion

- It is important to note that each individual is unique and may not practice or follow all the traditional beliefs of an organized religion. These examples are not meant to **stereotype** specific religions, but rather to give some generalizations to serve as a starting point in understanding. The goal is to gain insight into further understanding of some major beliefs. Always be sensitive to the needs of the person.
- **Christian** faith includes the Catholic faith as well as many different Protestant denominations. Most Christians believe that Jesus is the Son of God. Most believe in the Trinity (God is Father, Son, and Holy Spirit). By accepting Jesus Christ, a person is saved and will have eternal life. The Holy Bible is the sacred book for Christians.
- **Catholics** believe in sacraments and blessings. Baptism, Confession, Holy Communion, and Sacrament of the Sick are a few of these sacraments. Catholics who are unable to attend Mass may have Communion brought to them at a care center. When ill or near death, the Sacrament of the Sick (Last Rites) may be given by a priest. This sacrament can be given more than once. Catholics often abstain from meat on Fridays during Lent.
- **Jehovah's** Witness do not believe in receiving whole blood but may receive some blood products. They do not celebrate birthdays or many of the Christian holidays. Elders may pray and read scriptures to promote healing. Organ donation is a personal choice.
- **Church of Jesus Christ of Latter-Day Saints (Mormon)** believe in "laying on of hands" or blessings by church elders and the use of anointing oils for healing. Mormons believe in the teachings of both the Bible and the Book of Mormon. Special undergarments may be worn by some. Many fast on the first Sunday of the month. Most avoid tobacco and alcohol.
- **Hindus** are strictly vegetarian and fasting is a common practice. They are modest and may refuse care by someone of the opposite gender. They may

be reluctant to speak of genital or urinary issues if the spouse is present. After death, a family member of the same gender may be appointed to bathe the body. The act of washing is very important to them at certain times. They may use the right hand for "clean" tasks and the left hand for "unclean" tasks.
- The **Jewish** Sabbath is from sundown on Friday until sundown on Saturday. The person may refuse to perform tasks that could be considered "work" on these days or on religious holidays (Passover, Rosh Hashanah, and Yom Kippur). Fasting and dietary changes may also take place at these times. Many Jewish persons follow a kosher diet. They refrain from eating pork. Some Jewish persons wear a small cap on their head or a prayer shawl. The Torah is their holy book.
- **Muslim (Islam)** prayers are conducted five times a day. The person may kneel or bend to the floor (see Fig. 7.7). The holy book for Muslims is the Koran (Qur'an). Muslims do not eat pork or consume alcohol. Many follow a vegetarian diet. They are very modest in their dress. Many prefer that care is offered by someone of their same gender. During Ramadan, Muslims refrain from food and drink from dawn until sundown. They may see pain as spiritually enhancing and may refuse pain medication. Following death, family members may wish to bathe the body and to turn the bed toward Mecca.
- **Buddhism** believes that suffering is an inevitable part of life. Reincarnation is also a belief. Cleanliness is important, and these individuals may refuse medications that affect their mental awareness. They may also prefer care from a same-gender caregiver. After death, they believe the spirit resides in the body for some time. It may be necessary to keep the body as still as possible and avoid moving for a certain period of time.

❓ TIME TO REFLECT

Mrs. Younes is from the Middle East. She is very modest and prefers to have her daughter assist her with bathing. Today you come to her room to take Mrs. Younes's vital signs. As you leave the room, her daughter stops you near the doorway. She tells you that she noticed a lump in her mother's right breast. Your charge nurse today is Robert Long, a male RN. What are some considerations with this situation? What should happen from here?

▌ REVIEW QUESTIONS

Circle the BEST answer.
1. Which is *false*?
   a. Culture influences health and illness practices
   b. Culture and religion influence food practices
   c. Cultural and religious practices are allowed in nursing centers
   d. A person must follow all beliefs and practices of a culture or religion
2. An extended family includes
   a. Parents and their children
   b. Grandparents and grandchildren
   c. Parents and their siblings
   d. Parents, their children, grandparents, aunts, uncles, and cousins

3. Which will *not* benefit a person of a different culture or religion?
   a. Being sensitive to the beliefs of the person
   b. If a person refuses a certain food, trying to tell him how nutritious it is
   c. Being patient and listening attentively
   d. Treating his religious objects with respect
4. A resident plans to leave the center Sunday morning to attend church with her daughter. Which is incorrect?
   a. Remind her of the time she will be picked up
   b. Assist her to the entrance where she will meet her daughter
   c. Tell the resident you have many people to help besides her
   d. Make sure she has the appropriate clothing for the weather conditions

5. You are assisting Mr. Miller with putting on his shoes. His pastor knocks on the door of his room. You should
   a. Ask the pastor to come back later
   b. Sit down and visit with Mr. Miller and his pastor
   c. Leave the room immediately
   d. Finish putting on Mr. Miller's shoes, make sure his call signal is within reach, and then leave so they can talk in private

6. You come to Mrs. Garland's room to help her get ready for bed. She is sitting in her chair praying the rosary. You should
   a. Ask her to set her rosary aside because it is time for bed
   b. Pretend you did not notice she was praying
   c. Tell her to call you when she is finished
   d. Ask another assistant to help her

7. Mrs. Santi is Catholic. Today she became unresponsive. Her son has been at her bedside all evening and is very concerned. When you arrive to reposition Mrs. Santi, her son says, "I wish a priest could be called to pray with us and give my mom the sacrament of the sick." Which response is best?
   a. Call the priest for the family
   b. Report this to the nurse immediately
   c. Tell the son that things may be better in the morning
   d. Make Mrs. Santi comfortable and report this at the end of your shift

8. Which religion does not permit the use of whole blood transfusions?
   a. Catholic
   b. Jehovah's Witness
   c. Lutheran
   d. Seventh-Day Adventist

9. Mr. Khan is a practicing Muslim. Which of the following is *false*?
   a. He may offer prayers five times a day
   b. He does not eat pork
   c. He reads from the Holy Bible
   d. He follows the scriptures of the Koran (Qur'an)

10. Which dietary regulations does someone of the Jewish faith follow?
    a. A kosher diet
    b. A vegetarian diet
    c. No alcohol
    d. A seafood diet

11. Mrs. Sanchez speaks only Spanish. Which of the following will not be helpful?
    a. Using gestures
    b. Finding an interpreter
    c. Speaking loudly
    d. Using pictures

12. Which is the largest organized religion in the United States?
    a. Christianity
    b. Judaism
    c. Islam
    d. Hinduism

13. Lack of eye contact
    a. Always signifies disrespect
    b. May be a sign of modesty
    c. Means the person is not paying attention
    d. Shows the person is rude

14. A resident always keeps his Bible on the bedside table. Which is *true*?
    a. When he is out of the room, place it in a drawer
    b. Nothing should be placed on top of it
    c. It should be kept on a bookshelf
    d. Let another resident borrow it

15. Gestures
    a. Mean the same in every culture
    b. Should never be used
    c. Can easily be misinterpreted
    d. Are always offensive

16. Mrs. Chen is from Thailand. As you assist her at admission you offer her a handshake. Instead of shaking your hand, she bows and folds her own hands. Which is *true*?
    a. Mrs. Chen is showing rude behavior
    b. You should feel ashamed for offering a handshake
    c. Joke about this situation with a coworker
    d. Mrs. Chen is practicing a greeting that reflects her culture

See Appendix A for answers to these questions.

8

Body Structure and Function

OBJECTIVES

- Define the key terms and key abbreviations listed in this chapter.
- Identify the basic structures of the cell.
- Explain how cells divide.

- Describe four types of tissue.
- Identify the structures of each body system.
- Identify the functions of each body system.
- Explain how to promote quality of life.

KEY TERMS

artery A blood vessel that carries blood away from the heart

capillary A tiny blood vessel; food, oxygen, and other substances pass from the capillaries into the cells

cell The basic unit of body structure

digestion The process of physically and chemically breaking down food so it can be absorbed for use by the cells

hemoglobin The substance in red blood cells that carries oxygen and gives blood its color

hormone A chemical substance secreted by the endocrine glands into the bloodstream

immunity Protection against a disease or condition; the person will not get or be affected by the disease

menstruation The process in which the lining of the uterus breaks up and is discharged from the body through the vagina

metabolism The burning of food for heat and energy by the cells

organ Groups of tissues with the same function

peristalsis Involuntary muscle contractions in the digestive system that move food down the esophagus through the alimentary canal

respiration The process of supplying the cells with oxygen and removing carbon dioxide from them

system Organs that work together to perform special functions

tissue A group of cells with similar functions

vein A blood vessel that returns blood to the heart

KEY ABBREVIATIONS

GI Gastrointestinal
RBC Red blood cell

WBC White blood cell

You help residents meet basic needs. Their bodies do not work at peak levels because of illness, disease, or injury. Your care promotes comfort, healing, and recovery. You need to know the body's normal structure and function. It will help you understand signs, symptoms, and the reasons for care and procedures. You will give safe and more efficient care.

See Chapter 9 for changes in body structure and function that occur with aging.

CELLS, TISSUES, AND ORGANS

The basic unit of body structure is the cell. Cells have the same basic structure. Function, size, and shape may differ. Cells are very small. You need a microscope to see them. Cells need food, water, and oxygen to live and function.

Fig. 8.1 shows the cell and its structures. The cell membrane is the outer covering. It encloses the cell and helps it hold its shape. The *nucleus* is the control center of the cell. It directs the cell's activities. The nucleus is in the center of the cell. The *cytoplasm* surrounds the nucleus. Cytoplasm contains smaller structures that perform cell functions. Protoplasm means "living substance." It refers to all structures, substances, and water within the cell. *Protoplasm* is a semiliquid substance much like an egg white.

Chromosomes are threadlike structures in the nucleus. Each cell has 46 chromosomes. Chromosomes contain genes. *Genes* control the traits children inherit from their parents. Height, eye color, and skin color are examples.

The nucleus controls cell reproduction. Cells reproduce by dividing in half. The process of cell division is called *mitosis*. It is needed for tissue growth and repair. During mitosis, the 46 chromosomes arrange themselves in 23 pairs. As the cell divides, the 23 pairs are pulled in half. The two new cells are identical. Each has 46 chromosomes (Fig. 8.2).

Cells are the body's building blocks. Groups of cells with similar functions combine to form tissues:

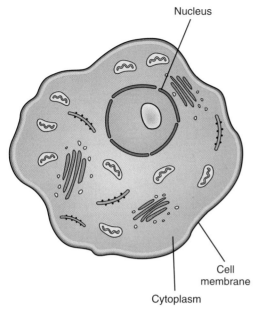

Fig. 8.1 Parts of a cell.

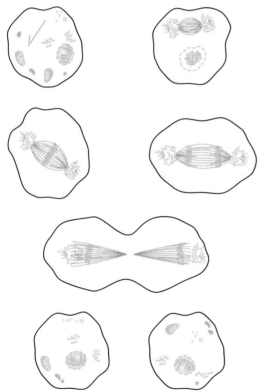

Fig. 8.2 Cell division.

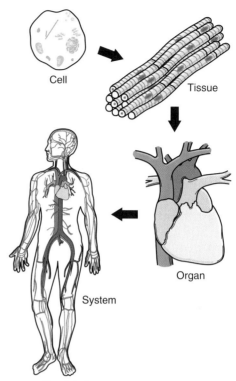

Fig. 8.3 Organization of the body.

- *Epithelial tissue* covers internal and external body surfaces. Tissue lining the nose, mouth, respiratory tract, stomach, and intestines is epithelial tissue. So are the skin, hair, nails, and glands.
- *Connective tissue* anchors, connects, and supports other tissues. It is in every part of the body. Bones, tendons, ligaments, and cartilage are connective tissue. Blood is a form of connective tissue.
- *Muscle tissue* stretches and contracts to let the body move.
- *Nerve tissue* receives and carries impulses to the brain and back to body parts.

Groups of tissue with the same function form organs. An organ has one or more functions. Examples of organs are the heart, brain, liver, lungs, and kidneys. Systems are formed by organs that work together to perform special functions (Fig. 8.3).

THE INTEGUMENTARY SYSTEM

The *integumentary system,* or *skin,* is the largest system. *Integument* means "covering." The skin covers the body. It has epithelial, connective, and nerve tissue. It also has oil glands and sweat glands. There are two skin layers (Fig. 8.4):
- The *epidermis* is the outer layer. It has living cells and dead cells. The dead cells were once deeper in the epidermis. They were pushed upward as the cells divided. Dead cells constantly flake off. They are replaced by living cells. Living cells also die and flake off. Living cells of the epidermis contain *pigment.* Pigment gives skin its color. The epidermis has no blood vessels and few nerve endings.
- The *dermis* is the inner layer. It is made up of connective tissue. Blood vessels, nerves, sweat glands, and oil glands are found in the dermis, as are hair roots.

The epidermis and dermis are supported by *subcutaneous tissue.* The subcutaneous tissue is a thick layer of fat and connective tissue.

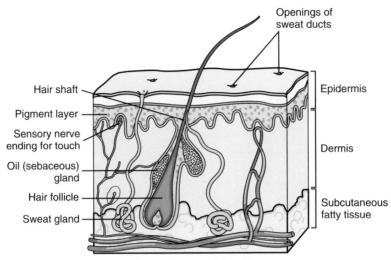

Fig. 8.4 Layers of the skin.

Oil glands and sweat glands, hair, and nails are skin appendages:

- *Hair*—covers the entire body, except the palms of the hands and the soles of the feet. Hair in the nose and ears and around the eyes protects these organs from dust, insects, and other foreign objects.
- *Nails*—protect the tips of the fingers and toes. Nails help fingers pick up and handle small objects.
- *Sweat glands*—help the body regulate temperature. Sweat consists of water, salt, and a small amount of wastes. Sweat is secreted through pores in the skin. The body is cooled as sweat evaporates.
- *Oil glands*—lie near the hair shafts. They secrete an oily substance into the space near the hair shaft. Oil travels to the skin surface. This helps keep the hair and skin soft and shiny.

The skin has many functions:

- It is the body's protective covering.
- It prevents microorganisms and other substances from entering the body.
- It prevents excess amounts of water from leaving the body.
- It protects organs from injury.
- Nerve endings in the skin sense both pleasant and unpleasant stimulation. Nerve endings are over the entire body. They sense cold, pain, touch, and pressure to protect the body from injury.
- It helps regulate body temperature. Blood vessels dilate (widen) when the temperature outside the body is high. More blood is brought to the body surface for cooling during evaporation. When blood vessels constrict (narrow), the body retains heat because less blood reaches the skin.

THE MUSCULOSKELETAL SYSTEM

The musculoskeletal system provides the framework for the body. It lets the body move. This system also protects and gives the body shape.

Bones

The human body has 206 bones (Fig. 8.5). There are four types of bones:

- *Long bones* bear the body's weight. Leg bones are long bones.
- *Short bones* allow skill and ease in movement. Bones in the wrists, fingers, ankles, and toes are short bones.
- *Flat bones* protect the organs. They include the ribs, skull, pelvic bones, and shoulder blades.
- *Irregular bones* are the vertebrae in the spinal column. They allow various degrees of movement and flexibility.

Bones are hard, rigid structures. They are made up of living cells. They are covered by a membrane called *periosteum*. Periosteum contains blood vessels that supply bone cells with oxygen and food. Inside the hollow centers of the bones is a substance called *bone marrow*. Blood cells are formed in the bone marrow.

Joints

A *joint* is the point at which two or more bones meet. Joints allow movement (Chapter 24). *Cartilage* is the connective tissue at the end of the long bones. It cushions the joint so that the bone ends do not rub together. The *synovial membrane* lines the joints. It secretes *synovial fluid*. Synovial fluid acts as a lubricant so the joint can move smoothly. Bones are held together at the joint by strong bands of connective tissue called *ligaments*.

There are three major types of joints (Fig. 8.6):

- *Ball-and-socket joint* allows movement in all directions. It is made up of the rounded end of one bone and the hollow end of another bone. The rounded end of one fits into the hollow end of the other. The joints of the hips and shoulders are ball-and-socket joints.
- *Hinge joint* allows movement in one direction. The elbow is a hinge joint.
- *Pivot joint* allows turning from side to side. A pivot joint connects the skull to the spine.

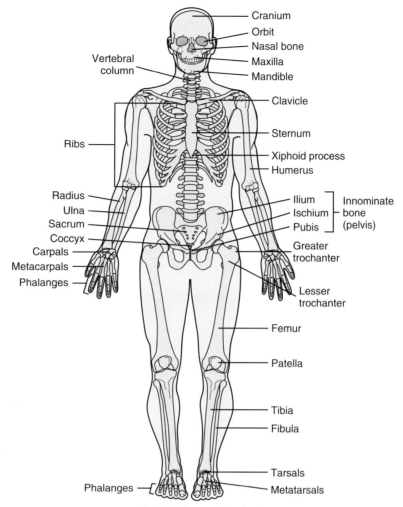

Fig. 8.5 Bones of the body.

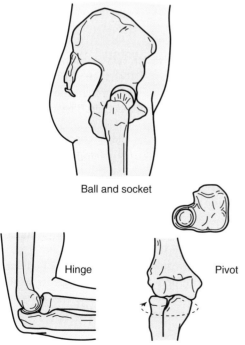

Ball and socket

Hinge   Pivot

Fig. 8.6 Types of joints.

Muscles

The human body has more than 500 muscles (Figs. 8.7 and 8.8). Some are voluntary; others are involuntary:

- *Voluntary muscles* can be consciously controlled. Muscles attached to bones *(skeletal muscles)* are voluntary. Arm muscles do not work unless you move your arm; likewise for leg muscles. Skeletal muscles are *striated*. That is, they look striped or streaked.
- *Involuntary muscles* work automatically. You cannot control them. They control the action of the stomach, intestines, blood vessels, and other body organs. Involuntary muscles also are called *smooth muscles.* They look smooth, not streaked or striped.
- *Cardiac muscle* is in the heart. It is an involuntary muscle. However, it appears striated like skeletal muscle.

Muscles have three functions:

- Movement of body parts
- Maintenance of posture
- Production of body heat

Strong, tough connective tissues called *tendons* connect muscles to bones. When muscles contract (shorten), tendons at

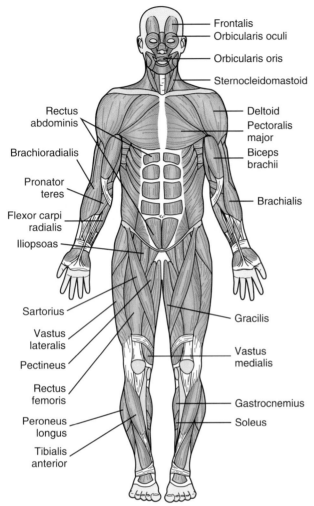

Fig. 8.7 Anterior view of the muscles of the body.

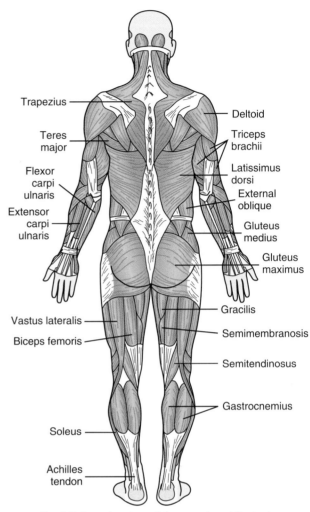

Fig. 8.8 Posterior view of the muscles of the body.

each end of the muscle cause the bone to move. The body has many tendons. See the Achilles tendon in Fig. 8.8. Some muscles constantly contract to maintain the body's posture. When muscles contract, they burn food for energy. Heat is produced. The more muscle activity, the greater the amount of heat produced. Shivering is how the body produces heat when exposed to cold. Shivering is from rapid, general muscle contractions.

THE NERVOUS SYSTEM

The nervous system controls, directs, and coordinates body functions. Its two main divisions are:
- The *central nervous system* (CNS). It consists of the brain and spinal cord (Fig. 8.9).
- The *peripheral nervous system*. It involves the *nerves* throughout the body (Fig. 8.10).

Nerves carry messages or impulses to and from the brain. Nerves connect to the spinal cord. They are easily damaged and take a long time to heal. Some nerve fibers have a protective covering called a *myelin sheath.* The myelin sheath also insulates the nerve fiber. Nerve fibers covered with myelin conduct impulses faster than those fibers without it.

The Central Nervous System

The *brain* and *spinal cord* make up the CNS. The brain is covered by the skull. The three main parts of the brain are the *cerebrum,* the *cerebellum,* and the *brainstem* (Fig. 8.11).

The cerebrum is the largest part of the brain. It is the center of thought and intelligence. The cerebrum is divided into two halves called the *right* and *left hemispheres.* The right hemisphere controls movement and activities on the body's left side. The left hemisphere controls the right side.

The outside of the cerebrum is called the *cerebral cortex.* It controls the highest functions of the brain. These include reasoning, memory, consciousness, speech, voluntary muscle movement, vision, hearing, sensation, and other activities.

The cerebellum regulates and coordinates body movements. It controls balance and the smooth movements of voluntary muscles. Injury to the cerebellum results in jerky movements, loss of coordination, and muscle weakness.

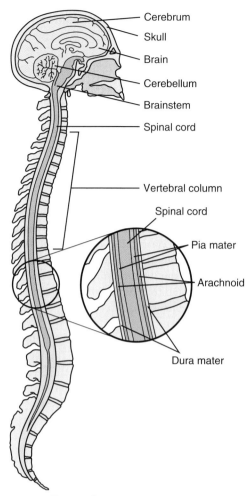

Fig. 8.9 Central nervous system.

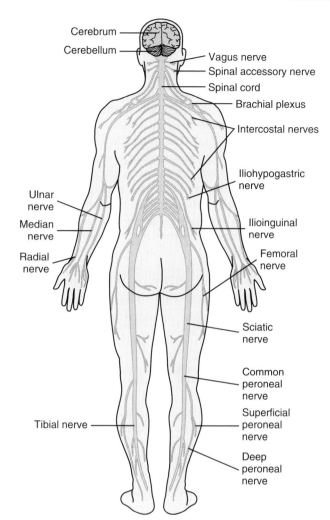

Fig. 8.10 Peripheral nervous system.

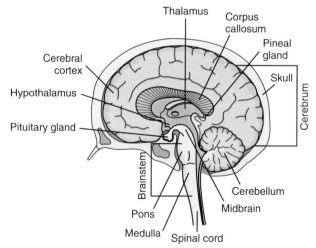

Fig. 8.11 The brain.

The brainstem connects the cerebrum to the spinal cord. The brainstem contains the *midbrain, pons,* and *medulla.* The midbrain and pons relay messages between the medulla and the cerebrum. The medulla is below the pons. The medulla controls heart rate, breathing, blood vessel size, swallowing, coughing, and vomiting. The brain connects to the spinal cord at the lower end of the medulla.

The spinal cord lies within the spinal column. The cord is 17 to 18 inches long. It contains pathways that conduct messages to and from the brain.

The brain and spinal cord are covered and protected by three layers of connective tissue called meninges:

- The outer layer lies next to the skull. It is a tough covering called the *dura mater.*
- The middle layer is the *arachnoid.*
- The inner layer is the *pia mater.*

The space between the middle layer (arachnoid) and inner layer (pia mater) is the *arachnoid space.* The space is filled with *cerebrospinal fluid.* It circulates around the brain and spinal cord. Cerebrospinal fluid protects the CNS. It cushions shocks that could easily injure brain and spinal cord structures.

The Peripheral Nervous System

The peripheral nervous system has 12 pairs of *cranial nerves* and 31 pairs of *spinal nerves.* Cranial nerves conduct impulses

between the brain and the head, neck, chest, and abdomen. They conduct impulses for smell, vision, hearing, pain, touch, temperature, and pressure. They also conduct impulses for voluntary and involuntary muscles. Spinal nerves carry impulses from the skin, extremities, and the internal structures not supplied by cranial nerves.

Some peripheral nerves form the *autonomic nervous system.* This system controls involuntary muscles and certain body functions. The functions include the heartbeat, blood pressure, intestinal contractions, and glandular secretions. These functions occur automatically.

The autonomic nervous system is divided into the *sympathetic nervous system* and the *parasympathetic nervous system.* They balance each other. The sympathetic nervous system speeds up functions. The parasympathetic nervous system slows functions. When you are angry, scared, excited, or exercising, the sympathetic nervous system is stimulated. The parasympathetic system is activated when you relax or when the sympathetic system is stimulated for too long.

The Sense Organs

The five senses are *sight, hearing, taste, smell,* and *touch.* Receptors for taste are in the tongue. They are called *taste buds.* Receptors for smell are in the nose. Touch receptors are in the dermis, especially in the toes and fingertips.

The Eye

Receptors for vision are in the *eyes* (Fig. 8.12). The eye is easily injured. Bones of the skull, eyelids and eyelashes, and tears protect the eyes from injury. The eye has three layers:

- The *sclera,* the white of the eye, is the outer layer. It is made of tough connective tissue.
- The *choroid* is the second layer. Blood vessels, the *ciliary muscle,* and the *iris* make up the choroid. The iris gives the eye its color. The opening in the middle of the iris is the *pupil.* Pupil size varies with the amount of light entering the eye. The pupil constricts (narrows) in bright light. It dilates (widens) in dim or dark places.
- The *retina* is the inner layer. It has receptors for vision and the nerve fibers of the *optic nerve.*

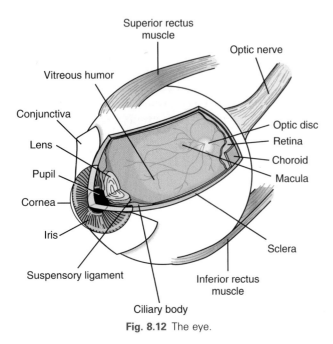

Fig. 8.12 The eye.

Light enters the eye through the *cornea.* It is the transparent part of the outer layer that lies over the eye. Light rays pass to the *lens,* which lies behind the pupil. The light is then reflected to the retina. Light is carried to the brain by the optic nerve.

The *aqueous chamber* separates the cornea from the lens. The chamber is filled with a fluid called *aqueous humor.* The fluid helps the cornea keep its shape and position. The *vitreous humor* is behind the lens. It is a gelatin-like substance that supports the retina and maintains the eye's shape.

The Ear

The *ear* is a sense organ (Fig. 8.13). It functions in hearing and balance. It has three parts: *external ear, middle ear,* and *inner ear.*

The external (outer) ear is called the *pinna* or *auricle.* Sound waves are guided through the external ear into the *auditory canal.* Glands in the auditory canal secrete a waxy substance called *cerumen.* The auditory canal extends about 1 inch to the *eardrum.* The eardrum *(tympanic membrane)* separates the external and middle ear.

The middle ear is a small space. It contains the *eustachian tube* and three small bones called *ossicles.* The eustachian tube connects the middle ear and the throat. Air enters the eustachian tube so that there is equal pressure on both sides of the eardrum. The ossicles amplify sound received from the eardrum and transmit the sound to the inner ear. The three ossicles are:

- The *malleus.* It looks like a hammer.
- The *incus.* It looks like an anvil.
- The *stapes.* It is shaped like a stirrup.

The inner ear consists of *semicircular canals* and the *cochlea.* The cochlea looks like a snail shell. It contains fluid. The fluid carries sound waves from the middle ear to the *acoustic nerve.* The acoustic nerve then carries the message to the brain.

The three semicircular canals are involved with balance. They sense the head's position and changes in position. They send messages to the brain.

THE CIRCULATORY SYSTEM

The circulatory system is made up of the *blood, heart,* and *blood vessels.* The heart pumps blood through the blood vessels. The circulatory system has many functions:

- Blood carries food, oxygen, and other substances to the cells.
- Blood removes waste products from the cells.
- Blood and blood vessels help regulate body temperature. The blood carries heat from muscle activity to other body parts. Blood vessels in the skin dilate to cool the body. They constrict to retain heat.
- The system produces and carries cells that defend the body from microbes that cause disease.

The Blood

The blood consists of blood cells and *plasma.* Plasma is mostly water. It carries blood cells to other body cells. Plasma also carries substances that cells need to function. This includes

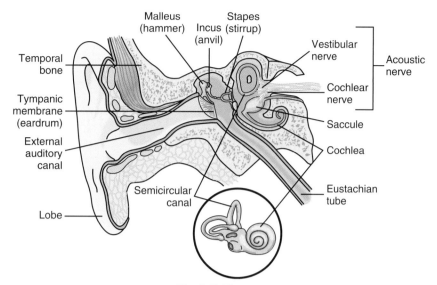

Fig. 8.13 The ear.

food (proteins, fats, and carbohydrates), hormones (p. ··), and chemicals.

Red blood cells (RBCs) are called *erythrocytes.* They give blood its red color because of a substance in the RBC called hemoglobin. As RBCs circulate through the lungs, hemoglobin picks up oxygen. Hemoglobin carries oxygen to the cells. When blood is bright red, hemoglobin in the RBCs is saturated (filled) with oxygen. As blood circulates through the body, oxygen is given to the cells. Cells release carbon dioxide (a waste product). It is picked up by the hemoglobin. RBCs saturated with carbon dioxide make the blood look dark red.

The body has about 25 trillion (25,000,000,000,000) RBCs. About 4.5 to 5 million cells are in 1 cubic millimeter of blood (the size of a tiny drop). RBCs live for 3 to 4 months. They are destroyed by the liver and spleen as they wear out. New RBCs are formed in the bone marrow. About 1 million RBCs are produced every second.

White blood cells (WBCs) are called *leukocytes.* They have no color. They protect the body against infection. There are about 5000 to 10,000 WBCs in 1 cubic millimeter of blood. At the first sign of infection, WBCs rush to the infection site. There they multiply rapidly. The number of WBCs increases when there is an infection. WBCs are formed by the bone marrow. They live about 9 days.

Platelets (thrombocytes) are needed for blood clotting. They are formed by the bone marrow. There are about 200,000 to 400,000 platelets in 1 cubic millimeter of blood. A platelet lives about 4 days.

The Heart

The heart is a muscle. It pumps blood through the blood vessels to the tissues and cells. The heart lies in the middle to lower part of the chest cavity toward the left side (Fig. 8.14). The heart is hollow and has three layers (Fig. 8.15):

- The *pericardium* is the outer layer. It is a thin sac covering the heart.

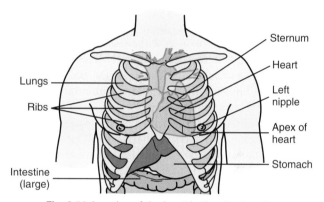

Fig. 8.14 Location of the heart in the chest cavity.

- The *myocardium* is the second layer. It is the thick, muscular part of the heart.
- The *endocardium* is the inner layer. A membrane, it lines the inner surface of the heart.

The heart has four chambers (see Fig. 8.15). Upper chambers receive blood and are called *atria.* The *right atrium* receives blood from body tissues. The *left atrium* receives blood from the lungs. Lower chambers are called *ventricles.* Ventricles pump blood. The *right ventricle* pumps blood to the lungs for oxygen. The *left ventricle* pumps blood to all parts of the body.

Valves are between the atria and ventricles. The valves allow blood flow in one direction. They prevent blood from flowing back into the atria from the ventricles. The *tricuspid valve* is between the right atrium and the right ventricle. The *mitral valve (bicuspid valve)* is between the left atrium and left ventricle.

Heart action has two phases:
- *Diastole* is the resting phase. Heart chambers fill with blood.
- *Systole* is the working phase. The heart contracts. Blood is pumped through the blood vessels when the heart contracts.

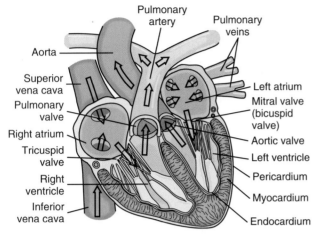

Fig. 8.15 Structures of the heart.

The Blood Vessels

Blood flows to body tissues and cells through the blood vessels. There are three groups of blood vessels: arteries, capillaries, and veins.

Arteries carry blood away from the heart. Arterial blood is rich in oxygen. The *aorta* is the largest artery. It receives blood directly from the left ventricle. The aorta branches into other arteries that carry blood to all parts of the body (Fig. 8.16). These arteries branch into smaller parts within the tissues. The smallest branch of an artery is an *arteriole*.

Arterioles connect to capillaries. Capillaries are very tiny blood vessels. Food, oxygen, and other substances pass from capillaries into the cells. The capillaries pick up waste products (including carbon dioxide) from the cells. Veins carry waste products back to the heart.

Veins return blood to the heart. They connect to the capillaries by *venules*. Venules are small veins. Venules branch together to form veins. The many veins also branch together as they near the heart to form two main veins (see Fig. 8.16). The two main veins are the *inferior vena cava* and the *superior vena cava*. Both empty into the right atrium. The inferior vena cava carries blood from the legs and trunk. The superior vena cava carries blood from the head and arms. Venous blood is dark red. It has little oxygen and a lot of carbon dioxide.

Blood flow through the circulatory system is shown in Fig. 8.15. The path of blood flow is as follows:

- Venous blood, poor in oxygen, empties into the right atrium.
- Blood flows through the tricuspid valve into the right ventricle.
- The right ventricle pumps blood into the lungs to pick up oxygen.
- Oxygen-rich blood from the lungs enters the left atrium.
- Blood from the left atrium passes through the mitral valve into the left ventricle.
- The left ventricle pumps the blood to the aorta. It branches off to form other arteries.
- Arterial blood is carried to the tissues by arterioles and to the cells by capillaries.

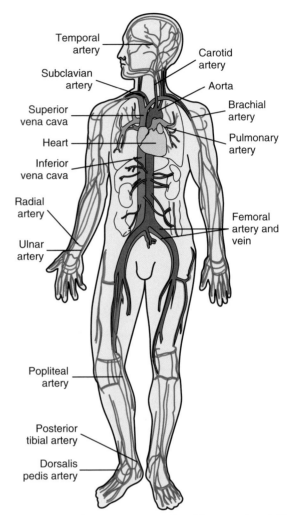

Fig. 8.16 Arterial and venous systems. Arterial system is red. Venous system is blue.

- Cells and capillaries exchange oxygen and nutrients for carbon dioxide and waste products.
- Capillaries connect with venules.
- Venules carry blood that has carbon dioxide and waste products.
- Venules form veins.
- Veins return blood to the heart.

THE RESPIRATORY SYSTEM

Oxygen is needed to live. Every cell needs oxygen. Air contains about 21% oxygen. This meets the body's needs under normal conditions. The respiratory system (Fig. 8.17) brings oxygen into the lungs and removes carbon dioxide. Respiration is the process of supplying the cells with oxygen and removing carbon dioxide from them. Respiration involves *inhalation* (breathing in) and *exhalation* (breathing out). The terms *inspiration* (breathing in) and *expiration* (breathing out) also are used.

Air enters the body through the *nose*. The air then passes into the *pharynx* (throat). It is a tube-shaped passageway for air and food. Air passes from the pharynx into the *larynx* (voice

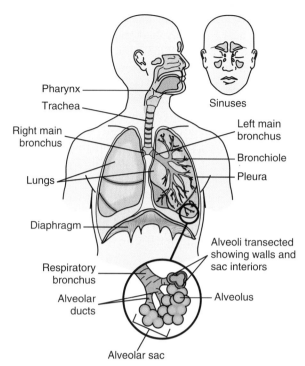

Fig. 8.17 Respiratory system.

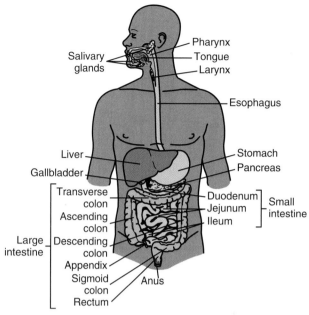

Fig. 8.18 Digestive system.

box). A piece of cartilage, the *epiglottis*, acts like a lid over the larynx. The epiglottis prevents food from entering the airway during swallowing. During inhalation the epiglottis lifts up to let air pass over the larynx. Air passes from the larynx into the *trachea* (windpipe).

The trachea divides at its lower end into the *right bronchus* and the *left bronchus*. Each bronchus enters a lung. Upon entering the lungs, the bronchi divide many times into smaller branches. The smaller branches are called *bronchioles*. Eventually the bronchioles subdivide. They end up in tiny one-celled air sacs called *alveoli*.

Alveoli look like small clusters of grapes. They are supplied by capillaries. Oxygen and carbon dioxide are exchanged between the alveoli and capillaries. Blood in the capillaries picks up oxygen from the alveoli. Then the blood is returned to the left side of the heart and pumped to the rest of the body. Alveoli pick up carbon dioxide from the capillaries for exhalation.

The lungs are spongy tissues. They are filled with alveoli, blood vessels, and nerves. Each lung is divided into lobes. The right lung has three lobes; the left lung has two. The lungs are separated from the abdominal cavity by a muscle called the *diaphragm*.

Each lung is covered by a two-layered sac called the *pleura*. One layer is attached to the lung and the other to the chest wall. The pleura secretes a very thin fluid that fills the space between the layers. The fluid prevents the layers from rubbing together during inhalation and exhalation. A bony framework made up of the ribs, sternum, and vertebrae protects the lungs.

THE DIGESTIVE SYSTEM

The digestive system breaks down food physically and chemically so it can be absorbed for use by the cells. This process is called digestion. The digestive system is also called the *gastrointestinal (GI) system.* The system also removes solid wastes from the body.

The digestive system involves the *alimentary canal (GI tract)* and the accessory organs of digestion (Fig. 8.18). The alimentary canal is a long tube. It extends from the mouth to the anus. Its major parts are the mouth, pharynx, esophagus, stomach, small intestine, and large intestine. Accessory organs are the teeth, tongue, salivary glands, liver, gallbladder, and pancreas.

Digestion begins in the *mouth.* The mouth also is called the *oral cavity.* It receives food and prepares it for digestion. Using chewing motions, the *teeth* cut, chop, and grind food into small particles for digestion and swallowing. The *tongue* aids in chewing and swallowing. Taste buds on the tongue's surface contain nerve endings. Taste buds allow sweet, sour, bitter, and salty tastes to be sensed. *Salivary glands* in the mouth secrete *saliva.* Saliva moistens food particles to ease swallowing and begin digestion. During swallowing, the tongue pushes food into the *pharynx.*

The pharynx (throat) is a muscular tube. Swallowing continues as the pharynx contracts. Contraction of the pharynx pushes food into the *esophagus.* The esophagus is a muscular tube about 10 inches long. It extends from the pharynx to the *stomach.* Involuntary muscle contractions called peristalsis move food down the esophagus through the alimentary canal.

The stomach is a muscular, pouchlike sac. It is in the upper left part of the abdominal cavity. Strong stomach muscles stir and churn food to break it up into even smaller particles. A mucous membrane lines the stomach. It contains glands that secrete *gastric juices.* Food is mixed and churned with the gastric juices to form a semiliquid substance called *chyme.* Through peristalsis, the chyme is pushed from the stomach into the small intestine.

The *small intestine* is about 20 feet long. It has three parts. The first part is the *duodenum*. There, more digestive juices are added to the chyme. One is called *bile*. Bile is a greenish liquid made in the *liver*. Bile is stored in the *gallbladder*. Juices from the *pancreas* and small intestine are added to the chyme. Digestive juices chemically break down food so it can be absorbed.

Peristalsis moves the chyme through the two other parts of the small intestine: the *jejunum* and the *ileum*. Tiny projections called *villi* line the small intestine. Villi absorb the digested food into the capillaries. Most food absorption takes place in the jejunum and the ileum.

Some chyme is not digested. Undigested chyme passes from the small intestine into the *large intestine (large bowel* or *colon)*. The colon absorbs most of the water from the chyme. The remaining semisolid material is called *feces*. Feces contain a small amount of water, solid wastes, and some mucus and germs. These are the waste products of digestion. Feces pass through the colon into the *rectum* by peristalsis. Feces pass out of the body through the *anus*.

THE URINARY SYSTEM

The digestive system rids the body of solid wastes. The lungs rid the body of carbon dioxide. Water and other substances leave the body through sweat. There are other waste products in the blood from cells burning food for energy. The urinary system (Fig. 8.19):

- Removes waste products from the blood.
- Maintains water balance within the body.

The *kidneys* are two bean-shaped organs in the upper abdomen. They lie against the back muscles on each side of the spine. They are protected by the lower edge of the rib cage.

Each kidney has over 1 million tiny *nephrons* (Fig. 8.20). Each nephron is the basic working unit of the kidney. Each nephron has a *convoluted tubule*, which is a tiny coiled tubule. Each convoluted tubule has a *Bowman capsule* at one end. The capsule partly surrounds a cluster of capillaries called a *glomerulus*. Blood passes through the glomerulus and is filtered by the capillaries. The fluid part of the blood is squeezed into the Bowman capsule. The fluid then passes into the tubule. Most of the water and other needed substances are reabsorbed by the blood. The rest of the fluid and the waste products form *urine* in the tubule. Urine flows through the tubule to a *collecting tubule*. All collecting tubules drain into the *renal pelvis* in the kidney.

A tube, called the *ureter*, is attached to the renal pelvis of the kidney. Each ureter is about 10 to 12 inches long. The ureters carry urine from the kidneys to the *bladder*. The bladder is a hollow, muscular sac. It lies toward the front in the lower part of the abdominal cavity.

Urine is stored in the bladder until the need to urinate is felt. This usually occurs when there is about a half pint (250 milliliters [mL]) of urine in the bladder. Urine passes from the bladder through the *urethra*. The opening at the end of the urethra is the *meatus*. Urine passes from the body through the meatus. Urine is a clear, yellowish fluid.

THE REPRODUCTIVE SYSTEM

Human reproduction results from the union of a male sex cell and a female sex cell. The male and female reproductive systems are different. This allows for the process of reproduction.

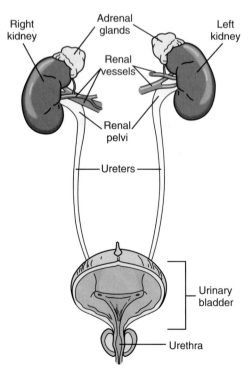

Fig. 8.19 Urinary system.

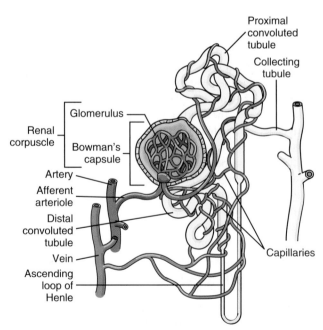

Fig. 8.20 A nephron.

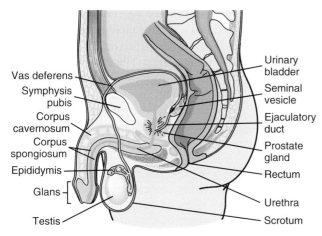

Fig. 8.21 Male reproductive system.

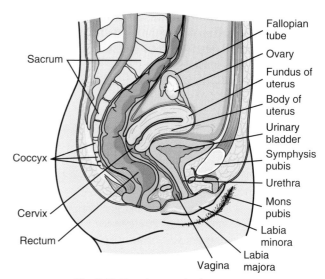

Fig. 8.22 Female reproductive system.

The Male Reproductive System

The male reproductive system is shown in Fig. 8.21. The *testes (testicles)* are the male sex glands. Sex glands also are called *gonads.* The two testes are oval or almond-shaped glands. Male sex cells are produced in the testes. Male sex cells are called *sperm* cells.

Testosterone, the male hormone, is produced in the testes. This hormone is needed for reproductive organ function. It also is needed for the development of the male secondary sex characteristics that include facial hair; pubic and axillary (underarm) hair; arm, chest, and leg hair; and increased neck and shoulder sizes.

The testes are suspended between the thighs in a sac called the *scrotum.* The scrotum is made of skin and muscle.

Sperm travel from a testis to the *epididymis.* The epididymis is a coiled tube on top and to the side of the testis. From the epididymis, sperm travel through a tube called the *vas deferens.* Each vas deferens joins a seminal vesicle. The two seminal vesicles store sperm and produce *semen.* Semen is a fluid that carries sperm from the male reproductive tract. The ducts of the seminal vesicles unite to form the *ejaculatory duct.* It passes through the *prostate gland.*

The prostate gland lies just below the bladder. It is shaped like a donut. The gland secretes fluid into the semen. As the ejaculatory ducts leave the prostate, they join the *urethra.* The urethra runs through the prostate gland. The urethra is the outlet for urine and semen. The urethra is contained within the *penis.*

The penis is outside of the body and has *erectile* tissue. When a man is sexually excited, blood fills the erectile tissue. The penis enlarges and becomes hard and erect. The erect penis can enter a female's vagina. The semen, which contains sperm, is released into the vagina.

The Female Reproductive System

Fig. 8.22 shows the female reproductive system. The female gonads are two almond-shaped glands called *ovaries.* An ovary is on each side of the uterus in the abdominal cavity.

The ovaries contain *ova* or eggs. Ova are the female sex cells. One ovum (egg) is released monthly during the woman's reproductive years. Release of an ovum is called *ovulation.*

The ovaries secrete the female hormones *estrogen* and *progesterone.* These hormones are needed for reproductive system function. They also are needed for the development of secondary sex characteristics in the female. These include increased breast size, pubic and axillary (underarm) hair, slight deepening of the voice, and widening and rounding of the hips.

When an ovum is released from an ovary, it travels through a *fallopian tube.* There are two fallopian tubes, one on each side. The tubes are attached at one end to the uterus. The ovum travels through the fallopian tube to the *uterus.*

The *uterus* is a hollow, muscular organ shaped like a pear. It is in the center of the pelvic cavity behind the bladder and in front of the rectum. The main part of the uterus is the *fundus.* The neck or narrow section of the uterus is the *cervix.* Tissue lining the uterus is called the *endometrium.* The endometrium has many blood vessels. If sex cells from the male and female unite into one cell, that cell implants into the endometrium. There the cell grows into a baby. The uterus serves as a place for the *fetus* (unborn baby) to grow and receive nourishment.

The cervix of the uterus projects into a muscular canal called the *vagina.* The vagina opens to the outside of the body. It is just behind the urethra. The vagina receives the penis during intercourse. It also is part of the birth canal. Glands in the vaginal wall keep it moistened with secretions. In young girls, the external vaginal opening is partially closed by a membrane called the *hymen.* The hymen ruptures when the female has intercourse for the first time.

The external female genitalia are called the *vulva* (Fig. 8.23):

* The *mons pubis* is a rounded, fatty pad over a bone called the *symphysis pubis.* The mons pubis is covered with hair in the adult female.
* The *labia majora* and *labia minora* are two folds of tissue on each side of the vaginal opening.
* The *clitoris* is a small organ composed of erectile tissue. It becomes hard when sexually stimulated.

The *mammary glands (breasts)* secrete milk after childbirth. The glands are on the outside of the chest. They are made up of glandular tissue and fat (Fig. 8.24). The milk drains into ducts that open onto the *nipple.*

Menstruation

The endometrium is rich in blood to nourish the cell that grows into a fetus. If pregnancy does not occur, the endometrium breaks up. It is discharged from the body through the vagina. This process is called menstruation. Menstruation occurs about every 28 days. Therefore it is called the *menstrual cycle.*

The first day of the menstrual cycle begins with menstruation. Blood flows from the uterus through the vaginal opening. Menstrual flow usually lasts 3 to 7 days. Ovulation occurs during the next phase. An ovum matures in an ovary and is released. Ovulation usually occurs on or about day 14 of the cycle.

Meanwhile, estrogen and progesterone (the female hormones) are secreted by the ovaries. These hormones cause the endometrium to thicken for pregnancy. If pregnancy does not occur, the hormones decrease in amount. This causes the blood supply to the endometrium to decrease. The endometrium breaks up. It is discharged through the vagina. Another menstrual cycle begins.

Fertilization

To reproduce, a male sex cell (sperm) must unite with a female sex cell (ovum). The uniting of the sperm and ovum into one cell is called *fertilization.* A sperm has 23 chromosomes. An ovum has 23 chromosomes. When the two cells unite, the fertilized cell has 46 chromosomes.

During intercourse, millions of sperm are deposited into the vagina. Sperm travel up the cervix, through the uterus, and into the fallopian tubes. If a sperm and an ovum unite in a fallopian tube, fertilization results. Pregnancy occurs. The fertilized cell travels down the fallopian tube to the uterus. After a short time, the fertilized cell implants in the thick endometrium and grows during pregnancy.

THE ENDOCRINE SYSTEM

The endocrine system is made up of glands called the *endocrine glands* (Fig. 8.25). The endocrine glands secrete chemical substances called hormones into the bloodstream. Hormones regulate the activities of other organs and glands in the body.

The *pituitary gland* is called the *master gland.* About the size of a cherry, it is at the base of the brain behind the eyes. The

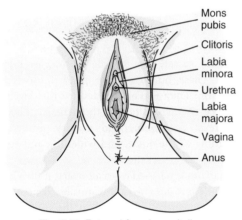

Fig. 8.23 External female genitalia.

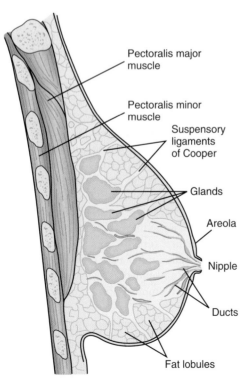

Fig. 8.24 The female breast.

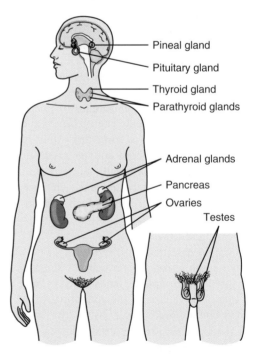

Fig. 8.25 Endocrine system.

pituitary gland is divided into the *anterior pituitary lobe* and the *posterior pituitary lobe.* The anterior pituitary lobe secretes:

- *Growth hormone (GH)*—needed for growth of muscles, bones, and other organs. It is needed throughout life to maintain normal-sized bones and muscles. Growth is stunted if a baby is born with deficient amounts of growth hormone. Too much of the hormone causes excessive growth.
- *Thyroid-stimulating hormone (TSH)*—needed for thyroid gland function.
- *Adrenocorticotropic hormone (ACTH)*—stimulates the adrenal gland.

The anterior lobe also secretes hormones that regulate growth, development, and function of the male and female reproductive systems.

The posterior pituitary lobe secretes *antidiuretic hormone (ADH)* and *oxytocin.* ADH prevents the kidneys from excreting excessive amounts of water. Oxytocin causes uterine muscles to contract during childbirth.

The *thyroid gland,* shaped like a butterfly, is in the neck in front of the larynx. *Thyroid hormone (TH, thyroxine)* is secreted by the thyroid gland. It regulates metabolism. Metabolism is the burning of food for heat and energy by the cells. Too little TH results in slowed body processes, slowed movements, and weight gain. Too much TH causes increased metabolism, excess energy, and weight loss. Some babies are born with deficient amounts of TH. Their physical growth and mental growth are stunted.

The four *parathyroid glands* secrete *parathyroid hormone.* Two lie on each side of the thyroid gland. parathyroid hormone regulates calcium use. Calcium is needed for nerve and muscle function. Insufficient amounts of calcium cause *tetany.* Tetany is a state of severe muscle contraction and spasm. If untreated, tetany can cause death.

There are two *adrenal glands.* An adrenal gland is on the top of each kidney. The adrenal gland has two parts: the *adrenal medulla* and the *adrenal cortex.* The adrenal medulla secretes *epinephrine* and *norepinephrine.* These hormones stimulate the body to quickly produce energy during emergencies. Heart rate, blood pressure, muscle power, and energy all increase.

The adrenal cortex secretes three groups of hormones needed for life:

- *Glucocorticoids*—regulate the metabolism of carbohydrates. They also control the body's response to stress and inflammation.
- *Mineralocorticoids*—regulate the amount of salt and water that is absorbed and lost by the kidneys.
- Small amounts of *male and female sex hormones*—pp. ·· and · · ·.

The *pancreas* secretes *insulin.* Insulin regulates the amount of sugar in the blood available for use by the cells. Insulin is needed for sugar to enter the cells. If there is too little insulin, sugar cannot enter the cells. If sugar cannot enter the cells, excess amounts of sugar build up in the blood. This condition is called *diabetes.*

The *gonads* are the glands of human reproduction. Male sex glands (testes) secrete *testosterone.* Female sex glands (ovaries) secrete *estrogen* and *progesterone.*

THE IMMUNE SYSTEM

The immune system protects the body from disease and infection. Abnormal body cells can grow into tumors. Sometimes the body produces substances that cause the body to attack itself. Microorganisms (bacteria, viruses, and other germs) can cause an infection. The immune system defends against threats inside and outside the body.

The immune system gives the body immunity. Immunity means that a person has protection against a disease or condition. The person will not get or be affected by the disease. There are two types of immunity:

- *Specific immunity* is the body's reaction to a certain threat.
- *Nonspecific immunity* is the body's reaction to anything it does not recognize as a normal body substance.

Special cells and substances function to produce immunity:

- *Antibodies*—normal body substances that recognize other substances. They are involved in destroying abnormal or unwanted substances.
- *Antigens*—substances that cause an immune response. Antibodies recognize and bind with unwanted antigens. This leads to the destruction of unwanted substances and the production of more antibodies.
- *Phagocytes*—WBCs that digest and destroy microorganisms and other unwanted substances.
- *Lymphocytes*—WBCs that produce antibodies. Lymphocyte production increases as the body responds to an infection.
- *B lymphocytes (B cells)*—cause the production of antibodies that circulate in the plasma. The antibodies react to specific antigens.
- *T lymphocytes (T cells)*—cells that destroy invading cells. *Killer T cells* produce poisons near the invading cells. Some T cells attract other cells. The other cells destroy the invaders.

When the body senses an antigen from an unwanted substance, the immune system acts. Phagocyte and lymphocyte production increases. Phagocytes destroy the invaders through digestion. The lymphocytes produce antibodies that identify and destroy the unwanted substances.

🧍 QUALITY OF LIFE

The human body is made up of systems. Each has its own structures and functions. The systems are related to and depend on each other to properly function and survive. Injury or disease of one part of a system affects the entire system and the whole body.

Basic knowledge of the body's normal structure and function should result in safe, quality care. It will help you better understand the reasons for the care you give. Always treat the person and the person's body with dignity and respect.

❓ TIME TO REFLECT

Ms. Chapman is suffering from a lung infection. The nurse tells you that blood will be drawn from her to check the WBC count. What is another name for a white blood cell? Would you expect this result to be elevated? What is the significance of obtaining accurate vital signs for Ms. Chapman? What other measures will you likely perform to help Ms. Chapman improve?

REVIEW QUESTIONS

Circle the BEST answer.

1. The basic unit of body structure is the
   a. Cell
   b. Neuron
   c. Nephron
   d. Ovum
2. The outer layer of the skin is called the
   a. Dermis
   b. Epidermis
   c. Integument
   d. Myelin
3. Which is *not* a function of the skin?
   a. Provides the protective covering for the body
   b. Regulates body temperature
   c. Senses cold, pain, touch, and pressure
   d. Provides the shape and framework for the body
4. Skeletal muscles
   a. Are under involuntary control
   b. Appear smooth
   c. Are under voluntary control
   d. Appear striped and smooth
5. The highest functions in the brain take place in the
   a. Cerebral cortex
   b. Medulla
   c. Brainstem
   d. Spinal nerves
6. The ear is involved with
   a. Regulating body movements
   b. Balance
   c. Smoothness of body movements
   d. Controlling involuntary muscles
7. The liquid part of the blood is the
   a. Hemoglobin
   b. Red blood cell
   c. Plasma
   d. White blood cell
8. Which part of the heart pumps blood to the body?
   a. Right atrium
   b. Left atrium
   c. Right ventricle
   d. Left ventricle
9. Which carry blood away from the heart?
   a. Capillaries
   b. Veins
   c. Venules
   d. Arteries
10. Oxygen and carbon dioxide are exchanged
    a. In the bronchi
    b. Between the alveoli and capillaries
    c. Between the lungs and pleura
    d. In the trachea
11. Digestion begins in the
    a. Mouth
    b. Stomach
    c. Small intestine
    d. Colon
12. Most food absorption takes place in the
    a. Stomach
    b. Small intestine
    c. Colon
    d. Large intestine
13. Urine is formed by the
    a. Jejunum
    b. Kidneys
    c. Bladder
    d. Liver
14. Urine passes from the body through the
    a. Ureters
    b. Urethra
    c. Anus
    d. Nephrons
15. The male sex gland is called the
    a. Penis
    b. Semen
    c. Testis
    d. Scrotum
16. The male sex cell is the
    a. Semen
    b. Ovum
    c. Gonad
    d. Sperm
17. The female sex gland is the
    a. Ovary
    b. Cervix
    c. Uterus
    d. Vagina
18. The discharge of the lining of the uterus is called
    a. The endometrium
    b. Ovulation
    c. Fertilization
    d. Menstruation
19. The endocrine glands secrete
    a. Hormones
    b. Mucus
    c. Semen
    d. Insulin
20. The immune system protects the body from
    a. Low blood sugar
    b. Disease and infection
    c. Loss of fluid
    d. Stunted growth

See Appendix A for answers to these questions.

9

The Older Person

OBJECTIVES

- Define the key terms and key abbreviations listed in this chapter.
- Identify the developmental tasks for each age group.
- Identify the psychologic and social changes common in older adulthood.
- Describe the physical changes from aging and the care required.
- Describe housing options for older persons.
- Explain how to promote quality of life.

KEY TERMS

development Changes in mental, emotional, and social function

developmental task A skill that must be completed during a stage of development

dysphagia Difficulty (*dys-*) swallowing (*-phagia*)

dyspnea Difficult, labored, or painful (*dys-*) breathing (*-pnea*)

geriatrics The care of aging people

gerontology The study of the aging process

growth The physical changes that are measured and that occur in a steady, orderly manner

menopause When menstruation stops and there has been at least 1 year without a menstrual period

podiatrist A medical professional who treats disorders of the foot, ankle, and related structures of the leg

presbyopia Age-related (*presby-*) farsightedness (*-opia* means "eye")

KEY ABBREVIATIONS

CCRC Continuing care retirement community

CMS Centers for Medicare & Medicaid Services

OBRA Omnibus Budget Reconciliation Act of 1987

People live longer than ever before. They are healthier and more active. US government reports show the following for the United States:

- In 2019, there were nearly 54.1 million people age 65 and older.
- In 2019, there were approximately 24.1 million men age 65 and older. There were approximately 30 million women age 65 and older.
- In 2020, there were more older men (70%) who were married than older women (48%) who were married.
- In 2019, there were 6.6 million people age 85 and older. In 2040, the number of people age 85 and older is expected to double to more than 14.4 million (a 118% increase).

Chronic illness is common in older persons. Disability often results. Most older persons have at least one disability. Disabilities increase and become more severe with aging. They can interfere with:

- Self-care—bathing, dressing, eating, elimination.
- Mobility and getting around one's home setting.
- Fixing meals, shopping, doing housework.
- Managing money.
- Using a phone.
- Taking medications.
- Leisure and recreational activities.

Still, most older people live in a family setting. They live with a partner, children, siblings, or other family. Some live alone or with friends. Still others live in nursing centers. The need for nursing center care increases with aging.

GROWTH AND DEVELOPMENT

Throughout life, people grow and develop. Growth is the physical changes that are measured and that occur in a steady, orderly manner. Growth is measured in height and weight. Changes in appearance and body functions also measure growth (Fig. 9.1).

Development relates to changes in mental, emotional, and social function. A person behaves and thinks in certain ways in each stage of development. A 2-year-old thinks in simple terms. A 40-year-old thinks in complex ways. The entire person is affected.

Growth and development occur in a sequence, order, and pattern. Certain skills must be completed during each stage. A developmental task is a skill that must be completed during a stage of development. A stage cannot be skipped. Each stage is the basis for the next stage. Each stage has its own characteristics and developmental tasks (Box 9.1).

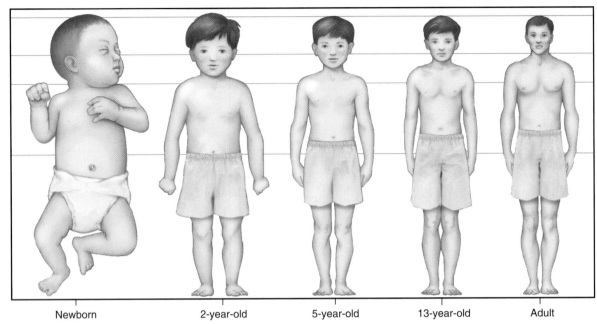

| Newborn | 2-year-old | 5-year-old | 13-year-old | Adult |

Fig. 9.1 Body appearance changes during growth. (From Thibodeau GA, Patton KT: *The human body in health & disease*, ed 5, St Louis, 2010, Mosby.)

BOX 9.1   Stages of Growth and Development

Infancy (Birth—1 Year)
- Learning to walk
- Learning to eat solid foods
- Beginning to talk and communicate with others
- Learning to trust
- Beginning to have emotional relationships with parents, brothers, and sisters
- Developing stable sleep and feeding patterns

Toddlerhood (1—3 Years)
- Tolerating separation from parents or primary caregivers
- Gaining control of bowel and bladder function
- Using words to communicate
- Becoming less dependent on parents or primary caregivers

Preschool (3—6 Years)
- Increasing the ability to communicate and understand others
- Performing self-care
- Learning gender (male, female) differences and developing sexual modesty
- Learning right from wrong and good from bad
- Learning to play with others
- Developing family relationships

School Age (6—9 or 10 Years)
- Developing social and physical skills needed for playing games
- Learning to get along with children of the same age and background (peers)
- Learning gender-appropriate behaviors and attitudes
- Learning basic reading, writing, and arithmetic skills
- Developing a conscience and morals
- Developing a good feeling and attitude about oneself

Late Childhood (9 or 10—12 Years)
- Becoming independent of adults and learning to depend on oneself
- Developing and keeping friendships with peers
- Understanding the physical, psychologic, and social roles of one's sex

- Developing moral and ethical behavior
- Developing greater muscular strength, coordination, and balance
- Learning how to study

Adolescence (12—18 Years)
- Accepting changes in the body and appearance
- Developing appropriate relationships with males and females of the same age
- Accepting the male or female role appropriate for one's age
- Becoming independent from parents and adults
- Preparing for marriage and family life
- Preparing for a career
- Developing the morals, attitudes, and values needed to function in society

Young Adulthood (18—40 Years)
- Choosing education and a career
- Selecting a partner
- Learning to live with a partner
- Becoming a parent and raising children
- Developing a satisfactory sex life

Middle Adulthood (40—65 Years)
- Adjusting to physical changes
- Having grown children
- Developing leisure time activities
- Adjusting to aging parents

Late Adulthood (65 Years and Older)
- Adjusting to decreased strength and loss of health
- Adjusting to retirement and reduced income
- Coping with a partner's death
- Developing new friends and relationships
- Preparing for one's own death

TABLE 9.1 Myths and Facts About Aging

Myth	Fact
All old people are the same.	Each person is unique. People age in different ways. Culture, religion, education, income, and life experiences affect aging. People develop throughout life.
Aging means illness and disability.	Older persons are at risk for health problems and disabilities. However, most are healthy. Not smoking, good nutrition, and exercise can reverse or slow many changes blamed on aging.
Older persons lose interest in sex.	Aging does not mean that sexual activity and expression must end. Many older people enjoy a fulfilling sex life. Sexuality is important throughout life. Intimacy, love, and companionship are needed.
Older people are lonely and isolated.	Most older people have frequent contact with their children. Older parents commonly live within 10 miles of their children. Most see a child at least once a week and take part in family activities. Regular contact with sisters and brothers is common. They can provide support and companionship. Many older persons have jobs, do volunteer work, and enjoy hobbies.
Mental function declines with age.	Older persons may receive and process information more slowly than younger people. However, people learn until very late in life. Many 90-year-olds have high levels of mental function.
Most older persons live in nursing centers.	Less than 5% of people 65 years and older live in long-term care settings.
Old people are crabby and rude.	Some old people are crabby and rude. So are people of all ages. Older persons who are crabby and rude were probably crabby and rude when younger.

Late Adulthood (65 Years and Older)

Late adulthood ranges from 65 years of age and older. The *oldest-old* are 85 years of age and older.

Gerontology is the study of the aging process. Geriatrics is the care of aging people. Aging is normal. It is not a disease. Normal changes occur in body structure and function. They increase the risk for illness, injury, and disability. Psychologic and social changes also occur. Often changes are slow. Most people adjust well to these changes. They lead happy, meaningful lives. The developmental tasks of late adulthood are listed in Box 9.1.

There are many myths about aging and older persons. A *myth* is a widely believed story that is not true. To provide good care, you need to know the facts about older persons and aging. Table 9.1 lists both common myths and facts.

PSYCHOLOGIC AND SOCIAL CHANGES

Graying hair, wrinkles, and slow movements are physical reminders of growing old. These changes affect self-esteem. They threaten self-image and feelings of self-worth. They also threaten independence.

Social roles also change. A parent may depend on an adult child for care. Retirees need activities to replace the work role. Adjusting to the death of a partner, family members, and friends is common. People face their own death.

People cope with aging in their own way. How they cope depends on health status, life experiences, finances, education, and social support systems.

Retirement

Age 65 is the usual retirement age. Some people retire earlier; others work into their 70s or 80s. Retirement is a reward for a lifetime of work. The person can relax and enjoy life (Fig. 9.2). Travel, leisure, and doing what one desires are retirement "benefits." Some people spend more time with existing hobbies. Some retired people develop new hobbies. Spending more time

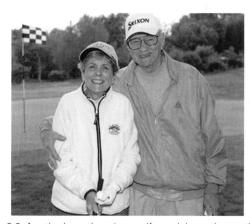

Fig. 9.2 A retired couple enjoys golf as a leisure time activity.

with grandchildren and other family members and friends is common. Many people enjoy retirement, but others are not so lucky. They may be ill or disabled. Poor health and medical bills can make retirement very hard.

Work helps people meet their needs for love, belonging, and self-esteem. They feel fulfilled and useful. Friendships form. Coworkers share daily events. Leisure time, recreation, and companionship often involve coworkers. Some retired people want to work. They have part-time jobs or do volunteer work (Fig. 9.3).

Reduced Income

Retirement usually means reduced income. Social security may provide the only income.

The retired person still has expenses. Rent or house payments continue. Food, clothing, utility bills, and taxes are other expenses. Car expenses, home repairs, medications, and health care are other costs. So are entertainment and gifts.

Reduced income may force lifestyle changes. Examples include:

- Limiting social and leisure events.
- Buying cheaper food, clothes, and household items.

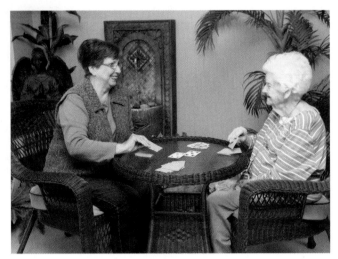

Fig. 9.3 This retired woman is a nursing center volunteer.

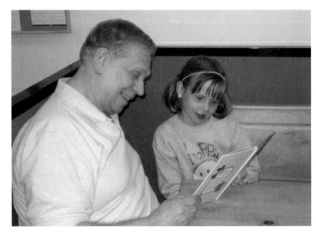

Fig. 9.5 An older man reads with his grandchild.

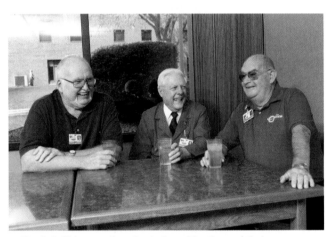

Fig. 9.4 Older people enjoy being with others of their own age.

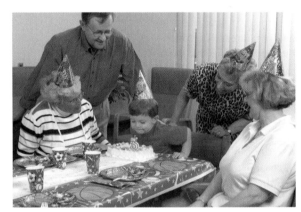

Fig. 9.6 An older couple takes part in family activities.

- Moving to cheaper housing.
- Living with children or other family.
- Avoiding health care or needed medications.
- Relying on children or other family for money or needed items.

Severe money problems can result. Some people plan for retirement. They have savings, investments, retirement plans, and insurance. They are financially comfortable during retirement.

Social Relationships

Social relationships change throughout life. Children grow up and leave home. They have their own families. Some live far away from parents. Older family members and friends die, move away, or are disabled. Yet most older people have regular contact with children, grandchildren, family, and friends. Others are lonely. Separation from children is a common cause. So is lack of companionship with people their own age (Fig. 9.4).

Many older people adjust to these changes. Hobbies, religious and community events, and new friends help prevent loneliness. Some community groups sponsor bus trips to ball games, shopping, plays, and concerts.

Grandchildren can bring great love and joy (Fig. 9.5). Family times help prevent loneliness. They help the older person feel useful and wanted (Fig. 9.6).

See *Focus on Communication: Social Changes.*

FOCUS ON COMMUNICATION

Social Changes

The social changes of aging can cause loneliness. If nursing center care is needed, the loneliness can seem even greater. The person may be in the same building with other people. However, those people do not replace relationships with family and friends. To help the person feel less lonely, you can:

- Suggest that the person call a family member or friend. Offer to assist with finding phone numbers and dialing.
- Keep the phone within the person's reach. This helps the person place or answer calls with ease.
- Suggest that the person read cards and letters. Offer to assist.
- Visit with the person a few times during your shift and explore the person's interests.
- Introduce new residents to other residents and staff. Perhaps arrange a "buddy" that might help a new resident settle in.

Children as Caregivers

Some children care for older parents. Parents and children change roles. The child cares for the parent. This helps some older persons feel more secure. Others feel unwanted, in the way, and useless. Some lose dignity and self-respect. Tensions may occur among the child, parent, and other household members. Lack of privacy is a cause. So are disagreements and criticisms about housekeeping, raising children, cooking, and friends.

Death of a Partner

As couples age, the chances increase that a partner will die. Women usually live longer than men. Therefore many women become widows.

A person may try to prepare for a partner's death. When death occurs, the loss is crushing. No amount of preparation is ever enough for the emptiness and changes that result. The person loses a lover, friend, companion, and confidant. Grief may be very great. The person's life will likely change. Serious physical and mental health problems may result. Some become depressed and lose the will to live. Some consider suicide. These individuals need a lot of support and understanding. There are support groups and therapists that often help people with their loss.

PHYSICAL CHANGES

Physical changes occur with aging (Box 9.2). They happen to everyone. Body processes slow down. Energy level and body efficiency decline. The rate and degree of change vary with each person. They depend on such factors as diet, health, exercise, stress, environment, and heredity. Changes are slow over many years. Often they are not seen for a long time.

Normal aging does not mean loss of health. Quality of life does not have to decline. The person can adjust to many of the changes.

The Integumentary System

The skin loses its elasticity, strength, and fatty tissue layer. The skin thins and sags. Wrinkles appear. Secretions from oil and sweat glands decrease. Dry skin and itching occur. The skin is fragile and easily injured. The skin's blood vessels are fragile. Skin breakdown, skin tears, and pressure injuries are risks (Chapters 31 and 32). So are bruising and delayed healing. This is because the skin's blood vessels are fragile.

Brown spots appear on sun-exposed areas. They are called "age spots" or "liver spots." They are common on the wrists and hands.

Loss of the skin's fatty tissue layer affects body temperature. The person is more sensitive to cold. Protect the person from drafts and cold. Sweaters, lap blankets, socks, and extra blankets are helpful, as are higher thermostat settings.

Dry skin causes itching. It is easily damaged. A shower or bath twice a week is enough for hygiene. Partial baths are taken at other times. Mild soaps or soap substitutes are used to clean the underarms, genitals, and under the breasts. Often soap is not used on the arms, legs, back, chest, and abdomen. Lotions and creams prevent drying and itching. Deodorants may not be needed because sweat gland secretion is decreased. See Chapter 18 for hygiene.

Nails become thick and tough. Feet usually have poor circulation. A nick or cut can lead to a serious infection. The services of a podiatrist (foot doctor) are often beneficial. See Chapter 19 for nail and foot care.

The skin has fewer nerve endings. This affects the sensing of heat, cold, pressure, and pain. Burns are great risks. Fragile skin, poor circulation, and decreased ability to sense heat and cold increase the risk of burns. Older persons often complain of cold feet. Socks provide warmth. Hot water bottles and heating pads are not used because of the risk for burns.

White or gray hair is common. Hair loss occurs in men. Hair thins on men and women. Thinning occurs on the head, in the pubic area, and under the arms. Women and men may choose to wear wigs. Some color hair to cover graying. Facial hair (lip and chin) may occur in women.

Hair is drier from decreases in scalp oils. Brushing promotes circulation and oil production. Shampoo frequency depends on personal choice. Usually it decreases with age. It is done as needed for hygiene and comfort.

Skin disorders increase with age. They rarely cause death if treated early. The risk of skin cancer increases with age. Prolonged sun exposure is a cause.

Skin changes can be seen. Gray hair, hair loss, brown spots, wrinkles, and sagging skin are some examples. These changes can affect self-esteem and body image.

The Musculoskeletal System

Muscle cells decrease in number. Muscles atrophy (shrink) and decrease in strength.

Bones lose minerals, especially calcium. Bones lose strength. They become brittle and break easily. Sometimes just turning in bed can cause fractures (broken bones).

Vertebrae shorten. Joints become stiff and painful. Hip and knee joints flex (bend) slightly. These changes cause gradual loss of height and strength. Mobility also decreases.

Older persons need to stay active. Activity, exercise, and diet help prevent bone loss and loss of muscle strength. Walking is good exercise. Exercise groups and range-of-motion exercises are helpful (Chapter 24). A diet high in protein, calcium, and vitamins is needed.

Bones can break easily. Protect the person from injury and prevent falls (Chapters 11 and 12). Turn and move the person gently and carefully (Chapter 15). Some persons need help and support getting out of bed. Some need help walking.

The Nervous System

Nerve cells are lost. Nerve conduction and reflexes slow. Responses are slower. For example, an older person slips. The message telling the brain of the slip travels slowly. The message from the brain to prevent the fall also travels slowly. The person falls.

BOX 9.2 Common Physical Changes During the Aging Process

Integumentary System
- Skin becomes less elastic
- Skin loses strength
- Brown spots ("age spots" or "liver spots") on the wrists and hands
- Fewer nerve endings
- Fewer blood vessels
- Fatty tissue layer is lost
- Skin thins and sags
- Skin is fragile and easily injured
- Folds, lines, and wrinkles appear
- Blood vessels in the dermis become more fragile
- Decreased secretion of oil and sweat glands
- Dry skin
- Itching
- Increased sensitivity to heat and cold
- Decreased sensitivity to pain
- Nails become thick and tough
- Whitening or graying hair
- Facial hair in some women
- Loss or thinning of hair
- Drier hair

Musculoskeletal System
- Muscles atrophy
- Strength, tone, and contractility decrease
- Bone mass decreases
- Bones become weaker
- Bones become brittle; can break easily
- Vertebrae shorten
- Joints become stiff and painful
- Hip and knee joints become flexed
- Gradual loss of height; trunk becomes shorter
- Decreased mobility

Nervous System
- Brain and spinal cord lose nerve cells
- Nerve cells send messages at a slower rate
- Reflexes slow
- Reduced blood flow to the brain
- Abnormal structures can form in the brain
- Brain tissue may shrink (atrophy)
- Changes in brain cells
- Shorter memory
- Forgetfulness
- Slower ability to respond
- Confusion
- Dizziness
- Sleep patterns change
- Reduced sensitivity to touch
- Reduced sensitivity to pain
- Smell and taste decrease
- Eyelids thin, wrinkle, and may droop
- Less tear secretion
- Pupils less responsive to light
- Decreased vision at night or in dark rooms
- Problems seeing green and blue colors
- Poor vision
- Changes in auditory nerve
- Eardrums atrophy
- High-pitched sounds are not heard
- Decreased earwax secretion
- Hearing loss

Circulatory System
- Heart pumps with less force
- Heart valves thicken and become stiff
- Heart rate may slow
- Abnormal heart rhythms may occur
- Heart may enlarge slightly
- Heart walls thicken
- Arteries narrow and become stiffer
- Less blood flows through narrowed arteries
- Weakened heart works harder to pump blood through narrowed vessels
- Number of red blood cells decreases

Respiratory System
- Respiratory muscles weaken
- Some lung tissue is lost
- Lung tissue becomes less elastic
- Chest is less able to stretch to breathe
- Difficulty breathing (dyspnea [p. ··])
- Decreased strength for coughing and clearing the airway

Digestive System
- Decreased saliva production
- Difficulty swallowing (dysphagia [p. ··])
- Decreased appetite
- Decreased secretion of digestive juices
- Difficulty digesting fried and fatty foods
- Indigestion
- Loss of teeth
- Decreased peristalsis causing flatulence and constipation

Urinary System
- Kidney function decreases
- Reduced blood supply to kidneys
- Kidneys atrophy
- Urine becomes concentrated
- Bladder tissue less able to stretch
- Bladder muscles weaken
- Bladder may not empty completely when urinating
- Urinary frequency
- Urinary urgency may occur
- Urinary incontinence may occur
- Nighttime urination may occur

Reproductive System
- Men:
  - Testosterone decreases slightly
  - Erections take longer
  - Longer phase between erection and orgasm
  - Less forceful orgasms
  - Erections lost quickly
  - Longer time between erections
- Women:
  - Menopause (p. ··)
  - Estrogen and progesterone decrease
  - Uterus, vagina, and genitalia shrink (atrophy)
  - Thinning of vaginal walls
  - Vaginal dryness
  - Arousal takes longer
  - Less intense orgasms
  - Quicker return to preexcitement state

Blood flow to the brain is reduced. Dizziness may occur. It increases the risk for falls. Practice measures to prevent falls (Chapter 12). Remind the person to get up slowly from bed or a chair. This helps prevent dizziness.

Changes occur in brain cells. This affects personality and mental function. So does reduced blood flow to the brain. Memory is shorter. Forgetfulness increases. Responses slow. Confusion, dizziness, and fatigue may occur. Older persons often remember events from long ago better than recent ones. Many older people are mentally active and involved in current events. They show fewer personality and mental changes. (See Chapter 40 for confusion and dementia.)

Sleep patterns change. Falling asleep is harder for older persons. Sleep periods are shorter. They wake often at night and have less deep sleep. Less sleep is needed. Loss of energy and decreased blood flow may cause fatigue. They may rest or nap during the day. They may go to bed early and get up early.

The Senses

Aging affects touch, smell, taste, sight, and hearing.

Touch. Touch and sensitivity to pain and pressure are reduced. So is sensing heat and cold. These changes increase the risk for injury. The person may not notice painful injuries or diseases. Or the person feels minor pain. You need to:

- Protect older persons from injury (Chapters 11 and 12).
- Follow safety measures for heat and cold (Chapter 31).
- Check for signs of skin breakdown (Chapters 18, 31, and 32).
- Give good skin care (Chapter 18).
- Prevent skin tears (Chapter 31) and pressure injuries (Chapter 32).

Taste and Smell. Taste and smell dull. Appetite decreases. Taste buds decrease in number. The tongue senses sweet, salty, bitter, and sour tastes. Sweet and salty tastes are lost first. Older people often complain that food has no taste or tastes bitter. They like more salt and sugar on food.

The Eye. Eyelids thin and wrinkle. Tear secretion is less. Dust and pollutants can irritate the eyes.

The pupil becomes smaller and responds less to light. Vision is poor at night or in dark rooms. The eye takes longer to adjust to lighting changes. Vision problems occur when going from a dark to a bright room. They also occur when going from a bright to a dark room.

Clear vision is reduced. Eyeglasses are needed. The lens of the eye yellows and becomes opaque. Therefore greens and blues are harder to see. Cataracts develop (Chapter 33) and the person may need surgery.

Older persons become more farsighted. This is called presbyopia. (*Presby-* relates to aging; *-opia* means "eye.") The lens becomes more rigid with age. It is harder for the eye to shift from far to near vision and from near to far vision. These changes increase the risk of falls and accidents. The risk is greater on stairs and where lighting is poor. Eyeglasses are worn as needed. Keep rooms well lit. Nightlights help in dark areas.

The Ear. Changes occur in the auditory nerve. Eardrums atrophy (shrink). High-pitched sounds are hard to hear. Severe hearing loss occurs if these changes progress. A hearing aid may be needed. It must be clean and placed correctly in the ear.

Wax secretion decreases. Wax becomes harder and thicker. It is easily impacted (wedged in the ear). This can cause hearing loss. A health care provider or nurse removes the wax.

The Circulatory System

The heart muscle weakens. It pumps blood with less force. Problems may not occur at rest. Activity, exercise, excitement, and illness increase the body's need for oxygen and nutrients. A damaged or weak heart cannot meet these needs.

Arteries narrow and are less elastic. Less blood flows through them. Poor circulation occurs in many body parts. A weak heart must work harder to pump blood through narrowed vessels.

Exercise helps maintain health and well-being. Many older persons exercise daily. They walk, jog, golf, and bicycle. They also hike, ski, play tennis, swim, and play other sports. Older persons need to be as active as possible.

Sometimes circulatory changes are severe. Rest is needed during the day. Overexertion is avoided. The person should not walk far, climb many stairs, or carry heavy things. Personal care items, TV, phone, and other needed items are kept nearby. Some exercise helps circulation. It also prevents blood clots in leg veins. Some persons need to stay in bed. They need range-of-motion exercises (Chapter 24). Health care providers may order certain exercises and activity limits.

The Respiratory System

Respiratory muscles weaken. Lung tissue becomes less elastic. Often lung changes are not noted at rest. Difficult, labored, or painful breathing, called dyspnea, may occur with activity. (*Dys-* means "difficult"; *-pnea* means "breathing.") The person may lack strength to cough and clear the airway of secretions. Respiratory infections and diseases may develop. These can threaten the older person's life.

Normal breathing is promoted. Avoid heavy bed linens over the chest. They prevent normal chest expansion. Turning, repositioning, and deep breathing are important. They help prevent respiratory complications from bedrest. Breathing usually is easier in the semi-Fowler position (Chapter 15). The person should be as active as possible.

The Digestive System

Salivary glands produce less saliva. This can cause difficulty swallowing, or dysphagia. (*Dys-* means "difficult"; *-phagia* means "swallowing"; see Chapter 20.) Dry foods may be hard to swallow, and taste and smell become dull. This decreases appetite.

Secretion of digestive juices decreases. As a result, fried and fatty foods are hard to digest. They may cause indigestion.

Loss of teeth and ill-fitting dentures cause chewing problems, which leads to digestion problems. Hard-to-chew foods are avoided. Ground or chopped meat is easier to chew and swallow.

Peristalsis decreases. The stomach and colon empty slower. Flatulence and constipation can occur (Chapter 23).

Dry, fried, and fatty foods are avoided. This helps swallowing and digestion problems. Oral hygiene and denture care improve taste. Some people do not have teeth or dentures. Their food is pureed or ground.

High-fiber foods help prevent constipation. However, they are hard to chew and can irritate the intestines. They include apricots, celery, and fruits and vegetables with skins and seeds. Persons with chewing problems or constipation often need foods that provide soft bulk. They include whole-grain cereals and cooked fruits and vegetables.

Fewer calories are needed. Energy and activity levels decline. More fluids are needed for chewing, swallowing, digestion, and kidney function. Foods are needed to prevent constipation and bone changes. High-protein foods are needed for tissue growth and repair. However, some older persons lack protein in their diets. High-protein foods (meat and fish) are costly.

The Urinary System

Kidney function decreases. The kidneys shrink (atrophy). Blood flow to the kidneys is reduced. Waste removal is less efficient. Urine is more concentrated.

The ureters, bladder, and urethra lose tone and elasticity. Bladder muscles weaken. Bladder size decreases. Therefore the bladder stores less urine. Urinary frequency or urgency may occur. Many older persons have to urinate during the night. Urinary incontinence (inability to control the passage of urine from the bladder) may occur (Chapter 22).

In men, the prostate gland enlarges. This puts pressure on the urethra. Difficulty urinating or frequent urination occurs.

Urinary tract infections are risks. Adequate fluids are needed. The person needs water, juices, milk, and gelatin. Provide fluids according to the care plan. Remind the person to drink. Offer fluids often to those who need help. Most fluids should be taken before 1700 (5:00 PM). This reduces the need to urinate during the night.

Persons with incontinence may need bladder training programs. Sometimes catheters are necessary.

The Reproductive System

Reproductive organs change with aging. For the effects of aging on sexuality, see Chapter 10.

- *Men.* The hormone *testosterone* decreases slightly. It affects strength, sperm production, and reproductive tissues. These changes affect sexual activity. An erection takes longer. The phase between erection and orgasm also is longer. Orgasm is less forceful than when younger. Erections are lost quickly. The time between erections also is longer. Older men may need the penis stimulated for arousal. Fatigue, overeating, and drinking too much alcohol affect erections. Some men fear performance problems. They may avoid closeness.
- *Women.* Menopause is when menstruation stops and there has been at least 1 year without a menstrual period. The woman can no longer have children. This occurs around 50 years of age. Female hormones (*estrogen* and *progesterone*) decrease. The uterus, vagina, and genitalia shrink (atrophy). Vaginal walls thin. There is vaginal dryness. These changes

make intercourse uncomfortable or painful. Arousal takes longer. Orgasm is less intense. The preexcitement state returns more quickly.

HOUSING OPTIONS

A person's home is more than a place to live. A home has family memories. It is a link to neighbors and the community. It brings pride and self-esteem. Aging can lead to changes in a person's home setting.

Most older people live in their own homes. Some choose smaller homes when children are gone. Some retire to warmer climates. Others move closer to children and family. Still others have to give up their homes. It is very difficult for many people to leave the home they have resided in for many years. Reduced income, taxes, home repairs, and yard work are factors. Some people cannot care for themselves.

Many housing options meet the needs of older people. A new home setting could maintain or improve the person's quality of life.

Living With Family

Sometimes older brothers, sisters, and cousins live together. They:

- Provide companionship.
- Share living expenses.
- Provide care during illness or disability.

Living with children is an option. The older parent (or parents) moves in with the child. Or the child moves to the parent's home. The parent may be healthy, may need some help, or may be ill or disabled. Some adult children give care to avoid nursing center care. A nursing center is an option if they cannot give needed care.

Living with an adult child is a social change. Everyone in the home must adjust. Sleeping plans may change if there is no spare bedroom. The parent may need a hospital bed. It can go in a family or living room, dining room, den, or bedroom.

The adult child's family needs time alone. Other family members may help give care. Respite care (Chapter 6) is an option for weekends and vacations. Home care agencies can provide nurses or home health care aides. Many community and church groups have volunteers who help give care.

Adult Day Care Centers

Many children need to work even though the parent cannot stay alone. Adult day care centers provide meals, supervision, and activities (Fig. 9.7). Some provide rides to and from the center. Some serve persons with dementia (Chapter 40).

Requirements vary. Some centers require that the person be able to walk. A cane or walker is used as needed. Others allow wheelchairs. Most require that the person perform some self-care.

Many activities are offered. Cards, board games, movies, crafts, dancing, walks, exercise groups, and lectures are common. Some provide bowling and swimming. All activities are supervised. Needed help is given.

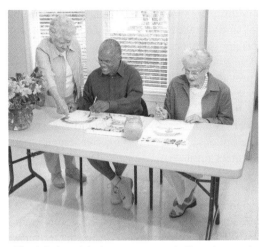

Fig. 9.7 An adult day care center. (©Getty Images.)

Some areas have intergenerational day care centers. Children and older persons are in the same center. They work together on some activities. They eat and play together. Young children bring much joy to older persons. They give older persons purpose, love, and affection. In turn, children learn about aging. They also receive love and affection from older persons.

Elder Cottage Housing Opportunity

Elder cottage housing opportunity (ECHO) homes are small homes designed for older and disabled persons. The portable home is placed in the yard of a single-family home. The older person lives independently but near family or friends.

Apartments

Some older persons live in apartments. They pay rent and utility bills. The owner provides maintenance, yard work, snow removal, and appliance repair. Older persons remain independent. They can keep personal items. Many older persons like to garden or do yard work (Fig. 9.8). Apartment living usually does not provide such activities.

An *accessory dwelling unit (ADU)* is a separate living area in a home. It has a kitchen, bedroom, and bathroom. Some have a small living room. The older person lives independently near other people. Some children have these apartments for older

parents. Or the older person's home may have an apartment. ADUs are also called *in-law apartments, accessory apartments*, and *second units.*

Residential Hotels

Some cities have residential hotels. Private rooms or small apartments are rented. Food services may include a dining room, cafeteria, or room service. Some provide recreational activities and emergency medical services. Most hotels are close to shopping, places of worship, and other civic services.

Congregate Housing

Congregate means a group, gathering, or cluster. In congregate housing, apartments are for older people. Buildings have wheelchair access, hand rails, elevators, and other safety features. Apartments are designed to meet the needs of older persons. Some are furnished.

Services are many. A doctor or nurse is on call. Someone checks on the person daily. A dining room is common. Rides are provided to places of worship, the doctor, or shopping areas. Tenants pay monthly rent.

Senior Citizen Housing

In many areas, state and federal funds support apartment complexes for older and disabled persons. Such persons have low to moderate incomes. Monthly rents are lower. The rent depends on the person's monthly income. It is common for persons living in this type of housing to also have services from home health care agencies.

Home Sharing

Two or more people may share a house or apartment. Each person has a bedroom. They share other living spaces—kitchen, bathroom, and living room. They share household chores and expenses. Or cooking, cleaning, and yard work are exchanged for rent.

Shared housing is a way to avoid living alone. It provides companionship. Some people feel safer when living with another person.

Assisted Living Residences

Assisted living residences are for persons who need help with daily living (Chapters 1 and 43). The person has social contact with others in a homelike setting. Health care and 24-hour oversight are provided. Complete nursing care is not provided.

Board and Care Homes

Board and care homes provide a room, meals, laundry, and supervision (Chapter 1). Some homes are for older persons. Others are for people with certain problems. Dementia, mental health disorders, and developmental disabilities are examples.

Homes vary in size—from housing 4 to 30 people or more. The care provided and rules vary from state to state. The person pays monthly rent. Some board and care homes receive government funds.

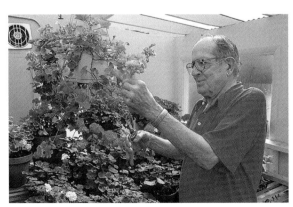

Fig. 9.8 This man enjoys gardening.

Adult Foster Care

Adult foster care can take two forms:
- An older person lives with a family.
- A single-family home serves four to five persons with special needs. They may be older, disabled, or mentally ill.

The person receives help with daily living. A room, meals, and laundry are provided. Help is given with shopping and transportation. The person receives needed health care.

Continuing Care Retirement Communities

Continuing care retirement communities (CCRCs) offer many services. They range from independent living units to 24-hour nursing care. A CCRC has housing, activity, and health care services. It meets the changing needs of older persons living alone or with a partner. CCRCs usually provide:
- Nursing care and other health care services.
- Meals (including special diets).
- Housekeeping.
- Transportation.
- Personal assistance.
- Recreational and educational activities.

Independent living units are small apartments. Residents perform self-care and take their own medications. Food service is provided. Help is nearby if needed. Many people have their own cars. They travel or drive about as desired. Rides are provided for those who need them.

Services are added as the person's needs change. Over time, some persons need nursing center care. They move into the nursing center within the CCRC. Many older couples find comfort in this plan. One partner needs nursing care. The other is close by and can visit often.

The person signs a contract with the CCRC. The contract is for a certain time or for the person's lifetime. The contract lists services provided and the required fees.

Nursing Centers

Some older persons cannot care for themselves. Nursing centers are options for them (Chapter 1). Some people stay in nursing centers until death. Others stay until they can return home. The nursing center is the person's temporary or permanent home. The setting is as homelike as possible (Fig. 9.9).

The person needing nursing center care may suffer some or all of these losses:
- Loss of identity as a productive member of a family and community
- Loss of possessions (e.g., home, household items, car)
- Loss of independence
- Loss of real-world experiences (e.g., shopping, traveling, cooking, driving, hobbies)
- Loss of health and mobility

The person may feel useless, powerless, and hopeless. The health team helps the person cope with loss and improve quality of life. Treat the person with dignity and respect. Also practice good communication skills. Follow the care plan.

Nursing centers serve to meet the needs of older and disabled persons. Physical changes of aging are considered in the center's design. So are safety needs. Programs and services meet the person's basic needs. Box 9.3 lists the features of a quality nursing center.

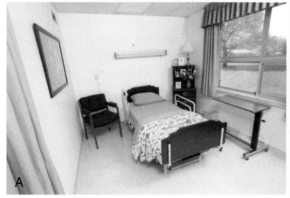 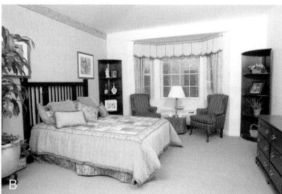

Fig. 9.9 (A) A nursing center is as homelike as possible. (B) Some centers allow residents to bring their own bed and furniture from home.

BOX 9.3 Features of a Quality Nursing Center

Basic Information
- The center is Medicare certified.
- The center is Medicaid certified.
- The center provides the level of care needed. Rehabilitation, dementia, and ventilator services are examples.
- The center is located close enough for family and friends to visit.

Resident Appearance
- Residents are clean and well groomed.
- Residents are dressed appropriately for the season or time of day.

Living Spaces
- The center is free from overwhelming, unpleasant odors.
- The center appears clean and well kept.
- The temperature is comfortable for the residents.
- The center has good lighting.
- Noise levels in the dining room are comfortable.
- Noise levels in common areas are comfortable.
- Smoking is not allowed. If allowed, it is restricted to certain areas.
- Furnishings are sturdy, comfortable, and attractive.

BOX 9.3   Features of a Quality Nursing Center—cont'd

Staff

- The relationship between the staff and residents appears to be warm, polite, and respectful.
- All staff wear name tags.
- Staff knock on the person's door before entering the room.
- Staff refer to residents by name.
- The center offers a training and continuing education program for all staff.
- The center does background checks on all staff.
- The center has licensed nurses on staff 24 hours a day. A registered nurse (RN) is present at least 8 hours a day, 7 days a week.
- The same nursing team (including nursing assistants) works with the same resident 4 to 5 days a week.
- Nursing assistants work with a reasonable number of residents.
- Nursing assistants take part in care planning meetings.
- The center has a full-time social worker on staff.
- A licensed health care provider is on staff, who is there regularly and can be reached at all times.
- The center's management team has worked together for at least 1 year. This includes the administrator and director of nursing.

Residents' Rooms

- Residents may have personal belongings in their rooms.
- Residents may have personal furniture in their rooms.
- Each resident has storage space (closet and drawers) in own room.
- Each resident has a window in own room.
- Residents have access to a personal telephone.
- Residents have access to a personal TV.
- Residents have a choice of roommates.
- The resident can reach own water pitcher.
- The center has policies and procedures to protect residents' belongings.

Hallways, Stairs, Lounges, and Bathrooms

- Exits are clearly marked.
- The center has quiet areas where residents can visit with family and friends.
- The center has smoke detectors and sprinklers.
- All common areas, resident rooms, and doorways are designed for wheel-chair use.
- The center has hand rails in the hallways.
- The center has grab bars in bathrooms.

Menus and Food

- Residents have a choice of food items at each meal.
- The person's favorite foods are served.
- Nutritious snacks are available upon request.
- Staff help residents eat and drink if help is needed.

Activities

- Residents may choose to take part in a variety of activities. This includes residents who cannot leave their rooms.
- The center has outdoor areas for resident use. Staff help residents to go outside.
- The center has an active volunteer program.

Safety and Care

- The center has an emergency evacuation plan.
- Regular fire drills are held. Residents, including the bedbound, are moved to safety.
- Residents receive preventive care to stay healthy. Yearly flu shots are an example.
- Residents may see their personal doctors.
- The center has an arrangement with a nearby hospital for emergencies.
- Care plan meetings are held with residents and family members.
- • The center has corrected all problems on its last state inspection report.

Modified from Centers for Medicare & Medicaid Services, *Your guide to choosing a nursing home or other long-term services & supports,* Baltimore, 2019, US Department of Health and Human Services.

Some center designs, programs, and services follow the *Eden Alternative*™. Animals, plants, and children play a key role in giving residents dignity and purpose. The center may have an aviary (Fig. 9.10), which provides bird-watching enjoyment to residents. Some centers may have a resident dog or cat. Others offer pet therapy through pet visits. House plants and outdoor garden spaces give residents enjoyment. Special events are arranged where groups of children come to sing or perform plays. The goal is to prevent residents from feeling lonely, helpless, and bored. *Household, neighborhood,* and *community* are other nursing center models and designs.

Most nursing centers receive Medicare or Medicaid funds. They must meet requirements of the Omnibus Budget Reconciliation Act of 1987 (OBRA). OBRA protects the person's rights and promotes quality of life. The Centers for Medicare & Medicaid Services (CMS) has rules and regulations for OBRA (Box 9.4). The CMS is a federal agency. It has the power to issue standards, rules, and regulations. These are called agency-made laws. Employers and employees must comply with them. Unannounced surveys are conducted to see if nursing centers are meeting OBRA and CMS requirements.

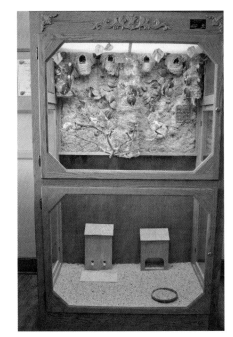

Fig. 9.10 An aviary offers residents the enjoyment of bird watching.

BOX 9.4   Environment Requirements

- The person's care equipment is clean and properly stored. This includes toothbrushes, dentures, denture cups, glasses and water pitchers, emesis basins, hair brushes and combs, bedpans, urinals, feeding tubes, leg bags and catheter bags, pads, and positioning devices.
- Bed linens are clean and in good condition.
- There are clean towels and washcloths for each person.
- The person has closet space with shelves. The person can reach the shelves.
- Lighting levels are comfortable and adequate.
- Temperature levels are comfortable and safe. The temperate is between 71 and 81 degrees Fahrenheit (°F).
- Sound levels are comfortable. Sound levels allow for hearing, privacy, and social interaction.
- Safety precautions are followed for persons who smoke (see Chapter 11).

- Hand rails, assist devices, and other surfaces are in good repair. They are free from sharp edges or other hazards.
- Furniture is appropriate for the residents.
- The person's setting is as free from accident hazards as possible:
  - Resident care equipment is used following the manufacturer's instructions.
  - Safety measures are practiced for hazardous substances (Chapter 11).
  - Safety measures are practiced to prevent burns from hot water temperatures (Chapter 11).
  - Safety measures are practiced to prevent equipment accidents (Chapter 11). This includes electrical safety.
  - Safety measures are practiced to prevent accidents from assist devices and equipment. This includes canes, walkers, wheelchairs, mechanical lifts, restraints, bed rails, mattresses, and so on.

Modified from Centers for Medicare & Medicaid Services, *State operations manual,* Baltimore, 2018, US Department of Health and Human Services.

QUALITY OF LIFE

Moving to a nursing center can cause feelings of loneliness and isolation. Making new friends helps the person adjust. It also improves quality of life. Some residents cannot visit with friends or get to activities without help. Offer to take them to visit in a friend's room or to an activity.

Some people are trying to cope with many losses. They may have a hard time talking to others. Encourage them to talk about losses. They may find that other residents have similar losses.

Urinary problems may cause older persons to avoid social events. Help them to the bathroom before the event or visit. Follow the care plan if other measures are needed.

Feeling good about one's appearance and setting is important to feel comfortable with others. These measures can help residents:

- Make sure their clothes and linens are clean and dry.
- Help them with grooming (e.g., shaving, makeup, hair care).
- Help them dress in clothes of their choice.
- Make sure dentures, eyeglasses, and hearing aids are in place.
- Keep their rooms clean and orderly.
- Help them display personal items if asked. Do not touch items without the person's permission.
- Treat each person as if you were in that person's home.
- Respect persons and their settings.

Some quiet, private persons avoid social contacts. Respect their wishes for privacy.

TIME TO REFLECT

Mrs. Charles has many chronic health problems. She had lived at home with her husband until he died recently from a heart attack. Mr. and Mrs. Charles had been married for over 60 years. Mrs. Charles's husband did most of the care for her, so now she needs to be cared for in a nursing center. You notice that Mrs. Charles appears depressed and is not adjusting well to her new environment. More than once she has mentioned that she is ready to die and "just wants to join her husband in heaven." One evening, as you place her eyeglasses in the top drawer of her bedside table, you notice several capsules partially wrapped in a tissue. She sees that you noticed them and she pleads, "Promise you won't tell anyone—I'm just saving those in case I can't stand this misery any longer." What should you do in this situation? What are some methods for meeting Mrs. Charles's needs? Do you understand how difficult it may be for some older people to adjust to living in a care center?

REVIEW QUESTIONS

Circle the BEST answer.

1. People age 85 and older are
   a. The young-old
   b. Old
   c. The oldest-old
   d. Elderly
2. The study of the aging process is called
   a. Geriatrics
   b. Dysphagia
   c. Gerontology
   d. Dyspnea
3. Retirement usually means
   a. Lowered income
   b. Changes from aging
   c. Less free time
   d. Financial security
4. Which does *not* cause loneliness in older persons?
   a. Children moving away
   b. The death of family and friends
   c. Problems communicating with others
   d. Contact with other older persons

5. Older persons may choose to live with family members. Which is *false*?
   a. They may share living expenses
   b. Family members may provide care when needed
   c. There is always a lack of companionship
   d. Family members may need to make adjustments to the new living arrangement
6. These statements are about a partner's death. Which is *false*?
   a. The person loses a lover, friend, companion, and confidant
   b. Preparing for the event lessens grief
   c. The survivor may develop health problems
   d. The survivor's life will likely change
7. Skin changes occur with aging. Care should include the following *except*
   a. Providing for warmth
   b. Applying lotion
   c. A daily bath with soap
   d. Providing good skin care
8. An older person complains of cold feet. You should
   a. Provide socks
   b. Apply a hot water bottle
   c. Soak the feet in hot water
   d. Apply a heating pad
9. Aging causes changes in the musculoskeletal system. Which is *false*?
   a. Bones become brittle and can break easily
   b. Bedrest is needed for loss of strength
   c. Joints become stiff and painful
   d. Exercise slows musculoskeletal changes
10. Changes occur in the nervous system. Which is *true*?
    a. Less sleep is needed than when younger
    b. The person forgets events from long ago
    c. Sensitivity to pain increases
    d. Confusion occurs in all older persons
11. Changes occur in the eye. Which is *false*?
    a. Night vision decreases
    b. Blue and green colors are easy to see
    c. Eyelids thin and wrinkle
    d. The eye is easily irritated by dust
12. Which is *not* a common cause of hearing loss in older persons?
    a. Changes in the auditory nerve
    b. Atrophy of the eardrums
    c. Impacted earwax
    d. Ear infections
13. Arteries narrow and lose their elasticity. These changes result in
    a. A slower heart rate
    b. Lower blood pressure
    c. Poor circulation to many body parts
    d. Less blood in the body
14. An older person has cardiovascular changes. Care includes the following *except*
    a. Placing needed items nearby
    b. A moderate amount of daily exercise
    c. Avoiding exertion
    d. Long walks
15. Respiratory changes occur with aging. Which is *false*?
    a. Heavy bed linens are avoided
    b. The person is turned often if on bedrest
    c. The side-lying position is best for breathing
    d. The person should be as active as possible
16. Older persons should avoid dry foods because of
    a. Decreases in saliva
    b. Loss of teeth or ill-fitting dentures
    c. Decreased amounts of digestive juices
    d. Decreased peristalsis
17. Changes occur in the digestive system. Older persons should eat
    a. Fruits and vegetables with skins and seeds
    b. Dry and fatty foods
    c. Raw apricots and celery
    d. Protein foods
18. Changes occur in the urinary system. Which is *true*?
    a. Kidneys increase in size
    b. Fluids are needed for kidney function
    c. The bladder becomes larger
    d. Blood flow to the kidneys increases
19. The doctor orders increased fluid intake for an older person. You should
    a. Give most of the fluid before 1700 (5:00 PM)
    b. Provide mostly juice
    c. Start a bladder training program
    d. Insert a catheter
20. Most older people live
    a. In nursing centers
    b. In their own homes
    c. With children
    d. In senior citizen housing
21. These statements are about adult day care centers. Which is *false*?
    a. They provide meals, supervision, and activities
    b. Usually the person must do some self-care
    c. All activities are supervised
    d. Total assistance with personal care is provided
22. Which housing option provides lodging, meals, and some help with personal care?
    a. Apartments
    b. Senior citizen housing
    c. Board and care homes
    d. Residential hotels

23. A continuing care retirement community provides the following *except*
    a. Independent living units
    b. A nursing center
    c. Adult foster care
    d. Meals, transportation, and recreational activities

24. A quality nursing center
    a. Provides the needed level of care
    b. Is owned by doctors and nurses
    c. Has independent living units
    d. Provides adult and child day care

    See Appendix A for answers to these questions.

10

Sexuality

OBJECTIVES

- Define the key terms and key abbreviations listed in this chapter.
- Describe sex, sexuality, and sexual relationships.
- Explain why sexuality is important throughout life.
- Explain how injury and illness can affect sexuality.
- Explain how aging can affect sexuality in older persons.
- Explain how the nursing team can promote sexuality.
- Explain why some persons become sexually aggressive.
- Describe how to deal with sexually aggressive persons.
- Explain how to promote quality of life.

KEY TERMS

bisexual A person who may be attracted to people of more than one gender.

erectile dysfunction (ED) See "impotence"

heterosexual A person who is attracted to members of the opposite sex

homosexual A person who is attracted to members of the same sex

impotence The inability of the male to have an erection; erectile dysfunction

mastectomy The surgical removal of a breast

natal sex A person's genital anatomy that is present at birth

sex Physical activities involving the reproductive organs; done for pleasure or to have children

sexuality The physical, emotional, social, cultural, and spiritual factors that affect a person's feelings and attitudes about one's own sex

transgender A broad term used to describe people who self-identify as a gender that does not match the natal sex

KEY ABBREVIATIONS

ED Erectile dysfunction

LGBTQ+ Lesbian, gay, bisexual, transgender, queer or questioning community

OBRA Omnibus Budget Reconciliation Act of 1987

Residents are viewed as whole persons. They have physical and safety needs, as well as the need for love and belonging, self-esteem, and self-actualization. Their physical, emotional, social, and spiritual needs are considered.

Sexuality involves the whole person. Illness, injury, and aging can affect sexuality.

SEX AND SEXUALITY

Sex is the physical activities involving the reproductive organs (Chapter 8). It is done for pleasure or to have children. Sexuality is the physical, emotional, social, cultural, and spiritual factors that affect a person's feelings and attitudes about one's own sex. Sexuality involves the personality and the body. It affects how a person behaves, thinks, dresses, and responds to others.

Sexuality often begins when a baby's gender is known. By the age of 3, children begin to identify as males or females. They learn male and female roles from adults (Fig. 10.1). Children learn that boys and girls each behave in certain ways.

As children grow older, interest increases about the body and how it works. Teens are more aware of sex and the body. Their bodies respond to stimulation. Some may engage in sexual behaviors. They kiss, embrace, pet, or may have intercourse. Pregnancy and sexually transmitted diseases (Chapter 38) are great risks.

Sex has more meaning as young adults mature. Attitudes and feelings are important. Partners are selected. They decide whether to have sex before marriage and about the use of birth control.

Sexuality is important throughout life. Attitudes and sex needs change with aging. They are affected by life events. These include divorce, death of a partner, injury, illness, and surgery.

SEXUAL RELATIONSHIPS

A heterosexual is a person who is attracted to members of the opposite sex. Men are attracted to women. Women are attracted to men. Sexual behavior is male-female.

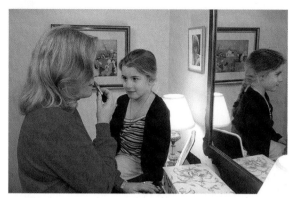

Fig. 10.1 This little girl is learning female roles from her mother.

Some people do not identify as heterosexual individuals. They may identify as lesbian, gay, bisexual, transgender, queer, or questioning community (LGBTQ+).

A homosexual is a person who is attracted to people of the same gender. Men are attracted to men. Women are attracted to women (*lesbian*). *Gay* refers to homosexuality. Before the 1960s and 1970s, many gay persons were secret about their sexual orientation. Now many gay persons openly express their sexual preferences and relationships. *Queer* is a term to describe anyone who is not heterosexual. In the past, it was a negative term, but the term is increasingly used to describe identities.

Bisexuals are attracted to both sexes. Some have same-gender and male-female behaviors. They often marry and have children. They may seek a same-gender relationship or experience outside of marriage.

A transgender person self-identifies as the opposite gender or gender that does not match the natal sex. The term also is used to describe persons who are undergoing hormone therapy or surgery for sexual reassignment (female to male; male to female).

INJURY, ILLNESS, AND SURGERY

Injury, illness, and surgery can affect sexual function. Sometimes the nervous, circulatory, and reproductive systems are involved. One or more systems may be affected. Sexual ability may change. Most chronic illnesses affect sexual function. Heart disease, stroke, diabetes, and chronic obstructive pulmonary disease are examples.

Reproductive system surgeries have physical and mental effects. Removal of the uterus, ovaries, or a breast affects women. A woman who has had a mastectomy (breast removal) may be very self-conscious during bathing. Always remember to provide privacy. Prostate or testes removal affects erections.

During bathing (Chapter 18) it is always best if residents can perform their own perineal care. Some residents are not able to do this. At times a male may have an erection when perineal care or bathing is performed. The man may be embarrassed. It is best to assure him that this happens at times. Quickly finish the task and give him privacy. For some new nursing assistants this can cause anxiety. Talk to your charge nurse if you have concerns.

Impotence (erectile dysfunction [ED]) is the inability of the natal male to have an erection. Diabetes, spinal cord injuries, multiple sclerosis, prostate problems, and alcoholism are causes. Heart and circulatory disorders, medications, drug abuse, and psychologic factors are other causes. Some medications for high blood pressure cause ED. There are forms of treatment for ED, including medications.

Emotional changes are common. The person may feel unclean, unwhole, or unattractive. Attitudes may change. The person may feel unfit for closeness and love. Therefore some problems are emotional. Time, understanding, and a caring partner are helpful. For some individuals, counseling may be helpful.

Changes in sexual function have a great impact on the person. Fear, anger, worry, and depression are common. They are seen in the person's behavior and comments. The person's feelings are normal and expected. Follow the care plan. It has measures to help the person deal with such feelings.

SEXUALITY AND OLDER PERSONS

Love, affection, and intimacy are needed throughout life (Fig. 10.2). Older persons love, fall in love, hold hands, and embrace. Many have intercourse.

Older persons have many losses. Children leave home. Family and friends die. People retire. Health problems occur. Strength decreases. Appearance changes. It helps to feel close to another person.

Reproductive organs change with aging (Chapter 9). Frequency of sex decreases for many older persons. Reasons relate

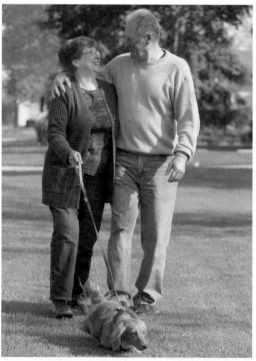

Fig. 10.2 Love and affection are important to persons of all ages.

to weakness, fatigue, and pain. Reduced mobility, aging, and chronic illness are factors.

Some older people do not have intercourse. This does not mean loss of sexual needs or desires. Often needs are expressed in other ways. They may hold hands, touch, caress, and embrace. These activities bring closeness and intimacy.

Sexual partners are lost through death, divorce, and relationship breakups. Or a partner needs hospital or nursing center care. These situations occur in adults of all ages.

MEETING SEXUAL NEEDS

The nursing team promotes the meeting of sexual needs. The measures in Box 10.1 may be part of the person's care plan.

❖   Married couples in nursing centers may share the same room if they wish. This option is a requirement of the Omnibus Budget Reconciliation Act of 1987 (OBRA). The couple may have lived together a long time. Long-term care is no reason to keep them apart. They can share the same bed if their conditions permit. A double, queen-size, or king-size bed is provided by the couple or the center. Some married couples may prefer separate rooms in nursing centers. For some couples, the level of care required may differ for each partner. For example, one

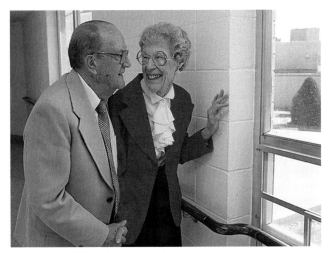

Fig. 10.3 Relationships develop in nursing centers.

partner may need health care center nursing services, whereas the other can live in an assisted living environment. Arrangements are often made for them to spend time together and ◆ share meals with each other.

Single persons may develop relationships. They are allowed time together, not kept apart (Fig. 10.3). Staff need to respect the request for private time.

THE SEXUALLY AGGRESSIVE PERSON

Some persons want the health team to meet their sexual needs. They flirt or make sexual advances or comments. Some expose themselves, masturbate, or touch the staff inappropriately. This can anger and embarrass staff members. These reactions are normal. Often there are reasons for the person's behavior. Understanding this helps you deal with the matter.

Sexually aggressive behaviors have many causes. They include:
- Nervous system disorders.
- Confusion, disorientation, and dementia.
- Medication side effects.
- Fever.
- Poor vision.

The person may confuse someone with a partner. Or the person cannot control behavior. The cause is a change in mental function. The healthy person controls sexual urges. Changes in the brain make control difficult. Sexual behavior in these cases is usually innocent.

Sometimes touch serves to gain attention. For example, Mr. Green cannot speak. He cannot move his right side. Your buttocks are near him. To get your attention, he touches your buttocks. His behavior is not sexual.

Sometimes masturbation is a sexually aggressive behavior. Some persons touch and fondle the genitals for sexual pleasure. However, urinary or reproductive system disorders can cause genital soreness or itching. So can poor hygiene and being wet or soiled from urine or feces. Touching genitals could signal a health problem.

BOX 10.1   Promoting Sexuality

- Let the person practice grooming routines. Assist as needed. For women, this includes applying makeup, nail polish, and cologne. Many women shave their legs and underarms and pluck eyebrows. Men may use aftershave lotion and cologne. Hair care is important to men and women.
- Let the person choose clothing. Hospital gowns embarrass both men and women. Street clothes are worn if the person's condition permits.
- Protect the right to privacy. Do not expose the person. Drape and screen the person. Be especially careful in bathing and shower rooms.
- Accept the person's sexual relationships. The person may not share your sexual attitudes, values, or practices. The person may have a homosexual, premarital, or extramarital relationship. The person may identify with LGBTQ+ community. Do not judge or gossip about relationships. Do not make assumptions about the person's sexual orientation.
- Allow privacy. You can usually tell when people want to be alone. If the person has a private room, close the door for privacy. Some centers have *DO NOT DISTURB* signs for doors. Let the person and partner know how much time they have alone. For example, remind them about meal times, medication administration, and treatments. Tell other staff members that the person wants time alone.
- Knock before you enter any room. This is a simple courtesy that shows respect for privacy.
- Consider the person's roommate. Privacy curtains provide little privacy. They do not block sound. Arrange for privacy when the roommate is out of the room. Sometimes roommates offer to leave for a while. If the roommate cannot leave, the nurse finds a private area.
- Allow privacy for masturbation. It is a normal form of sexual expression. Close the privacy curtain and the door. Knock before you enter any room. This saves you and the person embarrassment. Sometimes confused persons masturbate in public areas. Lead the person to a private area or provide a distraction with another activity.

Sometimes the purpose of touch is sexual. For example, some residents want to prove they are attractive and can perform sexually. You must be professional about the matter.

- Ask them not to touch you. State the places where you were touched.
- Tell them that you will not do what they want.
- Tell them what behaviors make you uncomfortable. Politely tell them not to act that way.
- Allow privacy if they become aroused. Provide for safety. Complete a safety check of the room (see the inside of the front cover). Tell them when you will return.
- Discuss such matters with the nurse. The nurse can help you understand the behavior.
- Follow the care plan. It has measures to deal with sexually aggressive behaviors. They are based on the cause of the behavior. Many centers have classes to help staff deal with such behavior.

See *Focus on Communication: The Sexually Aggressive Person.*

FOCUS ON COMMUNICATION

The Sexually Aggressive Person

Confronting the sexually aggressive person is difficult. This is true for young and older staff and for new and experienced staff. Ask yourself these questions:

- Does the person have a health problem that affects impulse control? If yes, the behavior may not have a sexual purpose.
- Is the person's behavior on purpose? Is the intent sexual? If yes, you must confront the behavior. Be direct and matter-of-fact. For example, you can say:
  - "You brushed your hand across my breast (or other body part) two times this morning. Please don't do that again."
  - "No, I cannot kiss you. I am your nursing assistant and our relationship is strictly professional."
  - "You exposed yourself to me again today. Please do not do that again."

Protecting the Person

The person must be protected from unwanted sexual comments and advances. This is sexual abuse (Chapter 2) and is very serious. Tell the nurse right away. No one should be allowed to sexually abuse another person. This includes staff members, residents, family members or other visitors, and volunteers.

SEXUALLY TRANSMITTED DISEASES

Some diseases are spread by sexual contact. They are discussed in Chapter 38.

The sexually aggressive person needs the nurse's attention. Discuss the matter with the nurse. Report what happened and when. Also report what you said and did. The nurse must deal with the problem. If other staff are reporting such behaviors, the nurse views the problem in a broader and different way.

QUALITY OF LIFE

Sexuality is part of the total person. Illness or injury does not make it of little concern. Nor does surgery or aging. How sexuality is expressed may change. To meet the person's sexual needs, follow the care plan. Always provide for privacy.

Do not judge or gossip about a person's sexuality. Healthy, pleasurable sexual relationships and intimacy enhance the quality of life for people of all ages.

TIME TO REFLECT

Mr. James is a 75-year-old resident who suffers from emphysema. When he was first admitted to the care center, he would often tell jokes and kid with the staff. Recently his jokes have turned sexual in nature and you find them offensive. Amy, a young and inexperienced nursing assistant, tells you that she is afraid to help Mr. James with his shower. She tells you that yesterday in the shower room she asked Mr. James to wash his perineal area. He refused and replied, "Aw, come on, it's more fun when you do it for me." How should this situation be handled from here?

REVIEW QUESTIONS

Circle the BEST answer.

1. Sex involves
   a. The organs of reproduction
   b. Attitudes and feelings
   c. Cultural and spiritual factors
   d. Masturbation
2. Sexuality is important to
   a. Young adults
   b. Middle-age adults
   c. Older adults
   d. Persons of all ages
3. Impotence is
   a. When menstruation stops
   b. A reaction to illness

c. Not being able to achieve an erection
   d. No sexual activity
4. A person who is attracted to members of the same gender is a
   a. Heterosexual
   b. Transvestite
   c. Transsexual
   d. Homosexual
5. Mr. and Mrs. Green live in a nursing center. Which will *not* promote their sexuality?
   a. Allowing their normal grooming routines
   b. Having them wear hospital gowns
   c. Allowing them privacy
   d. Accepting their relationship

6. Two residents are holding hands. Nursing staff should
   a. Keep them apart
   b. Report this to their families
   c. Allow them to do this
   d. Tease them about their relationship

7. Mr. and Mrs. Green want some time alone. The nursing team can do the following *except*
   a. Close the room door
   b. Put a "do not disturb" sign on the door
   c. Tell other staff that they want some time alone
   d. Close the privacy curtain so no one can hear them

8. Mr. and Mrs. Green are married. OBRA requires that
   a. They should have separate rooms
   b. They may share the same room
   c. They live in separate facilities
   d. Their meals are free

9. A person is masturbating in the dining room. You should do the following *except*
   a. Cover and quietly take the person to their room
   b. Scold the person
   c. Provide privacy
   d. Tell the nurse

10. A person touches you sexually and asks for a kiss. You should do the following *except*
   a. Discuss the matter with the nurse
   b. Ignore the person and hope that the behavior will stop
   c. Explain that the behaviors make you uncomfortable
   d. Ask the person not to touch you

   See Appendix A for answers to these questions.

11

Safety

OBJECTIVES

- Define the key terms and key abbreviations listed in this chapter.
- Describe accident risk factors.
- Explain why you identify a person before giving care.
- Explain how to correctly identify a person.
- Describe the safety measures to prevent burns, poisoning, and suffocation.
- Identify the signs and causes of choking.
- Explain how to prevent equipment accidents.
- Explain how to handle hazardous substances.
- Describe safety measures for fire prevention and oxygen use.

- Explain what to do during a fire.
- Give examples of natural and human-made disasters.
- Explain what to do during a tornado.
- Recognize where emergency procedure plans are located.
- Understand how to read evacuation maps.
- Explain how to report accidents and errors.
- Explain how to protect yourself from workplace violence.
- Describe your role in risk management.
- Perform the procedures described in this chapter.
- Explain how to promote quality of life.

KEY TERMS

anticoagulant Blood-thinning medication

coma A state of being unaware of one's surroundings and being unable to react or respond to people, places, or things

dementia The loss of cognitive and social function caused by changes in the brain

disaster A sudden catastrophic event in which people are injured and killed and property is destroyed

electric shock When electric current passes through the body

ground That which carries leaking electricity to the earth and away from an electrical item

hazard Anything in the person's setting that may cause injury or illness

hazardous substance Any chemical in the workplace that can cause harm

hemiplegia Paralysis on one side of the body

hemorrhage The excessive loss of blood in a short time

incident Any event that has harmed or could harm a resident, visitor, or staff member

paralysis Loss of muscle function, loss of sensation, or loss of both

paraplegia Paralysis in the legs and lower trunk

quadriplegia Paralysis in the arms, legs, and trunk; tetraplegia

suffocation When breathing stops from the lack of oxygen

tetraplegia See "quadriplegia"

workplace violence Violent acts (including assault and threat of assault) directed toward persons at work or while on duty

KEY ABBREVIATIONS

AED Automated external defibrillator

C Centigrade

CPR Cardiopulmonary resuscitation

EMS Emergency Medical Services

F Fahrenheit

FBAO Foreign-body airway obstruction

ID Identification

NOAA National Oceanic and Atmospheric Association

OBRA Omnibus Budget Reconciliation Act of 1987

OSHA Occupational Safety and Health Administration

PASS Pull the safety pin, aim low, squeeze the lever, sweep back and forth

PPE Personal Protective Equipment

RACE Rescue, alarm, confine, extinguish

SDS Safety Data Sheet

Safety is a basic need. Residents are at great risk for accidents and falls (Chapter 12). Some accidents and injuries cause death.

The health team must provide for safety. This includes you. Ordinary and sometimes extraordinary measures are needed to prevent accidents and keep residents safe. The goal is to decrease the person's risk of accidents and injuries without limiting mobility and independence.

The Omnibus Budget Reconciliation Act of 1987 (OBRA) requires that nursing centers follow safety policies and procedures, and accrediting agency standards. The intent is to keep residents, visitors, and staff safe. Measures to protect residents must not interfere with their rights (Chapter 2).

Common sense and simple safety measures can prevent most accidents. You must protect residents, visitors, yourself, and coworkers. The safety measures in this chapter apply to nursing and everyday life. The care plan lists other safety measures for the person.

A SAFE SETTING

In a safe setting, a person has little risk of illness or injury. The person's setting is free of hazards to the extent possible. A hazard is anything in the person's setting that may cause injury or illness.

The person feels safe and secure physically and mentally. The risk of infection, falls, burns, poisoning, and other injuries is low. Temperature and noise levels are comfortable. Smells are pleasant. There is enough room and light to move about safely. The person and personal property are safe from fire and intruders. The person is not afraid and has few worries and concerns.

The person must receive the right care and treatment. The person is protected from falls, burns, poisoning, suffocation, and infection. To protect the person from harm, follow the person's care plan. Also practice the safety measures in this chapter.

See *Teamwork and Time Management: A Safe Setting.*

TEAMWORK AND TIME MANAGEMENT

A Safe Setting

The entire health team must provide a safe setting. You may see something unsafe. Correct the matter right away if it is something you can do. For example:

- You see a water spill. Wipe up the spill right away. Do so even if you did not cause the spill.
- You see a person sliding out of a wheelchair. Position the person correctly in the chair. Do so even if a coworker is responsible for the person's care.
- A person is having problems holding a cup of coffee. Offer to help the person.
- Food is left unattended in a microwave oven. Turn off the device. Then tell your coworker the reason for your action.
- A grab bar is loose in the bathroom. Tell the nurse. Follow center policy for reporting the problem.

You cannot correct some safety issues. Follow center policy for reporting such problems. They include:

- Electrical outlets or switches coming out of the wall
- Electrical outlets that do not work
- Water leaks from windows, doors, ceilings, pipes, faucets, tubs, showers, toilets, hot water heaters, fountains, and other water sources
- Toilets that do not work properly
- Water from faucets that does not warm up or that is very hot
- Broken windows
- Windows and doors that do not work properly
- Knobs and handles that are broken or do not work properly
- Handrails and grab bars that are loose or need repair
- Odd smells and odors
- Odd sounds
- Signs of rodents, flies, or other pests
- Broken or damaged furniture
- Lights and lamps that do not work or have burnt-out bulbs
- Flooring (carpeting, tiles) in need of repair
- Ice on sidewalks and entryways

ACCIDENT RISK FACTORS

Some people cannot protect themselves. They present dangers to themselves and others. They rely on others for safety. Know the factors that increase a person's risk of accidents and injuries. Follow the person's care plan to provide for safety.

- *Age.* Changes from aging increase the risk for falls and other injuries. Older persons have decreased strength and move slowly. Some are unsteady. Often balance is affected. These changes prevent quick and sudden movements to avoid dangers and prevent falls. Older persons also are less sensitive to heat and cold. They have poor vision, hearing problems, and a dulled sense of smell. Confusion, poor judgment, memory problems, and disorientation may occur (Chapter 40).
- *Awareness of surroundings.* People need to know their surroundings to protect themselves from injury. Coma is a state of being unaware of one's surroundings and being unable to react or respond to people, places, or things. A coma can occur from illness or injury. The person in a coma relies on others for protection. Confused and disoriented persons may not understand what is happening to and around them. See *Residents with Dementia: Accident Risk Factors (Awareness of Surroundings).*
- *Agitated and aggressive behaviors.* Pain can cause these behaviors. So can confusion, decreased awareness of surroundings, and fear of what may happen.
- *Vision loss.* Persons with poor vision have problems seeing things. They can fall or trip over toys, rugs, equipment, furniture, and cords. Some have problems reading labels on cleaners and other containers. Poisoning can result. It also can result from taking the wrong medication or the wrong dose.
- *Hearing loss.* Persons with hearing loss have problems hearing explanations and instructions. They may not hear warning signals or fire alarms. Some cannot hear approaching meal carts, drug carts, stretchers, or people in wheelchairs. They do not know to move to safety.
- *Impaired smell and touch.* Illness and aging affect smell and touch. The person may not detect smoke or gas odors. When touch is reduced, burns are a risk. The person has problems sensing heat and cold. Some people have a decreased pain sense. They may be unaware of injury. For example, Mrs. Parks does not feel a blister from her shoes. She has poor circulation to her legs and feet. The blister can become a serious wound.
- *Impaired mobility.* Some diseases and injuries affect mobility. A person may know there is danger but cannot move to safety. Some persons cannot walk or propel wheelchairs. Some persons are paralyzed. Paralysis means loss of muscle function, loss of sensation, or loss of both. Paraplegia is paralysis in the legs and lower trunk. Quadriplegia (tetraplegia) is paralysis in the arms, legs, and trunk. Hemiplegia is paralysis on one side of the body.
- *Medications.* Medications have side effects. They include loss of balance, drowsiness, and lack of coordination. Reduced awareness, confusion, and disorientation can occur. The person may be fearful and uncooperative. Report behavior changes to the nurse. Also report the person's complaints.

RESIDENTS WITH DEMENTIA

Accident Risk Factors (Awareness of Surroundings)
Some persons suffer from dementia. Dementia is the loss of cognitive and social function caused by changes in the brain (Chapter 40). Memory and the ability to think and reason are lost. Dementia is caused by diseases and injuries.

Persons with dementia are confused and disoriented. Their awareness of surroundings is reduced. They may not understand what is happening to and around them. Judgment is poor. They no longer know what is safe and what are dangers. They may access closets, cupboards, or other unsafe and unlocked areas. They may eat or drink cleaning products, drugs, or poisons. Accidents and injuries are great risks. The health team must meet all safety needs.

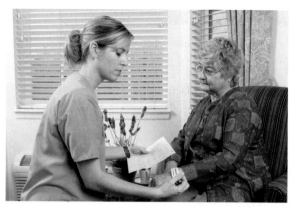

Fig. 11.2 The identification (ID) bracelet is checked against the assignment sheet to accurately identify the person.

IDENTIFYING THE PERSON

You will care for many people. Each has different treatments, therapies, and activity limits. You must give the right care to the right person. Life and health are threatened if the wrong care is given.

The person may receive an identification (ID) bracelet when admitted to the center (Fig. 11.1). The bracelet has the person's name, room and bed number, birth date, age, doctor, and center name. Other identifying information may include the person's ID number given by the center. Some centers include the person's religion.

You use the bracelet to identify the person before giving care. The assignment sheet states what care to give. To identify the person:

- Compare identifying information on the assignment sheet with that on the ID bracelet (Fig. 11.2). Carefully check the information. Some people have the same first and last names. For example, John Smith is a very common name.
- Use at least two identifiers. An identifier cannot be the person's room or bed number. Some centers require that the person state one's own name and birth date. Others require using the person's ID number. Always follow center policy.
- Call the person by name when checking the ID bracelet. This is a courtesy given as you touch the person and before giving care. Just calling the name is not enough to identify the person. Confused, disoriented, drowsy, hard-of-hearing, or distracted persons may answer to any name.

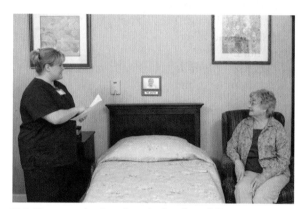

Fig. 11.3 The person's photo is at the headboard. Her name is under the photo. The nursing assistant is using the photo to identify the person.

Alert and oriented residents may choose not to wear ID bracelets. This is noted on the person's care plan. Follow center policy and the care plan to identify the person.

Some nursing centers have photo ID systems (Fig. 11.3). The person's photo is taken on admission. Then it is placed in the person's medical record. If your center uses such a system, learn to use it safely.

See *Promoting Safety and Comfort: Identifying the Person.*

PROMOTING SAFETY AND COMFORT

Identifying the Person
Safety
Always identify the person before you begin a task or procedure. Do not identify the person and then leave the room to collect supplies and equipment. You could go to the wrong room and give care to the wrong person. And the person for whom the care was intended would not receive it. This too could cause harm. It is also important to identify the correct resident in the dining room when serving meals. Some centers have a seating diagram or the residents' names placed at their table.

Sometimes ID bracelets become damaged from water, spilled food and fluids, and everyday wear and tear. Make sure you can read the information on the ID bracelet. If you cannot, tell the nurse. The nurse can have a new bracelet made for the person.

Comfort
Make sure the person's ID bracelet is not too tight. You should be able to slide one or two fingers under the bracelet. If it is too tight, tell the nurse.

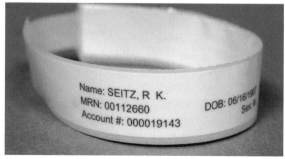

Name: SEITZ, R K.
MRN: 00112660
DOB: 06/16/19__
Account #: 000019143
Sex __

Fig. 11.1 Identification (ID) bracelet.

PREVENTING BURNS

Burns are a leading cause of death among children and older persons. Smoking, spilled hot liquids, electrical items, and very hot water (hand sinks, tubs, showers) are some causes in nursing centers. Risk factors for burns in older persons are decreased skin thickness, decreased sensitivity to heat, reduced reaction time, decreased mobility, communication problems, confusion, and dementia.

Burn severity depends on water temperature and length of exposure (Table 11.1). The person's condition also is a factor. The three degrees of burns are:

- *Superficial (first-degree) burn*—involves the epidermis (top layer of skin). Sunburn is an example. The skin is red and painful to touch. There may be mild swelling.
- *Partial-thickness (second-degree) burn*—involves the epidermis and dermis. The skin appears deep red. The person has pain and blisters. The skin may appear glossy from leaking fluid.
- *Full-thickness (third-degree) burn*—the epidermis and dermis, fat, muscle, and bone may be injured or destroyed.

These burns are not painful. Nerve endings are destroyed. The skin appears charred or has white, brown, or black patches.

The safety measures in Box 11.1 can prevent burns.

PREVENTING POISONING

Poisoning also is a health hazard and a major cause of death. Older persons are at risk. Medications and household products are common poisons. Poisoning in adults may be from carelessness, confusion, or poor vision when reading labels. As a result, a person may take too much of a medication. Chemicals should always be stored in their original containers. For example, never place a cleaning chemical in a beverage bottle or drinking cup. It could accidentally get swallowed. Sometimes poisoning is a suicide attempt.

The measures in Box 11.2 can prevent poisoning.

PREVENTING SUFFOCATION

Suffocation is when breathing stops from the lack of oxygen. Death occurs if the person does not start breathing. Common causes include choking, drowning, inhaling gas or smoke, strangulation, and electric shock (p. 127).

Carbon monoxide poisoning is another cause. Carbon monoxide is a colorless, odorless, and tasteless gas. It is produced by burning fuel. For example, motor vehicles, furnaces, gas water heaters, gas stoves, and gas dryers use fuel. These devices must be in good working order and used correctly. Otherwise, dangerous levels of carbon monoxide may result. Instead of breathing in oxygen, the person breathes in air filled with carbon monoxide. Headache, nausea, and dizziness are common. So are confusion, breathing problems, sleepiness, and cherry-pink skin. Death can occur.

Measures to prevent suffocation are listed in Box 11.3. Clear the airway if the person is choking.

TABLE 11.1 Water Temperature and Length of Exposure for a Third-Degree Burn		
Fahrenheit (F)	**Centigrade (C)**	**Time Required for a Third-Degree Burn to Occur**
155°F	68°C	1 second
148°F	64°C	2 seconds
140°F	60°C	5 seconds
133°F	56°C	15 seconds
127°F	52°C	1 minute
120°F	48°C	5 minutes
100°F	37°C	Usually a safe temperature for bathing

Modified from Centers for Medicare & Medicaid Services: *State operations manual*, Baltimore, 2022, US Department of Health and Human Services.

BOX 11.1 Safety Measures to Prevent Burns

Eating and Drinking
- Assist with eating and drinking as needed. Spilled hot food or fluids can cause burns.
- Be careful when carrying hot foods and fluids near older persons.

Water
- Turn on cold water first, then hot water. Turn off hot water first, then cold water.
- Measure bath or shower water temperature (Chapter 18). Check it before a person gets into the tub or shower.
- Check for "hot spots" in bath water. Move your hand back and forth.

Appliances
- See "Preventing Equipment Accidents" (p. 126).
- Do not allow the use of space heaters.
- Do not let the person sleep with a heating pad.
- Do not let the person use an electric blanket.
- Turn off curling irons, electric rollers, and hair dryers when not in use.

Smoking
- Be sure residents smoke only in smoking areas.
- Do not leave smoking materials at the bedside. They are only left at the bedside if the person is trusted to smoke alone in smoking areas. Follow the care plan.
- Supervise the smoking of persons who cannot protect themselves.
- Do not allow smoking in bed.
- Do not allow smoking where oxygen is used or stored (Chapter 26).
- Be alert to ashes that may fall onto an older person.

Other
- Follow safety guidelines when applying heat and cold.
- Do not allow candles or other open flames.

BOX 11.2   Safety Measures to Prevent Poisoning

- Keep harmful products in locked areas.
- Keep child-resistant caps on all harmful products.
- Store personal care items according to center policy. Soap, mouthwash, lotion, deodorant, and shampoo are examples. These items could cause harm when swallowed.
- Use and store harmful products according to the manufacturer instructions (p. 130).
- Do not leave harmful products unattended when in use.
- Make sure all harmful products are labeled (p. 129).
- Do not mix cleaning products.
- Read all labels carefully. Have good lighting.
- Keep harmful products in their original containers. Do not store them in food containers.
- Do not store harmful products near food.
- Discard harmful products that are outdated.
- Keep emergency numbers by the telephone: poison control center (1-800-222-1222, American Association of Poison Control Centers), police, ambulance, hospital, and doctor.

BOX 11.3   Safety Measures to Prevent Suffocation

- Cut food into bite-sized pieces for persons who cannot do so themselves.
- Make sure dentures fit properly and are in place.
- Make sure the person can chew and swallow the food served.
- Report loose teeth or dentures.
- Check the care plan for swallowing problems before providing food (including snacks) or fluids. The person may ask for something that he or she cannot swallow.
- Tell the nurse at once if the person has swallowing problems.
- Do not give oral food or fluids to persons with feeding tubes (Chapter 21).
- Follow aspiration precautions.
- Do not leave a person unattended in a bathtub or shower.
- Move all persons from the area if you smell smoke.
- Position the person in bed properly (Chapter 15).
- Use bed rails correctly (Chapter 12).
- Use restraints correctly (Chapter 13).
- Prevent entrapment in the bed system (Chapter 16).
- See "Preventing Equipment Accidents" (p.126).

Choking

Foreign bodies can obstruct the airway. This is called *choking* or *foreign-body airway obstruction (FBAO)*. Air cannot pass through the air passages to the lungs. The body does not get enough oxygen. It can lead to cardiac arrest. *Cardiac arrest* is when the heart stops suddenly and without warning (Chapter 44).

Choking often occurs during eating. A large, poorly chewed piece of meat is the most common cause. Weakness, dentures that fit poorly, dysphagia (difficulty swallowing), and chronic illness are also causes. So are laughing and talking while eating and excessive alcohol intake.

Unconscious persons can choke. Common causes are aspiration of vomitus and the tongue falling back into the airway. These also occur during cardiac arrest.

Foreign bodies can cause mild or *severe airway obstruction*. With *mild airway obstruction,* some air moves in and out of the lungs. The person is conscious and usually can speak. Often forceful coughing can remove the object. Breathing may sound like wheezing between coughs. For mild airway obstruction:

- Stay with the person.
- Encourage the person to keep coughing to expel the object.
- Do not interrupt the person's efforts to clear the airway. If breathing and coughing, abdominal thrusts are not needed.
- If the obstruction persists, call for help.

Difficulty breathing occurs with *severe airway obstruction*. Air does not move in and out of the lungs. The person may not be able to breathe, speak, or cough. If able to cough, the cough is of poor quality. When the person tries to inhale, there is no noise or a high-pitched noise. The person may appear pale and cyanotic (bluish color). Emergency care for severe airway obstruction is covered in Chapter 44.

CONTROLLING BLEEDING

When blood vessels are cut, bleeding can occur. Hemorrhage is the excessive loss of blood in a short time. The amount of bleeding depends on the type of vessel that was damaged and how many. Bleeding can come from arteries, veins, or capillaries (Chapter 8). Since arteries carry blood away from the heart, this bleeding is the most serious. Blood from an artery is usually bright red and spurts out of the body quickly. It must be stopped as soon as possible. Venous blood is usually darker and flows out slower. Blood from capillaries flows even slower and is usually easy to stop. Whatever the source of bleeding, always follow the rules for bloodborne pathogen exposure (Chapter 14). Control of bleeding is covered in detail in Chapter 44. Some centers have special bleeding control kits. For persons taking anticoagulants (blood-thinning medications), bleeding may be harder to control.

PREVENTING INFECTION

The spread of infection is a major hazard in nursing centers. Infections are caused by microorganisms that easily spread from one person to another. Infection is a risk for persons who are older, chronically ill, or disabled. Infections increase their health problems. They often cause death. Chapter 14 describes how to prevent infections.

PREVENTING EQUIPMENT ACCIDENTS

All equipment is unsafe if broken, not used correctly, or not working properly. This includes hospital beds. Inspect all equipment before use. Check glass and plastic items for cracks, chips, and sharp or rough edges. They can cause cuts, stabs, or scratches. Follow the bloodborne pathogen standard (Chapter 14).

Electric items must work properly and be in good repair. Frayed cords (Fig. 11.4) and overloaded electric outlets (Fig. 11.5) can cause fires, burns, and electric shocks. Electric shock is when electrical current passes through the body. It can burn the skin, muscles, nerves, and other tissues. It can affect the heart and cause death.

Three-pronged plugs (Fig. 11.6) are used on all electric items. Two prongs carry electric current. The third prong is the ground. Never remove the third prong of a three-prong plug to make it fit into an outlet. A ground carries leaking electricity to the earth and away from an electric item. If a ground is not used, leaking electricity can be conducted to the person. It can cause electric shocks and possible death. If you receive a shock, report it at once. Do not use the item.

Warning signs of a faulty electric item include:

- Shocks
- Loss of power or a power outage
- Dimming or flickering lights
- Sparks
- Sizzling or buzzing sounds
- Burning odor
- Loose plugs

Do not use or give damaged items to residents. Take the item to the nurse. The nurse will have you do one of the following:

- Discard the item following center policy.

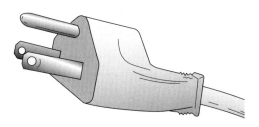

Fig. 11.6 A three-pronged plug.

- Tag the item and send it for repair following center policy.

Practice the safety measures in Box 11.4 when using equipment. An incident report (p. 142) is completed if a resident, visitor, or staff member has an equipment-related accident. The Safe Medical Devices Act requires that centers report equipment-related illnesses, injuries, and deaths.

WHEELCHAIR AND STRETCHER SAFETY

Some people cannot walk or have severe problems walking. A wheelchair may be useful (Fig. 11.8). If able, the person propels the chair using the hand rims. Some use the feet to move the chair. Other wheelchairs are propelled by motors. The person moves the chair with hand, chin, mouth, or other controls. If the person cannot propel the wheelchair, another person pushes it using the hand grips/push handles. When another person pushes a resident in a wheelchair, the seated person should always have the feet resting on the foot pedals.

Stretchers are used to transport persons who cannot use wheelchairs. When on a stretcher, they cannot sit up or must lie down.

Follow the safety measures in Box 11.5 when using wheelchairs and stretchers. The person can fall from the wheelchair or stretcher, or fall during transfers to and from the wheelchair or stretcher.

HANDLING HAZARDOUS SUBSTANCES

A hazardous substance is any chemical in the workplace that can cause harm. The Occupational Safety and Health Administration (OSHA) requires that health care employees:

- Understand the risks of hazardous substances.
- Know how to safely handle them.

Physical hazards can cause fires or explosions. *Health hazards* are chemicals that can cause acute or chronic health problems. Acute problems occur rapidly and last a short time. They usually are from short-term exposure. Chronic problems usually result from long-term exposure. They occur over a long time.

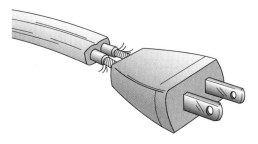

Fig. 11.4 A frayed electric cord.

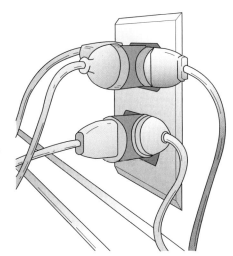

Fig. 11.5 An overloaded electric outlet.

BOX 11.4   Safety Measures to Prevent Equipment Accidents

General Safety

- Follow center policies and procedures.
- Follow the manufacturer instructions. Use equipment correctly.
- Read all caution and warning labels.
- Do not use an unfamiliar item. Ask for needed training. Also ask a nurse to supervise you the first time you use an item.
- Use an item only for its intended purpose.
- Make sure the item works before you begin.
- Make sure you have all needed equipment. For example, you need to plug in an item. There must be an outlet.
- Show a broken or damaged item to the nurse. Follow the nurse's instructions and center policies for discarding items or sending them for repair.
- Do not try to repair broken or damaged items.
- Do not use broken or damaged items.

Electric Safety

- Inspect electric cords and appliances for damage. Make sure they are in good repair.
- Use three-pronged plugs on all electric devices.
- Use extension cords for only one device. This prevents overloading a circuit.
- Do not use power strips for care equipment.
- Do not cover power cords with rugs, carpets, linens, or other materials. Do not run power cords under rugs.
- Connect a bed power cord directly to a wall outlet. Do not connect a bed power cord to an extension cord or outlet strip.
- Do not use electric items owned by the person until they are safety checked. The maintenance staff does this.
- Keep electric items away from water.
- Keep work areas clean and dry. Wipe up spills right away.
- Do not touch electrical items if you are wet, if your hands are wet, or if you are standing in water.
- Do not put a finger or any item into an outlet.

- Turn off equipment before unplugging it. Sparks occur when electrical items are unplugged while turned on.
- Hold on to the plug (not the cord) when removing it from an outlet (Fig. 11.7).
- Do not give showers or tub baths during electrical storms. Lightning can travel through pipes.
- Do not use electric items or phones during storms.
- Do not use water to put out an electrical fire. If possible, turn off or unplug the item.
- Do not touch a person who is experiencing an electrical shock. If possible, turn off or unplug the item. Call for help at once.
- Keep electrical cords away from heating vents and other heat sources.
- Turn off the electrical device when done using the item.
- Know where auxiliary outlets are located for emergency equipment (oxygen, etc.).
- Have battery-powered lighting available during power outages.
- Unplug all electrical devices when not in use.

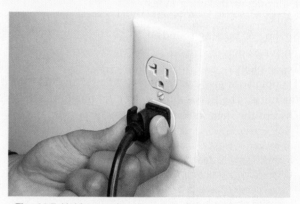

Fig. 11.7 Hold on to the plug to remove it from an outlet.

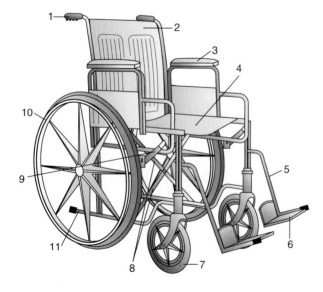

1. Handgrip/push handle
2. Back upholstery
3. Armrest
4. Seat upholstery
5. Front rigging
6. Footplate
7. Caster
8. Crossbrace
9. Wheel lock/brake
10. Wheel and handrim
11. Tipping lever

Fig. 11.8 Parts of a wheelchair.

Health hazards can:

- Cause cancer.
- Affect blood cell formation and function.
- Damage the kidneys, nervous system, lungs, skin, eyes, or mucous membranes.
- Cause birth defects, miscarriages, and fertility problems from reproductive system damage.

Exposure to hazardous substances can occur under normal working conditions. Hazardous chemicals could accidently splash on the skin or in the eyes. It also can happen during certain emergencies. Examples include equipment failures, container ruptures, or the uncontrolled release of a hazard into the workplace. Hazardous substances include the following:

- Medications used in cancer therapy (chemotherapy, anti-cancer medications)
- Anesthesia gases
- Gases used to sterilize equipment
- Oxygen
- Disinfectants and cleaning agents
- Radiation used for x-rays and cancer treatments
- Mercury (found in thermometers and blood pressure devices)

OSHA requires a hazard communication program. The program includes container labeling, Safety Data Sheets (SDSs),

BOX 11.5 Wheelchair and Stretcher Safety

Wheelchair Safety

- Check the wheel locks (brakes). Make sure you can lock and unlock them.
- Check for flat or loose tires. A wheel lock will not work on a flat or loose tire.
- Make sure the wheel spokes are intact. Damaged, broken, or loose spokes can interfere with moving the wheelchair or locking the wheels.
- Make sure the casters point forward. This keeps the wheelchair balanced and stable.
- Position the person's feet on the footplates.
- Make sure the person's feet are on the footplates before moving the chair. The person's feet must not touch or drag on the floor when the chair is moving. Never push a person in a wheelchair without feet resting on footplates.
- Push the chair forward when transporting the person. Do not pull the chair backward unless going through a doorway or entering an elevator.
- If going down a ramp or incline, always turn the wheelchair backward.
- Lock both wheels before you transfer a person to or from the wheelchair.
- Follow the care plan for keeping the wheels locked when not moving the wheelchair. Locking the wheels prevents the chair from moving if the person wants to move to or from the chair. (Locking the wheelchair may be viewed as a restraint. See Chapter 13.)
- Do not let the person stand on the footplates.
- Do not let the footplates fall back onto the person's legs.
- Make sure the person has needed wheelchair accessories—safety belt, pouch, tray, lapboard, cushion.
- Remove the armrests (if removable) when the person transfers to the bed, toilet, commode, tub, or car (Chapter 15).
- Swing front rigging out of the way for transfers to and from the wheelchair. Some front rigging detaches for transfers.
- Clean the wheelchair according to center policy.
- Ask a nurse or physical therapist to show you how to propel wheelchairs up steps and ramps and over curbs.
- Follow the safety measures to prevent equipment accidents (see Box 11.4).

Stretcher Safety

- Ask two coworkers to help you transfer the person to or from the stretcher (Chapter 15).
- Lock the stretcher wheels before the transfer.

- Fasten the safety straps when the person is properly positioned on the stretcher.
- Ask a coworker to help with the transport.
- Raise the side rails. Keep them up during the transport.
- Make sure the person's arms, hands, legs, and feet do not dangle through the side rail bars.
- Stand at the head of the stretcher. Your coworker stands at the foot of the stretcher.
- Move the stretcher feet first (Fig. 11.9).
- Do not leave the person alone.
- Follow the safety measures to prevent equipment accidents (see Box 11.4).

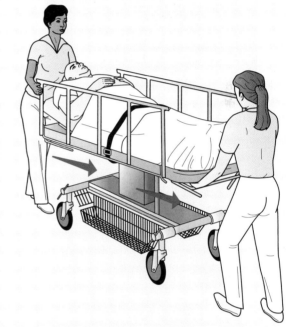

Fig. 11.9 A person is transported by stretcher. The stretcher is moved feet first.

and employee training. The center also posts signs of where eyewash stations are located (Fig 11.10). Be familiar with how the eyewash station operates (Fig 11.11). Total body wash stations may be located where hazardous substances are used.

Labeling

Hazardous substance containers include bags, barrels, bottles, boxes, cans, cylinders, drums, and storage tanks. All need warning labels (Fig. 11.12). The manufacturer supplies all labels. Warning labels identify:

- Physical and health hazards. Health hazards include the organs affected and potential health problems.
- Precaution measures (e.g., "Do not use near open flame" or "Avoid skin contact").
- What personal protective equipment to wear (e.g., gown, mask, gloves, goggles).
- How to use the substance safely.

- Storage and disposal information.

Words, pictures, and symbols communicate the warnings. A container must have a label. If a warning label is removed or damaged, do not use the substance. Take the container to the nurse and explain the problem. Do not leave the container unattended.

Safety Data Sheets

Every hazardous substance has an SDS. Previously this was called a Material Safety Data Sheet (MSDS). In the past these sheets contained valuable safety information, but they lacked a uniform format. The Globally Harmonized System of Classification ensures that all sheets have a standardized format. This will make it easier to find the necessary information quickly. The sheets provide detailed information about the substance:

- The chemical name and any common names
- The ingredients in the substance

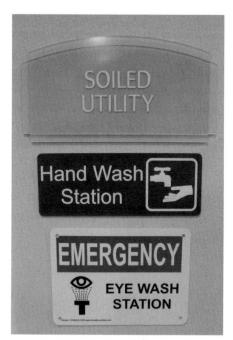

Fig 11.10 Sign for eyewash station

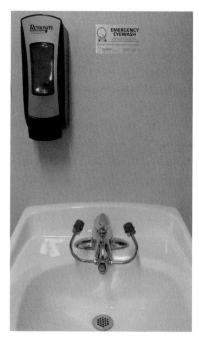

Fig 11.11 Eyewash station

- Physical and chemical characteristics (appearance, color, odor, boiling point, and others)
- Potential physical effects (fire, explosion)
- Conditions that could cause a chemical reaction
- How the chemical enters the body (inhalation, ingestion, skin contact, or absorption)
- Health hazards, including signs and symptoms
- Protective measures (how to use, handle, and store the substance)
- Emergency and first-aid procedures

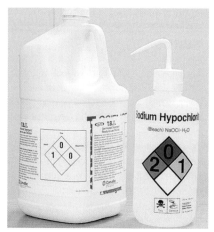

Fig. 11.12 Warning labels on hazardous substances.

- Explosion information and firefighting measures (including what type of fire extinguisher to use [p. ··])
- How to clean up a spill or leak
- Personal protective equipment needed during cleanup
- How to dispose of the hazardous substance
- Manufacturer information (name, address, and a telephone number for more information)

Employees must have ready access to SDSs. They are kept in a binder at a certain place on each nursing unit (Fig. 11.13). Some centers access SDSs through the Internet or an 800-hotline number. Check the SDSs before using a hazardous substance, cleaning up a leak or spill, or disposing of the substance. Tell the nurse about a leak or spill right away. Do not leave a leak or spill unattended.

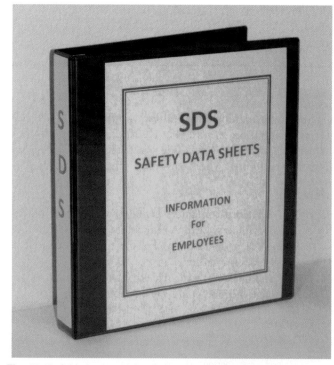

Fig. 11.13 A binder containing Safety Data Sheet information is readily available on the nursing unit.

BOX 11.6 **Safety Measures for Hazardous Substances**

- Read all warning labels.
- Follow the safety measures on the warning label and Safety Data Sheet (SDS).
- Make sure each container has a warning label that is not damaged.
- Use a leakproof container to carry or transport a hazardous substance.
- Wear personal protective equipment to clean spills and leaks. The warning label or SDS tells you what to wear (mask, gown, gloves, eye protection, safety boots).
- Clean up spills at once. Work from clean areas to dirty areas using circular motions.
- Dispose of hazardous waste in sealed bags or containers.
- Stand behind a lead shield during x-ray or radiation therapy procedures.
- Do not enter a room while a person is having x-rays or radiation therapy.
- Never allow food or beverages in areas where hazardous substances are present.
- Wash your hands after handling hazardous substances.
- Work in well-ventilated areas to avoid inhaling gases.
- Store a hazardous substance according to the SDS.
- Know the location of eyewash stations. Be familiar with their use.

Hazardous Substance Employee Training

Your employer provides hazardous substance training. You are told about hazards, exposure risks, and protection measures. You must know the location of eyewash stations and how to use them (p. 130). You learn to read and use warning labels and SDSs.

Each hazardous substance requires certain protection measures. Box 11.6 lists general rules to safely handle hazardous substances.

FIRE SAFETY

Fire is a constant danger. Faulty electrical equipment and wiring, overloaded electric circuits, and smoking are major causes of fires. The entire health team must prevent fires. They must act quickly and responsibly during a fire.

Fire and the Use of Oxygen

Three things are needed for a fire:
- Spark or flame
- Material that will burn
- Oxygen

Air has some oxygen. However, some people need extra oxygen (Chapter 26). Safety measures are needed where oxygen is used and stored:

- NO SMOKING signs are placed on the door and near the bed.
- The person and visitors are reminded not to smoke in the room.
- Smoking materials (cigarettes, cigars, and pipes), matches, and lighters are removed from the room.
- Electric items are turned off *before* being unplugged.
- Wool blankets and synthetic fabrics that cause static electricity are removed from the person's room.
- The person wears a cotton gown or pajamas.
- Electric items are in good working order. This includes electric shavers, TVs, radios, computers, and other electronic devices.
- Lit candles, incense, and other open flames are not allowed.
- Materials that ignite easily are removed from the room (e.g., oil, grease, nail polish remover).

Centers have no-smoking policies and smoke-free areas. No smoking is allowed inside the buildings. Signs are posted on all entry doors. Some people ignore such rules. Remind them about the no-smoking rules.

See *Focus on Communication: Fire and the Use of Oxygen.*

FOCUS ON COMMUNICATION

Fire and the Use of Oxygen

You may have to remind a resident or visitor not to smoke inside the center. You can simply say:

- "Mrs. Murphy, this is a smoke-free area. Here is an ashtray to put out your cigarette. If you want to smoke, I'll be happy to show you the smoking area outside."
- "Mr. Garcia, please don't smoke inside the center. We have a smoking area outside the back entrance on hallway 2. I'll be happy to show you the way."

Tell the nurse what happened, what you said, and what you did. The nurse may need to speak with the person about not smoking.

Preventing Fires

Fire prevention measures were described in relation to burns, equipment accidents, and oxygen use. Other fire prevention measures are listed in Box 11.7.

BOX 11.7 **Fire Prevention Measures**

- Follow the safety measures for oxygen use.
- Be familiar with the emergency policies for fires and take fire drills seriously.
- Smoke only where allowed to do so. Do not smoke in residents' rooms.
- Be sure all ashes, cigars, cigarettes, and other smoking materials are out before emptying ashtrays.
- Empty ashtrays into a metal container partially filled with sand or water. Do not empty ashtrays into plastic containers or wastebaskets lined with paper or plastic bags.
- Provide ashtrays for persons who are allowed to smoke.
- Supervise persons who smoke. This is very important for persons who are confused, disoriented, or sedated.
- Follow safety practices when using electric items.
- Keep matches, lighters, and flammable liquids and materials away from confused or disoriented persons.
- Do not leave cooking unattended on stoves, in ovens, or in microwave ovens.
- Store flammable liquids in their original containers. Keep the containers where residents cannot reach them.
- Do not smoke or light matches or lighters around flammable liquids or materials.
- Be aware of the presence of fire doors. When an alarm is activated these doors automatically close. You may need to evacuate residents to a safe area on the opposite side of the fire doors.
- Follow the safety measures to prevent equipment accidents (see Box 11.4).

What to Do During a Fire

Know your center's policies and procedures for emergencies (Fig. 11.14). Know where to find fire alarms, fire extinguishers, and emergency exits. Fire drills are held to practice emergency fire procedures. All staff must participate in drills so they will be able to act promptly in case of an actual fire. Remember the word *RACE* (Fig. 11.15).

R—for *rescue.* Rescue persons in immediate danger. Move them to a safe place.

A—for *alarm.* Sound the nearest fire alarm. Notify the operator.

C—for *confine.* Close doors and windows to confine the fire. Turn off oxygen or electric items used in the general area of the fire.

E—for *extinguish.* Use a fire extinguisher on a small fire that has not spread to a larger area.

Clear equipment from all normal and emergency exits. *Do not use elevators if there is a fire.*

See *Promoting Safety and Comfort: What to Do During a Fire.*

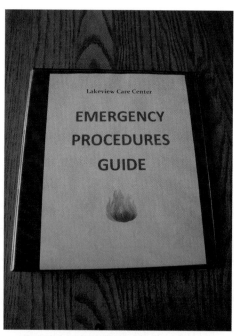

Fig 11.14 Emergency procedure manual

👤 **PROMOTING SAFETY AND COMFORT**

What to Do During a Fire
Safety
Touch doors before opening them. Do not open a hot door. Use another way out of the room or building.

If your clothing is on fire, do not run. Drop to the floor or ground. Cover your face. Roll to smother flames. If another person's clothing is on fire, get the person to the floor or ground. Roll the person, or cover the person with a blanket, bedspread, or coat. This smothers the flames.

If smoke is present, cover your nose and mouth with a damp cloth. Do the same for residents, visitors, and other staff. Have everyone crawl to the nearest exit.

Do the following if you cannot get out of the building because of flames or smoke:

- Call 911 or the fire department. Tell the operator where you are. Give exact information: center name, address, phone number, and where you are in the building.
- Cover your nose and mouth with a damp cloth. Do the same for residents, visitors, and other staff.
- Move away from the fire. Go to a room with a window. Close the room door. Stuff wet towels, blankets, sheets, or bedspreads at the bottom of the door.
- Open the window.
- Hang something from the window (towel, sheet, blanket, clothing). This helps firefighters find you.

✴ Using a Fire Extinguisher

Centers require that all employees demonstrate use of a fire extinguisher. Different extinguishers are used for different kinds of fires:

- Oil and grease fires
- Electrical fires
- Paper and wood fires

A general procedure for using a fire extinguisher is presented. Remember the word *PASS* used by the National Fire Protection Association:

P—for *pull the safety pin.* Doing so unlocks the handle on many types of fire extinguishers.

A—for *aim low.* Direct the hose or nozzle at the base of the fire. Do not try to spray the tops of the flames.

S—for *squeeze the lever.* Squeeze or push down on the lever, handle, or button to start the stream. Release the lever, handle, or button to stop the stream.

S—for *sweep back and forth.* Sweep the stream back and forth (side to side) at the base of the fire.

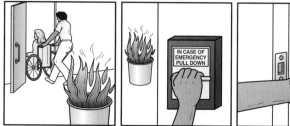
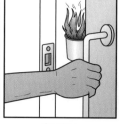
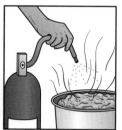

Rescue   Alarm   Confine   Extinguish

Fig. 11.15 During a fire, remember RACE: *Rescue, Alarm, Confine,* and *Extinguish.*

✤ USING A FIRE EXTINGUISHER

Procedure

1. Pull the fire alarm.
2. Get the nearest fire extinguisher.
3. Carry it upright.
4. Take it to the fire.
5. Follow the word *PASS*.
   - *P—for pull the safety pin* (Fig. 11.16A). This unlocks the handle.

- *A—for aim low* (Fig. 11.16B). Direct the hose or nozzle at the base of the fire. Do not try to spray the tops of the flames.
- *S—for squeeze the lever* (Fig. 11.16C). Squeeze or push down on the lever, handle, or button to start the stream. Release the lever, handle, or button to stop the stream.
- *S—for sweep back and forth* (Fig. 11.16D). Sweep the stream back and forth (side to side) at the base of the fire.

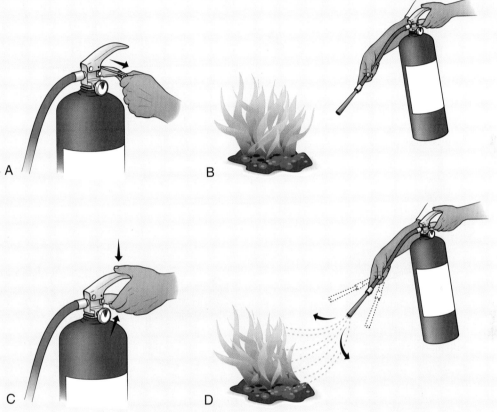

Fig. 11.16 Using a fire extinguisher. (A) *Pull* the safety pin. (B) *Aim* the hose at the base of the fire. (C) *Squeeze* the top handle down. (D) *Sweep* back and forth.

Evacuating

Some emergencies require evacuation. Centers have emergency evacuation policies and procedures. Know where these instructions are kept. Review them often. Evacuation routes are posted in the hallways (Fig. 11.17). If evacuation is necessary, residents closest to the fire are taken out first. Those who can walk are given blankets to wrap around themselves. A staff member takes them to a safe place. Most facilities have fire doors to separate larger areas. Helping residents to the other side of the fire door can save lives. Figs. 11.18 and 11.19 show how to rescue persons who cannot walk. Once firefighters arrive, they direct rescue efforts.

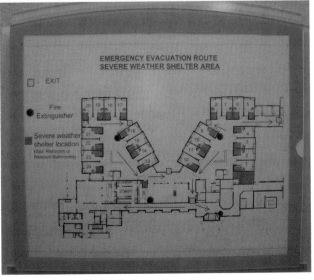

Fig 11.17 Evacuation route map

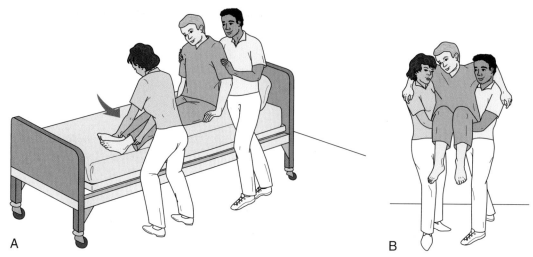

Fig. 11.18 Swing-carry technique. (A) Assist the person to a sitting position. A coworker grasps the person's ankles as you both turn the person so that he sits on the side of the bed. (B) Pull the person's arm over your shoulder. With one arm, reach across the person's back to your coworker's shoulder. Reach under the person's knees and grasp your coworker's arm. Your coworker does the same.

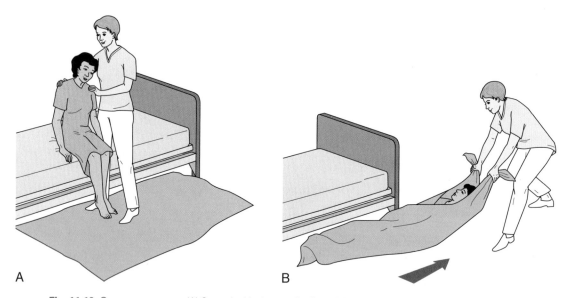

Fig. 11.19 One-rescuer carry. (A) Spread a blanket on the floor. Make sure the blanket will extend beyond the person's head. Assist the person to sit on the side of the bed. Grasp the person under the arms and cross your hands over her chest. Lower the person to the floor by sliding her down one of your legs. (B) Wrap the blanket around the person. Grasp the blanket over the head area. Pull the person to a safe area.

DISASTERS

A **disaster** is a sudden catastrophic event. People are injured and killed. Property is destroyed. Natural disasters include tornadoes, hurricanes, blizzards, earthquakes, volcanic eruptions, floods, and some fires. Human-made disasters include auto, bus, train, and airplane accidents. They also include fires, bombings, nuclear power plant accidents, riots, gas or chemical leaks, explosions, and wars.

The center has procedures for disasters that could occur in your area. Follow them to keep residents, visitors, staff, and yourself safe. Participate in fire and tornado drills. Know what to do in case these unfortunate events happen.

Communities, fire and police departments, and health care agencies have disaster plans. They include procedures to deal with the people needing treatment. The plan generally provides for the following:

- Discharging residents who can go home
- Assigning staff and equipment to an emergency area
- Assigning staff to transport persons from treatment areas
- Calling off-duty staff to work

A disaster may damage the center. The disaster plan includes evacuation procedures.

TORNADOES

Many facilities will have a method of notification of severe weather. This may be a NOAA (National Oceanic and Atmospheric Association) radio or automatic notification received through electronic means. The center will have an emergency procedure in place for tornadoes. Be familiar with this plan. Most agencies conduct drills on a regular basis. Some buildings have designated "safe rooms" where residents and staff will go. These areas have reinforced walls and ceilings. The safest area is an interior room on the lowest level of the building. It is very important, however, to remember that elevators cannot be used during tornadoes.

A *tornado watch* means weather conditions are favorable during the next few hours. A watch usually covers a large area. The National Weather Service issues a *tornado warning* when a tornado has been sighted or indicated by radar. A warning means that it is time to take action. There could be danger to life and property.

PROMOTING SAFETY AND COMFORT

What to Do During a Tornado
Safety
Be aware of changing weather conditions.
  When a *tornado watch* has been issued, do the following:
- Close privacy drapes around residents in bed.
- Remove glass and breakable items from surfaces near residents.
- Locate blankets, pillows, and battery-powered flashlights and radios.
- Talk with staff about a plan for moving residents to a safe place.
- Continue to monitor weather conditions.
  When a *tornado warning* has been issued, do the following:
- Stay calm. Reassure residents.
- Remember the safest place is an interior room on the lowest level of a building.
- Do not use elevators because of the risk of power failure.
- Move residents away from all windows if possible. It may be necessary to move them to a bathroom or an interior hallway.
- Instruct those who are able, to walk to the designated spot and remain seated.
- Move others by wheelchairs or transport entire beds to the hallway.
- Offer residents a pillow and blanket for protection from possible flying debris.
- Do not open any windows or doors.
- Remain in the safe area until the "all clear" notification has been given.

Power Failures

There may be times when severe weather causes the electricity to go out at the center. Most health care buildings have generators that provide auxiliary power. The generators may automatically cover vital functions for a time. Know where battery-powered lights are located. Be mindful of residents that may have medical equipment that must be plugged into an electrical supply. Oxygen equipment is an example. Falls can be a risk if there is not sufficient lighting.

Bomb Threats

Centers have procedures for bomb threats. You must follow them if a caller makes a bomb threat or if you find an item that looks or sounds strange. Often bomb threats are sent by phone, mail, email, messenger, or other means. Or the person can leave a bomb in the center. If you see a stranger in the center, tell the nurse at once. You cannot be too safe.

WORKPLACE VIOLENCE

Workplace violence is violent acts (including assault and threat of assault) directed toward persons at work or while on duty. It includes the following:
- Murders
- Beatings, stabbings, and shootings
- Rapes and sexual assaults
- Use of weapons (e.g., firearms, bombs, knives)
- Kidnapping
- Robbery
- Threats (e.g., obscene phone calls; threatening oral, written, or body language; and harassment of any nature [being followed, sworn at, or shouted at])

Workplace violence can occur in any place where an employee performs a work-related duty. It can be a permanent or temporary place. This includes buildings, parking lots, field sites, homes, and travel to and from work assignments. Workplace violence can occur anywhere in the center.

According to OSHA, more assaults occur in health care settings than in other industries. Nurses and nursing assistants are at risk. They have the most contact with residents and visitors. Risk factors include:
- People with weapons.
- Police holds—persons arrested or convicted of crimes.
- Acutely disturbed and violent persons seeking health care.
- Alcohol and drug abuse.
- Mentally ill persons who do not take needed drugs, do not have follow-up care, and are not in hospitals unless they are an immediate threat to themselves or others.
- Pharmacies that have medications and are a target for robberies.
- Gang members and substance abusers who are patients, residents, or visitors.
- Upset, agitated, and disturbed family and visitors.
- Long waits for emergency or other services.
- Being alone with the person during care or transport to other areas.
- Low staff levels during meals, emergencies, and at night.
- Poor lighting in hallways, rooms, parking lots, and other areas.
- Lack of training in recognizing and managing potentially violent situations.

OSHA has guidelines for violence prevention programs. The goal is to prevent or reduce employee exposure to situations that can cause death or injury. Worksite hazards are identified. Prevention measures are developed and followed. Also, employees receive safety and health training. You need to:

- Understand and follow your center's workplace violence prevention program.
- Understand and follow safety and security measures.
- Voice safety and security concerns.
- Report strange or suspicious persons right away.
- Report violent incidents promptly and accurately.
- Serve on health and safety committees that review workplace violence.

- Attend training programs that help you recognize and manage agitation, assaultive behavior, and criminal intent.

Active shooter incidents are on the rise. These incidents occur in schools, shopping malls, theaters, and health care facilities. Employees in care centers should not be fearful, but rather be prepared. The U.S. Department of Homeland Security promotes the "Run, Hide, Fight" program (Fig. 11.20). Training using videos and practice sessions help employees gain confidence to feel mentally and physically prepared. It is important to follow the guidelines that your workplace puts in place. Box 11.8 lists some measures to prevent or control workplace violence. Box 11.9 lists personal safety practices.

ACTIVE SHOOTER EVENTS

When an Active Shooter is in your vicinity, you must be prepared both mentally and physically to deal with the situation.

You have three options:

1 RUN

- Have an escape route and plan in mind
- Leave your belongings behind
- Evacuate regardless of whether others agree to follow
- Help others escape, if possible
- Do not attempt to move the wounded
- Prevent others from entering an area where the active shooter may be
- Keep your hands visible
- Call 911 when you are safe

2 HIDE

- Hide in an area out of the shooter's view
- Lock door or block entry to your hiding place
- Silence your cell phone (including vibrate mode) and remain quiet

3 FIGHT

- Fight as a last resort and only when your life is in imminent danger
- Attempt to incapacitate the shooter
- Act with as much physical aggression as possible
- Improvise weapons or throw items at the active shooter
- Commit to your actions . . . your life depends on it

The first officers to arrive on scene will not stop to help the injured. Expect rescue teams to follow initial officers. These rescue teams will treat and remove injured.

Once you have reached a safe location, you will likely be held in that area by law enforcement until the situation is under control, and all witnesses have been identified and questioned. Do not leave the area until law enforcement authorities have instructed you to do so.

Fig. 11.20 Steps to take for active shooter event. (From Department of Homeland Security Active Shooter Event Quick Reference Guide, https://www.cisa.gov/sites/default/files/publications/active-shooter-pamphlet-2017-508.pdf)

BOX 11.8 Measures to Prevent or Control Workplace Violence

Agitated or Aggressive Persons

- Stand away from the person. Judge the length of the person's arms and legs. Stand far enough away so that the person cannot hit or kick you.
- Stand close to the door. Do not become trapped in the room.
- Be aware of items in the room that can be used as weapons. Move away from such objects. Examples include vases, phones, radios, scissors, letter openers, paper weights, and belts.
- Know where to find panic buttons, call lights, alarms, closed-circuit monitors, and other security devices.
- Keep your hands free.
- Stay calm. Talk to the person in a calm manner. Do not raise your voice or argue, scold, or interrupt the person.
- Be aware of your body language. Do not point a finger or glare at the person. Do not put your hands on your hips.
- Do not touch the person.
- Tell the person that you will get the nurse to help.
- Leave the room as soon as you can. Make sure the person is safe.
- Tell the nurse or security officer about the matter. Report items in the room that can be used as weapons.

Safety Devices

- Alarm systems, closed-circuit video monitoring, panic buttons, handheld alarms, wireless phones, two-way radios, and phone systems are installed (Fig. 11.21). These systems have a direct line to security staff or the police.
- Metal detectors are at entrances to identify guns, knives, or other weapons.
- Curved mirrors are at hallway intersections and hard-to-see areas.
- Bullet-resistant, shatterproof glass is at nurses' stations.
- Staff do not turn off door alarms.
- Staff do not share security codes with anyone.

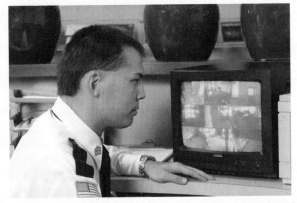

Fig. 11.21 People entering and leaving the center are monitored on closed-circuit TV.

Weapons

- Jewelry and scarves that can serve as weapons are not worn. For example, a person can grab earrings and bracelets. Or a person can strangle someone with a necklace or scarf.
- Long hair is worn up and off the collar. A person can pull long hair and cause head injuries.
- Keys, scissors, pens, or other items that can serve as weapons are not visible.
- Pictures, vases, and other items that can serve as weapons are few in number.
- Tools or items left by maintenance staff or visitors are removed if they can serve as weapons.

Family and Visitors

- Visitors sign in and receive a pass to access resident areas.
- Visiting hours and policies are enforced.
- A list of "restricted visitors" is made for residents with a history of violence or who are victims of violence.
- Waiting rooms and lounges are comfortable and reduce stress.
- Family and visitors are informed in a timely manner.

Building Safety and Security

- Unused doors are locked.
- Bright lights are inside and outside buildings.
- Broken lights, windows, and door locks are replaced or repaired.
- Staff restrooms lock and prevent access to visitors.
- Access to the pharmacy and drug storage areas is controlled.
- Furniture is placed to prevent entrapment. This includes furniture in resident rooms and in therapy areas, dining rooms, and lounges.
- Keys are not left unattended.

Staff Safety Measures

- Staff members are not alone when caring for persons with agitated or aggressive behaviors.
- Staff wear ID badges that prove employment.
- A "buddy system" is used when using elevators, stairways, restrooms, and low-traffic areas.
- Uniforms fit well. Tight uniforms limit running. An attacker can grab loose uniforms.
- Shoes have good soles. Shoes that cause slipping limit running.
- Vehicles are locked and in good repair.
- Security escort services are used for walking to vehicles, bus stops, or train stations.

Follow them all the time. Complete an incident report (p. 142) for any workplace violence.

The nurse assesses the behavior and the behavioral history of new and transferred residents. Restraints may be ordered if persons are a threat to themselves or others (Chapter 13). Persons with mental health disorders are supervised as they move throughout the center. Aggressive and agitated persons are treated in open areas. Privacy and confidentiality are maintained. Security officers deal with agitated, aggressive, or disruptive persons.

RISK MANAGEMENT

Risk management involves identifying and controlling risks and safety hazards affecting the center. The intent is to:

- Protect everyone in the center—residents, visitors, and staff.
- Protect center property from harm or danger.
- Protect the person's valuables.
- Prevent accidents and injuries.

Risk management deals with these and other safety issues:

- Accident and fire prevention
- Negligence and malpractice

BOX 11.9   Personal Safety Practices

General Measures

- Know the area where you are going. Ask questions about the area.
- Make a "dry run" of the area. Know the route in advance. The shortest route is not always the safest.
- Let someone know where you are at all times. Let someone know when you leave and when you arrive at your destination. If you do not call in when expected, the person knows something is wrong.
- Make it known that you do not carry drugs, needles, or syringes.
- Do not carry large amounts of money or valuables. Leave them at home or in the locked car trunk. If someone wants what you have, give it. The only thing of value is *you*.
- Carry wallets, purses, and backpacks safely. Men should carry wallets in an inside coat pocket or in a side pant pocket. Never carry a wallet in the rear pocket. Keep a firm grip on a purse. Keep it close to your body.
- Keep your cell phone in your hand.
- Carry a whistle or shriek alarm.
- Avoid automatic teller machines (ATMs) at night.
- Be careful when getting on elevators and when entering stairways.
- Do not approach a stranger or someone acting in a suspicious manner. Report the matter right away.

Home Settings

- Keep doors and windows to the home locked at all times.
- Do not open doors to strangers. Ask for identification.
- Do not let a stranger into the home to use a phone or bathroom. Offer to call the police if the person needs help.
- Do not give personal information to callers or people at the door.

Car Safety

- Have plenty of gas in your car.
- Keep your car in good working order.
- Keep these in your car—local map, flashlight with working batteries, flares, a fire extinguisher, and a first-aid kit.
- Raise the hood and use the flares if the car breaks down. Stay in the car. Call the police if you have a cell phone. If someone stops to help, ask that person to call the police.
- Lock your car. Sometimes you may want to leave it unlocked. If you need to get in the car fast, you do not want to fumble with keys. Use your judgment. Do not leave anything in the car if you leave it unlocked.
- Have your car key ready so you can get into the car quickly. Do not fumble for keys on the way to or at the car.
- Check under the car as you approach it. A person hiding under the car can grab your ankle or leg. Leave at once if someone is under the car. The person under the car may be working with a buddy who is waiting to attack you while you are being held or injured at the leg or ankle.
- Check the backseat before getting into the car. Make sure no one is in the car. Leave at once if someone is in the car.
- Lock car doors when you get in the car. Keep windows rolled up.
- Do not open the car door or window to talk to a person approaching your car.
- Do not get out of the car to remove something from the windshield.
- Keep purses, backpacks, and other valuables under the seat or near your side. Do not leave them on the seat. They are easy targets for smash-and-grab robbers.
- Do not hitchhike or pick up hitchhikers.
- If abducted and placed in the trunk of a car, feel for the emergency release lever to open the trunk. If the car is an older model, kick out the taillights and stick your hand through the opening.

Parking Your Car

- Check for places to park. Choose a well-lit area. If using a parking garage, park near entrances, exits, and on the lower level. Try to get close to the attendant if possible. The closest space to your destination is not always the safest for parking.
- Park your car so that you can leave quickly and easily. Park at street corners so no one can park in front of you. In parking lots, back in. You can see more from the front windshield than from the back window.

Walking

- Do not wear headphones or earbuds when walking. They keep you from hearing cars and people around you.
- Use well-lit and busy streets if you have to walk. Avoid vacant lots, alleys, wooded areas, and construction sites. The shortest way is not always the safest.
- Walk near the curb. Stay away from doorways, shrubs, and bushes.
- Carry a cell phone. Attach a small whistle to your key chain. Know your location and keep phone calls simple.
- Do not allow the use of cell phones to distract you from your surroundings.
- Go to a police or fire station or a store if you think someone is following you.

Public Transportation

- Carry money for bus, train, or taxi fares. Have money in your pocket to avoid fumbling with a purse or wallet.
- Stand with others and near the ticket booth. Sit near the driver or conductor.
- Keep your cell phone in your hand.
- Do not stand near the edge of a train or subway platform. People have been pushed into the path of a train.

If You Are Threatened or Attacked

- Scream as loud and as long as you can. Keep screaming. Men and women should scream.
- Yell "FIRE," not "help." Most people will respond to "FIRE."
- Use your car keys as a weapon. Carry them in your strong hand. Have one key extended (Fig. 11.22). Hold the key firmly. If you are attacked, aim for the person's face. Slash the person's face with the key. Do not use poking motions. Do not try for a certain target because you might miss. Do not be shy—your attacker will not be.
- Remember, you have two arms, two hands, two feet, and two knees. You can attack from more than one direction at once. Do not be shy—your attacker will not be. Push, pull, yank, and so on. You can attack a man's or woman's genitals.
- Use your thumbs as weapons. Aim for the person's eyes and push hard.
- Carry a travel-sized can of aerosol hairspray. Aim for the person's face.
- Carry a whistle.

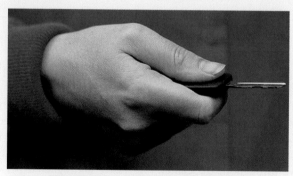

Fig. 11.22 A car key is used as a weapon.

- Resident abuse
- Workplace violence
- Federal and state requirements

Risk managers work with all center departments. They look for patterns and trends in incident reports, resident complaints, staff complaints, and accident and injury investigations. Risk managers look for and correct unsafe situations. They also make procedure changes and training recommendations as needed.

Color-Coded Wristbands

Some centers use color-coded wristbands to promote the person's safety and prevent harm. They quickly communicate an alert or warning (Fig. 11.23). The type of alert is printed on the band. The printing is useful in dim lighting and for persons who are color blind. Many states use these three colors:

- Red—means an "allergy alert." Red is a warning to "stop." A red wristband is used to warn of allergies to food, drugs, treatment supplies such as tape or latex gloves, dust, plants, grass, and so on. Allergies are not listed on the wristband. Some persons have too many allergies to list on the wristband.
- Yellow—means a "fall risk." Yellow implies "caution." The person is at risk for falling. Yellow wristbands are used for persons with a history of falls. Or they are used for persons at risk for falls because of dizziness, balance problems, confusion, and so on.
- Purple—means the person has a "Do Not Resuscitate (DNR)" order. See Chapter 45.

Some centers use other colors for other alerts. For example, pink is used for a "limb alert." This means that an arm or leg is not used for blood pressure measurements, blood draws, or intravenous infusions. To safely use color-coded wristbands:

- Know the wristband colors used in your center. Colors may vary among centers.
- Check the care plan and your assignment sheet when you see a color-coded wristband. You need to know the reason for the wristband and the care measures needed. Ask the nurse if you have questions.
- Do not confuse "social cause" bands with your center's color-coded wristbands.

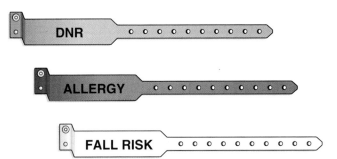

Fig. 11.23 Color-coded wristbands. The alert is printed on the band.

- Check for wristbands on persons transferred from another agency. That agency may use different colored wristbands. Or the colors' meanings may differ from those in your center. The nurse needs to remove wristbands from another agency. There is a national movement to standardize the color-coded wristbands so there is no confusion about their meaning.
- Tell the nurse if you think a person needs a color-coded wristband.

Personal Belongings

The person's belongings must be kept safe. Often they are sent home with the family. A personal belongings list is completed (Fig. 11.24). Each item is listed and described. The staff member and person sign the completed list.

A valuables envelope is used for jewelry and money. Each jewelry item is listed and described on the envelope. Describe what you see. For example, describe a ring as having a white stone with six prongs in a yellow setting. Do not assume the stone is a diamond in a gold setting. For valuables:

- Count money with the person.
- Put money and each jewelry item in the envelope with the person watching. Seal the envelope. Sign the envelope like a personal belongings list.
- Give the envelope to the nurse. The nurse takes it to the safe or sends it home with the family.

Dentures, eyeglasses, hearing aids, watches, some jewelry, radios, computers, cell phones, and other electronic devices are kept at the bedside. Items kept at the bedside are listed in the person's record. Some people keep money for newspapers and personal items. The amount kept is noted in the person's record.

Clothing and shoes are labeled with the person's name. So are other items brought from home.

Emergency Equipment and Training

A variety of equipment may be needed to respond to emergency situations. Box 11.10 lists examples of common life-saving equipment. Part of your new employee orientation will include knowing where these items are located. You may also have periodic training on the use of some of the equipment. It may be your job to retrieve a piece of equipment for the nurse to use in an emergency. For example, the nurse may ask you to bring the emergency cart (Fig.11. 25) to a resident's room.

Many centers have a safety committee. The members of the committee meet regularly and tour the facility and grounds to ensure a safe environment. Equipment must be inspected routinely to make sure it is in working order. Fire extinguishers are checked monthly, as part of the routine, among other things. Never borrow supplies from emergency or first-aid kits.

Firefighters, paramedics, and other professionals may offer training at the center. Inservice sessions may be offered to review emergency procedures or to train staff about new equipment. Always take training seriously. It may help you to save a life.

INVENTORY LIST

QTY.	ARTICLES	QTY.	APPLIANCES	QTY.	PROSTHETIC DEVICES	ACQUIRED AFTER ADMISSION	
	Belts		T.V. - Ser. #:		Dentures: ☐ Upper		
	Blouses		Radio - Ser. #:		☐ Lower ☐ Partial	Date	Item
	Coats		Hair Dryer		Eye Wear		
	Dresses		Electric Razor		Cane		
	Gloves				Walker - Ser. #:		
	Hats				W/chair - Ser. #:		
	Housecoats - Robes		JEWELRY		Brace		
	Jackets		Ring (Describe)				
	Nightgowns - Pajamas						
	Purses		Watch (Describe)		OTHER		
	Shaving Kit						
	Shoes		Other				
	Shorts						
	Slacks						
	Slippers						
	Slips		FURNITURE				
	Socks/Hose						
	Suitcases						
	Suits				VALUABLES RELEASED FROM SAFE		
	Sweaters						
	Ties						
	Undershirts						
	Underwear						

(Left margin vertical label: ON DISCHARGE)

I received on discharge in satisfactory condition the above articles and a copy of this list.
Disposition of belongings: _____

▶ _____ _____ ▶ _____ _____
Signature of Patient/Resp. Party   Date   Signature of Facility Representative   Date

NOTE ▶ Patient/Responsible Party is responsible for assuring that all personal belongings are properly marked. All items brought in after admission are added to this inventory at the request of Patient/Responsible Party.

QTY.	ARTICLES	QTY.	APPLIANCES	QTY.	PROSTHETIC DEVICES	ACQUIRED AFTER ADMISSION	
	Belts		T.V. - Ser. #:		Dentures: ☐ Upper		
	Blouses		Radio - Ser. #:		☐ Lower ☐ Partial	Date	Item
	Coats		Hair Dryer		Eye Wear		
	Dresses		Electric Razor		Cane		
	Gloves				Walker - Ser. #:		
	Hats				W/chair - Ser. #:		
	Housecoats - Robes		JEWELRY		Brace		
	Jackets		Ring (Describe)				
	Nightgowns - Pajamas						
	Purses		Watch (Describe)		OTHER		
	Shaving Kit						
	Shoes		Other				
	Shorts						
	Slacks						
	Slippers						
	Slips		FURNITURE				
	Socks/Hose						
	Suitcases						
	Suits				VALUABLES LOCKED IN SAFE		
	Sweaters						
	Ties						
	Undershirts						
	Underwear						

(Left margin vertical label: ON ADMISSION)

I certify that this is a correct list of my clothes and belongings which I wish to retain in my possession and for which I take ENTIRE RESPONSIBILITY. I have received a copy of this list.

▶ _____ _____ ▶ _____ _____
Signature of Patient/Resp. Party   Date   Signature of Facility Representative   Date

If the patient is unable to sign, state reason: _____

▶ Signature of Witness: _____

PATIENT NAME—LAST	FIRST	MIDDLE	HOSP. NO.	ROOM

INVENTORY LIST

Form 883/2   BRIGGS, Des Moines, Iowa 50306 PRINTED IN U.S.A.

Fig. 11.24 Personal belongings list. *QTY*, Quantity; *Resp. Party*, responsible party; *W/chair*, wheelchair. (Courtesy Briggs Corp., Des Moines, IA.)

BOX 11.10   Emergency Equipment

Know the location of the following equipment in your work area:
- Emergency procedure manual
- Fire extinguishers
- Fire pull alarms
- Automated external defibrillator (AED)
- Bleeding control kit
- First-aid kit
- Emergency cart
- Portable emergency suction
- Oxygen equipment
- CPR masks
- Emergency evacuation equipment
- Emergency evacuation maps (wall mounted)
- NOAA weather radio
- Sharps container
- Biohazard disposal receptacle
- Eyewash station
- Battery-powered flashlights
- PPE

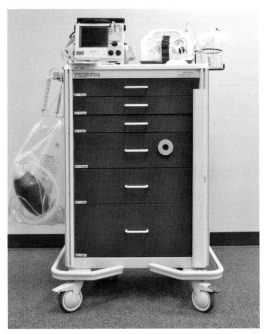

Fig. 11.25 Emergency cart. (From Niedzwiecki B: *Kinn's medical assisting fundamentals: administrative and clinical competencies with anatomy & physiology*, ed 2, St. Louis, 2021, Elsevier.)

Reporting Incidents

An incident is any event that has harmed or could harm a resident, visitor, or staff member. It includes accidents and errors in giving care. Box 11.11 provides examples.

Report accidents and errors at once. This includes:

- Accidents involving residents, visitors, or staff.
- Errors in care. This includes giving the wrong care, giving care to the wrong person, or not giving care.
- Broken or lost items owned by the person. Dentures, hearing aids, and eyeglasses are examples.
- Lost money or clothing.
- Hazardous substance incidents.
- Workplace violence incidents.

An *incident report* (Fig. 11.26) is completed as soon as possible after the incident. The following information is required:

- Names of those involved
- Date and time of the accident or error
- Location of the accident or error
- A complete description of what happened
- Names of witnesses
- Any other requested information

Not part of the medical record, incident reports are reviewed by risk management and a committee of health care workers. They look for patterns and trends of accidents or errors. For example, are falls occurring on the same shift and on the same unit? Are lost or missing items being reported on the same shift or same unit? Are residents being injured on the same shift or same unit? There may be new policies and procedures to prevent future incidents.

BOX 11.11 Common Incidents

- A resident's dentures are found broken in the laundry.
- A confused resident is found sleeping in bed with another resident.
- An agitated resident strikes another person.
- A resident is sitting on the porch of a house four blocks from the center.
- A resident is sleeping in a visitor's car.
- A visitor slips and falls on a wet floor.
- A housekeeper drops and breaks a resident's clock while dusting.
- A resident is found sitting on the floor by the bed.
- A nurse gives the wrong medication to a resident.
- A resident is burned while taking a bath.
- A resident receives a severe sunburn from sitting on the patio all afternoon.
- A resident drops a hearing aid into the toilet.
- A resident suffers a skin tear while resisting staff efforts to assist with dressing.
- A nursing assistant wears a ring with a large stone. A resident is scratched during care.
- A resident bites a staff member.
- A nurse leaves a needle on a resident's bed. A nursing assistant receives a needlestick injury when making the bed.
- A resident is given the wrong meal tray. The error is found after the person is done eating.
- The maintenance staff left tools in a resident's room. The person is injured on the tools.
- A resident is bruised from a restraint.
- A resident falls in the hallway.
- A resident was not repositioned for 6 hours. A pressure injury develops.
- A nursing assistant receives an electrical shock from a bed.
- The housekeeper splashes a cleaning chemical in her eye.
- A resident's dentures drop and break.
- Visitors are shouting in the hallway. Security is called.
- A resident reports missing money and jewelry.

QUALITY OF LIFE

Most accidents can be prevented. Remember, persons who are older and disabled are at great risk for accidents. To promote safety:

- Know the common safety hazards.
- Know the causes of accidents.
- Know who you need to protect.
- Use common sense.

The entire health team must provide a safe setting. You may see something unsafe. Do what you can to correct the matter.

Chronic illness, advanced age, disability, drugs, strange settings, and special equipment increase a person's risk for injury. Practice safety measures. Use safety devices as needed. Follow the person's care plan to give safe care.

Always identify the person before giving care. You can threaten a person's life and health if you give the wrong care or omit care. Use the ID bracelet to correctly identify the person. Two residents could have the same last name. Some may have the same first and last names.

To prevent fires, follow the safety measures for smoking and electric items. Extra measures are needed when oxygen is used. Residents who smoke present fire safety concerns. Ask the nurse if the person can have smoking materials at the bedside. Know where to find fire alarms, fire extinguishers, and emergency exits. Also know your center's procedure for a fire.

Follow procedures for handling hazardous substances. Physical hazards can cause fires and explosions. Some chemicals can cause acute or chronic health problems.

Workplace violence is a danger in health care settings. Practice measures to prevent and control workplace violence. Everyone must keep the center safe for residents, visitors, and staff.

INCIDENT/ACCIDENT REPORT

PERSON INVOLVED	(Last name)	(First name)	(Middle initial)				
			Adult ❑ Child ❑ Male ❑ Female ❑ Age _____				

Date of incident/accident	Time of incident/accident AM ❑ PM ❑	Exact location of incident/accident
		Resident's room _____ Hallway ❑ Bathroom ❑ Other ❑ Specify _____

RESIDENT ❑
List diagnosis if contributed to incident/accident

Resident's condition before incident/accident

Normal ❑   Confused ❑   Disoriented ❑   Sedate ❑   (Drug _____ Dose _____ Time _____)   Other ❑   Specify _____

Were bed rails ordered?	Were bed rails present?	If yes,	Was height of bed adjustable?	If yes,
Yes ❑ No ❑	Yes ❑ No ❑	Up ❑ Down ❑	Yes ❑ No ❑	Up ❑ Down ❑

Was a restraint in use? Yes ❑ No ❑

Physical restraint ❑   Type _____   Chemical restraint ❑   Specify _____

EMPLOYEE ❑	Department	Job title	Length of time in this position

VISITOR ❑ **OTHER ❑**	Home address	Home telephone
	Occupation	Reason for presence at this facility

Equipment involved ❑
Property involved ❑   Describe

Was person authorized to be at location of incident/accident
Yes ❑ No ❑

Describe exactly what happened; why it happened; what the causes were. If an injury, state part of body injured. If property or equipment damaged, describe damage.

TYPE OF INJURY
1. Laceration ❑
2. Hematoma ❑
3. Abrasion ❑
4. Burn ❑
5. Swelling ❑
6. None apparent ❑
7. Other (specify below) ❑

Indicate on diagram location of injury:

Vital signs (if applicable) when the resident is supine and at 1 and 3 minutes after standing (if unable to stand, use supine to sitting position)

Vital signs	Initial Incident supine	One minute after standing	Three minutes after standing
Temperature			
Pulse			
Respirations			
Blood pressure			

LEVEL OF CONSCIOUSNESS

Name of physician notified	Time of notification _____ AM/PM Time responded _____ AM/PM
Name and relationship of family member/resident representative notified	Time of notification _____ AM/PM Time responded _____ AM/PM
Was person involved seen by a physician? Yes ❑ No ❑ If yes, physician's name	Where? Date Time AM ❑ PM ❑
Was first aid administered? Yes ❑ No ❑ If yes, type of care provided and by whom?	Where? Date Time AM ❑ PM ❑
Was person involved taken to a hospital? Yes ❑ No ❑ If yes, hospital name?	By whom? Date Time AM ❑ PM ❑
Name, title (if applicable), address and telephone number of witnesses	Additional comments and/or steps taken to prevent recurrence:

SIGNATURE/TITLE/DATE	**SIGNATURE/TITLE/DATE**
Person preparing report	Medical Director
Director of Nursing	Administrator

Courtesy Briggs Corporation, Des Moines, IA.

Fig. 11.26 Incident report. (From Briggs Corporation, Des Moines, IA)

TIME TO REFLECT

Mrs. Sanchez is 89 years old and is a resident in the health care center. Recently she has experienced lower back pain. The doctor has ordered pain medication, but she does not seem to get much relief. As you approach her bed to help her to the bathroom, you notice an extension cord on the floor. As you get closer, you notice she is lying on a heating pad that is plugged into the extension cord. She tells you, "I had my daughter bring my trusty heating pad from home. It always seemed to help me sleep at night." What safety concerns exist with this situation? How will you proceed?

REVIEW QUESTIONS

Circle the BEST answer.

1. Who provides a safe setting for residents and visitors?
   a. The health team
   b. The nursing team
   c. The administrator
   d. The risk manager
2. Which is *not* a risk factor for accidents?
   a. Needing eyeglasses
   b. Hearing problems
   c. Memory problems
   d. Oriented to person, time, and place
3. A person in a coma
   a. Has suffered an electric shock
   b. Has dementia
   c. Is unaware of surroundings
   d. Has stopped breathing
4. A person with dementia
   a. Cannot think and reason
   b. Is not aware of own surroundings
   c. Is paralyzed
   d. Has suffered an electric shock
5. A person with dementia
   a. Is at high risk for accidents and injuries
   b. Knows what is safe
   c. Knows when to move away from danger
   d. Is agitated and aggressive
6. A person with quadriplegia is paralyzed
   a. From the waist down
   b. From the neck down
   c. On the right side of the body
   d. On the left side of the body
7. To identify a person, you
   a. Call the person by name
   b. Ask the person his or her name
   c. Compare information on the ID bracelet against your assignment sheet
   d. Ask both roommates their names
8. Burns are caused by the following *except*
   a. Smoking
   b. Spilled hot liquids
   c. Very hot bath water
   d. Oxygen
9. Safety measures to prevent poisoning include the following *except*
   a. Keeping harmful products in low storage areas
   b. Keeping child-resistant caps on harmful products
   c. Making sure all harmful products have labels
   d. Storing harmful products away from food
10. Which can cause suffocation?
   a. Reporting loose teeth or dentures
   b. Using electric items that are in good repair
   c. Cutting food into bite-sized pieces
   d. Restraints
11. The most common cause of choking in adults is
   a. A loose denture
   b. Meat
   c. Marbles
   d. Candy
12. Which is true during a tornado?
   a. The safest level of the building is the lowest level or basement
   b. Open windows a crack
   c. Take the elevator to the basement
   d. Evacuate the building as quickly as possible
13. Which source of bleeding is the most serious?
   a. Capillary
   b. Arterial
   c. Venous
   d. Superficial vessel
14. You need to shave a new resident. Before using the person's electric shaver
   a. You need to inspect it
   b. The maintenance staff must do a safety check
   c. You need to check for a frayed cord
   d. You need an electric outlet
15. You are using equipment. Which measure is *not* safe?
   a. Following the manufacturer instructions
   b. Keeping electric items away from water and spills
   c. Pulling on the cord to remove a plug from an outlet
   d. Turning off electric items after using them
16. A person uses a wheelchair. Which measure is *not* safe?
   a. The wheels are locked for transfers.
   b. The chair is pulled backward to transport the person.
   c. The feet are positioned on the footplates.
   d. The casters point forward.

17. Stretcher safety involves the following *except*
    a. Locking the wheels for transfers
    b. Fastening the safety straps
    c. Raising the side rails
    d. Moving the stretcher head first
18. You spilled a hazardous substance. You should do the following *except*
    a. Read the Safety Data Sheet
    b. Cover the spill and go tell the nurse
    c. Wear personal protective equipment to clean up the spill
    d. Complete an incident report
19. The fire alarm sounds. The following is done *except*
    a. Turning off oxygen
    b. Using elevators
    c. Closing doors and windows
    d. Moving residents to a safe place
20. Your clothing is on fire. You should do the following *except*
    a. Run to get help
    b. Drop to the floor or ground
    c. Cover your face
    d. Roll to smother the flames
21. A severe weather alert was issued for your area. What should you do?
    a. Take cover
    b. Follow the center's disaster plan
    c. Make sure your family is safe
    d. Pull the fire alarm
22. A person is agitated and aggressive. You should do the following *except*
    a. Stand away from the person
    b. Stand close to the door
    c. Use touch to show you care
    d. Talk to the person without raising your voice
23. A person has a yellow wristband. This means that the person
    a. Is at risk for bleeding
    b. Has an allergy
    c. Is at risk for falling
    d. Has an acute illness
24. You work the night shift. Which is *unsafe*?
    a. Parking in a well-lit area
    b. Locking your car
    c. Finding your keys after getting into the car
    d. Checking under the car and in your backseat
25. A resident brought a radio from home. Which helps prevent property loss?
    a. Allowing a roommate to use it
    b. Labeling the item with the person's name
    c. Putting the item in a safe
    d. Using a wheelchair pouch for the item
26. You gave a person the wrong treatment. Which is *true*?
    a. Report the error at the end of the shift
    b. Take action only if the person was injured
    c. You are guilty of negligence
    d. You must complete an incident report

See Appendix A for answers to these questions.

12

Preventing Falls

OBJECTIVES

- Define the key terms and key abbreviations listed in this chapter.
- Identify the causes and risk factors for falls.
- Describe the safety measures that help prevent falls.
- Explain how to use bed rails safely.
- Explain the purpose of handrails and grab bars.

- Explain how to use wheel locks safely.
- Describe how to use transfer/gait belts.
- Explain how to help the person who is falling.
- Perform the procedures described in this chapter.
- Explain how to promote quality of life.

KEY TERMS

bed rail A device that serves as a guard or barrier along the side of the bed; side rail

gait belt See "transfer belt"

orthostatic hypotension A form of low blood pressure that happens when standing up from sitting or lying position

transfer belt A device used to support a person who is unsteady or disabled; gait belt

KEY ABBREVIATIONS

CMS Centers for Medicare & Medicaid Services

OBRA Omnibus Budget Reconciliation Act of 1987

The risk of falling increases with age. Often falling is a sign of other health problems. Persons older than 65 years are at risk. A history of falls increases the risk of falling again. Falls are the most common accidents in nursing centers.

According to the Centers for Disease Control and Prevention (CDC):

- About 1800 nursing center residents die each year from falls.
- Nursing center falls can cause serious injury, including fractures. Fractures of the spine, hip, forearm, leg, ankle, pelvis, upper arm, and hand are the most common. Hip fractures and head trauma increase the risk of death.
- Falls result in disability, decline in function, and reduced quality of life.
- Fear of falling can cause further loss of function, depression, feelings of helplessness, and social isolation. This may increase the person's risk of falling again.

CAUSES OF AND RISK FACTORS FOR FALLS

Most falls occur in resident rooms and bathrooms. Poor lighting, cluttered floors, incorrect bed height, and out-of-place furniture are causes. So are wet and slippery floors, bathtubs, and showers. Wheelchairs can cause falls if they do not fit the person or are in poor repair. Needing to use the bathroom, usually to urinate, is a major cause of falls. For example, Mrs. Hines has an urgent need to urinate. She falls trying to get to the bathroom.

Most falls occur between 1600 (4:00 PM) and 2000 (8:00 PM). Falls also are more likely during shift changes. During shift changes, staff are busy going off and coming on duty. Confusion can occur about who gives care and answers call lights. Shift changes vary among centers. They often occur between these hours:

- 0600 (6:00 AM) and 0800 (8:00 AM)
- 1400 (2:00 PM) and 1600 (4:00 PM)
- 2200 (10:00 PM) and 2400 (midnight)

The accident risk factors described in Chapter 11 can lead to falls. The problems listed in Box 12.1 also increase a person's risk of falling.

See *Teamwork and Time Management: Causes of and Risk Factors for Falls.*

FALL PREVENTION PROGRAMS

Nursing centers have fall prevention programs. The measures listed in Box 12.2 are part of such programs and the person's care plan. The care plan also lists measures for the person's specific risk factors.

> **TEAMWORK AND TIME MANAGEMENT**
>
> **Causes of and Risk Factors for Falls**
> The entire health team must protect the person from harm. If you see something unsafe, tell the nurse at once. Do not assume the nurse knows or that someone is tending to the matter.
>
> Answer all call lights promptly. This includes the call lights of residents assigned to coworkers.
>
> Know your role during shift changes. Nursing staff going off duty and those coming on shift must work together to prevent falls.

BOX 12.1 Factors Increasing the Risk of Falls

Care Setting
- Bed: incorrect height
- Care equipment: intravenous (IV) poles, drainage tubes and bags, and others
- Cluttered floors
- Furniture out of place
- Lighting: poor
- Setting: strange and unfamiliar
- Throw rugs
- Wet and slippery floors, bathtubs, and showers
- Wheelchairs, walkers, canes, and crutches: improper use or fit

The Person
- Alcohol: overuse
- Balance problems
- Blood pressure: low or high
- Confusion
- Depression
- Disorientation
- Dizziness; dizziness on standing
- Elimination needs
- Falls: history of
- Foot problems
- Incontinence: urinary and fecal
- Joint pain and stiffness
- Judgment: poor
- Lightheadedness
- Medication side effects:
  - Low blood pressure when standing or sitting
  - Drowsiness
  - Fainting
  - Dizziness
  - Coordination: poor
  - Unsteadiness
  - Urination: frequent
  - Diarrhea
  - Confusion and disorientation
- Memory problems
- Mobility: decreased
- Muscle weakness
- Reaction time: slow
- Shoes that fit poorly
- Vision problems
- Weakness

BOX 12.2 Safety Measures to Prevent Falls

Basic Needs
- Fluid needs are met.
- Eyeglasses and hearing aids are worn as needed. Reading glasses are not worn when up and about.
- Tasks are explained before and while performing them.
- Help is given with elimination needs. It is given at regular times and when requested. Assist the person to the bathroom. Or provide the bedpan, urinal, or commode.
- The bedpan, urinal, or commode is kept within easy reach if the person can use the device without help.
- A warm drink, soft lights, or a back massage is used to calm the person who is agitated.
- Barriers are used to prevent wandering (Fig. 12.1).
- The person is properly positioned when in bed, a chair, or a wheelchair. Use pillows, wedge pads, or seats as the nurse and care plan direct (Chapter 15).
- Correct procedures are used for transfers (Chapter 15).
- The person is involved in meaningful activities.
- Exercise programs are followed. They help improve balance, strength, walking, and physical function.

Bathrooms and Shower/Tub Rooms
- Tubs and showers have nonslip surfaces or nonslip bathmats.
- Grab bars (safety bars) are in showers. They also are by tubs and toilets.
- Bathrooms have grab bars.
- Shower chairs are used (Chapter 18).
- Safety measures for tub baths and showers are followed (Chapter 18).

Floors
- Carpeting (if used) is wall-to-wall or tacked down.
- Scatter, area, and throw rugs are not used.
- Floor covers are one color. Bold designs can cause dizziness in older persons.
- Floors have nonglare, nonslip surfaces.
- Nonskid wax is used on hardwood, tiled, or linoleum floors.
- Loose floorboards and tiles are reported, as are frayed rugs and carpets.
- Floors and stairs are free of clutter, cords, and other items that can cause tripping.
- Floors are free of spills. Wipe up spills at once. Put a wet floor sign by the wet area.
- Floors are free of excess furniture and equipment.
- Electrical and extension cords are out of the way, including power strips.
- Equipment and supplies are kept on one side of the hallway.

Furniture
- Furniture is placed for easy movement.
- Furniture is kept in place. It is not rearranged.
- Chairs have armrests. Armrests give support when standing or sitting.
- Automatic lift chairs are used with caution. For persons with dementia the control device may be placed behind (out of sight) if there is a possibility of falling when raised to the upright position.
- A phone, lamp, and personal belongings are within the person's reach.

Beds and Other Equipment
- The bed is at the correct height for the person.
- The bed is in the lowest horizontal position, except when giving bedside care. The distance from the bed to the floor is reduced if the person falls or gets out of bed.
- Bed rails are used according to the care plan (p. 148).
- A mattress, special mat, or floor cushion is placed on the floor beside the bed (Fig. 12.2). This reduces the chance of injury if the person falls or gets out of bed.
- Wheelchairs, walkers, canes, and crutches fit properly. They are in good repair. Another person's equipment is not used.

BOX 12.2 Safety Measures to Prevent Falls—cont'd

- Crutches, canes, and walkers have nonskid tips.
- Correct equipment is used for transfers (Chapter 15). Follow the care plan.
- Positioning devices are used as directed (Chapter 15).
- Wheelchair and stretcher safety is followed (Chapter 11).
- Wheel locks on beds (p. 149), wheelchairs, and stretchers are in working order.
- Bed and wheelchair or stretcher wheels are locked for transfers.
- Linens are checked for sharp objects and for the person's property (dentures, eyeglasses, hearing aids, etc.).

Lighting

- Rooms, hallways, and stairways have good lighting, as do bathrooms and shower/tub rooms.
- Light switches (including those in bathrooms) are within reach and easy to find.
- Nightlights are in bedrooms, hallways, and bathrooms.

Shoes and Clothing

- Nonskid footwear is worn. Socks, bedroom slippers, and long shoelaces are avoided.
- Clothing fits properly. Clothing is not loose. It does not drag on the floor. Belts are tied or secured in place.
- Some centers will designate one color of hospital gowns for those persons who are in the high fall risk category.

Call Lights and Alarms

- The person is taught how to use the call light (Chapter 16).
- The call light is always within the person's reach. This includes when sitting in the chair or on the commode and when in the bathroom and tub/shower room.
- The person is asked to call for assistance when help is needed:
  - With getting out of bed or a chair
  - With walking
  - With getting to or from the bathroom or commode
  - With getting on or off the bedpan
- Call lights are answered promptly. The person may need help right away. The person may not wait for help.

- Bed, chair, door, floor mat, and belt alarms are used. They sense when the person tries to get up, get out of bed, or open a door (Fig. 12.3).
- Alarms are responded to at once.

Other

- Color-coded alerts are used to warn of a fall risk. Yellow is the common color for a fall alert. Besides wristbands (Chapter 11), some centers also use color-coded blankets, color-coded gowns, nonskid footwear, socks, and magnets or stickers to place on room doors.
- The person is checked often. This may be every 15 minutes or as required by the care plan. Careful and frequent observation is important.
- Frequent checks are made on persons with poor judgment or memory. This may be every 15 minutes or as required by the care plan.
- Persons at risk for falling are close to the nurses' station.
- Small video monitors may be placed to observe if the person attempts to get up without help.
- Handrails are on both sides of stairs and hallways.
- The person uses handrails when walking or using stairs.
- The person uses grab bars in bathrooms and shower/tub rooms.
- Family and friends are asked to visit during busy times. Mealtimes and shift changes are examples. They also are asked to visit during the evening and night shifts.
- Companions are provided. Sitters, companions, or volunteers are with the person.
- Nonslip strips are intact on the floor next to the bed and in the bathroom.
- Caution is used when turning corners, entering corridor intersections, and going through doors. You could injure a person coming from the other direction.
- Pull (do not push) wheelchairs, stretchers, carts, and other wheeled equipment through doorways. This allows you to lead the way and to see where you are going.
- A safety check is made of the room after visitors leave. (See the inside of the front cover.) They may have lowered a bed rail, removed a call light, or moved a walker out of reach. Or they may have brought and left an item that could harm the person.

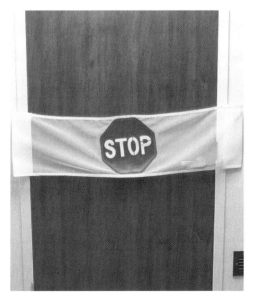

Fig. 12.1 Barriers are used to prevent wandering.

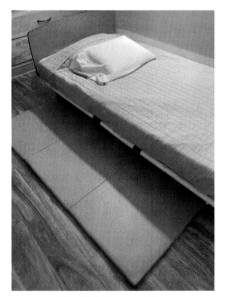

Fig. 12.2 Floor cushion.

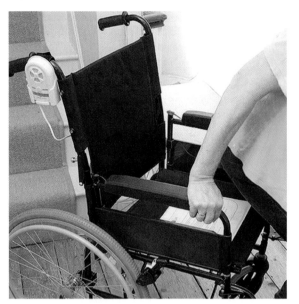

Fig. **12.3** Wheelchair alarm. (From Williams P: *Fundamental concepts and skills for nursing*, ed 6, St. Louis, 2021, Elsevier.)

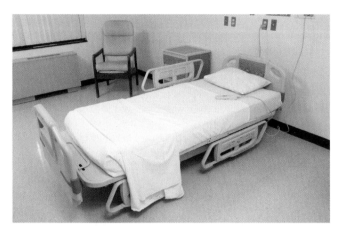

Fig. **12.4** Bed rails. The far bed rail is raised. The near bed rail is lowered.

 FOCUS ON COMMUNICATION

Fall Prevention Programs

Often falls occur when the person tries to get needed items. The person has to reach too far and falls out of bed or from a chair. Or the person tries to get up without help. Prevent falls by asking the person these questions:

- "What things would you like near you?"
- "Can I move this closer to you?"
- "Can you reach the call light?"
- "Can you reach your cane [walker/wheelchair]?"
- "Do you need to use the bathroom now?"
- "Is there anything else you need before I leave the room?"

PROMOTING SAFETY AND COMFORT

Fall Prevention Programs

Safety

Some people are visually impaired or blind. Besides the measures in Box 12.2, other safety measures are needed to protect them from falling. See Chapter 33.

Common sense and simple safety measures can prevent many falls. The health team works with the person and family to reduce the risk of falls. The goal is to prevent falls without decreasing the person's quality of life.

See *Focus on Communication: Fall Prevention Programs.*

See *Promoting Safety and Comfort: Fall Prevention Programs.*

Bed Rails

A bed rail *(side rail)* is a device that serves as a guard or barrier along the side of the bed. Bed rails are raised and lowered (Fig. 12.4). They lock in place with levers, latches, or buttons. Bed rails are half, three-quarters, or the full length of the bed.

When half-length rails are used, each side may have two rails. One is for the upper part of the bed, the other for the lower part.

The nurse and care plan tell you when to raise bed rails. They are needed by persons who are unconscious or sedated with medications. Some confused or disoriented people need them. If a person needs bed rails, keep them up at all times except when giving bedside nursing care.

❖ Bed rails present hazards.

The person can fall when trying to climb over them. Or the person cannot get out of bed or use the bathroom. *Entrapment* is a risk (Chapter 16). That is, the person can get caught, trapped, entangled, or strangled.

Bed rails prevent the person from getting out of bed. They are considered restraints by the Omnibus Budget Reconciliation Act of 1987 (OBRA) and the Centers for Medicare & Medicaid Services (CMS) if:

- The person cannot get out of bed.
- The person cannot lower them without help.

Bed rails cannot be used unless needed to treat a person's medical symptoms. Some people feel safer with bed rails up. Others use them to change positions in bed. The person or legal representative must give consent for raised bed rails. The need for bed rails is carefully noted in the person's medical record and the care plan.

Accrediting agency standards and federal and state laws affect bed rail use. They are allowed when the person's condition requires them. Bed rails must be in the person's best interests.

The procedures in this book include using bed rails. This helps you learn to use them correctly. The nurse, the care plan, and your assignment sheet tell you which people use bed rails. If a person does not use them, omit the "raise bed rails" or "lower bed rails" steps.

If a person uses bed rails, check the person often. Report to the nurse that you checked the person. If you are allowed to chart, record when you checked the person and your observations (Fig. 12.5).

See *Promoting Safety and Comfort: Bed Rails.*

Date	Time	Nursing Margin	Other Depts Margin
11/10	0900	I turned Mr. Adams from his back to his L side. One pillow placed	
		under his head, one against his back, and one supporting his R leg.	
		Full bed rails raised according to the care plan. Bed lowered to its	
		lowest position. Water pitcher and filled water glass c̄ straw placed	
		on the overbed table within Mr. Adam's reach. Phone and box of	
		tissue on the bedside table within reach. Urinal hung on the bed rail	
		per Mr. Adam's request. Signal light attached to the bed rail within	
		reach. Mr. Adams states he is comfortable and that needed items are	
		within his reach. I told him that I would be checking on him every 15	
		minutes and that he should use the signal light if he needed anything.	
		Gwen Rider, CNA.	

Fig. 12.5 Charting sample.

PROMOTING SAFETY AND COMFORT

Bed Rails

Safety

You raise the bed to give care. Follow these safety measures to prevent the person from falling:

- *For a person who uses bed rails.* Always raise the far bed rail if you are working alone. Raise both bed rails if you need to leave the bedside for any reason.
- *For the person who does not use bed rails.* Ask a coworker to help you. The coworker stands on the far side of the bed. This protects the person from falling.
- Never leave the person alone when the bed is raised.
- Always lower the bed to its lowest position when you are done giving care.

Comfort

The person has to reach over raised bed rails for items on the bedside stand and overbed table. Such items include the water pitcher and cup, tissues, phone, and TV and light controls. Adjust the overbed table so it is within the person's reach. Ask if the person wants other items nearby. Place them on the overbed table, too. Always ensure needed items, including the call light, are within the person's reach.

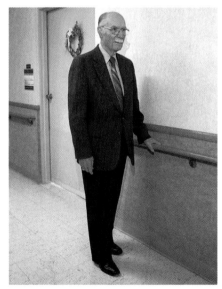

Fig. 12.6 Handrails provide support when walking.

Handrails and Grab Bars

Handrails are in hallways and stairways (Fig. 12.6). They give support to persons who are weak or unsteady when walking.

Grab bars (safety bars) are in bathrooms and in shower/tub rooms (Fig. 12.7). They provide support for sitting down or getting up from a toilet (Fig. 12.8). They also are used for getting in and out of the shower or tub.

Wheel Locks

Bed legs have wheels. They let the bed move easily. Each wheel has a lock to prevent the bed from moving (Fig. 12.9). Wheels are locked at all times except when moving the bed. Make sure bed wheels are locked:

- When giving bedside care.
- When you transfer a person to and from the bed.

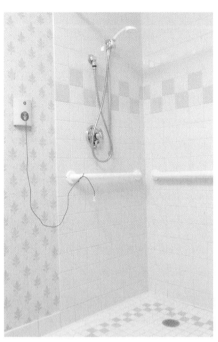

Fig. 12.7 Grab bars in a shower.

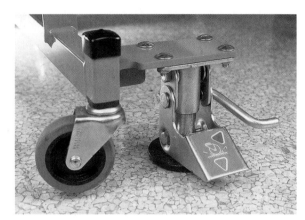

Fig. 12.9 Lock on a bed wheel.

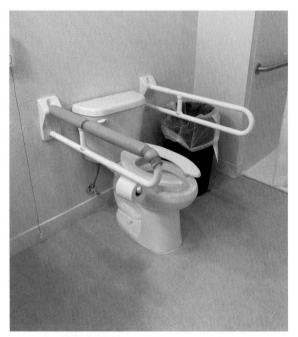

Fig. 12.8 Support bars next to toilet

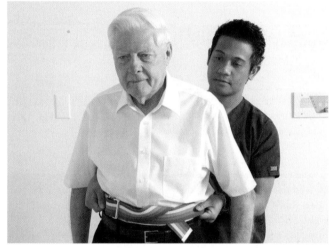

Fig. 12.10 Transfer/gait belt. The belt buckle is positioned off center. Excess strap is tucked under the belt. The nursing assistant grasps the belt from underneath.

Wheelchair and stretcher wheels also are locked during transfers (Chapters 11 and 15). You or the person can be injured if the bed, wheelchair, or stretcher moves.

TRANSFER/GAIT BELTS

A **transfer belt (gait belt)** is a device used to support a person who is unsteady or disabled (Fig. 12.10). It helps prevent falls

and injuries. When used to transfer a person (Chapter 15), it is called a *transfer belt*. When used to help a person walk, it is called a *gait belt*.

The belt is applied snugly around the person's waist. Grasp under the belt to support the person during the transfer or when assisting the person to walk.

See *Promoting Safety and Comfort: Transfer/Gait Belts*.

THE FALLING PERSON

A person may start to fall when standing or walking. The person may be weak, lightheaded, or dizzy. Fainting may occur. (See p. 146 for the risk factors for falls.)

Do not try to prevent the fall. You could injure yourself and the person while twisting and straining to prevent the fall. Balance is lost as the person falls. If you try to prevent the fall, you could lose your balance. Thus both you and the person could fall or cause the other person to fall, injuring the head, wrist, arm, hip, knee, or other area.

PROMOTING SAFETY AND COMFORT

Transfer/Gait Belts
Safety

Transfer/gait belts are routinely used in nursing centers. They help to stabilize the person and prevent falls. If the person needs help, a belt is required. To use one safely, always follow the manufacturer instructions.

Transfer/gait belts may have different types of fasteners, including Velcro, plastic clasps, or metal buckles. Some transfer/gait belts have a quick-release buckle. Position the quick-release buckle at the back where the person cannot reach it. This prevents the person from releasing the buckle during the procedure. Injury could result if the buckle is released.

Do not leave excess strap dangling. Tuck the excess strap under the belt.

Remove the belt after the procedure. Do not leave the person alone when wearing a transfer/gait belt.

Using a transfer/gait belt is unsafe for some persons. The belt could cause pressure or rub against care equipment. Check with the nurse and the care plan before using a transfer/gait belt if the person has any of the following:

- An ostomy—colostomy, ileostomy, urostomy (Chapters 23 and 38)
- A gastrostomy tube (Chapter 21)
- Chronic obstructive pulmonary disease (Chapter 36)
- An abdominal wound, incision, or drainage tube (Chapter 31)
- A chest wound, incision, or drainage tube
- Monitoring equipment
- A hernia—part of an organ that protrudes or projects through an opening in a muscle wall. Hernias often involve a loop of bowel or the stomach.
- Other conditions or care equipment involving the chest or abdomen.

Comfort
A transfer/gait belt is always applied over clothing. It is never applied over bare skin. Also, it is applied under the breasts. Breasts must not be caught under the belt. The belt buckle is never positioned over the person's spine.

APPLYING A TRANSFER/GAIT BELT

Quality of Life
Remember to:
- Knock before entering the person's room.
- Address the person by name.
- Introduce yourself by name and title.
- Explain the procedure to the person before beginning and during the procedure.
- Protect the person's rights during the procedure.
- Handle the person gently during the procedure.

Procedure
1. See *Promoting Safety and Comfort: Transfer/Gait Belts.*
2. Practice hand hygiene.
3. Identify the person. Check the identification (ID) bracelet against the assignment sheet. Also call the person by name.
4. Provide for privacy.
5. Assist the person to a sitting position.
6. Apply the belt around the person's waist over clothing. Do not apply it over bare skin.
7. Secure the buckle. The buckle is in front.
8. Tighten the belt so it is snug. It should not cause discomfort or impair breathing. You should be able to slide your open, flat hand under the belt. The belt will not be helpful if it is too loose.
9. Make sure that a woman's breasts are not caught under the belt.
10. Turn the belt so the quick-release buckle is at the person's back. The buckle is not over the spine.
11. Tuck any excess strap under the belt.

If starting to fall, ease the person to the floor. This lets you control the direction of the fall. You can also protect the person's head. Do not let the person move or get up before the nurse checks for injuries. Calmly explain that the nurse will check for injuries such as broken bones.

If you find a person on the floor, do not move the person. Stay with the person and call for the nurse.

An incident report is completed after all falls. The nurse may ask you to help with the report.

See *Residents with Dementia: The Falling Person.*

RESIDENTS WITH DEMENTIA

The Falling Person
Some older persons are confused. A confused person may not understand how to safely use the controls of an automatic lift chair. The person could raise the chair to its highest position and then fall to the floor. The control for the chair may need to be placed behind the person. The call light, however, should always be within reach. A confused person also may not understand the reason for not moving or getting up after a fall. Forcing a person not to move may injure the person and you. You may need to let the person move to keep both of you safe. Never use force to hold a person down. Stay calm and protect the person from injury. Talk to the person in a quiet, soothing voice. Call for help.

✳ HELPING THE FALLING PERSON

Procedure

1. Stand behind the person with your feet apart. Keep your back straight.
2. Bring the person close to your body as fast as possible. Use the transfer/gait belt (Fig. 12.11A). Or wrap your arms around the person's waist. If necessary (but not preferred), you can also hold the person under the arms.
3. Move your leg so the person's buttocks rest on it (see Fig. 12.11B). Move the leg near the person.
4. Lower the person to the floor. The person slides down your leg to the floor (see Fig. 12.11C). Bend at your hips and knees as you lower the person.
5. Call a nurse to check the person. Stay with the person.
6. Help the nurse return the person to bed. Ask other staff to help if needed.

Postprocedure

7. Provide for comfort. (See the inside of the front cover.)
8. Place the call light within reach.
9. Raise or lower bed rails. Follow the care plan.
10. Complete a safety check of the room. (See the inside of the front cover.)
11. Report and record the following:
    - How the fall occurred
    - How far the person walked
    - How activity was tolerated before the fall
    - Complaints before the fall
    - How much help the person needed while walking
12. Complete an incident report.

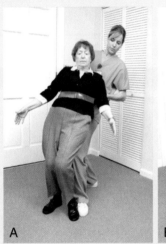 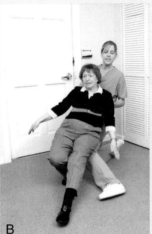 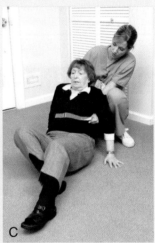

Fig. 12.11 The falling person. (A) The falling person is supported with the gait belt. (B) The person's buttocks rest on the nursing assistant's leg. (C) The person is eased to the floor on the nursing assistant's leg.

🌼 QUALITY OF LIFE

Older persons have fragile bones that break easily. The risk of a fracture is great. A fall can seriously affect a person's quality of life. For example, Ms. Polk has a broken wrist from a fall. She cannot fasten undergarments, button her blouse, pull up her pants, or tie her shoes. She cannot wipe herself after urinating or having a bowel movement. She depends on others to help her.

You must help prevent falls. However, you must not interfere with the person's rights. Sometimes preventing falls and the right to personal choice are in conflict. For example, Ms. Polk wants to wear socks without nonskid footwear. The socks could cause her to slip and fall. You need to respect her choice but also explain why it is best to wear nonskid shoes. Then have her choose what shoes to wear.

Sometimes safety measures to prevent falls are time consuming. Perhaps you cannot find a transfer belt. Or you need to get a walker. Or you must put on the person's shoes. Resist the urge to take shortcuts. Take the time to:

- Find and use assist devices.
- Put proper footwear on the person.
- Change the person's position gradually. (Moving too quickly may cause **orthostatic hypotension**)

- Raise or lower the bed and side rails as appropriate.
- Lock wheels on beds, stretchers, and wheelchairs.
- Ask others to help if needed.

Residents have the right to feel safe. Fear of falling does not make a person feel safe. Before moving a person, explain what you are going to do and what the person needs to do. Give step-by-step instructions as you progress. Do not move the person without prior notice. These measures increase the person's comfort. See Chapter 15 for how to safely handle, move, and transfer the person. Good communication promotes comfort. It supports the person's right to safety and security.

Some persons may feel restricted by the use of safety devices. They may feel it limits their independence. For example, Ms. Mills does not like having her bed rails up. She says, "I feel trapped. Do those have to be up?" Ms. Mills has fallen out of bed at night. The care plan includes having bed rails up while she is in bed.

Listen to the person's concerns. Kindly explain the reason for the safety device. If the person still refuses, tell the nurse. Do not let the person talk you out of performing a safety measure or using a safety device. Safety is always a priority.

Steven, a nursing assistant, is getting ready to shower Mr. Bryant in the bathing room. You are getting ready to assist Mr. Green in the same room but on the other side of a privacy curtain. You observe Steven getting ready to transfer Mr. Bryant from his wheelchair to the shower chair. Mr. Bryant is a large, tall man and slightly unsteady on his feet. The tile floor is wet, and you notice that Mr. Bryant is barefoot. Steven does not have a transfer belt near him. What would you do?

REVIEW QUESTIONS

Circle the BEST answer.

1. Most falls occur in
   a. Dining rooms
   b. Resident rooms and bathrooms
   c. Lounges
   d. Hallways

2. Most falls occur
   a. In the morning
   b. At lunchtime
   c. In the afternoon
   d. During the evening

3. A person's care plan includes fall prevention measures. Which should you question?
   a. Assist with elimination needs
   b. Keep phone, lamp, and TV controls within reach
   c. Check the person every 4 hours
   d. Complete a safety check after visitors leave the room

4. You observe the following in the person's room. Which is *not* safe?
   a. The lamp cord is by the chair
   b. The chair has armrests
   c. The nightlight works
   d. The bed is in the lowest horizontal position

5. You note the following after a person got dressed. Which is safe?
   a. The person is wearing nonskid shoes
   b. Pant cuffs are dragging on the floor
   c. The belt is not fastened
   d. The shirt is too big

6. A coworker is helping Mr. Yee today. His chair alarm goes off. What should you do?
   a. Find your coworker
   b. Tell the nurse
   c. Assist Mr. Yee
   d. Wait for someone to respond to the alarm

7. To help prevent falls, you need to report
   a. Equipment and supplies being on one side of the hallway
   b. A mattress on the floor beside the bed
   c. A coworker pulling a wheelchair through a doorway
   d. Clutter on stairways

8. Bed rails are used
   a. When you think they are needed
   b. When the bed is raised
   c. According to the care plan
   d. To support persons who are weak or unsteady

9. You are going to transfer a weak person from the bed to a chair.
   a. Bed wheels must be locked
   b. The person does not need footwear
   c. The bed is in the highest position
   d. A transfer belt is not needed

10. A transfer/gait belt is applied
    a. To the skin
    b. Over clothing
    c. Over the breasts
    d. Under the robe

11. To safely use a transfer/gait belt, you must
    a. Follow the manufacturer instructions
    b. Raise the bed rails
    c. Lock the bed wheels
    d. Set the bed alarm

12. You apply a transfer/gait belt. What should you do with the excess strap?
    a. Cut it off
    b. Wrap it around the person's waist
    c. Tuck it under the belt
    d. Let it dangle

13. A person starts to fall. Your first action is to
    a. Try to prevent the fall
    b. Call for help
    c. Bring the person close to your body as fast as possible
    d. Lower the person to the floor

14. You found a person lying on the floor. What should you do?
    a. Call for the nurse
    b. Help the person back to bed
    c. Apply a transfer belt
    d. Lock the bed wheels

15. Mr. Sikorski's blood pressure drops when he stands up too quickly. This is called
    a. Hypertension
    b. Orthostatic hypotension
    c. Tachycardia
    d. Hypothermia

See Appendix A for answers to these questions.

13

Restraint Alternatives and Safe Restraint Use

OBJECTIVES

- Define the key terms and key abbreviations listed in this chapter.
- Describe the purpose of restraints.
- Identify the complications from restraint use.
- Identify restraint alternatives.

- Explain the legal aspects of restraint use.
- Explain how to use restraints safely.
- Perform the procedure described in this chapter.
- Explain how to promote quality of life.

KEY TERMS

chemical restraint Any medication that is used for discipline or convenience and not required to treat medical symptoms

freedom of movement Any change in place or position of the body or any part of the body that the person is physically able to control

medical symptom An indication or characteristic of a physical or psychologic condition

physical restraint Any manual method or physical or mechanical device, material, or equipment attached to or near

the person's body that the person cannot remove easily and that restricts freedom of movement or normal access to one's body

remove easily The manual method, device, material, or equipment used to restrain the person that can be removed intentionally by the person in the same manner as it was applied by the staff

KEY ABBREVIATIONS

CMS Centers for Medicare & Medicaid Services
FDA Food and Drug Administration

OBRA Omnibus Budget Reconciliation Act of 1987
TJC The Joint Commission

Chapters 11 and 12 discuss many safety measures. However, some persons need extra protection. They may present dangers to themselves or others (including staff). For example:

- Mrs. Perez forgets to call for help when getting up and with walking. Falling is a risk.
- Mrs. Wilson tries to pull out her feeding tube. The tube is part of her treatment.
- Ms. Walsh scratches and picks at a wound. This can damage her skin or the wound.
- Mr. Ross wanders. He may wander into traffic or get lost in neighborhoods, parks, forests, or other areas. Exposure to hot or cold weather presents other dangers.
- Mr. Winters tries to hit, pinch, and bite the staff. They are at risk for harm.

❖   The Centers for Medicare & Medicaid Services (CMS) has rules for using restraints. Like the Omnibus Budget Reconciliation Act of 1987 (OBRA), CMS rules protect the person's rights and safety. This includes the right to be free from restraint or seclusion. Restraints may be used only to treat a medical symptom or for the immediate physical safety of the person or others. Restraints may be used only when less restrictive measures fail to protect the person or others. They must be discontinued at the earliest possible time.

The CMS uses these terms:

- *Physical restraint*—any manual method or physical or mechanical device, material, or equipment attached to or near the person's body that the person cannot remove easily and that restricts freedom of movement or normal access to one's body.
- *Chemical restraint*—any medication that is used for discipline or convenience and not required to treat medical symptoms. The medication or dosage is not a standard treatment for the person's condition.
- *Freedom of movement*—any change in place or position of the body or any part of the body that the person is physically able to control.
- *Remove easily*—the manual method, device, material, or equipment used to restrain the person can be removed intentionally by the person in the same manner as it was applied by the staff. For example, the person can put bed rails down, untie a knot, or unclasp a buckle. ◆

To meet the person's safety needs, a resident care conference is held. The health team reviews and updates the person's care plan. Every attempt is made to protect the person without using restraints. Sometimes they are needed. Restraints are used only as a *last resort* to protect persons from harming themselves or others.

HISTORY OF RESTRAINT USE

Restraints were once thought to *prevent* falls. Research shows that restraints *cause* falls. Falls occur when people try to get free of the restraints. Injuries are more serious from falls by restrained individuals than by those not restrained.

Restraints also were used to prevent wandering or interfering with treatment. They were often used for persons who showed confusion, poor judgment, or behavior problems. Older persons were restrained more often than younger persons. Restraints were viewed as necessary devices to protect a person. However, they can cause serious harm (Box 13.1). They can even cause death.

Besides the CMS, the Food and Drug Administration (FDA), state agencies, and The Joint Commission (TJC—an accrediting agency) have guidelines for the use of restraints. They do not forbid the use of restraints; however, *they require considering or trying all other appropriate alternatives first.*

Every center has policies and procedures about restraints. They include identifying persons at risk for harm, harmful behaviors, restraint alternatives, and proper restraint use. Staff training is required.

RESTRAINT ALTERNATIVES

Often there are causes and reasons for harmful behaviors. Knowing and treating the cause can prevent restraint use. The nurse tries to find out what the behavior means. This is very important for persons who have speech or cognitive problems. The focus is on these questions:

- Is the person in pain, ill, or injured?
- Is the person short of breath? Are cells getting enough oxygen (Chapter 26)?
- Is the person afraid in a new setting?
- Does the person need to use the bathroom?
- Is a dressing tight or causing other discomfort (Chapter 31)?
- Is clothing tight or causing other discomfort?
- Is the person's position uncomfortable?
- Are body fluids, secretions, or excretions causing skin irritation?
- Is the person too hot or too cold?
- Is the person hungry or thirsty?
- What are the person's lifelong habits at this time of day?
- Does the person have problems communicating?
- Is the person seeing, hearing, or feeling things that are not real (Chapter 39)?
- Is the person confused or disoriented (Chapter 40)?
- Are medications causing the behaviors?

Restraint alternatives for the person are identified (Box 13.2). They become part of the care plan. Care plan changes are made as needed. Restraint alternatives may not protect the person. The doctor may need to order restraints (Fig. 13.2).

SAFE RESTRAINT USE

Restraints can cause serious injury and even death. *CMS, OBRA, FDA, and TJC guidelines are followed. So are state laws.* They are part of your center's policies and procedures for restraint use.

Restraints are not used to discipline a person. They are not used for staff convenience. Discipline is any action that punishes or penalizes a person. Convenience is any action that:

- Controls or manages the person's behavior.
- Requires less effort by the center.
- Is not in the person's best interests.

Restraints are used only when necessary to treat a person's medical symptoms. The CMS defines a medical symptom as an indication or characteristic of a physical or psychologic condition. Symptoms may relate to physical, emotional, or behavioral problems. Sometimes restraints are needed to protect the person or others. That is, a person may have violent or aggressive behaviors that are harmful to self or others.

Physical and Chemical Restraints

According to the CMS, a *physical restraint:*

- May be any manual method, physical or mechanical device, material, or equipment.
- Is attached to or next to the person's body.
- Cannot be easily removed by the person.
- Restricts freedom of movement or normal access to one's body.

BOX 13.1 Risks of Restraint Use

- Agitation
- Anger
- Constipation
- Contractures
- Cuts and bruises
- Decline in physical function (ability to walk, muscle condition)
- Dehydration
- Delirium
- Depression
- Dignity: loss of
- Embarrassment and humiliation
- Falls
- Fractures
- Head trauma
- Incontinence
- Infections: pneumonia and urinary tract
- Mistrust
- Nerve injuries
- Pressure injuries
- Self-respect: loss of
- Social contact: reduced
- Strangulation
- Withdrawal

BOX 13.2   Alternatives to Restraint Use

- Diversion is provided (e.g., TV, videos, music, games, puzzles, relaxation tapes).
- Lifelong habits and routines are in the care plan (e.g., showers before breakfast, reads in the bathroom, walks outside before lunch, watches TV after lunch).
- Family and friends make videos of themselves for the person to watch.
- Videos are made of visits with family and friends for the person to watch.
- Time is spent in supervised areas (dining room, lounge, near the nurses' station).
- Pillows, wedge cushions, and posture and positioning aids are used.
- The call light is within reach.
- Call lights are answered promptly.
- Food, fluid, hygiene, and elimination needs are met.
- The bedpan, urinal, or commode is within the person's reach.
- Back massages are given.
- Family, friends, and volunteers visit.
- The person has companions or sitters.
- Time is spent with the person.
- Extra time is spent with a person who is restless.
- Reminiscing is done with the person.
- A calm, quiet setting is provided.
- The person wanders in safe areas.
- The entire staff is aware of persons who tend to wander. This includes staff in housekeeping, maintenance, the business office, dietary, and so on.
- Exercise programs are provided.
- Outdoor time is planned during nice weather.
- The person does agreed upon jobs or tasks.
- Warning devices are used on beds, chairs, and doors.
- Knob guards are used on doors.
- Padded hip protectors are worn under clothing (Fig. 13.1).
- Low beds are used.
- Floor cushions are placed next to beds (Chapter 12).
- Roll guards are attached to the bed frame.
- Falls are prevented (Chapter 12).
- The person's furniture meets needs (lower bed, reclining chair, rocking chair).
- Walls and furniture corners are padded.
- Observations and visits are made at least every 15 minutes, or as often as noted in the care plan.
- The person is moved to a room close to the nurses' station.
- Procedures and care measures are explained.
- Frequent explanations are given about equipment or devices.
- Confused persons are oriented to person, time, and place. Calendars and clocks are provided.
- Light is adjusted to meet the person's basic needs and preferences.
- Staff assignments are consistent.
- Sleep is not interrupted.
- Noise levels are reduced.

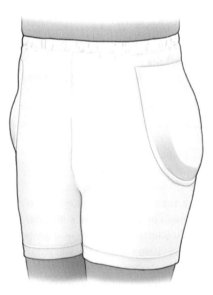

Fig. 13.1 Hip protector. (From Remmert LN, Sorrentino SA: *Mosby's essentials for nursing assistants,* ed 7, St. Louis, 2023, Elsevier.)

- Physical restraints are applied to the chest, waist, elbows, wrists, hands, or ankles. They confine the person to a bed or chair. Or they prevent movement of a body part. Some furniture or barriers also prevent freedom of movement:
- A device used with a chair that the person cannot remove easily. The device prevents the person from rising. Trays, tables, bars, and belts are examples (Fig. 13.3).

- Any chair that prevents the person from rising.
- Any bed or chair placed so close to the wall that the person cannot get out of the bed or chair.
- Bed rails (Chapter 12) that prevent the person from getting out of bed. For example, four half-length bed rails are raised. They are restraints if the person cannot lower them.
- Tucking in or using Velcro to hold a sheet, fabric, or clothing so tightly that freedom of movement is restricted.

Medications or medication dosages are *chemical restraints* if they:
- Control behavior or restrict movement.
- Are not standard treatment for the person's condition.

Medications cannot be used for discipline or staff convenience. They cannot be used if not required for the person's treatment. They cannot be used if they affect physical or mental function.

Sometimes medications can help persons who are confused or disoriented. They may be anxious, agitated, or aggressive. The doctor may order medications to control these behaviors. The medications should not make the person sleepy and unable to function at the highest level possible.

Complications of Restraint Use

Box 13.1 lists the many complications from restraints. Injuries occur as the person tries to get free of the restraint. Injuries also occur from using the wrong restraint, applying it incorrectly, or keeping it on too long. Cuts, bruises, and fractures are common. *The most serious risk is death from strangulation.*

There are also mental effects. Restraints affect dignity and self-esteem. See Box 13.1.

Date	Time	Nursing Margin	Other Depts Margin
4-16	1340	Resident's chair alarm sounded as he tried to get out of his wheelchair.	
		He repeated "I need to get up" over and over. I assisted him to the	
		bathroom. He voided 275mL. Then I pushed him around the enclosed	
		garden for 15 minutes. He talked about the flowers he used to grow	
		in his garden. After the walk, I positioned his wheelchair across from	
		the nurses' station and locked the wheels. I told him to ask for help if he	
		needs anything. He said "I will." I explained that to prevent him from	
		falling, his chair alarm would sound if he tried to get up without help. I	
		gave him a drink of water per his request. I gave him a magazine on	
		gardening. He states "I'm OK." He appears calm and relaxed. I told him I	
		would check on him in 15 minutes. I asked R. Carico, RN, and M. Herron	
		at the nurses' station to observe him. Lynn Larson, CNA ←	

Fig. 13.2 Charting sample.

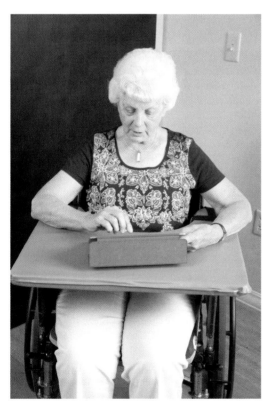

Fig. 13.3 This laptop tray is a restraint alternative. It is a restraint when used to prevent freedom of movement. (From Remmert LN, Sorrentino SA: *Mosby's essentials for nursing assistants*, ed 7, St. Louis, 2023, Elsevier.)

Restraints are medical devices. The Safe Medical Devices Act ❖ applies if a restraint causes illness, injury, or death. Also, CMS requires the reporting of any death that occurs:

- While a person is in a restraint.
- Within 24 hours after a restraint was removed.
- Within 1 week after a restraint was removed. This is done if the restraint may have contributed directly or indirectly to the person's death. ◆

Legal Aspects

Laws applying to restraint use must be followed. Remember the following:

- Restraints must protect the person. *They are not used for staff* ❖ *convenience or to discipline a person.* Restraining someone is not easier than properly supervising and observing the person. A restrained person requires more staff time for care, supervision, and observation. A restraint is used only when it is the best safety measure for the person. Restraints are not used to punish or penalize uncooperative persons.
- A doctor's order is required. *OBRA, CMS, state laws, FDA warnings, TJC, and other accrediting agencies protect persons from unnecessary restraint.* If restraints are needed for medical reasons, a doctor's order is required. The doctor gives the reason for the restraint, what body part to restrain, what to use, and how long to use it. This information is on the care plan and your assignment sheet. In an emergency, the nurse can decide to apply restraints before getting a doctor's order.

- The least restrictive method is used. It allows the greatest amount of movement or body access possible. Some restraints attach to the person's body and to a fixed (nonmovable) object. It restricts freedom of movement or body access. Vest, jacket, ankle, wrist, hand, and some belt restraints are examples. Other restraints are near but not directly attached to the person's body (bed rails or wedge cushions). They do not totally restrict freedom of movement. They allow access to certain body parts and are the least restrictive.
- Restraints are used only after other measures fail to protect the person (see Box 13.2). Some people can harm themselves or others. The care plan must include measures to protect the person and prevent harm to others. Many fall prevention measures are restraint alternatives (Chapter 12).
- Unnecessary restraint is false imprisonment (Chapter 2). You must understand the reason for the restraint and its risk. If not, politely ask about its use. If you apply an unneeded restraint, you could face charges of false imprisonment.
- Informed consent is required. The person must understand the reason for the restraint. The person is told how the restraint will help the planned medical treatment. The person is told about the risks of restraint use. If unable to give consent, the person's legal representative is given the information. Either the person or the legal representative must give consent before a restraint can be used. The doctor or nurse provides the necessary information and obtains the consent.

See *Focus on Communication: Legal Aspects.*

🗒 FOCUS ON COMMUNICATION

Legal Aspects

You may not know the reason for a restraint. If so, politely ask the nurse why it is needed. For example:
- "Why does Mr. Reed need a restraint?"
- "I don't understand. Why did the doctor order the restraint?"

Safety Guidelines

The restrained person must be kept safe. Follow the safety measures in Box 13.3. Also remember these key points:
- *Observe for increased confusion and agitation.* Restraints can increase confusion and agitation. Whether confused or alert, people are aware of restricted movements. They may try to get out of the restraint or to struggle or pull at it. Some restrained persons beg others to free or to help release them. These behaviors often are viewed as signs of confusion. Some people become more confused because they do not understand what is happening to them. Restrained persons need repeated explanations and reassurance. Spending time with them has a calming effect.

BOX 13.3 Safety Measures for Using Restraints

Before Applying Restraints
- Do not use sheets, towels, tape, rope, straps, bandages, Velcro, or other items to restrain a person.
- Apply a restraint only after being instructed about its proper use.
- Demonstrate proper application of the restraint before applying it.
- Use the restraint noted in the care plan. Use the correct size. Small restraints are tight. They cause discomfort and agitation. They also restrict breathing and circulation. Strangulation is a risk from big or loose restraints.
- Use only restraints that have manufacturer instructions and warning labels.
- Read the manufacturer warning labels. Note the front and back of the restraint.
- Follow the manufacturer instructions. Some restraints are safe for bed, chair, and wheelchair use. Others are used only with certain equipment.
- Use intact restraints. Look for broken stitches, tears, cuts, or frayed fabric or straps. Look for missing or loose buckles, locks, hooks, loops, or straps or other damage. The restraint must hold securely.
- Test zippers, buckles, locks, hooks, and other closures. The device must fasten securely.
- Do not use a restraint near a fire, a flame, or smoking materials.

Applying Restraints
- Do not use restraints to position a person on a toilet.
- Do not use restraints to position a person on furniture that does not allow for correct application. Follow the manufacturer instructions.
- Follow center policies and procedures.
- Position the person in good alignment before applying the restraint (Chapter 15).
- Pad bony areas and the skin as instructed by the nurse. This prevents pressure and injury from the restraint.

- Secure the restraint. It should be snug but allow some movement of the restrained part. Follow the manufacturer instructions to check for snugness. For example:
  - *If applied to the chest or waist*—Make sure that the person can breathe easily. A flat hand should slide between the restraint and the person's body (Fig. 13.4). Check with the nurse if you have very small or very large hands. Small or large hands could cause the restraint to be too tight or too loose.
  - *For wrist and mitt restraints*—You should be able to slide one finger under the restraint. Check with the nurse if you have very small or very large fingers. Small or large fingers could cause the restraint to be too tight or too loose.
- Criss-cross vest or jacket restraints in front (Fig. 13.5). Do not criss-cross restraints in the back unless part of the manufacturer instructions (Fig. 13.6). Criss-crossing vests or jackets in the back can cause death from strangulation.
- Buckle or tie restraints according to center policy. The policy should follow the manufacturer instructions and allow for quick release in an emergency. Quick-release buckles are used (Fig. 13.7). So are quick-release ties (Fig. 13.8).
- Secure straps out of the person's reach.
- Leave 1 to 2 inches of slack in the straps (if directed to do so by the nurse). This allows some movement of the part.
- Secure the restraint to the movable part of the bed frame at waist level (see Fig. 13.8). The restraint will not tighten or loosen when the head or foot of the bed is raised or lowered. For chairs, secure straps under the seat of the wheelchair or chair (Fig. 13.9).
- Make sure the straps cannot tighten, loosen, slip, or cause too much slack.

BOX 13.3 Safety Measures for Using Restraints—cont'd

- Make sure that straps will not slide in any direction. If straps slide, they change the restraint's position. The person can get suspended off the mattress or chair (Figs. 13.10 and 13.11). Strangulation can result.
- Never secure restraints to the bed rails. The person can reach bed rails to release knots or buckles. Also, injury to the person is likely when raising or lowering bed rails.
- Use bed rail covers or gap protectors according to the nurse's instructions (Fig. 13.12). They prevent entrapment between the rails or the bed rail bars (see Fig. 13.10). Entrapment can occur between:
  - The bars of a bed rail
  - The space between half-length (split) bed rails
  - The bed rail and mattress
  - The headboard or footboard and mattress
- Position the person in semi-Fowler position (Chapter 15) when using a vest, jacket, or belt restraint.
- Position the person in a chair so the hips are well to the back of the chair.
- Apply a belt restraint at a 45-degree angle over the thighs (Fig. 13.13).

After Applying Restraints

- Keep full bed rails up when using a vest, jacket, or belt restraint. Also use bed rail covers or gap protectors. Otherwise the person could fall off the bed and strangle on the restraint. If half-length bed rails are used, the person can get caught between them.
- Do not use back cushions when a person is restrained in a chair. If the cushion moves out of place, slack occurs in the straps. Strangulation could result if the person slides forward or down from the extra slack (see Fig. 13.11).
- Do not cover the person with a sheet, blanket, bedspread, or other covering. The restraint must be within plain view at all times.
- Check the person at least every 15 minutes for safety, comfort, and signs of injury.
- Check the person's circulation at least every 15 minutes if mitt, wrist, or ankle restraints are applied. You should feel a pulse at a pulse site below the restraint (Chapter 27). Fingers or toes should be warm and pink. Tell the nurse at once if:
  - You cannot feel a pulse.
  - Fingers or toes are cold, pale, or blue in color.
  - The person complains of pain, numbness, or tingling in the restrained part.
  - The skin is red or damaged.
- Check the person at least every 15 minutes if a belt, jacket, or vest restraint is used. The person should be able to breathe easily. Also check the position of the restraint, especially in the front and back.
- Monitor persons in the supine position constantly. They are at great risk for aspiration if vomiting occurs (Chapters 20 and 21). Call for the nurse at once.
- Keep scissors in your pocket. In an emergency, cutting the tie may be faster than untying a knot. Never leave scissors at the bedside where the person can reach them. Make sure the person cannot reach the scissors in your pocket.
- Remove or release the restraint and reposition the person every 2 hours or as often as noted in the care plan. The restraint is removed or released for at least 10 minutes. Meet the person's basic needs. You need to:
  - Measure vital signs.
  - Meet elimination needs.
  - Offer food and fluids.
  - Meet hygiene needs.
  - Give skin care.
  - Perform range-of-motion exercises or help the person walk. Follow the care plan.
  - Provide for physical and emotional comfort. (See the inside of the front cover.)
- Keep the call light within the person's reach. (Chart that this was done.)
- Complete a safety check before leaving the room. (See the inside of the front cover.)
- Report to the nurse every time you checked the person and removed or released the restraint. Report your observations and the care given. Follow center policy for recording.

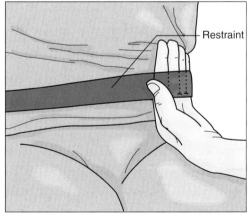

Fig. 13.4 A flat hand slides between the restraint and the person.

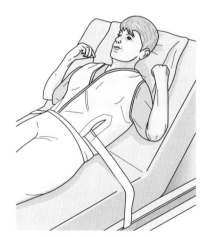

Fig. 13.5 The vest restraint criss-crosses in front. (Note: The bed rails are raised after the restraint is applied.)

- *Protect the person's quality of life.* Restraints are used for as short a time as possible. The care plan must show how to reduce restraint use. The person's needs are met with as little restraint as possible. You must meet the person's physical, emotional, and social needs. Visit with the person and explain the reason for the restraints.

- *Follow the manufacturer instructions.* They explain how to apply and secure the restraint for the person's safety. The restraint must be snug and firm but not tight. Tight restraints affect circulation and breathing. The person must be comfortable and able to move the restrained part to a

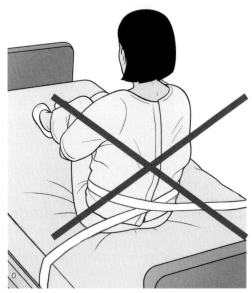

Fig. 13.6 Never criss-cross vest or jacket straps in back. (From Sorrentino SA, Remmert LN: *Mosby's textbook for long-term care nursing assistants*, ed 10, St. Louis, 2021, Elsevier.)

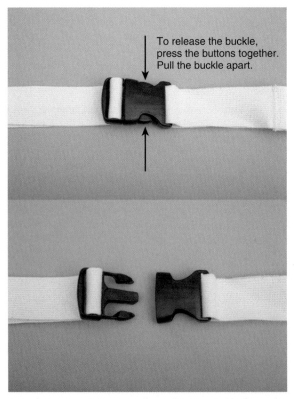

To release the buckle, press the buttons together. Pull the buckle apart.

Fig. 13.7 Quick-release buckle. (From Remmert LN, Sorrentino SA: *Mosby's essentials for nursing assistants*, ed 7, St. Louis, 2023, Elsevier.)

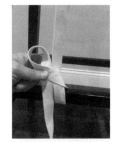

1   Wrap the strap around an area out of the person's reach—a movable part of the bed frame or below the chair or wheelchair seat.

Cross the loose end over the front of the strap.

Make a loop.

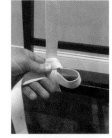

2   Pass the loop through the area where the strap crosses.

Pull to tighten.

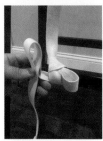

3   Make a second loop with the loose end.

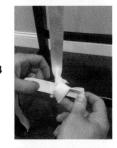

4   Pass the second loop through the first loop.

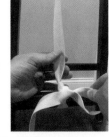

5   Pull to tighten.

Check that the strap is secure.

To untie, pull the loose end.

Fig. 13.8 Quick-release tie. (From Remmert LN, Sorrentino SA: *Mosby's essentials for nursing assistants*, ed 7, St. Louis, 2023, Elsevier.)

limited and safe extent. You could be negligent if you do not apply or secure a restraint properly.

- *Apply restraints with enough help to protect the person and staff from injury.* Persons in immediate danger of harming themselves or others are restrained quickly. Combative and agitated people can hurt themselves and the staff when restraints are applied. Enough staff members are needed to complete the task safely and quickly.

- *Observe the person at least every 15 minutes or as often as noted in the care plan.* Restraints are dangerous. Injuries and death can result from improper restraint use and poor observation. Prevent complications. Interferences with breathing and circulation are examples.

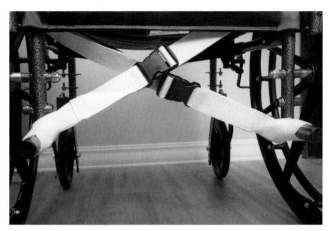

Fig. 13.9 The restraint straps are secured to the wheelchair frame. (From Remmert LN, Sorrentino SA: *Mosby's essentials for nursing assistants*, ed 7, St. Louis, 2023, Elsevier.)

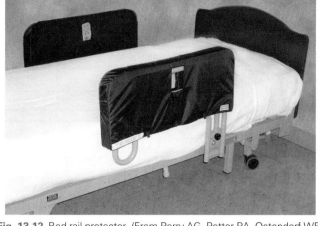

Fig. 13.12 Bed rail protector. (From Perry AG, Potter PA, Ostendorf WR: *Clinical nursing skills & techniques*, ed 9, St. Louis, 2018, Elsevier.)

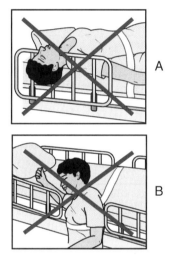

Fig. 13.10 (A) A person can get suspended and caught between bed rail bars. (B) The person can get suspended and caught between half-length bed rails. (From Sorrentino SA, Remmert LN: *Mosby's textbook for long-term care nursing assistants*, ed 10, St. Louis, 2021, Elsevier.)

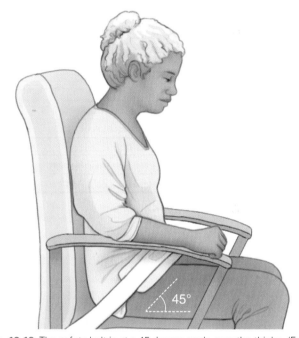

Fig. 13.13 The safety belt is at a 45-degree angle over the thighs. (From Remmert LN, Sorrentino SA: *Mosby's essentials for nursing assistants*, ed 7, St. Louis, 2023, Elsevier.)

- *Remove or release the restraint, reposition the person, and meet basic needs at least every 2 hours or as often as noted in the care plan.* The restraint is removed or released for at least 10 minutes. Provide for food, fluid, comfort, safety, hygiene, and elimination needs and give skin care. Perform range-of-motion exercises or help the person walk (Chapter 24). Follow the care plan.

  See *Focus on Communication: Safety Guidelines.*

  See *Teamwork and Time Management: Safety Guidelines.*

Reporting and Recording

Information about restraints is recorded in the person's medical record (Fig. 13.14). You might apply restraints or care for a restrained person. Report and record the following:
- Type of restraint applied
- Body part or parts restrained

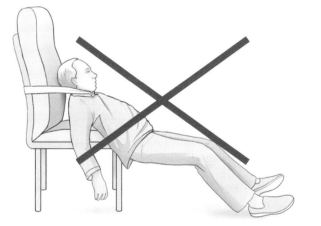

Fig. 13.11 Strangulation could result if the person slides forward or down in the chair because of extra slack in the restraint. (From Remmert LN, Sorrentino SA: *Mosby's essentials for nursing assistants*, ed 7, St. Louis, 2023, Elsevier.)

RESTRAINT MONITORING

Restraint Type and Location

☐ Limb holder		☒ Mitt		☐ Elbow splint
☐ Right wrist	☐ Right ankle	☒ Right wrist		☐ Right arm
☐ Left wrist	☐ Left ankle	☒ Left wrist		☐ Left arm

☐ Belt	☐ Vest	☐ Jacket	☐ Other:

Care Measures

☒ Restraints released/removed	☒ Food/fluid needs met	☒ Comfort measures
Duration: 15 minutes	☒ ROM/exercise/activity	☒ Skin care
☒ Restraints re-applied	☒ Urinary/bowel elimination	☒ Hygiene
☐ Measures refused	☒ Positioning	☐ Other:
Notified nurse: E. Scott, RN	☒ Call light and needed items in reach	

Vital Signs

Temp 98.4 °F	Pulse 70	R 14	BP 116 / 72 mmHg	Pain 0 /10

Circulation Observations (Normal in blue)

Color: ☒ Pink ☐ Pale ☐ Cyanotic (bluish)	**Tell the nurse at once if any observations are abnormal.**
Temperature: ☐ Hot ☒ Warm ☐ Cool ☐ Cold	
Sensation: ☒ Good sensation ☐ Numbness/tingling ☐ No sensation	Notified nurse:
Movement: ☒ Able to move extremities - ☐ Unable to move extremities	
Pulses: ☒ Pulses present in all extremities ☐ Pulse faint/absent in any extremity	

Behavior Observations

☒ Alert	☐ Agitated	☐ Restless	☐ Drowsy
☒ Calm/cooperative	☐ Aggressive	☐ Confused	☐ Sleeping

Fig. 13.14 Charting sample. (From Sorrentino SA, Remmert LN: *Mosby's textbook for long-term care nursing assistants*, ed 10, St. Louis, 2021, Elsevier.)

- Reason for the application
- Safety measures taken (e.g., bed rails padded and up, call light within reach)
- The time you applied the restraint
- The time you removed or released the restraint and for how long
- Person's vital signs
- The care given when the restraint was removed or released
- Skin color and condition
- Condition of the limbs
- Pulse felt in the restrained part

TEAMWORK AND TIME MANAGEMENT

Safety Guidelines

You may not be assigned to a restrained person. However, you must still help the nursing team keep the person safe. Make sure you know who is restrained on your unit. Every time you walk past the person or the person's room, check to see if the person is safe and comfortable. Answer the person's call light promptly.

FOCUS ON COMMUNICATION

Safety Guidelines

Restraints can increase confusion. Remind the person why the restraint is necessary and to call for help when it is needed. Repeat the following as often as needed:

- "Dr. Monroe ordered this restraint so you don't hurt yourself. If you need to get up, please call for help. I'll check on you every 15 minutes. Other staff will check on you, too."
- "How does the restraint feel? Is it too tight? Is it too loose?"
- "Please put your call light on. I want to make sure that you can reach and use it with the restraint on."
- "Please call for help right away if the restraint is too tight."
- "Please call for help right away if you feel pain in your fingers or hands. Also call for help if you feel numbness or tingling."
- "Please call for help right away if you are having problems breathing."
- Changes in the person's behavior
- Complaints of discomfort; a tight restraint; difficulty breathing; or pain, numbness, or tingling in the restrained part. (Report these complaints to the nurse at once.)

Applying Restraints

Restraints are made of cloth or leather. Cloth restraints (soft restraints) are mitts, belts, straps, jackets, and vests. They are applied to the wrists, ankles, hands, waist, and chest. Leather restraints are applied to the wrists and ankles. Leather restraints are used for extreme agitation and combativeness.

Wrist Restraints

Wrist restraints (limb holders) limit arm movement (Fig. 13.15). They may be used when a person continually tries to pull out

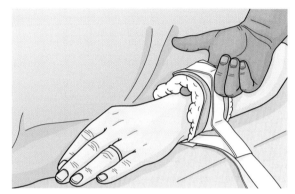

Fig. 13.15 Wrist restraint. The soft part is toward the skin. Note that one finger fits between the restraint and the wrist.

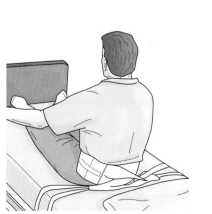

Fig. 13.16 Mitt restraint. (From Remmert LN, Sorrentino SA: *Mosby's essentials for nursing assistants*, ed 7, St. Louis, 2023, Elsevier.)

tubes used for life-saving treatment (intravenous infusion, feeding tube). Or the person scratches at, pulls at, or peels the skin, a wound, or a dressing. This can damage the skin or the wound.

Mitt Restraints

Hands are placed in mitt restraints. They prevent finger use. They allow hand, wrist, and arm movements. They are used for the same reasons as wrist restraints. Most mitts are padded (Fig. 13.16).

Belt Restraints

The belt restraint (Fig. 13.17) is used when injuries from falls are risks or for positioning during a medical treatment. The person cannot get out of bed or out of a chair. However, a roll belt allows the person to turn from side to side or sit up in bed.

The belt is applied around the waist and secured to the bed or chair (lap belt). It is applied over a garment. The person can release the quick-release type. It is less restrictive than those that only staff members can release.

Vest Restraints and Jacket Restraints

Vest and jacket restraints are applied to the chest. They may be used to prevent injuries from falls, and they may be used for persons who need positioning for a medical treatment. The person cannot turn in bed or get out of a chair.

A jacket restraint is applied with the opening in the back (Fig. 13.18). For a vest restraint, the vest crosses in front (see Fig. 13.5). *The straps of vest and jacket restraints always cross in the front.* They must *never* cross in the back. Vest and jacket restraints are never worn backward. Strangulation or other injury could occur if the person slides down in the bed or chair. The restraint is always applied over a garment. (*NOTE: A vest or jacket restraint may have a positioning slot in the back. Criss-cross the straps following the manufacturer instructions.*)

Vest and jacket restraints have life-threatening risks. Death can occur from strangulation. If the person gets caught in the restraint, it can become so tight that the person's chest cannot expand to inhale air. The person quickly suffocates and dies. Correctly applying vest and jacket restraints is critical. You are advised to

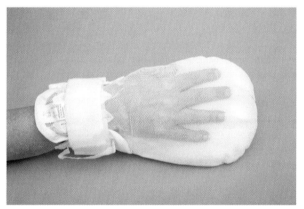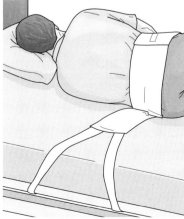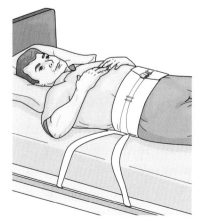

Fig. 13.17 Belt restraint. (NOTE: The bed rails are raised after the restraint is applied.)

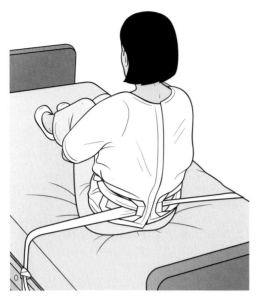

Fig. 13.18 Jacket restraint. (NOTE: The bed rails are raised after the restraint is applied.)

only assist the nurse in applying them. The nurse should assume full responsibility for applying a vest or jacket restraint.

RESIDENTS WITH DEMENTIA

Applying Restraints

Restraints may increase confusion and agitation in persons with dementia. Such persons do not understand what you are doing. They may resist your efforts to apply a restraint. They may actively try to get free from the restraint. Serious injuries and death are risks.

Never use force to apply a restraint. If a person is confused or agitated, ask a coworker to help apply the restraint. Report problems to the nurse at once.

FOCUS ON COMMUNICATION

Applying Restraints

The nurse may ask you to apply a restraint you have not used before. If you do not know how to apply a certain restraint, do not do so. Tell the nurse. Ask the nurse to show you the correct application. You can say, "I've never applied a restraint like this before. Would you please show me how and then watch me apply it?" Then thank the nurse for helping you.

When applying a restraint, explain to the person what you are going to do. Then tell the person what you are doing during each step. Always check for safety and comfort. You can ask, "How does the restraint feel? Is it too tight? Is it too loose?"

Make sure the person can communicate with you after you leave the room. Place the call light in reach. Make sure the person can use it with the restraint on. Remind the person to call if the person becomes uncomfortable or needs anything.

See *Residents with Dementia: Applying Restraints.*
See *Focus on Communication: Applying Restraints.*
See *Delegation Guidelines: Applying Restraints.*
See *Promoting Safety and Comfort: Applying Restraints.*

DELEGATION GUIDELINES

Applying Restraints

Before applying a restraint, you need this information from the nurse and the care plan:
- Why the doctor ordered the restraint
- What type and size to use
- Where to apply the restraint
- How to safely apply the restraint (Have the nurse show you how to apply it. Then show correct application back to the nurse.)
- How to correctly position the person
- What bony areas to pad and how to pad them
- If bed rail covers or gap protectors are needed
- If bed rails are up or down
- What special equipment is needed
- If the person needs to be checked more often than every 15 minutes
- When to apply and release the restraint
- What observations to report and record (p. ··)
- When to report observations
- What specific resident concerns to report at once

PROMOTING SAFETY AND COMFORT

Applying Restraints

Safety

Restraints can cause serious harm, even death. Always follow the manufacturer instructions. Manufacturers have many types of restraints. The instructions for one type may not apply to another. Also, the manufacturer may have instructions for applying restraints on persons who are agitated.

Never use force to apply a restraint. Ask a coworker to help apply a restraint on a person who is confused and agitated. Report problems to the nurse at once.

Check the person at least every 15 minutes or more often as instructed by the nurse and the care plan. Make sure the call light is within reach. Ask the person to use the call light at the first sign of problems or discomfort.

Never use a restraint as a seat belt in a car or other vehicle.

Comfort

The person's comfort is always important. It is more important when restraints are used. Remember, restraints limit movement. This affects position changes and reaching needed items. Position the person in good alignment before applying a restraint (Chapter 15). Also ensure the person can reach needed items (e.g., call light, water, tissues, phone, bed controls).

APPLYING RESTRAINTS

Quality of Life

Remember to do the following:

- Knock before entering the person's room
- Address the person by name
- Introduce yourself by name and title
- Explain the procedure to the person before beginning and during the procedure
- Protect the person's rights during the procedure
- Handle the person gently during the procedure

Preprocedure

1. Follow Delegation Guidelines: Applying Restraints. See Promoting Safety and Comfort: Applying Restraints.
2. Collect the following as instructed by the nurse:
- Correct type and size of restraints
- Padding for skin and bony areas
- Bed rail pads or gap protectors (if needed)
3. Practice hand hygiene.
4. Identify the person. Check the identification (ID) bracelet against the assignment sheet. Also call the person by name.
5. Provide for privacy.

Procedure

6. Make sure the person is comfortable and in good alignment.
7. Put the bed rail pads or gap protectors (if needed) on the bed if the person is in bed. Follow the manufacturer instructions.
8. Pad bony areas. Follow the nurse's instructions and the care plan.
9. Read the manufacturer instructions. Note the front and back of the restraint.
10. *For wrist restraints:*
   a. Apply the restraint following the manufacturer instructions. Place the soft or foam part toward the skin.
   b. Secure the restraint so it is snug but not tight. Make sure you can slide one finger under the restraint (see Fig. 13.15). Follow the manufacturer instructions. Adjust the straps if the restraint is too loose or too tight. Check for snugness again.
   c. Buckle or tie the straps to the movable part of the bed frame out of the person's reach. Use a quick-release tie.
   d. Repeat steps 10a–c for the other wrist.
11. For mitt restraints:
   a. Make sure the person's hands are clean and dry.
   b. Apply the mitt restraint. Follow the manufacturer instructions.
   c. Secure the restraint to the bed if directed to do so by the nurse. Buckle or tie the straps to the movable part of the bed frame. Use a quick-release tie.
   d. Make sure the restraint is snug. Slide one finger between the restraint and the wrist. Follow the manufacturer instructions. Adjust the straps if the restraint is too loose or too tight. Check for snugness again.
   e. Repeat steps 11b–d for the other hand.
12. *For a belt restraint:*
   a. Assist the person to a sitting position.
   b. Apply the restraint with your free hand. Follow the manufacturer instructions.
   c. Remove wrinkles or creases from the front and back of the restraint.
   d. Bring the ties through the slots in the belt.
   e. Position the straps at a 45-degree angle between the wheelchair seats and sides. Help the person lie down if in bed.
   f. Make sure the person is comfortable and in good alignment.
   g. Buckle or tie the straps to the movable part of the bed frame out of the person's reach. For a wheelchair, criss-cross and secure the straps as in Fig. 13.9. Use a quick-release tie.
   h. Ensure the belt is snug. Slide an open hand between the restraint and the person. Adjust the restraint if it is too loose or too tight. Check for snugness again.

13. *For a vest restraint:*
   a. Assist the person to a sitting position.
   b. Apply the restraint with your free hand. Follow the manufacturer instructions. The "V" part of the vest crosses in front.
   c. Bring the straps through the slots.
   d. Position the straps at a 45-degree angle between the wheelchair seats and sides. (Omit this step if the person is in bed.)
   e. Make sure the vest is free of wrinkles in the front and back.
   f. Help the person lie down if in bed.
   g. Make sure the person is comfortable and in good alignment.
   h. Buckle or tie the straps to the movable part of the bed frame. Use a quick-release tie. The buckle or tie is out of the person's reach. For a wheelchair, criss-cross and secure the straps as in Fig. 13.9.
   i. Ensure the vest is snug. Slide an open hand between the restraint and the person. Adjust the restraint if it is too loose or too tight. Check for snugness again.
14. *For a jacket restraint:*
   a. Assist the person to a sitting position.
   b. Apply the restraint with your free hand. Follow the manufacturer instructions. The jacket opening goes in the back.
   c. Close the back with the zipper, ties, or hook and loop closures.
   d. Make sure the side seams are under the arms. Remove any wrinkles in the front and back.
   e. Position the straps at a 45-degree angle between the wheelchair seat and sides. Help the person lie down if in bed.
   f. Make sure the person is comfortable and in good alignment.
   g. Buckle or tie the straps to the movable part of the bed frame. Use a quick-release tie. The buckle or tie is out of the person's reach. For a wheelchair, criss-cross and secure straps as in Fig. 13.9.
   h. Ensure the jacket is snug. Slide an open hand between the restraint and the person. Adjust the restraint if it is too loose or too tight. Check for snugness again.

Postprocedure

15. Position the person as the nurse directs.
16. Provide for comfort. (See the inside of the front cover.)
17. Place the call light within the person's reach.
18. Raise or lower bed rails. Follow the care plan and the manufacturer instructions for the restraint.
19. Unscreen the person.
20. Complete a safety check of the room. (See the inside of the front cover.)
21. Decontaminate your hands.
22. Check the person and the restraint at least every 15 minutes. Report and record your observations.
   a. *For wrist or mitt restraints:* Check the pulse, color, and temperature of the restrained parts.
   b. *For a vest, jacket, or belt restraint:* Check the person's breathing. *Call for the nurse at once if the person is not breathing or is having problems breathing.* Make sure the restraint is properly positioned in the front and back.
23. Do the following at least every 2 hours for at least 10 minutes:
   a. Remove or release the restraint.
   b. Measure vital signs.
   c. Reposition the person.
   d. Meet food, fluid, hygiene, and elimination needs.
   e. Give skin care.
   f. Perform range-of-motion exercises or help the person walk. Follow the care plan.
   g. Provide for physical and emotional comfort. (See the inside of the front cover.)
   h. Reapply the restraints.
24. Complete a safety check of the room. (See the inside of the front cover.)
25. Report and record your observations and the care given.

QUALITY OF LIFE

Because restraints lessen the person's dignity, they are ordered only for a specific medical symptom. The restrained person depends on others for basic needs.

Imagine the following:

- Your nose itches, but your hands and arms are restrained. You cannot scratch your nose.
- You need to use the bathroom, but your hands and arms are restrained so you cannot get up. You cannot reach your call light. You soil yourself with urine or a bowel movement.
- Your phone is ringing, but you cannot answer it because your hands and arms are restrained.
- You are not wearing your eyeglasses. You cannot identify people coming into and going out of your room. And you cannot speak because of a stroke. You have a vest restraint. You cannot move or turn in bed.
- You are thirsty. The water glass is within your reach, but your hands and arms are restrained.
- You hear the fire alarm. You have on a restraint. You cannot get up to move to a safe place. You must wait until someone rescues you.

What would you try to do? Would you calmly lie or sit there? Would you try to get free from the restraint? Would you cry out for help? What would the nursing staff think? Would they think that you are uncomfortable? Or would they think that you are agitated and uncooperative? Would they think your behavior is improving or getting worse? Would you feel anger, embarrassment, or humiliation?

Try to put yourself in the person's situation. Then you can better understand how the person feels. Treat the person like you would want to be treated—with kindness, caring, respect, and dignity.

You can promote quality of life by:

- *Providing for comfort.* The person's comfort is always important. It is especially important when the person is restrained. The person must be in good alignment and in a comfortable position. The restraint must allow for some movement. It must be snug, but not tight. If tight, the restraint can interfere with breathing and circulation. Also ensure that any needed items are within the person's reach.
- *Meeting safety and security needs.* The call light must always be within the person's reach. This safety measure also promotes physical and mental comfort. It promotes physical comfort because the person can call for help. Being able to call for help promotes mental comfort. So does knowing what is happening and why. The nurse explains the reason for the restraint to the person. You need to remind the person why the restraint is needed. When applying restraints, always explain what you are going to do. Tell the person what you are doing at each step. The person needs to feel safe and secure.
- *Promoting independence.* Mitt and hand restraints limit hand and arm use. Belt, vest, and jacket restraints allow hand and arm use. Make sure needed items are within the person's reach (e.g., water, tissues, bed and TV controls). Let the person do as much for oneself as safely possible.
- *Allowing personal choice.* Restraints are removed at least every 2 hours. Food, fluid, hygiene, and elimination needs are met. The person walks or range-of-motion exercises are done. Let the person choose to either use the bathroom first or walk first. Let the person choose where to walk and what to eat or drink. Allow choices that are safe for the person. Personal choices promote independence, dignity, and self-esteem.

TIME TO REFLECT

Mr. Sanderson has a feeding tube. At times he is confused. Recently, on two separate occasions, he has pulled out his feeding tube. The doctor has ordered that mitt restraints be applied to both hands. When Mr. Sanderson's wife comes to visit the first time after the mitts have been applied, she becomes very upset. She pleads with you to remove them. How should this situation be handled?

REVIEW QUESTIONS

Circle the BEST answer.

1. Which is *not* a restraint alternative?
   a. Positioning the person's chair close to the wall
   b. Answering call lights promptly
   c. Taking the person outside in nice weather
   d. Padding walls and corners of furniture

2. Physical restraints
   a. Can be removed easily by the person
   b. Are not allowed by OBRA
   c. Restrict freedom of movement
   d. Are safer than chemical restraints

3. The following can occur because of restraints. Which is the *most* serious?
   a. Fractures
   b. Strangulation
   c. Pressure injuries
   d. Urinary tract infections

4. A belt restraint is applied to a person in bed. Where should you secure the straps?
   a. To the bed rails
   b. To the headboard
   c. To the movable part of the bed frame
   d. To the footboard

5. A person has a restraint. You should check the person and the position of the restraint at least every
   a. 15 minutes
   b. 30 minutes
   c. Hour
   d. 2 hours

6. A person has mitt restraints. Which of these is especially important to report to the nurse?
   a. The heart rate
   b. The respiratory rate
   c. Why the restraints were applied
   d. If you felt a pulse in the restrained extremities

7. The doctor ordered mitt restraints for a person. You need the following information from the nurse *except*
   a. What size to use
   b. What other equipment is needed
   c. What medications the person is taking
   d. When to apply and release the restraints

8. A person has a vest restraint. It is not too tight or too loose if you can slide
   a. A fist between the vest and the person
   b. One finger between the vest and the person
   c. An open hand between the vest and the person
   d. Two fingers between the vest and the person

9. The correct way to apply any restraint is to follow the
   a. Nurse's directions
   b. Doctor's orders
   c. Care plan
   d. Manufacturer instructions

10. Unnecessary restraint is
    a. Neglect
    b. False imprisonment
    c. Invasion of privacy
    d. Battery

11. How often are restraints removed to reposition the person?
    a. At least every 2 hours
    b. At least every 4 hours
    c. Every shift
    d. When the staff have time

12. Which of the following statements is *false*?
    a. A doctor's order is needed
    b. Informed consent is required
    c. The least restrictive method must be used
    d. They are used to punish uncooperative persons

See Appendix A for answers to these questions.

14

Preventing Infection

OBJECTIVES

- Define the key terms and key abbreviations listed in this chapter.
- Identify what microbes need to live and grow.
- List the signs and symptoms of infection.
- Explain the chain of infection.
- Describe health care-associated infections and the persons at risk.
- Describe the practices of medical asepsis.

- Describe disinfection and sterilization methods.
- Explain how to care for equipment and supplies.
- Describe Standard Precautions and Transmission-Based Precautions.
- Explain the Bloodborne Pathogen Standard.
- Explain the principles and practices of surgical asepsis.
- Perform the procedures described in this chapter.
- Explain how to promote quality of life.

KEY TERMS

asepsis Being free of disease-producing microbes

asymptomatic Without symptoms

biohazardous waste Items contaminated with blood, body fluids, secretions, or excretions; *bio-* means "life" and *hazardous* means "dangerous or harmful"

carrier A human or animal that is a reservoir for microbes but does not have the signs and symptoms of infection

clean technique See "medical asepsis"

communicable disease A disease caused by pathogens that spreads easily; contagious disease

contagious disease See "communicable disease"

contamination The process of becoming unclean

disinfection The process of destroying pathogens

epidemic A sudden outbreak of disease in a certain geographic area

germicide A disinfectant applied to the skin, tissues, or nonliving objects

health care-associated infection (HAI) An infection that develops in a person cared for in any setting where health care is given; the infection is related to receiving health care

immunity Protection against a certain disease

infection A disease state resulting from the invasion and growth of microbes in the body

infection control Practices and procedures that prevent the spread of infection

medical asepsis Practices used to remove or destroy pathogens and to prevent their spread from one person or place to another person or place; clean technique

microbe See "microorganism"

microorganism A small *(micro-)* living plant or animal *(organism)* seen only with a microscope; microbe

nonpathogen A microbe that does not usually cause an infection

normal flora Microbes that live and grow in a certain area

norovirus A very contagious virus that causes vomiting and diarrhea

pandemic An outbreak of disease that spreads easily and extends across several countries or continents

pathogen A microbe that is harmful and can cause an infection

reservoir The environment in which a microbe lives and grows; host

spore A bacterium protected by a hard shell

sterile The absence of all microbes

sterile field A work area free of all pathogens and nonpathogens (including spores)

sterile technique See "surgical asepsis"

sterilization The process of destroying all microbes

surgical asepsis The practices that keep items free of all microbes; sterile technique

vaccination Giving a vaccine to produce immunity against an infectious disease

vaccine A preparation containing dead or weakened microbes

KEY ABBREVIATIONS

ABHR Alcohol-based hand rub

AIIR Airborne infection isolation room

CDC Centers for Disease Control and Prevention

C. diff Clostridium difficile

cm Centimeter

COVID-19 Coronavirus disease 2019

HAI Health care-associated infection

HBV Hepatitis B virus

HIV Human immunodeficiency virus

MDRO Multidrug-resistant organism

MRSA Methicillin-resistant *Staphylococcus aureus*
NIOSH National Institute for Occupational Safety and Health
OPIM Other potentially infectious materials
OSHA Occupational Safety and Health Administration
PHE Public Health Emergency

PPE Personal protective equipment
SARS Severe acute respiratory syndrome
TB Tuberculosis
VRE Vancomycin-resistant Enterococcus
WHO World Health Organization

An infection is a disease state resulting from the invasion and growth of microbes in the body. Infection is a major safety and health hazard. Minor infections cause short illnesses. Some infections are serious and can cause death. Older and disabled persons are at risk. The health team follows certain practices and procedures to prevent the spread of infection. Called infection control, such practices and procedures protect residents, visitors, and staff from infection. CMS requires that all facilities establish and maintain an infection prevention and control program. This program is designed to provide a safe, sanitary, and comfortable environment. It works to help prevent the development and transmission of communicable diseases and infections. One or more persons are designated as infection preventionists.

MICROORGANISMS

A microorganism (microbe) is a living thing that is too small to be seen with the naked eye. It is seen only with a microscope. Microbes are everywhere—in the mouth, nose, respiratory tract, stomach, and intestines. They are on the skin and in the air, soil, water, and food. They are on animals, clothing, and furniture.

Some microbes are helpful to the body. They are called nonpathogens and do not usually cause an infection. Some microbes are harmful and can cause infections. They are called pathogens.

Types of Microbes

There are five types of microbes.

- *Bacteria*—single-celled organisms that multiply rapidly. Often called *germs*. They can cause an infection in any body system.
- *Fungi*—plantlike organisms that live on other plants or animals. Mushrooms, yeasts, and molds are common fungi. Fungi can infect the mouth, vagina, skin, feet, and other body areas.
- *Protozoa*—one-celled animals. They can infect the blood, brain, intestines, and other body areas.
- *Rickettsiae*—found in fleas, lice, ticks, and other insects. They are spread to humans by insect bites. Rocky Mountain spotted fever is an example. The person has fever, chills, headache, rash, and other signs and symptoms.
- *Viruses*—grow in living cells. They cause many diseases. The common cold, herpes, acquired immunodeficiency syndrome (AIDS), coronavirus, influenza, and hepatitis are examples.

Requirements of Microbes

Microbes need a reservoir to live and grow. The reservoir *(host)* is the environment in which a microbe lives and grows. People, plants, animals, the soil, food, and water are common reservoirs. Microbes need *water* and *nourishment* from the reservoir. Most need *oxygen* to live. A *warm* and *dark* environment is needed. Most grow best at body temperature. They are destroyed by heat and light.

Normal Flora

Normal flora are microbes that live and grow in a certain area. Certain microbes are in the respiratory tract, in the intestines, and on the skin. They are nonpathogens when in or on a natural reservoir. When a nonpathogen is transmitted from its natural site to another site or host, it becomes a pathogen. *Escherichia coli (E. coli)* is found in the colon. If it enters the urinary system, it can cause an infection.

Multidrug-Resistant Organisms

Multidrug-resistant organisms (MDROs) are microbes that can resist the effects of antibiotics. *Antibiotics* are medications that kill microbes that cause infections. Some microbes can change their structures. This makes them harder to kill. They can survive in the presence of antibiotics. Therefore, the infections they cause are hard to treat.

MDROs are caused by doctors prescribing antibiotics when they are not needed (overprescribing). Not taking antibiotics for the length of time prescribed is another cause.

Three common MDROs are resistant to many antibiotics:

- *Methicillin-resistant* Staphylococcus aureus *(MRSA)*. Staphylococcus aureus ("staph") is a bacterium normally found in the nose and on the skin. MRSA is resistant to antibiotics often used for staph infections. It can cause serious wound and bloodstream infections and pneumonia.
- *Vancomycin-resistant* Enterococcus *(VRE)*. Enterococcus is a bacterium normally found in the intestines and in feces. It can be transmitted to others by contaminated hands, toilet seats, care equipment, and other items that the hands touch. When not in their natural site (the intestines), enterococci can cause urinary tract, wound, pelvic, and other infections. Vancomycin is an antibiotic often used to treat such infections. Enterococci resistant to vancomycin are called vancomycin-resistant enterococci.

- *Clostridium difficile (C. diff or C. difficile). C. diff* is another bacterium that causes illness usually related to individuals taking antibiotics. In recent years it has become more frequent and more difficult to treat. It commonly affects older adults in long-term care facilities. The most common symptoms are watery diarrhea and abdominal cramping. *C. diff* bacteria are passed in feces and spread to food, surfaces, and objects when people do not wash their hands properly. The bacteria produce spores that can stay on a surface for a long time. Alcohol-based hand sanitizers are not effective in destroying these spores. When caring for these individuals it is important to wash your hands thoroughly with soap and warm water.

INFECTION

A *local infection* is in a body part. A *systemic infection* involves the whole body. (*Systemic* means one or more body systems are affected.) The person has some or all of the signs and symptoms listed in Box 14.1.

Infection in Older Persons

The immune system protects the body from disease and infection (Chapter 8). Like other body systems, changes occur in the immune system with aging, thus putting older persons at risk. Infections are a major cause of death in older adults despite advances in antibiotic therapy. They account for one-third of all deaths in people 65 years and older. As the population of older adults increases, there are increasing numbers of cases of infectious disease in older adults. This is especially true with health care-associated infections (HAI).

An infection can become life threatening before the older person has obvious signs and symptoms. During an infection, an older person may not show the signs and symptoms listed in Box 14.1. The person may be **asymptomatic** (without symptoms). The person may have only a slight fever or no fever. Redness and swelling may be very slight. The person may not complain of pain. The person's mobility may be lessened, or the person may fall. Confusion and delirium may occur (Chapter 40). You must be alert to the most minor changes in the person's behavior, condition, or vital signs (Chapter 27). Report any concerns to the nurse at once.

Healing takes longer than when younger. Therefore, an infection can prolong the rehabilitation process. Independence and quality of life are affected.

The Chain of Infection

The chain of infection (Fig. 14.1) is a process involving several things:
- Infectious agent
- Reservoir
- Portal of exit
- Mode of transmission
- Portal of entry
- Host

The infectious agent or *source* is a pathogen. It must have a *reservoir* where it can grow and multiply. Humans and animals are reservoirs. If they do not have signs and symptoms of infection, they are carriers. A **carrier** is a human or animal that is a reservoir for microbes but does not have the signs and symptoms of infection. Carriers can pass the pathogen to others. To leave the reservoir, the pathogen needs a *portal of exit*. Exits are the respiratory, gastrointestinal (GI), urinary, and reproductive tracts; breaks in the skin; and the blood.

After leaving the reservoir, the pathogen must be *transmitted* to another host (Fig. 14.2). The pathogen enters the body through a *portal of entry*. Portals of entry and exit are the same (respiratory, GI, urinary, and reproductive tracts; breaks in the skin; blood). A *host* is needed for the microbe to grow and

BOX 14.1 Signs and Symptoms of Infection

- Fever (elevated body temperature)
- Chills
- Pulse rate: increased
- Respiratory rate: increased
- Pain or tenderness
- Fatigue and loss of energy
- Loss of sense of smell
- Appetite: loss of (anorexia)
- Nausea
- Vomiting
- Diarrhea
- Rash
- Sores on mucous membranes
- Redness and swelling of a body part
- Discharge or drainage from the infected area
- Heat or warmth in a body part
- Limited use of a body part
- Headache
- Muscle aches
- Joint pain
- Confusion

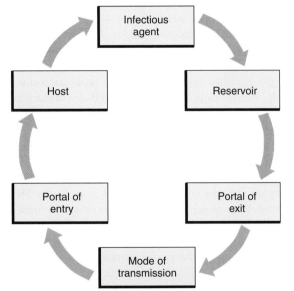

Fig. 14.1 The chain of infection. (From Potter PA, Perry AG: *Fundamentals of nursing*, ed. 10, St. Louis, 2021, Elsevier.)

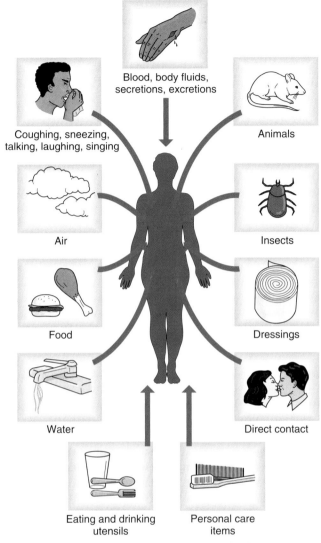

Fig. 14.2 Methods of transmitting microbes.

multiply. Susceptible hosts are persons at risk for infection. They include persons who:

- Are very young or who are older.
- Are ill.
- Were exposed to the pathogen.
- Do not follow infection control practices.

The human body can protect itself from infection. The ability to resist infection relates to age, nutrition, stress, fatigue, and health. Medications, disease, and injury also are factors.

Health Care-Associated Infection

A health care-associated infection (HAI) is an infection that develops in a person cared for in any setting where health care is given. The infection is related to receiving health care. Hospitals, nursing centers, clinics, and home care settings are examples. HAIs also are called *nosocomial infections.* (*Nosocomial* comes from the Greek word for hospital.) HAIs are caused by normal flora, or they are caused by microbes transmitted to the person from other sources.

For example, *E. coli* is normally in the colon. Feces contain *E. coli.* Poor wiping after bowel movements can cause *E. coli* to enter the urinary system. The hands can transmit *E. coli* to other body areas. If hand washing is poor, *E. coli* spreads to any body part or anything the hands touch. It also can be transmitted to other people.

Microbes can enter the body through equipment used in treatments, therapies, and tests. Such items must be free of microbes. Staff can transfer microbes from one person to another and from themselves to others. Common sites for HAIs are:

- The urinary system.
- The respiratory system.
- Wounds.
- The bloodstream.

Older persons have a hard time fighting infections. The health team must prevent the spread of infection. HAIs are prevented by:

- Medical asepsis, including hand hygiene.
- Surgical asepsis.
- Standard Precautions.
- Transmission-Based Precautions.
- The Bloodborne Pathogen Standard.

There may be times when certain infections spread through a nursing center. When a Public Health Emergency (PHE) takes place, new guidelines and recommendations are issued by the CDC and CMS. Examples of types of illnesses are influenza (flu), coronavirus, pneumonia, norovirus, and gastroenteritis. When these occur, it may be necessary to practice additional measures to keep residents safe. This was the case in late 2019 when COVID-19 began to spread. In March 2020 the World Health Organization (WHO) declared a state of pandemic. A pandemic is when infection spreads quickly and over a large area. The elderly population was at great risk. The CDC, CMS, and local health agencies issued guidelines for long-term care facilities. These infection control measures were quickly put in place. Box 14.2 lists examples of measures taken.

Viruses can mutate (change) and cause new illnesses. Precautions to protect the elderly must respond to these new illnesses. Changes are put into place for the safety and protection of the residents, staff, volunteers, and visitors. It may be necessary to wear additional PPE and practice social distancing. Workers may be required to undergo periodic testing to keep residents protected from transmission of infection. Vaccination requirements may be put into place. There may be changes to visitation policies.

Many older persons receive an annual "flu" vaccine. They may also receive vaccinations to prevent pneumonia, coronavirus, or shingles. The center may also require the workers and volunteers to receive certain vaccinations each year. If workers have signs and symptoms of illness, they should not come to the workplace. They could expose the residents and other employees to the illness. Many centers require employees to have annual tuberculosis (TB) tests. The center may also require the employees to give copies of documents that show proof of immunization and a recent physical exam.

BOX 14.2 **Examples of Infection Control Policies During COVID-19**

Employees

- All staff are required to wear masks (covering mouth and nose) at all times. Some facilities require (and provide) N-95 masks and face shields (Fig.14.17).
- Employees are screened upon arrival to work.
- Employees are tested for COVID-19 on frequent basis.
- Employees are required to isolate at home if tested positive.
- All employees are encouraged to be vaccinated.
- Physical distancing is at least 6 feet between people, in accordance with CDC guidance.
- Frequent hand hygiene is advised (use of alcohol-based hand rub is preferred).

Residents

- All residents are encouraged to accept vaccination.
- All residents are tested frequently according to CDC guidelines.
- No communal activities are allowed.
- Residents' temperatures are taken daily.
- Residents are served meals in their rooms.
- Residents are required to wear masks when not in rooms.
- If a resident leaves the facility for an appointment, an isolation period is required upon return.

Visitors

- Visitors may not enter the facility except in compassionate care visit situations.
- Outdoor visitation settings are arranged (weather permitting).
- Window visitation is arranged.
- Electronic devices (tablets, laptop computers, cellular phones, etc.) are available for virtual visits with family and friends. Assistance is offered by staff.

Facility

- Staff and visitors enter and exit the building from a single entrance and must be screened.
- Instructional signage is displayed throughout the facility, and proper visitor education on COVID-19 signs and symptoms, infection control precautions is provided.
- Hand sanitizing stations are located in convenient places throughout facility.
- Cleaning and disinfecting high-frequency touched surfaces in the facility are a priority.
- Appropriate staff use of PPE.
- Plexiglass barriers are used.
- Separate areas are dedicated to caring for residents who test positive for COVID-19.
- Residents testing positive for COVID-19 reside in private rooms, and doors are kept closed.

MEDICAL ASEPSIS

Asepsis is being free of disease-producing microbes. Microbes are everywhere. Measures are needed to achieve asepsis. Medical asepsis (clean technique) is the practice used to:

- Remove or destroy pathogens. The number of pathogens is reduced.
- Prevent pathogens from spreading from one person or place to another person or place.

Microbes cannot be present during surgery or when instruments are inserted into the body. Open wounds (cuts, burns, incisions) require the absence of microbes. They are portals of entry for microbes. Surgical asepsis (sterile technique) is the practice that keeps items free of *all* microbes. Sterile means the absence of *all* microbes—pathogens and nonpathogens. Sterilization is the process of destroying *all* microbes (pathogens and nonpathogens).

Contamination is the process of becoming unclean. In medical asepsis, an item or area is clean when it is free of pathogens. The item or area is contaminated if pathogens are present. A sterile item or area is contaminated when pathogens or nonpathogens are present.

Common Aseptic Practices

Aseptic practices break the chain of infection. To prevent the spread of microbes, wash your hands at these times:

- After urinating or having a bowel movement
- After changing tampons or sanitary pads
- After contact with your own or another person's blood, body fluids, secretions, or excretions. (This includes saliva, vomitus, urine, feces, vaginal discharge, mucus, semen, wound drainage, pus, and respiratory secretions.)
- After coughing, sneezing, or blowing your nose
- Before and after handling, preparing, or eating food
- After smoking a cigarette, cigar, or pipe
  Also do the following:
- Provide all persons with their own linens and personal care items.
- Cover your nose and mouth when coughing, sneezing, or blowing your nose. If tissues are not available, cough or sneeze into your upper arm. Do not cough or sneeze into your hands.
- Bathe, wash hair, and brush your teeth regularly.
- Wash fruits and raw vegetables before eating or serving them.
- Wash cooking and eating utensils with soap and water after use.
  See *Residents with Dementia: Common Aseptic Practices.*

RESIDENTS WITH DEMENTIA

Common Aseptic Practices

Persons with dementia do not understand aseptic practices. Others must protect them from infection. Assist them with hand washing at these times:

- After elimination
- After coughing, sneezing, or blowing the nose
- Before or after they eat or handle food
- Any time their hands are soiled

Check and clean their hands and fingernails often. They may not or cannot tell you when soiling occurs.

✳ Hand Hygiene

Hand hygiene is the easiest and most important way to prevent the spread of infection. Your hands are used for almost everything. They are easily contaminated. They can spread microbes to other persons or items. *Practice hand hygiene before and after giving care.* Box 14.3 provides the rules of hand hygiene.

See *Promoting Safety and Comfort: Hand Hygiene.*

👤 PROMOTING SAFETY AND COMFORT

Hand Hygiene

Safety

You use your hands in almost every task. They can pick up microbes from one person, place, or thing. Your hands transfer them to other people, places, and things. That is why hand hygiene is so very important. You must practice hand hygiene before and after giving care.

Comfort

You will practice hand hygiene very often during your shift. Hand lotions and hand creams help prevent chapping and dry skin. Apply hand lotion or cream as often as needed. Use a center-approved lotion or cream.

Supplies and Equipment

Most health care equipment is disposable. Single-use items are discarded after use. A person uses multiple-use items many times. These include bedpans, urinals, wash basins, water pitchers, drinking cups, and glasses. Do not "borrow" such items for another person. Disposable items help prevent the spread of infection.

Nondisposable items are cleaned, disinfected, and sometimes sterilized.

Cleaning

Cleaning reduces the number of microbes present. It also removes organic matter such as blood, body fluids, secretions, and excretions. To clean equipment:

- Wear personal protective equipment (PPE) when cleaning items contaminated with blood, body fluids, secretions, or excretions. PPE includes gloves, a mask, a gown, and goggles or a face shield.
- Rinse the item to remove organic matter. Use cold water. Heat makes organic matter thick, sticky, and hard to remove.
- Wash the item with soap and hot water.
- Scrub thoroughly. Use a brush if necessary.
- Rinse the item in warm water.
- Dry the item.
- Disinfect or sterilize the item.
- Disinfect equipment and the sink used in the cleaning procedure.
- Discard PPE.
- Practice hand hygiene.

BOX 14.3 Rules of Hand Hygiene

- Wash your hands (with soap and water) when they are visibly dirty or soiled with blood, body fluids, secretions, or excretions.
- Wash your hands (with soap and water) before eating and after using a restroom.
- Wash your hands (with soap and water) if exposure to *Clostridium difficile* or the anthrax spore is suspected or proven.
- Use an alcohol-based hand rub to decontaminate your hands if they are not visibly soiled. (If an alcohol-based hand rub is not available, wash your hands with soap and water.) Follow this rule in the following situations:
  - Before having direct contact with a person
  - After contact with the person's intact skin (e.g., after taking a pulse or blood pressure or after moving a person)
  - After contact with body fluids or excretions, mucous membranes, non-intact skin, and wound dressings if hands are not visibly soiled
  - When moving from a contaminated body site to a clean body site during care activities
  - After contact with objects (including equipment) in the person's care setting
  - After removing gloves
- Follow these rules for washing your hands with soap and water (see *Hand Washing*, p. ··):
  - Wash your hands under warm running water. Do not use hot water.
  - Stand away from the sink. Do not let your hands, body, or uniform touch the sink. The sink is contaminated (see Fig. 14.3).
  - Do not touch the inside of the sink at any time.
  - Keep your hands and forearms lower than your elbows. Your hands are dirtier than your elbows and forearms. If you hold your hands and forearms up, dirty water runs from your hands to your elbows. Those areas become contaminated.
- Rub your palms together to work up a good lather (see Fig. 14.4). The rubbing action helps remove microbes and dirt.
- Pay attention to areas often missed during hand washing—thumbs, knuckles, sides of the hands, little fingers, and under the nails.
- Clean fingernails by rubbing the fingertips against your palms (see Fig. 14.5).
- Use a nail file or orangewood stick to clean under fingernails (see Fig. 14.6). Microbes easily grow under the fingernails.
- Wash your hands for at least 20 seconds. Wash your hands longer if they are dirty or soiled with blood, body fluids, secretions, or excretions. Use your judgment and follow center policy.
- Use a clean, dry paper towel to dry your hands.
- Dry your hands starting at the fingertips. Work up to your forearms. You will dry the cleanest area first.
- Use a clean, dry paper towel for each faucet to turn the water off (see Fig. 14.7). Faucets are contaminated. The paper towels prevent clean hands from becoming contaminated again.
- Follow these rules when decontaminating your hands with an alcohol-based hand rub:
  - Apply the product to the palm of one hand. Follow the manufacturer instructions for the amount to use (see Fig. 14.8).
  - Rub your hands together.
  - Make sure you cover all surfaces of your hands and fingers.
  - Continue rubbing your hands together until your hands are dry.
  - Apply hand lotion or cream after hand hygiene. This prevents the skin from chapping and drying. Skin breaks can occur in chapped and dry skin. Skin breaks are portals of entry for microbes.

Modified from Centers for Disease Control and Prevention: Guideline for hand hygiene in health care settings. *MMWR Recomm Rep* 51(RR-16):1—45, 2002.

Nursing centers have "clean" and "dirty" utility rooms. Equipment is cleaned in the "dirty" utility room. Then it is disinfected or sterilized in the "clean" utility room. Single-use supplies are often stored in the "clean" utility room.

✳ HAND WASHING (NATCEP)

Procedure

1. See *Promoting Safety and Comfort: Hand Hygiene*.
2. Make sure you have soap, paper towels, an orangewood stick or nail file, and a wastebasket. Collect missing items.
3. Push your watch up your arm 4 to 5 inches. If your uniform sleeves are long, push them up too.
4. Stand away from the sink so your clothes do not touch the sink. Stand so the soap and faucet are easy to reach (Fig. 14.3). Do not touch the inside of the sink at any time.
5. Turn on and adjust the water until it feels warm.
6. Wet your wrists and hands. Keep your hands lower than your elbows. Be sure to wet the area 3 to 4 inches above your wrists.
7. Apply about 1 teaspoon of soap to your hands.
8. Rub your palms together and interlace your fingers to work up a good lather (Fig. 14.4). This step should last at least 20 seconds. (*NOTE:* Some state competency tests require that you wash your hands for 20–30 seconds. Know what is required in your state.)
9. Wash each hand and wrist thoroughly. Clean well between the fingers.
10. Clean under the fingernails. Rub your fingertips against your palms (Fig. 14.5).
11. Clean under the fingernails with a nail file or orangewood stick (Fig. 14.6). This step is done for the first hand washing of the day and when your hands are very soiled.
12. Rinse your wrists and hands well. Water flows from the arms to the hands.
13. Repeat steps 7 through 12, if needed.
14. Dry your wrists and hands with a clean, dry paper towel. Pat dry starting at your fingertips.
15. Discard the paper towel into the wastebasket.
16. Turn off faucets with clean, dry paper towels. This prevents you from contaminating your hands (Fig. 14.7). Use a clean paper towel for each faucet.
17. Discard the paper towels in the wastebasket.

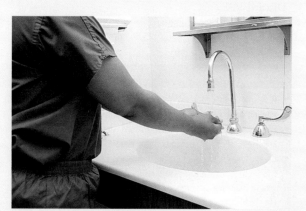

Fig. 14.3 The uniform does not touch the sink. Soap and water are within reach. Hands are lower than the elbows. Hands do not touch the inside of the sink.

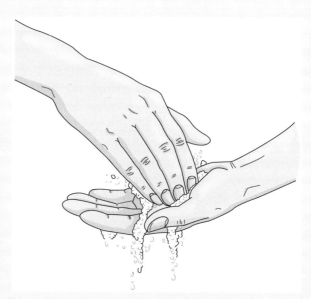

Fig. 14.5 The fingertips are rubbed against the palms to clean under the fingernails.

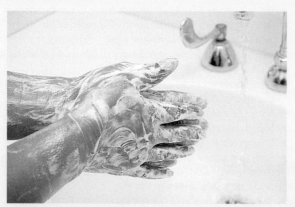

Fig. 14.4 The palms are rubbed together to work up a good lather.

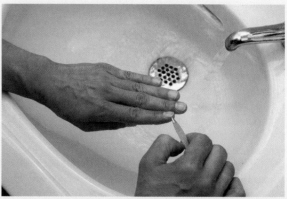

Fig. 14.6 A nail file is used to clean under the fingernails.

✳ HAND WASHING (NATCEP)—cont'd

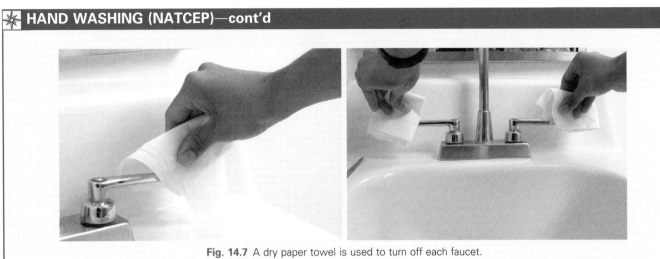

Fig. 14.7 A dry paper towel is used to turn off each faucet.

✳ HAND HYGIENE USING AN ALCOHOL-BASED HAND RUB (ABHR) (NATCEP)

Procedure

1. See *Promoting Safety and Comfort: Hand Hygiene.*
2. Apply the product to the palm of one hand. Follow the manufacturer instructions for the amount to use (Fig. 14.8A).
3. Rub palms together in a circular manner (see Fig. 14.8B).
4. Interlace fingers to spread hand rub on all surfaces of fingers (see Fig. 14.8C and D).
5. Rub tips of fingers up and down on palm of opposite hand (see Fig. 14.8E).

6. Coat surface of each thumb with hand rub (see Fig. 14.8F).
7. Rub fingertips in palm of opposite hand using circular motions (see Fig. 14.8G).
8. Continue rubbing in product until hands are dry (at least 15 seconds or according to manufacturer recommendation). There is no need to use water or paper towels when using alcohol-based hand rubs (ABHR).
9. Apply hand lotion or cream after hand hygiene. This prevents the skin from chapping and drying.

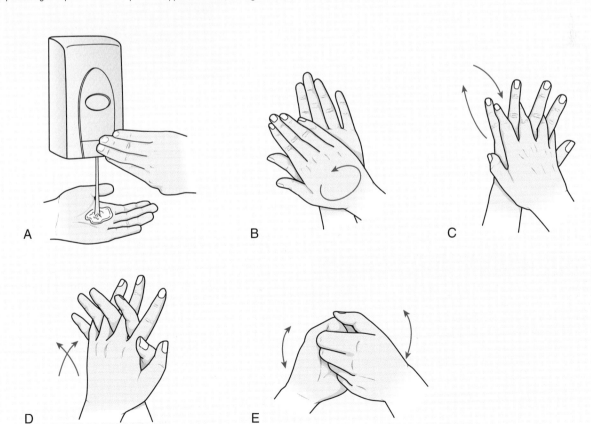

Fig. 14.8 (A) Applying alcohol-based hand rub. (B) Rubbing palms together. (C, D) Interlacing fingers. (E) Rubbing fingertips against palms.

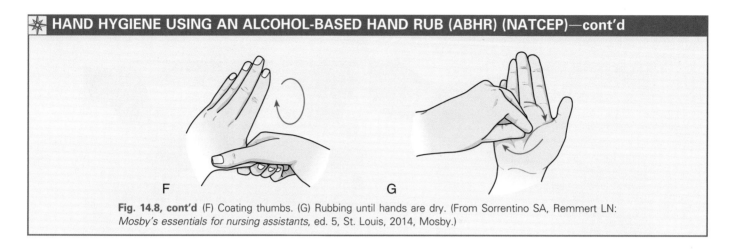

F   G

Fig. 14.8, cont'd (F) Coating thumbs. (G) Rubbing until hands are dry. (From Sorrentino SA, Remmert LN: *Mosby's essentials for nursing assistants*, ed. 5, St. Louis, 2014, Mosby.)

Disinfection

Disinfection is the process of destroying pathogens. Spores are not destroyed. Spores are bacteria protected by a hard shell. Spores are killed by very high temperatures.

Germicides are disinfectants applied to skin, tissues, and nonliving objects. Alcohol is a common germicide.

Chemical disinfectants are used to clean surfaces. Counters, tubs, and showers are examples. They also are used to clean reusable items. Such items include:

- Blood pressure cuffs.
- Commodes and metal bedpans.
- Wheelchairs and stretchers.
- Furniture.
  See *Promoting Safety and Comfort: Disinfection.*

Sterilization

Sterilizing destroys all nonpathogens and pathogens, including spores. Very high temperatures are used because microbes are destroyed by heat.

Boiling water, radiation, liquid or gas chemicals, dry heat, and *steam under pressure* are sterilization methods. An *autoclave* (Fig. 14.9) is a pressure steam sterilizer. Glass, surgical items, and metal objects are autoclaved. High temperatures destroy plastic and rubber items. They are not autoclaved. Steam under pressure sterilizes objects in 30 to 45 minutes.

👤 PROMOTING SAFETY AND COMFORT

Disinfection

Safety

Chemical disinfectants can burn and irritate the skin. Wear utility gloves or rubber household gloves to prevent skin irritation. These gloves are waterproof. Do not wear disposable gloves.

Some chemical disinfectants have special measures for use and storage. Check the Safety Data Sheet (SDS) before handling a disinfectant. See Chapter 11.

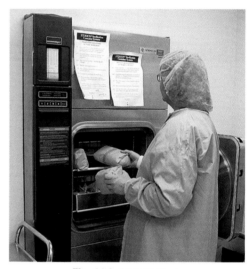

Fig. 14.9 An autoclave.

Other Aseptic Measures

Hand hygiene, cleaning, disinfection, and sterilization are important aseptic measures. So are the measures listed in Box 14.4. They are useful in home, work, and everyday life.

ISOLATION PRECAUTIONS

Blood, body fluids, secretions, and excretions can transmit pathogens. Sometimes barriers are needed to prevent their escape. The pathogens are kept within a certain area. Usually the area is the person's room. This requires isolation precautions.

The *2007 Guideline for Isolation Precautions: Preventing Transmission of Infectious Agents in Healthcare Settings* is followed. The guideline was issued by the Centers for Disease Control and Prevention (CDC) in 2007 and was updated in 2017.

BOX 14.4 Aseptic Measures

Controlling Reservoirs (Hosts—You or the Person)
- Provide for the person's hygiene needs (Chapter 18).
- Wash contaminated areas with soap and water. Feces, urine, and blood can contain microbes, as can body fluids, secretions, and excretions.
- Use leakproof plastic bags for soiled tissues, linens, and other materials.
- Keep tables, counters, wheelchair trays, and other surfaces clean and dry.
- Label bottles with the person's name and the date the bottle was opened.
- Keep bottles and fluid containers tightly capped or covered.
- Keep drainage containers below the drainage site (Chapters 22 and 31).
- Empty drainage containers and dispose of drainage following center policy. Usually, drainage containers are emptied every shift. Follow the nurse's directions.

Controlling Portals of Exit
- Cover your nose and mouth when coughing or sneezing.
- Provide the person with tissues to use when coughing or sneezing.
- Wear PPE as needed (p. ··).

Controlling Transmission
- Make sure all persons have their own personal care equipment. This includes wash basins, bedpans, urinals, commodes, and eating and drinking utensils.
- Do not take equipment from one person's room to use for another person. Even if the item is unused, do not take it from one room to another.
- Hold equipment and linens away from your uniform (Fig. 14.10).
- Practice hand hygiene (see Box 14.3).
- Assist the person with hand washing:
  - Before and after eating.
  - After elimination.
  - After changing tampons, sanitary napkins, or other personal hygiene products.
  - After contact with blood, body fluids, secretions, or excretions.
- Prevent dust movement. Do not shake linens or equipment. Use a damp cloth for dusting.
- Clean from the cleanest area to the dirtiest. This prevents soiling a clean area.
- Clean away from your body. Do not dust, brush, or wipe toward yourself. Otherwise, you transmit microbes to your skin, hair, and clothing.

- Flush urine and feces down the toilet. Avoid splatters and splashes.
- Pour contaminated liquids directly into sinks or toilets. Avoid splashing onto other areas.
- Do not sit on the person's bed and do not sit on the floor. You will pick up microbes. You will transfer them to the next surface that you sit on.
- Do not use items that are on the floor. The floor is contaminated.
- Clean tubs, showers, and shower chairs after each use. Follow the center's disinfection procedures.
- Clean bedpans, urinals, and commodes after each use. Follow the center's disinfection procedures.
- Report pests (e.g., ants, spiders, mice).

Controlling Portals of Entry
- Provide for good skin care (Chapter 18). This promotes intact skin.
- Provide for good oral hygiene (Chapter 18). This promotes intact mucous membranes.
- Do not let the person lie on tubes or other items. This protects the skin from injury.
- Make sure linens are dry and wrinkle free (Chapter 17). This protects the skin from injury.
- Turn and reposition the person as directed by the nurse and care plan (Chapter 15). This protects the skin from injury.
- Assist with or clean the genital area after elimination (Chapter 18). Wipe and clean from the urethra (the cleanest area) to the rectum (the dirtiest area). This helps prevent urinary tract infections.
- Make sure drainage tubes are properly connected. This prevents microbes from entering the drainage system.

Protecting the Susceptible Host
- Follow the care plan to meet hygiene needs. This protects the skin and mucous membranes.
- Follow the care plan to meet nutrition and fluid needs (Chapter 20). This helps prevent infection.
- Assist with deep-breathing and coughing exercises as directed (Chapter 26). This helps prevent respiratory infections.

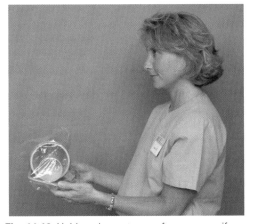

Fig. 14.10 Hold equipment away from your uniform.

Isolation precautions prevent the spread of communicable diseases (contagious diseases). They are diseases caused by pathogens that spread easily.

Isolation precautions are based on *clean* and *dirty*. *Clean* areas or objects are free of pathogens. They are not contaminated. *Dirty* areas or objects are contaminated with pathogens. If a *clean* area or object has contact with something *dirty*, the

clean area is now dirty. *Clean* and *dirty* also depend on how the pathogen is spread.

The CDC's isolation precautions guideline has two tiers of precautions:
- Standard Precautions
- Transmission-Based Precautions
  See *Focus on Communication: Isolation Precautions.*
  See *Delegation Guidelines: Isolation Precautions.*
  See *Promoting Safety and Comfort: Isolation Precautions.*
  See *Teamwork and Time Management: Isolation Precautions.*

Standard Precautions

Standard Precautions are part of the CDC's isolation precautions (Box 14.5). They reduce the risk of spreading pathogens. They also reduce the risk of spreading known and unknown infections. *Standard Precautions are used for all persons whenever care is given.* They prevent the spread of infection from:
- Blood.
- All body fluids, secretions, and excretions (except sweat) even if blood is not visible. Sweat is not known to spread infection.
- Nonintact skin (skin with open breaks).
- Mucous membranes.

BOX 14.5 Standard Precautions

Hand Hygiene
- Follow the rules for hand hygiene (see Box 14.3).
- Avoid unnecessary touching of surfaces close to the person. This prevents contamination of clean hands from environmental surfaces. It also prevents the transmission of pathogens from contaminated hands to other surfaces.
- Do not wear fake nails or nail extenders if you will have contact with persons at risk for infection or other adverse outcomes. (*NOTE:* Some centers do not allow fake nails or nail extenders.)

Personal Protective Equipment
- Wear PPE when contact with blood or body fluids is likely.
- Do not contaminate your clothing or skin when removing PPE.
- Remove and discard PPE before leaving the person's room or care setting.

Gloves
- Wear gloves when contact with the following is likely:
  - Blood
  - Potentially infectious materials (e.g., body fluids, secretions, excretions)
  - Mucous membranes
  - Nonintact skin
  - Skin that may be contaminated (e.g., a person is incontinent of feces or urine)
- Wear gloves that fit and are appropriate for the task:
  - Wear disposable gloves to provide direct care to the person.
  - Wear disposable gloves or utility gloves for cleaning equipment or care settings.
- Remove gloves after contact with the person or the person's care setting. The care setting includes equipment used in the person's care.
- Remove gloves after contact with care equipment.
- Do not wear the same pair of gloves to care for more than one person. Remove gloves after contact with a person and before going to another person.
- Do not wash gloves for reuse with different persons.
- Change gloves during care if your hands will move from a contaminated body site to a clean body site.

Gowns
- Wear a gown that is appropriate to the task.
- Wear a gown to protect your skin and clothing when contact with blood, body fluids, secretions, or excretions is likely.
- Wear a gown for direct contact with a person who has uncontained secretions or excretions.
- Remove the gown and perform hand hygiene before leaving the person's room or care setting.
- Do not reuse gowns, even for repeat contacts with the same person.

Mouth, Nose, and Eye Protection
- Wear PPE (masks, goggles, face shield) for procedures and tasks that are likely to cause splashes and sprays of blood, body fluids, secretions, or excretions.
- Wear PPE (mask, goggles, face shield) appropriate for the procedure or task.
- Wear gloves, a gown, and one of the following for procedures that are likely to cause sprays of respiratory secretions:
  - Face shield that fully covers the front and sides of the face
  - Mask with attached shield
  - Mask and goggles

Respiratory Hygiene and Cough Etiquette
- Instruct persons with respiratory symptoms to:
  - Cover the nose and mouth when coughing or sneezing.
  - Use tissues to contain respiratory secretions.
  - Dispose of tissues in the nearest waste container after use.
  - Perform hand hygiene after contact with respiratory secretions.
  - Provide visitors with masks according to center policy.

Care Equipment
- Wear appropriate PPE when handling care equipment that is visibly soiled with blood, body fluids, secretions, or excretions.
- Wear appropriate PPE when handling care equipment that may have been in contact with blood, body fluids, secretions, or excretions.
- Remove organic material before disinfection and sterilization procedures. Use cleaning agents according to center policy.

Care of the Environment
- Follow center policies and procedures for cleaning and maintaining surfaces (e.g., environmental surfaces and care equipment). Surfaces near the person may need more frequent cleaning and maintenance (e.g., doorknobs, bed rails, overbed tables, toilet surfaces, and areas).
- Clean and disinfect multiple-use electronic equipment according to center policy. This includes:
  - Items used by residents.
  - Items used to give care.
  - Mobile devices that are moved in and out of resident rooms.
- Follow these rules for toys used by children and toys in waiting areas:
  - Select toys that can be easily cleaned and disinfected.
  - Do not allow use of stuffed furry toys if they will be shared.
  - Clean and disinfect large stationary toys at least weekly and whenever visibly soiled.
  - Clean and disinfect a toy immediately when it requires cleaning, or store the toy in a labeled container away from toys that are clean and ready for use.

Textiles and Laundry
- Handle used textiles and fabrics (linens) with minimum agitation. This is done to avoid contamination of air, surfaces, and other persons.

Worker Safety
- Protect yourself and others from exposure to bloodborne pathogens. This includes knowing how to handle needles and other sharps. Follow federal and state standards and guidelines. See the Bloodborne Pathogen Standard (p. 190).
- Use a mouthpiece, resuscitation bag, or other ventilation device during resuscitation to prevent contact with the person's mouth and oral secretions (Chapter 44).

Resident Placement
- A private room is preferred if the person is at risk for transmitting the infection to others.
- Follow the nurse's instructions if a private room is not available.

Modified from Siegel JD, Rhinehart E, Jackson M, et al.: Healthcare Infection Control Practices Advisory Committee: 2007 Guideline for isolation precautions: preventing transmission of infectious agents in health care settings, Atlanta, 2007, Centers for Disease Control and Prevention.

FOCUS ON COMMUNICATION

Isolation Precautions

Some centers require visitors to wear PPE when visiting a person needing isolation precautions. Visitors may question the need for PPE. They do not wear PPE in the person's home or outside the center. They do not understand why it is needed. Some visitors ignore signs or requests to wear PPE. It is important to communicate with the person and visitors about PPE. You can politely say:

- "Your visitors will need to wear a gown and gloves while in your room."
- "Please wear this mask. It is our policy to protect you, your family member, and others."

Tell the nurse if the person or visitors have more questions. Also tell the nurse if someone refuses to follow isolation precautions.

DELEGATION GUIDELINES

Isolation Precautions

You may assist in the care of persons who require isolation precautions. If so, review the type used with the nurse. You also need this information from the nurse and the care plan:

- What PPE to use
- What special safety measures are needed

PROMOTING SAFETY AND COMFORT

Isolation Precautions

Safety

Preventing the spread of infection is important. Isolation precautions protect everyone—residents, visitors, staff, and you. If you are careless, everyone's safety is at risk.

Comfort

Persons requiring isolation precautions usually must stay in their rooms. The person may feel lonely, especially if visitors are few. You can help the person by:

- Remembering that the pathogen is undesirable, not the person.
- Treating the person with respect, kindness, and dignity.
- Providing newspapers, magazines, books, and other reading material.
- Providing hobby materials or puzzles if possible.
- Placing a clock in the room.
- Urging the person to call family and friends.
- Assisting the person with a virtual visit (tablet, laptop, etc.) with family or friends.
- Organizing your work so you can stay to visit with the person.
- Saying "hello" from the doorway often.

Items brought into the person's room become contaminated. Disinfect or discard the items according to center policy.

TEAMWORK AND TIME MANAGEMENT

Isolation Precautions

Donning (putting on) and removing PPE take time and effort. Once you don PPE, you must remove it before leaving the room. Therefore, you need to plan your time and work so that you do not need to leave the room. Meet the needs of other residents first. Ask a coworker to answer their call lights for you. Ask politely and thank your coworker for helping you. Then gather the care items that you need to bring to the room. Before leaving the room, make sure the person's needs are met. Complete a safety check of the room. Also tell the person when you will return to the room.

Offer to help a coworker care for a person needing isolation precautions. Bring items to the room as needed. Also answer call lights for your coworker. Be sure to tell the coworker what you did for the person and what you observed.

Transmission-Based Precautions

Some infections require Transmission-Based Precautions (Box 14.6). You must understand how certain infections are spread (see Fig. 14.2). This helps you understand the types of Transmission-Based Precautions.

Protective Measures

Center policies may differ from those in this text. Current epidemic conditions may require specific measures. The rules in Box 14.7 are a general guide for giving safe care when using isolation precautions.

Isolation precautions involve wearing PPE (e.g., gloves, gown, mask, goggles, face shield).

Removing linens, trash, and equipment from the room may require double-bagging. Follow center procedures when collecting specimens and transporting persons.

See *Promoting Safety and Comfort: Protective Measures.*

BOX 14.6 **Transmission-Based Precautions**

Contact Precautions

- Used for persons with known or suspected infections or conditions that increase the risk of contact transmission.
- Resident placement: a single room is preferred.
- Do the following if a room is shared with another person who is not infected with the same agent:
  - Keep the privacy curtain between the beds closed.
  - Change PPE and perform hand hygiene between contact with persons in the same room. Do so regardless of whether one or both persons are on contact precautions.
- Gloves:
  - Don gloves upon entering the person's room or care setting.

- Wear gloves whenever touching the person's intact skin.
- Wear gloves whenever touching surfaces or items near the person.
- Gowns:
  - Wear a gown whenever clothing may have direct contact with the person.
  - Wear a gown whenever contact is likely with surfaces or equipment near the person.
  - Don the gown upon entering the person's room or care setting.
  - Remove the gown and perform hand hygiene before leaving the person's room or care setting.
  - Make sure your clothing and skin do not touch potentially contaminated surfaces after removing the gown.

BOX 14.6   Transmission-Based Precautions—cont'd

- Resident transport:
  - Limit transport and movement of the person outside the room to medically necessary purposes.
  - Cover the area of the person's body that is infected.
  - Remove and discard contaminated PPE and perform hand hygiene before transporting the person.
  - Don clean PPE to handle the person at the transport destination.
- Care equipment:
  - Follow Standard Precautions.
  - Use disposable equipment when possible. If possible, leave non-disposable equipment in the person's room.
  - Clean and disinfect nondisposable and multiple-use equipment before use on another person.

Droplet Precautions

- Used for persons known or suspected to be infected with pathogens transmitted by respiratory droplets. Such droplets are generated by a person who is coughing, sneezing, or talking.
- Resident placement: a single room is preferred.
- Do the following if a room is shared with another person who is not infected with the same agent:
  - Keep the privacy curtain between the beds closed.
  - Change PPE and perform hand hygiene between contact with persons in the same room. Do so regardless of whether one or both persons are on Droplet Precautions.
- Personal protective equipment: Don a mask upon entering the person's room or care setting.

- Resident transport:
  - Limit transport and movement of the person outside the room to medically necessary purposes.
  - Have the person wear a mask.
  - Instruct the person to follow "Respiratory Hygiene and Cough Etiquette" (see Box 14.4).

Airborne Precautions

- Used for persons known or suspected to be infected with pathogens transmitted person to person by the airborne route. Tuberculosis (TB), measles, chickenpox, smallpox, and severe acute respiratory syndrome (SARS), and COVID-19 are examples.
- The resident is placed in an airborne infection isolation room (AIIR) if available.
- Health team members susceptible to the infection are restricted from entering the room if immune staff members are available.
- Personal protective equipment:
  - An approved respirator is worn on entering the room or home of a person with TB.
  - Respiratory protection is recommended for all health team members when caring for persons with smallpox.
- Resident transport:
  - Limit transport and movement of the person outside the room to medically necessary purposes.
  - Have the person wear a surgical mask.
  - Instruct the person to follow "Respiratory Hygiene and Cough Etiquette" (see Box 14.5).
  - Cover skin lesions infected with the microbe.

Modified from Siegel JD, Rhinehart E, Jackson M, et al.: Healthcare Infection Control Practices Advisory Committee: 2007 Guideline for isolation precautions: preventing transmission of infectious agents in health care settings, Atlanta, 2007, Centers for Disease Control and Prevention.

BOX 14.7   Rules for Isolation Precautions

- Collect all needed items before entering the room.
- Prevent contamination of equipment and supplies. Floors are contaminated, as is any object on the floor or that falls to the floor.
- Use mops wetted with a disinfectant solution to clean floors. Floor dust is contaminated.
- Prevent drafts. Some microbes are carried in the air by drafts.
- Use paper towels to handle contaminated items.
- Remove items from the room in leakproof plastic bags.
- Double-bag items if the outer part of the bag is or can be contaminated (p. 188).
- Follow center policy for removing and transporting disposable and reusable items.
- Return reusable dishes, drinking vessels, eating utensils, and trays to the food service (dietary) department. Discard disposable dishes,

drinking vessels, eating utensils, and trays in the waste container in the person's room.
- Do not touch your hair, nose, mouth, eyes, or other body parts.
- Do not touch any clean area or object if your hands are contaminated.
- Wash your hands if they are visibly dirty or contaminated with blood, body fluids, secretions, or excretions.
- Place clean items on paper towels.
- Do not shake linens.
- Use paper towels to turn faucets on and off.
- Use a paper towel to open the door to the person's room. Discard it as you leave.
- Tell the nurse if you have any cuts, open skin areas, a sore throat, vomiting, or diarrhea.

PROMOTING SAFETY AND COMFORT

Protective Measures

Safety

The PPE needed for Standard Precautions depends on what tasks, procedures, and care measures you will do while in the room. The PPE needed also depends on the type of Transmission-Based Precautions ordered for the person. Sometimes only gloves are needed. The nurse tells you when other PPE is needed.

According to the CDC's isolation guideline, gloves are always worn when gowns are worn. Sometimes other PPE is needed when gowns are worn. The isolation guideline shows PPE donned and removed in the following order:
- Donning PPE (Fig. 14.11A):

- Gown
- Mask or respirator
- Eyewear (goggles or face shield)
- Gloves
- Removing PPE (removed at the doorway before leaving the person's room) (see Fig. 14.11B):
  - Gloves
  - Eyewear (goggles or face shield)
  - Gown
  - Mask or respirator

SEQUENCE FOR PUTTING ON PERSONAL PROTECTIVE EQUIPMENT (PPE)

The type of PPE used will vary based on the level of precautions required, such as standard and contact, droplet or airborne infection isolation precautions. The procedure for putting on and removing PPE should be tailored to the specific type of PPE.

1. GOWN

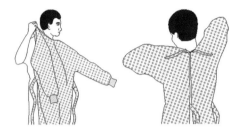

- Fully cover torso from neck to knees, arms to end of wrists, and wrap around the back
- Fasten in back of neck and waist

2. MASK OR RESPIRATOR

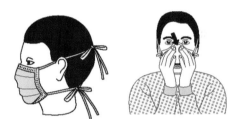

- Secure ties or elastic bands at middle of head and neck
- Fit flexible band to nose bridge
- Fit snug to face and below chin
- Fit-check respirator

3. GOGGLES OR FACE SHIELD

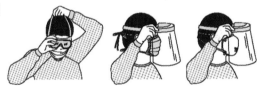

- Place over face and eyes and adjust to fit

4. GLOVES

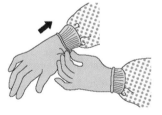

- Extend to cover wrist of isolation gown

USE SAFEWORK PRACTICES TO PROTECT YOURSELF AND LIMIT THE SPREAD OF CONTAMINATION

- Keep hands away from face
- Limit surfaces touched
- Change gloves when torn or heavily contaminated
- Perform hand hygiene

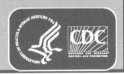

A

Fig. 14.11 (A) Donning personal protective equipment. (B) Removing personal protective equipment. (C) Method 2 removing PPE. (From Centers for Disease Control and Prevention, U.S. Department of Health and Human Services, National Institute for Occupational Safety and Health, https://www.cdc.gov/niosh/npptl/)

HOW TO SAFELY REMOVE PERSONAL PROTECTIVE EQUIPMENT (PPE) EXAMPLE 1

There are a variety of ways to safely remove PPE without contaminating your clothing, skin, or mucous membranes with potentially infectious materials. Here is one example. **Remove all PPE before exiting the patient room** except a respirator, if worn. Remove the respirator **after** leaving the patient room and closing the door. Remove PPE in the following sequence:

1. GLOVES

- Outside of gloves are contaminated!
- If your hands get contaminated during glove removal, immediately wash your hands or use an alcohol-based hand sanitizer
- Using a gloved hand, grasp the palm area of the other gloved hand and peel off first glove
- Hold removed glove in gloved hand
- Slide fingers of ungloved hand under remaining glove at wrist and peel off second glove over first glove
- Discard gloves in a waste container

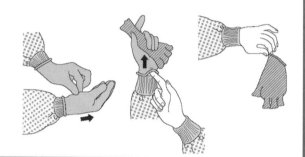

2. GOGGLES OR FACE SHIELD

- Outside of goggles or face shield are contaminated!
- If your hands get contaminated during goggle or face shield removal, immediately wash your hands or use an alcohol-based hand sanitizer
- Remove goggles or face shield from the back by lifting head band or ear pieces
- If the item is reusable, place in designated receptacle for reprocessing. Otherwise, discard in a waste container

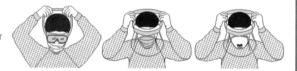

3. GOWN

- Gown front and sleeves are contaminated!
- If your hands get contaminated during gown removal, immediately wash your hands or use an alcohol-based hand sanitizer
- Unfasten gown ties, taking care that sleeves don't contact your body when reaching for ties
- Pull gown away from neck and shoulders, touching inside of gown only
- Turn gown inside out
- Fold or roll into a bundle and discard in a waste container

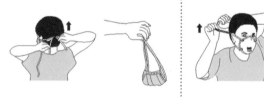

4. MASK OR RESPIRATOR

- Front of mask/respirator is contaminated — DO NOT TOUCH!
- If your hands get contaminated during mask/respirator removal, immediately wash your hands or use an alcohol-based hand sanitizer
- Grasp bottom ties or elastics of the mask/respirator, then the ones at the top, and remove without touching the front
- Discard in a waste container

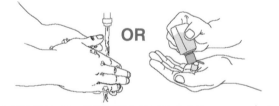

5. WASH HANDS OR USE AN ALCOHOL-BASED HAND SANITIZER IMMEDIATELY AFTER REMOVING ALL PPE

OR

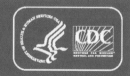

PERFORM HAND HYGIENE BETWEEN STEPS IF HANDS BECOME CONTAMINATED AND IMMEDIATELY AFTER REMOVING ALL PPE

CS250672-E

B

Fig. 14.11, cont'd

HOW TO SAFELY REMOVE PERSONAL PROTECTIVE EQUIPMENT (PPE) EXAMPLE 2

Here is another way to safely remove PPE without contaminating your clothing, skin, or mucous membranes with potentially infectious materials. **Remove all PPE before exiting the patient room** except a respirator, if worn. Remove the respirator **after** leaving the patient room and closing the door. Remove PPE in the following sequence:

1. GOWN AND GLOVES

- Gown front and sleeves and the outside of gloves are contaminated!
- If your hands get contaminated during gown or glove removal, immediately wash your hands or use an alcohol-based hand sanitizer
- Grasp the gown in the front and pull away from your body so that the ties break, touching outside of gown only with gloved hands
- While removing the gown, fold or roll the gown inside out into a bundle
- As you are removing the gown, peel off your gloves at the same time, only touching the inside of the gloves and gown with your bare hands. Place the gown and gloves into a waste container

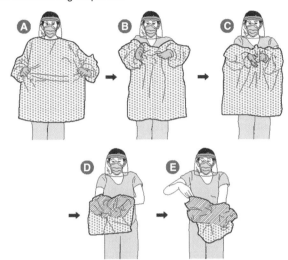

2. GOGGLES OR FACE SHIELD

- Outside of goggles or face shield are contaminated!
- If your hands get contaminated during goggle or face shield removal, immediately wash your hands or use an alcohol-based hand sanitizer
- Remove goggles or face shield from the back by lifting head band and without touching the front of the goggles or face shield
- If the item is reusable, place in designated receptacle for reprocessing. Otherwise, discard in a waste container

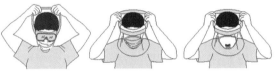

3. MASK OR RESPIRATOR

- Front of mask/respirator is contaminated — DO NOT TOUCH!
- If your hands get contaminated during mask/respirator removal, immediately wash your hands or use an alcohol-based hand sanitizer
- Grasp bottom ties or elastics of the mask/respirator, then the ones at the top, and remove without touching the front
- Discard in a waste container

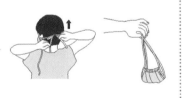

4. WASH HANDS OR USE AN ALCOHOL-BASED HAND SANITIZER IMMEDIATELY AFTER REMOVING ALL PPE

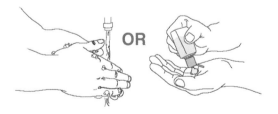

OR

PERFORM HAND HYGIENE BETWEEN STEPS IF HANDS BECOME CONTAMINATED AND IMMEDIATELY AFTER REMOVING ALL PPE

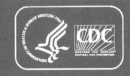

CS250672-E

C

Fig. 14.11, cont'd

✳ Gloves

The skin is a natural barrier. It prevents microbes from entering the body. Small skin breaks on the hands and fingers are common. Some are very small and hard to see. Disposable gloves act as a barrier. They protect you from pathogens in the person's blood, body fluids, secretions, and excretions. They also protect the person from microbes on your hands.

Wear gloves whenever contact with blood, body fluids, secretions, excretions, mucous membranes, or nonintact skin is likely. Contact may be direct; or contact may be indirect with items or surfaces contaminated with blood, body fluids, secretions, or excretions.

Wearing gloves is the most common protective measure used with Standard Precautions and Transmission-Based Precautions. Remember the following when using gloves:

- The outside of gloves is contaminated.
- Gloves are easier to put on when your hands are dry.
- Do not tear gloves when putting them on. Carelessness, long fingernails, and rings can tear gloves. Blood, body fluids, secretions, and excretions can enter the glove through the tear. This contaminates your hand.
- You need a new pair for every person.
- Remove and discard torn, cut, or punctured gloves at once. Practice hand hygiene. Then put on a new pair.
- Wear gloves once. Discard them after use.
- Put on clean gloves just before touching mucous membranes or nonintact skin.
- Put on new gloves whenever gloves become contaminated with blood, body fluids, secretions, or excretions. A task may require more than one pair of gloves.
- Change gloves whenever moving from a contaminated body site to a clean body site.
- Change gloves if interacting with the person involves touching portable computer keyboards or other mobile equipment that is transported from room to room.
- Put on gloves last when they are worn with other PPE.
- Make sure gloves cover your wrists. If you wear a gown, gloves cover the cuffs (Fig. 14.12).
- Remove gloves so the inside part is on the outside. The inside is *clean.*
- Decontaminate your hands after removing gloves.
  See *Promoting Safety and Comfort: Gloves.*

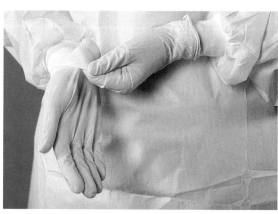

Fig. 14.12 The gloves cover the cuffs of the gown.

Gowns

Gowns prevent the spread of microbes. They protect your clothes and body from contact with blood, body fluids, secretions, and excretions. They also protect against splashes and sprays.

👤 PROMOTING SAFETY AND COMFORT

Gloves

Safety

No special method is needed to put on nonsterile gloves. To remove gloves, see *Removing Gloves.*

Most facilities are now using only latex-free gloves. In the past, some gloves were made of latex (a rubber product). Latex allergies are common. If skin rashes and breathing problems occur, report these to the nurse at once.

Comfort

Many nurses and nursing assistants wear gloves for every resident contact. Remember, gloves are needed whenever contact with blood, body fluids, secretions, excretions, mucous membranes, or nonintact skin is likely. You do not need to wear gloves when such contact is not likely. Back massages and brushing and combing hair are examples, unless the person has open areas on the skin or scalp.

✳ REMOVING GLOVES (NATCEP)

Procedure

1. See *Promoting Safety and Comfort: Gloves.*
2. Make sure that glove touches only glove.
3. Grasp a glove just below the cuff (Fig. 14.13A). Grasp it on the outside.
4. Pull the glove down over your hand so it is inside out (see Fig. 14.13B).
5. Hold the removed glove with your other gloved hand.
6. Reach inside the other glove. Use the first two fingers of the ungloved hand (see Fig. 14.13C).
7. Pull the glove down (inside out) over your hand and the other glove (see Fig. 14.13D).
8. Discard the gloves. Follow center policy.
9. Decontaminate your hands.

✳ REMOVING GLOVES (NATCEP)—cont'd

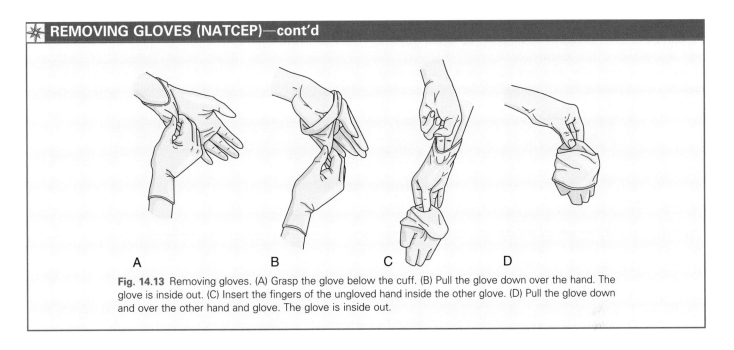

Fig. 14.13 Removing gloves. (A) Grasp the glove below the cuff. (B) Pull the glove down over the hand. The glove is inside out. (C) Insert the fingers of the ungloved hand inside the other glove. (D) Pull the glove down and over the other hand and glove. The glove is inside out.

✳ DONNING AND REMOVING A GOWN (NATCEP)

Procedure

1. Remove your watch and all jewelry.
2. Roll up uniform sleeves.
3. Practice hand hygiene.
4. Hold a clean gown out in front of you. Let it unfold. Do not shake the gown.
5. Put your hands and arms through the sleeves (see Fig. 14.11A).
6. Make sure the gown covers you from your neck to your knees. It must cover your arms to the end of your wrists.
7. Tie the strings at the back of the neck (see Fig. 14.11A).
8. Overlap the back of the gown. Make sure it covers your uniform. The gown should be snug, not loose. (If the gown does not cover your back, you may need to take a second gown and put it on with the opening in the front.)
9. Tie the waist strings. Tie them at the back or the side. Do not tie them in front.
10. Put on other PPE:
    a. Mask or respirator (if needed)
    b. Goggles or face shield (if needed)
    c. Gloves (ensure gloves cover gown cuffs)
11. Provide care.
12. Remove and discard the gloves.
13. Remove and discard goggles or face shield if worn.
14. Remove the gown. Do not touch the outside of the gown.
    a. Untie the neck and waist strings (see Fig. 14.11B).
    b. Pull the gown down from each shoulder toward the same hand (see Fig. 14.11).
    c. Turn the gown inside out as it is removed. Hold it at the inside shoulder seams and bring your hands together (Fig. 14.14).
15. Hold and roll up the gown away from you (see Fig. 14.11). Keep it inside out.
16. Discard the gown.
17. Remove and discard the mask if worn.
18. Decontaminate your hands.

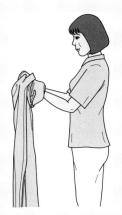

Fig. 14.14 The gown is turned inside out as it is removed.

Gowns must completely cover you from your neck to your knees. The long sleeves have tight cuffs. The gown opens at the back. It is tied at the neck and waist. The gown front and sleeves are considered to be *contaminated*.

Gowns are used once. A wet gown is contaminated. It is removed and a dry one put on. Disposable gowns are discarded after use.

✳ Masks and Respiratory Protection

You wear masks for these reasons:

- For protection from contact with infectious materials from the resident. Respiratory secretions and sprays of blood or body fluids are examples.
- To protect the person from infectious agents that you could possibly be carrying in your mouth or nose.

Masks are disposable. A wet or moist mask is contaminated. Breathing can cause masks to become wet or moist. Apply a new mask when contamination occurs.

A mask fits snugly over your nose and mouth. Practice hand hygiene before putting on a mask. When removing a mask, touch only the ties or the elastic bands. The front of the mask is contaminated.

There are several types of masks. Figure 14.15 compares a surgical mask and an N-95 mask. The National Institute for Occupational Safety and Health (NIOSH) tests and approves

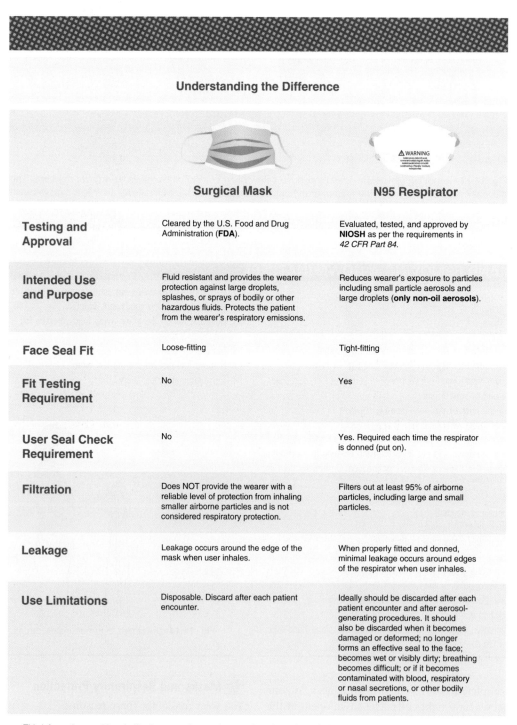

Understanding the Difference

	Surgical Mask	N95 Respirator
Testing and Approval	Cleared by the U.S. Food and Drug Administration (**FDA**).	Evaluated, tested, and approved by **NIOSH** as per the requirements in *42 CFR Part 84.*
Intended Use and Purpose	Fluid resistant and provides the wearer protection against large droplets, splashes, or sprays of bodily or other hazardous fluids. Protects the patient from the wearer's respiratory emissions.	Reduces wearer's exposure to particles including small particle aerosols and large droplets (**only non-oil aerosols**).
Face Seal Fit	Loose-fitting	Tight-fitting
Fit Testing Requirement	No	Yes
User Seal Check Requirement	No	Yes. Required each time the respirator is donned (put on).
Filtration	Does NOT provide the wearer with a reliable level of protection from inhaling smaller airborne particles and is not considered respiratory protection.	Filters out at least 95% of airborne particles, including large and small particles.
Leakage	Leakage occurs around the edge of the mask when user inhales.	When properly fitted and donned, minimal leakage occurs around edges of the respirator when user inhales.
Use Limitations	Disposable. Discard after each patient encounter.	Ideally should be discarded after each patient encounter and after aerosol-generating procedures. It should also be discarded when it becomes damaged or deformed; no longer forms an effective seal to the face; becomes wet or visibly dirty; breathing becomes difficult; or if it becomes contaminated with blood, respiratory or nasal secretions, or other bodily fluids from patients.

This information provides clarification regarding respirator and mask use in workplaces in which employees are exposed to respiratory hazards. It is not specific for the COVID-19 pandemic.

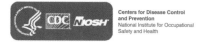

Centers for Disease Control and Prevention
National Institute for Occupational Safety and Health

Fig. 14.15 Surgical mask vs. N-95 mask. (From Understanding the Difference, Centers for Disease Control and Prevention, U.S. Department of Health and Human Services, National Institute for Occupational Safety and Health, https://www.cdc.gov/niosh/npptl/)

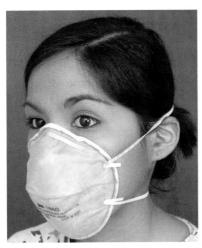

Fig. 14.16 Tuberculosis respirator.

N-95 masks. Tuberculosis respirators (Fig. 14.16) are worn when caring for persons with TB (Chapter 36). Follow the policy of your center. If you have questions about which type of mask should be worn, ask the nurse.

Goggles and Face Shields

Goggles and face shields protect your eyes, mouth, and nose from splashing or spraying of blood, body fluids, secretions, and excretions. Splashes and sprays can occur when giving care, cleaning items, or disposing of fluids. Figure 14.17 shows a face shield and an N-95 mask worn by the nursing assistant. A face shield could also be attached to a mask (Fig 14.18).

The front of goggles or a face shield is contaminated. The ties, earpieces, or headband used to secure the device are considered "clean." Use them to remove the device after hand hygiene. They are safe to touch with bare hands.

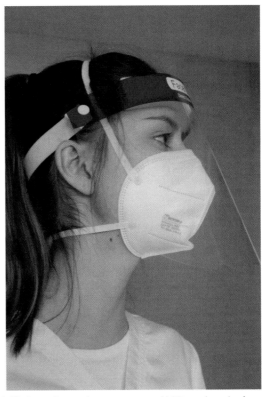

Fig. 14.17 A nursing assistant wears an N-95 mask and a face shield.

Discard disposable goggles or face shields after use. Reusable eyewear is cleaned before reuse. It is washed with soap and water. Then a disinfectant is used.

See *Promoting Safety and Comfort: Goggles and Face Shields.*

PROMOTING SAFETY AND COMFORT

Goggles and Face Shields
Safety
Eyeglasses and contact lenses do not provide eye protection. If you wear eyeglasses, use a face shield that fits over your glasses with minimal gaps.

Goggles do not provide splash or spray protection to other parts of your face.

DONNING AND REMOVING A MASK

Procedure
1. Practice hand hygiene.
2. Put on a gown if required.
3. Pick up a mask by its upper ties. Do not touch the part that will cover your face.
4. Place the mask over your nose and mouth (see Fig. 14.18A).
5. Place the upper strings above your ears. Tie them at the back in the middle of your head (see Fig. 14.18B).
6. Tie the lower strings at the back of your neck (see Fig. 14.18C). The lower part of the mask is under your chin.
   (Some types of masks have elastic that slips over the ears instead of ties. Secure these over both ears. Others may have elastic bands that slip over the head.)
7. Pinch the metal band around your nose. The top of the mask must be snug over your nose. If you wear eyeglasses, the mask must be snug under the bottom of the eyeglasses.
8. Make sure the mask is snug over your face and under your chin.
9. Put on goggles or a face shield if needed and if not part of the mask.
10. Put on gloves.
11. Provide care. Avoid coughing, sneezing, and unnecessary talking.
12. Change the mask if it becomes wet or contaminated.
13. Remove the mask (see Fig. 14.11B):
    a. Remove the gloves.
    b. Remove the goggles or face shield and gown if worn.
    c. Untie the lower strings of the mask.
    d. Untie the top strings.
    e. Hold the top strings or elastic straps. Remove the mask.
14. Discard the mask.
15. Decontaminate your hands.

✦ **DONNING AND REMOVING A MASK—cont'd**

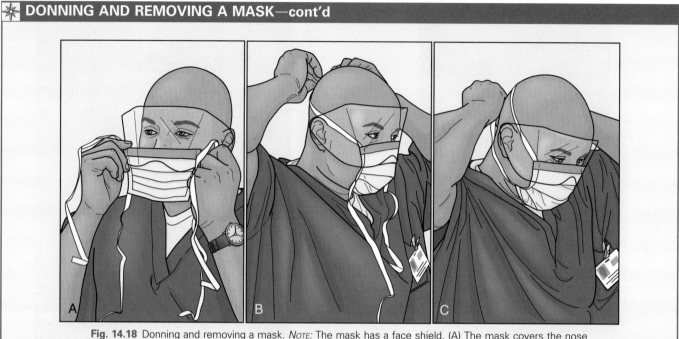

Fig. 14.18 Donning and removing a mask. *Note:* The mask has a face shield. (A) The mask covers the nose and mouth. (B) Upper strings are tied at the back of the head. (C) Lower strings are tied at the back of the neck.

Bagging Items

Contaminated items are bagged to remove them from the person's room. Leakproof plastic bags are used. They have the *BIOHAZARD* symbol (Fig. 14.19). Biohazardous waste are items contaminated with blood, body fluids, secretions, or excretions. (*Bio* means "life"; *hazardous* means "dangerous or harmful.")

Bag and transport linens following center policy. Laundry bags with contaminated linen need a *BIOHAZARD* symbol. Meltaway bags are common. They dissolve in hot water. Once soiled linen is bagged, no one needs to handle it. Do not overfill the bag. Tie the bag securely, then place it in a laundry hamper lined with a biohazard plastic bag.

Trash is placed in a container labeled with the *BIOHAZARD* symbol. Follow center policy for bagging and transporting trash, equipment, and supplies.

Usually one bag is needed. Double-bagging involves two bags. Double-bagging is not needed unless the outside of the bag is wet, soiled, or may be contaminated. Two staff members are needed.

- One is inside the room.
- The other is at the doorway outside the room.
- The person in the room places contaminated items in a bag, then the bag is sealed.
- The person outside the room holds open another bag. This bag is *clean*. A wide cuff is made on the clean bag to protect the hands from contamination (Fig. 14.20).
- The contaminated bag is placed into the clean bag at the doorway.

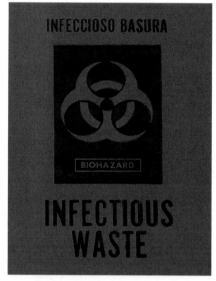

Fig. 14.19 *BIOHAZARD* symbol.

Collecting Specimens

Blood, body fluids, secretions, and excretions often require laboratory testing (Chapter 29). Specimens are transported to the laboratory in biohazard specimen bags. To collect a specimen:

- Label the specimen container and biohazard specimen bag. Apply warning labels according to center policy.
- Don PPE as required. Gloves are worn.
- Put the specimen container and lid in the person's bathroom on a paper towel.

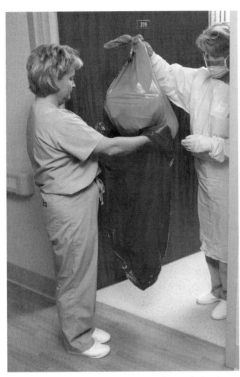

Fig. 14.20 Double bagging. One nursing assistant is in the room by the doorway. The other is outside the doorway. The *dirty* bag is placed inside the *clean* bag.

- Collect the specimen. Do not contaminate the outside of the container. Also avoid contamination when transferring the specimen from the collecting vessel to the specimen container.
- Put the lid on securely.
- Remove the PPE. Decontaminate your hands.
- Use a paper towel to pick up and take the container outside the room.
- Put the container in the biohazard bag.
- Discard the paper towels.
- Follow center policy for storing the specimen.
- Decontaminate your hands.

Transporting Persons

Persons on Transmission-Based Precautions usually do not leave their rooms. Sometimes they go to other areas for treatments or tests.

Transporting procedures vary among centers. Some require transport by bed. This prevents contaminating wheelchairs and stretchers. Others use wheelchairs and stretchers.

A safe transport means that other persons are protected from the infection. Follow center procedures and these guidelines:

- Have the person wear a clean gown or pajamas and an isolation gown.
- Have the person wear a mask as required by the Transmission-Based Precautions used.
- Cover any draining wounds.
- Give the person tissues and a leakproof bag. Used tissues are placed in the bag.

- Wear PPE as required.
- Place an extra layer of sheets and absorbent pads on the stretcher or wheelchair. This protects against draining body fluids.
- Do not let anyone else on the elevator. This reduces exposure to infection.
- Alert staff in the receiving area about the Transmission-Based Precautions. They wear gloves and PPE as needed.
- Disinfect the stretcher or wheelchair after use.

Meeting Basic Needs

The person has needs for love, belonging, and self-esteem. Often, these needs are unmet when Transmission-Based Precautions are used. Visitors and staff often avoid the person. They may need to put on gowns, masks, goggles or face shields, and gloves. These tasks take extra effort before entering the room. Some are not sure what they can touch. They may fear getting the disease.

The person may feel lonely, unwanted, and rejected. Self-esteem suffers. The person knows the disease can be spread to others. The person may feel dirty and undesirable. Without intending to, visitors and staff can make the person feel ashamed and guilty for having a contagious disease.

The nurse helps the person, visitors, and staff understand the need for Transmission-Based Precautions and how they affect the person. You can help meet the person's needs for love, belonging, and self-esteem. See *Promoting Safety and Comfort: Isolation Precautions* earlier in the chapter.

During periods of intense spread of infection, it may be necessary to restrict visitors. Some LTC facilities declare a state of "lockdown" to curb the spread of infection. This isolation is very hard on people. They miss their family and friends. It is difficult for many to understand why their loved ones are not allowed to visit. It is also difficult for the family and friends. Alternatives to in-person visits may help. These might include using electronic devices for virtual visits, phone calls, window visits. Outdoor visits may be another option if weather permits.

Persons with poor vision need to know who you are. Let them see your face before you put on a mask or goggles or a face shield. State your name and explain what you are going to do. Then put on PPE.

See *Focus on Communication: Meeting Basic Needs.*
See *Residents with Dementia: Meeting Basic Needs.*

📋 FOCUS ON COMMUNICATION

Meeting Basic Needs

Without intending to, people can make the person feel ashamed and guilty for having a contagious disease. Be careful what you say. For example, do not say:

- "What were you doing?"
- "How did you get that?"
- "I'm afraid to touch you."
- "Don't breathe on me."

Always treat the person with respect, kindness, and dignity.

RESIDENTS WITH DEMENTIA

Meeting Basic Needs

Persons with dementia do not understand the need for isolation precautions. Masks, gowns, goggles, and face shields may increase confusion and cause fear and agitation. These measures can help:

- Let the person see your face before putting on PPE if possible.
- Tell the person who you are and what you are going to do.
- Use a calm, soothing voice.
- Do not hurry the person.
- Use touch to reassure the person.
- Follow the care plan and the nurse's instructions for other measures to help the person.
- Report signs of increased confusion or behavior changes.

BLOODBORNE PATHOGEN STANDARD

The human immunodeficiency virus (HIV) and the hepatitis B virus (HBV) are major health concerns (Chapters 34 and 38). The health team is at risk for exposure to these viruses. The Bloodborne Pathogen Standard is intended to protect them from exposure. It is a regulation of the Occupational Safety and Health Administration (OSHA). Box 14.8 lists terms used in the standard.

HIV and HBV are found in the blood. They are bloodborne pathogens. They exit the body through blood. They are spread to others by blood. Other potentially infectious materials (OPIM) also spread the viruses (see Box 14.8).

Exposure Control Plan

The center must have an exposure control plan. It identifies staff at risk for exposure to blood or OPIM. All caregivers and the laundry, central supply, and housekeeping staffs are at risk. The plan includes actions to take for an exposure incident.

Staff at risk receive free training. Training occurs upon employment and then yearly. Training is also required for new or changed tasks involving exposure to bloodborne pathogens. Training must include:

- An explanation of the standard and where to get a copy.
- The causes, signs, and symptoms of bloodborne diseases.
- How bloodborne pathogens are spread.
- An explanation of the exposure control plan and where to get a copy.
- How to know which tasks might cause exposure.
- The use and limits of safe work practices, engineering controls, and PPE.
- Information about hepatitis B vaccination.

BOX 14.8   Bloodborne Pathogen Standard Terms

blood Human blood, human blood components, and products made from human blood

bloodborne pathogens Pathogens present in human blood and that can cause disease in humans; they include but are not limited to the hepatitis B virus (HBV) and human immunodeficiency virus (HIV)

contaminated The presence or reasonably anticipated presence of blood or other potentially infectious materials on an item or surface

contaminated laundry Laundry soiled with blood or other potentially infectious materials or that may contain sharps

contaminated sharps Any contaminated object that can penetrate the skin (e.g., needles, scalpels, broken glass, broken capillary tubes, exposed ends of dental wires)

decontamination The use of physical or chemical means to remove, inactivate, or destroy bloodborne pathogens on a surface or item to the point where infectious particles can no longer be transmitted and the surface or item is safe for handling, use, or disposal

engineering controls Controls that isolate or remove the bloodborne pathogen hazard from the workplace (sharps disposal containers, self-sheathing needles)

exposure incident Eye, mouth, other mucous membrane, nonintact skin, or parenteral contact with blood or other potentially infectious materials that results from an employee's duties

hand washing facilities The adequate supply of running water, soap, single-use towels, or hot-air drying machines

HBV hepatitis B virus

HIV human immunodeficiency virus

occupational exposure Reasonably anticipated skin, eye, mucous membrane, or parenteral contact with blood or other potentially infectious materials that may result from an employee's duties

other potentially infectious materials (OPIM):

- Human body fluids—semen, vaginal secretions, cerebrospinal fluid, synovial fluid, pleural fluid, pericardial fluid, peritoneal fluid, amniotic fluid, saliva in dental procedures, any bodily fluid that is visibly contaminated with blood,

and all body fluids when it is difficult or impossible to differentiate between them

- Any tissue or organ (other than intact skin) from a human (living or dead)
- HIV-containing cell or tissue cultures, organ cultures, and HIV- or HBV-containing culture medium or other solutions; blood, organs, or other tissues from experimental animals infected with HIV or HBV

parenteral Piercing mucous membranes or the skin barrier through needlesticks, human bites, cuts, abrasions, and so on

personal protective equipment (PPE) The clothing or equipment worn by an employee for protection against a hazard

regulated waste:

- Liquid or semiliquid blood or OPIM
- Contaminated items that would release blood or OPIM in a liquid or semiliquid state if compressed
- Items caked with dried blood or OPIM that can release these materials during handling
- Contaminated sharps
- Pathologic and microbiologic wastes containing blood or OPIM

source individual Any person (living or dead) whose blood or OPIM may be a source of occupational exposure to employees; examples include but are not limited to:

- Hospital and clinic patients
- Clients in agencies for the developmentally disabled
- Trauma victims
- Clients of drug and alcohol treatment agencies
- Hospice and nursing center residents
- Human remains
- Persons who donate or sell blood or blood components

sterilize The use of a physical or chemical procedure to destroy all microbes, including spores

work practice controls Controls that reduce the likelihood of exposure by changing the way the task is performed

- Who to contact and what to do in an emergency.
- Information on reporting an exposure incident, postexposure evaluation, and follow-up.
- Information on warning labels and color coding.

Preventive Measures

Preventive measures reduce the risk of exposure. Such measures follow.

Hepatitis B Vaccination

Hepatitis B is a liver disease. It is caused by the hepatitis B virus (HBV). HBV is spread by blood and sexual contact.

The hepatitis B vaccine produces immunity against hepatitis B. Immunity means that a person has protection against a certain disease and therefore will not get the disease.

A vaccination involves giving a vaccine to produce immunity against an infectious disease. A vaccine is a preparation containing dead or weakened microbes. The hepatitis B vaccination involves three injections (shots). The second injection is given 1 month after the first. The third injection is given 6 months after the second one. The vaccination can be given before or after exposure to HBV.

You can receive the hepatitis B vaccination within 10 working days of being hired. The center pays for it. You can refuse the vaccination. If so, you must sign a statement refusing the vaccine. You can have the vaccination at a later date.

Engineering and Work Practice Controls

Engineering controls reduce employee exposure in the workplace. Special containers for contaminated sharps (needles, broken glass) and specimens remove and isolate the hazard from staff. Containers are puncture resistant, leakproof, and color coded in red. They have the *BIOHAZARD* symbol.

Work practice controls also reduce exposure risks. All tasks involving blood or OPIM are done in ways to limit splatters, splashes, and sprays. Producing droplets also is avoided. OSHA requires these work practice controls:

- Do not eat, drink, smoke, apply cosmetics or lip balm, or handle contact lenses in areas of occupational exposure.
- Do not store food or drinks where blood or OPIM are kept.
- Practice hand hygiene after removing gloves.
- Wash hands as soon as possible after skin contact with blood or OPIM.
- Never recap, bend, or remove needles by hand. When recapping, bending, or removing contaminated needles is required, use mechanical means (forceps) or a one-handed method.
- Never shear or break contaminated needles.
- Discard contaminated needles and sharp instruments (such as razors) in containers that are closable, puncture resistant, and leakproof (Fig. 14.21). Containers are color coded in red

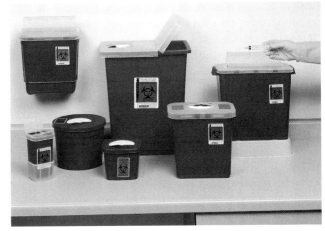

Fig. 14.21 Sharps containers. (Courtesy Lab Safety Supply, Janesville, WI.)

and have the *BIOHAZARD* symbol. Containers must be upright and not allowed to overfill.

Personal Protective Equipment

PPE includes gloves, goggles, face shields, masks, laboratory coats, gowns, shoe covers, and surgical caps. Blood or OPIM must not pass through them. They protect your clothes, undergarments, skin, eyes, mouth, and hair.

PPE is free to employees. Correct sizes are available. The center makes sure that PPE is cleaned, laundered, repaired, replaced, or discarded. OSHA requires these measures for the safe handling and use of PPE:

- Remove PPE before leaving the work area.
- Remove PPE when a garment becomes contaminated.
- Place used PPE in marked areas or containers when being stored, washed, decontaminated, or discarded.
- Wear gloves when you expect contact with blood or OPIM.
- Wear gloves when handling or touching contaminated items or surfaces.
- Replace worn, punctured, or contaminated gloves.
- Never wash or decontaminate disposable gloves for reuse.
- Discard utility gloves that show signs of cracking, peeling, tearing, or puncturing. Utility gloves are decontaminated for reuse if the process will not ruin them.

Equipment

Contaminated equipment is cleaned and decontaminated. Decontaminate work surfaces with a proper disinfectant:

- Upon completing tasks.
- At once when there is obvious contamination.
- After any spill of blood or OPIM.
- At the end of the work shift when surfaces became contaminated since the last cleaning.

Use a brush and dustpan or tongs to clean up broken glass. Never pick up broken glass with your hands, not even with gloves. Discard broken glass into a puncture-resistant container.

Waste

Special measures are used to discard regulated waste:

- Liquid or semiliquid blood or OPIM
- Items contaminated with blood or OPIM
- Items caked with blood or OPIM
- Contaminated sharps

Closable, puncture-resistant, and leakproof containers are used. Containers are color coded in red. They have the *BIOHAZARD* symbol.

Housekeeping

The center must be kept clean and sanitary. A cleaning schedule is required. It includes decontamination methods and the tasks and procedures to be done.

Laundry

OSHA requires these measures for contaminated laundry:

- Handle it as little as possible.
- Wear gloves or other needed PPE.
- Bag contaminated laundry where it is used.
- Mark laundry bags or containers with the *BIOHAZARD* symbol for laundry sent offsite.
- Place wet, contaminated laundry in leakproof containers before transport. The containers are color coded in red or have the *BIOHAZARD* symbol.

Exposure Incidents

An *exposure incident* is any eye, mouth, other mucous membrane, nonintact skin, or parenteral contact with blood or OPIM. *Parenteral* means piercing the mucous membranes or the skin barrier. Piercing occurs through needlesticks, human bites, cuts, and abrasions.

Report exposure incidents at once. Medical evaluation, follow-up, and required tests are free. Your blood is tested for HIV and HBV. If you refuse testing, the blood sample is kept for at least 90 days. Testing is done later if you change your mind.

Confidentiality is important. You are told of the evaluation results. You also are told of any medical conditions that may need treatment. You receive a written opinion of the medical evaluation within 15 days after its completion.

The *source individual* is the person whose blood or body fluids are the source of an exposure incident. This person's blood is tested for HIV or HBV. The center informs you of laws affecting the source's identity and test results.

SURGICAL ASEPSIS

Surgical asepsis (sterile technique) is the practice that keeps equipment and supplies free of all microbes. Recall that *sterile* means the absence of all microbes, including spores. Surgical asepsis is required any time the skin or sterile tissues are

entered. If a break occurs in sterile technique, microbes can enter the body. Infection is a risk.

Assisting with Sterile Procedures

You can assist nurses with sterile procedures. Some states let nursing assistants perform certain sterile procedures. A sterile dressing change is an example.

See *Delegation Guidelines: Assisting with Sterile Procedures.*

See *Promoting Safety and Comfort: Assisting with Sterile Procedures.*

DELEGATION GUIDELINES

Assisting with Sterile Procedures

A nurse may ask you to assist with a sterile procedure. If so, you need this information from the nurse:

- The name of the procedure and the reason for it
- What gloves to wear—sterile or nonsterile
- What you are expected to do
- When to report observations
- What you can and cannot touch
- What specific resident concerns to report at once

PROMOTING SAFETY AND COMFORT

Assisting with Sterile Procedures
Safety

Do not perform a sterile procedure unless:

- Your state allows you to perform the procedure.
- The procedure is in your job description.
- You received the necessary education and training.
- You review the procedure with the nurse.
- A nurse is available for questions and guidance.

Principles of Surgical Asepsis

All items in contact with the person are kept sterile. If an item is contaminated, infection is a risk. A sterile field is needed. A sterile field is a work area free of *all* pathogens and nonpathogens (including spores). Box 14.9 lists the principles and practices of surgical asepsis. Follow them to maintain a sterile field.

✳ Sterile Gloving

You might need sterile gloves when assisting with a sterile procedure. The sterile field is set up first. Then sterile gloves are put on. After sterile gloves are on, you can handle sterile items within the sterile field. Do not touch anything outside the sterile field.

BOX 14.9   Principles and Practices for Surgical Asepsis

- A sterile item can touch only another sterile item:
  - If a sterile item touches a clean item, the sterile item is contaminated.
  - If a clean item touches a sterile item, the sterile item is contaminated.
  - A sterile package that is open, torn, punctured, wet, or moist is contaminated.
  - A sterile package is contaminated when the expiration date has passed.
  - Place only sterile items on a sterile field.
  - Use sterile gloves or sterile forceps to handle other sterile items (Fig. 14.22).
  - Consider any item as contaminated if unsure of its sterility.
  - Do not use contaminated items. They are discarded or resterilized.
- A sterile field or sterile items are always kept within your vision and above your waist:
  - If you cannot see an item, the item is contaminated.
  - If the item is below your waist, the item is contaminated.
  - Keep sterile-gloved hands above your waist and within your sight.
  - Do not leave a sterile field unattended.
  - Do not turn your back on a sterile field.
- Airborne microbes can contaminate sterile items or a sterile field:
  - Prevent drafts. Close the door and avoid extra movements. Ask other staff in the room to avoid extra movements.
  - Avoid coughing, sneezing, talking, or laughing over a sterile field. Turn your head away from the sterile field if you must talk.
  - Wear a mask if you need to talk during the procedure.
- Do not perform or assist with sterile procedures if you have a respiratory infection.
- Do not reach over a sterile field.
- Fluid flows downward, in the direction of gravity:
  - Hold wet items down (see Fig. 14.22). If held up, fluid flows down into a contaminated area. The contaminated fluid flows back into the sterile field when the item is held down.
- The sterile field is kept dry, unless the area below it is sterile:
  - The sterile field is contaminated if it gets wet and the area below it is not sterile.
  - Avoid spilling and splashing when pouring sterile fluids into sterile containers.
- The edges of a sterile field are contaminated:
  - A 1-inch (2.5-cm) margin around the sterile field is considered contaminated (Fig. 14.23).
  - Place all sterile items inside the 1-inch (2.5-cm) margin of the sterile field.
  - Items outside the 1-inch (2.5-cm) margin are contaminated.
- Honesty is essential to sterile technique:
  - You know when you contaminate an item or sterile field. Be honest with yourself even if other staff members are not present.
  - Remove the contaminated item and correct the matter. If necessary, start over with sterile supplies.
  - Report the contamination to the nurse.

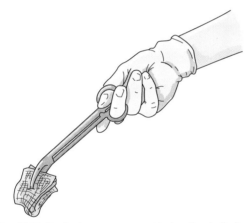

Fig. 14.22 Sterile forceps are used to handle sterile items.

Fig. 14.23 A 1-inch (2.5-cm) margin around the sterile field is considered contaminated. The shading and slash marks show that the 1-inch margin is contaminated.

✳ STERILE GLOVING

Procedure

1. Follow *Delegation Guidelines: Assisting with Sterile Procedures* (p. ··). See *Promoting Safety and Comfort*:
   a. *Assisting with Sterile Procedures* (p. ··)
   b. *Sterile Gloving*
2. Practice hand hygiene.
3. Inspect the package of sterile gloves for sterility:
   a. Check the expiration date.
   b. See if the package is dry.
   c. Check for tears, holes, punctures, and watermarks.
4. Arrange a work surface:
   a. Make sure you have enough room.
   b. Arrange the work surface at waist level and within your vision.
   c. Clean and dry the work surface.
   d. Do not reach over or turn your back on the work surface.
5. Open the package. Grasp the flaps. Gently peel them back.
6. Remove the inner package. Place it on your work surface.
7. Read the manufacturer instructions on the inner package. It may be labeled with *left*, *right*, *up*, and *down*.

✳ STERILE GLOVING—cont'd

8. Arrange the inner package for left, right, up, and down. The left glove is on your left. The right glove is on your right. The cuffs are near you with the fingers pointing away from you.

9. Grasp the folded edges of the inner package. Use the thumb and index finger of each hand.

10. Fold back the inner package to expose the gloves (Fig. 14.24A). Do not touch or otherwise contaminate the inside of the package or the gloves. The inside of the inner package is a sterile field.

11. Note that each glove has a cuff about 2 to 3 inches wide. The cuffs and insides of the gloves are *not considered sterile.*

12. Put on the right glove if you are right handed. Put on the left glove if you are left handed.
   a. Pick up the glove with your other hand. Use your thumb and index and middle fingers (see Fig. 14.24B).
   b. Touch only the cuff and inside of the glove.
   c. Turn the hand to be gloved palm side up.
   d. Lift the cuff up. Slide your fingers and hand into the glove (see Fig. 14.24C).

   e. Pull the glove up over your hand. If some fingers get stuck, leave them that way until the other glove is on. *Do not use your ungloved hand to straighten the glove. Do not let the outside of the glove touch any non-sterile surface.*
   f. Leave the cuff turned down.

13. Put on the other glove. Use your gloved hand.
   a. Reach under the cuff of the second glove. Use the four fingers of your gloved hand (see Fig. 14.24D). Keep your gloved thumb close to your gloved palm.
   b. Pull on the second glove (see Fig. 14.24E). Your gloved hand cannot touch the cuff or any surface. Hold the thumb of your first gloved hand away from the gloved palm.

14. Adjust each glove with the other hand. The gloves should be smooth and comfortable (see Fig. 14.24F).

15. Slide your fingers under the cuffs to pull them up (see Fig. 14.24G).

16. Touch only sterile items.

17. Remove the gloves (see Fig. 14.13).

18. Decontaminate your hands.

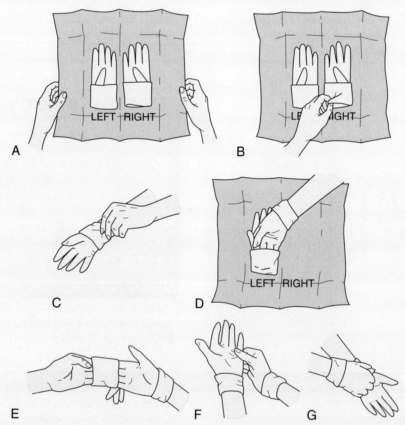

Fig. 14.24 Sterile gloving. (A) Open the inner wrapper to expose the gloves. (B) Pick up the glove at the cuff with your thumb and index and middle fingers. (C) Slide your fingers and hand into the glove. (D) Reach under the cuff of the other glove with your fingers. (E) Pull on the second glove. (F) Adjust each glove for comfort. (G) Slide your fingers under the cuffs to pull them up.

Sterile gloves are disposable. They come in many sizes so they fit snugly. The insides are powdered for ease in donning the gloves. The right and left gloves are marked on the package.

See *Promoting Safety and Comfort: Sterile Gloving.*

PROMOTING SAFETY AND COMFORT

Sterile Gloving

Safety

Always keep sterile gloved hands above your waist and within your vision. Touch only items within the sterile field. If you contaminate the gloves, remove them. Tell the nurse what happened. Decontaminate your hands and put on a new pair. Replace gloves that are torn, cut, or punctured.

Comfort

If you or the nurse contaminates your gloves, they must be removed. This means leaving the bedside to get another pair. Care is delayed. The person's comfort is affected if the care is painful or involves an uncomfortable position. When collecting supplies, get an extra pair of gloves. The gloves are in the room if the first pair is contaminated. Care can continue with little delay.

QUALITY OF LIFE

The health team must prevent the spread of microbes and infection. You must be very careful about your work. Staff and residents assume that you will practice medical asepsis. They also assume that you will follow Standard Precautions and Transmission-Based Precautions.

Even one careless act can spread microbes. It affects the person's safety. The reverse is also true. You can catch the person's infection. Practicing hand hygiene before and after resident contact greatly reduces the spread of microbes.

TIME TO REFLECT

Mrs. Newton has diabetes and is unable to reposition herself. You go to her room to turn her onto her side. As you are rolling her over, a sharp object pierces your index finger. You look down to see an insulin syringe resting on the sheets. (The nurse carelessly left the syringe in the bed instead of putting it in a sharps container.) What should you do first? What steps will need to be taken next? Are you required to report this incident? How could this have been prevented?

REVIEW QUESTIONS

Circle the BEST answer.

1. Most pathogens need the following to grow *except*
   a. Water
   b. Light
   c. Oxygen
   d. Nourishment

2. Signs and symptoms of infection include the following *except*
   a. Fever, nausea, vomiting, rash, and/or sores
   b. Pain or tenderness, redness, and/or swelling
   c. Fatigue, loss of appetite, and/or a discharge
   d. A wound and/or bleeding

3. Which is *not* a portal of exit?
   a. Respiratory tract
   b. Blood
   c. Reproductive system
   d. Intact skin

4. Which does *not* prevent health care-associated infections?
   a. Hand hygiene before and after giving care
   b. Sterilizing all care items
   c. Surgical asepsis
   d. Standard Precautions

5. Your hands are soiled with blood. What should you do?
   a. Wash your hands with soap and water
   b. Decontaminate your hands
   c. Rinse your hands
   d. Use hand sanitizer

6. During care, you move from a contaminated body site to a clean body site. Your hands are not visibly soiled. What should you do?
   a. Wash your hands
   b. Decontaminate your hands
   c. Rinse your hands
   d. Put on sterile gloves

7. You are going to decontaminate your hands with an alcohol-based hand rub. Which action is *not* correct?
   a. Wash your hands before applying the hand rub
   b. Rub your hands together
   c. Cover all surfaces of your hands and fingers
   d. Rub your hands together until they are dry

8. When cleaning equipment, do the following *except*
   a. Rinse the item in cold water before cleaning
   b. Wash the item with soap and hot water
   c. Use a brush if necessary
   d. Work from dirty to clean areas

9. Isolation precautions
   a. Prevent infection
   b. Destroy pathogens
   c. Keep pathogens within a certain area
   d. Destroy all microbes

10. Standard Precautions
    a. Are used for all persons
    b. Prevent the spread of pathogens through the air
    c. Require gowns, masks, gloves, and goggles
    d. Require a doctor's order

11. You wear utility gloves for contact with
    a. Blood
    b. Body fluids
    c. Secretions and excretions
    d. Cleaning solutions

12. A mask
    a. Can be reused
    b. Is clean on the inside
    c. Is contaminated when moist
    d. Should fit loosely for breathing

13. These statements are about PPE. Which is *false?*
    a. Wash disposable gloves for reuse
    b. Remove PPE before leaving the work area
    c. Discard cracked or torn utility gloves
    d. Wear gloves when touching contaminated items or surfaces
14. Contaminated surfaces are cleaned at the following times *except*
    a. After completing a task
    b. When there is obvious contamination
    c. After blood is spilled
    d. After removing gloves
15. Goggles or a face shield is worn
    a. When using Standard Precautions
    b. When splashing body fluids is likely
    c. If you have an eye infection
    d. When assisting with sterile procedures
16. According to the Bloodborne Pathogen Standard, you should *not*
    a. Wear gloves
    b. Discard sharp items into a biohazard container
    c. Store food and blood in different places
    d. Eat and drink in care settings

17. You were exposed to a bloodborne pathogen. Which is *true?*
    a. You do not have to report the exposure
    b. You pay for required tests
    c. You can refuse HIV and HBV testing
    d. The source individual can refuse testing
18. These statements are about surgical asepsis. Which is *false?*
    a. A sterile item can touch only another sterile item
    b. Wet items are held up
    c. If you cannot see an item, it is considered contaminated
    d. Sterile items are kept above your waist
19. You have on sterile gloves. You can touch
    a. Anything on the sterile field
    b. Anything on your work surface
    c. Anything below your waist
    d. Any part of your uniform
20. Which of the following does *not* require wearing gloves?
    a. Assisting with perineal care
    b. Changing a brief
    c. Giving a back massage
    d. Helping a person who has a nosebleed

See Appendix A for answers to these questions.

15

Body Mechanics and Safe Resident Handling, Positioning, and Transfers

OBJECTIVES

- Define the key terms and key abbreviations listed in this chapter.
- Explain the purpose and rules of body mechanics.
- Explain how ergonomics can prevent work-related injuries.
- Identify the causes, signs, and symptoms of back injuries.
- Position persons in the basic bed positions and in a chair.
- Identify comfort and safety measures for handling, moving, and transferring the person.

- Explain how to prevent work-related injuries when handling, moving, and transferring persons.
- Describe four levels of dependence.
- Identify the information needed from the nurse and care plan before handling, moving, and transferring persons.
- Perform the procedures described in this chapter.
- Explain how to promote quality of life.

KEY TERMS

base of support The area on which an object rests

body alignment The way the head, trunk, arms, and legs are aligned with one another; posture

body mechanics Using the body in an efficient and careful way

dorsal recumbent position See "supine position"

ergonomics The science of designing a job to fit the worker

Fowler position A semi-sitting position; the head of the bed is raised between 45 and 60 degrees

friction The rubbing of one surface against another

lateral position The person lies on one side or the other; side-lying position

left semiprone position A lateral position in which the upper leg (right leg) is sharply flexed so it is not on the lower leg

(left leg) and the lower arm (left arm) is behind the person. Used for rectal procedures.

logrolling Turning the person as a unit, in alignment, with one motion

posture See "body alignment"

prone position Lying on the abdomen with the head turned to one side

shearing When skin sticks to a surface while muscles slide in the direction the body is moving

side-lying position See "lateral position"

supine position The back-lying position; dorsal recumbent position

transfer Moving the person from one place to another

KEY ABBREVIATIONS

ID Identification
MSD Musculoskeletal disorder

OSHA Occupational Safety and Health Administration

Body mechanics means using the body in an efficient and careful way. It involves good posture, balance, and using your strongest and largest muscles for work. Fatigue, muscle strain, and injury can result from the improper use and positioning of the body during activity or rest. Focus on the person's and your own body mechanics. Good body mechanics reduce the risk of injury.

PRINCIPLES OF BODY MECHANICS

Body alignment (posture) is the way the head, trunk, arms, and legs are aligned with one another. Good alignment lets the body move and function with strength and efficiency. Standing, sitting, and lying down require good alignment.

Base of support is the area on which an object rests. A good base of support is needed for balance (Fig. 15.1). When standing, your feet are your base of support. Stand with your feet apart for a wider base of support and more balance.

Your strongest and largest muscles are in the shoulders, upper arms, hips, and thighs. Use these muscles to handle and move persons and heavy objects. Otherwise, you place strain and exertion on smaller and weaker muscles. This causes fatigue and injury. *Back injuries are a major risk.* For good body mechanics:

- Bend your knees and squat to lift a heavy object (Fig. 15.2). Do not bend from your waist. Bending from the waist places strain on small back muscles.

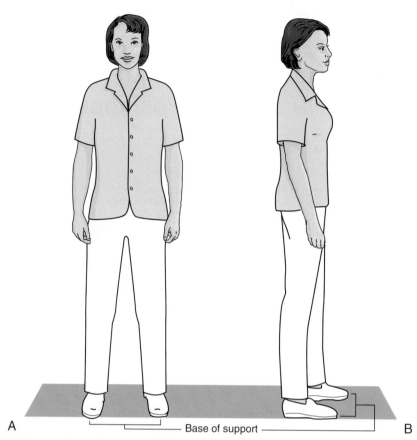

Fig. 15.1 (A) Anterior (front) view of an adult in good body alignment. The feet are apart for a wide base of support. (B) Lateral (side) view of an adult with good posture and alignment.

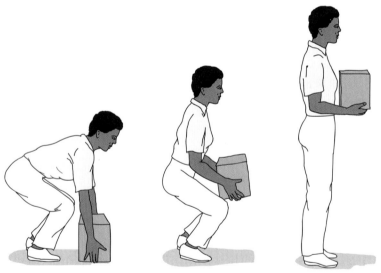

Fig. 15.2 Picking up a box using good body mechanics.

- Hold items close to your body and base of support (see Fig. 15.2). This involves upper arm and shoulder muscles. Holding objects away from your body places strain on small muscles in your lower arms.

All activities require good body mechanics. You must safely and efficiently handle and move persons and heavy objects. Follow the rules in Box 15.1.

ERGONOMICS

Ergonomics is the science of designing a job to fit the worker. (*Ergo-* means "work"; *-nomos* means "law.") It involves changing the task, workstation, equipment, and tools to help reduce stress on the worker's body. The goal is to eliminate a serious and disabling work-related

BOX 15.1 Rules for Body Mechanics

- Keep your body in good alignment with a wide base of support.
- Use an upright working posture. Bend your legs. Do not bend your back.
- Use the stronger and larger muscles in your shoulders, upper arms, thighs, and hips.
- Keep objects close to your body when you lift, move, or carry them (see Fig. 15.2).
- Avoid unnecessary bending and reaching. Raise the bed so it is close to your waist. Adjust the overbed table so it is at your waist level.
- Face your work area. This prevents unnecessary twisting.
- Push, slide, or pull heavy objects when you can rather than lifting them. Pushing is easier than pulling.
- Widen your base of support when pushing or pulling. Move your front leg forward when pushing. Move your rear leg back when pulling (Fig. 15.3).
- Use both hands and arms to lift, move, or carry objects.
- Turn your whole body when changing the direction of your movement. Move and turn your feet in the direction of the turn instead of twisting your body.
- Work with smooth and even movements. Avoid sudden or jerky motions.
- Do not lean over a person to give care.
- Get help from a coworker to move heavy objects. Do not lift or move them by yourself.
- Bend your hips and knees to lift heavy objects from the floor (see Fig. 15.2). Straighten your back as the object reaches thigh level. Your leg and thigh muscles work to raise the item off the floor and to waist level.
- Do not lift objects higher than chest level. Do not lift above your shoulders. Use a step stool or ladder to reach an object higher than chest level.

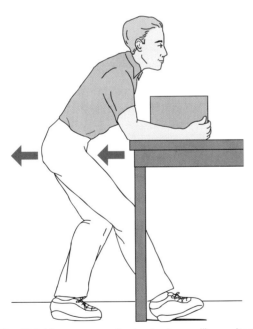

Fig. 15.3 Move your rear leg back when pulling an item.

musculoskeletal disorder (MSD). MSDs are caused or made worse by the work setting.

Work-Related MSDs

MSDs are injuries and disorders of the muscles, tendons, ligaments, joints, and cartilage. They also can involve the nervous system. The arms and back are often affected. So are the hands, fingers, neck, wrists, legs, and shoulders. MSDs are painful and disabling. They can develop slowly over weeks, months, and years. Or they can occur from one event. Pain, numbness, tingling, stiff joints, difficulty moving, and muscle loss can occur. Sometimes there is paralysis.

MSDs are workplace health hazards. Early signs and symptoms include pain, limited joint movement, or soft tissue swelling. Time off work is often needed. According to the U.S. Department of Labor, nursing assistants are at great risk for MSDs.

Always report a work-related injury as soon as possible. Early attention can help prevent the problem from becoming worse. Also, injuries are often less serious and less costly to treat if they receive early attention. In later stages, the problem can become more serious and harder and more costly to treat.

The following nursing tasks are known to be high risk for MSDs:
- Transfers—to and from beds, chairs, wheelchairs, Geri-chairs, toilets, stretchers, and bathtubs
- Trying to stop a person from falling
- Picking up a person from the floor to the bed
- Lifting alone
- Lifting persons who are confused or uncooperative
- Lifting persons who cannot support their own weight
- Lifting heavy persons
- Weighing a person
- Moving a person up in bed
- Repositioning a person in a bed or in a chair
- Changing an incontinence product
- Making beds
- Dressing and undressing a person
- Feeding a person in bed
- Giving a bed bath
- Applying antiembolism stockings

The Occupational Safety and Health Administration (OSHA) has identified risk factors for MSDs in nursing team members. The risk of an MSD increases if risk factors are combined. For example, a task involves both force and repeating actions.
- *Force*—the amount of physical effort needed to perform a task. Lifting or transferring heavy residents, preventing falls, and unexpected or sudden motions are examples.
- *Repeating action*—performing the same motion or series of motions continually or frequently. Repositioning residents and transfers to and from beds, chairs, and commodes without adequate rest breaks are examples. So is frequently cranking manual beds.
- *Awkward postures*—assuming positions that place stress on the body. Examples include reaching above shoulder height, kneeling, squatting, leaning over a bed, bending, or twisting the torso while lifting.
- *Heavy lifting*—manually lifting residents who cannot move themselves.

OSHA requires a safe work setting. The setting must be free of hazards that cause or are likely to cause death or serious physical harm to employees. The employer must make reasonable attempts to prevent or reduce the hazard. OSHA inspection teams enforce this law.

Back Injuries

Back injuries are major threats. Back injuries can occur from repeated activities or from one event. Signs and symptoms include:

- Pain when trying to assume a normal posture.
- Decreased mobility.
- Pain when standing or rising from a seated position.
- These and other factors can lead to back disorders:
- Reaching while lifting
- Poor posture when sitting or standing
- Staying in one position too long
- Poor body mechanics when lifting, pushing, pulling, or carrying objects
- Poor physical condition—not having the strength or endurance to perform tasks without strain
- Repeated lifting of awkward items, equipment, or persons
- Shifting weight when a person loses balance or strength while moving
- Twisting while lifting
- Bending while lifting
- Maintaining a bent posture such as leaning over a bed
- Reaching over raised bed rails
- Working in a confined, crowded, or cluttered area (rooms, bathrooms, hallways)
- Fatigue
- Poor footing such as on slippery floors
- Lifting with forceful movement

Follow the rules in Box 15.1. They help prevent back injuries. Also, be extra careful when performing tasks associated with back injuries.

See *Promoting Safety and Comfort: Back Injuries.*

👤 PROMOTING SAFETY AND COMFORT

Back Injuries

Safety

According to OSHA, these activities are associated with back injuries in nursing centers:

- Moving a person who totally depends on others for care
- Moving a person who is combative
- Transferring a person who is on the floor to the bed or a chair
- Repositioning a person in bed or in a chair
- Transferring a person from bed to chair or from chair to bed
- Transferring a person from one chair to another (includes transfers to and from the wheelchair and toilet)
- Bending to bathe, dress, or feed a person
- Bending to make a bed or change linens
- Weighing a person
- Changing an incontinence product
- Trying to stop a person from falling

Use good body mechanics to protect yourself from injury. Do not work alone. Avoid lifting when possible.

POSITIONING THE PERSON

The person must be properly positioned at all times. Regular position changes and good alignment promote comfort and well-being. Breathing is easier. Circulation is promoted. Pressure ulcers and contractures are prevented.

You move and turn when in bed or in a chair for your comfort. Many residents do too. Some need reminding to adjust their positions. Others need help. Still others depend entirely on the nursing team for position changes.

Whether in bed or chair, the person is repositioned at least every 2 hours. Some people are repositioned more often. You must follow the nurse's instructions and the care plan. To safely position a person:

- Use good body mechanics.
- Ask a coworker to help you if needed.
- Explain the procedure to the person.
- Be gentle when moving the person.
- Provide for privacy.
- Use pillows as directed by the nurse for support and alignment.
- Provide for comfort after positioning. (See the inside of the front cover.)
- Place the call light within reach after positioning.
- Complete a safety check before leaving the room. (See the inside of the front cover.)

See *Focus on Communication: Positioning the Person.*
See *Delegation Guidelines: Positioning the Person.*
See *Promoting Safety and Comfort: Positioning the Person.*

📋 FOCUS ON COMMUNICATION

Positioning the Person

Moving is painful for many persons. Some older persons have painful joints. Most persons have pain after surgery or an injury. Make sure that you do not cause pain when positioning the person. Tell the person what you are going to do before and during the procedure. Move the person slowly and gently. Give the person time to tell you if a movement is painful. Make sure the person is comfortable. You can say:

- "Am I hurting you?"
- "Please tell me if I'm moving you too fast."
- "Please tell me if you feel pain or discomfort."
- "Do you need a pillow adjusted?"
- "Are you comfortable?"
- "How can I help make you more comfortable?"

📄 DELEGATION GUIDELINES

Positioning the Person

You are often delegated tasks that involve positioning and repositioning. You need this information from the nurse and the care plan:

- Position or positioning limits ordered by the doctor
- How often to turn and reposition the person
- How many staff members need to help you
- What assist devices to use
- What skin care measures to perform (Chapter 18)

- What range-of-motion exercises to perform (Chapter 24)
- Where to place pillows
- What positioning devices are needed and how to use them (Chapter 24)
- What observations to report and record
- When to report observations
- What specific resident concerns to report at once

Fowler Position

Fowler position is a semi-sitting position. The head of the bed is raised between 45 and 60 degrees (Fig. 15.4). The knees may be slightly elevated. For good alignment:

- The spine is straight.
- The head is supported with a small pillow.
- The arms are supported with pillows.

👤 PROMOTING SAFETY AND COMFORT

Positioning the Person

Safety

Pressure injuries (Chapter 32) are serious threats from lying or sitting too long in one place. Wet, soiled, and wrinkled linens are other causes. Whenever you reposition a person, make sure linens are clean, dry, and wrinkle free. Change or straighten linens as needed.

Contractures can develop from staying in one position too long (Chapter 24). A contracture is the lack of joint mobility caused by abnormal shortening of a muscle. Repositioning, exercise, and activity help prevent contractures.

Comfort

Pillows and positioning devices are used to position the person. They support body parts and keep the person in good alignment. This promotes comfort. Place pillows and positioning devices as directed by the nurse and the care plan.

Most older persons do not tolerate the prone position. They have limited range of motion in their necks. The left semiprone position usually is not comfortable for them. Check with the nurse before placing any older person in the prone or semiprone position.
- The upper leg (right leg) is supported with a pillow.
- A pillow is under the upper arm (right arm) and hand (right hand).

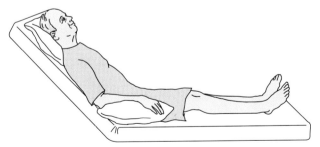

Fig. 15.4 Fowler position.

The nurse may ask you to place small pillows under the lower back, thighs, and ankles. Persons with heart and respiratory disorders usually breathe easier in Fowler position.

Supine Position

The supine position (dorsal recumbent position) is the back-lying position (Fig. 15.5). For good alignment:
- The bed is flat.
- The head and shoulders are supported on a pillow.
- Arms and hands are at the sides. You can support the arms with regular pillows. Or you can support the hands upon small pillows with the palms down.

The nurse may ask you to place a folded or rolled towel under the lower back and a small pillow under the thighs. A pillow under the lower legs lifts the heels off the bed. This prevents them from rubbing on the sheets.

Prone Position

A person in the prone position lies on the abdomen with the head turned to one side. For good alignment:
- The bed is flat.
- Small pillows are placed under the head, abdomen, and lower legs (Fig. 15.6).
- Arms are flexed at the elbows with the hands near the head.

You also can position a person with the feet hanging over the end of the mattress (Fig. 15.7). A pillow is not needed under the feet.

Lateral Position

A person in the lateral position (side-lying position) lies on one side or the other (Fig. 15.8). For good alignment:
- The bed is flat.
- A pillow is under the head and neck.
- The upper leg is in front of the lower leg. (The nurse may ask you to position the upper leg behind the lower leg, not on top of it.)
- The ankle, upper leg, and thigh are supported with pillows.
- A small pillow is positioned against the person's back. The person rolls back against the pillow so that the back is at a 45-degree angle with the mattress.
- A small pillow is under the upper hand and arm.

Left Semiprone Position

The left semiprone position is a left side-lying position. This position is often used for administering enemas and suppositories. It is also used for rectal exams and rectal temperatures. The upper leg (right leg) is sharply flexed so it is not on the lower leg (left leg). The lower arm (left arm) is behind the person (Fig. 15.9). For good alignment:
- The bed is flat.
- A pillow is under the person's head and shoulder.

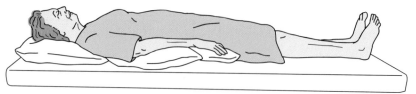

Fig. 15.5 Supine position.

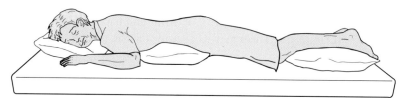

Fig. 15.6 Prone position.

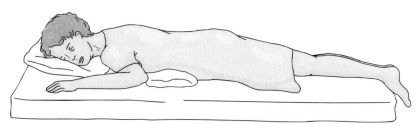

Fig. 15.7 Prone position with the feet hanging over the edge of the mattress.

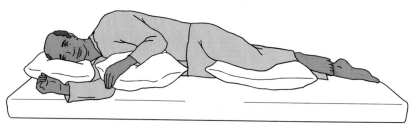

Fig. 15.8 Lateral position.

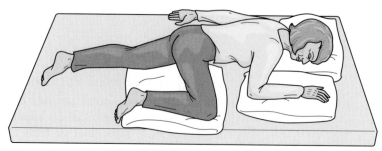

Fig. 15.9 Left semiprone position.

Chair Position

Persons who sit in chairs must hold their upper bodies and heads erect. If not, poor alignment results. For good alignment:

- The person's back and buttocks are against the back of the chair.
- Feet are flat on the floor or wheelchair footplates. Never leave feet unsupported.

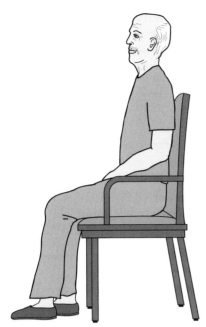

Fig. 15.10 The person is positioned in a chair. The person's feet are flat on the floor; the calves do not touch the chair. The back is straight and against the back of the chair.

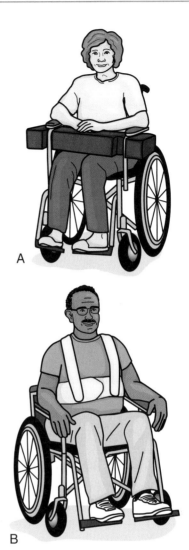

Fig. 15.11 Postural supports. (A) Pelvic holder. (B) Torso support.

- Backs of the knees and calves are slightly away from the edge of the seat (Fig. 15.10).

The nurse may ask you to put a small pillow between the person's lower back and the chair. This supports the lower back. *Remember, a pillow is not used behind the back if restraints are used* (Chapter 13).

Paralyzed arms are supported on pillows. Some persons have special positioners ordered. Ask the nurse about their proper use. Wrists are positioned at a slight upward angle.

Some people require postural supports if they cannot keep the upper body erect (Fig. 15.11A and B). Postural supports help keep them in good alignment. The health team selects the best product for the person's needs. The person's safety, dignity, and function are considered.

You will turn and reposition persons often. You move them in bed. You transfer them to and from beds, chairs, wheelchairs, stretchers, and toilets. To transfer a person means moving the person from one place to another. During these and other tasks, you must use your body correctly. This protects you and the person from injury.

See *Focus on Communication: Safe Resident Handling, Moving, and Transfers.*

See *Promoting Safety and Comfort: Safe Resident Handling, Moving, and Transfers.*

See *Teamwork and Time Management: Safe Resident Handling, Moving, and Transfers.*

📋 FOCUS ON COMMUNICATION

Safe Resident Handling, Moving, and Transfers

Handling, moving, and transfers can be very painful following an injury or surgery. Many older persons have painful joints. The fears of pain and falling are common. Always explain what you are going to do before starting the procedure. Then explain what you are doing step by step. This promotes comfort. When giving step-by-step directions:

- Speak slowly and clearly.
- Talk loudly enough for the person to hear you.
- Give directions calmly and kindly. Do not yell at or insult the person.
- Face the person and use eye contact when possible.
- Give one direction at a time.

You must ensure that the person is comfortable and you are not causing pain. You can say:

- "Am I hurting you?"
- "Please tell me when you feel pain or discomfort."
- "Do you need a pillow adjusted?"
- "Are you comfortable?"
- "How can I help make you more comfortable?"

PROMOTING SAFETY AND COMFORT

Safe Resident Handling, Moving, and Transfers

Safety

Many older persons have osteoporosis or arthritis (Chapter 35). They have fragile bones and joints. To prevent injuries:

- Follow the rules of body mechanics.
- Always have help when moving a person.
- Be aware of equipment and tubing involved in the person's care. Urinary catheters and oxygen, intravenous, drainage, and nasogastric tubes are examples.
- Move the person carefully to prevent injury or pain.
- Keep the person in good alignment.
- Position the person in good alignment after handling, moving, or transferring.
- Make sure the person's face, nose, and mouth are not obstructed by a pillow or other device.

Comfort

To promote mental comfort when handling, moving, or transferring the person:

- Always explain what you are going to do and how the person can help.
- Always screen and cover the person to protect the right to privacy.
  To promote physical comfort:
- Keep the person in good alignment.
- Make sure the person's head does not hit the headboard when being moved up in bed. If the person can be without a pillow, place it upright against the headboard.
- Use pillows to position the person as directed by the nurse and the care plan. If a pillow is allowed under the person's head, make sure it is under the head and shoulders.
- Use other positioning devices as directed by the nurse and the care plan.
- Ask persons how they would like their sheets and blankets placed. For example, some people like blankets pulled all the way up to their neck. Others like to have their arms on top of the blankets.

TEAMWORK AND TIME MANAGEMENT

Safe Resident Handling, Moving, and Transfers

Residents need to be moved, turned, transferred, and repositioned. These tasks and procedures are best done by at least two staff members.

Friendships are common among coworkers; and some working relationships are better than others. Do not just ask your friends or those with whom you work well to help you. Include all coworkers. Do not just help your friends or those with whom you work well. Assist anyone who asks for your help. This includes new staff members and those from other units.

PREVENTING WORK-RELATED INJURIES

You must prevent work-related injuries when handling, moving, and transferring residents. Follow the rules in Box 15.2. OSHA recommends that manual lifting:

- Be minimized in all cases.
- Be eliminated when possible.

To safely handle, move, and transfer the person, the nurse and health team determine:

- *The person's dependence level.* Dependence levels relate to the ability to move without help. Some persons do not need help

moving. Others totally depend on the staff. You need to know the person's dependence level before you handle, move, or transfer a person (Box 15.3).

- *The amount of assistance needed.* This depends on the person's height, weight, cognitive function, and dependence level. Some persons only need help from one staff member. Others need help from at least two or three staff members.
- *What procedure to use.* This chapter includes handling, moving, and transfer procedures. The nurse and care plan tell you what procedure to use.
- *The equipment needed.* Assist equipment and devices are useful to safely handle, move, and transfer persons. They are presented throughout this chapter. Long-term care centers are recognizing the importance of preventing work-related injuries. Newer and safer devices are utilized to prevent injuries. The nurse and care plan tell you what to use. Always follow the manufacturer instructions. Ask for any needed training to use the equipment and devices safely.

See *Residents with Dementia: Preventing Work-Related Injuries.*

See *Teamwork and Time Management: Preventing Work-Related Injuries.*

See *Delegation Guidelines: Preventing Work-Related Injuries.*

RESIDENTS WITH DEMENTIA

Preventing Work-Related Injuries

Some older persons have dementia. They may not understand what you are doing. They may resist your handling, moving, and transfer efforts. The person may shout at you, grab you, or try to hit you. Always get a coworker to help you. Do not force the person. The rules and guidelines in Box 15.3 apply. The person's care plan also has measures for providing safe care. For example:

- Proceed slowly.
- Use a calm, pleasant voice.
- Divert the person's attention. For example, let the person hold on to a washcloth or other soft object. This helps distract the person and keeps the person's hands busy.

Tell the nurse at once if you have problems handling, moving, or transferring the person.

TEAMWORK AND TIME MANAGEMENT

Preventing Work-Related Injuries

Some centers have "lift teams." These teams perform most of the lifting, moving, and transfer procedures. They use assist equipment and do not manually lift or move residents unless necessary.

The nurse advises the lift team of scheduled procedures. The team is called by beeper, pager, wireless phone, or other device for unscheduled transfers.

Do not assume that the lift team will lift, move, or transfer your assigned residents. Follow center policy for checking or adding to the lift team's schedule. Do not neglect or omit a procedure because the center has a lift team. If the person is on the team's schedule, always ensure that the procedure was done. Sometimes the team can get delayed because of unscheduled or unexpected events. Always thank the team for the work that they do. Their work protects residents and you from injury.

BOX 15.2 Preventing Work-Related Injuries

General Guidelines

- Wear shoes that provide good traction. Avoid shoes with worn-down soles. Good traction can help prevent slips or falls.
- Use assist equipment and devices when possible instead of lifting and moving the person manually. Follow the person's care plan.
- Get help from other staff. The nurse and care plan tell you how many staff members are needed to complete the task.
- Plan and prepare for the task (e.g., know what equipment you will need, where to place chairs or wheelchairs, and what side of the bed to work on).
- Schedule harder tasks early in your shift.
- Balance lighter and harder tasks. Plan your work so that you can complete a lighter task after a harder one.
- Lock bed wheels and wheelchair or stretcher wheels.
- Tell the person what assistance is needed. Give clear, simple instructions. Give the person time to respond.
- Do not hold or grab the person under the underarms.
- Do not let the person hold or grasp you around your neck.

Manual Lifting

- Use good body mechanics:
  - Stand with good posture. Keep your back straight.
  - Bend your legs, not your back.
  - Use your legs to do the work.
  - Face the person.
  - Do not twist or turn. Pick up your feet and pivot your whole body in the direction of the move.
- Try to keep what you are moving close to you (e.g., the person, equipment, or supplies).
- Move the person toward you, not away from you.
- Use slides and lateral transfers instead of manual lifting.
- Use a wide, balanced base of support. Stand with one foot slightly ahead of the other.
- Lower the person slowly by bending your legs. Do not bend your back. Return to an erect position as soon as possible.
- Use smooth, even movements. Avoid jerking movements.
- Lift on "the count of 3" when lifting with others. Everyone should lift at the same time.

Lateral Transfers

- Position surfaces as close as possible to each other (bed and chair; bed and stretcher).
- Adjust surfaces so that they are at about waist height. The receiving surface should be slightly lower to take advantage of gravity (e.g., when transferring the person from bed to a chair, the chair surface is lower than the bed).
- Make sure bed rails are down. Make sure side rails on stretchers are down.
- Use drawsheets, turning pads, large incontinence pads, or other friction-reducing devices. Such devices include slide boards, slide sheets, and low-friction mattress covers.
- Get a good handhold. Roll up drawsheets, turning pads, and incontinence pads, or use assist devices with handles.
- Kneel on the bed or stretcher to help prevent extended reaches and bending the back.
- Have staff on both sides of the bed or other surface. Move the person on "the count of 3." Use a smooth, push-pull motion. Do not reach across the person.

Gait/Transfer Belts

- Keep the person as close to you as possible.

- Avoid bending, reaching, or twisting when:
  - Attaching or removing a belt.
  - Lowering the person to a chair, the bed, the toilet, or the floor.
  - Assisting the person with ambulation.
- Use a gentle rocking motion to assist the person to stand. The rocking motion gives strength and force as you pull the person to standing position.

Stand-Pivot Transfers

- Use assist devices as directed. Follow the care plan.
- Use a gait/transfer belt with handles.
- Keep your feet at least shoulder width apart.
- Lower the bed so the person can place the feet on the floor.
- Plan the transfer so that the person moves the strong side first.
- Get the person close to the edge of the bed or the chair. Ask the person to lean forward when standing.
- Block the person's weak leg with your legs or knees. If the position is awkward, do the following:
  - Use a transfer belt with handles.
  - Straddle your legs around the person's weak leg.
- Bend your legs. Do not bend your back.
- Pivot with your feet to turn.
- Use a gentle rocking motion to assist the person to stand. The rocking motion gives strength and force as you pull the person to a standing position.

Lifting or Moving the Person in Bed

- Adjust the height of the bed, stretcher, or other surface so that it is at waist level.
- Lower the bed rail or the stretcher side rail.
- Work on the side where the person will be closest to you.
- Place equipment or other items close to you and at waist level.
- Use drawsheets, turning pads, large incontinence pads, or slide sheets.

Transporting Residents and Equipment

- Push, do not pull.
- Keep the load close to your body.
- Use an upright posture.
- Push with your whole body, not just your arms.
- Move down the center of the hallway, to help avoid collisions.
- Watch out for door handles and high thresholds on floors, which can cause abrupt stops.

Transferring the Person from the Floor

- Use a mechanical lift if possible (p. ··). If not, place a sling, blanket, drawsheet, cot, or other assist device under the person as directed by the nurse.
- Position at least two staff members on each side of the person. More staff is needed if the person is large.
- Bend at your knees, not your back. Do not twist.
- Roll the person onto the side to position the assist device. Do not reach across the person.
- Lower the boom (if using a mechanical lift) to attach the sling. The boom should be low enough so that you can easily attach the sling.
- Do the following for a manual lift:
  - Kneel on one knee.
  - Grasp the blanket, drawsheet, cot, or other device.
  - Lift smoothly with your legs as you stand on "the count of 3." Do not bend your back.

Modified from Cal/OSHA: *A back injury prevention guide for health care providers*, Sacramento, CA, revised November 1997, and referenced in Occupational Safety and Health Administration: *Ergonomics: guidelines for nursing homes*, revised March 2009.

BOX 15.3   Levels of Dependence

Code 4: Total Dependence. The person cannot help with the transfer. The task or procedure is done by the staff.
- The person should be lifted and transferred using a full-sling mechanical lift (Figs. 15.36 and 15.37A and B). The mechanical lift is used for transfers between beds, chairs, and toilets. It is also used for transfers to and from bathtubs and weighing scales.

Code 3: Extensive Assistance. The person can bear some weight, can sit up with help, and may be able to pivot to transfer.
- The person should be lifted and transferred using a mechanical lift. The mechanical lift is used for transfers between beds, chairs, and toilets. It is also used for transfers to and from bathtubs and weighing scales. The type of lift to use is noted on the person's care plan—full-sling mechanical lift (Fig. 15.36), ceiling-mounted mechanical lift (Fig. 15.37), or stand-assist lift (Figs. 15.12 and 15.13).

Code 2: Limited Assistance. The person is highly involved in the moving or transfer procedure. The person needs some help moving the legs. The person can stand (bear weight). The person has upper body strength and can sit up. The person is able to pivot to transfer.
- Stand-assist devices may be needed. These can be attached to the bed or chair (Fig. 15.14). Other stand-assist devices include walkers (Chapter 24) and gait/transfer belts with handles.
- Sliding boards are useful for transfers to and from beds and chairs (Fig. 15.15).
- Pivot discs may be useful for transfers to chairs or toilets (Fig. 15.16).

Code 1: Supervision. The staff needs to look after, encourage, or cue the person. To cue means to remind the person what to do.
- The devices for Code 2 may be needed.

Code 0: Independent. The person can walk without help. Sometimes the person may need limited assistance.
- Mechanical assistance is not normally required for transfers, lifting, or repositioning.

Modified from Nelson AL: *Patient care ergonomics resource guide: safe patient handling and movement*, Tampa, FL, 2005, Patient Safety Center of Inquiry, Veterans Health Administration and Department of Defense.

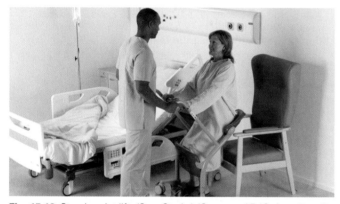

Fig. 15.12 Stand-assist lift. (Sara Stedy.) (Courtesy ARJO, Inc., Roselle, IL [800]323-1245.)

📄 DELEGATION GUIDELINES

Preventing Work-Related Injuries

Many delegated tasks involve handling, moving, and transferring persons. Before doing so, you need this information from the nurse and the care plan:
- The person's height and weight
- The person's dependence level (see Box 15.3)
- The person's physical abilities (e.g., Can the person sit up, stand up, or walk without help? Does the person have enough arm strength?)
- If the person has a weak side (and if yes, which side is weak?)
- If the person has a medical condition that increases the risk of injury (e.g., dizziness, confusion, hearing or vision problems, recent surgery, fragile skin)
- Any doctor's orders for handling, moving, or transferring the person
- The person's ability to follow directions
- If behavior problems are likely (e.g., combative, agitated, uncooperative, unpredictable behaviors)
- The amount of assistance needed

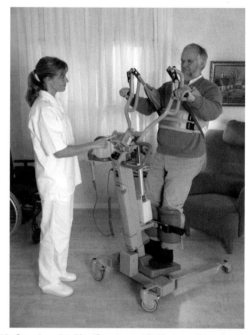

Fig. 15.13 Stand-assist lift. (Courtesy ARJO, Inc., Roselle, IL [800]323-1245.)

- How many staff members are needed to complete the task safely
- What procedure to use
- What equipment to use

See *Promoting Safety and Comfort: Preventing Work-Related Injuries.*

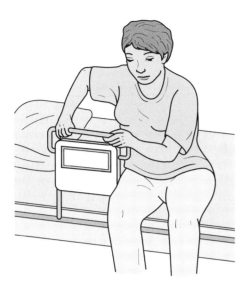

Fig. 15.14 Stand-assist bed attachment.

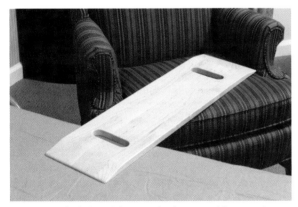

Fig. 15.15 Slide board for transferring to and from surfaces.

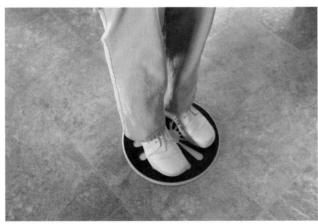

Fig. 15.16 Pivot disc.

PROMOTING SAFETY AND COMFORT

Preventing Work-Related Injuries
Safety

Decide how to move the person before starting the procedure. If you need help from other staff members, ask them to help before you begin. Also plan how to protect drainage tubes or containers connected to the person.

Beds are raised to move persons in bed. This reduces bending and reaching. You must:

• Use the bed correctly.
• Protect the person from falling when the bed is raised.
• Follow the rules of body mechanics.

MOVING PERSONS IN BED

Some persons can move and turn in bed. Others need help from at least one person. Those who are weak, unconscious, paralyzed, or in casts need help. Sometimes two or three people or a mechanical lift is needed.

• A dependence level of *Code 4: Total Dependence*—use a mechanical lift or friction-reducing device and at least two staff members.
• A dependence level of *Code 3: Extensive Assistance*—use a mechanical lift or friction-reducing device and at least two staff members.
• The person weighs less than 200 pounds—two to three staff members and a friction-reducing device are needed.
• If the person weighs more than 200 pounds—at least three staff members and a friction-reducing device are needed.
See *Delegation Guidelines: Moving Persons in Bed.*

Protecting the Skin

Older persons have fragile skin that is easily damaged. Protect their skin during handling, moving, and transfer procedures. Friction and shearing injure the skin. Both cause infection and pressure injuries (Chapter 32).

• Friction is the rubbing of one surface against another. When moved in bed, the person's skin rubs against the sheet.
• Shearing is when the skin sticks to a surface while muscles slide in the direction the body is moving (Fig. 15.17). It occurs when the person slides down in bed or is moved in bed. Reduce friction and shearing when moving the person in bed. Do so by:

• Rolling the person.
• Using friction-reducing devices. Such devices include a lift sheet (turning sheet). A cotton drawsheet (Chapter 17) serves as a lift sheet (turning sheet). Turning pads, large incontinence products, slide boards, and slide sheets are other friction-reducing devices.

✸ Raising the Person's Head and Shoulders

You may have to raise the person's head and shoulders to give care. Simply turning or removing a pillow requires this procedure. You can raise the person's head and shoulders easily and

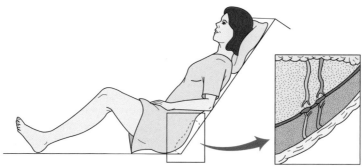

Fig. 15.17 Shearing. When the head of the bed is raised to a sitting position, skin on the buttocks stays in place. However, internal structures move forward as the person slides down in bed. This causes the skin to be pinched between the mattress and the hip bones.

safely by locking arms with the person. *Do not pull on the person's arm or shoulder.* It is best to have help with older persons and with those who are heavy or hard to move. This protects the person and you from injury.

📄 DELEGATION GUIDELINES

Moving Persons in Bed

Many delegated tasks involve moving the person in bed. Before moving a person, you need this information from the nurse and the care plan:

- What procedure to use
- How many workers are needed to safely move the person
- Position limits and restrictions
- How far you can lower the head of the bed
- Any limits in the person's ability to move or be repositioned
- What pillows can be removed before moving the person
- What equipment is needed—trapeze, lift sheet, slide sheet, mechanical lift
- How to position the person
- If the person uses bed rails

What observations to report and record:

- Who helped you with the procedure
- How much help the person needed
- How the person tolerated the procedure
- How you positioned the person
- Complaints of pain or discomfort
- When to report observations
- What specific resident concerns to report at once

🙌 RAISING THE PERSON'S HEAD AND SHOULDERS

Quality of Life

Remember to:

- Knock before entering the person's room.
- Address the person by name.
- Introduce yourself by name and title.
- Explain the procedure to the person before beginning and during the procedure.
- Protect the person's rights during the procedure.
- Handle the person gently during the procedure.

Preprocedure

1. Follow Delegation Guidelines:
   a. Preventing Work-Related Injuries, p. ··
   b. Moving Persons in Bed
2. See Promoting Safety and Comfort:
   a. Safe Resident Handling, Moving, and Transfers, p. ··
   b. Preventing Work-Related Injuries
3. Ask a coworker to assist if you need help.
4. Practice hand hygiene.
5. Identify the person. Check the identification (ID) bracelet against the assignment sheet. Also call the person by name.
6. Provide for privacy.
7. Lock the bed wheels.
8. Raise the bed for body mechanics. Bed rails are up if used.

Procedure

9. Ask your coworker to stand on the other side of the bed. Lower the bed rails if up.

10. Ask the person to put the near arm under your near arm and behind your shoulder. The person's hand rests on top of your shoulder. If you are standing on the right side, the person's right hand rests on your right shoulder (Fig. 15.18A). The person does the same with your coworker. The person's left hand rests on your coworker's left shoulder (Fig. 15.19A).
11. Put your arm nearest to the person under the arm. Your hand is on the person's shoulder. Your coworker does the same.
12. Put your free arm under the person's neck and shoulders (see Fig. 15.18B). Your coworker does the same (see Fig. 15.19B). Support the neck.
13. Help the person raise to a sitting or semi-sitting position on "the count of 3" (see Figs. 15.18C and 15.19C).
14. Use the arm and hand that supported the person's neck and shoulders to give care (see Fig. 15.18D). Your coworker supports the person (see Fig. 15.19D).
15. Help the person lie down. Provide support with your locked arm. Support the person's neck and shoulders with your other arm. Your coworker does the same.

Postprocedure

16. Provide for comfort. (See the inside of the front cover.)
17. Place the call light within reach.
18. Lower the bed to its lowest position.
19. Raise or lower bed rails. Follow the care plan.
20. Unscreen the person.
21. Complete a safety check of the room. (See the inside of the front cover.)
22. Decontaminate your hands.
23. Report and record your observations.

RAISING THE PERSON'S HEAD AND SHOULDERS—cont'd

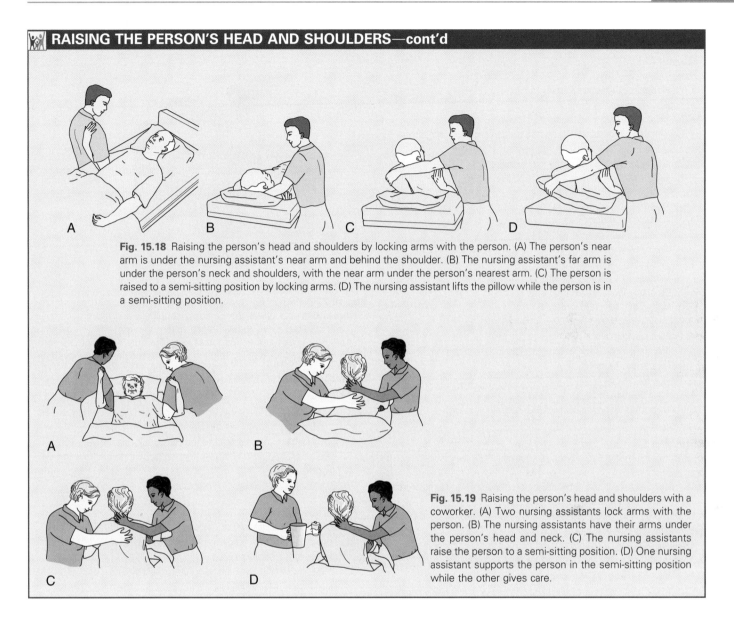

Fig. 15.18 Raising the person's head and shoulders by locking arms with the person. (A) The person's near arm is under the nursing assistant's near arm and behind the shoulder. (B) The nursing assistant's far arm is under the person's neck and shoulders, with the near arm under the person's nearest arm. (C) The person is raised to a semi-sitting position by locking arms. (D) The nursing assistant lifts the pillow while the person is in a semi-sitting position.

Fig. 15.19 Raising the person's head and shoulders with a coworker. (A) Two nursing assistants lock arms with the person. (B) The nursing assistants have their arms under the person's head and neck. (C) The nursing assistants raise the person to a semi-sitting position. (D) One nursing assistant supports the person in the semi-sitting position while the other gives care.

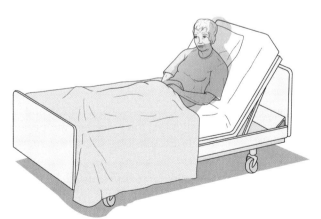

Fig. 15.20 A person in poor alignment after sliding down in bed.

✳ Moving the Person Up in Bed

When the head of the bed is raised, it is easy to slide down toward the middle and foot of the bed (Fig. 15.20). The person is moved up in bed for good alignment and comfort.

👤 PROMOTING SAFETY AND COMFORT

Moving the Person Up in Bed
Safety
This procedure is best done with at least two staff members. Assist devices are used as directed by the nurse and the care plan.
   Perform this procedure alone only if:
* The person is small in size.
* The person can follow directions.
* The person can assist with much of the moving.
* The person uses a trapeze.
* The person can push against the mattress with the feet.
* The nurse says it is safe to do so.
* You are comfortable doing so.
   Follow the nurse's directions and the care plan. Ask any questions before you begin the procedure.

✳ MOVING THE PERSON UP IN BED

Quality of Life

Remember to:
- Knock before entering the person's room.
- Address the person by name.
- Introduce yourself by name and title.
- Explain the procedure to the person before beginning and during the procedure.
- Protect the person's rights during the procedure.
- Handle the person gently during the procedure.

Preprocedure

1. Follow Delegation Guidelines:
    a. Preventing Work-Related Injuries, p. ··
    b. Moving Persons in Bed, p. ··
2. See Promoting Safety and Comfort:
    a. Safe Resident Handling, Moving, and Transfers, p. ··
    b. Preventing Work-Related Injuries, p. ··
    c. Moving the Person Up in Bed
3. Ask a coworker to help you.
4. Practice hand hygiene.
5. Identify the person. Check the ID bracelet against the assignment sheet. Also call the person by name.
6. Provide for privacy.
7. Lock the bed wheels.
8. Raise the bed for body mechanics. Bed rails are up if used.

Procedure

9. Lower the head of the bed to a level appropriate for the person. It is as flat as possible.
10. Stand on one side of the bed. Your coworker stands on the other side.
11. Lower the bed rails if up.
12. Remove pillows as directed by the nurse. Place a pillow upright against the headboard if the person can be without it.
13. Stand with a wide base of support. Point the foot near the head of the bed toward the head of the bed. Face the head of the bed.
14. Bend your hips and knees. Keep your back straight.
15. Place one arm under the person's shoulder and one arm under the thighs. Your coworker does the same. Grasp each other's forearms (Fig. 15.21).
16. Ask the person to grasp the trapeze.
17. Have the person flex both knees.
18. Explain the following:
    a. You will count "1, 2, 3."
    b. The move will be on "3."

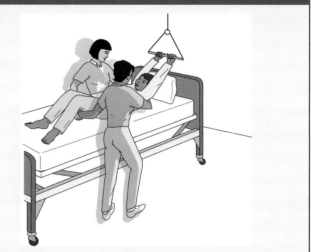

Fig. 15.21 A person is moved up in bed by two nursing assistants. Each has one arm under the person's shoulders and the other under the thighs. They have locked arms under the person. The person grasps the trapeze and flexes the knees. The nursing assistants shift their weight from the rear leg to the front leg as the person is moved up in bed.

c. On "3," the person pushes against the bed with the feet if able. And the person pulls up with the trapeze.
19. Move the person to the head of the bed on the count of "3." Shift your weight from your rear leg to your front leg (see Fig. 15.21). Your coworker does the same.
20. Repeat steps 13 through 19 if necessary.

Postprocedure

21. Put the pillow under the person's head and shoulders. Straighten linens.
22. Position the person in good alignment. Raise the head of the bed to a level appropriate for the person.
23. Provide for comfort. (See the inside of the front cover.)
24. Place the call light within reach.
25. Lower the bed to its lowest position.
26. Raise or lower bed rails. Follow the care plan.
27. Unscreen the person.
28. Complete a safety check of the room. (See the inside of the front cover.)
29. Decontaminate your hands.
30. Report and record your observations.

This skill also covered in *Clinical Skills: Nurse Assisting*.

You can sometimes move lightweight adults up in bed alone if they can assist and use a trapeze. However, it is best to have help and to use an assist device—lift sheet, large incontinence product, slide sheet (p. ··). Two or more staff members are needed to move heavy, weak, and very old persons up in bed. Always protect the person and yourself from injury.

See *Promoting Safety and Comfort: Moving the Person Up in Bed.*

✳ Moving the Person Up in Bed with an Assist Device

Assist devices are used to move some persons up in bed. Such assist devices include a drawsheet (lift sheet), flat sheet folded in half, turning pad (Fig. 15.22), slide sheet (Fig. 15.23), and large incontinence pad product. With these devices, the person is moved more evenly; and the devices reduce shearing and friction.

The device is placed under the person from the head to above the knees or lower. At least two staff members are needed. This procedure is used for most residents. It is used:

- Following the guidelines for "Moving Persons in Bed," p. ··.
- For persons recovering from spinal cord surgery or spinal cord injuries.
- For older persons.

See *Promoting Safety and Comfort: Moving the Person Up in Bed with an Assist Device.*

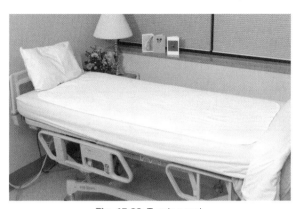

Fig. 15.22 Turning pad.

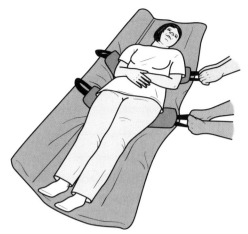

Fig. 15.23 Slide sheet.

PROMOTING SAFETY AND COMFORT

Moving the Person Up in Bed with an Assist Device

Safety

Not all incontinence pad products can be used as assist devices. Disposable, single-use underpads are not strong enough to hold the person's weight during the move. Reusable underpads are stronger. For safety, the underpad must:

- Be strong enough to support the person's weight.
- Extend from under the person's head to above the knees or lower.

- Be wide enough for you and other staff to get a firm grip for the lift.

Check with the nurse to ensure the person's underpad is safe to use as an assist device.

If using a slide sheet, you will need to place it under the person. See procedure: Making an Occupied Bed in Chapter 17 for this step. After moving the person up in bed, remove the slide sheet. The person is in danger of sliding down in bed or off the bed if the slide sheet is not removed.

MOVING THE PERSON UP IN BED WITH AN ASSIST DEVICE

Quality of Life

Remember to:
- Knock before entering the person's room.
- Address the person by name.
- Introduce yourself by name and title.
- Explain the procedure to the person before beginning and during the procedure.
- Protect the person's rights during the procedure.
- Handle the person gently during the procedure.

Preprocedure

1. Follow Delegation Guidelines:
   a. Preventing Work-Related Injuries, p. ··
   b. Moving Persons in Bed, p. ··
2. See Promoting Safety and Comfort:
   a. Safe Resident Handling, Moving, and Transfers, p. ··
   b. Preventing Work-Related Injuries, p. ··
   c. Moving the Person Up in Bed, p. ··
   d. Moving the Person Up in Bed with an Assist Device
3. Ask a coworker to help you.
4. Practice hand hygiene.
5. Identify the person. Check the ID bracelet against the assignment sheet. Also call the person by name.
6. Provide for privacy.
7. Lock the bed wheels.
8. Raise the bed for body mechanics. Bed rails are up if used.

Procedure

9. Lower the head of the bed to a level appropriate for the person. It is as flat as possible.
10. Stand on one side of the bed. Your coworker stands on the other side.
11. Lower the bed rails if up.

12. Remove pillows as directed by the nurse. Place a pillow upright against the headboard if the person can be without it.
13. Stand with a broad base of support. Point the foot near the head of the bed toward the head of the bed. Face that direction.
14. Roll the sides of the assist device up close to the person. (*Note:* Omit this step if the device has handles.)
15. Grasp the rolled-up assist device firmly near the person's shoulders and hips (Fig. 15.24). Or grasp it by the handles. Support the head.
16. Bend your hips and knees.
17. Move the person up in bed on "the count of 3." Shift your weight from your rear leg to your front leg.
18. Repeat steps 13 through 17 if necessary.
19. Unroll the assist device. (*Note:* Omit this step if the device has handles.)

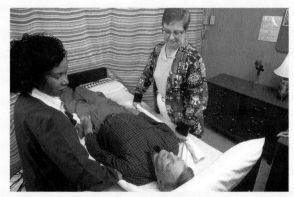

Fig. 15.24 A drawsheet is used to move the person up in bed. It extends from the person's head to above the knees. Rolled close to the person, the drawsheet is held near the shoulders and hips.

Continued

❋ MOVING THE PERSON UP IN BED WITH AN ASSIST DEVICE—cont'd

Postprocedure

20. Put the pillow under the person's head and shoulders.
21. Position the person in good alignment. Raise the head of the bed to a level appropriate for the person.
22. Provide for comfort. (See the inside of the front cover.)
23. Place the call light within reach.

24. Lower the bed to its lowest position.
25. Raise or lower bed rails. Follow the care plan.
26. Unscreen the person.
27. Complete a safety check of the room. (See the inside of the front cover.)
28. Decontaminate your hands.
29. Report and record your observations.

This skill also covered in *Clinical Skills: Nurse Assisting.*

 Moving the Person to the Side of the Bed

Repositioning and care procedures require moving the person to the side of the bed. The person is moved to the side of the bed before turning. Otherwise, after turning, the person lies on the side of the bed—not in the middle.

Sometimes you have to reach over the person, such as when giving a bed bath. You reach less if the person is close to you.

One method involves moving the person in segments (Fig. 15.25). Sometimes one person can do this. Use a mechanical lift (p. ··) or the assist device method:

- Following the guidelines for "Moving Persons in Bed," p. ···.

- For older persons.
- For persons with arthritis.
- For persons recovering from spinal cord injuries or spinal cord surgery.

Assist devices for this procedure include a drawsheet (lift sheet), flat sheet folded in half, turning pad, slide sheet, slide board, and large incontinence pad product. Using an assist device helps prevent pain and skin damage. It also helps prevent injury to the bones, joints, and spinal cord.

See *Promoting Safety and Comfort: Moving the Person to the Side of the Bed.*

👤 PROMOTING SAFETY AND COMFORT

Moving the Person to the Side of the Bed

Safety

Use the method and equipment that are best for the person. Get this information from the nurse and the care plan when delegated tasks involve moving the person to the side of the bed. Such tasks include repositioning, bedmaking, bathing, and range-of-motion exercises.

The wrong method could seriously injure a person. This is very important for persons who are very old, have arthritis, or have spinal cord involvement.

When using an assist device, you need at least one coworker to help you. Depending on the person's size, three staff members may be needed. You will need to ask two coworkers to help you.

If using a slide board or slide sheet, you will need to place it under the person. After moving the person up in bed, remove the device.

To move the person in segments, move the person toward you, not away from you. This helps protect you from injury.

Comfort

After moving the person to the side of the bed, move the pillow too. Make sure the pillow is positioned correctly. It should be under the person's head and shoulders.

❋ MOVING THE PERSON TO THE SIDE OF THE BED

Quality of Life

Remember to:

- Knock before entering the person's room.
- Address the person by name.
- Introduce yourself by name and title.
- Explain the procedure to the person before beginning and during the procedure.
- Protect the person's rights during the procedure.
- Handle the person gently during the procedure.

Preprocedure

1. Follow Delegation Guidelines:
   a. Preventing Work-Related Injuries, p. ··
   b. Moving Persons in Bed, p. ··
2. See Promoting Safety and Comfort:
   a. Safe Resident Handling, Moving, and Transfers, p. ··
   b. Preventing Work-Related Injuries, p. ··
   c. Moving the Person to the Side of the Bed, p. ··
3. Ask a coworker to help you if using an assist device.

4. Practice hand hygiene.
5. Identify the person. Check the ID bracelet against the assignment sheet. Also call the person by name.
6. Provide for privacy.
7. Lock the bed wheels.
8. Raise the bed for body mechanics. Bed rails are up if used.

Procedure

9. Lower the head of the bed to a level appropriate for the person. It is as flat as possible.
10. Stand on the side of the bed to which you will move the person.
11. Lower the bed rail near you if bed rails are used. (Both bed rails are lowered for step 16.)
12. Remove pillows as directed by the nurse.
13. Stand with your feet about 12 inches apart. One foot is in front of the other. Flex your knees.
14. Cross the person's arms over the person's chest.
15. Method 1—*Moving the person in segments:* (This method is **not** used for persons with back or spinal injuries.)

❋ MOVING THE PERSON TO THE SIDE OF THE BED—cont'd

a. Place your arm under the person's neck and shoulders. Grasp the far shoulder.
b. Place your other arm under the midback.
c. Move the upper part of the person's body toward you. Rock backward and shift your weight to your rear leg (see Fig. 15.25A).
d. Place one arm under the person's waist and one under the thighs.
e. Rock backward to move the lower part of the person toward you (see Fig. 15.25B).
f. Repeat the procedure for the legs and feet (see Fig. 15.25C). Your arms should be under the person's thighs and calves.

16. Method 2—Moving the person with a drawsheet:
a. Roll up the drawsheet close to the person (see Fig. 15.24).
b. Grasp the rolled-up drawsheet near the person's shoulders and hips. Your coworker does the same. Support the person's head.
c. Rock backward on "the count of 3," moving the person toward you. Your coworker rocks backward slightly and then forward toward you while keeping the arms straight.
d. Unroll the drawsheet. Remove any wrinkles.

Postprocedure

17. Position the person in good alignment.
18. Provide for comfort. (See the inside of the front cover.)
19. Place the call light within reach.
20. Lower the bed to its lowest position.
21. Raise or lower bed rails. Follow the care plan.
22. Unscreen the person.
23. Complete a safety check of the room. (See the inside of the front cover.)
24. Decontaminate your hands.
25. Report and record your observations.

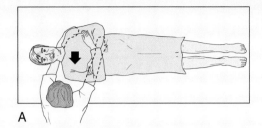

A

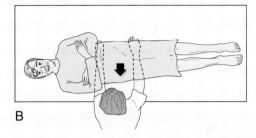

B

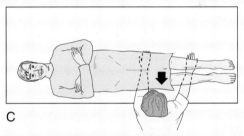

C

Fig. 15.25 Moving the person to the side of the bed in segments. (A) The upper part of the body is moved. (B) The lower part of the body is moved. (C) The legs and feet are moved.

This skill also covered in *Clinical Skills: Nurse Assisting.*

❋ TURNING PERSONS

Turning persons onto their side helps prevent complications from bedrest (Chapter 24). Certain procedures and care measures also require the side-lying position. The person is turned toward you or away from you. The direction depends on the person's condition and the situation.

After turning, position the person in good alignment. Use pillows to support the person in the side-lying position.

Some persons can turn and reposition themselves in bed. Others need help. Some totally depend on the nursing staff for care. Make sure the person's face, nose, and mouth are not obstructed by a pillow or other device.

Many older persons suffer from arthritis in their spine, hips, and knees. When turning these persons, logrolling is preferred. Logrolling may be less painful for these persons.

See *Delegation Guidelines: Turning Persons.*
See *Promoting Safety and Comfort: Turning Persons.*

DELEGATION GUIDELINES

Turning Persons

Before turning and repositioning a person, you need this information from the nurse and the care plan:

- The person's dependency level (see Box 15.3)
- How much help the person needs
- How many staff members are needed to safely complete the procedure
- The person's comfort level and what body parts are painful
- Which procedure to use
- What assist devices to use
- What supportive devices are needed for positioning (Chapter 24)
- Where to place pillows
- What observations to report and record:
  - Who helped you with the procedure
  - How much help the person needed
  - How the person tolerated the procedure
  - How you positioned the person
  - Complaints of pain or discomfort
  - When to report observations
  - What specific resident concerns to report at once

PROMOTING SAFETY AND COMFORT

Turning Persons
Safety
Use good body mechanics when turning a person in bed. Follow the rules in Box 15.2.

The person must be in good alignment. Otherwise, musculoskeletal injuries, skin breakdown, or pressure injuries could occur.

If using an assist device, ask a coworker to help you.

Do not turn a person away from you with the far bed rail down. Raise the bed rail on the side near you. Then go to the other side of the bed. Lower that bed rail if up. Turn the person toward you.

Comfort
After turning, position the person in good alignment. Use pillows as directed to support the person in the side-lying position.

✳ Logrolling

Logrolling is turning the person as a unit, in alignment, with one motion. The spine is kept straight. The procedure is used to turn:
- Older persons with arthritic spines or knees.
- Persons recovering from hip fractures.

- Persons with spinal cord injuries (the spine is kept straight at all times after spinal cord injury).
- Persons recovering from spinal surgery (the spine is kept straight at all times after spinal surgery).
  See *Promoting Safety and Comfort: Logrolling.*

✳ TURNING AND REPOSITIONING THE PERSON (NATCEP)

Quality of Life
Remember to:
- Knock before entering the person's room.
- Address the person by name.
- Introduce yourself by name and title.
- Explain the procedure to the person before beginning and during the procedure.
- Protect the person's rights during the procedure.
- Handle the person gently during the procedure.

Preprocedure
1. Follow Delegation Guidelines:
   a. Preventing Work-Related Injuries, p. ··
   b. Moving Persons in Bed, p. ··
   c. Turning Persons
2. See Promoting Safety and Comfort:
   a. Safe Resident Handling, Moving, and Transfers, p. ··
   b. Preventing Work-Related Injuries, p. ··
   c. Moving the Person to the Side of the Bed, p. ··
   d. Turning Persons
3. Practice hand hygiene.

4. Identify the person. Check the ID bracelet against the assignment sheet. Also call the person by name.
5. Provide for privacy.
6. Lock the bed wheels.
7. Raise the bed for body mechanics. Bed rails are up.

Procedure
8. Lower the head of the bed to a level appropriate for the person. It is as flat as possible.
9. Stand on the side of the bed opposite to where you will turn the person.
10. Lower the bed rail near you.
11. Move the person to the side near you. (See procedure: Moving the Person to the Side of the Bed, p. ··.)
12. Cross the person's arms over the chest. Cross the leg near you over the far leg.
▶ 13. Turning the person away from you:
   a. Stand with a wide base of support. Flex the knees.
   b. Place one hand on the person's shoulder. Place the other on the hip near you.
   c. Roll the person gently away from you toward the raised bed rail (Fig. 15.26A). Shift your weight from your rear leg to your front leg.

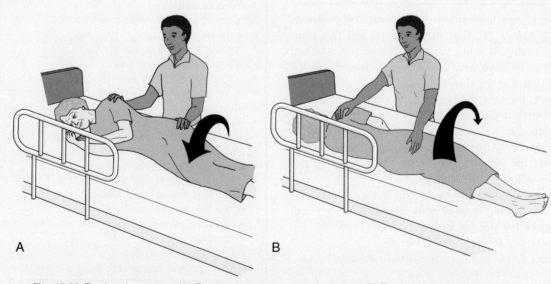

A   B

Fig. 15.26 Turning the person. (A) Turning the person away from you. (B) Turning the person toward you. *NOTE:* Nonstandard bed rails are used to show positioning and hand placement.

TURNING AND REPOSITIONING THE PERSON (NATCEP)—cont'd

14. Turning the person toward you:
    a. Raise the bed rail.
    b. Go to the other side of the bed. Lower the bed rail.
    c. Stand with a wide base of support. Flex your knees.
    d. Place one hand on the person's far shoulder. Place the other on the far hip.
    e. Roll the person toward you gently (see Fig. 15.26B).
15. Position the person. Follow the nurse's directions and the care plan. The following is common:
    a. Place a pillow under the head and neck.
    b. Adjust the shoulder. The person should not lie on an arm.
    c. Place a small pillow under the upper hand and arm.
    d. Position a pillow against the back.

    e. Flex the upper knee. Position the upper leg in front of the lower leg.
    f. Support the upper leg and thigh on pillows. Make sure the ankle is supported.

Postprocedure
16. Provide for comfort. (See the inside of the front cover.)
17. Place the call light within reach.
18. Lower the bed to its lowest position.
19. Raise or lower bed rails. Follow the care plan.
20. Unscreen the person.
21. Complete a safety check of the room. (See the inside of the front cover.)
22. Decontaminate your hands.
23. Report and record your observations.

PROMOTING SAFETY AND COMFORT

Logrolling

Safety

Two or three staff members are needed to logroll a person. Three are needed if the person is tall or heavy. Sometimes an assist device is needed—drawsheet, turning pad, large incontinence product, or slide sheet.

Comfort

After spinal cord injury or surgery, the spine must be kept straight. This includes the person's neck. Therefore, a pillow is usually not allowed under the head and neck. Follow the nurse's directions and the care plan for positioning the person and using pillows.

LOGROLLING THE PERSON

Quality of Life

Remember to:
- Knock before entering the person's room.
- Address the person by name.
- Introduce yourself by name and title.
- Explain the procedure to the person before beginning and during the procedure.
- Protect the person's rights during the procedure.
- Handle the person gently during the procedure.

Preprocedure

1. Follow Delegation Guidelines:
   a. Preventing Work-Related Injuries, p. ··
   b. Moving Persons in Bed, p. ··
   c. Turning Persons, p. ··
2. See Promoting Safety and Comfort:
   a. Safe Resident Handling, Moving, and Transfers, p. ··
   b. Preventing Work-Related Injuries, p. ··

   c. Turning Persons, p. ··
   d. Logrolling
3. Ask a coworker to help you.
4. Practice hand hygiene.
5. Identify the person. Check the ID bracelet against the assignment sheet. Also call the person by name.
6. Provide for privacy.
7. Lock the bed wheels.
8. Raise the bed for body mechanics. Bed rails are up if used.

Procedure

9. Make sure the bed is flat.
10. Stand on the side opposite to which you will turn the person. Your coworker stands on the other side.
11. Lower the bed rails if used.
12. Move the person as a unit to the side of the bed near you. Use the assist device. (If the person has a spinal cord injury, assist the nurse as directed.)

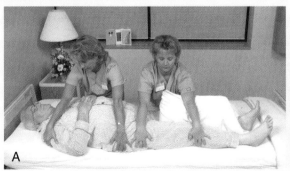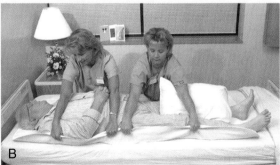

Fig. 15.27 Logrolling. (A) A pillow is between the person's legs. The arms are crossed on the chest. The person is on the far side of the bed. (B) The assist device is used to logroll the person.

Continued

✳ LOGROLLING THE PERSON—cont'd

13. Place the person's arms across the chest. Place a pillow between the knees.
14. Raise the bed rail if used.
15. Go to the other side.
16. Stand near the shoulders and chest. Your coworker stands near the hips and thighs.
17. Stand with a broad base of support. One foot is in front of the other.
18. Ask the person to hold the body rigid.
19. Roll the person toward you (Fig. 15.27A). Or use the assist device (see Fig. 15.27B). Turn the person as a unit.
20. Position the person in good alignment. Use pillows as directed by the nurse and the care plan. The following is common (unless the spinal cord is involved):
    a. One pillow against the back for support

b. One pillow under the head and neck if allowed
c. One pillow or a folded bath blanket between the legs
d. A small pillow under the upper arm and hand

Postprocedure
21. Provide for comfort. (See the inside of the front cover.)
22. Place the call light within reach.
23. Lower the bed to its lowest position.
24. Raise or lower bed rails. Follow the care plan.
25. Unscreen the person.
26. Complete a safety check of the room. (See the inside of the front cover.)
27. Decontaminate your hands.
28. Report and record your observations.

This skill also covered in *Clinical Skills: Nurse Assisting.*

✳ SITTING ON THE SIDE OF THE BED (DANGLING)

Residents sit on the side of the bed *(dangle)* for many reasons. Many older persons become dizzy or faint when getting out of bed too fast. They may need to sit on the side of the bed for 1 to 5 minutes before walking or transferring. Some persons increase activity in stages—bedrest, to sitting on the side of the bed, and then to sitting in a chair. Walking is the next step.

While dangling the legs, the person coughs and deep breathes. The person moves the legs back and forth in circles. This stimulates circulation.

Two staff members may be needed. A person with balance and coordination problems needs support. If dizziness or fainting occurs, lay the person down.

See *Delegation Guidelines: Dangling.*
See *Promoting Safety and Comfort: Dangling.*

📋 DELEGATION GUIDELINES

Dangling

The nurse may ask you to help a person sit on the side of the bed. The procedure is part of other tasks—assisting the person to stand, transferring from bed to chair, partial bath, and others. When delegated the dangling procedure or tasks that involve dangling, you need this information from the nurse and the care plan:
- Areas of weakness. For example, if the arms are weak, the person cannot hold on to the side of the mattress for support. If the left side is weak, turn the person onto the stronger right side. The person can use the right arm to help move from the lying to sitting position.
- The person's dependence level (see Box 15.3).
- The amount of help the person needs.
- If you need a coworker to help you.
- If the bed is raised or in its lowest position.
- How long the person needs to sit on the side of the bed.
- What exercises the person needs to perform while dangling:

- Range-of-motion exercises (Chapter 24)
- Deep-breathing and coughing exercises (Chapter 26)
- If the person will walk or transfer to a chair after dangling. If yes, the bed is in its lowest position.
  - What observations to report and record (Fig. 15.28):
  - Pulse and respiratory rates (Chapter 27)
  - Pale or bluish skin color (cyanosis)
  - Complaints of dizziness, lightheadedness, or difficulty breathing
  - Who helped you with the procedure
  - How well the activity was tolerated
  - The length of time the person dangled
  - The amount of help needed
  - Other observations and complaints
- When to report observations.
- What specific resident concerns to report at once.

Date	Time	Nursing Margin	Other Depts Margin
9/9	0900	Assisted to sit on the side of the bed with assistance of one.	
		Active leg exercises performed. Tolerated procedure without	
		complaints of pain or discomfort. No c/o dizziness. BP-130/78 L	
		arm sitting, P-74 regular rate and rhythm, R-20 unlabored. Color	
		good. Assisted to lie down after 5 minutes. Positioned on L side.	
		Bed in low position, call light within reach. Adam Aims, CNA ———	

Fig. 15.28 Charting sample. BP, Blood pressure; c/o, complaints of; L, left; P, pulse; R, respirations.

PROMOTING SAFETY AND COMFORT

Dangling

Safety

This procedure is not used for persons with these dependence levels:
- Code 4: Total Dependence
- Code 3: Extensive Assistance

Problems with sitting and balance often occur after illness, injury, surgery, and bedrest. Some persons who are disabled also have problems sitting and with balance. Provide support when the person is sitting on the side of the bed. It is best to have a coworker help you. This protects the person from falling and other injuries.

Comfort

Provide for the person's warmth during the dangling procedure. Help the person put on a robe, or cover the person's shoulders and back with a bath blanket.

The person may want to perform simple hygiene measures while sitting on the side of the bed. Oral hygiene and washing the face and hands are examples. These measures refresh the person and stimulate circulation. Follow the nurse's directions and the care plan.

SITTING ON THE SIDE OF THE BED (DANGLING)

Quality of Life

Remember to:
- Knock before entering the person's room.
- Address the person by name.
- Introduce yourself by name and title.
- Explain the procedure to the person before beginning and during the procedure.
- Protect the person's rights during the procedure.
- Handle the person gently during the procedure.

Preprocedure

1. Follow Delegation Guidelines:
   a. Preventing Work-Related Injuries, p. ··
   b. Dangling
2. See Promoting Safety and Comfort:
   a. Safe Resident Handling, Moving, and Transfers, p. ··
   b. Preventing Work-Related Injuries, p. ··
   c. Dangling
3. Ask a coworker to help you if the person will dangle.
4. Practice hand hygiene.
5. Identify the person. Check the ID bracelet against the assignment sheet. Also call the person by name.
6. Provide for privacy.
7. Decide what side of the bed to use.
8. Move furniture to provide moving space.
9. Lock the bed wheels.
10. Raise the bed for body mechanics. Bed rails are up if used.

Procedure

11. Lower the bed rail if up.
12. Position the person in a side-lying position facing you. The person lies on the strong side.
13. Raise the head of the bed to a sitting position.
14. Stand by the person's hips. Face the foot of the bed.
15. Stand with your feet apart. The foot near the head of the bed is in front of the other foot.
16. Slide one arm under the person's neck and shoulders. Grasp the far shoulder. Place your other hand over the thighs near the knees (Fig. 15.29A).
17. Pivot toward the foot of the bed while moving the person's legs and feet over the side of the bed. As the legs go over the edge of the mattress, the trunk is upright (see Fig. 15.29B).
18. Ask the person to hold on to the edge of the mattress. This supports the person in the sitting position. If possible, raise a half-length bed rail for the person to grasp. Raise the bed rail on the person's strong side. Have your coworker support the person at all times.
19. Do not leave the person alone. Provide support at all times.
20. Check the person's condition:
    a. Ask how the person feels. Ask if the person feels dizzy or lightheaded.
    b. Check the pulse and respirations.
    c. Check for difficulty breathing.
    d. Note if the skin is pale or bluish in color (cyanosis).
21. Reverse the procedure to return the person to bed. (Or prepare to transfer the person to a chair or wheelchair. Lower the bed to its lowest position so the person's feet are flat on the floor. Support the person at all times.)
22. Lower the head of the bed after the person returns to bed. Help the person move to the center of the bed.
23. Position the person in good alignment.

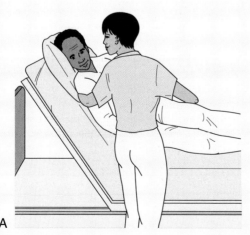
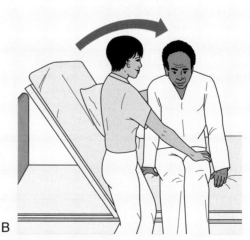

Fig. 15.29 Helping the person sit on the side of the bed. (A) The person's shoulders and thighs are supported. (B) The person sits upright as the legs and feet are pulled over the edge of the bed.

✳ SITTING ON THE SIDE OF THE BED (DANGLING)—cont'd

Postprocedure

24. Provide for comfort. (See the inside of the front cover.)
25. Place the call light within reach.
26. Lower the bed to its lowest position.
27. Raise or lower bed rails. Follow the care plan.

28. Return furniture to its proper place.
29. Unscreen the person.
30. Complete a safety check of the room. (See the inside of the front cover.)
31. Decontaminate your hands.
32. Report and record your observations.

TRANSFERRING PERSONS

Residents are moved to and from beds, chairs, wheelchairs, shower chairs, commodes, toilets, and stretchers. The amount of help needed and the method used vary with the person's dependency level (see Box 15.3). Some persons transfer by themselves or need little help. Some persons need help from at least one to three people.

The rules of body mechanics apply to transfers. So follow the guidelines in Box 15.2. Arrange the room so there is enough space for a safe transfer. Correct placement of the chair, wheelchair, or other device also is needed for a safe transfer.

See *Delegation Guidelines: Transferring Persons.*
See *Promoting Safety and Comfort: Transferring Persons.*
See *Teamwork and Time Management: Transferring Persons.*

TRANSFER BELTS

Transfer belts were discussed in Chapter 12. Also called gait belts, they are used to support residents during transfers. They also are used to reposition persons in chairs and wheelchairs (p. ··).

Wider belts have padded handles. They are easier to grip and allow better control should the person fall.

✳ Bed to Chair or Wheelchair Transfers

Safety is important for chair, wheelchair, commode, and shower chair transfers. Help the person out of bed on the person's strong side. If the left side is weak and the right side is strong, get the person out of bed on the right side. In transferring, the strong side moves first. It pulls the weaker side along. Transfers from the weak side are awkward and unsafe.

📄 DELEGATION GUIDELINES

Transferring Persons
When delegated transferring procedures, you need this information from the nurse and the care plan:
- What procedure to use
- The person's dependency level (see Box 15.3)
- The amount of help the person needs
- What equipment to use—transfer belt, wheelchair, mechanical assist device, positioning devices, wheelchair cushion, and so on

- The person's height and weight
- How many staff members are needed to complete the task safely
- Areas of weakness (for example, if the arms are weak, the person cannot hold on to the mattress for support; if there is a weak left side, the person gets out of bed on the stronger right side; the person uses the right arm to help move from the lying to sitting position)
- What observations to report and record:
  - Pulse rate before and after the transfer (Chapter 27)
  - Complaints of lightheadedness, pain, discomfort, difficulty breathing, weakness, or fatigue
  - The amount of help needed to transfer the person
  - Who helped you with the procedure
  - How the person helped with the transfer
  - How you positioned the person
- When to report observations.
- What specific resident concerns to report at once.

👤 PROMOTING SAFETY AND COMFORT

Transferring Persons
Safety
The person wears nonskid footwear for transfers. Such footwear protects the person from falls. Slipping and sliding are prevented. Tie shoelaces securely to prevent the person from trips and falls.

Check the length of the person's gown or robe if necessary. Long gowns and robes can cause falls. Also, avoid robes with long ties. The person can trip and fall.

Lock bed and wheelchair wheels and wheels on other devices. This prevents the bed and the device from moving during the transfer. Otherwise, the person can fall. You also are at risk for injury.

Comfort
After the transfer, position the person in good alignment. Make sure needed items are within reach.

👥 TEAMWORK AND TIME MANAGEMENT

Transferring Persons
Mechanical assist devices are used to transfer some residents. After using such a device, return it to the storage area. It needs to be available for use by other staff. Do not leave a device in a person's room or other care setting. Your coworkers should not have to assume that an assist device is in use or take time looking for one.

Many mechanical assist devices are battery operated. The battery must be charged for the device to work properly. Follow center policy for charging or replacing batteries.

You may need help from one or two coworkers to safely transfer a person. Politely ask coworkers to help you. Tell them what time you need the help and for how long. This helps them plan their own work. Always thank your co-workers for helping you. Willingly help them when asked.

The following stand and pivot transfers are used if:

- The person's legs are strong enough to bear some or all body weight.
- The person is cooperative and can follow directions.
- The person can assist with the transfer.

See *Promoting Safety and Comfort: Bed to Chair or Wheelchair Transfers.*

PROMOTING SAFETY AND COMFORT

Bed to Chair or Wheelchair Transfers
Safety

The chair, wheelchair, or other device must support the person's weight. The number of staff members needed for a transfer depends on the person's abilities, condition, and size. For some persons, you will use mechanical assist devices (p. ··).

The person must not put the arms around your neck. Otherwise, the person can pull you forward or cause you to lose your balance. Neck, back, and other injuries from falls are possible.

If not using a mechanical assist device, using a gait/transfer belt is the preferred method for chair or wheelchair transfers. It is safer for the person and you. Putting your arms around the person and grasping the shoulder blades is the other method. It can cause the person discomfort. And it can be stressful for you. Use this method only if instructed to do so by the nurse and the care plan.

Bed and wheelchair wheels are locked for a safe transfer. After the transfer, unlock the wheelchair wheels to position the wheelchair as the person prefers. After positioning the chair, lock the wheels or keep them unlocked according to the care plan. Locked wheels may be viewed as restraints if the person cannot unlock them to move the wheelchair (Chapter 13). However, falls and other injuries are risks if the person tries to stand when the wheelchair wheels are unlocked.

Comfort

Most wheelchairs and bedside chairs have vinyl seats and backs. Vinyl holds body heat. The person becomes warm and perspires more. You can cover the back and seat with a folded bath blanket to increase the person's comfort in the chair. Some people have wheelchair cushions or positioning devices. Ask the nurse how to use and place the devices. Also follow the manufacturer instructions.

TRANSFERRING THE PERSON TO A CHAIR OR WHEELCHAIR (NATCEP)

Quality of Life
Remember to:

- Knock before entering the person's room.
- Address the person by name.
- Introduce yourself by name and title.
- Explain the procedure to the person before beginning and during the procedure.
- Protect the person's rights during the procedure.
- Handle the person gently during the procedure.

Preprocedure
1. Follow Delegation Guidelines:
   a. Preventing Work-Related Injuries, p. ··
   b. Transferring Persons, p. ··
2. See Promoting Safety and Comfort:
   a. Transfer/Gait Belts (Chapter 12)
   b. Safe Resident Handling, Moving, and Transfers, p. ··
   c. Preventing Work-Related Injuries, p. ··
   d. Transferring Persons
   e. Bed to Chair or Wheelchair Transfers
3. Collect:
   - Wheelchair or armchair
   - Bath blanket
   - Lap blanket
   - Robe and nonskid footwear
   - Paper or sheet
   - Transfer belt (if needed)
   - Seat cushion (if needed)
4. Practice hand hygiene.
5. Identify the person. Check the ID bracelet against the assignment sheet. Also call the person by name.
6. Provide for privacy.
7. Decide which side of the bed to use. Move furniture for a safe transfer.

Procedure
8. Position the chair.
   a. The chair is near the head of the bed on the person's strong side.
   b. The chair faces the foot of the bed.
   c. The arm of the chair almost touches the bed.
9. Place a folded bath blanket or cushion on the seat (if needed).
10. Lock the wheelchair wheels. Raise the footplates. Remove or swing the front rigging out of the way.
11. Lower the bed to its lowest position. Lock the bed wheels.
12. Fan-fold top linens to the foot of the bed.
13. Place the paper or sheet under the person's feet. (This protects the person's linens from the footwear.) Put footwear on the person.
14. Help the person sit on the side of the bed (p. ··). The feet touch the floor.
15. Help the person put on a robe.
16. Apply the transfer belt if needed (Chapter 12).
17. Method 1: Using a transfer belt:
   a. Stand in front of the person.
   b. Have the person hold on to the mattress.
   c. Make sure the person's feet are flat on the floor.
   d. Have the person lean forward.
   e. Grasp the transfer belt at each side. Grasp the handles or grasp the belt from underneath. See Chapter 12.
   f. Prevent the person from sliding or falling by doing one of the following:
      (1) Brace your knees against the person's knees (Fig. 15.30). Block the person's feet with your feet.
      (2) Use the knee and foot of one leg to block the person's weak leg or foot. Place your other foot slightly behind you for balance.
      (3) Straddle your legs around the person's weak leg.

Continued

✳ TRANSFERRING THE PERSON TO A CHAIR OR WHEELCHAIR (NATCEP)—cont'd

g. Explain the following:
   (1) You will count "1, 2, 3."
   (2) The move will be on "3."
   (3) On "3," the person pushes down on the mattress and stands.
h. Ask the person to push down on the mattress and to stand on "the count of 3." Pull the person to a standing position as you straighten your knees (Fig. 15.31).

18. Method 2: No transfer belt: (*Note:* Use this method only if directed by the nurse and the care plan.)
   a. Follow steps 17a–c.

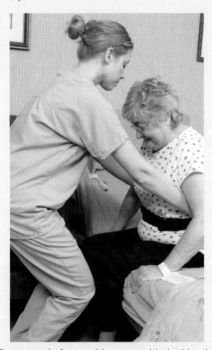

Fig. 15.30 The person's feet and knees are blocked by the nursing assistant's feet and knees. This prevents the person from sliding or falling.

b. Place your hands under the person's arms. Your hands are around the person's shoulder blades (Fig. 15.32).
c. Have the person lean forward.
d. Prevent the person from sliding or falling by doing one of the following:
   (1) Brace your knees against the person's knees. Block the person's feet with your feet.
   (2) Use the knee and foot of one leg to block the person's weak leg or foot. Place your other foot slightly behind you for balance.
   (3) Straddle your legs around the person's weak leg.
e. Explain the "count of 3." See step 17g.
f. Ask the person to push down on the mattress and to stand on "the count of 3." Pull the person up into a standing position as you straighten your knees.

19. Support the person in the standing position. Hold the transfer belt or keep your hands around the person's shoulder blades. Continue to prevent the person from sliding or falling.
20. Turn the person to grasp the far arm of the chair. The legs will touch the edge of the chair (Fig. 15.33).
21. Continue to turn the person until the other armrest is grasped.
22. Lower the person into the chair as you bend your hips and knees. The person assists by leaning forward and bending the elbows and knees (Fig. 15.34).
23. Make sure the hips are to the back of the seat. Position the person in good alignment.
24. Attach the wheelchair front rigging. Position the person's feet on the wheelchair footplates.
25. Cover the person's lap and legs with a lap blanket. Keep the blanket off the floor and the wheels.
26. Remove the transfer belt if used.
27. Position the chair as the person prefers. Lock the wheelchair wheels according to the care plan.

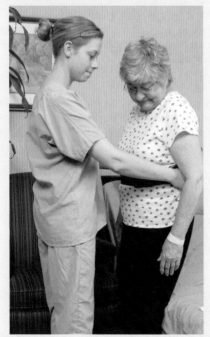

Fig. 15.31 The person is pulled up to a standing position and supported by holding the transfer belt and blocking the person's knees and feet.

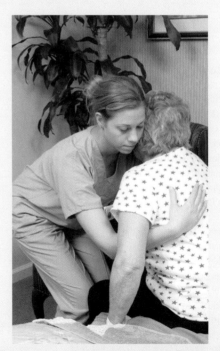

Fig. 15.32 The person is being prepared to stand. The hands are placed under the person's arms and around the shoulder blades.

✳ TRANSFERRING THE PERSON TO A CHAIR OR WHEELCHAIR (NATCEP)—cont'd

Postprocedure

28. Provide for comfort. (See the inside of the front cover.)
29. Place the call light and other needed items within reach.
30. Unscreen the person.
31. Complete a safety check of the room. (See the inside of the front cover.)
32. Decontaminate your hands.
33. Report and record your observations.
34. See procedure: Transferring the Person from a Chair or Wheelchair to Bed (p. ··) to return the person to bed.

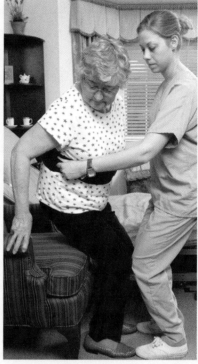

Fig. 15.34 The person holds the armrests, leans forward, and bends the elbows and knees while being lowered into the chair.

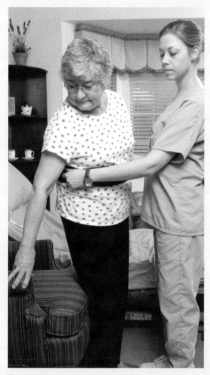

Fig. 15.33 The person is supported while grasping the far arm of the chair. The legs are against the chair.

This skill also covered in *Clinical Skills: Nurse Assisting.*

Chair or Wheelchair to Bed Transfers

Chair or wheelchair to bed transfers have the same rules as bed to chair transfers. If the person is weak on one side, transfer the person so that the strong side moves first. Or the chair or wheelchair is positioned so the person's strong side is near the bed so it moves first.

For example, Mrs. Lee's right side is weak. Her left side is strong. To transfer her from bed to chair, the chair was on the left side of the bed. This allowed her left side (strong side) to move first. Now you will transfer Mrs. Lee back to bed. If the chair is on the left side of the bed, her right side—the weak side—is near the bed. It is not safe to move the weak side first. You need to move the chair to the other side of the bed or turn the chair around. Mrs. Lee's stronger left side will be near the bed. The stronger side moves first for a safe transfer.

✳ TRANSFERRING THE PERSON FROM A CHAIR OR WHEELCHAIR TO BED

Quality of Life

Remember to:

- Knock before entering the person's room.
- Address the person by name.
- Introduce yourself by name and title.
- Explain the procedure to the person before beginning and during the procedure.
- Protect the person's rights during the procedure.
- Handle the person gently during the procedure.

Preprocedure

1. Follow Delegation Guidelines:
   a. Preventing Work-Related Injuries, p. ··
   b. Transferring Persons, p. ··
2. See Promoting Safety and Comfort:
   a. Transfer/Gait Belts (Chapter 12)
   b. Safe Resident Handling, Moving, and Transfers, p. ··
   c. Preventing Work-Related Injuries, p. ··
   d. Transferring Persons, p. ··

Continued

✦ TRANSFERRING THE PERSON FROM A CHAIR OR WHEELCHAIR TO BED—cont'd

    e. Bed to Chair or Wheelchair Transfers, p. ··
3. Collect a transfer belt if needed.
4. Practice hand hygiene.
5. Identify the person. Check the ID bracelet against the assignment sheet. Also call the person by name.
6. Provide for privacy.

Procedure
7. Move furniture for moving space.
8. Raise the head of the bed to a sitting position. The bed is in the lowest position.
9. Move the call light so it is on the strong side when the person is in bed.
10. Position the chair or wheelchair so the person's strong side is next to the bed (Fig. 15.36). Have a coworker help you if necessary.
11. Lock the wheelchair and bed wheels.
12. Remove and fold the lap blanket.
13. Remove the person's feet from the footplates. Raise the footplates. Remove or swing the front rigging out of the way. (The person has on nonskid footwear.)
14. Apply the transfer belt (if needed).
15. Make sure the person's feet are flat on the floor.
16. Stand in front of the person.
17. Ask the person to hold on to the armrests. (If the nurse directs you to do so, place your arms under the person's arms. Your hands are around the shoulder blades.)
18. Have the person lean forward.
19. Grasp the transfer belt on each side if using it. Grasp underneath the belt.
20. Prevent the person from sliding or falling. Do one of the following:
    a. Brace your knees against the person's knees. Block the person's feet with your feet.
    b. Use the knee and foot of one leg to block the person's weak leg or foot. Place your other foot slightly behind you for balance.
    c. Straddle your legs around the person's weak leg.
21. Explain "the count of 3." (See procedure: Transferring the Person to a Chair or Wheelchair, p. ···.)
22. Ask the person to push down on the armrests on "the count of 3." Pull the person into a standing position as you straighten your knees.

23. Support the person in the standing position. Hold the transfer belt or keep your hands around the person's shoulder blades. Continue to prevent the person from sliding or falling.
24. Turn the person to reach the edge of the mattress. The legs will touch the mattress.
25. Continue to turn the person to reach the mattress with both hands.
26. Lower the person onto the bed as you bend your hips and knees. The person assists by leaning forward and bending the elbows and knees.
27. Remove the transfer belt.
28. Remove the robe and footwear.
29. Help the person lie down.

Postprocedure
30. Provide for comfort. (See the inside of the front cover.)
31. Place the call light and other needed items within reach.
32. Raise or lower bed rails. Follow the care plan.
33. Arrange furniture to meet the person's needs.
34. Unscreen the person.
35. Complete a safety check of the room. (See the inside of the front cover.)
36. Decontaminate your hands.
37. Report and record your observations.

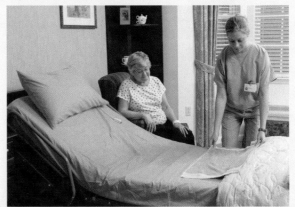

Fig. 15.35 To transfer the person from chair to bed, the chair is positioned so the person's strong side is near the bed.

Mechanical Lifts

Persons who cannot help themselves are transferred with mechanical lifts (Fig. 15.36). So are persons too heavy for the staff to transfer. The devices are used for transfers to and from beds, chairs, stretchers, tubs, shower chairs, toilets, commodes, whirlpools, or vehicles.

    There are manual, battery-operated, and electric lifts. Some lifts have tracks mounted on the ceiling (Fig 15.37).

Slings

The type of sling (Fig 15.38) used depends on the person's size, condition, and other needs. Slings are padded, unpadded, or made of mesh.
- *Standard full sling*—used for normal transfers.

- *Extended length sling*—used for persons with extra-large thighs.
- *Bathing sling*—used to transfer the person directly from the bed or chair into a bathtub. The sling is left in place and attached to the lift during the bath.
- *Toileting sling*—the sling bottom is open. For infection control, each person should have own toileting sling.
- *Amputee sling*—used for the person who has had both legs amputated (double amputee).
- Follow center policy and the manufacturer instructions for washing slings. Also follow center policy for handling and washing contaminated slings. A sling is contaminated if it:
- Has any visible sign of blood, body fluids, secretions, or excretions.
- Is used on a person's bare skin.
- Is used to bathe a person.

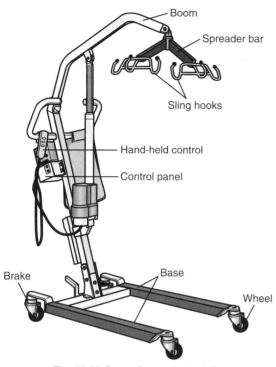

Fig. 15.36 Parts of a mechanical lift.

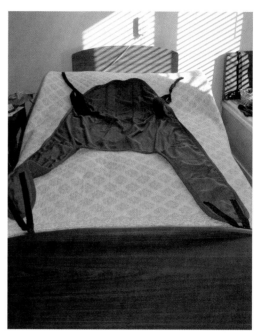

Fig. 15.38 A sling for use with mechanical lift.

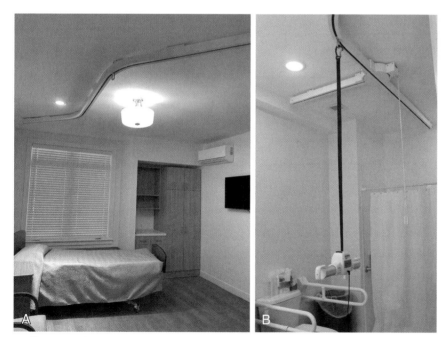

Fig. 15.37 A ceiling-mounted mechanical lift. (A) The ceiling track. (B) The controller.

✳ Using a Mechanical Lift

Before using a lift:
- You must be trained in its use.
- You must be at least 18 years of age.
- It must be in good working condition.
- The sling, straps, hooks, and chains must be in good repair.
- The person's weight must not exceed the lift's capacity.
- At least two staff members are needed.

There are different types of mechanical lifts. Always follow the manufacturer instructions. Many facilities will have periodic employee training sessions for the safe use of mechanical lifts. Follow the center's policy for use of mechanical lifts. The U.S. Department of Labor requires that all operators of mechanical lifts be at least 18 years of age. The following procedure is used as a guide.

See *Delegation Guidelines: Using a Mechanical Lift.*

See *Promoting Safety and Comfort: Using a Mechanical Lift.*

DELEGATION GUIDELINES

Using a Mechanical Lift
When delegated tasks that involve using a mechanical lift, you need this information from the nurse and the care plan:
- The person's dependency level (see Box 15.3)
- What lift to use
- What sling to use—full, extended length, bathing, toileting, amputee
- What size sling to use
- If you should use a padded, unpadded, or mesh sling
- How many staff members are needed to perform the task safely (minimum of two)

PROMOTING SAFETY AND COMFORT

Using a Mechanical Lift
Safety
Always follow the manufacturer instructions. Knowing how to use one lift does not mean that you know how to use others.

If you have questions, ask the nurse. If you have not used a certain lift before, ask for needed training. Ask the nurse to help you until you are comfortable using the lift.

Ensure that the operator of the lift is at least 18 years of age.

Mechanical lifts must be in good working order. Tell the nurse when a lift needs repair or is not working properly.

Some mechanical lifts are powered by batteries. The batteries must be well charged. Many centers will have two batteries for each unit so one can be charged while the other is in use. Follow the manufacturer instructions.

Comfort
The person will be lifted up and off the bed or chair. Falling from the lift is a common fear. To promote the person's mental comfort, always explain the procedure before you begin. Also show the person how the lift works.

Transferring the Person to and from the Toilet
Using the bathroom for elimination promotes dignity, self-esteem, and independence. It also is more private than using a bedpan, urinal, or bedside commode. However, getting to the toilet is hard for persons who use wheelchairs. Bathrooms are often small. There is little room for you or a wheelchair. Therefore, transfers involving wheelchairs and toilets are often hard. Falls and work-related injuries are risks.

Sometimes mechanical lifts are used to transfer the person to and from a toilet. A slide board (see Fig. 15.15) may be used if:
- The wheelchair armrests are removable.
- The person has upper body strength.

TRANSFERRING THE PERSON USING A MECHANICAL LIFT

Quality of Life
Remember to:
- Knock before entering the person's room.
- Address the person by name.
- Introduce yourself by name and title.
- Explain the procedure to the person before beginning and during the procedure.
- Protect the person's rights during the procedure.
- Handle the person gently during the procedure.

Preprocedure
1. Follow Delegation Guidelines:
   a. Preventing Work-Related Injuries, p. ··
   b. Transferring Persons, p. ··
   c. Using a Mechanical Lift
2. See Promoting Safety and Comfort:
   a. Safe Resident Handling, Moving, and Transfers, p. ··
   b. Preventing Work-Related Injuries, p. ··
   c. Transferring Persons, p. ··
   d. Using a Mechanical Lift, p. ··
3. Ask a coworker to help you.
4. Collect:
   - Mechanical lift and sling
   - Armchair or wheelchair
   - Footwear
   - Bath blanket or cushion
   - Lap blanket
5. Practice hand hygiene.

6. Identify the person. Check the ID bracelet against the assignment sheet. Also call the person by name.
7. Provide for privacy.

Procedure
8. Raise the bed for body mechanics. Bed rails are up if used.
9. Lower the head of the bed to a level appropriate for the person. It is as flat as possible.
10. Stand on one side of the bed. Your coworker stands on the other side.
11. Lower the bed rails if up.
12. Center the sling under the person (Fig. 15.39A). To position the sling, turn the person from side to side as if making an occupied bed (Chapter 17). Position the sling according to the manufacturer instructions.
13. Position the person in semi-Fowler position.
14. Place the chair at the head of the bed. It is even with the headboard and about 1 foot away from the bed. Place a folded bath blanket or cushion in the chair.
15. Lock the bed wheels. Lower the bed to its lowest position.
16. Raise the lift so you can position it over the person.
17. Position the lift over the person (see Fig. 15.39B).
18. Lock the lift wheels in position.
19. Attach the sling to the sling hooks (see Fig. 15.39C).
20. Raise the head of the bed to a sitting position.
21. Cross the person's arms over the chest.
22. Raise the lift high enough until the person and sling are free of the bed (see Fig. 15.39D).
 23. Have your coworker support the person's legs as you move the lift and the person away from the bed (see Fig. 15.39E).

✦ TRANSFERRING THE PERSON USING A MECHANICAL LIFT—cont'd

24. Position the lift so the person's back is toward the chair.
25. Position the chair so you can lower the person into it.
26. Lower the person into the chair. Guide the person into the chair (see Fig. 15.39F).
27. Lower the spreader bar to unhook the sling. Remove the sling from under the person unless otherwise indicated.
28. Put footwear on the person. Position the person's feet on the wheelchair footplates.
29. Cover the person's lap and legs with a lap blanket. Keep it off the floor and wheels.
30. Position the chair as the person prefers. Lock the wheelchair wheels according to the care plan.

Postprocedure
31. Provide for comfort. (See the inside of the front cover.)
32. Place the call light and other needed items within the person's reach.
33. Unscreen the person.
34. Complete a safety check of the room. (See the inside of the front cover.)
35. Decontaminate your hands.
36. Report and record your observations.
37. Reverse the procedure to return the person to bed.

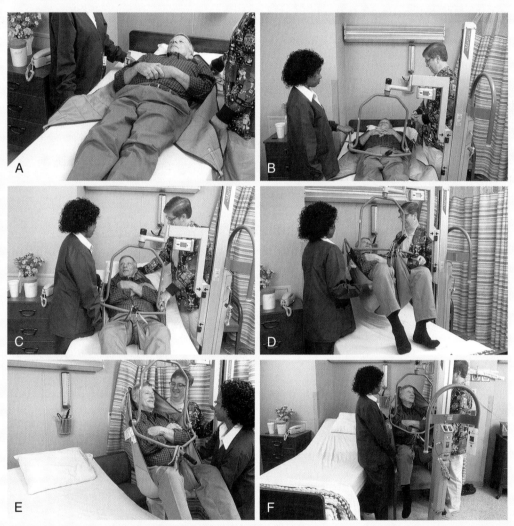

Fig. 15.39 Using a mechanical lift. (A) The sling is positioned under the person. (B) The lift is over the person. (C) The sling is attached to the spreader bar. (D) The lift is raised until the sling and person are off the bed. (E) The person's legs are supported as the person and lift are moved away from the bed. (F) The person is guided into a chair.

This skill also covered in *Clinical Skills: Nurse Assisting.*

- The person has good sitting balance.
- There is enough room to position the wheelchair next to the toilet.

The following procedure can be used if the person can stand and pivot from the wheelchair to the toilet.

See *Promoting Safety and Comfort: Transferring the Person to and from the Toilet.*

PROMOTING SAFETY AND COMFORT

Transferring the Person to and from the Toilet
Safety
Make sure the person has a raised toilet seat. The toilet seat and wheelchair are at the same level.

Check the grab bars by the toilet. If they are loose, tell the nurse. Do not transfer the person to the toilet if the grab bars are not secure.

Follow Standard Precautions and the Bloodborne Pathogen Standard. Wear gloves if the person is incontinent of urine or feces.

Moving the Person to a Stretcher

Stretchers (gurneys) are used to transport persons to other areas. They are used for persons who:

- Cannot sit up.
- Must stay in a lying position.
- Are seriously ill.

The stretcher is covered with a folded flat sheet or bath blanket. A pillow and extra blankets are on hand. With the nurse's permission, raise the head of the stretcher to a Fowler or semi-Fowler position to increase the person's comfort.

TRANSFERRING THE PERSON TO AND FROM THE TOILET

Quality of Life
Remember to:

- Knock before entering the person's room.
- Address the person by name.
- Introduce yourself by name and title.
- Explain the procedure to the person before beginning and during the procedure.
- Protect the person's rights during the procedure.
- Handle the person gently during the procedure.

Preprocedure

1. Follow Delegation Guidelines:
   a. Preventing Work-Related Injuries, p. ··
   b. Transferring Persons, p. ··
2. See Promoting Safety and Comfort:
   a. Transfer/Gait Belts (Chapter 12)
   b. Safe Resident Handling, Moving, and Transfers, p. ··
   c. Preventing Work-Related Injuries, p. ··
   d. Transferring Persons, p. ··
   e. Bed to Chair or Wheelchair Transfers, p. ··
   f. Transferring the Person to and from the Toilet
3. Practice hand hygiene.

Procedure

4. Have the person wear nonskid footwear.
5. Position the wheelchair next to the toilet if there is enough room. If not, position the chair at a right (90-degree) angle to the toilet (Fig. 15.40). It is best if the person's strong side is near the toilet.
6. Lock the wheelchair wheels.
7. Raise the footplates. Remove or swing the front rigging out of the way.
8. Apply the transfer belt.
9. Help the person unfasten clothing.
10. Use the transfer belt to help the person stand and turn to the toilet. (See procedure: Transferring the Person to a Chair or Wheelchair, p. ··.) The person uses the grab bars to turn to the toilet.
11. Support the person with the transfer belt while the person lowers clothing. Or have the person hold on to the grab bars for support. Lower the person's pants and undergarments.
12. Use the transfer belt to lower the person onto the toilet seat. Make sure the person is properly positioned on the toilet.
13. Tell the person you will stay nearby. Remind the person to use the call light or to call for you when help is needed. Stay with the person if required by the care plan.
14. Close the bathroom door to provide for privacy.

15. Stay near the bathroom. Complete other tasks in the person's room. Check on the person every 5 minutes.
16. Knock on the bathroom door when the person calls for you.
17. Help with wiping, perineal care (Chapter 18), flushing, and hand washing as needed. Wear gloves and practice hand hygiene after removing the gloves.
18. Use the transfer belt to help the person stand.
19. Help the person raise and secure clothing.
20. Use the transfer belt to transfer the person to the wheelchair. (See procedure: Transferring the Person to a Chair or Wheelchair, p. ··.)
21. Make sure the person's buttocks are to the back of the seat. Position the person in good alignment.
22. Position the person's feet on the footplates.
23. Remove the transfer belt.
24. Cover the person's lap and legs with a lap blanket. Keep the blanket off the floor and wheels.
25. Position the chair as the person prefers. Lock the wheelchair wheels according to the care plan.

Postprocedure

26. Provide for comfort. (See the inside of the front cover.)
27. Place the call light and other need items within the person's reach.
28. Unscreen the person.
29. Complete a safety check of the room. (See the inside of the front cover.)
30. Practice hand hygiene.
31. Report and record your observations.

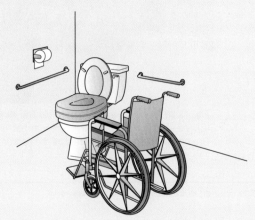

Fig. 15.40 The wheelchair is placed at a right (90-degree) angle to the toilet.

A drawsheet, turning pad, large incontinence underpad, slide sheet, or slide board is used. At least two or three staff members are needed for a safe transfer. OSHA recommends the following:

- If the person weighs less than 100 pounds—use a lateral sliding aid and two staff members
- If the person weighs 100 to 200 pounds—use a lateral sliding aid or a friction-reducing device and two staff members
- If the person weighs more than 200 pounds, use one of the following:
- A lateral sliding aid and three staff members
- A friction-reducing device or lateral transfer device and two staff members
- A mechanical lateral transfer device with a built-in slide board

Safety straps are used when the person is on the stretcher. The stretcher side rails are kept up during the transport. The stretcher is moved feet first, so the staff member at the head of the stretcher can watch the person's breathing and color during the transport. Never leave a person on a stretcher alone.

See *Promoting Safety and Comfort: Moving the Person to a Stretcher.*

PROMOTING SAFETY AND COMFORT

Moving the Person to a Stretcher
Safety
Protect yourself and the person from injury:
- Position the stretcher and bed surfaces as close as possible to each other.
- Avoid extended reaches and bending your back. You may need to kneel on the bed or stretcher.
- Follow the rules for stretcher safety (Chapter 11).
- Make sure the bed and stretcher wheels are locked.
- Practice good body mechanics and follow the guidelines in Box 15.2.
- Keep the person in good alignment.
- Make sure you have enough help.
- Hold the person securely. You must not drop the person onto the floor.

MOVING THE PERSON TO A STRETCHER

Quality of Life
Remember to:
- Knock before entering the person's room.
- Address the person by name.
- Introduce yourself by name and title.
- Explain the procedure to the person before beginning and during the procedure.
- Protect the person's rights during the procedure.
- Handle the person gently during the procedure.

Preprocedure
1. Follow Delegation Guidelines:
   a. Preventing Work-Related Injuries, p. ··
   b. Transferring Persons, p. ··
2. See Promoting Safety and Comfort:
   a. Safe Resident Handling, Moving, and Transfers, p. ··
   b. Preventing Work-Related Injuries, p. ··
   c. Transferring Persons, p. ··
   d. Moving the Person to a Stretcher
3. Ask one or two staff members to help you.
4. Collect:
   - Stretcher covered with a sheet or bath blanket
   - Bath blanket
   - Pillow(s) if needed
   - Slide sheet, slide board, drawsheet, or other assist device
5. Practice hand hygiene.
6. Identify the person. Check the ID bracelet against the assignment sheet. Also call the person by name.
7. Provide for privacy.
8. Raise the bed and stretcher for body mechanics.

Procedure
9. Position yourself and coworkers.
   a. One or two workers stand on the side of the bed where the stretcher will be.
   b. One worker stands on the other side of the bed.
10. Lower the head of the bed. It is as flat as possible.
11. Lower the bed rails if used.
12. Cover the person with a bath blanket. Fan-fold top linens to the foot of the bed.
13. Position the assist device. Or loosen the drawsheet on each side.
14. Use the assist device to move the person to the side of the bed. This is the side where the stretcher will be.
15. Protect the person from falling. Hold the far arm and leg.
16. Have your coworkers position the stretcher next to the bed. They stand behind the stretcher (Fig. 15.41A).
17. Lock the bed and stretcher wheels.
18. Grasp the assist device (see Fig. 15.41B).
19. Transfer the person to the stretcher on "the count of 3." Center the person on the stretcher.
20. Place a pillow(s) under the person's head and shoulders if allowed. Raise the head of the stretcher if allowed.
21. Cover the person. Provide for comfort.
22. Fasten the safety straps. Raise the side rails.
23. Unlock the stretcher wheels. Transport the person.

Postprocedure
24. Decontaminate your hands.
25. Report and record:
   - The time of the transport
   - Where the person was transported to
   - Who went with the person
   - How the transfer was tolerated
26. Reverse the procedure to return the person to bed.

Continued

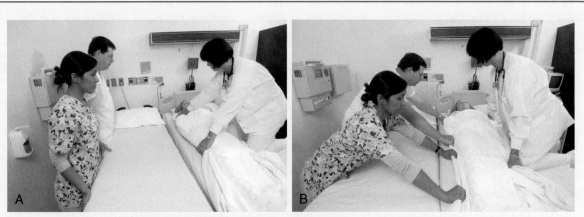

Fig. 15.41 Transferring the person to a stretcher. (A) The stretcher is against the bed and is held in place. (B) A drawsheet is used to transfer the person from the bed to a stretcher.

This skill also covered in *Clinical Skills: Nurse Assisting.*

REPOSITIONING IN A CHAIR OR WHEELCHAIR

The person can slide down into the chair. For good alignment and safety, the person's back and buttocks must be against the back of the chair.

Some persons can help with repositioning. Others need help. If the person cannot help, a mechanical lift is needed to reposition the person. Follow the nurse's directions and the care plan for the best way to reposition a person in a chair or wheelchair. *Do not pull the person from behind the chair or wheelchair.*

If the person's chair reclines, do the following:
- Ask a coworker to help you.
- Lock the wheels.
- Recline the chair.
- Position a friction-reducing device (drawsheet or slide sheet) under the person.
- Use the device to move the person up. See procedure: *Moving the Person Up in Bed with an Assist Device*, p. ⋯.

The following method can be used if the person is alert and cooperative. The person must be able to follow directions and have the strength to help.
- Lock the wheelchair wheels.
- Remove or swing the front rigging out of the way.
- Position the person's feet flat on the floor.
- Apply a transfer belt.
- Position the person's arms on the armrests.
- Stand in front of the person. Block the person's knees and feet with your knees and feet.
- Grasp the transfer belt on each side while the person leans forward.
- Ask the person to push with the feet and arms on "the count of 3."
- Move the person back into the chair on the count of "3" as the person pushes with the feet and arms (Fig. 15.42).

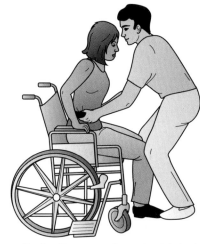

Fig. 15.42 Repositioning the person in a wheelchair. A transfer belt is used to move the person to the back of the chair.

🧑 QUALITY OF LIFE

Nursing centers provide care in a manner that maintains and improves each person's quality of life, health, and safety. Proper body mechanics protect the person from injuries that could affect health and ability to function.

Remaining independent to the extent possible promotes dignity, self-esteem, and pride. Talk with the person during the moving process. Ask about the person's preferences. Doing so promotes comfort, independence, and social interaction.

The person's rights also are protected by allowing personal choice when possible. If safety is not affected, let the person choose such things as bed positions, where the chair or wheelchair is positioned, and when to get up or go back to bed. Always check with the nurse and the care plan to make sure the person's choices are safe. Also let the person help with moving and transferring to the extent possible.

The person has the right to be free from restraint. Restraints are used only with the person's consent. Many procedures involve raising the bed for good body mechanics. Always check with the nurse and the care plan about using bed rails. If the person does not use bed rails and you need to raise the bed, you need to have a coworker help you. Your coworker stands on the other side of the bed to protect the person from falling from that side. When you use bed rails, always explain to the person why you are using them.

When moving or transferring, always respect the person's privacy. Properly cover the person. For example, a person is wearing a gown that is open in the back. The person's back is exposed. Apply a robe or another gown to cover the person's backside. Use a covering that is safe during the transfer. Avoid long robes or robes with long ties. These could get caught or cause the person to fall. Expose only the body part involved in the procedure. Close window coverings as needed.

Persons who need help moving and transferring have limited independence. They cannot turn or move in bed alone, sit up in a chair alone, or go to the bathroom alone. They may feel embarrassed or helpless. To promote independence:

- Focus on the person's abilities.
- Encourage the person.
- Let the person help as much as safely possible.
- Tell the person when you notice even small improvements. Such motivation can improve self-esteem and aid in healing.

❓ TIME TO REFLECT

You normally work the day shift but have agreed to work a week of overnight shifts to cover for a staff member who is on vacation. You are familiar with Mr. Rodriguez, an elderly man who is dependent for all his care. During the day you routinely help him change position at least every 2 hours. While working the night shift, you ask another assistant to help you turn Mr. Rodriguez. The assistant replies, "We usually don't disturb Mr. Rodriguez much at night—he gets angry if awakened. If you turn him once during the shift, that will be good." How would you respond in this situation?

REVIEW QUESTIONS

Circle the BEST answer.

1. Good body mechanics involve the following *except*
   a. Good posture
   b. Balance
   c. Using the strongest and largest muscles
   d. Having the job fit the worker

2. Good alignment means
   a. The area on which an object rests
   b. Having the head, trunk, arms, and legs aligned with one another
   c. Using muscles, tendons, ligaments, and joints correctly
   d. The back-lying or supine position

3. These actions are about body mechanics. Which action is *not* correct?
   a. Hold objects away from your body when lifting, moving, or carrying them
   b. Face the direction you are working to prevent twisting
   c. Push, pull, or slide heavy objects
   d. Use both hands and arms to lift, move, or carry heavy objects

4. You are turning a person in bed. Which action is *not* correct?
   a. Explain the procedure to the person
   b. Keep the far bed rail down
   c. Position the person in good alignment
   d. Have pillows ready to support the back

5. Residents are repositioned at least every
   a. 30 minutes
   b. 1 hour
   c. 2 hours
   d. 3 hours

6. The back-lying position is called
   a. Fowler position
   b. Supine position
   c. Prone position
   d. Lateral position

7. Breathing is usually easier in
   a. Fowler position
   b. Supine position
   c. Lateral position
   d. Prone position

8. A pillow is placed against the person's back in
   a. Fowler position
   b. Prone position
   c. Lateral position
   d. Supine position

9. A person's skin rubs against the sheet. This is called
   a. Shearing
   b. Friction
   c. Ergonomics
   d. Posture

10. Which occurs when a person slides down in bed?
    a. Shearing
    b. Friction
    c. Ergonomics
    d. Posture

11. Before side-turning a person, you
    a. Move the person to the side of the bed where the back will be
    b. Move the person to the middle of the bed
    c. Lock arms with the person
    d. Position pillows for comfort

12. The logrolling procedure
    a. Is used after spinal cord injuries or surgeries
    b. Requires a transfer belt
    c. Requires a mechanical lift
    d. Involves a stretcher and a drawsheet

13. When getting ready to dangle a person, you need to know
    a. Which side is stronger
    b. If bed rails are used
    c. If a mechanical lift is needed
    d. If a transfer belt is needed

14. For chair and wheelchair transfers, the person must
    a. Have a drawsheet or other assist device
    b. Have the bed rails up
    c. Use a mechanical lift
    d. Wear nonskid footwear
15. When transferring the person to bed, a chair, or the toilet
    a. The person's strong side moves first
    b. The person's weak side moves first
    c. Pillows are used for support
    d. The transfer belt is removed
16. You are going to use a mechanical lift. You must do the following *except*
    a. Follow the manufacturer instructions
    b. Make sure the lift works
    c. Compare the person's weight to the lift's weight limit
    d. Use a transfer belt

17. To safely transfer a person with a mechanical lift, at least
    a. One worker is needed
    b. Two workers are needed
    c. Three workers are needed
    d. Four workers are needed
18. These statements are about transfers to and from a stretcher? Which is *false*?
    a. The bed and stretcher wheels must be locked
    b. The stretcher's side rails are raised when the person is on the stretcher
    c. Once on the stretcher, the person can be left alone
    d. At least two workers are needed for a safe transfer

See Appendix A for answers to these questions.

16

The Resident's Unit

OBJECTIVES

- Define the key terms and key abbreviations listed in this chapter.
- Identify the room temperatures required by OBRA and the CMS.
- Describe how to protect the person from drafts.
- List ways to prevent or reduce odors and noise.
- Explain how lighting affects comfort.
- Describe the basic bed positions.
- Identify the persons at risk for entrapment in the hospital bed system.

- Identify hospital bed system entrapment zones.
- Explain how to use the furniture and equipment in the person's unit.
- Describe how a bathroom is equipped for the person's use.
- Describe how to provide for safety, privacy, and comfort in the person's unit.
- Explain how to maintain the person's unit.
- Describe OBRA and CMS requirements for resident rooms.
- Explain how to promote quality of life.

KEY TERMS

Fowler position A semi-sitting position; the head of the bed is raised between 45 and 60 degrees

full visual privacy Having the means to be completely free from public view while in bed

high-Fowler position A semi-sitting position; the head of the bed is raised between 60 and 90 degrees

resident unit The personal space, furniture, and equipment provided for the person by the nursing center

reverse Trendelenburg position The head of the bed is raised, and the foot of the bed is lowered

semi-Fowler position The head of the bed is raised 30 degrees; or the head of the bed is raised 30 degrees, and the knee portion is raised 15 degrees

Trendelenburg position The head of the bed is lowered, and the foot of the bed is raised

KEY ABBREVIATIONS

CMS Centers for Medicare & Medicaid Services

F Fahrenheit

FDA Food and Drug Administration

OBRA Omnibus Budget Reconciliation Act of 1987

Nursing centers are designed to provide comfort, safety, and privacy. The intent is to have resident units be as personal and homelike as possible. A resident unit is the personal space, furniture, and equipment provided for the person by the nursing center (Fig. 16.1).

Some residents have private rooms. Others share a room with another person. This area is private. It is treated like the person's home.

Residents bring some furniture and personal items from home. As space allows, the person chooses where to place personal items. This promotes dignity and self-esteem. However, a resident cannot take or use another person's space. Doing so violates the other person's rights.

COMFORT

Age, illness, and activity affect comfort. So do temperature, ventilation, odors, noise, and lighting. These factors are controlled to meet the person's needs.

Temperature and Ventilation

Heating and air-conditioning systems maintain a comfortable temperature. Most healthy people are comfortable when the temperature is 68°F (Fahrenheit) to 74°F. This range may be too hot or too cold for others. Older persons and those who are ill may need higher temperatures for comfort. Nursing centers maintain a temperature range of 71°F to 81°F. This is a requirement of the Omnibus Budget Reconciliation Act of 1987 (OBRA) and the Centers for Medicare & Medicaid Services (CMS).

Persons who are less active usually do not like cool areas. Nor do those who need help moving about. They must be dressed warmly. They also need warm room temperatures. You may find the rooms rather warm.

Stale room air and lingering odors affect comfort and rest. Ventilation systems provide fresh air and move room air. Drafts occur as air moves. Older persons and those who are ill are sensitive to drafts. To protect them from drafts:

- Make sure they wear the correct clothing.

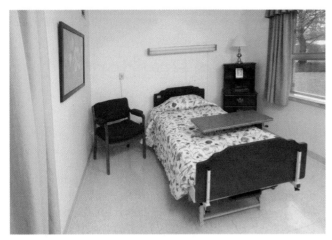

Fig. 16.1 Furniture and equipment in a resident's unit.

- Make sure they wear enough clothing. Many wear sweaters during warm weather.
- Offer lap robes to those in chairs and wheelchairs. Lap robes cover the legs.
- Provide enough blankets for warmth.
- Cover them with bath blankets when giving care.
- Move them from drafty areas.

Odors

Many odors occur in nursing centers. Food aromas and flower scents are pleasant. Bowel movements and urine have embarrassing odors, as do draining wounds and vomitus. Body, breath, and smoking odors may offend others.

Some people are very sensitive to odors. They may become nauseated. Good nursing care, ventilation, and housekeeping practices help prevent odors. To reduce odors:

- Empty, clean, and disinfect bedpans, urinals, commodes, and kidney basins promptly.
- Check to make sure toilets are flushed.
- Check incontinent persons often (Chapters 22 and 23).
- Clean persons who are wet or soiled from urine, feces, vomitus, or wound drainage.
- Change wet or soiled linens and clothing promptly.
- Keep laundry containers closed.
- Follow center policy for wet or soiled linens and clothing.
- Dispose of incontinence and ostomy products promptly (Chapters 22 and 23).
- Remove plastic trash can liners promptly, tie off bag, and transport to soiled utility area.
- Provide good hygiene to prevent body and breath odors (Chapter 18).
- Use room deodorizers as needed and allowed by center policy. Sometimes odors remain after removing the cause. Do not use sprays around persons with breathing problems. Ask the nurse if you are unsure.

Smoke odors present special problems. Residents, visitors, and staff smoke only in the areas allowed. If you smoke, follow the center's policy. Practice hand washing after handling smoking materials and before giving care. Give careful attention to your uniforms, hair, and breath because of smoke odors.

The center is the person's home. Keep it free of unpleasant odors.

Noise

❖ The CMS requires comfortable sound levels. A "comfortable" sound level:
- Does not interfere with a person's hearing.
- Promotes privacy when privacy is desired.
◆ • Allows the person to take part in social activities.

Many older and ill persons are sensitive to noises and sounds. Common health care sounds may disturb them. Examples include the following:
- The clanging of equipment
- The clatter of dishes and meal trays
- Loud voices
- Ringing phones, televisions, radios, among other communication devices
- Intercom systems and call lights
- Equipment needing repair
- Wheels on stretchers, wheelchairs, carts, and other items needing oil
- Cleaning equipment such as vacuum cleaners
- Alarms on exit doors or personal sensor alarms

Loud talking and laughter in hallways and at the nurses' station are common. Residents may think that the staff is talking and laughing about them.

People want to know the cause and meaning of new sounds. This relates to safety and security needs. Residents may find sounds dangerous, frightening, or irritating. They may become upset, anxious, and uncomfortable. What is noise to one person may not be noise to another. For example, a teenager enjoys loud music, but it may bother adults.

Nursing centers are designed to reduce noise. Window coverings, carpets, and acoustical tiles absorb noise. Plastic items make less noise than metal equipment (bedpans, urinals, wash basins). To decrease noise:
- Control your voice.
- Handle equipment carefully.
- Keep equipment in good working order.
- Answer phones, call lights, and intercoms promptly.
  See *Residents with Dementia: Noise.*
  See *Focus on Communication: Noise.*

Lighting

❖ The CMS requires comfortable lighting. Such lighting:
- Lessens glares.
- Allows the resident to control the intensity, location, and direction of light.
- Allows persons who are visually impaired to maintain or increase independent
◆ functioning.

Good lighting is needed for safety and comfort. Glares, shadows, and dull lighting can cause falls, headaches, and eyestrain. A bright room is cheerful. Dim light is better for relaxing and rest.

RESIDENTS WITH DEMENTIA

Noise

Persons with dementia do not understand what is happening around them. They do not react to common, everyday sounds as other people do. For example, a ringing phone may frighten a person with dementia. The person may not know or understand the sound and may have an extreme reaction to the sound (Chapter 40). The reaction may be more severe at night. This is likely when the sound awakens the person suddenly. A dark, strange room can make the problem worse.

How do you feel when a strange sound wakes you? Do you feel safe and secure? Or are you afraid?

FOCUS ON COMMUNICATION

Noise

Reducing noise requires cooperation from all staff members. To reduce noise:
- Do not talk loudly in the hallways or nurses' station.
- If necessary, politely ask others to speak more softly.
- Avoid unnecessary conversation. Always be professional. Do not discuss inappropriate topics at work. Others may overhear and become offended.

Adjust lighting to meet the person's changing needs. Window coverings are adjusted as needed. The overbed light can provide soft, medium, or bright lighting. Some centers have ceiling lights. They provide soft to very bright light.

Persons with poor vision need bright light. This is very important at mealtime and when moving about in the room and center. Bright lighting also helps the staff perform procedures.

Always keep light controls within the person's reach. This protects the right to personal choice.

See *Residents with Dementia: Lighting.*

RESIDENTS WITH DEMENTIA

Lighting

In dementia care units, lighting is adjusted to help control agitated and aggressive behaviors. Soft, nonglare lights are relaxing. They can decrease agitation. Brighter lighting may improve orientation because the person can see surroundings more clearly.

ROOM FURNITURE AND EQUIPMENT

Rooms are furnished and equipped to meet basic needs. The room has furniture and equipment for comfort, sleep, elimination, nutrition, hygiene, and activity. There is equipment to communicate with staff, family, and friends. The right to privacy is considered.

The Bed

Beds have electrical or manual controls. Beds are raised horizontally to give care. This reduces bending and reaching. The lowest horizontal position lets the person get out of bed with ease (Fig. 16.2). The head of the bed is flat or raised varying degrees.

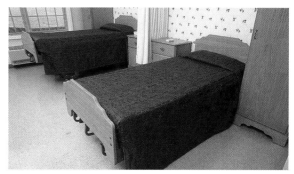
Fig. 16.2 One bed is in the highest horizontal position. The other bed is in the lowest horizontal position.

Electric beds are common. Controls are on a side panel, bed rail, or the footboard (Fig. 16.3A). Some controls are handheld devices (see Fig. 16.3B). Alert and oriented residents are taught to use the controls safely. They are warned not to raise the bed to the high position or to adjust the bed to harmful positions. They are told of any position limits or restrictions.

Most electric beds "lock" into any position by the staff. The person cannot adjust the bed to unsafe positions. Persons restricted to certain positions may need their beds locked. So may persons with confusion or dementia.

Manual beds have cranks at the foot of the bed (Fig. 16.4):
- Left crank—raises or lowers the head of the bed
- Right crank—adjusts the knee portion
- Center crank—raises or lowers the entire bed horizontally

The cranks are pulled up for use. They are kept down at all other times. Cranks in the "up" position are safety hazards. Anyone walking past may bump into them.

See *Promoting Safety and Comfort: The Bed.*

PROMOTING SAFETY AND COMFORT

The Bed

Safety

Beds have bed rails and wheels. Bed wheels (Chapter 11) are locked at *all* times except when moving the bed. They must be locked when you:
- Give bedside care.
- Transfer the person to and from the bed. The person can be injured if the bed moves, and so can you.

Use bed rails as the nurse and care plan direct. Otherwise the person could suffer injury or harm.

Comfort

Some persons spend a lot of time in bed. Make sure the bed is adjusted to meet the person's needs. Tell the nurse if the person complains about the bed or mattress.

Bed Positions

The six basic bed positions are:
- *Flat*—This is the usual sleeping position. The position is used after spinal cord injury or surgery and for cervical traction.

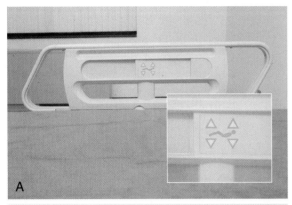

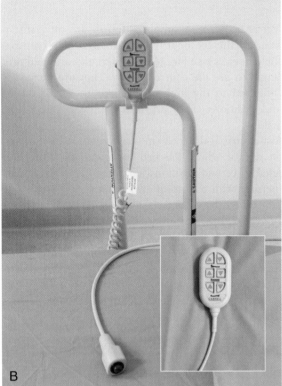

Fig. 16.3 Controls for an electric bed. (A) Controls in the bed rail. (B) Handheld bed control *(see inset)* can be attached to the bed rail.

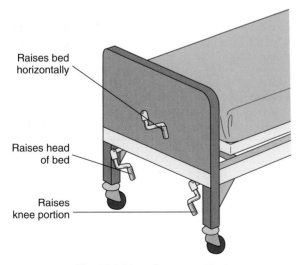

Raises bed horizontally

Raises head of bed

Raises knee portion

Fig. 16.4 Manually operated bed.

- *Fowler position*—Fowler position is a semi-sitting position. The head of the bed is raised between 45 and 60 degrees (Fig. 16.5). See Chapter 15.
- *High-Fowler position*—High-Fowler position is a semi-sitting position. The head of the bed is raised between 60 and 90 degrees (Fig. 16.6).
- *Semi-Fowler position*—In semi-Fowler position, the head of the bed is raised 30 degrees (Fig. 16.7). Some centers define semi-Fowler position as when the head of the bed is raised 30 degrees and the knee portion is raised 15 degrees. This position is comfortable and prevents sliding down in bed. However, raising the knee portion can interfere with circulation in the legs. To give safe care, know the definition used by your center. Also check with the nurse before using this position.
- *Trendelenburg position*—In Trendelenburg position, the head of the bed is lowered and the foot of the bed is raised (Fig. 16.8). A doctor orders the position. It is used in emergency situations when a person experiences shock. Blocks are placed under the legs at the foot of the bed, or the bed frame is tilted.
- *Reverse Trendelenburg position*—In reverse Trendelenburg position, the head of the bed is raised and the foot of the

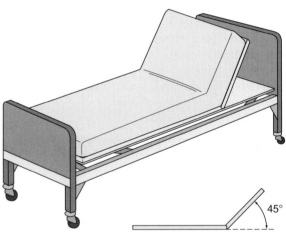

45°

Fig. 16.5 Fowler position.

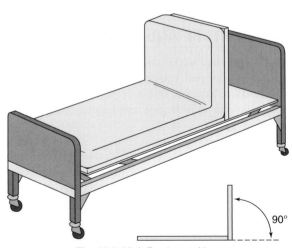

90°

Fig. 16.6 High-Fowler position.

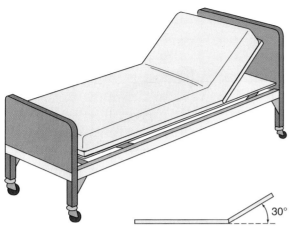

Fig. 16.7 Semi-Fowler position.

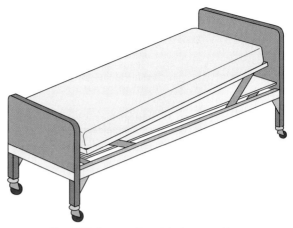

Fig. 16.9 Reverse Trendelenburg position.

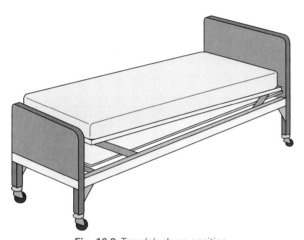

Fig. 16.8 Trendelenburg position.

bed is lowered (Fig. 16.9). Blocks are placed under the legs at the head of the bed, or the bed frame is tilted. This position requires a doctor's order.

Bed Safety

Bed safety involves the *hospital bed system*. The Food and Drug Administration (FDA) defines the hospital bed system as the bed frame and its parts. The parts include the mattress, bed rails, headboard and footboard, and bed attachments. Some nursing centers use beds that have removable bed rails. Many individuals need no bed rails at all. *Entrapment* within parts of the hospital bed system is a risk. That is, the person can get caught, trapped, or entangled in spaces created by bed rails, the mattress, the bed frame, the headboard, or the footboard. Serious injuries and deaths have occurred from head, neck, and chest entrapment. Arm and leg entrapment also can occur. Persons at greatest risk include those who:

- Are older.
- Are frail.
- Are confused or disoriented.
- Are restless.
- Have uncontrolled body movements.

- Have poor muscle control.
- Are small.
- Are restrained (Chapter 13).

Hospital bed systems have seven entrapment zones (Figs. 16.10 and 16.11). You may feel that a person is at risk for entrapment. Report your concerns to the nurse at once. Also, always check the person for entrapment. If a person is caught, trapped, or entangled in the bed or any of its parts, try to release the person. Also call for the nurse at once.

The Overbed Table

The overbed table (see Fig. 16.1) is placed over the bed by sliding the base under the bed. It is raised or lowered for the person in bed or in a chair. Turn the handle or push the lever to adjust the table. It is used for meals, writing, reading, and other activities.

Many overbed tables have a storage area under the top for beauty, hair care, shaving, or other personal items. Many also have a flip-up mirror for grooming.

The nursing team uses the overbed table as a work area. Only clean and sterile items are placed on the table. Never place bedpans, urinals, or soiled linen on the overbed table. Clean the table after using it for a work surface. Also clean it before serving meal trays.

The Bedside Stand

The bedside stand is next to the bed. It is used to store personal items and personal care equipment. It has a top drawer and a lower cabinet with shelves or drawers (Fig. 16.12). The top drawer is used for money, eyeglasses, dentures, hearing aids, books, among other items.

The top shelf or middle drawer is used for the wash basin. The wash basin holds personal items—soap and soap dish, powder, lotion, deodorant, towels, washcloth, bath blanket, and sleepwear. An emesis basin or kidney basin (shaped like a kidney) holds oral hygiene items. The kidney basin is stored in the top drawer, middle drawer, or on the top shelf. The bedpan and its cover, the urinal, and toilet paper are stored on the lower shelf or in the bottom drawer.

Zone 1: Within the rail

Zone 2: Between the top of the compressed mattress and the bottom of the rail, between the supports

Zone 3: Between the rail and the mattress

Zone 4: Between the top of the compressed mattress and the bottom of the rail, at the end of the rail

Zone 5: Between the split bed rails

Zone 6: Between the end of the rail and the side edge of the head-board or foot-board

Zone 7: Between the head- or foot-board and the mattress end

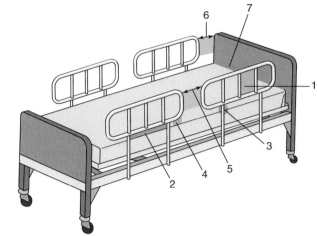

Fig. 16.10 Hospital bed system entrapment zones. (Redrawn from US Food and Drug Administration: *Hospital bed system dimensional and assessment guidance to reduce entrapment*, Silver Spring, MD, 2006, Author.)

The top of the stand is often used for tissues and other personal items. A radio, clock, photos, phone, flowers, cards, and gifts are examples. Some stands have a side or back rod for towels and washcloths.

Place only clean and sterile items on the bedside stand. Never place bedpans, urinals, or soiled linens on the top of the stand. Clean the bedside stand after using it for a work surface.

Chairs

The person's unit has at least one chair for personal and visitor use (see Fig. 16.1). The chair is usually upholstered with arm-rests. It must be comfortable and sturdy. It must not move or tip during transfers. The person should be able to get in and out of the chair with ease. It should not be too low or too soft. Nursing center residents may bring chairs from home. Some residents may have a reclining chair or an electric reclining/lift chair.

Privacy Curtains

❖ *OBRA and the CMS require that rooms be equipped and designed for full visual privacy.* Full visual privacy is having the means to be completely free from public view while in bed. The privacy curtain helps provide full visual privacy. It extends around the bed.

The curtain is pulled around the bed to provide privacy for the person (Chapter 2). Rooms with more than one bed have a privacy curtain between the units. *Always pull the curtain completely around the bed before giving care.*

Privacy curtains prevent others from seeing the person. They do not block sound or voices. Others in the room can hear sounds or talking behind the curtain.

Personal Care Items

Personal care items are used for hygiene and elimination. A bedpan and urinal are provided. The center also provides a wash basin, kidney basin, water pitcher and cup, and soap and a soap dish (Fig. 16.13). Some provide powder, lotion, tooth-brush, toothpaste, mouthwash, tissues, and a comb.

Often residents bring their own oral hygiene equipment, hair care supplies, and deodorant. Some also prefer their own soap, lotion, and powder. Respect the person's choices in personal care products.

The Call System

❖ *The CMS requires a resident call system. When in their rooms, using the toilet, or in a bathing area, residents must be able to contact the staff at the nurses' station.* The call system lets the person signal for help. The call light may be at the end of a long cord (Fig. 16.14A). In resident units, it may be attached to the bed or chair. (See p. 238 for call lights in bathrooms.) Some are cordless models and may be placed on a table near the person (see Fig. 16.14B). Always keep the call light within the person's reach—in the room, bathroom, and shower or tub room. In some centers the residents wear the call signal around their neck like a pendant (see Fig. 16.14C).

To get help, the person presses a button on the call light. In some centers the call light at the bedside (bathroom, shower or tub room) is connected to a light above the room door. The call light also connects to a light panel or intercom system at the nurses' station (Fig. 16.15). These tell the staff that the person needs help. In some nursing centers, the signal is transmitted to receiving pagers that the nursing assistants wear or carry in

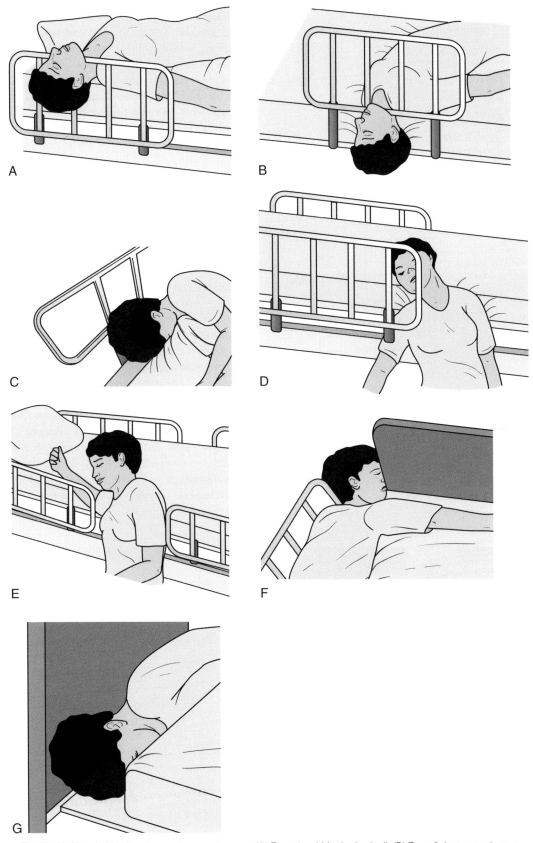

Fig. 16.11 Hospital bed system entrapment zones. (A) Zone 1: within the bed rail. (B) Zone 2: between the top of the compressed mattress and the bottom of the bed rail and between the rail supports. (C) Zone 3: between the bed rail and the mattress. (D) Zone 4: between the top of the compressed mattress and the bottom of the bed rail and at the end of the bed rail. (E) Zone 5: between the split bed rails. (F) Zone 6: between the end of the bed rail and the side edge of the headboard or footboard. (G) Zone 7: between the headboard or footboard and the end of the mattress. (Redrawn from US Food and Drug Administration: *Hospital bed system dimensional and assessment guidance to reduce entrapment,* Silver Spring, MD, 2006, Author.)

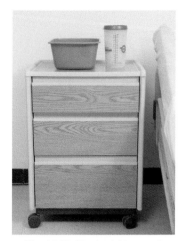

Fig. 16.12 The bedside stand.

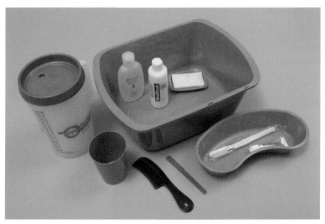

Fig. 16.13 Personal care items.

their pockets. The staff member shuts off the light at the bedside when responding to the call for help.

An intercom system lets the staff talk with the person from the nurses' station. The person tells what is needed. Then the light is turned off at the station. Persons who are hard of hearing may have problems using an intercom. Be careful when using an intercom. Remember confidentiality. Persons nearby can hear what you and the person say.

Some call lights are turned on by tapping them with a hand or fist (Fig. 16.16). They are useful for persons with limited hand mobility.

The person is taught how to use the call system when admitted to the center. Some people cannot use call lights. Examples are persons who are confused or in a coma. The care plan lists special communication measures. Check these persons often. Make sure their needs are met.

The term "call light" is used in this book when referring to the call system. You must:

- Keep the call light within the person's reach. Even if the person cannot use the call light, keep it within reach for use by visitors and staff. They may need to signal for help.
- Place the call light on the person's strong side.
- Remind the person to signal when help is needed.
- Answer call lights promptly. The person signals when help is needed. For example, the person may have an urgent need to use the bathroom. Promptly helping the person to the bathroom prevents embarrassing problems. You also help prevent infection, skin breakdown, pressure ulcers, and falls.
- Answer bathroom and shower or tub room call lights at once.

See *Teamwork and Time Management: The Call System.*
See *Focus on Communication: The Call System.*

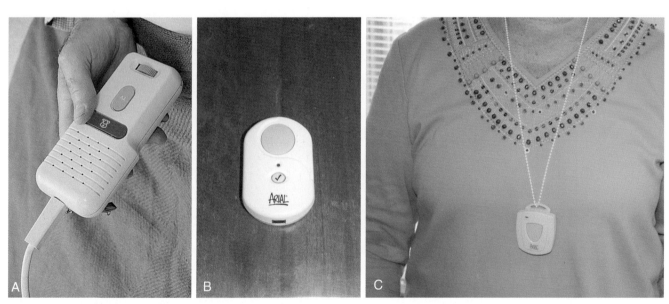

Fig. 16.14 (A) The call light button is pressed when help is needed. (B) A wireless call button. (C) A pendant call button.

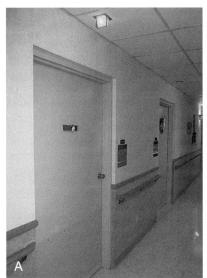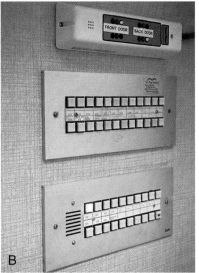

Fig. 16.15 (A) Light above the room door. (B) Light panel and intercom at the nurses' station.

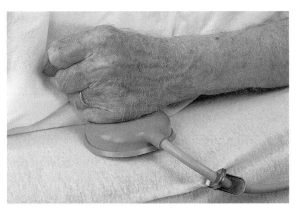

Fig. 16.16 Call light for a person with limited hand mobility.

- "Mr. Duncan, I'll be happy to take your meal tray. I'll tell your nursing assistant what you ate."
- "Mrs. Palmer, do you use the bathroom or the bedpan?"

Sometimes a resident may use the call light often to ask for help. Do not delay in meeting the person's needs. Never take the person's call light away. This is not safe. Avoid statements that make the person feel like a burden. For example, do not say:

- "I just helped you to the bathroom. Can't you wait?"
- "I was just in your room. What do you want now?"

Do not discourage the person from asking for help. The person may try to do something alone. This could cause injury. Tell the nurse. Your coworkers can help you meet the person's needs.

TEAMWORK AND TIME MANAGEMENT

The Call System

Residents use their call lights when they need help. A person may put on a call light when you are with another person. The same may happen to another nursing team member. If nursing team members answer call lights for each other, lights are answered promptly. Residents receive quality care. Everyone is responsible for answering call lights even if not assigned to the person.

FOCUS ON COMMUNICATION

The Call System

You will answer call lights for coworkers. You may not know the residents and they may not know you. To promote quality of life and promote safe care, you can say:

- "My name is Kate Hines. I'm a nursing assistant. How can I help you?"
- "Mrs. Janz, I'll need to check your care plan before I bring you more salt. I'll be right back but is there anything else I can do before I leave?"

The Bathroom

❖ *All resident rooms must be equipped with or near toilet facilities.* Many centers have a bathroom in each room. Some have a bathroom between two rooms. A toilet, sink, call system, and mirror are standard equipment (Fig. 16.17A). Some bathrooms have showers (Fig. 16.17B).

Grab bars are by the toilet for safety. The person uses them for support when lowering to or raising from the toilet. Some bathrooms have raised toilet seats. The higher toilets make wheelchair transfers easier. They also are helpful for persons with joint problems.

Towel racks, toilet paper, soap, paper towel dispenser, and a wastebasket are in the bathroom. They are placed within easy reach of the person.

Usually the call light is next to the toilet. Pressing a button or pulling a cord turns on the call light. When the bathroom call light is used, the light flashes above the room door and at the nurses' station. The sound at the nurses' station is different from call lights in rooms. These differences alert the staff that the person is in the bathroom. Someone must respond at once when a person needs help in a bathroom.

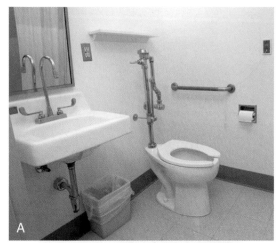

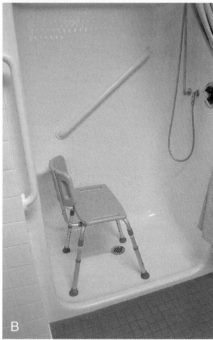

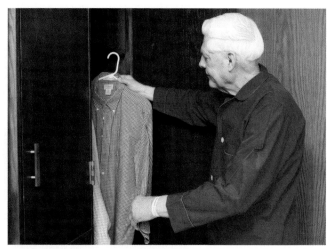

Fig. 16.18 The resident can reach items in his closet.

Fig. 16.17 (A) Bathroom adjoining a resident's room in a nursing center. (B) Private walk-in shower. (B, From *Firestein & Kelley's textbook of rheumatology*, ed 11, Philadelphia, 2020, Elsevier.)

Closet and Drawer Space

❖ Closet and drawer space are provided for clothing. *OBRA and the CMS require that nursing centers provide each person with closet space. The closet space must have shelves and a clothes rack* (Fig. 16.18). *The person must have free access to the closet and its contents.*

Items in closets and drawers are the person's private property. You must have the person's permission to open or search closets or drawers.

Sometimes people hoard items (e.g., medications, napkins, straws, food, sugar, salt, pepper). Hoarding can cause safety or health risks. Center staff can inspect a person's closet or drawers if hoarding is suspected. The person is informed of the inspection and is present when it takes place.

See *Promoting Safety and Comfort: Closet and Drawer Space.*

🧍 PROMOTING SAFETY AND COMFORT

Closet and Drawer Space
Safety
The nurse may ask you to inspect a person's closet, drawers, or personal items. If so, the person must be present. Also have a coworker with you. Your coworker is a witness to what you are doing. This protects you if the person claims that something was stolen or damaged.

Other Equipment

Some nursing centers provide wall-mounted televisions. Residents may be allowed to bring furniture and other items from home. Televisions, radios, clocks, photos, and other small items help residents feel "at home" in their units. Some centers have a policy to inspect electrical appliances for safety before they can be used. Phones and Internet access are available in some centers.

See *Promoting Safety and Comfort: Other Equipment.*
See *Focus on Rehabilitation: Other Equipment.*

🧍 PROMOTING SAFETY AND COMFORT

Other Equipment
Safety
The resident is allowed personal choice in arranging items. The choices must be safe and not cause falls or other accidents. Some nursing centers require any electrical appliances brought from home to be inspected by their maintenance staff to make sure they are safe to use. Also, the person's choices must not interfere with the rights of others. You may have to help the person choose the best place for personal items.

🍃 FOCUS ON REHABILITATION

Other Equipment
Rehabilitation centers usually have more medical equipment and supplies to manage complex health care needs. Some rooms have blood pressure equipment mounted on the wall. Some beds have IV (intravenous) poles for IV

therapy (Chapter 21). The poles are stored in the bed frame. If not part of the bed, an IV pole is brought to the bedside when needed. Some units have wall outlets for oxygen and suction. Some beds have an overhead trapeze attached to the frame (Chapter 24). This assists the person to reposition in bed.

GENERAL RULES

Everyone involved in the person's care must keep the unit clean, neat, safe, and comfortable. To maintain the person's unit, follow the rules in Box 16.1.

QUALITY OF LIFE

Nursing center residents have left their homes. Each had furniture, appliances, a private bathroom, and many personal items and treasures. Now the person lives in a strange place. The person may have a roommate. Leaving one's home is a hard part of growing old with poor health. It is important to make the person's unit as homelike as possible.

Residents may bring some furniture and personal items from home. A chair, footstool, lamp, and small table are often allowed. Some centers provide televisions. In others, the residents may bring their own from home. They can bring photos, religious items, and books. Some have plants to care for. Personal choice is allowed in arranging items. You can help the person choose the best place for them. Some centers allow residents to have a small pet in their room. Special arrangements must be made concerning the care of the pet. Many long-term care facilities do not allow pets. The health team must make sure that the person's choices:

- Are safe.
- Will not cause falls or other accidents.
- Do not interfere with the rights of others.

The center is the person's home. You must help the person feel safe, secure, and comfortable. A homelike setting is important for quality of life. OBRA and the CMS serve to promote quality of life. Box 16.2 lists OBRA and CMS requirements for resident rooms.

TIME TO REFLECT

Mr. Peterson has a favorite upholstered chair that he brought from home. He enjoys sitting in it every day as he watches television. One day he pressed his call light to ask for help to go into the bathroom. Unfortunately, none of the staff responded in a timely manner and Mr. Peterson became incontinent of urine. His daughter is upset that her father's chair now has an odor and is ruined. How do you think this situation should be handled from here? What steps can be taken to prevent this from happening again?

BOX 16.2 OBRA and CMS Requirements for Resident Rooms

- Rooms are designed for one to four persons.
- Rooms have a direct access to an exit corridor.
- Rooms are designed or equipped for full visual privacy (i.e., ceiling-suspended privacy curtain that extends around the bed, movable screens, window coverings, doors).
- Rooms have at least one window to the outside.
- Each person has closet space with racks and shelves.
- Toilet facilities are in the room or nearby (includes bathing facilities).
- Rooms, bathrooms, and bathing areas have a functioning call system.
- The person has a bed of proper height and size.
- The person has a clean, comfortable mattress.
- Bed and bath linens (towels and washcloths) are clean and in good condition.
- Bed linens are appropriate to the weather and climate.
- The room has furniture for clothing, personal items, and a chair for visitors.
- Rooms are clean and orderly.
- Room temperature levels are between 71°F and 81°F.
- Ventilation, humidity, and odor levels are acceptable.
- Nonsmoking areas are identified.
- Sound levels are comfortable.
- Lighting is adequate and comfortable with little glare.
- Rooms have clean, orderly drawers and shelves for personal items.
- The room is free of pests and rodents.
- Handrails are in good repair.
- Floors are clean and dry.
- The person's setting is free of clutter.
- Personal supplies and items are labeled and stored appropriately.
- Items are within reach for use in bed or bathroom.
- There is space for wheelchair or walker use.
- A raised toilet seat is available (if needed).

BOX 16.1 Maintaining the Person's Unit

- Keep the call light within the person's reach at all times.
- Meet the needs of persons who cannot use the call system.
- Make sure the person can reach the overbed table and the bedside stand.
- Arrange personal items as the person prefers. Make sure they are easy to reach.
- Make sure the person can reach the phone, TV, and bed and light controls.
- Protect the person's eyeglasses, hearing aids, and dentures. These should be kept in their own containers and stored in the top drawer of the bedside table when not being used.
- Provide the person with enough tissues and toilet paper.
- Adjust lighting, temperature, and ventilation for the person's comfort.
- Handle equipment carefully to prevent noise.
- Explain the causes of strange noises.
- Empty wastebaskets in the person's room and bathroom. Empty them every shift or at least once a day. Empty them more often if they become full.
- Respect the person's belongings. An item may not have importance or value to you, yet it has great meaning for the person. Even a scrap of paper can have great meaning to the person.
- Do not throw away any items belonging to the person.
- Do not move furniture or the person's belongings. Persons with poor vision rely on memory or feel for the location of items.
- Straighten bed linens and towels as often as needed.
- Complete a safety check before leaving the room. (See the inside of the front cover.)

REVIEW QUESTIONS

Circle the BEST answer.

1. Which room temperature range is required by OBRA and the CMS?
   a. 61°F to 68°F
   b. 68°F to 74°F
   c. 71°F to 81°F
   d. 76°F to 81°F

2. Which does *not* protect a person from drafts?
   a. Wearing enough clothing
   b. Being covered with enough blankets
   c. Being moved from a drafty area
   d. Sitting by a fan

3. Which does *not* prevent or reduce odors?
   a. Placing flowers in the room
   b. Emptying bedpans promptly
   c. Using room deodorizers
   d. Practicing good hygiene

4. To prevent odors, you need to do the following *except*
   a. Check incontinent persons often
   b. Dispose of ostomy products at the end of your shift
   c. Keep laundry containers closed
   d. Clean persons who are wet or soiled

5. Which does *not* control noise?
   a. Using plastic items
   b. Handling dishes with care
   c. Speaking softly
   d. Talking with others in the hallway

6. Beds are raised horizontally to
   a. Prevent bending and reaching when giving care
   b. Let the person get in and out of bed with ease
   c. Raise the head of the bed
   d. Lock the bed in position

7. The head of the bed is raised 30 degrees. This is called
   a. Fowler position
   b. Semi-Fowler position
   c. Trendelenburg position
   d. Reverse Trendelenburg position

8. These statements are about hospital bed system entrapment. Which is *false?*
   a. Serious injuries and death can occur
   b. Older, frail, and confused persons are at risk
   c. The head, neck, and chest are areas of entrapment
   d. Bed rails present the only risk for entrapment

9. The overbed table is *not* used
   a. For eating
   b. As a working surface
   c. For the urinal
   d. To store shaving items

10. The bedpan is stored in the
    a. Closet
    b. Bedside stand
    c. Overbed table
    d. Bookshelf

11. Call lights are answered
    a. When you have time
    b. At the end of your shift
    c. Promptly
    d. When you are near the person's room

12. To maintain the person's unit, you can do the following *except*
    a. Clean the surface of the overbed table
    b. Provide enough tissues and toilet paper
    c. Place personal items as you choose
    d. Straighten bed linens as needed

13. Which promotes relaxation?
    a. Loud music
    b. Soft, dim lighting
    c. Cold room temperature
    d. Bright sunlight from windows

14. The nurse asks you to inspect a resident's drawers. Which is true?
    a. The resident does not need to be present
    b. Have a coworker present as a witness
    c. You have the right to throw away belongings
    d. It is best to do this when the resident is sleeping

15. Which is *not* true about privacy curtains?
    a. They provide full visual privacy
    b. They must be present in rooms with more than one bed
    c. They provide privacy from public view
    d. They block sound and voices

16. The head of the bed is lower than the feet (as in the emergency position for a person in shock). This is called
    a. Fowler
    b. Trendelenburg
    c. Supine
    d. Reverse Trendelenburg

See Appendix A **for answers to these questions.**

17

Bedmaking

OBJECTIVES

- Define the key terms listed in this chapter.
- Describe open, closed, occupied, and surgical beds.
- Explain when to change linens.
- Explain how to use drawsheets.
- Handle linens following the rules of medical asepsis.
- Perform the procedures described in this chapter.
- Explain how to promote quality of life.

KEY TERMS

cotton drawsheet A drawsheet made of cotton; it helps keep the mattress and bottom linens clean

drawsheet A small sheet placed over the middle of the bottom sheet

waterproof drawsheet A drawsheet made of plastic, rubber, or absorbent material used to protect the mattress and bottom linens from dampness and soiling

Most residents are up during the day. Some are always in bed. Food, fluid, hygiene, and elimination needs are met while in bed. Some persons are incontinent of urine or feces. Clean, dry, wrinkle-free linens are important for all residents to:

- Promote comfort.
- Prevent skin breakdown and pressure ulcers.

Beds are made every day. They are usually made in the morning after baths. Or they are made while the person is in the chair or out of the room. Beds are made and rooms are straightened before visitors arrive.

To keep beds neat and clean:

- Straighten linens when loose or wrinkled.
- Straighten loose or wrinkled linens at bedtime.
- Check for and remove food and crumbs after meals.
- Check linens for dentures, eyeglasses, hearing aids, sharp objects, and other items.
- Change linens when they become wet, soiled, or damp.
- Follow Standard Precautions and the Bloodborne Pathogen Standard; contact with blood, body fluids, secretions, or excretions is likely.

TYPES OF BEDS

Beds are made in these ways:

- A *closed bed* is not used until bedtime (Fig. 17.1), or the bed is ready for a new resident. Top linens are not folded back.
- An *open bed* is in use. Top linens are fan-folded back so the person can get into bed. A closed bed becomes an open bed by fan-folding back the top linens (Fig. 17.2).
- An *occupied bed* is made with the person in it (Fig. 17.3).
- A *surgical bed* is made to transfer a person from a stretcher (Fig. 17.4). This bed also is made for persons who arrive by ambulance.

LINENS

In nursing centers, linens are not changed every day. The center is the person's home. People do not change linens every day at home. A complete linen change is usually done on the person's bath day. This may be once or twice a week. Pillowcases, top and bottom sheets, and drawsheets (if used) are changed twice a week. Linens are always changed if wet, damp, soiled, or very wrinkled.

Handling Linens

When handling linens and making beds, practice medical asepsis. Your uniform is considered dirty. Always hold linens away from your body and uniform. Never shake linens. Shaking spreads microbes. Place clean linens on a clean surface. Never put clean or dirty linens on the floor.

Collect enough linens. If the person has two pillows, get two pillowcases. The person may need extra blankets for warmth. Do not bring unneeded linens to a person's room. Once in the person's room, extra linens are considered contaminated. Do not use it for another person.

Collect linens in the order you will use them:

- Mattress pad (if needed)
- Bottom sheet (flat or fitted)
- Waterproof drawsheet or waterproof pad (if needed)
- Cotton drawsheet (if needed)
- Top sheet
- Blanket
- Bedspread
- Pillowcase(s)
- Bath towel(s)
- Hand towel
- Washcloth
- Gown or pajamas
- Bath blanket

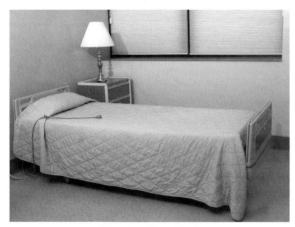

Fig. 17.1 Closed bed.

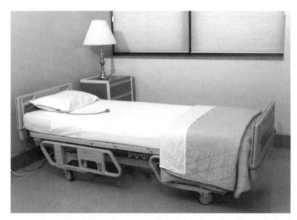

Fig. 17.2 Open bed. Top linens are fan-folded to the foot of the bed.

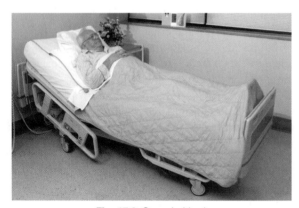

Fig. 17.3 Occupied bed.

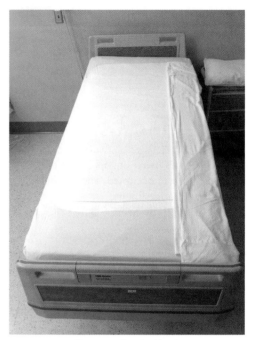

Fig. 17.4 Surgical bed.

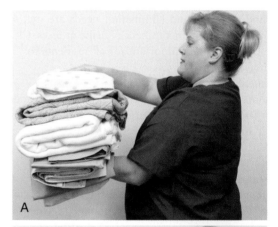

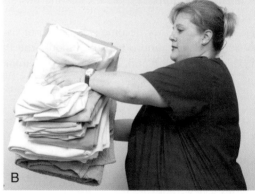

Fig. 17.5 Collecting linens. Linens are held away from the body and uniform. (A) The arm is placed over the top of the stack of linens. (B) The stack of linens is turned onto the arm. Note that the linens are held away from the body.

Use one arm to hold the linens. Use your other hand to pick them up. The first item to use is at the bottom of your stack. (You picked up the mattress pad first. It is at the bottom. The bath blanket is on top.) You need the mattress pad first. To get it on top, place your arm over the bath blanket. Then turn the stack over onto the arm on the bath blanket (Fig. 17.5). The arm that held the linens is now free. Place the clean linens on a clean surface.

Remove dirty linens one piece at a time. Roll each piece away from you. The side that touched the person is inside the roll and away from you (Fig. 17.6).

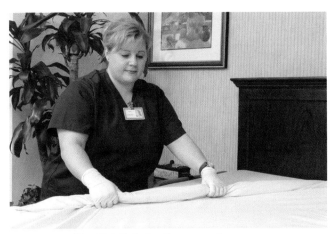

Fig. 17.6 Roll dirty linen away from you.

Drawsheets

A drawsheet is a small sheet placed over the middle of the bottom sheet.

- A cotton drawsheet is made of cotton. It helps keep the mattress and bottom linens clean.
- A waterproof drawsheet is made of plastic, rubber, or absorbent material. It protects the mattress and bottom linens from dampness and soiling. Some are rubber or plastic on one side—the waterproof side. The waterproof side is placed down, away from the person. The other side is cotton. It is placed up, toward the person. Other waterproof drawsheets are disposable. They are discarded when wet, soiled, or wrinkled.

The cotton drawsheet protects the person from contact with plastic or rubber and absorbs moisture. However, discomfort and skin breakdown may occur. Plastic and rubber retain heat. Waterproof drawsheets are hard to keep tight and wrinkle free. Many centers use incontinence products (Chapter 22) to keep the person and linens dry. Others use waterproof pads or disposable bed protectors (Fig. 17.7).

Cotton drawsheets are often used without waterproof drawsheets. Plastic-covered mattresses cause some persons to perspire heavily. This causes discomfort. A cotton drawsheet reduces heat retention and absorbs moisture. Cotton drawsheets are often used as assist devices to move and transfer persons in bed (Chapter 15). If used as an assist device, do not tuck it in at the sides.

The procedures that follow include waterproof and cotton drawsheets. This is so you learn how to use them. Ask the nurse about the type used in your center.

MAKING BEDS

Safety and medical asepsis are important for bedmaking. Follow the rules in Box 17.1.

See *Delegation Guidelines: Making Beds.*
See *Promoting Safety and Comfort: Making Beds.*
See *Teamwork and Time Management: Making Beds.*

📋 DELEGATION GUIDELINES

Making Beds

Before making a bed, you need this information from the nurse and the care plan:

- What type of bed to make—closed, open, occupied, or surgical
- If you need to use a cotton drawsheet
- If you need to use a waterproof drawsheet, waterproof pad, or incontinence product
- Position restrictions or limits in the person's movement or activity
- If the person uses bed rails
- The person's treatment, therapy, and activity schedule (e.g., Mr. Smith needs a treatment in bed, so change linens after the treatment; make Mrs. Carter's bed while she is in physical therapy)
- How to position the person and the positioning devices needed
- If the bed needs to be locked into a certain position (Chapter 16)
- When to report observations
- What specific resident concerns to report at once

👤 PROMOTING SAFETY AND COMFORT

Making Beds

Safety

You need to raise the bed for body mechanics. The bed also must be flat. If the bed is locked, unlock it. Then adjust the bed. Return the bed to the correct position when you are done. Then lock the bed.

Wear gloves when removing linens from the person's bed. Also follow other aspects of Standard Precautions and the Bloodborne Pathogen Standard. Linens may contain blood, body fluids, secretions, or excretions. Follow the center's policy for placement of linens that contain blood or other body fluids or wastes.

After making a bed, lower the bed to a level appropriate for the person. Follow the care plan. For an occupied bed, raise or lower bed rails according to the care plan.

Comfort

For an occupied bed, cover the person with a bath blanket before removing the top sheet. Do not leave the person uncovered when making the bed. The bath blanket provides for warmth and privacy.

If the person uses a pillow, adjust it as needed during the procedure. After the procedure, position the person as directed by the nurse and the care plan. Always make sure linens are straight and wrinkle free.

👥 TEAMWORK AND TIME MANAGEMENT

Making Beds

To save time and energy, make beds with a coworker. Make one side of the bed while your coworker makes the other.

Making beds with a coworker is faster, easier, and safer for residents, you, and your coworker. Always thank your coworker for helping you. Also help your coworker make beds when asked to do so.

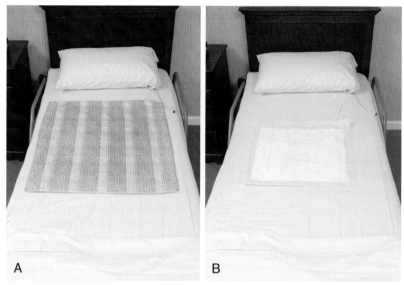

Fig. 17.7 (A) Waterproof pad. (B) Disposable bed protector.

BOX 17.1   Rules for Bedmaking

- Use good body mechanics at all times (Chapter 15).
- Follow the rules in Chapter 15 to safely handle, move, and transfer the person.
- Follow the rules of medical asepsis.
- Follow Standard Precautions and the Bloodborne Pathogen Standard.
- Follow the center policy for bedmaking. Not all centers use the same types of linens.
- Practice hand hygiene before handling clean linens.
- Practice hand hygiene after handling dirty linens.
- Bring enough linens to the person's room. Do not bring extra linens.
- Bring only the linens that you will need. You cannot use extra linens for another person.
- Place clean linens on a clean surface. Use the bedside chair, overbed table, or bedside stand. Place a barrier (towel, paper towels) between the clean surface and the linens if required by center policy.

- Do not use extra linens in the person's room for another resident. Extra linens are considered contaminated. Put them with the dirty laundry.
- Do not use torn or frayed linens.
- Never shake linens. Shaking spreads microbes.
- Hold linens away from your body and uniform. Do not let dirty or clean linens touch your uniform.
- Never put dirty linens on the floor or on clean linens. Follow center policy for dirty linens.
- Keep bottom linens tucked in and wrinkle free.
- Cover a waterproof drawsheet with a cotton drawsheet. Plastic or rubber must not touch the person's body.
- Straighten and tighten loose sheets, blankets, and bedspreads as needed.
- Make as much of one side of the bed as possible before going to the other side. This saves time and energy.
- Change wet, damp, and soiled linens right away.

✳ The Closed Bed

Closed beds are made for:

- Residents who are up for most or all of the day. Top linens are folded back at bedtime. Clean linens are used as needed.

- For new residents. The bed is made after the bed frame and mattress are cleaned and disinfected. Clean linens are needed for the entire bed.

✳ MAKING A CLOSED BED

Quality of Life

Remember to:

- Knock before entering the person's room.
- Address the person by name.
- Introduce yourself by name and title.
- Explain the procedure to the person before beginning and during the procedure.
- Protect the person's rights during the procedure.
- Handle the person gently during the procedure.

Preprocedure

1. Follow *Delegation Guidelines: Making Beds,* p. · · ·. See *Promoting Safety and Comfort: Making Beds,* p. · ·.
2. Practice hand hygiene.
3. Collect clean linens:
   - Mattress pad (if needed)
   - Bottom sheet (flat sheet or fitted sheet)
   - Waterproof drawsheet or waterproof pad (if needed)
   - Cotton drawsheet (if needed)

✳ MAKING A CLOSED BED—cont'd

- Top sheet
- Blanket
- Bedspread
- A pillowcase for each pillow
- Bath towel(s)
- Hand towel
- Washcloth
- Gown or pajamas
- Bath blanket
- Gloves
- Laundry bag
- Paper towels (if you need a barrier for clean linens)

4. Place linens on a clean surface. Use the paper towels as a barrier between the clean surface and clean linens if required by center policy.
5. Raise the bed for body mechanics. Bed rails are down.

Procedure

6. Put on the gloves.
7. Remove linens. Roll each piece away from you. Place each piece in a laundry bag. (*Note:* Discard incontinence products or disposable bed protectors in the trash. Do not put them in the laundry bag.)
8. Clean the bed frame and mattress (if this is your job).
9. Remove and discard gloves. Decontaminate your hands.
10. Move the mattress to the head of the bed.
11. Put the mattress pad on the mattress. It is even with the top of the mattress.
12. Place the bottom sheet on the mattress pad (Fig. 17.8). Unfold it lengthwise. Place the center crease in the middle of the bed. If using a flat sheet:
    a. Position the lower edge even with the bottom of the mattress.
    b. Place the large hem at the top and the small hem at the bottom.
    c. Face hemstitching downward, away from the person.
13. Open the sheet. Fan-fold it to the other side of the bed (Fig. 17.9).

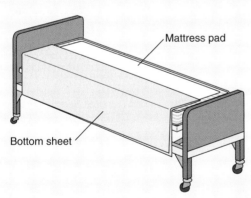

Fig. 17.8 The bottom sheet is on the bed with the center crease in the middle. The lower edge of the sheet is even with the bottom of the mattress.

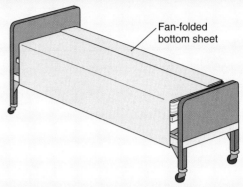

Fig. 17.9 The bottom sheet is fan-folded to the other side of the bed.

14. Tuck the corners of a fitted sheet over the mattress at the top and then the foot of the bed. If using a flat sheet, tuck the top of the sheet under the mattress. The sheet is tight and smooth.
15. Make a mitered corner if using a flat sheet (Fig. 17.10).
16. Place the waterproof drawsheet on the bed. It is in the middle of the mattress, or put the waterproof pad on the bed.
17. Open the waterproof drawsheet. Fan-fold it to the other side of the bed.
18. Place a cotton drawsheet over the waterproof drawsheet. It covers the entire waterproof drawsheet (Fig. 17.11).
19. Open the cotton drawsheet. Fan-fold it to the other side of the bed.
20. Tuck both drawsheets under the mattress, or tuck each in separately.
21. Go to the other side of the bed.
22. Miter the top corner of the flat bottom sheet.
23. Pull the bottom sheet tight so there are no wrinkles. Tuck in the sheet.
24. Pull the drawsheets tight so there are no wrinkles. Tuck both in together or separately (Fig. 17.12).
25. Go to the other side of the bed.
26. Put the top sheet on the bed. Unfold it lengthwise. Place the center crease in the middle. Do the following if using a flat sheet:
    a. Place the large hem even with the top of the mattress.
    b. Open the sheet. Fan-fold it to the other side.
    c. Face hemstitching outward, away from the person.
    d. Do not tuck the bottom in yet.
    e. Never tuck top linens in on the sides.
27. Place the blanket on the bed:
    a. Unfold it so the center crease is in the middle.
    b. Put the upper hem about 6 to 8 inches from the top of the mattress.
    c. Open the blanket. Fan-fold it to the other side.
    d. If steps 33 and 34 are not done, turn the top sheet down over the blanket. Hemstitching is down, away from the person.
28. Place the bedspread on the bed:
    a. Unfold it so the center crease is in the middle.
    b. Place the upper hem even with the top of the mattress.
    c. Open and fan-fold the bedspread to the other side.
    d. Make sure the bedspread facing the door is even. It covers all top linens.

Continued

✦ MAKING A CLOSED BED—cont'd

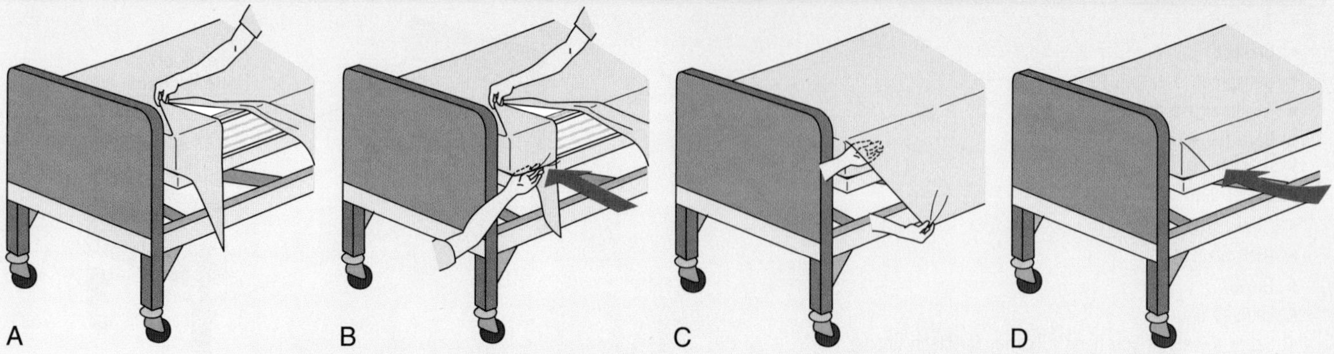

Fig. 17.10 Making a mitered corner. (A) The bottom sheet is tucked under the mattress at the head of the bed. The side of the sheet is raised onto the mattress. (B) The remaining portion of the sheet is tucked under the mattress. (C) The raised portion of the sheet is brought off the mattress. (D) The entire side of the sheet is tucked under the mattress.

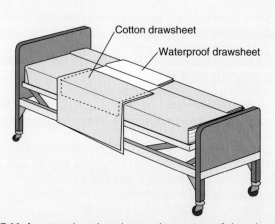

Fig. 17.11 A cotton drawsheet is over the waterproof drawsheet. The cotton drawsheet completely covers the waterproof drawsheet.

Cotton drawsheet

Waterproof drawsheet

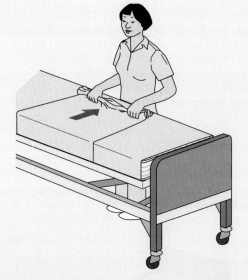

Fig. 17.12 The drawsheet is pulled tight to remove wrinkles.

29. Tuck in top linens together at the foot of the bed so they are smooth and tight. Make a mitered corner.
30. Go to the other side.
31. Straighten all top linens. Work from the head of the bed to the foot.
32. Tuck in top linens together at the foot of the bed. Make a mitered corner.
33. Turn the top hem of the bedspread under the blanket to make a cuff (Fig. 17.13).

34. Turn the top sheet down over the bedspread. Hemstitching is down. (Steps 33 and 34 are not done in some centers. The bedspread covers the pillow. If so, tuck the bedspread under the pillow.)
35. Put the pillowcase on the pillow as in Fig. 17.14 or 17.15. Fold extra material under the pillow at the seam end of the pillowcase.
36. Place the pillow on the bed. The open end of the pillowcase is away from the door. The seam is toward the head of the bed.

✳ MAKING A CLOSED BED—cont'd

Postprocedure

37. Provide for comfort. (See the inside of the front cover.) *NOTE:* Omit this step if the bed is prepared for a new resident.
38. Attach the call light to the bed or place it within the person's reach.
39. Lower the bed to its lowest position. Lock the bed wheels.
40. Put the towels, washcloth, gown or pajamas, and bath blanket in the bedside stand.
41. Complete a safety check of the room. (See the inside of the front cover.)
42. Follow center policy for dirty linens.
43. Decontaminate your hands.

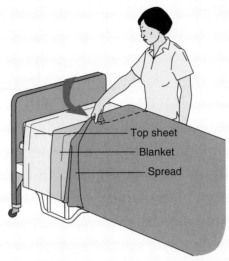

Fig. 17.13 The top hem of the bedspread is turned under the top hem of the blanket to make a cuff.

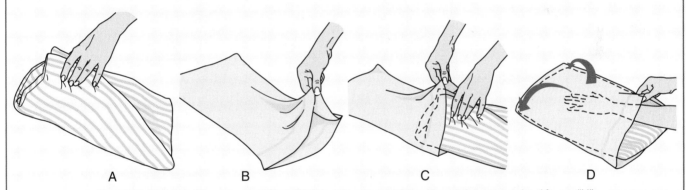

A   B   C   D

Fig. 17.14 Putting a pillowcase on a pillow. (A) Grasp the corners of the pillow at the seam end and form a "V" with the pillow. (B) Open the pillowcase with your free hand. (C) Guide the "V" end of the pillow into the pillowcase. (D) Let the "V" end of the pillow fall into the corners of the pillowcase.

Continued

✷ MAKING A CLOSED BED—cont'd

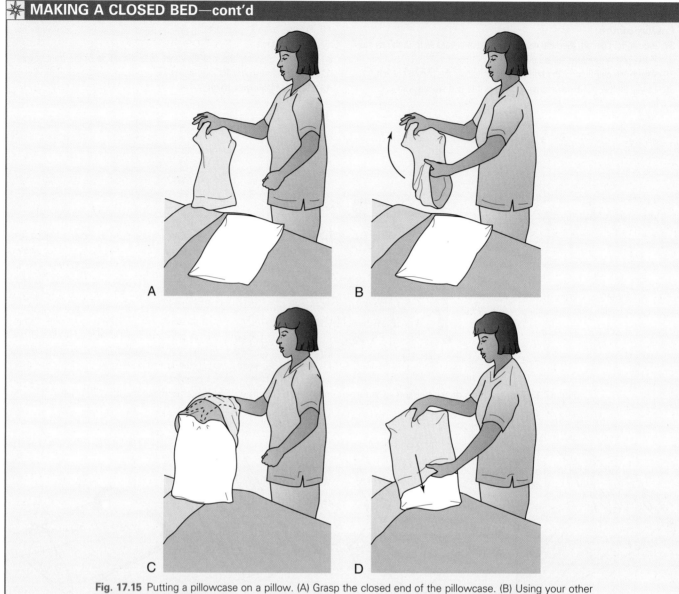

Fig. 17.15 Putting a pillowcase on a pillow. (A) Grasp the closed end of the pillowcase. (B) Using your other hand, gather up the pillowcase. The pillowcase should cover your hand holding the closed end. (C) Grasp the pillow with the hand covered by the pillowcase. (D) Pull the pillowcase down over the pillow with your other hand.

This skill is also covered in *Clinical Skills: Nurse Assisting.*

✷ The Open Bed

A closed bed becomes an open bed by fan-folding back the top linen. The open bed lets the person get into bed with ease. Make this bed for:

- Newly admitted persons arriving by wheelchair.
- Persons who are getting ready for bed.
- Persons who are out of bed for a short time.

✷ MAKING AN OPEN BED

Quality of Life

Remember to:

- Knock before entering the person's room.
- Address the person by name.
- Introduce yourself by name and title.
- Explain the procedure to the person before beginning and during the procedure.

- Protect the person's rights during the procedure.
- Handle the person gently during the procedure.

Procedure

1. Follow *Delegation Guidelines: Making Beds*, p. ⋯ See *Promoting Safety and Comfort: Making Beds*, p. ⋯.
2. Practice hand hygiene.

✳ MAKING AN OPEN BED—cont'd

3. Collect linens for a closed bed.
4. Make a closed bed. See procedure: *Making a Closed Bed*, pp. ··—··.
5. Fan-fold top linens to the foot of the bed (see Fig. 17.2).
6. Attach the call light to the bed.
7. Lower the bed to its lowest position.
8. Put towels, washcloth, gown or pajamas, and the bath blanket in the bedside stand.

Postprocedure

9. Provide for comfort. (See the inside of the front cover.)
10. Place the call light within the person's reach.
11. Complete a safety check of the room. (See the inside of the front cover.)
12. Follow center policy for dirty linen.
13. Decontaminate your hands.

This skill is also covered in *Clinical Skills: Nurse Assisting*.

✳ The Occupied Bed

You make an occupied bed when the person stays in bed. Keep the person in good alignment. Follow restrictions or limits in the person's movement or position.

Explain each procedure step to the person before it is done. This is important even if the person cannot respond to you or is in a coma.

See *Focus on Communication: The Occupied Bed.*
See *Promoting Safety and Comfort: The Occupied Bed.*

📋 FOCUS ON COMMUNICATION

The Occupied Bed

After making an occupied bed, make sure the person is comfortable. You can ask:

- "Are you comfortable?"
- "How can I make you more comfortable?"
- "Are you warm enough?"
- "Can I adjust your pillow?"

After making the bed, thank the person for cooperating.

👤 PROMOTING SAFETY AND COMFORT

The Occupied Bed
Safety

The person lies on one side of the bed and then the other. Protect the person from falling out of bed. If bed rails are used, the far bed rail is up. If the person does not use bed rails, have a coworker help you. You work on one side of the bed; your coworker works on the other.

Comfort

To make an occupied bed, the person lies on the side. You tuck dirty bottom linens under the person. Then you put clean linens on the bed. These, too, are tucked under the person. The tucked linens create a "bump" in the middle of the bed. To make the other side, the person rolls over the "bump" to the other side of the bed. To promote comfort, make the "bump" as low as possible. Do this by fan-folding dirty and clean bottom linens neatly and flatly.

✳ MAKING AN OCCUPIED BED

Quality of Life
Remember to:

- Knock before entering the person's room.
- Address the person by name.
- Introduce yourself by name and title.
- Explain the procedure to the person before beginning and during the procedure.
- Protect the person's rights during the procedure.
- Handle the person gently during the procedure.

Preprocedure

1. Follow *Delegation Guidelines: Making Beds*, p. ··. See *Promoting Safety and Comfort:*
   a. *Making Beds*, p. ··
   b. *The Occupied Bed*
2. Practice hand hygiene.
3. Collect the following:
   - Gloves
   - Laundry bag
   - Clean linens (see procedure: *Making a Closed Bed*, pp. ··—··)
   - Paper towels (if you need a barrier for clean linens)
4. Place linens on a clean surface. Place the paper towels between the clean surface and clean linens if a barrier is required by center policy.

5. Identify the person. Check the ID (identification) bracelet against the assignment sheet. Also call the person by name.
6. Provide for privacy.
7. Remove the call light.
8. Raise the bed for body mechanics. Bed rails are up if used. Bed wheels are locked.
9. Lower the head of the bed. It is as flat as possible.

Procedure

10. Decontaminate your hands. Put on gloves.
11. Loosen top linens at the foot of the bed.
12. Lower the bed rail near you if up.
13. Remove the bedspread (Fig. 17.16). Then remove the blanket in the same way. Place each over the chair.
14. Cover the person with a bath blanket. Use the blanket in the bedside stand.
    a. Unfold the bath blanket over the top sheet.
    b. Ask the person to hold on to the bath blanket. If the person cannot, tuck the top part under the person's shoulders.
    c. Grasp the top sheet under the bath blanket at the shoulders. Bring the sheet down to the foot of the bed. Remove the sheet from under the blanket (Fig. 17.17).
15. Position the person on the side of the bed away from you. Adjust the pillow for comfort.

✳ MAKING AN OCCUPIED BED—cont'd

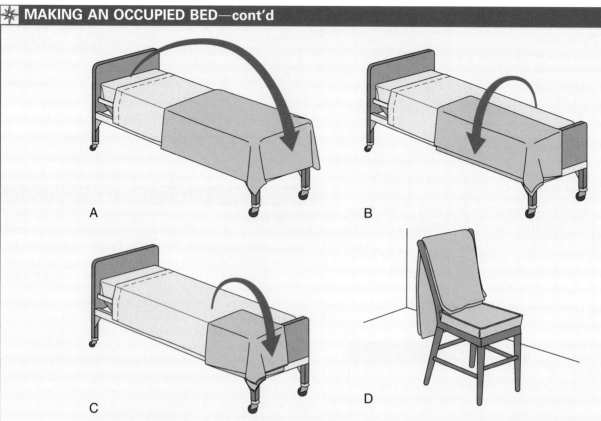

Fig. 17.16 Folding linen for reuse. (A) Fold the top edge of the bedspread down to the bottom edge. (B) Fold the bedspread from the far side of the bed to the near side. (C) Fold the top edge of the bedspread down to the bottom edge again. (D) Place the folded bedspread over the back of the chair.

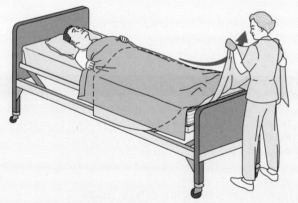

Fig. 17.17 The person holds on to the bath blanket. The top sheet is removed from under the bath blanket.

16. Loosen bottom linens from the head to the foot of the bed.
17. Fan-fold bottom linens one at a time toward the person. Start with the cotton drawsheet (Fig. 17.18). If reusing the mattress pad, do not fan-fold it.
⏵ 18. Place a clean mattress pad on the bed. Unfold it lengthwise. The center crease is in the middle. Fan-fold the top part toward the person. If reusing the mattress pad, straighten and smooth any wrinkles.
19. Place the bottom sheet on the mattress pad. Hemstitching is away from the person. Unfold the sheet so the crease is in the middle. If using a flat sheet, the small hem is even with the bottom of the mattress. Fan-fold the top part toward the person.
20. Tuck the corners of a fitted sheet over the mattress. If using a flat sheet, make a mitered corner at the head of the bed. Tuck the sheet under the mattress from the head to the foot.

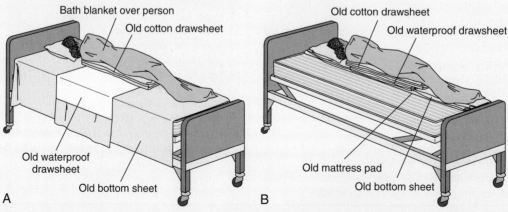

Fig. 17.18 Occupied bed. (A) The cotton drawsheet is fan-folded and tucked under the person. (B) All bottom linens are tucked under the person.

MAKING AN OCCUPIED BED—cont'd

21. Pull the waterproof drawsheet toward you over the bottom sheet. Tuck excess material under the mattress. Do the following for a clean waterproof drawsheet (Fig. 17.19).
    a. Place the waterproof drawsheet on the bed. It is in the middle of the mattress.
    b. Fan-fold the top part toward the person.
    c. Tuck in excess fabric.
22. Place the cotton drawsheet over the waterproof drawsheet. It covers the entire waterproof drawsheet. Fan-fold the top part toward the person. Tuck in excess fabric.
23. Explain and assure that the person will roll over a "bump" but will not fall.
24. Help the person turn to the other side. Adjust the pillow for comfort.
25. Raise the bed rail. Go to the other side and lower the bed rail.
26. Loosen bottom linens. Remove one piece at a time. Place each piece in the laundry bag. (*Note:* Discard disposable bed protectors and incontinence products in the trash. Do not put them in the laundry bag.)
27. Remove and discard the gloves. Decontaminate your hands.
28. Straighten and smooth the mattress pad.

29. Pull the clean bottom sheet toward you. Tuck the corners of a fitted sheet over the mattress. If using a flat sheet, make a mitered corner at the top. Tuck the sheet under the mattress from the head to the foot of the bed.
30. Pull the drawsheets tightly toward you. Tuck both under together or separately.
31. Position the person supine in the center of the bed. Adjust the pillow for comfort.
32. Put the top sheet on the bed. Unfold it lengthwise. The crease is in the middle. The large hem is even with the top of the mattress. Hemstitching is on the outside.
33. Ask the person to hold the top sheet so you can remove the bath blanket, or tuck the top sheet under the person's shoulders. Remove and discard the bath blanket.
34. Place the blanket on the bed. Unfold it so the crease is in the middle and it covers the person. The upper hem is 6 to 8 inches from the top of the mattress.
35. Place the bedspread on the bed. Unfold it so the center crease is in the middle and it covers the person. The top hem is even with the mattress top.
36. Turn the top hem of the bedspread under the blanket to make a cuff.
37. Bring the top sheet down over the bedspread to form a cuff.
38. Go to the foot of the bed.
39. Make a toe pleat. Make a 2-inch pleat across the foot of the bed. The pleat is about 6 to 8 inches from the foot of the bed.
40. Lift the mattress corner with one arm. Tuck all top linens under the mattress. Make a mitered corner.
41. Raise the bed rail. Go to the other side and lower the bed rail.
42. Straighten and smooth top linens.
43. Tuck all top linens under the mattress. Make a mitered corner.
44. Change the pillowcase(s).

Postprocedure
45. Provide for comfort. (See the inside of the front cover.)
46. Place the call light within reach.
47. Lower the bed to its lowest position. Bed wheels are locked.
48. Raise or lower bed rails. Follow the care plan.
49. Put the clean towels, washcloth, gown or pajamas, and bath blanket in the bedside stand.
50. Unscreen the person.
51. Complete a safety check of the room. (See the inside of the front cover.)
52. Follow center policy for dirty linens.
53. Decontaminate your hands.

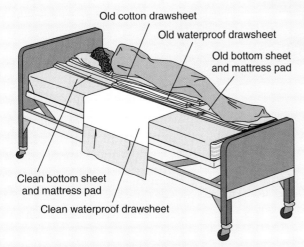

Old cotton drawsheet
Old waterproof drawsheet
Old bottom sheet and mattress pad
Clean bottom sheet and mattress pad
Clean waterproof drawsheet

Fig. 17.19 A clean bottom sheet and waterproof drawsheet are on the bed with both fan-folded and tucked under the person.

This skill is also covered in *Clinical Skills: Nurse Assisting*.

The Surgical Bed

The surgical bed also is called a *recovery bed* or *postoperative bed*. It is a form of the open bed. Top linens are folded to transfer the person from a stretcher to the bed. These beds are made for persons who:

- Arrive at the center by ambulance. A complete linen change is needed if the person is a new resident or is returning to the center from the hospital.
- Go by stretcher to treatment or therapy areas. A complete linen change is not needed.
- Use portable tubs. Because the person has a bath, a complete linen change is needed.
  See *Promoting Safety and Comfort: The Surgical Bed.*

PROMOTING SAFETY AND COMFORT

The Surgical Bed
Safety
To safely transfer a person from a stretcher to a surgical bed, see procedure: *Moving the Person to a Stretcher* in Chapter 15. Also follow the rules for stretcher safety (Chapter 11). After the transfer, lower the bed to its lowest position. Make sure the bed wheels are locked. Raise or lower bed rails according to the care plan.

✳ MAKING A SURGICAL BED

Procedure

1. Follow *Delegation Guidelines: Making Beds*, p. ·· . See *Promoting Safety and Comfort*.
   a. *Making Beds*, p. ··
   b. *The Surgical Bed*
2. Practice hand hygiene.
3. Collect the following:
   - Clean linens (see procedure: *Making a Closed Bed*, pp. ··—··)
   - Gloves
   - Laundry bag
   - Equipment requested by the nurse
   - Paper towels (if you need a barrier for clean linens)
4. Place linens on a clean surface. Place the paper towels between the clean surface and clean linens if a barrier is required by center policy.
5. Remove the call light.
6. Raise the bed for body mechanics.
7. Remove all linens from the bed. Wear gloves. Decontaminate your hands after removing them.

8. Make a closed bed (see procedure: *Making a Closed Bed*, pp. ··—··). Do not tuck top linens under the mattress.
9. Fold all top linens at the foot of the bed back onto the bed. The fold is even with the edge of the mattress (Fig. 17.20A).
10. Fan-fold linen lengthwise to the side of the bed farthest from the door (see Fig. 17.20B).
11. Put the pillowcase(s) on the pillow(s).
12. Place the pillow(s) on a clean surface.
13. Leave the bed in its highest position.
14. Leave both bed rails down.
15. Put the clean towels, washcloth, gown or pajamas, and bath blanket in the bedside stand.
16. Move furniture away from the bed. Allow room for the stretcher and the staff.
17. Do not attach the call light to the bed.
18. Complete a safety check of the room. (See the inside of the front cover.)
19. Follow center policy for soiled linen.
20. Decontaminate your hands.

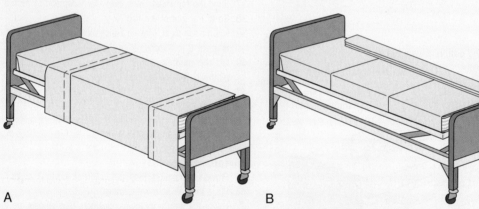

Fig. 17.20 Surgical bed. (A) The bottom of the top linens is folded back onto the bed. The fold is even with the bottom edge of the mattress. (B) Top linens are fan-folded lengthwise to the opposite side of the bed.

This skill is also covered in *Clinical Skills: Nurse Assisting*.

👥 QUALITY OF LIFE

The bed is the largest item in the resident's unit. The person, family, and visitors question the quality of care if the bed is unmade, messy, or dirty. They also question the person's quality of life. The bed must be neat, clean, and well made. It helps provide an orderly and pleasant setting. If the person stays in bed, straighten and tighten sheets and other linens as needed.

Some persons bring bedspreads, pillows, blankets, comforters, and quilts from home. Use these when making the bed if they prefer. Such items are the person's property. Handle them with care and respect. Make sure they are labeled with the person's name. This protects them from loss. It also prevents them from becoming confused with the property of others.

Allow personal choice when possible. The center may use colored or printed linens. If so, let the person choose which linens to use. Also, let the person decide how many pillows or blankets to use. If possible, the person chooses when the bed is made. The more choices allowed, the greater the person's sense of control and quality of life.

👤 TIME TO REFLECT

Mrs. Davis is a large person who is dependent for all her care. The doctor has ordered complete bedrest for her. You have just finished giving her a complete bed bath and are preparing to make an occupied bed. What should be the order of the clean linens that you have stacked ready to use? The bottom sheets were soiled with feces. How would you proceed with changing her bed so that the new linens will not become soiled by the previous dirty linens?

REVIEW QUESTIONS

Circle the BEST answer.

1. Which requires a linen change?
   a. The person will have visitors
   b. Wet linen
   c. Wrinkled linen
   d. Crumbs in the bed

2. You will transfer a person from a stretcher to the bed. Which bed should you make?
   a. Closed bed
   b. Open bed
   c. Occupied bed
   d. Surgical bed

3. When handling linens
   a. Put dirty linens on the floor
   b. Hold linens away from your body and uniform
   c. Shake linens to unfold them
   d. Take extra linens to another person's room

4. A resident is out of the bed most of the day. Which bed should you make?
   a. Closed bed
   b. Open bed
   c. Occupied bed
   d. Surgical bed

5. A complete linen change is done when
   a. The bottom linens are wet or soiled
   b. The bed is made for a new person
   c. The person will transfer from a stretcher to a bed
   d. Linens are loose or wrinkled

6. You are using a waterproof drawsheet. Which is *true*?
   a. A cotton drawsheet must completely cover the waterproof drawsheet
   b. Waterproof pads are needed
   c. The person's consent is needed
   d. The plastic or rubber is in contact with the person's skin

7. To make an occupied bed, you do the following *except*
   a. Cover the person with a bath blanket
   b. Screen the person
   c. Raise the far bed rail
   d. Fan-fold top linens to the foot of the bed

8. A surgical bed is kept
   a. In Fowler position
   b. In the lowest position
   c. In the highest position
   d. In the supine position

9. Mrs. Sanders is comatose. Which is correct when making her bed?
   a. Place the soiled linen on the floor
   b. Make an open bed
   c. Talk to her and explain what steps you are taking
   d. Place extra linen in her closet

10. Which is incorrect when changing a pillowcase?
    a. Hold the pillow under your chin
    b. Fold the corners of the pillow and guide it in the opening
    c. Change the pillowcase on a clean surface
    d. Place the open end of the pillowcase away from the door

11. Ms. Rodriguez always likes a blanket on her bed for warmth. Where is the best place for this to be place?
    a. On top of the bottom sheet
    b. Between the top sheet and bed spread
    c. Folded under the pillow
    d. On top of the bedspread

12. Ms. Rodriguez asks her daughter to bring her favorite comforter from home. Which is incorrect?
    a. She is told this is not allowed
    b. It may have special meaning for her
    c. It will be labeled with her name to prevent loss
    d. It will be handled carefully to prevent damage

See Appendix A for answers to these questions.

18

Hygiene

OBJECTIVES

- Define the key terms and key abbreviations listed in this chapter.
- Explain why personal hygiene is important.
- Describe the care given before and after breakfast, after lunch, and in the evening.
- Describe the rules for bathing.
- Identify safety measures for tub baths and showers.
- Explain the purposes of a back massage.
- Explain the purposes of perineal care.
- Identify the observations to report and record when assisting with hygiene.
- Perform the procedures described in this chapter.
- Explain how to promote quality of life.

KEY TERMS

AM care See "early morning care"

aspiration Breathing fluid, food, vomitus, or an object into the lungs

denture An artificial tooth or a set of artificial teeth

early morning care Care given before breakfast; AM care

evening care Care given in the evening at bedtime; PM care

HS care See "evening care"

morning care Care given after breakfast; hygiene measures are more thorough at this time

oral hygiene Mouth care

pericare See "perineal care"

perineal care Cleaning the genital and anal areas; pericare

plaque A thin film that sticks to the teeth; it contains saliva, microbes, and other substances

PM care See "evening care"

tartar Hardened plaque

KEY ABBREVIATIONS

C Centigrade
F Fahrenheit

ID Identification

Hygiene promotes comfort, safety, and health. The skin is the body's first line of defense against disease. Intact skin prevents microbes from entering the body and causing an infection. Likewise, mucous membranes of the mouth, genital area, and anus must be clean and intact. Besides cleansing, good hygiene prevents body and breath odors. It is relaxing and increases circulation.

Culture and personal choice affect hygiene. See *Caring About Culture: Personal Hygiene.* Some people take showers. Others take tub baths. Some bathe at bedtime. Others bathe in the morning. Bathing frequency also varies. Some bathe once or twice a day—before work and after work or exercise. Some people prefer to not have staff members of the opposite sex assist with their bathing. Some people do not have water for bathing. Others cannot afford soap, deodorant, shampoo, toothpaste, or other hygiene products.

Many factors affect hygiene needs—perspiration, elimination, vomiting, drainage from wounds or body openings, bedrest, and activity. Illness and aging changes can affect self-care abilities. Some people need help with hygiene. The nurse uses the nursing process to meet the person's hygiene needs. Follow the nurse's directions and the care plan.

Some older persons resist your efforts to assist with hygiene. Illness, disability, dementia, and personal choice are common reasons. Follow the care plan to meet the person's needs.

See *Residents with Dementia: Hygiene.*

See *Focus on Communication: Hygiene.*

See *Focus on Rehabilitation: Hygiene.*

DAILY CARE

Most people have hygiene routines and habits. For example, teeth are brushed and the face and hands washed after sleep. These and other hygiene measures are often done before and after meals and at bedtime.

Weak and disabled persons need help with hygiene. Routine care is given during the day and evening. You assist with hygiene when it is needed. You must protect the person's right to privacy and to personal choice.

RESIDENTS WITH DEMENTIA

Hygiene

Persons with dementia may resist your efforts to assist with hygiene. Follow the care plan to meet the person's needs. Also see Chapter 40.

 FOCUS ON COMMUNICATION

Hygiene

During hygiene procedures, make sure that the person is warm enough. You can ask:

- "Is the water warm enough? Is it too hot? Is it too cold?"
- "Are you warm enough?"
- "Do you need another bath blanket?"
- "Is the water starting to cool?"
- "Is the room warm enough?"

 FOCUS ON REHABILITATION

Hygiene

Bending and reaching may be hard for older and disabled persons. Some have weak hand grips. They cannot hold soap or a washcloth. For independence, the person may use an adaptive device for hygiene (Fig. 18.1). Remember to let the person do as much self-care as safely as possible.

Before Breakfast

Routine care given before breakfast is called early morning care or AM care. Night shift or day shift staff members give AM care. They get residents ready for breakfast or morning tests. AM care includes the following:

- Assisting with elimination
- Cleaning incontinent persons
- Changing wet or soiled linens and garments
- Assisting with hygiene—face and hand washing, oral hygiene
- Assisting with dressing and hair care

- Positioning persons for breakfast—dining room, bedside chair, or in bed
- Making beds and straightening units

After Breakfast

Morning care is given after breakfast. Hygiene measures are more thorough at this time. They usually involve:

- Assisting with elimination.
- Cleaning incontinent persons.
- Changing wet or soiled linens and garments.
- Assisting with hygiene—face and hand washing, oral hygiene, bathing, back massage, and perineal care.
- Assisting with grooming—hair care, shaving, dressing, and undressing.
- Assisting with activity—range-of-motion exercises and ambulation.
- Making beds and straightening units.

Afternoon Care

Routine hygiene is done after lunch and before the evening meal. It is done before the person takes a nap, has visitors, or attends activity programs. Afternoon care involves:

- Assisting with elimination before and after naps.
- Cleaning incontinent persons before and after naps.
- Changing wet or soiled linens before and after naps.
- Changing wet or soiled garments before and after naps.
- Assisting with hygiene and grooming—face and hand washing, oral hygiene, and hair care.
- Assisting with activity—range-of-motion exercises and ambulation.
- Straightening beds and units.

Evening Care

Care given in the evening at bedtime is called evening care, PM care, or HS care. Evening care is relaxing and promotes comfort. Measures performed before sleep include the following:

- Assisting with elimination

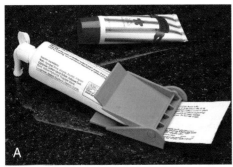
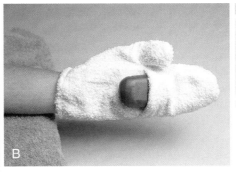
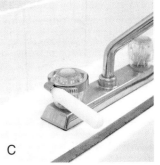
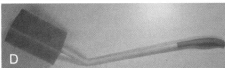

Fig. 18.1 Adaptive devices for hygiene. (A) Tube squeezer for toothpaste. (B) The wash mitt holds a bar of soap. (C) A tap turner makes round knobs easy to turn. (D) A long-handled sponge is used for hard-to-reach body parts.

- Cleaning incontinent persons
- Changing wet or soiled linens and garments
- Assisting with hygiene—face and hand washing, oral hygiene, and back massages
- Helping persons change into sleepwear
- Straightening beds and units

ORAL HYGIENE

Oral hygiene (mouth care) does the following:
- Keeps the mouth and teeth clean
- Prevents mouth odors and infections
- Increases comfort
- Makes food taste better
- Reduces the risk for *cavities (dental caries)* and *periodontal disease*
- Reduces the risk of heart disease

Periodontal disease *(gum disease, pyorrhea)* is an inflammation of tissues around the teeth. Plaque and tartar build up from poor oral hygiene. Plaque is a thin film that sticks to the teeth. It contains saliva, microbes, and other substances. Plaque causes tooth decay *(cavities)*. When plaque hardens, it is called tartar. Tartar builds up at the gum line near the neck of the tooth. Tartar buildup causes periodontal disease. The gums are red and swollen and bleed easily. As the disease progresses, bone is destroyed and teeth loosen. Tooth loss is common.

Illness, disease, and some medications often cause:
- A bad taste in the mouth.
- A whitish coating in the mouth and on the tongue.
- Redness and swelling in the mouth and on the tongue.
- Dry mouth; dry mouth also is common from oxygen, smoking, decreased fluid intake, and anxiety.

The nurse assesses the person's need for mouth care. The speech-language pathologist and the dietitian may also do so.

Flossing

Dental floss is a soft thread used to clean between the teeth. Flossing removes plaque and tartar from the teeth. These substances cause periodontal disease. Flossing also removes food from between the teeth. Usually done after brushing, it can be done at other times. Some people floss after meals. If done once a day, bedtime is the best time to floss.

You need to floss for persons who cannot do so themselves. Some older persons do not floss their teeth. For some older persons flossing may not be helpful. They may have loose teeth or swollen gums, which would prevent flossing from being performed. Never attempt to floss dentures. Follow the care plan.

Equipment

A toothbrush, toothpaste, dental floss, and mouthwash are needed. A toothbrush with soft bristles is best. Persons with dentures need a denture cleaner, denture cup, and denture brush or toothbrush. Use only denture cleaning products. Otherwise, you could damage dentures.

Sponge swabs are used for persons with sore, tender mouths. They also are used for unconscious persons. Use sponge swabs

with care. Check the foam pad to make sure it is tight on the stick. The person could choke on the foam pad if it comes off the stick.

You also need a kidney basin, water glass or cup, straw, tissues, towels, and gloves. Many persons bring oral hygiene equipment from home.

See *Delegation Guidelines: Oral Hygiene.*
See *Promoting Safety and Comfort: Oral Hygiene.*

📋 DELEGATION GUIDELINES

Oral Hygiene

To assist with oral hygiene, you need this information from the nurse and the care plan:
- The type of oral hygiene to give. See procedures:
  - *Assisting the Person to Brush and Floss the Teeth,* p. 259
  - *Brushing and Flossing the Person's* Teeth, pp 259-260
  - *Providing Mouth Care for the Unconscious Person,* pp 261-262
  - *Providing Denture Care,* pp 263-264
- If flossing is needed
- What cleaning agent and equipment to use
- If lubricant is applied to the lips; if so, what lubricant to use
- How often to give oral hygiene
- How much help the person needs
- What observations to report and record:
  - Dry, cracked, swollen, or blistered lips
  - Mouth or breath odor
  - Redness, swelling, irritation, sores, or white patches in the mouth or on the tongue
  - Bleeding, swelling, or redness of the gums
  - Loose teeth
  - Rough, sharp, or chipped areas on dentures
- When to report observations
- What specific resident concerns to report at once

👤 PROMOTING SAFETY AND COMFORT

Oral Hygiene

Safety

Follow Standard Precautions and the Bloodborne Pathogen Standard when giving oral hygiene. You have contact with the person's mucous membranes. Gums may bleed during mouth care. Also, the mouth has many microbes. Pathogens spread through sexual contact may be in the mouths of some persons.

Comfort

Assist with oral hygiene after sleep, after meals, and at bedtime. Many people practice oral hygiene before meals. Some persons need mouth care every 2 hours or more often. Always follow the care plan.

✳ Brushing and Flossing Teeth

Many people perform oral hygiene themselves. Others need help gathering and setting up equipment for oral hygiene. You may have to perform oral hygiene for persons who:
- Are very weak.
- Cannot move or use their arms.
- Are too confused to brush their teeth.

ASSISTING THE PERSON TO BRUSH AND FLOSS THE TEETH

Quality of Life

Remember to:

- Knock before entering the person's room.
- Address the person by name.
- Introduce yourself by name and title.
- Explain the procedure to the person before beginning and during the procedure.
- Protect the person's rights during the procedure.
- Handle the person gently during the procedure.

Preprocedure

1. Follow *Delegation Guidelines: Oral Hygiene*, p. 258. See *Promoting Safety and Comfort: Oral Hygiene.*
2. Practice hand hygiene.
3. Collect the following:
   - Toothbrush
   - Toothpaste
   - Mouthwash (or solution noted on the care plan)
   - Dental floss (if used)
   - Water glass with cool water
   - Straw
   - Kidney basin
   - Hand towel
   - Paper towels

   Gloves
4. Place the paper towels on the overbed table. Arrange items on top of them.
5. Identify the person. Check the ID (identification) bracelet against the assignment sheet. Also call the person by name.

6. Provide for privacy.
7. Lower the bed rail near you if up.

Procedure

8. Position the person to brush with ease.
9. Place the towel over the person's chest. This protects garments and linens from spills.
10. Adjust the overbed table in front of the person.
11. Let the person perform oral hygiene. This includes brushing the teeth and tongue, rinsing the mouth, flossing, and using mouthwash or other solution.
12. Remove the towel when the person is done.
13. Move the overbed table to the side of the bed.

Postprocedure

14. Provide for comfort. (See the inside of the front cover.)
15. Place the call light within reach.
16. Raise or lower bed rails. Follow the care plan.
17. Clean and return items to their proper place. Wear gloves.
18. Wipe off the overbed table with the paper towels. Discard the paper towels.
19. Remove the gloves. Decontaminate your hands.
20. Unscreen the person.
21. Complete a safety check of the room. (See the inside of the front cover.)
22. Follow center policy for dirty linens.
23. Decontaminate your hands.
24. Report and record your observations.

This skill is also covered in *Clinical Skills: Nurse Assisting.*

BRUSHING AND FLOSSING THE PERSON'S TEETH

Quality of Life

Remember to:

- Knock before entering the person's room.
- Address the person by name.
- Introduce yourself by name and title.
- Explain the procedure to the person before beginning and during the procedure.
- Protect the person's rights during the procedure.
- Handle the person gently during the procedure.

Preprocedure

1. Follow *Delegation Guidelines: Oral Hygiene*, p. 258. See *Promoting Safety and Comfort: Oral Hygiene*, p. 258.
2. Practice hand hygiene.
3. Collect the following:
   - Toothbrush with soft bristles
   - Toothpaste
   - Mouthwash (or solution noted on the care plan)
   - Dental floss (if used)
   - Water glass with cool water
   - Straw
   - Kidney basin
   - Hand towel
   - Paper towels
   - Gloves
4. Place the paper towels on the overbed table. Arrange items on top of them.
5. Identify the person. Check the ID bracelet against the assignment sheet. Also call the person by name.

6. Provide for privacy.
7. Raise the bed for body mechanics. Bed rails are up if used.

Procedure

8. Lower the bed rail near you if up.
9. Assist the person to a sitting position or to a side-lying position near you.
10. Place the towel across the person's chest.
11. Adjust the overbed table so you can reach it with ease.
12. Decontaminate your hands. Put on the gloves.
13. Hold the toothbrush over the kidney basin. Pour some water over the brush.
14. Apply toothpaste to the toothbrush.
15. Brush the teeth gently (Fig. 18.2).
16. Brush the tongue gently.
17. Let the person rinse the mouth with water. Hold the kidney basin under the person's chin (Fig. 18.3). Repeat this step as needed.
18. Floss the person's teeth (optional).
    a. Break off an 18-inch piece of dental floss from the dispenser.
    b. Hold the floss between the middle fingers of each hand (Fig. 18.4A).
    c. Stretch the floss with your thumbs.
    d. Start at the upper back tooth on the right side. Work around to the left side.
    e. Move the floss gently up and down between the teeth (see Fig. 18.4B). Move the floss up and down against the side of the tooth. Work from the top of the crown to the gum line.
    f. Move to a new section of floss after every second tooth.
    g. Floss the lower teeth. Use up-and-down motions as for the upper teeth. Start on the right side. Work around to the left side.

BRUSHING AND FLOSSING THE PERSON'S TEETH—cont'd

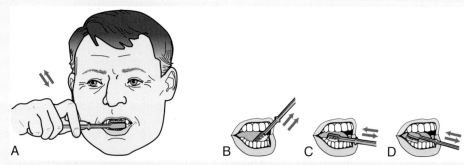

Fig. 18.2 Brushing teeth. (A) The brush is held at a 45-degree angle to the gums. Teeth are brushed with short strokes. (B) The brush is at a 45-degree angle against the inside of the front teeth. Teeth are brushed from the gum to the crown of the tooth with short strokes. (C) The brush is held horizontally against the inner surfaces of the teeth. The teeth are brushed back and forth. (D) The brush is positioned on the biting surfaces of the teeth. The teeth are brushed back and forth.

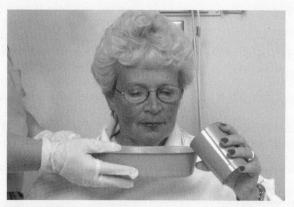

Fig. 18.3 The kidney basin is held under the person's chin.

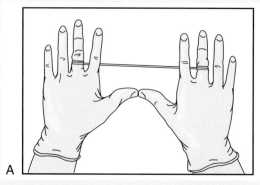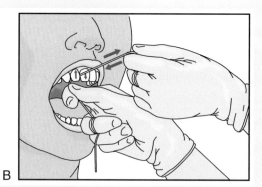

Fig. 18.4 Flossing. (A) Floss is wrapped around the middle fingers. (B) Floss is moved in up-and-down motions between the teeth. Floss is moved up and down from the crown to the gum line.

19. Let the person use mouthwash or other solution. Hold the kidney basin under the chin.
20. Wipe the person's mouth. Remove the towel.
21. Remove and discard the gloves. Decontaminate your hands.

Postprocedure

22. Provide for comfort. (See the inside of the front cover.)
23. Place the call light within reach.
24. Lower the bed to its lowest position.

25. Raise or lower bed rails. Follow the care plan.
26. Clean and return equipment to its proper place. Wear gloves.
27. Wipe off the overbed table with the paper towels. Discard the paper towels.
28. Unscreen the person.
29. Complete a safety check of the room. (See the inside of the front cover.)
30. Follow center policy for dirty linens.
31. Remove the gloves. Decontaminate your hands.
32. Report and record your observations.

This skill is also covered in *Clinical Skills: Nurse Assisting.*

Mouth Care for the Unconscious Person

Unconscious persons cannot eat or drink. They may breathe with their mouth open. Many receive oxygen. These factors cause mouth dryness. They also cause crusting on the tongue and mucous membranes. Oral hygiene keeps the mouth clean and moist. It also helps prevent infection.

The care plan tells you what cleaning agent to use. Use sponge swabs to apply the cleaning agent. Apply a lubricant (check the care plan) to the lips after cleaning. It prevents cracking of the lips.

Unconscious persons usually cannot swallow. Protect them from choking and aspiration. *Aspiration* is breathing fluid, food, vomitus, or an object into the lungs. It can cause pneumonia and death. To prevent aspiration:

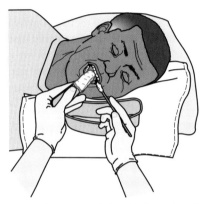

Fig. 18.5 The unconscious person's head is turned well to the side to prevent aspiration. A padded tongue blade is used to keep the mouth open while cleaning the mouth with swabs.

- Position the person on one side with the head turned well to the side (Fig. 18.5). In this position, excess fluid runs out of the mouth.
- Use only a small amount of fluid to clean the mouth.
- Do not insert dentures. Dentures are not worn when the person is unconscious.

PROMOTING SAFETY AND COMFORT

Mouth Care for the Unconscious Person

Safety

Use sponge swabs with care. Make sure the sponge pad is tight on the stick. The person could choke or aspirate on the sponge if it comes off the stick.

Comfort

Unconscious persons are repositioned at least every 2 hours. To promote comfort, combine mouth care with skin care, repositioning, and other comfort measures.

Keep the person's mouth open with a padded tongue blade (Fig. 18.6). Do not use your fingers. The person can bite down on them. The bite breaks the skin and creates a portal of entry for microbes. Infection is a risk.

Unconscious persons cannot speak or respond to you. However, some can hear. Always assume that unconscious persons can hear. Explain what you are doing step by step. Also tell the person when you are done, when you are leaving the room, and when you will return.

Mouth care is given at least every 2 hours. Follow the nurse's directions and the care plan.

See *Promoting Safety and Comfort: Mouth Care for the Unconscious Person.*

PROVIDING MOUTH CARE FOR THE UNCONSCIOUS PERSON

Quality of Life

Remember to:
- Knock before entering the person's room.
- Address the person by name.
- Introduce yourself by name and title.
- Explain the procedure to the person before beginning and during the procedure.
- Protect the person's rights during the procedure.
- Handle the person gently during the procedure.

Preprocedure

1. Follow *Delegation Guidelines: Oral Hygiene*, p. 258. See *Promoting Safety and Comfort:*
   a. *Oral Hygiene*, p. 258
   b. *Mouth Care for the Unconscious Person*
2. Practice hand hygiene.
3. Collect the following:
   - Cleaning agent (check the care plan)
   - Sponge swabs
   - Padded tongue blade
   - Water glass or cup with cool water
   - Hand towel
   - Kidney basin
   - Lip lubricant
   - Paper towels

- Gloves
4. Place the towels on the overbed table. Arrange items on top of them.
5. Identify the person. Check the ID bracelet against the assignment sheet. Also call the person by name.
6. Provide for privacy.
7. Raise the bed for body mechanics. Bed rails are up if used.

Procedure

8. Lower the bed rail near you if up.
9. Decontaminate your hands. Put on the gloves.
10. Position the person in a side-lying position near you. Turn the person's head well to the side.
11. Place the towel under the person's face.
12. Place the kidney basin under the chin.
13. Separate the upper and lower teeth. Use the padded tongue blade. Be gentle. Never use force. If you have problems, ask the nurse for help.
14. Clean the mouth using sponge swabs moistened with the cleaning agent (see Fig. 18.5).
    a. Clean the chewing and inner surfaces of the teeth.
    b. Clean the gums and outer surfaces of the teeth.
    c. Swab the roof of the mouth, inside of the cheeks, and the lips.
    d. Swab the tongue.
    e. Moisten a clean swab with water. Swab the mouth to rinse.
    f. Place used swabs in the kidney basin.
15. Remove the kidney basin and supplies.

Continued

✳ PROVIDING MOUTH CARE FOR THE UNCONSCIOUS PERSON—cont'd

16. Wipe the person's mouth. Remove the towel.
17. Apply lubricant to the lips.
18. Remove and discard the gloves. Decontaminate your hands.

Postprocedure

19. Provide for comfort. (See the inside of the front cover.)
20. Place the call light within reach.
21. Lower the bed to its lowest position.
22. Raise or lower bed rails. Follow the care plan.

23. Clean and return equipment to its proper place. Discard disposable items. (Wear gloves.)
24. Wipe off the overbed table with paper towels. Discard the paper towels.
25. Unscreen the person.
26. Complete a safety check of the room. (See the inside of the front cover.)
27. Tell the person when you are leaving the room, and when you will return.
28. Follow center policy for dirty linens.
29. Remove the gloves. Decontaminate your hands.
30. Report and record your observations.

This skill is also covered in *Clinical Skills: Nurse Assisting.*

✳ Denture Care

A **denture** is an artificial tooth or a set of artificial teeth (Fig. 18.7). They are often called "false teeth." Dentures replace missing teeth. People lose teeth because of gum disease, tooth decay, or injury. Dentures are expensive. Assistants must handle them with care. Full and partial dentures are common:

- *Full denture.* The person has no upper or no lower natural teeth. Dentures replace the upper or lower teeth.
- *Partial denture.* The person has some natural teeth. The partial denture replaces the missing teeth.

Mouth care is given and dentures cleaned as often as natural teeth. Dentures are slippery when wet. They easily break or chip if dropped onto a hard surface (floors, sinks, counters). Hold them firmly when removing or inserting them. During cleaning, firmly hold them over a basin of water lined with a towel. This prevents them from falling onto a hard surface.

To use a cleaning agent, follow the manufacturer instructions. They tell how to use the cleaning agent and what water temperature to use. Hot water causes dentures to lose their shape (warp). If not worn after cleaning, store dentures in a container with cool water or a denture soaking solution. Otherwise, they can dry out and warp.

Dentures are usually removed at bedtime. Some people do not wear their dentures. Others wear dentures for eating and remove them after meals. Remind them not to wrap dentures in tissues or napkins. Otherwise, they are easily discarded.

Many people clean their own dentures. Some need help collecting items used to clean dentures. They may need help getting to the bathroom. You clean dentures for those who cannot do so.

See *Promoting Safety and Comfort: Denture Care.*

👤 PROMOTING SAFETY AND COMFORT

Denture Care

Safety

Dentures are the person's property. They are costly. Handle them very carefully. Label the denture cup with the person's name and room and bed number. Report lost or damaged dentures to the nurse at once. Losing or damaging dentures is negligent conduct.

Never carry dentures in your hands. Always use a denture cup or kidney basin. You could easily drop the dentures as you move from the bedside to the bathroom. Or you could drop them when moving from the bathroom to the bedside.

Comfort

Many people do not like being seen without their dentures. Privacy is important. Allow privacy when the person cleans dentures. If you clean dentures, return them to the person as quickly as possible.

Persons with dentures may have some natural teeth. They need to brush and floss the natural teeth. See procedure: *Assisting the Person to Brush and Floss the Teeth*, p. 259. Or see procedure: *Brushing and Flossing the Person's Teeth*, pp. 259-260.

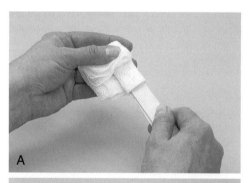
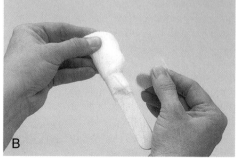

Fig. 18.6 Making a padded tongue blade. (A) Place two wooden tongue blades together. Wrap gauze around the top half. (B) Tape the gauze in place.

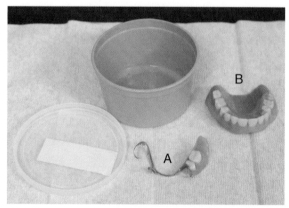

Fig. 18.7 Dentures. (A) Partial denture. (B) Full denture.

✳ PROVIDING DENTURE CARE (NATCEP)

Quality of Life

Remember to:

- Knock before entering the person's room.
- Address the person by name.
- Introduce yourself by name and title.
- Explain the procedure to the person before beginning and during the procedure.
- Protect the person's rights during the procedure.
- Handle the person gently during the procedure.

Preprocedure

1. Follow *Delegation Guidelines: Oral Hygiene*, p. 258. See *Promoting Safety and Comfort*:
   a. *Oral Hygiene*, p. 258
   b. *Denture Care*, p. 262
2. Practice hand hygiene.
3. Collect the following:
   - Denture brush or toothbrush (for cleaning dentures)
   - Denture cup labeled with the person's name and room and bed number
   - Denture cleaning agent
   - Soft-bristled toothbrush or sponge swabs (for oral hygiene)
   - Toothpaste
   - Water glass with cool water
   - Straw
   - Mouthwash (or other noted solution)
   - Kidney basin
   - Two hand towels
   - Gauze squares
   - Paper towels
   - Gloves
4. Place the paper towels on the overbed table. Arrange items on top of them.
5. Identify the person. Check the ID bracelet against the assignment sheet. Also call the person by name.
6. Provide for privacy.
7. Raise the bed for body mechanics.

Procedure

8. Lower the bed rail near you if used.
9. Decontaminate your hands. Put on the gloves.
10. Place a towel over the person's chest.
11. Ask the person to remove the dentures. Carefully place them in the kidney basin.
12. Remove the dentures if the person cannot do so. Use gauze squares to get a good grip on the slippery dentures.
    a. Grasp the denture with your thumb and index finger (Fig. 18.8). Move it up and down slightly to break the seal. Gently remove the denture. Place it in the kidney basin.
    b. Grasp and remove the lower denture with your thumb and index finger. Turn it slightly and lift it out of the person's mouth. Place it in the kidney basin.
13. Follow the care plan for raising bed rails.
14. Take the kidney basin, denture cup, denture brush, and denture cleaning agent to the sink.
15. Line the sink with a towel. Fill the sink halfway with water.
16. Rinse each denture under cool or warm running water. Follow center policy for water temperature.
17. Return dentures to the kidney basin or denture cup.
18. Apply the denture cleaning agent to the brush.
19. Brush the dentures as in Fig. 18.9. Brush the inner, outer, and chewing surfaces.

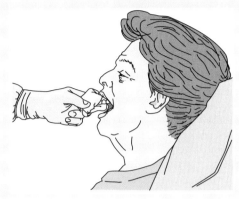

Fig. 18.8 Remove the upper denture by grasping it with the thumb and index finger of one hand. Use a piece of gauze to grasp the slippery denture.

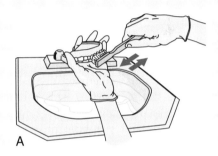

A

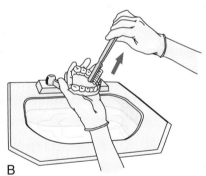

B

Fig. 18.9 Cleaning dentures. (A) Brush the outer surfaces of the denture with back-and-forth motions. The denture is held over the sink. The sink is filled halfway with water and is lined with a towel. (B) Position the brush vertically to clean the inner surfaces of the denture. Use upward strokes.

20. Rinse the dentures under running water. Use warm or cool water as directed by the cleaning agent manufacturer. (Some state competency tests require cool water.)
21. Rinse the denture cup and lid. Place dentures in the denture cup. Cover the dentures with cool or warm water. Follow center policy for water temperature.
22. Clean the kidney basin.
23. Take the denture cup and kidney basin to the overbed table.
24. Lower the bed rail if up.
25. Position the person for oral hygiene.
26. Clean the person's gums and tongue. Use toothpaste and the toothbrush (or sponge swabs).

✳ PROVIDING DENTURE CARE (NATCEP)—cont'd

27. Have the person use mouthwash (or noted solution). Hold the kidney basin under the chin.
28. Ask the person to insert the dentures. Insert them if the person cannot.
    a. Hold the upper denture firmly with your thumb and index finger. Raise the upper lip with the other hand. Insert the denture. Gently press on the denture with your index fingers to make sure it is in place.
    b. Hold the lower denture with your thumb and index finger. Pull the lower lip down slightly. Insert the denture. Gently press down on it to make sure it is in place.
29. Place the denture cup in the top drawer of the bedside stand if the dentures are not worn. The dentures must be in water or in a denture soaking solution.
30. Wipe the person's mouth. Remove the towel.
31. Remove the gloves. Decontaminate your hands.

Postprocedure

32. Assist with hand washing.

33. Provide for comfort. (See the inside of the front cover.)
34. Place the call light within reach.
35. Lower the bed to its lowest position.
36. Raise or lower bed rails. Follow the care plan.
37. Remove the towel from the sink. Drain the sink.
38. Clean and return equipment to its proper place. Discard disposable items. Wear gloves for this step.
39. Wipe off the overbed table with the paper towels. Discard the paper towels.
40. Unscreen the person.
41. Complete a safety check of the room. (See the inside of the front cover.)
42. Follow center policy for dirty linens.
43. Remove the gloves. Decontaminate your hands.
44. Report and record your observations.

This skill is also covered in *Clinical Skills: Nurse Assisting.*

BATHING

Bathing cleans the skin. It also cleans the mucous membranes of the genital and anal areas. Microbes, dead skin, perspiration, and excess oils are removed. A bath is refreshing and relaxing. Circulation is stimulated and body parts exercised. Observations are made and you have time to talk to the person.

Complete or partial baths, tub baths, or showers are given. The method depends on the person's condition, self-care abilities, and personal choice. In nursing centers, bathing usually occurs after breakfast or the evening meal. The person's choice of type of bath and time of day is respected when possible.

Bathing frequency is a personal matter. Some people bathe daily. Others bathe once or twice a week. Personal choice, weather, activity, and illness affect bathing frequency. Ill persons may have fevers and perspire heavily. They need frequent bathing. Other illnesses and dry skin may limit bathing to every 2 or 3 days.

Dry skin occurs with aging. Soap also dries the skin. Dry skin is easily damaged. Therefore older persons usually need a complete bath or shower twice a week. Partial baths are taken on the other days. Some bathe daily but not with soap. Thorough rinsing is needed when using soap. Lotions and oils help keep the skin soft. Some people may have allergies to skin care products. Always follow the care plan if certain products are to be used or avoided.

The rules for bed baths, showers, and tub baths are listed in Box 18.1. Table 18.1 describes common skin care products.

See *Focus on Communication: Hygiene*, p. 257.
See *Residents with Dementia: Bathing*, p. 265.
See *Delegation Guidelines: Bathing*, p. 266.
See *Promoting Safety and Comfort: Bathing*, p. 266.

BOX 18.1   Rules for Bathing

- Follow the care plan for bathing method and skin care products.
- Allow personal choice when possible.
- Follow Standard Precautions and the Bloodborne Pathogen Standard.
- Collect needed items before starting the procedure.
- Provide for privacy. Screen the person. Close doors and window coverings (drapes, shades, blinds, shutters, etc.).
- Assist the person with elimination. Bathing stimulates the need to urinate. Comfort and relaxation increase if urination needs are met.
- Remove and safely store the person's hearing aids and eyeglasses.
- If the person has a bandage or dressing, check with the nurse to see if it must be kept dry or have the nurse remove it before bathing.
- Cover the person for warmth and privacy.
- Reduce drafts. Close doors and windows.
- Protect the person from falling.
- Use good body mechanics at all times.
- Follow the rules to safely handle, move, and transfer the person (Chapter 15).

- Know what water temperature to use. See *Delegation Guidelines: Bathing*, p. 266.
- Keep bar soap in the soap dish between latherings. This prevents soapy water. It also reduces the chances of slipping and falls in showers and tubs. Bar soap should not be shared between persons. Many centers use liquid soap dispensers.
- Wash from the cleanest areas to the dirtiest areas.
- Encourage the person to help as much as is safely possible.
- Rinse the skin thoroughly. You must remove all soap.
- Pat the skin dry to avoid irritating or breaking the skin. Do not rub the skin. Warm towels and bath blankets offer extra comfort.
- Dry under the breasts, between skin folds, in the perineal area, and between the toes.
- Bathe skin when urine or feces are present. This prevents skin breakdown and odors.

TABLE 18.1 Skin Care Products

Type	Purpose	Care Considerations
Soaps	• Clean the skin • Remove dirt, dead skin, skin oil, some microbes, and perspiration	• Tend to dry and irritate the skin • Dry skin is easily injured and causes itching and discomfort • Skin must be thoroughly rinsed to remove all soap • Not needed for every bath; plain water can clean the skin • Plain water is often used for older persons due to dry skin • People with dry skin may use soaps containing bath oils • Not used if a person has very dry skin
Bath oils	• Keep the skin soft • Prevent dry skin	• Some soaps contain bath oil • Liquid bath oil can be added to bath water • Showers and tubs become slippery from bath oils; safety measures are needed to prevent falls
Creams and lotions	• Protect the skin from the drying effect of air and evaporation	• Do not feel greasy but leave an oily film on the skin • Lotion applied to body areas after bathing to prevent skin breakdown (back, elbows, knees, and heels) • Lotion used for back massages • Most are scented
Powders	• Absorb moisture • Prevent friction when two skin surfaces rub together	• Usually applied under the breasts, under the arms, and in the groin area, and sometimes between the toes • Applied to dry skin in a thin, even layer • Excessive amounts cause caking and crusts that can irritate the skin
Deodorants	• Mask and control body odors	• Applied to the underarms • Not applied to irritated skin • Do not take the place of bathing
Antiperspirants	• Reduce the amount of perspiration	• Applied to the underarms • Not applied to irritated skin • Do not take the place of bathing

RESIDENTS WITH DEMENTIA

Bathing

Bathing procedures can threaten persons with dementia. They do not understand what is happening or why. And they may fear harm or danger. Confusion can increase. Therefore they may resist care and become agitated and combative. They may shout at you and cry out for help. You must be calm, patient, and soothing.

The nurse assesses the person's behaviors and routines. The person may be calmer and less confused or agitated during a certain time of the day. Bathing is scheduled for the person's calm times. The nurse decides if a bed bath, tub bath, shower, or towel bath (p. 270) is best for the person.

The rules in Box 18.1 apply when bathing these persons. The care plan also includes measures to help the person through the bath. Such measures may include:

- Use terms such as "cleaned up" or "washed" rather than "shower" or "bath."
- Complete preprocedure activities (e.g., ready supplies and linens). Make sure you have everything that you need.
- Provide for warmth. Increase the room temperature before starting the bath or shower. Have extra towels and a robe nearby. Warm towels or a bath blanket can offer comfort.
- Play soft music to help the person relax.
- Provide for safety:
  - Use a handheld shower nozzle.
  - Have the person use a shower chair or shower bench.
- Do not use bath oil. It can make the tub or shower slippery, and it may cause a urinary tract infection.
- Do not leave the person alone in the tub or shower.
- Draw bath water ahead of time. Test the water temperature. Add warm or cold water as necessary.
- Tell the person what you are doing step by step. Use clear, simple statements.
- Let the person help as much as possible (e.g., provide a washcloth and ask the person to wash the arms; if the person does not know what to do, still let the person hold the washcloth if it is safe to do so).
- Put a towel over the person's shoulder or lap (tub or shower). This helps the person feel less exposed.
- Do not rush the person.
- Use a calm, pleasant voice.
- Divert the person's attention if necessary.
- Calm the person.
- Handle the person gently.
- Try giving a partial bath if a shower or tub bath agitates the person.
- Try the bath later if the person continues to resist care.

Persons with dementia may respond well to a *towel bath*. An oversized towel is used. It covers the body from the neck to the feet. The towel is wet with a solution—water, cleaning agent, and skin-softening agent. It also has a drying agent so the person's body dries fast. The nurse and care plan tell you when to use a towel bath. To give a towel bath, follow center policy.

DELEGATION GUIDELINES

Bathing

To assist with bathing, you need this information from the nurse and the care plan:

- What bath to give—complete bed bath, partial bath, tub bath, shower, towel bath, or bag bath
- How much help the person needs
- The person's activity or position limits
- What water temperature to use. Bath water cools rapidly. Heat is lost to the bath basin, overbed table, washcloth, and your hands. Therefore water temperature for complete bed baths and partial bed baths is usually between 110°F and 115°F (Fahrenheit) (43.3°C and 46.1°C [Centigrade]) for adults. Older persons have fragile skin. They need lower water temperatures.
- What skin care products to use and what the person prefers
- What observations to report and record:

- The color of the skin, lips, nail beds, and sclera (whites of the eyes)
- The location and description of rashes
- Dry skin
- Bruises or open skin areas
- Pale or reddened areas, particularly over bony parts
- Any body part that cannot get wet or bandages, dressings, or casts that must stay dry
- Drainage or bleeding from wounds or body openings
- Swelling of the feet and legs
- Corns or calluses on the feet
- Skin temperature
- Complaints of pain or discomfort
- When to report observations
- What specific resident concerns to report at once

✵ The Complete Bed Bath

The *complete bed bath* involves washing the person's entire body in bed. You give complete bed baths to persons who cannot bathe themselves. Bed baths are usually needed by persons who are:

- Unconscious.
- Paralyzed.
- In casts or traction.
- Weak from illness or surgery.

A bed bath is new to some people. Some are embarrassed to have others see their body. Some fear exposure. Explain how the bed bath is given. Also explain how you cover the body for privacy.

PROMOTING SAFETY AND COMFORT

Bathing

Safety

Hot water can burn delicate and fragile skin. Measure water temperature according to center policy. If unsure whether the water is too hot, ask the nurse to check it.

Protect the person from falls and other injuries. Practice the safety measures presented in Chapters 11 and 12. Also protect the person from drafts.

Use caution when applying powder. Do not use powders near persons with respiratory disorders. Inhaling powder can irritate the airway and lungs. Before applying powder, check with the nurse and the care plan. Do not shake or sprinkle powder onto the person. To safely apply powder:

- Turn away from the person.
- Sprinkle a small amount of powder onto your hands or a cloth.
- Apply the powder in a thin layer.
- Make sure powder does not get on the floor. Powder is slippery and can cause falls.

Beds are made after baths. After making the bed, lower the bed to its lowest position. Then lock the bed wheels. For an occupied bed, raise or lower bed rails according to the care plan.

Protect the person and yourself from infection. When giving baths and making beds, contact with blood, body fluids, secretions, and excretions is likely. Follow Standard Precautions and the Bloodborne Pathogen Standard.

Comfort

Before bathing, allow the person to meet elimination needs (Chapters 22 and 23). Bathing stimulates the need to urinate. The person is more comfortable if the bladder is empty. Also, bathing is not interrupted.

Many people perform oral hygiene as part of their bathing routine. Some do so before the bathing procedure; others do so after. Allow personal choice and follow the person's care plan.

Provide for warmth. Cover the person with a bath blanket. Many centers have blanket warmers (Fig. 18.10) for towels and bath blankets. Make sure the water is warm enough for the person. Cool water causes chilling.

Remove the person's gown or pajamas after washing the eyes, face, ears, and neck. Waiting to remove sleepwear at this time helps the person feel less exposed and more comfortable with the bath. If the person prefers, you can remove the sleepwear before washing the eyes, face, ears, and neck.

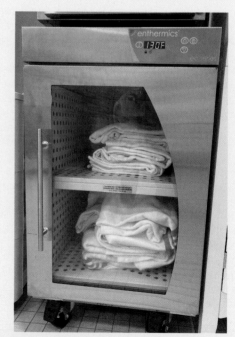

Fig. 18.10 A blanket warmer located in the bathing room.

✳ GIVING A COMPLETE BED BATH (NATCEP)

Quality of Life

Remember to:

- Knock before entering the person's room.
- Address the person by name.
- Introduce yourself by name and title.
- Explain the procedure to the person before beginning and during the procedure.
- Protect the person's rights during the procedure.
- Handle the person gently during the procedure.

Preprocedure

1. Follow *Delegation Guidelines: Bathing*, p. 266. See *Promoting Safety and Comfort: Bathing*.
2. Practice hand hygiene.
3. Identify the person. Check the ID bracelet against the assignment sheet. Also call the person by name.
4. Collect clean linens for a closed bed. See procedure: *Making a Closed Bed* in Chapter 17. Place linens on a clean surface.
5. Collect the following:
   - Wash basin
   - Soap
   - Bath thermometer
   - Orangewood stick or nail file
   - Washcloth
   - Two bath towels and two hand towels
   - Bath blanket
   - Clothing or sleepwear
   - Lotion
     - Powder
     - Deodorant or antiperspirant
     - Brush and comb
     - Other grooming items as requested
     - Paper towels
     - Gloves
6. Cover the overbed table with paper towels. Arrange items on the overbed table. Adjust the height as needed.
7. Provide for privacy.
8. Raise the bed for body mechanics. Bed rails are up if used.

Procedure

9. Remove the call light.
10. Decontaminate your hands. Put on gloves.
11. Cover the person with a bath blanket (warm if possible). Remove top linens (see procedure: *Making an Occupied Bed* in Chapter 17).
12. Lower the head of the bed. It is as flat as possible. The person has at least one pillow.
13. Fill the wash basin two-thirds full with water. Follow the care plan for water temperature. Water temperature is usually 110°F to 115°F (43.3°C to 46.1°C) for adults. Measure water temperature. Use the bath thermometer. Or test the water by dipping your elbow or inner wrist into the basin.
14. Lower the bed rail near you if up.
15. Ask the person to check the water temperature. Adjust the water temperature if it is too hot or too cold. Raise the bed rail before leaving the bedside. Lower it when you return.
16. Place the basin on the overbed table.
17. Remove the sleepwear. Do not expose the person.
18. Place a hand towel over the person's chest.
19. Make a mitt with the washcloth (Fig. 18.11). Use a mitt for the entire bath.
20. Wash around the person's eyes with water. Do not use soap.
    a. Clean the far eye. Gently wipe from the inner to the outer aspect of the eye with a corner of the mitt (Fig. 18.12).
    b. Clean around the eye near you. Use a clean part of the washcloth for each stroke.
21. Ask the person if you should use soap to wash the face.
22. Wash the face, ears, and neck. Rinse and pat dry with the towel on the chest.
23. Help the person move to the side of the bed near you.
24. Expose the far arm. Place a bath towel lengthwise under the arm. Apply soap to the washcloth.
25. Support the arm with your palm under the person's elbow. The person's forearm rests on your forearm.
26. Wash the arm, shoulder, and underarm. Use long, firm strokes (Fig. 18.13). Rinse and pat dry.

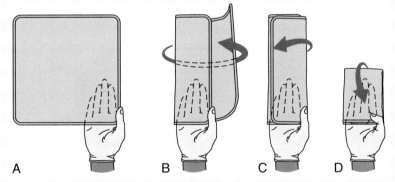

Fig. 18.11 Making a mitted washcloth. (A) Grasp the near side of the washcloth with your thumb. (B) Bring the washcloth around and behind your hand. (C) Fold the side of the washcloth over your palm as you grasp it with your thumb. (D) Fold the top of the washcloth down and tuck it under next to your palm.

✳ GIVING A COMPLETE BED BATH (NATCEP)—cont'd

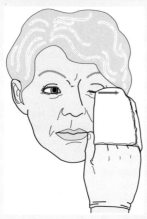

Fig. 18.12 Wash the person's eyes with a mitted washcloth. Wipe from the inner to the outer aspect of the eye.

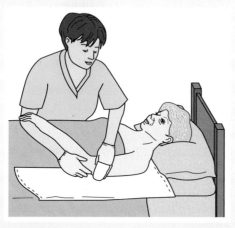

Fig. 18.13 The person's arm is washed with firm, long strokes using a mitted washcloth.

27. Place the basin on the towel. Put the person's hand into the water (Fig. 18.14). Wash it well. Clean under the fingernails with an orangewood stick or nail file.
28. Have the person exercise the hand and fingers.
29. Remove the basin. Dry the hand well. Cover the arm with the bath blanket.
30. Repeat steps 24 to 29 for the near arm.
31. Place a bath towel over the chest crosswise. Hold the towel in place. Pull the bath blanket from under the towel to the waist. Apply soap to the washcloth.
32. Lift the towel slightly and wash the chest (Fig. 18.15). Do not expose the person. Rinse and pat dry, especially under the breasts.
33. Move the towel lengthwise over the chest and abdomen. Do not expose the person. Pull the bath blanket down to the pubic area. Apply soap to the washcloth.
34. Lift the towel slightly and wash the abdomen (Fig. 18.16). Rinse and pat dry.
35. Pull the bath blanket up to the shoulders, covering both arms. Remove the towel.
36. Change soapy or cool water. Measure bath water temperature as in step 13. If bed rails are used, raise the bed rail near you before leaving the bedside. Lower it when you return.
37. Uncover the far leg. Do not expose the genital area. Place a towel lengthwise under the foot and leg. Apply soap to the washcloth.

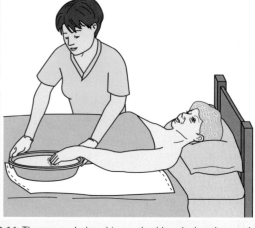

Fig. 18.14 The person's hand is washed by placing the wash basin on the bed.

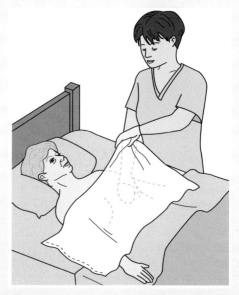

Fig. 18.15 The person's breasts are not exposed during the bath. A bath towel is placed crosswise over the chest area. The towel is lifted slightly to reach under to wash the breasts and chest.

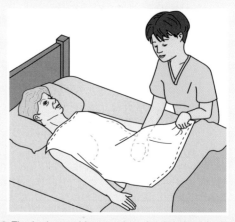

Fig. 18.16 The bath towel is turned so that it is lengthwise to cover the breasts and abdomen. The towel is lifted slightly to bathe the abdomen. The bath blanket covers the pubic area.

Continued

GIVING A COMPLETE BED BATH (NATCEP)—cont'd

38. Bend the knee and support the leg with your arm. Wash it with long, firm strokes. Rinse and pat dry.
39. Place the basin on the towel near the foot.
40. Lift the leg slightly. Slide the basin under the foot.
41. Place the foot in the basin (Fig. 18.17). Use an orangewood stick or nail file to clean under toenails if necessary. If the person cannot bend the knees:
    a. Wash the foot. Carefully separate the toes. Rinse and pat dry.
    b. Clean under the toenails with an orangewood stick or nail file if necessary.
42. Remove the basin. Dry the leg and foot. Apply lotion to the foot if directed by the nurse and care plan. Cover the leg with the bath blanket. Remove the towel.
43. Repeat steps 37 to 42 for the near leg.
44. Change the water. Measure water temperature as in step 13. If bed rails are used, raise the bed rail near you before leaving the bedside. Lower it when you return.
45. Turn the person onto the side away from you. The person is covered with the bath blanket.
46. Uncover the back and buttocks. Do not expose the person. Place a towel lengthwise on the bed along the back. Apply soap to the washcloth.
47. Wash the back. Work from the back of the neck to the lower end of the buttocks. Use long, firm, continuous strokes (Fig. 18.18). Rinse and dry well.
48. Give a back massage (p. 274). The person may want the back massage after the bath.
49. Turn the person onto the back.
50. Change the water for perineal care (p. 276). For water temperature, see step 14 in procedure: *Giving Female Perineal Care*, pp 277-279. (Some state competency tests also require changing gloves and hand hygiene at this time.) If bed rails are used, raise the bed rail near you before leaving the bedside. Lower it when you return.

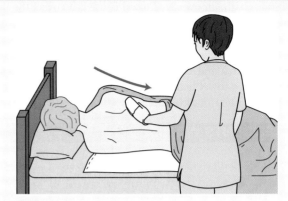

Fig. 18.18 The back is washed with long, firm, continuous strokes. Note that the person is in a side-lying position. A towel is placed lengthwise on the bed to protect the linens from water.

51. Let the person wash the genital area. Adjust the overbed table so the person can reach the wash basin, soap, and towels with ease. Place the call light within reach. Ask the person to signal when finished. Make sure the person understands what to do.
52. Remove the gloves. Decontaminate your hands.
53. Answer the call light promptly. Knock before entering the room. Provide perineal care if the person cannot do so (pp 277-279). (Decontaminate your hands and wear gloves for perineal care.)
54. Give a back massage if you have not already done so.
55. Apply deodorant or antiperspirant. Apply lotion and powder as requested. See *Promoting Safety and Comfort: Bathing*, p. 266.
56. Put clean garments on the person.
57. Comb and brush the hair (Chapter 19).
58. Make the bed.

Postprocedure
59. Provide for comfort. (See the inside of the front cover.)
60. Place the call light within reach.
61. Lower the bed to its lowest position.
62. Raise or lower bed rails. Follow the care plan.
63. Put on clean gloves.
64. Empty, clean, and dry the wash basin. Return it and other supplies to their proper place.
65. Wipe off the overbed table with paper towels. Discard the paper towels.
66. Unscreen the person.
67. Complete a safety check of the room. (See the inside of the front cover.)
68. Follow center policy for dirty linens.
69. Remove the gloves. Decontaminate your hands.
70. Report and record your observations.

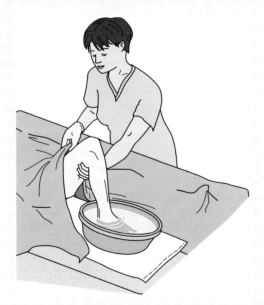

Fig. 18.17 The foot is washed by placing it in the wash basin on the bed.

This skill is also covered in *Clinical Skills: Nurse Assisting.*

Towel Baths

For a towel bath, an oversized towel is used. It covers the body from the neck to the feet. The towel is completely wet with a solution—water and cleaning, skin-softening, and drying agents. The drying agent promotes fast drying of the person's body. The nurse and care plan tell you when to use a towel bath. To give a towel bath, follow center policy.

See *Residents with Dementia: Towel Baths.*

RESIDENTS WITH DEMENTIA

Towel Baths

The towel bath is quick, soothing, and relaxing. Persons with dementia often respond well to this type of bath. The nurse and care plan tell you when to use the towel bath.

Bag Baths

Bag baths are commercially prepared or prepared at the center. A plastic bag has 8 to 10 washcloths. They are moistened with a cleaning agent that does not need rinsing. To give a bag bath:

- Warm the washcloths in a microwave oven. Follow the manufacturer instructions for what microwave setting to use. (Some nursing centers have warming units that the prepared bath packages are kept in at a constant warm temperature.)
- Use a new washcloth for each body part.
- Let the skin air-dry. You do not need towels.

✳ The Partial Bath

The *partial bath* involves bathing the face, hands, axillae (underarms), back, buttocks, and perineal area. Odors or discomfort occurs if these areas are not clean. Some persons bathe themselves in bed or at the sink. You assist as needed. Most need help washing the back. You give partial baths to persons who cannot bathe themselves.

The rules for bathing apply (see Box 18.1). So do the complete bed bath considerations.

✳ ASSISTING WITH THE PARTIAL BATH

Quality of Life

Remember to:

- Knock before entering the person's room.
- Address the person by name.
- Introduce yourself by name and title.
- Explain the procedure to the person before beginning and during the procedure.
- Protect the person's rights during the procedure.
- Handle the person gently during the procedure.

Preprocedure

1. Follow *Delegation Guidelines: Bathing*, p. 266. See *Promoting Safety and Comfort: Bathing*, p. 266.
2. Follow steps 2 through 7 in procedure: *Giving a Complete Bed Bath*, p. 267.

Procedure

3. Make sure the bed is in the lowest position.
4. Decontaminate your hands. Put on gloves.
5. Cover the person with a bath blanket. Remove top linens.
6. Fill the wash basin two-thirds full with water. Water temperature is usually 110°F to 115°F (43.3°C to 46.1°C) or as directed by the nurse. Measure water temperature with the bath thermometer. Or test bath water by dipping your elbow or inner wrist into the basin.
7. Ask the person to check the water temperature. Adjust the water temperature if it is too hot or too cold.
8. Place the basin on the overbed table.
9. Position the person in Fowler position, or assist the person to sit at the bedside.
10. Adjust the overbed table so the person can reach the basin and supplies.
11. Help the person undress. Provide for privacy and warmth with the bath blanket.
12. Ask the person to wash easy-to-reach body parts (Fig. 18.19). Explain that you will wash the back and areas the person cannot reach.
13. Place the call light within reach. Ask the person to signal when help is needed or bathing is complete.
14. Decontaminate your hands. Then leave the room.

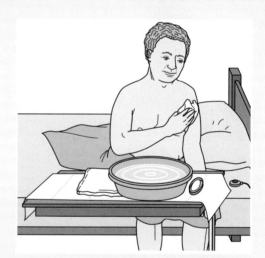

Fig. 18.19 The person is bathing oneself while sitting on the side of the bed. Necessary equipment is within reach.

15. Return when the call light is on. Knock before entering. Decontaminate your hands.
16. Change the bath water. Measure bath water temperature as in step 6.
17. Raise the bed for body mechanics. The far bed rail is up if used.
18. Ask what was washed. Put on gloves. Wash and dry areas the person could not reach. The face, hands, underarms, back, buttocks, and perineal area are washed for the partial bath.
19. Remove the gloves. Decontaminate your hands.
20. Give a back massage (p. 275).
21. Apply lotion, powder, and deodorant or antiperspirant as requested.
22. Help the person put on clean garments.
23. Assist with hair care and other grooming needs.
24. Assist the person to a chair. (Lower the bed if the person transfers to a chair.) Or turn the person onto the side away from you.
25. Make the bed. (Raise the bed for body mechanics.)

Continued

✳ ASSISTING WITH THE PARTIAL BATH—cont'd

Postprocedure

26. Provide for comfort. (See the inside of the front cover.)
27. Place the call light within reach.
28. Lower the bed to its lowest position.
29. Raise or lower bed rails. Follow the care plan.
30. Put on clean gloves.
31. Empty, clean, and dry the bath basin. Return the basin and supplies to their proper place.

32. Wipe off the overbed table with the paper towels. Discard the paper towels.
33. Unscreen the person.
34. Complete a safety check of the room. (See the inside of the front cover.)
35. Follow center policy for dirty linens.
36. Remove the gloves. Decontaminate your hands.
37. Report and record your observations.

This skill is also covered in *Clinical Skills: Nurse Assisting.*

Tub Baths and Showers

Some people like tub baths. Others like showers. Falls, burns, and chilling from water are risks. Safety is important (Box 18.2). The measures in Box 18.1 also apply. If other measures are needed, follow the nurse's directions and the care plan.

Some bathrooms have showers. If not, reserve the shower or tub room for the person.

🧍 PROMOTING SAFETY AND COMFORT

Tub Baths and Showers

Safety

Some persons are very weak. At least two persons are needed to safely assist them with tub baths and showers. If the person is heavy, three staff members may be needed.

The person may use a tub with a side entry door, a shower chair, a shower trolley, or other device. Always follow the manufacturer instructions.

Protect the person from falls, chilling, and burns. Follow the safety measures in Chapters 11 and 12. Remember to measure water temperature.

Clean and disinfect the tub or shower before and after use. This prevents the spread of microbes and infection.

Comfort

Warmth and privacy promote comfort during tub baths and showers. You need to:
- Make sure the tub or shower room is warm.
- Provide for privacy. Close the room door, screen the person, and close window coverings.
- Make sure water temperature is warm enough for the person.
- Have the person remove clothing or robe and footwear just before getting into the tub or shower. Do not let the person remain exposed longer than necessary.
- Have warm towels or bath blanket ready to gently dry the person.

Tub Baths

Tub baths are relaxing. A tub bath can make a person feel faint, weak, or tired. These are great risks for persons who were on bedrest. A tub bath lasts no longer than 20 minutes.

The person may need one of these devices to get in and out of the tub:
- Transfer bench (Fig. 18.20)
- A tub with a side entry door (Fig. 18.21)
- Wheelchair or stretcher lift. The person is transferred to the tub room by wheelchair or stretcher. Then the device and person are lifted into the tub (Fig. 18.22).
- Mechanical lift (Chapter 15)

Whirlpool tubs have a cleansing action. You wash the upper body. Carefully wash under the breasts and between skin folds.

Also wash the perineal area. Pat dry the person with towels after the bath.

Showers

Some people can stand and use a regular shower. They use the grab bars for support during the shower. Like tubs, showers have nonskid surfaces. If not, a bathmat is used. Never let weak or unsteady persons stand in the shower. They need to use one of the following:

- *Shower chairs.* Water drains through an opening (Fig. 18.23). You use the chair to transport the person to and from the shower. Lock the wheels during the shower to prevent the chair from moving.
- *Shower stalls or cabinets.* The person walks into the device or is wheeled in on a wheelchair (Fig. 18.24). Use the handheld nozzle.
- *Shower trolleys (portable tubs).* The person has a shower lying down (Fig. 18.25). You lower the sides to transfer the person from the bed to the trolley. Raise the side rails after the transfer. Then transport the person to the tub or shower room. Use the handheld nozzle to give the shower in the usual manner.

Some shower rooms have two or more stations. Provide for privacy. The person has the right not to be exposed to others. Properly screen and cover the person. Also close doors and the shower curtain.

See *Delegation Guidelines: Tub Baths and Showers.*
See *Promoting Safety and Comfort: Tub Baths and Showers.*
See *Teamwork and Time Management: Tub Baths and Showers.*

📄 DELEGATION GUIDELINES

Tub Baths and Showers

Before assisting with a tub bath or shower, you need this information from the nurse and the care plan:
- If the person takes a tub bath or shower
- If the person will have the hair shampooed
- What water temperature to use (usually 105°F [40.5°C])
- What equipment is needed (e.g., shower chair, shower cabinet, shower trolley)
- How much help the person needs
- If the person can bathe oneself
- What observations to report and record:
  - Dizziness
  - Lightheadedness
  - *See Delegation Guidelines: Bathing,* p. 266
- When to report observations
- What specific resident concerns to report at once

BOX 18.2   Safety Measures for Tub Baths and Showers

- Know what water temperature to use. See *Delegation Guidelines: Tub Baths and Showers*, p. 271.
- Clean and disinfect the tub or shower before and after use.
- Dry the tub or shower room floor.
- Check handrails, grab bars, hydraulic lifts, and other safety aids. They must be in working order.
- Place a bathmat in the tub or on the shower floor. This is not needed if there are nonskid strips or a nonskid surface.
- Cover the person for warmth and privacy. This includes during transport to and from the shower or tub room.
- Place needed items within the person's reach.
- Place the call light within the person's reach.
- Show the person how to use the call light in the shower or tub room.
- Have the person use the grab bars when getting in and out of the tub. The person must not use towel bars for support.
- Turn cold water on first, then hot water. Turn hot water off first, then cold water.
- Adjust water temperature and pressure to prevent chilling or burns. Do this before the person gets into the shower. If a shower chair is used, position it first.
- Direct water away from the person while adjusting water temperature and pressure.
- Fill the tub before the person gets into it.
- Measure the water temperature. For showers and tub baths, use the digital display. Or you can use a bath thermometer for a tub bath.
- Keep the water spray directed toward the person during the shower. This helps keep the person warm. (*Note:* Do not direct the water spray toward the person's face. This can frighten the person.)
- Bar soap is used for only one person. It cannot be shared. Keep bar soap in the soap dish between latherings. This prevents soapy water. It reduces the risk of slipping and falls in showers and tubs. Many centers use liquid soap dispensers.
- Avoid using bath oils. They make tub and shower surfaces slippery.
- Do not leave weak, unsteady, or confused persons unattended.
- Stay within hearing distance if the person can be left alone. Wait outside the shower curtain or door. You will be nearby if the person calls for you or has an accident.
- Drain the tub before the person gets out of the tub. Turn off the shower before the person gets out of the shower. Cover the person to provide privacy and prevent chilling.

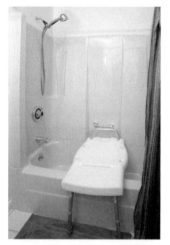

Fig. 18.20 A transfer bench is positioned for the person's use in getting into and out of the tub. A floor mat is in front of the tub.

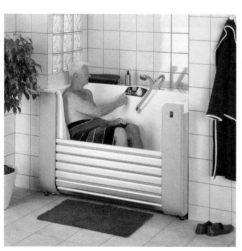

Fig. 18.21 Tub with a side entry door. (Courtesy ARJO, Inc., Roselle, IL [800] 323-1245.)

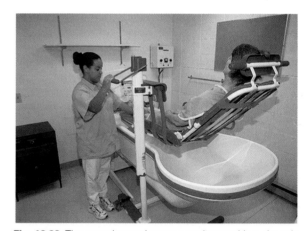

Fig. 18.22 The stretcher and person are lowered into the tub.

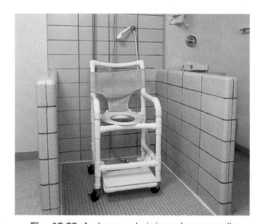

Fig. 18.23 A shower chair in a shower stall.

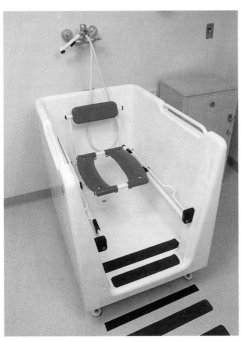

Fig. 18.24 A shower cabinet.

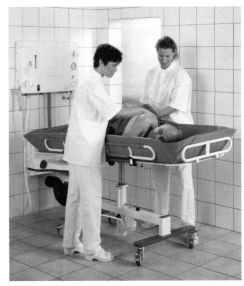

Fig. 18.25 Shower trolley. The sides are lowered for transfers into and out of the trolley. (Courtesy ARJO, Inc., Roselle, IL [800]323-1245.)

TEAMWORK AND TIME MANAGEMENT

Tub Baths and Showers

Most centers do not have tub and shower equipment for each person. You need to reserve the room and needed equipment for the person. Your coworkers do the same for their residents. Consider the needs of others. For example, you reserve the shower room from 0945 to 1030. Do your very best to follow the schedule. Make sure the shower room is clean and ready for the next person, or you and a coworker schedule something for the same time. Plan a new schedule with your coworker.

All bed linens are changed on the person's bath or shower day. Ask coworkers to make the person's bed while you assist with the tub bath or shower. Also ask coworkers to straighten the person's unit. The person returns to a clean bed and unit. Return the favor when your coworkers are assisting with tub baths, showers, or other care measures.

ASSISTING WITH A TUB BATH OR SHOWER

Quality of Life

Remember to:

- Knock before entering the person's room.
- Address the person by name.
- Introduce yourself by name and title.
- Explain the procedure to the person before beginning and during the procedure.
- Protect the person's rights during the procedure.
- Handle the person gently during the procedure.

Preprocedure

1. Follow *Delegation Guidelines*:
   a. *Bathing*, p. 266
   b. *Tub Baths and Showers*, p. 271
2. *See Promoting Safety and Comfort:*
   a. *Bathing*, p. 266
   b. *Tub Baths and Showers*, p. 271
3. Reserve the bathtub or shower.

4. Practice hand hygiene.
5. Identify the person. Check the ID bracelet against the assignment sheet. Also call the person by name.
6. Collect the following:
   - Two washcloths and two bath towels
   - Soap
   - Bath thermometer (for a tub bath)
   - Clothing or sleepwear
   - Grooming items as requested
   - Robe and nonskid footwear
   - Rubber bathmat if needed
   - Disposable bathmat
   - Gloves
   - Wheelchair, shower chair, transfer bench, and so on as needed

Procedure

7. Place items in the tub or shower room. Use the space provided or a chair.
8. Clean and disinfect the tub or shower.

✴ ASSISTING WITH A TUB BATH OR SHOWER—cont'd

9. Place a rubber bathmat in the tub or on the shower floor. Do not block the drain.
10. Place the disposable bathmat on the floor in the front of the tub or shower.
11. Put the occupied sign on the door.
12. Return to the person's room. Provide for privacy. Decontaminate your hands.
13. Help the person sit on the side of the bed.
14. Help the person put on a robe and nonskid footwear, or the person can leave on clothing.
15. Assist or transport the person to the tub room or shower.
16. Provide a chair to sit on if the person walked to the tub or shower room.
17. Provide for privacy.
18. *For a tub bath:*
    a. Fill the tub halfway with warm water (usually 105°F [40.5°C]). Follow the care plan for water temperature.
    b. Measure water temperature. Use the bath thermometer or check the digital display.
    c. Ask the person to check the water temperature. Adjust the water temperature if it is too hot or too cold.
19. *For a shower:*
    a. Turn on the shower.
    b. Adjust water temperature and pressure. Check the digital display.
    c. Ask the person to check the water temperature. Adjust the water temperature if it is too hot or too cold.
20. Help the person undress and remove footwear.
21. Help the person into the tub or shower. Position the shower chair and lock the wheels.
22. Ask the person about shampooing the hair. If yes, perform this before washing the body. After shampooing, cover the head with a towel to prevent chilling.
23. Assist with washing as necessary. Wear gloves.
24. Ask the person to use the call light when done or when help is needed. Remind the person that a tub bath lasts no longer than 20 minutes.
25. Place a towel across the chair.
26. Leave the room if the person can bathe alone. If not, stay in the room or nearby. Remove the gloves and decontaminate your hands if you will leave the room.
27. Check on the person at least every 5 minutes.
28. Return when the person signals for you. Knock before entering. Decontaminate your hands.
29. Turn off the shower or drain the tub. Cover the person while the tub drains.
30. Help the person out of the shower or tub and onto the chair.
31. Help the person dry off. Pat gently. Dry under the breasts, between skin folds, in the perineal area, and between the toes.
32. Assist with lotion and other grooming items as needed.
33. Help the person dress and put on footwear.
34. Help the person return to the room. Provide for privacy.
35. Assist the person to a chair or into bed.
36. Provide a back massage if the person returns to bed.
37. Assist with hair care and other grooming needs.

Postprocedure

38. Provide for comfort. (See the inside of the front cover.)
39. Place the call light within reach.
40. Raise or lower bed rails. Follow the care plan.
41. Unscreen the person.
42. Complete a safety check of the room. (See the inside of the front cover.)
43. Clean and disinfect the tub or shower. Remove soiled linen. Wear gloves.
44. Discard disposable items. Put the unoccupied sign on the door. Return supplies to their proper place.
45. Follow center policy for dirty linens.
46. Remove the gloves. Decontaminate your hands.
47. Report and record your observations.

This skill is also covered in *Clinical Skills: Nurse Assisting*.

✴ THE BACK MASSAGE

The back massage (back rub) relaxes muscles and stimulates circulation. You give back massages after baths and showers and with evening care. You also give them at other times. Examples include after repositioning or helping the person to relax.

Back massages last 3 to 5 minutes. Observe the skin before the massage. Look for breaks in the skin, bruises, reddened areas, and other signs of skin breakdown.

Lotion reduces friction during the massage. It is warmed before being applied. To warm lotion, do one of the following:

- Rub some lotion between your hands
- Place the bottle in the bath water
- Hold the bottle under warm water

Use firm strokes. Also keep your hands in contact with the person's skin. After the massage, apply some lotion to the elbows, knees, and heels. This keeps the skin soft. These bony areas are at risk for skin breakdown.

See *Delegation Guidelines: The Back Massage.*
See *Promoting Safety and Comfort: The Back Massage.*

DELEGATION GUIDELINES

The Back Massage

Before giving a back massage, you need this information from the nurse and the care plan:

- If the person can have a back massage (see *Promoting Safety and Comfort: The Back Massage*)
- How to position the person
- If the person has position limits
- When the person is to receive a back massage
- If the person needs frequent back massages for comfort and to relax
- What observations to report and record:
  - Breaks in the skin
  - Bruising
  - Reddened areas
  - Signs of skin breakdown
- When to report observations
- What specific resident concerns to report at once

PROMOTING SAFETY AND COMFORT

The Back Massage

Safety

Back massages are dangerous for persons with certain heart and kidney diseases, back injuries, back and other surgeries, skin diseases, and lung disorders. Check with the nurse and the care plan before giving back massages to persons with these conditions.

Do not massage reddened bony areas. Reddened areas signal skin breakdown and pressure ulcers. Massage can lead to more tissue damage.

Wear gloves if the person's skin is not intact. Always follow Standard Precautions and the Bloodborne Pathogen Standard.

Comfort

The prone position is best for a massage. The side-lying position is often used. Older and disabled persons usually find the side-lying position more comfortable.

The back massage involves stroking down the back and over the buttocks. Some persons may not want the buttocks exposed and touched for massage. Explain the procedure to the person. Obtain the person's consent to expose and touch the buttocks. If the person does not give consent, modify the procedure as in step 14 in procedure: *Giving a Back Massage*.

✳ GIVING A BACK MASSAGE

Quality of Life

Remember to:

- Knock before entering the person's room.
- Address the person by name.
- Introduce yourself by name and title.
- Explain the procedure to the person before beginning and during the procedure.
- Protect the person's rights during the procedure.
- Handle the person gently during the procedure.

Preprocedure

1. Follow *Delegation Guidelines: The Back Massage*. See *Promoting Safety and Comfort: The Back Massage*.
2. Practice hand hygiene.
3. Identify the person. Check the ID bracelet against the assignment sheet. Also call the person by name.
4. Collect the following:
   - Bath blanket
   - Bath towel
   - Lotion
5. Provide for privacy.
6. Raise the bed for body mechanics. Bed rails are up if used.

Procedure

7. Lower the bed rail near you if up.
8. Position the person in the prone or side-lying position. The back is toward you.
9. Expose the back, shoulders, upper arms, and buttocks. Cover the rest of the body with the bath blanket. Expose the buttocks only if the person gives consent.
10. Lay the towel on the bed along the back. Do this if the person is in a side-lying position.
11. Warm the lotion.
12. Explain that the lotion may feel cool and wet.
13. Apply lotion to the lower back area.
14. Stroke up from the buttocks to the shoulders. Then stroke down over the upper arms. Stroke up the upper arms, across the shoulders, and down the back to the buttocks (Fig. 18.26). Use firm strokes. Keep your hands in contact with the person's skin. If the person does not want the buttocks exposed, stroke down the back to the waist and up the back to the shoulders.
15. Repeat step 14 for at least 3 minutes.
16. Knead the back (Fig. 18.27).
    a. Grasp the skin between your thumb and fingers.
    b. Knead half of the back. Start at the buttocks and move up to the shoulder. Then knead down from the shoulder to the buttocks.
    c. Repeat on the other half of the back.
17. Apply lotion to bony areas. Use circular motions with the tips of your index and middle fingers. (Do not massage reddened bony areas.)
18. Use fast movements to stimulate. Use slow movements to relax the person.
19. Stroke with long, firm movements to end the massage. Tell the person you are finishing.

GIVING A BACK MASSAGE—cont'd

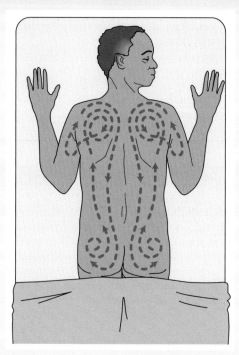

Fig. 18.26 The person lies in the prone position for a back massage. Stroke upward from the buttocks to the shoulders, down over the upper arms, back up the upper arms, across the shoulders, and down the back to the buttocks.

20. Straighten and secure clothing or sleepwear.
21. Cover the person. Remove the towel and bath blanket.

Postprocedure
22. Provide for comfort. (See the inside of the front cover.)
23. Place the call light within reach.

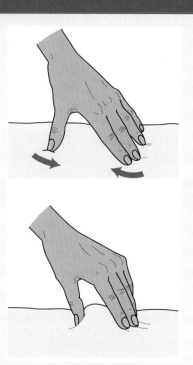

Fig. 18.27 Kneading is done by picking up tissue between the thumb and fingers.

24. Lower the bed to its lowest position.
25. Raise or lower bed rails. Follow the care plan.
26. Return lotion to its proper place.
27. Unscreen the person.
28. Complete a safety check of the room. (See the inside of the front cover.)
29. Follow center policy for dirty linens.
30. Decontaminate your hands.
31. Report and record your observations.

This skill is also covered in *Clinical Skills: Nurse Assisting.*

PERINEAL CARE

Perineal care (pericare) involves cleaning the genital and anal areas. These areas provide a warm, moist, and dark place for microbes to grow. Cleaning prevents infection and odors and it promotes comfort.

Perineal care is done daily during the bath. It also is done whenever the area is soiled with urine or feces. Perineal care is very important for persons who:

- Have urinary catheters (Chapter 22).
- Have had rectal or genital surgery.
- Are menstruating (Chapter 8).
- Are incontinent of urine or feces.
- Are uncircumcised. Being *circumcised* means that the fold of skin (foreskin) covering the head of the penis was surgically removed. Being *uncircumcised* means that the person has foreskin covering the head of the penis.

The person does perineal care if able. Otherwise, it is given by the nursing staff. This procedure embarrasses many people and nursing staff, especially when it involves the other sex.

Perineal and *perineum* are not common terms. Most people understand *privates, private parts, crotch, genitals,* or the *area between the legs.* Use terms the person understands. The term must be in good taste professionally.

FOCUS ON COMMUNICATION

Perineal Care

Talking to the person about perineal care may be difficult. You may be embarrassed. However, you must explain the procedure to the person.

When a person performs own perineal care, you can say:

- "Mrs. Bell, I'll give you some privacy while you finish your bath. Can you reach everything you need? Please call me if you need help. Here is your call light."
- "Mr. Monroe, I'll give you time to finish your bath. Please wash your genital and rectal areas. Signal for me when you're done or need help."
- If you provide perineal care for the person, you can say:
- "Mrs. Allan, next I'll clean between your legs. I'll keep you covered with the bath blanket. I'll tell you before I touch you. Please tell me if you feel any pain or discomfort."
- "Mr. Scott, I'll clean your private parts now. Please let me know if you feel any pain or discomfort."

Standard Precautions, medical asepsis, and the Blood-borne Pathogen Standard are followed. Work from the cleanest area to the dirtiest. This is commonly called cleaning from "front to back." The urethral area (the front) is the cleanest. The anal area (the back) is the dirtiest. Therefore clean from the urethra to the anal area. This prevents the transmission of bacteria from the anal area to the vagina and urinary system.

DELEGATION GUIDELINES

Perineal Care

Before giving perineal care, you need this information from the nurse and the care plan:
- When to give perineal care
- What terms the person understands (*perineum, privates, private parts, crotch, genitals, area between the legs,* etc.)
- How much help the person needs

- What water temperature to use—usually 105°F to 109°F (40.5°C to 42.7°C). Water in a basin cools rapidly.
- What cleaning agent to use
- Any position restrictions or limits
- What observations to report and record:
  - Odors
  - Redness, swelling, discharge, bleeding, or irritation
  - Complaints of pain, burning, or other discomfort
  - Signs of urinary or fecal incontinence
- When to report observations
- What specific resident concerns to report at once

The perineal area is delicate and easily injured. Use warm water, not hot. Use washcloths, towelettes, cotton balls, or swabs according to center policy. Rinse thoroughly. Pat dry after rinsing. This reduces moisture and promotes comfort.

See *Focus on Communication: Perineal Care.*
See *Delegation Guidelines: Perineal Care.*
See *Promoting Safety and Comfort: Perineal Care.*

PROMOTING SAFETY AND COMFORT

Perineal Care

Safety

Hot water can burn delicate perineal tissues. To prevent burns, measure water temperature according to center policy. If the water seems too hot, ask the nurse to check it.

Protect yourself and the person from infection. Contact with blood, body fluids, secretions, or excretions is likely during perineal care. Follow Standard Precautions and the Bloodborne Pathogen Standard.

Persons who are incontinent need perineal care. Protect the person and dry garments and linens from the wet or soiled items. After cleaning and drying the perineal area, remove the wet or soiled incontinence products, garments, and linen. Then apply clean, dry ones.

Comfort

To avoid embarrassment, it is best if the person does perineal care. If you provide this care, explain how privacy is protected. Act in a professional manner at all times.

Perineal care involves touching the genital and anal areas. The person may prefer that someone of the same sex provide this care. Or the person may fear sexual assault. Always obtain the person's consent before providing perineal care. For mental comfort, the person may want a family member or another staff member present to witness the procedure. Ask if the person wants someone present and that person's name.

GIVING FEMALE PERINEAL CARE (NATCEP)

Quality of Life

Remember to:
- Knock before entering the person's room.
- Address the person by name.
- Introduce yourself by name and title.
- Explain the procedure to the person before beginning and during the procedure.
- Protect the person's rights during the procedure.
- Handle the person gently during the procedure.

Preprocedure

1. *Follow Delegation Guidelines: Perineal Care.* See *Promoting Safety and Comfort: Perineal Care.*
2. Practice hand hygiene.
3. Collect the following:
   - Soap or other cleaning agent as directed
   - At least four washcloths
   - Bath towel
   - Bath blanket
   - Bath thermometer
   - Wash basin

- Waterproof pad
- Gloves
- Paper towels

4. Cover the overbed table with paper towels. Arrange items on top of them.
5. Identify the person. Check the ID bracelet against the assignment sheet. Also call the person by name.
6. Provide for privacy.
7. Raise the bed for body mechanics. Bed rails are up if used.

Procedure

8. Lower the bed rail near you if up.
9. Decontaminate your hands. Put on gloves.
10. Cover the person with a bath blanket. Move top linens to the foot of the bed.
11. Position the person on the back.
12. Drape the person as in Fig. 18.28.
13. Raise the bed rail if used.
14. Fill the wash basin. Water temperature is usually 105°F to 109°F (40.5°C to 42.7°C). Follow the care plan for water temperature. Measure water temperature according to center policy.

GIVING FEMALE PERINEAL CARE (NATCEP)—cont'd

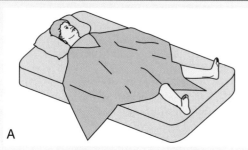
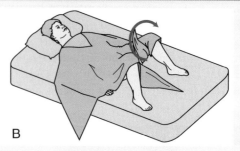

Fig. 18.28 Draping for perineal care. (A) Position the bath blanket like a diamond: One corner is at the neck, there is a corner at each side, and one corner is between the person's legs. (B) Wrap the blanket around the leg by bringing the corner around under the leg and over the top. Tuck the corner under the hip.

15. Ask the person to check the water temperature. Adjust the water temperature if it is too hot or too cold. Raise the bed rail before leaving the bedside. Lower it when you return.
16. Place the basin on the overbed table.
17. Lower the bed rail if up.
18. Help the person flex her knees and spread her legs. Or help her spread her legs as much as possible with the knees straight.
19. Place a waterproof pad under her buttocks. Protect the person and dry linens from the wet or soiled incontinence product.
20. Fold the corner of the bath blanket between her legs onto her abdomen.
21. Wet the washcloths.
22. Squeeze out excess water from a washcloth. Make a mitted washcloth. Apply soap.
23. Separate the labia. Clean downward from front to back with one stroke (Fig. 18.29).
24. Repeat steps 22 and 23 until the area is clean. Use a clean part of the washcloth for each stroke. Use more than one washcloth if needed.
25. Rinse the perineum with a clean washcloth. Separate the labia. Stroke downward from front to back. Repeat as necessary. Use a clean part of the washcloth for each stroke. Use more than one washcloth if needed.

26. Pat the area dry with the towel. Dry from front to back.
27. Fold the blanket back between her legs.
28. Help the person lower her legs and turn onto her side away from you.
29. Apply soap to a mitted washcloth.
30. Clean the rectal area. Clean from the vagina to the anus with one stroke (Fig. 18.30).
31. Repeat steps 29 and 30 until the area is clean. Use a clean part of the washcloth for each stroke. Use more than one washcloth if needed.
32. Rinse the rectal area with a washcloth. Stroke from the vagina to the anus. Repeat as necessary. Use a clean part of the washcloth for each stroke. Use more than one washcloth if needed.
33. Pat the area dry with the towel. Dry from front to back.
34. Remove any wet or soiled incontinence product. Remove the waterproof pad.
35. Remove and discard the gloves. Decontaminate your hands. Put on clean gloves.
36. Provide clean and dry linens and incontinence products as needed.

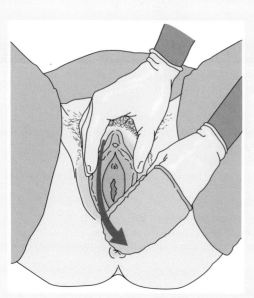

Fig. 18.29 Separate the labia with one hand. Use a mitted washcloth to cleanse between the labia with downward strokes.

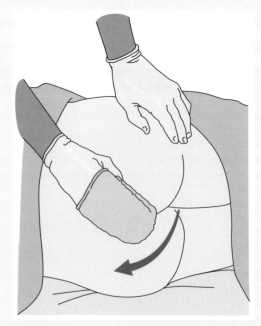

Fig. 18.30 The rectal area is cleaned by wiping from the vagina to the anus. The side-lying position allows the anal area to be cleaned more thoroughly.

Continued

✳ GIVING FEMALE PERINEAL CARE (NATCEP)—cont'd

Postprocedure

37. Cover the person. Remove the bath blanket.
38. Provide for comfort. (See the inside of the front cover.)
39. Place the call light within reach.
40. Lower the bed to its lowest position.
41. Raise or lower bed rails. Follow the care plan.
42. Empty, clean, and dry the wash basin.
43. Return the basin and supplies to their proper place.

44. Wipe off the overbed table with the paper towels. Discard the paper towels.
45. Unscreen the person.
46. Complete a safety check of the room. (See the inside of the front cover.)
47. Follow center policy for dirty linens.
48. Remove the gloves. Decontaminate your hands.
49. Report and record your observations.

This skill is also covered in *Clinical Skills: Nurse Assisting.*

✳ GIVING MALE PERINEAL CARE

Quality of Life

Remember to:
- Knock before entering the person's room.
- Address the person by name.
- Introduce yourself by name and title.
- Explain the procedure to the person before beginning and during the procedure.
- Protect the person's rights during the procedure.
- Handle the person gently during the procedure.

Procedure

1. Follow steps 1 through 17 in procedure: *Giving Female Perineal Care,* pp 277-279. Drape the person as in Fig. 18.28.
2. Place a waterproof pad under his buttocks. Protect the person and dry linens from the wet or soiled incontinence product.
3. Retract the foreskin if the person is uncircumcised (Fig. 18.31).
4. Grasp the penis.
5. Clean the tip. Use a circular motion. Start at the meatus of the urethra and work outward (Fig. 18.32). Repeat as needed. Use a clean part of the washcloth each time.

6. Rinse the area with another washcloth.
7. Return the foreskin to its natural position immediately after rinsing.
8. Clean the shaft of the penis. Use firm downward strokes. Rinse the area.
9. Help the person flex his knees and spread his legs. Or help him spread his legs as much as possible with his knees straight.
10. Clean the scrotum. Rinse well. Observe for redness and irritation of the skin folds.
11. Pat dry the penis and the scrotum. Use the towel.
12. Fold the bath blanket back between his legs.
13. Help him lower his legs and turn onto his side away from you.
14. Clean the rectal area (see procedure: *Giving Female Perineal Care,* pp 277-279). (*Note:* For males, clean from the scrotum to the anus.) Rinse and dry well.
15. Remove any wet or soiled incontinence product. Remove the waterproof pad.
16. Remove and discard the gloves. Decontaminate your hands. Put on clean gloves.
17. Provide clean and dry linens and incontinence products.

Postprocedure

18. Follow steps 37 through 49 in procedure: *Giving Female Perineal Care,* pp 277-279.

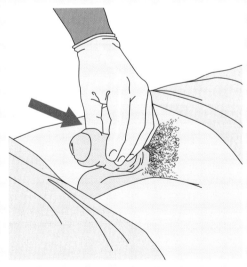

Fig. 18.31 The foreskin of the uncircumcised male is pulled back for perineal care. It is returned to the normal position immediately after cleaning and rinsing.

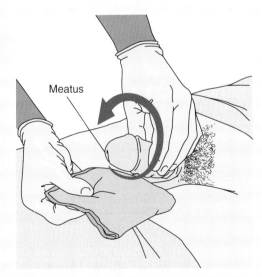

Meatus

Fig. 18.32 The penis is cleaned with circular motions starting at the meatus.

This skill is also covered in *Clinical Skills: Nurse Assisting.*

Activities-of-Daily-Living Flow Sheet

ORDER/INSTRUCTION	TIME	JAN 1	FEB 2	MAR 3	APR 4	MAY 5	JUN 6	JUL 7	AUG 8	SEP 9	OCT 10	NOV 11	DEC 12	13	14	15	16	17	18	19	20	21	22	23	24	25	26	27	28	29	30	31
Oral Care Own/Dentures/None I=Independent S=Set up A=Assist	11-7																															
	7-3	S	S	S																												
	3-11	S	S	S																												
Hygiene, Washing Face and Hands I=Independent S=Set up A=Assist T=Total Care	11-7	/	/	/																												
	7-3	/	/	/																												
	3-11	/	/	/																												
Bath and Shampoo every _Monday_ and _Thurs_ on _7-3_ shift T=Tub S=Shower B=Bed bath	11-7																															
	7-3	T																														
	3-11																															
Back massage daily	11-7																															
	7-3																															
	3-11	✓	✓	✓																												
Pericare I=Independent S=Set up A=Assist T=Total Care	11-7	A	A	A																												
	7-3																															
	3-11	A	A	A																												

Fig. 18.33 Charting sample.

REPORTING AND RECORDING

You make many observations while assisting with hygiene. Report the following at once:

- Bleeding
- Signs of skin breakdown
- Discharge from the vagina or urinary tract
- Unusual odors
- Changes from prior observations

Also report and record the care given (Fig. 18.33). If care is not recorded, it is assumed that care was not given. This can cause serious legal problems.

QUALITY OF LIFE

Residents' rights serve to improve the person's quality of life, health, and safety. You must provide hygiene in a way that maintains or improves the person's quality of life, health, and safety. You must protect the person's rights when giving care.

To protect the right to privacy:

- Do not expose the person.
- Ask visitors to leave the room before you give care. A family member or friend may want to help. The person must consent to this.
- Close doors, privacy curtains, and window coverings.
- Expose only the body part involved in the procedure.
- Cover persons who are taken to and from tub or shower rooms. In some centers, residents wear their clothes to the shower or tub room. They put on clean clothes in the shower or tub room after the procedure.

- Protect the person from exposure when others are present. Some centers have more than one shower station.

Residents have the right to personal choice. They have the right to be involved in planning care and treatment. Hygiene is a very personal matter. Residents have a voice about when and how hygiene is done. Personal choice is allowed in such matters as bath time, products used, what to wear, and hair styling.

Residents have the right to keep and use personal items. You will handle the person's property during hygiene procedures. Protect dentures and eyeglasses from loss or breakage. If jewelry or religious items are removed for care, protect them from loss, damage, or theft.

Freedom from restraint is another resident right. Sometimes bed rails are restraints (Chapter 13). Follow the person's care plan for bed rail use.

TIME TO REFLECT

It is shortly after dinner and Mrs. Carson is sitting in her recliner chair. Suddenly she begins to feel nauseated and rushes into her bathroom. While there she vomits into the toilet. She pulls her call light for assistance. When you arrive, you knock on the bathroom door and begin to help Mrs. Carson get cleaned up. She is distraught and tearful and tells you that her dentures accidently fell into the toilet when she vomited. (She has not flushed the toilet.) What action would you take with this situation? Do you think the dentures can be saved? What are some infection control principles that would be involved?

REVIEW QUESTIONS

Circle the BEST answer.

1. Oral hygiene does the following *except*
   a. Prevent mouth odors
   b. Prevent infection
   c. Increase comfort
   d. Coat and dry the mouth

2. You brush a person's teeth and note the following. Which is *not* reported to the nurse?
   a. Bleeding, swelling, or redness of the gums
   b. Irritations, sores, or white patches in the mouth or on the tongue
   c. Lips that are dry, cracked, swollen, or blistered
   d. Food between the teeth

3. How do you position the unconscious person for oral hygiene?
   a. Prone position
   b. On the side with head also side turned
   c. Prone position
   d. High Fowler position

4. Which is true about dentures?
   a. They can be worn when the person is unconscious
   b. They are cleaned with hot water
   c. They are removed at bedtime
   d. They are stored in a clean dry container

5. The resident cannot remove her own dentures. What do you use to remove the denture?
   a. Tongue blade
   b. Wash cloth
   c. Your ungloved finger
   d. Gauze squares

6. Which is *not* a purpose of bathing?
   a. Increasing circulation
   b. Promoting drying of the skin
   c. Exercising body parts
   d. Refreshing and relaxing the person

7. Soaps do the following *except*
   a. Remove dirt and dead skin
   b. Soften the skin
   c. Remove skin oil
   d. Dry the skin

8. Which action is *wrong* when bathing a person?
   a. Covering the person for warmth and privacy
   b. Rinsing the skin thoroughly to remove all soap
   c. Washing from the dirtiest to the cleanest area
   d. Patting the skin dry

9. Water for a complete bed bath is at least
   a. 100°F
   b. 105°F
   c. 110°F
   d. 120°F

10. You are going to give a back massage. Which is *false?*
    a. It should last 3 to 5 minutes
    b. Lotion is warmed before being applied
    c. Your hands are always in contact with the skin
    d. The person is placed in the supine position

11. Which type of bath is usually given to the unconscious person?
    a. Shower
    b. Complete bed bath
    c. Tub bath
    d. Partial bath

12. Which of the following does *not* ensure the person's privacy while bathing?
    a. Close the room door
    b. Pull the privacy curtain
    c. Keep window shades open
    d. Remove clothing just before getting in the tub

13. Which position do older persons usually find most comfortable for a back massage?
    a. Side-lying
    b. Prone
    c. Supine
    d. Sitting

14. You are giving a tub bath to a person with dementia. You realize you forgot to bring the person's clean clothing into the bathing room. Which is correct?
    a. Leave the person momentarily and go get the clothing
    b. Complete the bath and dress the person in the soiled clothing
    c. Use the call signal and ask a coworker to bring clean clothing
    d. Cover the resident with a bath blanket when the bath is finished and then return to the person's room

15. Mrs. Dean has dementia. She is frightened of bathing. She can be uncooperative when attempts are made to assist her with bathing. Which type of bath might she respond to best?
    a. Towel bath
    b. Shower
    c. Whirlpool bath
    d. Complete bed bath

    See Appendix A for answers to these questions.

19

Grooming

OBJECTIVES

- Define the key terms and key abbreviations listed in this chapter.
- Explain why grooming is important.
- Identify the factors that affect hair care.
- Explain how to care for matted and tangled hair.
- Describe how to shampoo hair.
- Describe the measures practiced when shaving a person.
- Explain why nail and foot care are important.
- Describe the rules for changing clothing and gowns.
- Perform the procedures described in this chapter.
- Explain how to promote quality of life.

KEY TERMS

alopecia Hair loss

anticoagulant A medication that prevents or slows (*anti-*) blood clotting (*coagulate*)

bed bugs Small, flat, red-brown insects that may live around or near areas where people sleep and that feed on the blood of people and animals

dandruff Excessive amounts of dry, white flakes from the scalp

hirsutism Excessive body hair

lice See "pediculosis"

mite A very small, spiderlike organism

pediculosis Infestation with wingless insects; lice

pediculosis capitis Infestation of the scalp (capitis) with lice; head lice

pediculosis corporis Infestation of the body (corporis) with lice

pediculosis pubis Infestation of the pubic (pubis) hair with lice

KEY ABBREVIATIONS

C Centigrade	ID Identification
F Fahrenheit	IV Intravenous

Hair care, shaving, and nail and foot care are important to many residents. Like hygiene, these grooming measures prevent infection and promote comfort. They also affect love, belonging, and self-esteem needs.

People differ in their grooming measures. Some want only clean hair. Others want a certain hairstyle. Some want only clean hands. Others want clean, manicured, and polished nails. Many men shave and groom their beards. Likewise, many women shave their legs and underarms. Some women have facial hair. They may shave or use other hair removal methods.

See *Focus on Rehabilitation: Grooming.*

See *Teamwork and Time Management: Grooming.*

HAIR CARE

How the hair looks and feels affects mental well-being. Some people cannot perform hair care. You assist with hair care when needed.

> ### 📋 FOCUS ON COMMUNICATION
>
> **Grooming**
>
> As with hygiene, the person should tend to grooming measures to the extent possible. This promotes the person's independence and quality of life. The person may use adaptive devices for hair care and dressing. See Fig. 19.1 for examples.

> ### 👥 TEAMWORK AND TIME MANAGEMENT
>
> **Grooming**
>
> Some equipment for grooming procedures is shared among residents. Shampoo trays, electric shavers, and whirlpool foot baths are examples. Let other team members know when you need to use an item. Schedule use of the item according to center policy. After the procedure, clean and promptly return the item to its proper place. Do not make your coworkers look for or clean an item.

The nursing process reflects the person's culture, personal choice, skin and scalp condition, health history, and self-care ability. Many nursing centers have beauty and barber shops

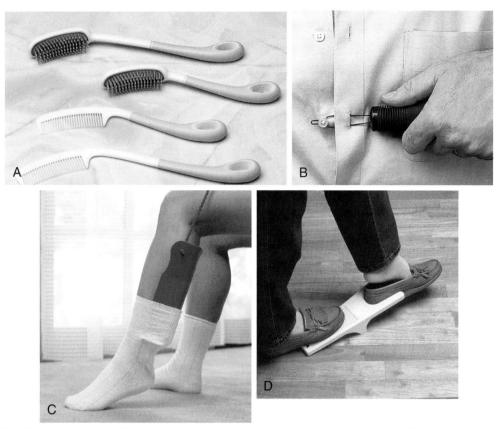

Fig. 19.1 Grooming aids. (A) Long-handled combs and brushes are used for hair care. (B) A button hook is used to button and zip clothing. (C) A sock assist is used to pull on socks and stockings. (D) A shoe remover is used to take off shoes. (From North Coast Medical Inc., Morgan Hill, CA.)

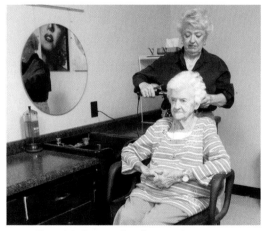

Fig. 19.2 Beauty shop in a nursing center.

for residents (Fig. 19.2). Residents can have their hair shampooed, cut, and styled. Men also can have their mustaches and beards groomed.

Skin and Scalp Conditions

Skin and scalp conditions include hair loss, excessive body hair, dandruff, lice, and scabies.

See *Focus on Communication: Skin and Scalp Conditions.*

FOCUS ON COMMUNICATION

Skin and Scalp Conditions

Some skin or scalp conditions may alarm you. Remain professional. Do not make statements that may embarrass the person.

Tell the nurse if you notice an abnormal skin or scalp condition. Describe what you saw as best as you can. For example:

- "I saw some small red spots on Mr. Martin's right underarm when I gave him his bath. Would you please take a look at them?"
- "I was getting ready to wash Ms. Miller's hair. I saw some small white specks. Would you please look at them before I wash her hair?"

Alopecia, Hirsutism, and Dandruff

Alopecia means "hair loss." Hair loss may be complete or partial. Male-pattern baldness occurs with aging. It results from heredity. Hair also thins in some women with aging. Cancer treatments (radiation therapy to the head and chemotherapy) often cause alopecia in males and females. Skin disease is another cause. Stress, poor nutrition, pregnancy, some medications, and hormone changes are other causes. Except for hair loss from aging, hair usually grows back.

Hirsutism is excessive body hair. It can occur in women and children. It results from heredity and abnormal amounts of male hormones.

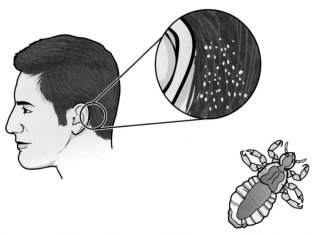

Fig. 19.3 Head lice. (Redrawn from MedlinePlus: Head lice, Bethesda, MD, National Institutes of Health.)

Dandruff is the excessive amount of dry, white flakes from the scalp. Itching often occurs. Sometimes eyebrows and ear canals are involved. Medicated shampoos correct the problem.

Lice

Pediculosis (lice) is the infestation with wingless insects *(lice)* (Fig. 19.3). *Infestation* means being in or on a host. Lice attach their eggs *(nits)* to hair shafts. Nits are oval and yellow to white in color. They hatch in about 1 week.

After hatching, lice feed on blood to live. Therefore, they bite the scalp or skin. Adult lice are about the size of a sesame seed. They are tan to gray-white in color. Lice bites cause severe itching in the affected body area.

- **Pediculosis capitis** is the infestation of the scalp *(capitis)* with lice. It is commonly called "head lice."
- **Pediculosis pubis** is the infestation of the pubic *(pubis)* hair with lice. This form of lice is also called "crabs."
- **Pediculosis corporis** is the infestation of the body *(corporis)* with lice.

Lice easily spread to others through clothing, head coverings, furniture, beds, towels, bed linens, and sexual contact. They also are spread by sharing combs and brushes. Lice are treated with medicated shampoos, lotions, and creams. Thorough bathing is needed. So is washing clothing and linens in hot water.

Report signs and symptoms of lice to the nurse at once:
- Complaints of a tickling feeling or something moving in the hair
- Itching
- Irritability
- Sores on the head or body caused by scratching
- Rash

Scabies

Scabies is a skin disorder caused by a female mite (Fig. 19.4). A **mite** is a very small spiderlike organism (Fig. 19.5). The female mite burrows into the skin and lays eggs. When the eggs hatch, the females produce more eggs. The person becomes infested with mites.

The person has a rash and intense itching. Common sites are between the fingers, around the wrists, in the underarm area, on the thighs, and in the genital area. Other sites include the breasts, waist, and buttocks.

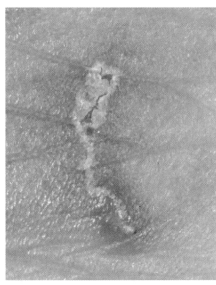

Fig. 19.4 Scabies. (From Marks JG, Miller JJ: *Lookingbill and Marks' principles of dermatology*, ed. 4, St. Louis, 2006, Saunders.)

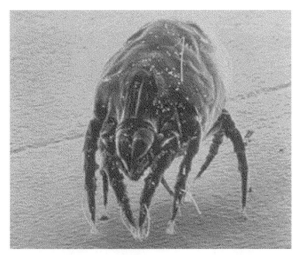

Fig. 19.5 Dust mite. (From Cook G: Putting your finger on the asthma trigger: allergens or irritants: what's making your asthma worse? *Asthma* 7(6):23–25, 2000.)

Scabies is highly contagious. It is transmitted to others by close contact. Persons living in crowded living settings are at risk. So are persons with weakened immune systems. Special creams are ordered to kill the mites. The person's room is cleaned. Clothing and linens are washed in hot water.

Bed Bugs

Bed bugs are small, flat, red-brown insects that may live around or near areas where people sleep (Fig. 19.6). They feed on the blood of people or animals. There has been a recent surge in bed bug infestations in many different settings, including long-term care centers and hospitals. Bed bugs can travel in luggage, bedding, furniture, and clothing. It is difficult to spot bed bugs during the day. They often hide in places like the seams of mattresses, headboards, tables, and cracks in walls. They are usually within 8 feet of where people sleep. Most people do not realize when they are bitten. It is not until reddened marks appear that they realize they may have been bitten. The marks look like mosquito bites and are very itchy. It is difficult to

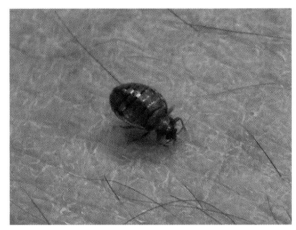

Fig. 19.6 Bed bug. (Courtesy Dr. Harold Harlan.)

control infestations of bed bugs. If you see bed bugs in a person's linens or surroundings, report this immediately. Often, professional pesticide companies are hired to get rid of the insects. High heat, chemical pesticides, and thorough cleaning may be used to kill bed bugs.

✳ Brushing and Combing Hair

Brushing and combing hair are part of early morning care, morning care, and afternoon care. And they are done when needed. Some people also brush and comb their hair at bedtime. Make sure you complete hair care before visitors arrive.

Encourage residents to do their own hair care. Assist as needed. Perform hair care for those who cannot do so. The person chooses how to brush, comb, and style hair.

Brushing increases blood flow to the scalp, and it brings scalp oils along the hair shaft. Scalp oils help keep hair soft and shiny. Brushing and combing prevent tangled and matted hair. When brushing and combing hair, start at the scalp. Then brush or comb to the hair ends.

Long hair easily mats and tangles. Daily brushing and combing prevent the problem. So does braiding. You need the person's consent to braid hair. *Never cut matted or tangled hair. Never cut hair for any reason.* Tell the nurse if the person has matted or tangled hair. The nurse may have you comb or brush through the matting and tangling.

Special measures are needed for curly, coarse, and dry hair. Use a wide-tooth comb for curly hair. Start at the neckline. Working upward, lift and fluff hair outward. Continue to the forehead. Wet hair or apply conditioner, petroleum jelly, or the person's special hair product as directed. This makes combing easier.

The person may have certain hair care practices and products. They are part of the care plan. Also, let the person guide you when giving hair care. Have a mirror handy so the person can see what you are doing. Try to follow the person's directions to promote pride in appearance.

See *Caring About Culture: Brushing and Combing Hair.*
See *Delegation Guidelines: Brushing and Combing Hair.*
See *Promoting Safety and Comfort: Brushing and Combing Hair.*

📋 DELEGATION GUIDELINES

Brushing and Combing Hair
To brush and comb hair, you need this information from the nurse and the care plan:
- How much help the person needs
- What to do if hair is matted or tangled
- What to do for curly, coarse, or dry hair
- What hair care products to use
- The person's preferences and routine hair care measures
- What observations to report and record:
  - Scalp sores
  - Flaking
  - Itching
  - The presence of nits or lice
- Nits (lice eggs attached to hair shafts)—oval and yellow to white in color
- Lice—about the size of a sesame seed and gray-white in color:
  - Patches of hair loss
  - Hair falling out in patches
  - Very dry or very oily hair
  - Matted or tangled hair
- When to report observations
- What specific resident concerns to report at once

👤 PROMOTING SAFETY AND COMFORT

Brushing and Combing Hair
Safety
Sharp bristles can injure the scalp, as can a comb with sharp or broken teeth. Tell the nurse if you have concerns about the person's brush or comb.

Comfort
When giving hair care, place a towel across the person's back and shoulders to protect garments from falling hair. If the person is in bed, give hair care before changing linens and the pillowcase. If done after a linen change, place a towel across the pillow to collect falling hair.

✳ BRUSHING AND COMBING THE PERSON'S HAIR

Quality of Life
Remember to:
- Knock before entering the person's room.
- Address the person by name.
- Introduce yourself by name and title.
- Explain the procedure to the person before beginning and during the procedure.
- Protect the person's rights during the procedure.
- Handle the person gently during the procedure.

Preprocedure
1. Follow *Delegation Guidelines: Brushing and Combing Hair.* See *Promoting Safety and Comfort: Brushing and Combing Hair.*
2. Practice hand hygiene.
3. Identify the person. Check the ID (identification) bracelet against the assignment sheet. Also call the person by name.
4. Ask the person how to style hair.

✳ BRUSHING AND COMBING THE PERSON'S HAIR—cont'd

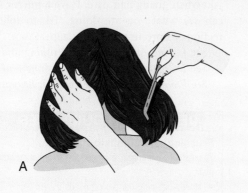

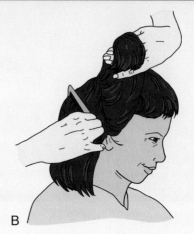

Fig. 19.7 Part hair. (A) Part hair down the middle. Divide it into two sides. (B) Then part one side into two smaller sections.

5. Collect the following:
   - Comb and brush
   - Bath towel
   - Other hair care items as requested
6. Arrange items on the bedside stand.
7. Provide for privacy.

Procedure
8. Lower the bed rail if up.
9. Help the person to the chair. The person puts on a robe and nonskid footwear when up. (If the person is in bed, raise the bed for body mechanics. Bed rails are up if used. Lower the bed rail near you. Assist the person to a semi-Fowler position if allowed.)
10. Place a towel across the person's back and shoulders or across the pillow.
11. Ask the person to remove eyeglasses. Put them in the eyeglass case. Put the case inside the bedside stand.
12. *Brush and comb hair that is* not *matted or tangled*:
    a. Use the comb to part the hair.
       (1) Part hair down the middle into two sides (Fig. 19.7A).
       (2) Divide one side into two smaller sections (see Fig. 19.7B).
    b. Brush one of the small sections of hair. Start at the scalp and brush toward the hair ends (Fig. 19.8). (For course or very curly hair, it may be easier to start at the neck.) Do the same for the other small section of hair.
    c. Repeat steps 12a(2) and 12b for the other side.
13. *Brush and comb matted and tangled hair*:
    a. Take a small section of hair near the ends.
    b. Comb or brush through to the hair ends.
    c. Add small sections of hair as you work up to the scalp.
    d. Comb or brush through each longer section to the hair ends.
    e. Brush or comb from the scalp to the hair ends.
14. Style the hair as the person prefers.

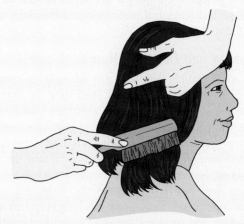

Fig. 19.8 Brush hair by starting at the scalp. Brush down to the hair ends.

15. Remove the towel.
16. Let the person put on the eyeglasses.

Postprocedure
17. Provide for comfort. (See the inside of the front cover.)
18. Place the call light within reach.
19. Lower the bed to its lowest position.
20. Raise or lower bed rails. Follow the care plan.
21. Clean and return hair care items to their proper place.
22. Unscreen the person.
23. Complete a safety check of the room. (See the inside of the front cover.)
24. Follow center policy for dirty linens.
25. Decontaminate your hands.

This skill also covered in *Clinical Skills: Nurse Assisting*.

✳ SHAMPOOING

Oil gland secretion decreases with aging. Therefore, older persons have dry hair. Shampooing frequency depends on the person's needs and preferences. Usually shampooing is done weekly on the person's bath day.

Some persons use certain shampoos and conditioners. Others used medicated products ordered by the doctor.

Residents usually need help with shampooing. If a woman's hair is done by a hairdresser, do not shampoo her hair. She wears a shower cap during the tub bath or shower.

The shampoo method depends on the person's condition, safety factors, and personal choice. The health team decides on the method to use.

- *Shampoo during the shower or tub bath.* The person shampoos in the shower. You use a handheld nozzle for those using shower chairs or taking tub baths. You direct a spray of water at the hair.
- *Shampoo at the sink.* The person sits facing away from the sink. A folded towel is placed over the sink edge to protect the neck. The person's head is tilted back over the edge of the sink. You use a water pitcher or handheld nozzle to wet and rinse the hair.

- *Shampoo on a stretcher.* The stretcher is in front of the sink. A towel is placed under the neck. The head is tilted over the edge of the sink (Fig. 19.9). You use a water pitcher or handheld nozzle to wet and rinse the hair.
- *Shampoo in bed.* The person's head and shoulders are moved to the edge of the bed if possible. A shampoo tray is placed under the head to protect the linens and mattress from water. The tray drains into a basin placed on a chair by the bed (Fig. 19.10). You use a water pitcher to wet and rinse the hair. This method is used for persons who need complete bed baths. It also is used for persons who cannot use a chair, wheelchair, or stretcher.

✳ SHAMPOOING THE PERSON'S HAIR

Quality of Life

Remember to:
- Knock before entering the person's room.
- Address the person by name.
- Introduce yourself by name and title.
- Explain the procedure to the person before beginning and during the procedure.
- Protect the person's rights during the procedure.
- Handle the person gently during the procedure.

Preprocedure

1. Follow *Delegation Guidelines: Shampooing*, p. 288. See *Promoting Safety and Comfort: Shampooing*, p. 288.
2. Practice hand hygiene.
3. Collect the following:
   - Two bath towels
   - Washcloth
   - Shampoo
   - Hair conditioner (if requested)
   - Bath thermometer
   - Pitcher or handheld nozzle (if needed)
   - Shampoo tray (if needed)
   - Basin or pan (if needed)
   - Waterproof pad (if needed)
   - Gloves (if needed)
   - Comb and brush
   - Hair dryer
4. Arrange items nearby.
5. Identify the person. Check the ID bracelet against the assignment sheet. Also call the person by name.
6. Provide for privacy.
7. Remove any hearing aids and eyeglasses.
8. Raise the bed for body mechanics for a shampoo in bed. Bed rails are up if used.
9. Decontaminate your hands.

Procedure

10. Lower the bed rail near you if up.
11. Cover the person's chest with a bath towel.
12. Brush and comb the hair to remove snarls and tangles.
13. Position the person for the method you will use. To shampoo the person in bed:
    a. Lower the head of the bed and remove the pillow.
    b. Place the waterproof pad and shampoo tray under the head and shoulders.
    c. Support the head and neck with a folded towel if necessary.
14. Raise the bed rail if used.
15. Obtain water. Water temperature is usually 105°F (40.5°C). Test water temperature according to center policy. Also ask the person to check the

water. Adjust water temperature as needed. Raise the bed rail before leaving the bedside.
16. Lower the bed rail near you if up.
17. Put on gloves (if needed).
18. Ask the person to hold a washcloth over the eyes. It should not cover the nose and mouth. (*Note:* A damp washcloth is easier to hold. It will not slip. However, some state competency tests require a dry washcloth.)
19. Use the pitcher or nozzle to wet the hair.
20. Apply a small amount of shampoo.
21. Work up a lather with both hands. Start at the hairline. Work toward the back of the head.
22. Massage the scalp with your fingertips. Do not scratch the scalp.
23. Rinse the hair until the water runs clear.
24. Repeat steps 20 through 23.
25. Apply conditioner according to directions on the container.
26. Squeeze water from the person's hair.
27. Cover the hair with a bath towel.
28. Remove the shampoo tray, basin, and waterproof pad.
29. Dry the person's face with the towel. Use the towel on the person's chest.
30. Help the person raise the head if appropriate. For the person in bed, raise the head of the bed.
31. If using a disposable shampoo cap:
    a. Comb hair to remove any tangles
    b. Open package, apply cap, and tuck all hair in cap.
    c. Massage head through cap, check that cap is fitted properly.
    d. Massage for 2 to 4 minutes or as directed on package.
    e. Remove cap and discard in trash.
32. Rub the hair and scalp with the towel. Use the second towel if the first one is wet.
33. Comb the hair to remove snarls and tangles.
34. Dry and style hair as quickly as possible.
35. Remove and discard the gloves (if used). Decontaminate your hands.

Postprocedure

36. Provide for comfort. (See the inside of the front cover.)
37. Assist person to replace hearing aids and eyeglasses.
38. Place the call light within reach.
39. Lower the bed to its lowest position.
40. Raise or lower bed rails. Follow the care plan.
41. Unscreen the person.
42. Complete a safety check of the room. (See the inside of the front cover.)
43. Clean, dry, and return equipment to its proper place. Remember to clean the brush and comb. Discard disposable items.
44. Follow center policy for dirty linens.
45. Decontaminate your hands.
46. Report and record your observations.

This skill is also covered in *Clinical Skills: Nurse Assisting.*

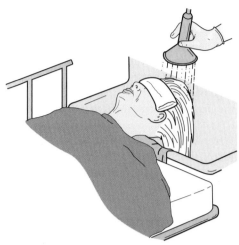

Fig. 19.9 Shampooing while the person is on a stretcher. The stretcher is in front of the sink.

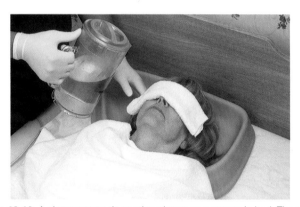

Fig. 19.10 A shampoo tray is used to shampoo a person in bed. The tray is directed to the side of the bed so water drains into a collecting basin.

- *Shampoo using disposable shampoo cap.* The prepackaged shampoo cap is placed over the person's head while sitting in a chair or in bed. The head is massaged through the cap for several minutes. (Fig. 19.11)

Dry and style hair as quickly as possible after the shampoo. Women may want hair curled or rolled up before drying. Check with the nurse before doing so.

See *Delegation Guidelines: Shampooing.*

See *Promoting Safety and Comfort: Shampooing.*

📄 DELEGATION GUIDELINES

Shampooing

Before shampooing a person's hair, you need this information from the nurse and the care plan:

- When to shampoo the person's hair
- What method to use
- What shampoo and conditioner to use
- The person's position restrictions or limits
- What water temperature to use—usually 105°F (Fahrenheit) (40.5°C [Centigrade])
- If hair is curled or rolled up before drying
- What observations to report and record:
  - Scalp sores
  - Flaking
  - Itching

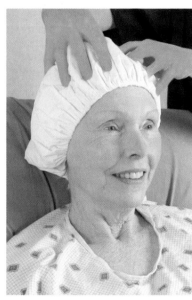

Fig. 19.11 A disposable shampoo cap. (From Perry AG et al.: *Clinical nursing skills and techniques*, ed. 10, St. Louis, 2022, Elsevier.)

- The presence of nits or lice
- Patches of hair loss
- Hair falling out in patches
- Very dry or very oily hair
- Matted or tangled hair
- How the person tolerated the procedure
- When to report observations
- What specific resident concerns to report at once

👤 PROMOTING SAFETY AND COMFORT

Shampooing

Safety

Keep shampoo away from and out of the eyes. Have the person hold a washcloth over the eyes. When rinsing, cup your hand at the person's forehead. This keeps soapy water from running down the person's forehead and into the eyes.

Return medicated products to the nurse. Never leave them at the bedside unless instructed to do so.

Wear gloves if the person has scalp sores. Follow Standard Precautions and the Bloodborne Pathogen Standard.

For a shampoo on a stretcher, follow the rules for stretcher use (Chapter 11). To safely transfer the person to and from the stretcher, see procedure: *Moving the Person to a Stretcher* (Chapter 15). Lock the stretcher wheels and use the safety straps and side rails. The far side rail is raised during the procedure.

Some people can shampoo themselves during a tub bath or shower. Place an extra towel, shampoo, and hair conditioner within the person's reach. Assist as needed.

Comfort

When shampooing during the tub bath or shower, the person tips the head back to keep shampoo and water out of the eyes. Support the back of the person's head with one hand. Shampoo with your other hand. Some persons cannot tip their head back. They lean forward and hold a folded washcloth over the eyes. Support the forehead with one hand as you shampoo with the other. Make sure that the person can breathe easily.

Many people have limited range of motion in their neck. They are not shampooed at the sink or on a stretcher.

BOX 19.1 Rules for Shaving

- Use electric shavers for persons taking anticoagulants. Never use safety razors.
- Never use a resident's shaver for anyone else. This is the resident's private property.
- If the person wears dentures, have those in place in the mouth.
- If the person is receiving oxygen therapy (Chapter 26), operate the shaver on battery power.
- Protect bed linens. Place a towel under the part being shaved, or place a towel across the person's chest and shoulders to protect clothing.
- Soften the skin before shaving. Apply a wet washcloth or towel to the face for a few minutes.
- Encourage the person to do as much as safely possible.
- Hold the skin taut as needed.
- Shave in the correct direction:

- Shaving the face with a safety razor—shave in the direction of hair growth.
- Shaving the underarms with a safety razor—shave in the direction of hair growth.
- Shaving the legs with a safety razor—shave up from the ankles. This is against hair growth.
- Using an electric shaver—move the shaver in small circles over the face if using a rotary-type shaver. For a straight-type electric shaver, shave against the direction of hair growth. (*NOTE:* Your state and agency may require shaving in the direction of hair growth. Follow the manufacturer instructions and the rules in your state and agency.)
- Do not cut, nick, or irritate the skin.
- Rinse the body part thoroughly.
- Apply direct pressure to nicks or cuts (Chapter 44).
- Report nicks, cuts, or irritation to the nurse at once.

✳ SHAVING

Many men shave for comfort and mental well-being. Many women shave their legs and underarms. Women with coarse facial hair may shave or they may use other hair removal methods. See Box 19.1 for shaving rules.

Safety razors or electric shavers are used (Fig. 19.12). Usually residents are required to have their own electric shavers. If the center's shaver is used, clean it after every use. Follow the manufacturer instructions for brushing out whiskers. Also follow center policy for cleaning electric shavers.

Safety razors (blade razors) involve razor blades. They can cause nicks and cuts. Older persons with wrinkled skin are at risk for nicks and cuts. Therefore, safety razors are not used on persons who have healing problems or for those who take anticoagulants. An anticoagulant is a medication that prevents or slows down *(anti-)* blood clotting *(coagulate)*. Bleeding occurs easily and is hard to stop. A nick or cut can cause serious bleeding. Electric shavers are used.

Soften the beard before using an electric shaver or safety razor. Do so by applying a moist, warm washcloth or towel for a few minutes. Then pat dry the face and apply talcum powder if using an electric shaver. If using a safety razor, lather the face with soap and water or shaving cream.

See *Residents with Dementia: Shaving.*
See *Delegation Guidelines: Shaving.*
See *Promoting Safety and Comfort: Shaving.*

Caring for Mustaches and Beards

Mustaches and beards need daily care. Food can collect in the whiskers. So can mouth and nose drainage. Daily washing and combing are needed. Ask the person how to groom the mustache or beard. *Never trim a mustache or beard without the person's consent.*

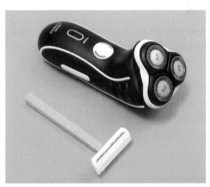

Fig. 19.12 Electric shaver *(top)* and safety razor *(bottom)*.

🧍 RESIDENTS WITH DEMENTIA

Shaving

Safety razors are not used to shave persons with dementia. They may not understand what you are doing. They may resist care and move suddenly. Serious nicks and cuts can occur. Use electric shavers for these persons.

📋 DELEGATION GUIDELINES

Shaving

Before shaving a person, you need this information from the nurse and the care plan:

- What shaver to use—electric or safety
- If the person takes anticoagulants
- When to shave the person
- What facial hair to shave
- The location of tender or sensitive areas on the person's face
- What observations to report and record:
  - Nicks (report at once)
  - Cuts (report at once)
  - Bleeding (report at once)
  - Irritation
- When to report observations
- What specific resident concerns to report at once

PROMOTING SAFETY AND COMFORT

Shaving

Safety

Safety razors are very sharp. Protect the person and yourself from nicks or cuts. Prevent contact with blood. If using an electric shaver, follow safety measures for electrical equipment (Chapter 11).

Rinse the safety razor often during the shaving procedure. Rinsing removes whiskers and lather. Then wipe the razor. To protect yourself from cuts:

- Place several thicknesses of tissues or paper towels on the overbed table. Do not hold them in your hand.
- Wipe the razor on the tissues or paper towels.

Follow Standard Precautions and the Bloodborne Pathogen Standard. Discard used razor blades and disposable shavers in the sharps container (Chapter 14). Do not recap the razor.

Comfort

Some residents have tender and sensitive skin. Usually the neck area below the jaw is tender and sensitive. Some electric shavers become very warm or hot while in use. Such heat can irritate the skin. Shave tender areas first while the shaver is cool. Then move to the other areas of the face.

Some people apply lotion or aftershave to the skin after shaving. Lotion softens the skin. Aftershave closes skin pores. Heat is applied before shaving to soften the skin. It also opens pores.

Shaving Legs and Underarms

Many women shave their legs and underarms. This practice varies among cultures. Some women shave only the lower legs; others shave to midthigh or the entire leg.

Legs and underarms are shaved after bathing. The skin is soft at this time. Soap and water, shaving cream, or lotion is used for lather. Collect shaving items with bath items. Use the kidney basin to rinse the razor. Do not use the bath water. Follow the rules in Box 19.1.

SHAVING THE PERSON'S FACE WITH A SAFETY RAZOR

Quality of Life

Remember to:

- Knock before entering the person's room.
- Address the person by name.
- Introduce yourself by name and title.
- Explain the procedure to the person before beginning and during the procedure.
- Protect the person's rights during the procedure.
- Handle the person gently during the procedure.

Preprocedure

1. Follow *Delegation Guidelines: Shaving.* See *Promoting Safety and Comfort: Shaving,* This page.
2. Practice hand hygiene.
3. Collect the following:
   - Wash basin
   - Bath towel
   - Hand towel
   - Washcloth
   - Safety razor
   - Mirror
   - Shaving cream, soap, or lotion
   - Shaving brush
   - Aftershave or lotion
   - Tissues
   - Paper towels
   - Gloves
4. Arrange paper towels and supplies on the overbed table.
5. Identify the person. Check the ID bracelet against the assignment sheet. Also call the person by name.
6. Provide for privacy.
7. Raise the bed for body mechanics. Bed rails are up if used.

Procedure

8. Fill the wash basin with warm water.
9. Place the basin on the overbed table.
10. Lower the bed rail near you if up.
11. Decontaminate your hands. Put on gloves.

12. Assist the person to semi-Fowler position if allowed or to the supine position.
13. Adjust lighting to clearly see the person's face.
14. Place the bath towel over the person's chest and shoulders.
15. Adjust the overbed table for easy reach.
16. Tighten the razor blade to the shaver if necessary.
17. Wash the person's face. Do not dry.
18. Wet the washcloth or towel. Wring it out.
19. Apply the washcloth or towel to the face for a few minutes.
20. Apply shaving cream with your hands or use a shaving brush to apply lather.
21. Hold the skin taut with one hand.
22. Shave in the direction of hair growth. Use shorter strokes around the chin and lips (Fig. 19.13).
23. Rinse the razor often. Wipe it with tissues or paper towels.
24. Apply direct pressure to any bleeding areas (Chapter 44).

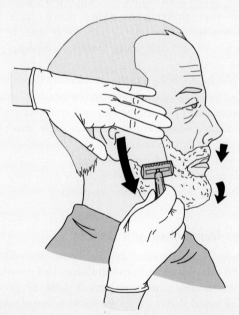

Fig. 19.13 Shave in the direction of hair growth. Use longer strokes on the larger areas of the face. Use short strokes around the chin and lips.

Continued

✖ SHAVING THE PERSON'S FACE WITH A SAFETY RAZOR—cont'd

25. Wash off any remaining shaving cream or soap. Pat dry with a towel.
26. Apply aftershave or lotion if requested. (If there are nicks or cuts, do not apply aftershave or lotion.)
27. Remove the towel and gloves. Decontaminate your hands.

Postprocedure
28. Provide for comfort. (See the inside of the front cover.)
29. Place the call light within reach.
30. Lower the bed to its lowest position.
31. Raise or lower bed rails. Follow the care plan.

32. Clean and return equipment and supplies to their proper place. Discard a razor blade or a disposable razor into the sharps container. Discard other disposable items. Wear gloves.
33. Wipe off the overbed table with paper towels. Discard the paper towels.
34. Unscreen the person.
35. Complete a safety check of the room. (See the inside of the front cover.)
36. Follow center policy for dirty linens.
37. Remove the gloves. Decontaminate your hands.
38. Report nicks, cuts, irritation, or bleeding to the nurse at once. Also report and record other observations.

This skill is also covered in *Clinical Skills: Nurse Assisting.*

✖ SHAVING THE PERSON'S FACE WITH AN ELECTRIC SHAVER

Quality of Life
Remember to:
- Knock before entering the person's room.
- Address the person by name.
- Introduce yourself by name and title.
- Explain the procedure to the person before beginning and during the procedure.
- Protect the person's rights during the procedure.
- Handle the person gently during the procedure.

Preprocedure
1. Follow *Delegation Guidelines: Shaving.* See *Promoting Safety and Comfort: Shaving.*
2. Practice hand hygiene.
3. Collect the following:
   - Wash basin
   - Bath towel
   - Hand towel
   - Washcloth
   - Person's own electric shaver
   - Mirror
   - Soap
   - Preshave or aftershave lotion
   - Tissues
   - Paper towels
   - Gloves
4. Arrange paper towels and supplies on the overbed table.
5. Identify the person. Check the ID bracelet against the assignment sheet. Also call the person by name.
6. Provide for privacy.
7. If the person wears dentures, be sure they are being worn.
8. Do not use an electric shaver if the person is using oxygen. Can use shaver on battery power if the shaver has this option.
9. Raise the bed for body mechanics. Bed rails are up if used.

Procedure
10. Fill the wash basin with warm water.
11. Place the basin on the overbed table.
12. Lower the bed rail near you if up.
13. Decontaminate your hands. Put on gloves.
14. Assist the person to semi-Fowler position if allowed or to the supine position.
15. Adjust lighting to clearly see the person's face.
16. Place the bath towel over the person's chest and shoulders.
17. Adjust the overbed table for easy reach.
18. Wash the person's face and rinse. The beard may be softened by leaving a moist, warm washcloth or towel in place for a few minutes. Pat dry.

19. Apply preshave lotion or talcum powder if desired.
20. For a rotary-type shaver, hold the skin taut with one hand as you shave in circular motions (Fig. 19.14). For a straight-type electric shaver, gently press the shaving edge against the skin and shave against the direction of the hair growth. (*NOTE:* Your state and agency may require shaving in the direction of hair growth. Follow the manufacturer instructions and the rules in your state and agency.)
21. Shave the cheek area first, then around the mouth.
22. Shave the neck area last. Have the person tilt the head back if able.
23. Apply direct pressure to any bleeding areas (Chapter 44).
24. Apply aftershave lotion if requested. (If there are nicks or cuts, do not apply aftershave lotion.)
25. Remove the towel and gloves. Decontaminate your hands.

Postprocedure
26. Provide for comfort. (See the inside of the front cover.)
27. Place the call light within reach.
28. Lower the bed to its lowest position.
29. Raise or lower bed rails. Follow the care plan.
30. Clean equipment and put in proper place. Clean shaver by removing head and using a soft brush to remove the whiskers. Wipe off head with alcohol prep. Put shaver back in case.
31. Wipe off the overbed table with paper towels. Discard the paper towels.
32. Unscreen the person.
33. Complete a safety check of the room. (See the inside of the front cover.)
34. Follow center policy for dirty linens.
35. Remove the gloves. Decontaminate your hands.
36. Report nicks, cuts, irritation, or bleeding to the nurse at once. Also report and record other observations.

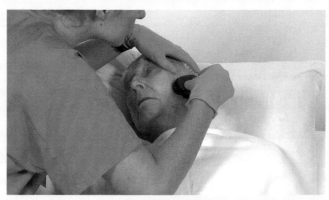

Fig. 19.14 Shave in a circular motion. Hold the skin taut with one hand.

NAIL AND FOOT CARE

Nail and foot care prevents infection, injury, and odors. Hangnails, ingrown nails (nails that grow in at the side), and nails torn away from the skin cause skin breaks. These breaks are portals of entry for microbes. Long or broken nails can scratch skin or snag clothing.

The feet are easily infected and injured. Dirty feet, socks, or stockings harbor microbes and cause odors. Shoes and socks provide a warm, moist environment for microbes to grow. Injuries occur from stubbing toes, stepping on sharp objects, or being stepped on. Shoes that fit poorly cause blisters.

Poor circulation prolongs healing. Diabetes and vascular diseases are common causes of poor circulation. Infections or foot injuries are very serious for older persons and persons with circulatory disorders. Gangrene and amputation are serious complications (Chapter 35). Trimming and clipping toenails can easily cause injuries.

Nails are easier to trim and clean right after soaking or bathing. Use nail clippers to cut fingernails. *Never use scissors.* Use extreme caution to prevent damage to nearby tissues.

Some states do not allow nursing assistants to cut or trim fingernails or toenails. Some centers do not allow nursing assistants to cut or trim fingernails or toenails. Some centers also do not allow nursing assistants to push back cuticles. Always follow center policy and what is allowed in your state.

See *Delegation Guidelines: Nail and Foot Care.*
See *Promoting Safety and Comfort: Nail and Foot Care.*
See *Teamwork and Time Management: Nail and Foot Care.*

DELEGATION GUIDELINES

Nail and Foot Care

Before giving nail and foot care, you need this information from the nurse and the care plan:

- What water temperature to use
- How long to soak fingernails (usually 5 to 10 minutes)
- How long to soak feet (usually 15 to 20 minutes)
- Who will trim the nails
- What observations to report and record:

- Reddened, irritated, or calloused areas
- Breaks in the skin
- Corns (Chapter 31) on top of and between the toes
- Very thick nails
- Loose nails
- When to report observations
- What specific resident concerns to report at once

PROMOTING SAFETY AND COMFORT

Nail and Foot Care

Safety

Many states have regulations about nursing assistants trimming fingernails and toenails. Always follow the policy at your center and the rules for your state. Nursing assistants never cut or trim nails if a person:

- Has diabetes
- Has poor circulation
- Takes medications that affect blood clotting
- Has very thick nails or ingrown toenails

The RN or podiatrist (foot *[pod-]* doctor) cuts toenails and provides foot care for these persons.

Check between the toes for cracks and sores. These areas are often overlooked. If left untreated, a serious infection could occur.

The feet are easily burned. Persons with decreased sensation or circulatory problems may not feel hot temperatures.

After soaking, apply lotion or petroleum jelly to the feet. This can cause slippery feet. Help the person put on nonskid footwear before you transfer the person or let the person walk.

Breaks in the skin and bleeding can occur. Follow Standard Precautions and the Bloodborne Pathogen Standard.

Comfort

Sometimes just fingernail care is done. Sometimes just foot care is given. Sometimes both are done. When both are done, the person sits at the overbed table (Fig. 19.15). Make sure the person is warm and comfortable.

Promote your own comfort when giving nail and foot care. Sit in front of the overbed table when cleaning and trimming fingernails. When giving foot care, rest the person's lower leg and foot on your lap, or you can kneel on the floor. Lay a towel across your lap or on the floor to protect your uniform. Remember to use good body mechanics. In whatever way you position yourself, you must also support the person's foot and ankle when giving foot care.

TEAMWORK AND TIME MANAGEMENT

Nail and Foot Care

Use your time well when giving nail and foot care. The fingernails soak for 5 to 10 minutes. The feet soak for 15 to 20 minutes. You can make the person's bed or straighten the person's unit while the fingernails and feet soak. Or you could assist with brushing and combing hair. Check your assignment sheet for other ways to meet the person's needs.

✳ GIVING NAIL AND FOOT CARE (NATCEP)

Quality of Life

Remember to:

- Knock before entering the person's room.
- Address the person by name.
- Introduce yourself by name and title.
- Explain the procedure to the person before beginning and during the procedure.
- Protect the person's rights during the procedure.
- Handle the person gently during the procedure.

Preprocedure

1. Follow *Delegation Guidelines: Nail and Foot Care*. See *Promoting Safety and Comfort: Nail and Foot Care*.
2. Practice hand hygiene.
3. Collect the following:
   - Wash basin or whirlpool foot bath
   - Soap
   - Bath thermometer
   - Bath towel
   - Hand towel
   - Washcloth
   - Kidney basin
   - Nail clippers
   - Orangewood stick
   - Emery board or nail file
   - Lotion for the hands
   - Lotion or petroleum jelly for the feet
   - Paper towels
   - Bathmat
   - Gloves
4. Arrange paper towels and other items on the overbed table.
5. Identify the person. Check the ID bracelet against the assignment sheet. Also call the person by name.
6. Provide for privacy.
7. Assist the person to the bedside chair. Place the call light within reach.

Procedure

8. Place the bathmat under the feet.
9. Fill the wash basin or whirlpool foot bath two-thirds full with water. The nurse tells you what water temperature to use. (Measure water temperature with a bath thermometer or test it by dipping your elbow or inner wrist into the basin. Follow center policy.) Also ask the person to check the water temperature. Adjust the water temperature as needed.
10. Place the basin or foot bath on the bathmat.
11. Put on gloves.
12. Help the person put the feet into the basin or foot bath. Make sure both feet are completely covered by water.
13. Adjust the overbed table in front of the person.
14. Fill the kidney basin two-thirds full with water. See step 9 for water temperature.
15. Place the kidney basin on the overbed table.
16. Place the person's fingers into the basin. Position the arms for comfort (see Fig. 19.15).
17. Let the fingers soak for 5 to 10 minutes. Let the feet soak for 15 to 20 minutes. Rewarm water as needed.
18. Remove the kidney basin.
19. Clean under the fingernails with the flat end of the orangewood stick. Use a towel to wipe the orangewood stick after each nail.
20. Dry the hands and between the fingers thoroughly.
21. Clip fingernails straight across with the nail clippers (Fig. 19.16). (Follow center policy.)

22. Shape nails with an emery board or nail file. Nails are smooth with no rough edges. Check each nail for smoothness. File as needed (Fig. 19.17).
23. Gently push cuticles back with the orangewood stick or a washcloth. (Follow center policy.)
24. Apply lotion to the hands. Warm lotion before applying it.
25. Move the overbed table to the side.
26. Lift a foot out of the water. Support the foot and ankle with one hand. With your other hand, wash the foot and between the toes with soap and a washcloth. Return the foot to the water for rinsing. Make sure you rinse between the toes.
27. Repeat step 26 for the other foot.
28. Remove the feet from the basin or foot bath. Dry thoroughly, especially between the toes.

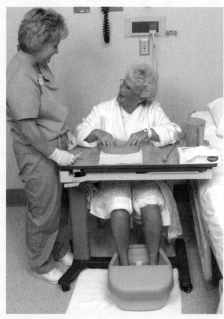

Fig. 19.15 Nail and foot care. The feet soak in a whirlpool foot bath. The fingers soak in a kidney basin.

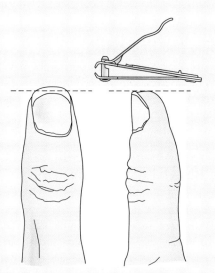

Fig. 19.16 Clip fingernails straight across. Use a nail clipper.

Continued

✳ GIVING NAIL AND FOOT CARE (NATCEP)—cont'd

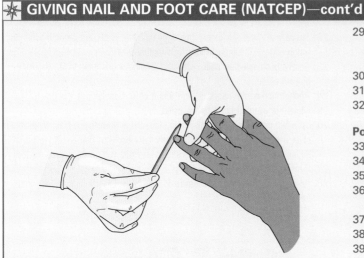

Fig. 19.17 Smooth the rough edges of the nail with an emery board or nail file.

29. Apply lotion or petroleum jelly to the tops and soles of the feet. Do not apply between the toes. Warm lotion or petroleum jelly before applying it. Remove excess lotion or petroleum jelly with a towel.
30. Remove and discard the gloves. Decontaminate your hands.
31. Assist the person to put on stockings.
32. Help the person put on nonskid footwear.

Postprocedure
33. Provide for comfort. (See the inside of the front cover.)
34. Place the call light within reach.
35. Raise or lower bed rails. Follow the care plan.
36. Clean, dry, and return equipment and supplies to their proper place. Discard disposable items. Wear gloves for this step.
37. Unscreen the person.
38. Complete a safety check of the room. (See the inside of the front cover.)
39. Follow center policy for dirty linens.
40. Remove the gloves. Decontaminate your hands.
41. Report and record your observations.

This skill is also covered in *Clinical Skills: Nurse Assisting*.

CHANGING CLOTHING AND HOSPITAL GOWNS

Residents change from sleepwear into clothing after morning care. They undress and put on sleepwear at bedtime. Garments are changed when wet or soiled. These activities are easier for those who can move their arms and legs. You may need to assist with changing clothes and hospital gowns. Follow these rules:

- Provide for privacy. Do not expose the person.
- Encourage the person to do as much as possible.
- Let the person choose what to wear. Make sure the right undergarments are chosen.
- Remove clothing from the strong or "good" side first. This is often called the *unaffected side.*
- Put clothing on the weak side first. This is often called the *affected side.*
- Support the arm or leg when removing or putting on a garment.

See *Residents with Dementia: Changing Clothing and Hospital Gowns.*

✳ Dressing and Undressing

Most residents wear street clothes during the day. Some dress and undress themselves. Others need help. Personal choice is a resident right. Let the person choose what to wear. Follow the rules for changing clothing and hospital gowns.

See *Focus on Communication: Dressing and Undressing.*
See *Delegation Guidelines: Dressing and Undressing.*

Changing Hospital Gowns Procedure

Some residents wear hospital gowns. Gowns are usually worn for IV (intravenous) therapy (Chapter 21). Some centers have special gowns for IV therapy. They open along the sleeve and close with ties, snaps, or Velcro (Fig. 19.18). Sometimes standard gowns are used. Some residents may wear hospital gowns only at night. This makes changing incontinent products easier when in bed.

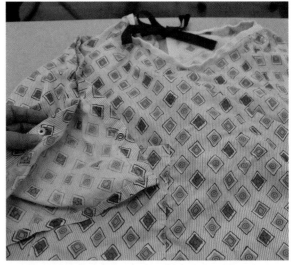

Fig. 19.18 A hospital gown with snaps at shoulder.

👤 RESIDENTS WITH DEMENTIA

Changing Clothing and Hospital Gowns
Persons with dementia may not want to change clothes, or they may not know how. For example, a person may try to put slacks on over the head. The Alzheimer's Disease Education and Referral Center (ADEAR) suggests the following:

- Try to assist with dressing and undressing at the same time each day. The person learns to expect these tasks as a part of own daily routine.
- Let the person dress oneself to the extent possible. Allow extra time for this task. Do not rush the person.
- Let the person choose what to wear from two or three outfits. If the person has a favorite outfit, the family may buy several of the same outfit. This makes dressing easier if the person insists on wearing the same outfit.
- Choose clothes that are comfortable to wear and easy to get on and off. Garments with elastic waistbands and Velcro closures are examples. The person does not have to handle zippers, buttons, hooks, snaps, or other closures.
- Stack clothes in the order they are put on. The person sees one item at a time. For example, underpants or undershorts are put on first. The item is on top of the stack.
- Give clear, simple, step-by-step directios.

📋 **FOCUS ON COMMUNICATION**

Dressing and Undressing

Allow for personal choice and independence when assisting with dressing and undressing. You can ask:

- "What would you like to wear today?"
- "There's a concert today in the lounge. Do you want to wear something special?"
- "Can I help you with those buttons?"
- "Would you like me to help you with that zipper?"

📄 **DELEGATION GUIDELINES**

Dressing and Undressing

Before assisting with dressing and undressing, you need this information from the nurse and the care plan:

- How much help the person needs
- Which side is the person's strong side
- If the person needs to wear certain garments
- What observations to report and record:
  - How much help was given
  - How the person tolerated the procedure
  - Any complaints by the person
  - Any changes in the person's behavior
- When to report observations
- What specific resident concerns to report at once

✴ UNDRESSING THE PERSON

Quality of Life

Remember to:

- Knock before entering the person's room.
- Address the person by name.
- Introduce yourself by name and title.
- Explain the procedure to the person before beginning and during the procedure.
- Protect the person's rights during the procedure.
- Handle the person gently during the procedure.

Preprocedure

1. Follow *Delegation Guidelines: Dressing and Undressing.*
2. Practice hand hygiene.
3. Collect a bath blanket and clothing requested by the person.
4. Identify the person. Check the ID bracelet against the assignment sheet. Also call the person by name.
5. Provide for privacy.
6. Raise the bed for body mechanics. Bed rails are up if used.
7. Lower the bed rail on the person's weak side.
8. Position the person supine.
9. Cover the person with a bath blanket. Fan-fold linens to the foot of the bed.

Procedure

10. Remove garments that open in the back.
    a. Raise the head and shoulders. Or turn the person onto the side away from you.
    b. Undo buttons, zippers, ties, or snaps.
    c. Bring the sides of the garment to the sides of the person (Fig. 19.19). If in a side-lying position, tuck the far side under the person. Fold the near side onto the chest (Fig. 19.20).

    d. Position the person supine.
    e. Slide the garment off the shoulder on the strong side. Remove it from the arm (Fig. 19.21).
    f. Remove the garment from the weak side.
11. Remove garments that open in the front.
    a. Undo buttons, zippers, ties, or snaps.
    b. Slide the garment off the shoulder and arm on the strong side.
    c. Assist the person to sit up or raise the head and shoulders. Bring the garment over to the weak side (Fig. 19.22).

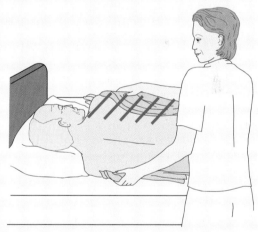

Fig. 19.20 A garment that opens in the back is removed from the person in the side-lying position. The far side of the garment is tucked under the person. The near side is folded onto the person's chest. (Note that the "weak" side is indicated by *slash marks.*)

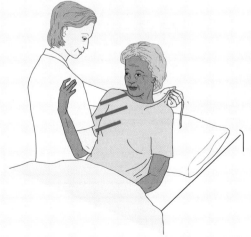

Fig. 19.19 The sides of the garment are brought from the back to the sides of the person. (Note that the "weak" side is indicated by *slash marks.*)

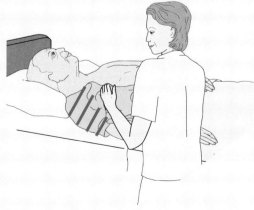

Fig. 19.21 The garment is removed from the strong side first. (Note that the "weak" side is indicated by *slash marks.*)

✳ UNDRESSING THE PERSON—cont'd

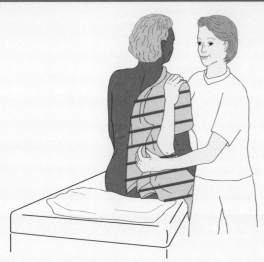

Fig. 19.22 A front-opening garment is removed with the person's head and shoulders raised. The garment is removed from the strong side first. Then it is brought around the back to the weak side. (Note that the "weak" side is indicated by *slash marks*.)

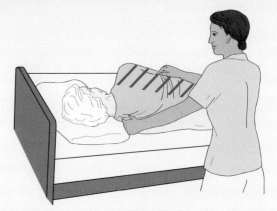

Fig. 19.23 A pullover garment is removed from the strong side first. Then the garment is brought up to the person's neck so it can be removed from the weak side. (Note that the "weak" side is indicated by *slash marks*.)

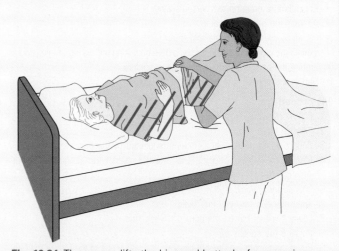

Fig. 19.24 The person lifts the hips and buttocks for removing the pants. The pants are slid down over the hips and buttocks. (Note that the "weak" side is indicated by *slash marks*.)

    d. Lower the head and shoulders. Remove the garment from the weak side.

    e. If you cannot raise the head and shoulders:

       (1) Turn the person toward you. Tuck the removed part under the person.

       (2) Turn the person onto the side away from you.

       (3) Pull the side of the garment out from under the person. Make sure the person will not lie on it when supine.

       (4) Return the person to the supine position.

       (5) Remove the garment from the weak side.

12. Remove pullover garments.

    a. Undo any buttons, zippers, ties, or snaps.

    b. Remove the garment from the strong side.

    c. Raise the head and shoulders, or turn the person onto the side away from you. Bring the garment up to the person's neck (Fig. 19.23).

    d. Remove the garment from the weak side.

    e. Bring the garment over the person's head.

    f. Place the person in the supine position.

13. Remove pants or slacks.

    a. Remove footwear and socks.

    b. Position the person supine.

    c. Undo buttons, zippers, ties, snaps, or buckles.

    d. Remove the belt.

    e. Ask the person to lift the buttocks off the bed. Slide the pants down over the hips and buttocks (Fig. 19.24). Have the person lower the hips and buttocks.

    f. If the person cannot raise the hips off the bed:

       (1) Turn the person toward you.

       (2) Slide the pants off the hip and buttock on the strong side (Fig. 19.25).

       (3) Turn the person away from you.

       (4) Slide the pants off the hip and buttock on the weak side (Fig. 19.26).

    g. Slide the pants down the legs and over the feet.

14. Dress the person. See procedure: *Dressing the Person*, pp 297-298.

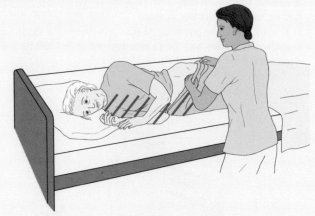

Fig. 19.25 Pants are removed in the side-lying position. They are removed from the strong side first. They are slid over the hip and buttock. (Note that the "weak" side is indicated by *slash marks*.)

Continued

✴ UNDRESSING THE PERSON—cont'd

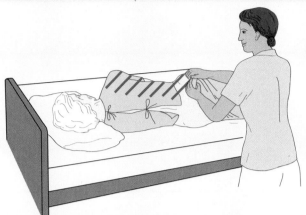

Fig. 19.26 The person is turned onto the strong side. The pants are removed from the weak side. (Note that the "weak" side is indicated by *slash marks*.)

Postprocedure
15. Provide for comfort. (See the inside of the front cover.)
16. Place the call light within reach.
17. Lower the bed to its lowest position.
18. Raise or lower bed rails. Follow the care plan.
19. Unscreen the person.
20. Complete a safety check of the room. (See the inside of the front cover.)
21. Follow center policy for soiled clothing.
22. Decontaminate your hands.
23. Report and record your observations.

This skill is also covered in *Clinical Skills: Nurse Assisting.*

✴ DRESSING THE PERSON (NATCEP)

Quality of Life
Remember to:
- Knock before entering the person's room.
- Address the person by name.
- Introduce yourself by name and title.
- Explain the procedure to the person before beginning and during the procedure.
- Protect the person's rights during the procedure.
- Handle the person gently during the procedure.

Preprocedure
1. Follow *Delegation Guidelines: Dressing and Undressing*, p. 295.
2. Practice hand hygiene.
3. Ask the person to choose what to wear.
4. Get a bath blanket and clothing requested by the person.
5. Identify the person. Check the ID bracelet against the assignment sheet. Also call the person by name.
6. Provide for privacy.
7. Raise the bed for body mechanics. Bed rails are up if used.
8. Lower the bed rail (if up) on the person's strong side.
9. Position the person supine.
10. Cover the person with a bath blanket. Fan-fold linens to the foot of the bed.
11. Undress the person. (See procedure: *Undressing the Person*, pp 295-297.)

Procedure
12. Put on garments that open in the back.
    a. Slide the garment onto the arm and shoulder of the weak side.
    b. Slide the garment onto the arm and shoulder of the strong side.
    c. Raise the person's head and shoulders.
    d. Bring the sides to the back.
    e. If you cannot raise the person's head and shoulders:
       (1) Turn the person toward you.
       (2) Bring one side of the garment to the person's back (Fig. 19.27A).
       (3) Turn the person away from you.
       (4) Bring the other side to the person's back (see Fig. 19.27B).
    f. Fasten buttons, zippers, snaps, or other closures.
    g. Position the person supine.

13. Put on garments that open in the front.
    a. Slide the garment onto the arm and shoulder on the weak side.
    b. Raise the head and shoulders. Bring the side of the garment around to the back. Lower the person down. Slide the garment onto the arm and shoulder of the strong arm.
    c. If the person cannot raise the head and shoulders:
       (1) Turn the person away from you.
       (2) Tuck the garment under him or her.
       (3) Turn the person toward you.
       (4) Pull the garment out from underneath the person.
       (5) Turn the person back to the supine position.
       (6) Slide the garment over the arm and shoulder of the strong arm.
    d. Fasten buttons, zippers, ties, snaps, or other closures.
14. Put on pullover garments.
    a. Position the person supine.
    b. Bring the neck of the garment over the head.
    c. Slide the arm and shoulder of the garment onto the weak side.
    d. Raise the person's head and shoulders.
    e. Bring the garment down.
    f. Slide the arm and shoulder of the garment onto the strong side.
    g. If the person cannot assume a semi-sitting position:
       (1) Turn the person away from you.
       (2) Tuck the garment under the person.
       (3) Turn the person toward you.
       (4) Pull the garment out from underneath the person.
       (5) Position the person supine.
       (6) Slide the arm and shoulder of the garment onto the strong side.
    h. Fasten buttons, zippers, ties, snaps, or other closures.
15. Put on pants or slacks.
    a. Slide the pants over the feet and up the legs.
    b. Ask the person to raise the hips and buttocks off the bed.
    c. Bring the pants up over the buttocks and hips.
    d. Ask the person to lower the hips and buttocks.
    e. If the person cannot raise the hips and buttocks:
       (1) Turn the person onto the strong side.
       (2) Pull the pants over the buttock and hip on the weak side.
       (3) Turn the person onto the weak side.

Continued

✳ DRESSING THE PERSON (NATCEP)—cont'd

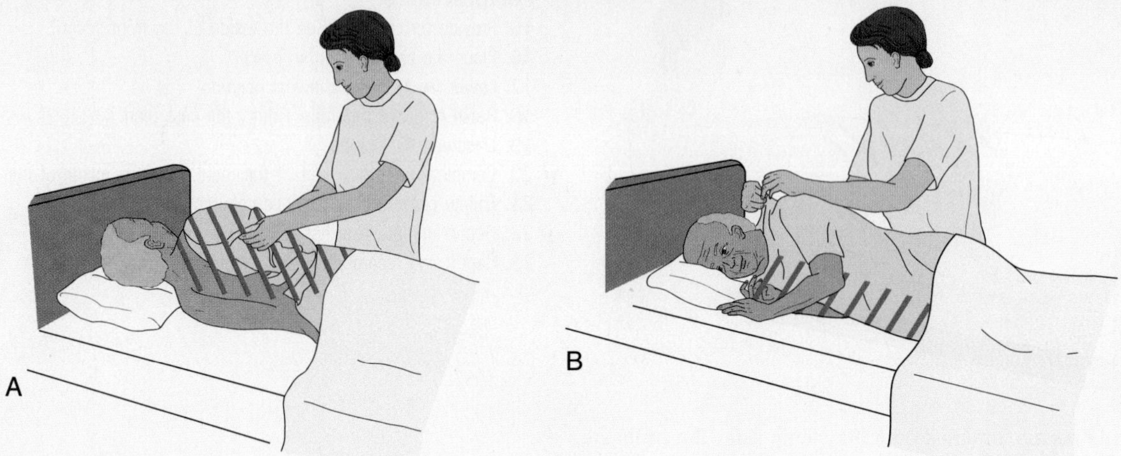

Fig. 19.27 Dressing a person. (A) The side-lying position can be used to put on garments that open in the back. Turn the person toward you after the garment is put on the arms. The side of the garment is brought to the person's back. (B) Then turn the person away from you. The other side of the garment is brought to the back and fastened. (Note that the "weak" side is indicated by *slash marks*.)

(4) Pull the pants over the buttock and hip on the strong side.

(5) Position the person supine.

 f. Fasten buttons, zippers, ties, snaps, a belt buckle, or other closures.

16. Put socks and nonskid footwear on the person. Make sure socks are up all the way and smooth.

17. Help the person get out of bed. If the person will stay in bed, cover the person. Remove the bath blanket.

Postprocedure

18. Provide for comfort. (See the inside of the front cover.)

19. Place the call light within reach.

20. Lower the bed to its lowest position.

21. Raise or lower bed rails. Follow the care plan.

22. Unscreen the person.

23. Complete a safety check of the room. (See the inside of the front cover.)

24. Follow center policy for soiled clothing.

25. Decontaminate your hands.

26. Report and record your observations.

📋 DELEGATION GUIDELINES

Changing Hospital Gowns

Before changing a gown, you need this information from the nurse and the care plan:

- Which arm has the IV
- If the person has an IV pump (see *Promoting Safety and Comfort: Changing Hospital Gowns*)

If there is injury or paralysis, the gown is removed from the strong arm first. Support the weak arm while removing the gown. Put the clean gown on the weak arm first and then on the strong arm.

 See *Delegation Guidelines: Changing Hospital Gowns.*

 See *Promoting Safety and Comfort: Changing Hospital Gowns.*

👤 PROMOTING SAFETY AND COMFORT

Changing Hospital Gowns

Safety

IV pumps control how fast fluid enters a vein. This is called the flow rate. If the person has an IV pump and a standard gown, do not use the following procedure. The arm with the IV is not put through the sleeve.

 If the person has an IV, changing the gown can cause the flow rate to change. Always ask the nurse to check the flow rate after you change a gown.

 Do not disconnect or remove any part of the IV setup.

Comfort

Some hospital gowns are secured with ties at the upper back. The back and buttocks are exposed when the person stands. Other gowns overlap in the back and tie at the side. These gowns provide more privacy. Because they tie at the side, uncomfortable bows and knots at the back are avoided.

CHANGING THE GOWN OF THE PERSON WITH AN IV

Quality of Life

Remember to:

- Knock before entering the person's room.
- Address the person by name.
- Introduce yourself by name and title.
- Explain the procedure to the person before beginning and during the procedure.
- Protect the person's rights during the procedure.
- Handle the person gently during the procedure.

Preprocedure

1. Follow *Delegation Guidelines: Changing Hospital Gowns.* See *Promoting Safety and Comfort: Changing Hospital Gowns.*
2. Practice hand hygiene.
3. Get a clean gown and a bath blanket.
4. Identify the person. Check the ID bracelet against the assignment sheet. Also call the person by name.
5. Provide for privacy.
6. Raise the bed for body mechanics. Bed rails are up if used.

Procedure

7. Lower the bed rail near you (if up).
8. Cover the person with a bath blanket. Fan-fold linens to the foot of the bed.
9. Untie the gown. Free parts that the person is lying on.
10. Remove the gown from the arm with *no IV.*
11. Gather up the sleeve of the arm *with the IV.* Slide it over the IV site and tubing. Remove the arm and hand from the sleeve (Fig. 19.28A).

12. Keep the sleeve gathered. Slide your arm along the tubing to the bag (see Fig. 19.28B).
13. Remove the bag from the pole. Slide the bag and tubing through the sleeve (see Fig. 19.28C). Do not pull on the tubing. Keep the bag above the person.
14. Hang the IV bag on the pole.
15. Gather the sleeve of the clean gown that will go on the arm with the IV infusion.
16. Remove the bag from the pole. Slip the sleeve over the bag at the shoulder part of the gown (see Fig. 19.28D). Hang the bag.
17. Slide the gathered sleeve over the tubing, hand, arm, and IV site. Then slide it onto the shoulder.
18. Put the other side of the gown on the person. Fasten the gown.
19. Cover the person. Remove the bath blanket.

Postprocedure

20. Provide for comfort. (See the inside of the front cover.)
21. Place the call light within reach.
22. Lower the bed to its lowest position.
23. Raise or lower bed rails. Follow the care plan.
24. Unscreen the person.
25. Complete a safety check of the room. (See the inside of the front cover.)
26. Follow center policy for dirty linen.
27. Decontaminate your hands.
28. Ask the nurse to check the flow rate.
29. Report and record your observations.

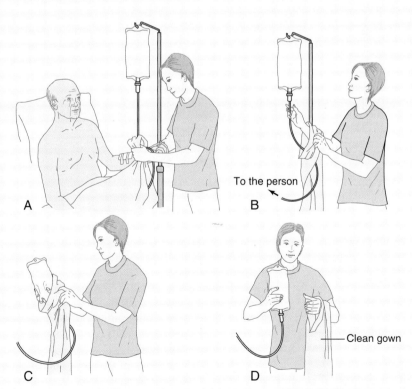

Fig. 19.28 Changing a gown. (A) The gown is removed from the arm with no IV. The sleeve on the arm with the IV is gathered up, slipped over the IV site and tubing, and removed from the arm and hand. (B) The gathered sleeve is slipped along the IV tubing to the bag. (C) The IV bag is removed from the pole and passed through the sleeve. (D) The gathered sleeve of the clean gown is slipped over the IV bag at the shoulder part of the gown.

Activities-of-Daily-Living Flow Sheet

ORDER/INSTRUCTION	TIME	1	2	3	4	5	6	7	8	9	10	11	12	13	14	15	16	17	18	19	20	21	22	23	24	25	26	27	28	29	30	31
Dressing	11-7																															
I=Independent S=Set up A=Assist T=Total Care	7-3	SS	SS	BG																												
	3-11																															
Grooming, Combing Hair	11-7																															
I=Independent S=Set up A=Assist T=Total Care	7-3	SS	SS	BG																												
	3-11																															
Shave Men Daily	11-7																															
Shave Women every __2__ days	7-3	SS		BG																												
	3-11																															
Trim Fingernails Weekly	11-7																															
	7-3																															
	3-11		ME																													

Fig. 19.29 Charting sample.

QUALITY OF LIFE

Grooming measures promote comfort. They also help the person's body image and self-esteem needs. Clean hair, nails, and garments all help mental well-being. So does a clean-shaven face or a well-groomed beard or mustache. A person's pride may be boosted by a visit to the hair salon. It may be your responsibility to transport the person by wheelchair if the salon is a distance.

The person may not have energy for some procedures. The nurse tells you what care to give and when to give it. Encourage and allow personal choice when possible. Grooming practices vary from person to person. Always assist as needed.

Carefully handle the person's grooming products, shaver, hair dryer, brush and comb, perfumes, and other personal care items. Garments also need your attention. Do not break zippers, tear clothing, lose buttons, or cause other damage. Treat the person's property with care and respect.

Respect the person's privacy by helping with putting on a robe over a hospital gown when walking in hallways. This prevents the person from exposing the backside inadvertently.

Sometimes family members want to help with grooming. For example, they want to help style the person's hair. Or they want to apply lotion to the person's hands and feet. With the person's permission, allow family members to assist with grooming measures as much as safely possible. This promotes social interaction. It also involves the family in the person's care.

Report your observations to the nurse. Also record your observations and the care given according to center policy (Fig. 19.29). This information is needed to meet the person's needs.

TIME TO REFLECT

Mrs. Martin is a retired beautician who resides at the nursing center. She has recently suffered a stroke and has right-sided weakness. She always takes pride in her personal appearance. You are working the day shift and have many residents to help with morning care and transport to the dining room before breakfast is served. Mrs. Martin refuses to let you transport her by wheelchair to the dining room table until her hair is fixed and her makeup is applied. How could you approach this situation?

REVIEW QUESTIONS

Circle the BEST answer.

1. A person has alopecia. This is
   a. Excessive body hair
   b. Dry, white flakes from the scalp
   c. An infestation with lice
   d. Hair loss

2. Which prevents hair from matting and tangling?
   a. Bedrest
   b. Daily brushing and combing
   c. Daily shampooing
   d. Cutting hair

3. A person's hair is not matted or tangled. When brushing hair, start at the
   a. Forehead and brush backward
   b. Hair ends
   c. Scalp
   d. Back of the neck and brush forward

4. Brushing keeps the hair
   a. Soft and shiny
   b. Clean
   c. Free of lice
   d. Long

5. A person requests a shampoo. You should
   a. Shampoo the hair during the person's shower
   b. Shampoo hair at the sink
   c. Shampoo the person in bed
   d. Follow the care plan
6. When shaving a person's face with a safety razor, do the following *except*
   a. Practice Standard Precautions
   b. Follow the Bloodborne Pathogen Standard
   c. Shave in the direction of hair growth
   d. Shave when the skin is dry
7. A person is nicked during shaving. Your first action is to
   a. Wash your hands
   b. Apply direct pressure
   c. Tell the nurse
   d. Apply a bandage
8. Mr. Carlson receives oxygen through a nasal cannula. He owns an electric shaver. What is the best option when assisting him?
   a. Set the shaver to battery power
   b. Plug the cord into the electrical outlet
   c. Ask the nurse to shave him
   d. Encourage him to grow a beard
9. Clean under fingernails with a(n)
   a. Emery board
   b. Flat end of an orangewood stick
   c. Washcloth
   d. Cotton ball
10. Ms. Sweeney has diabetes. Which are you *not* allowed to perform?
    a. Clean under her fingernails
    b. File her fingernails
    c. Trim her fingernails
    d. Soak her hands
11. Mr. Melnyk has limited use of his hands but refuses assistance with dressing. Which would not be helpful for him?
    a. Pants with an elastic waistband
    b. Slip-on shoes
    c. Shirt with small buttons
    d. Slipover sweatshirt
12. It is common for a foot doctor to make visits at care centers to provide services. What is another name for a foot doctor?
    a. Pediatrician
    b. Podiatrist
    c. Pathologist
    d. Manicurist

See Appendix A for answers to these questions.

20

Nutrition and Fluids

OBJECTIVES

- Define the key terms and key abbreviations listed in this chapter.
- Explain the purpose and use of the MyPlate symbol.
- Explain how to use the *Dietary Guidelines for Americans, 2020-2025*.
- Describe the functions and sources of nutrients.
- Explain how to read and use food labels.
- Describe the factors that affect eating and nutrition.
- Describe the OBRA requirements for serving food.
- Describe the special diets and between-meal snacks.
- Identify the signs, symptoms, and precautions for aspiration.
- Describe fluid requirements and the causes of dehydration.
- Explain what to do when the person has special fluid orders.
- Explain the purpose of intake and output records.
- Identify what is counted as fluid intake.
- Explain how to assist with food and fluid needs.
- Explain how to assist with calorie counts.
- Explain how to safely provide drinking water.
- Explain how to prevent foodborne illnesses.
- Perform the procedures described in this chapter.
- Explain how to promote quality of life.

KEY TERMS

anorexia The loss of appetite

aspiration Breathing fluid, food, vomitus, or an object into the lungs

calorie The fuel or energy value of food

Daily Value (DV) How a serving fits into the daily diet; expressed in a percentage (%) based on a daily diet of 2000 calories

dehydration A decrease in the amount of water in body tissues

dysphagia Difficulty (*dys-*) swallowing (*-phagia*)

edema The swelling of body tissues with water

graduate A measuring container for fluid

intake The amount of fluid taken in

nutrient A substance that is ingested, digested, absorbed, and used by the body

nutrition The processes involved in the ingestion, digestion, absorption, and use of foods and fluids by the body

output The amount of fluid lost

KEY ABBREVIATIONS

CMS Centers for Medicare & Medicaid Services
DV Daily Value
F Fahrenheit
FDA Food and Drug Administration
GI Gastrointestinal
ID Identification
IDDSI International Dysphagia Diet Standardisation Initiative
I&O Intake and output

mg Milligram
mL Milliliter
NDD National Dysphagia Diet
NPO *Non per os*; nothing by mouth
OBRA Omnibus Budget Reconciliation Act of 1987
oz Ounce
USDA United States Department of Agriculture

Food and water are physical needs. They are necessary for life. The person's diet affects physical and mental well-being. A poor diet and poor eating habits:

- Increase the risk for infection.
- Increase the risk of acute and chronic diseases.
- Cause chronic illnesses to become worse.
- Cause healing problems.
- Affect physical and mental function, increasing the risk for accidents and injuries.

Eating and drinking provide pleasure. They often are part of social times with family and friends. A friendly, social setting for meals is important. Otherwise, the person may eat poorly.

Many factors affect dietary practices. They include culture, finances, and personal choice. See Chapter 7 for religious and cultural considerations related to diet. Dietary practices also include selecting, preparing, and serving food. The health team considers these factors when planning to meet the person's nutrition needs.

❖   The Centers for Medicare & Medicaid Services (CMS) requires that the health team assess the resident's nutritional status. This will include the following:

- Medications that affect taste or cause dry mouth, nausea, and confusion
- Weight and height (Chapter 28)
- Appearance
- Food intake and fluid intake (p. 314)
- Factors affecting eating and nutrition (pp. 308-309)

The health team then must develop a care plan to meet the person's nutritional needs. CMS surveyors may ask you about the following. You will learn how to answer their questions as you study this chapter.

- How the person's food and fluid intake is observed and reported
- How the person's eating ability is observed and reported
- How the person's weight is measured and reported
- What measures are taken to prevent or meet changes in the person's nutritional needs (e.g., snacks, frequent meals)
- The goals for nutrition in the person's care plan

BASIC NUTRITION

Nutrition is the processes involved in the ingestion, digestion, absorption, and use of foods and fluids by the body. Good nutrition is needed for growth, healing, and body functions. A well-balanced diet and correct calorie intake are needed.

A high-fat and high-calorie diet causes weight gain and obesity. Weight loss occurs with a low-calorie diet.

Foods and fluids contain nutrients. A nutrient is a substance that is ingested, digested, absorbed, and used by the body. Nutrients are grouped into fats, proteins, carbohydrates, vitamins, minerals, and water.

Fats, proteins, and carbohydrates give the body fuel for energy. The amount of energy provided by a nutrient is measured in calories. A calorie is the fuel or energy value of food.

- 1 gram of fat—9 calories
- 1 gram of protein—4 calories
- 1 gram of carbohydrate—4 calories

Older persons need fewer calories than younger people. Energy and activity levels are lower.

Dietary Guidelines

The *Dietary Guidelines for Americans, 2020-2025* (Box 20.1) is for persons 2 years of age and older. It is also for persons at risk for chronic disease. Certain diseases are linked to poor diet and lack of physical activity. Table 20.1 addresses health conditions related to nutrition. These include cardiovascular disease, hypertension (high blood pressure), diabetes, obesity, osteoporosis, and some cancers. The *Dietary Guidelines* help people:

- Attain and maintain a healthy weight.
- Reduce the risk of chronic disease.
- Promote overall health.

BOX 20.1   Key Recommendations From Dietary Guidelines for Americans, 2020-2025

Balancing Calories to Manage Weight

- Prevent and/or reduce overweight and obesity through improved eating and physical activity behaviors.
- Control total calorie intake to manage body weight. For people who are overweight or obese, this will mean consuming fewer calories from foods and beverages.
- Increase physical activity and reduce time spent in sedentary behaviors.
- Maintain appropriate calorie balance during each stage of life—childhood, adolescence, adulthood, pregnancy and breastfeeding, and older age.

Food and Food Components to Reduce

- Reduce daily sodium intake to less than 2300 milligrams (mg) and further reduce intake to 1500 mg among persons who are 51 and older and those of any age who are Black or have hypertension, diabetes, or chronic kidney disease. The 1500 mg recommendation applies to about half of the US population, including children and the majority of adults.
- Consume less than 10% of calories from saturated fatty acids by replacing them with monounsaturated and polyunsaturated fatty acids.
- Consume less than 300 mg per day of dietary cholesterol.
- Keep *trans* fatty acid consumption as low as possible by limiting foods that contain synthetic sources of *trans* fats, such as partially hydrogenated oils, and by limiting other solid fats.
- Reduce the intake of calories from solid fats and added sugars.
- Limit the consumption of foods that contain refined grains, especially refined grain foods that contain solid fats, added sugars, and sodium.
- If alcohol is consumed, it should be consumed in moderation—up to one drink per day for women and two drinks per day for men—and only by adults of legal drinking age.

Food and Nutrients to Increase

Individuals should meet the following recommendations as part of a healthy eating pattern while staying within their calorie needs:

- Increase vegetable and fruit intake
- Eat a variety of vegetables, especially dark green, red, and orange vegetables and beans and peas
- Consume at least half of all grains as whole grains (Fig. 20.1); increase whole-grain intake by replacing refined grains with whole grains
- Increase intake of fat-free or low-fat milk and milk products, such as milk, yogurt, cheese, or fortified soy beverages
- Choose a variety of protein foods, which include seafood, lean meat, and poultry, eggs, beans, and peas, soy products, and unsalted nuts and seeds
- Increase the amount and variety of seafood consumed by choosing seafood in place of meat and poultry
- Replace protein foods that are higher in solid fats with choices that are lower in solid fats and calories and/or are sources of oils
- Use oils to replace solid fats where possible
- Choose foods that provide more potassium, dietary fiber, calcium, and vitamin D, which are nutrients of concern in American diets; these foods include vegetables, fruits, whole grains, and milk and milk products

Recommendations for Specific Population Groups
Women Capable of Becoming Pregnant

- Choose foods that supply heme iron, which is more readily absorbed by the body, additional iron sources, and enhancers of iron absorption such as vitamin C–rich foods.
- Consume 400 micrograms (mcg) per day of synthetic folic acid (from fortified foods and/or supplements) in addition to food forms of folate from a varied diet.

BOX 20.1   Key Recommendations From Dietary Guidelines for Americans, 2020-2025—cont'd

Women Who Are Pregnant or Breastfeeding
- Consume 8 to 12 oz of seafood per week from a variety of seafood types.
- Due to their high methyl mercury content, limit white (albacore) tuna to 6 oz per week and do not eat the following four types of fish: tilefish, shark, swordfish, and king mackerel.
- If pregnant, take an iron supplement, as recommended by an obstetrician or other health care provider.

Individuals Ages 50 Years and Older
- Consume foods fortified with vitamin B_{12}, such as fortified cereals, or dietary supplements.

Building Healthy Eating Patterns
- Select an eating pattern that meets nutrient needs over time at an appropriate calorie level.
- Account for all foods and beverages consumed and assess how they fit within a total healthy eating pattern.
- Follow food safety recommendations when preparing and eating foods to reduce the risk of foodborne illnesses (Fig. 20.2).

From US Department of Agriculture: *Dietary guidelines for Americans, 2020*, Washington, DC, 2020, Author.

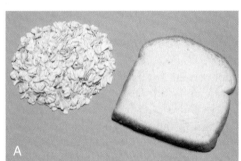 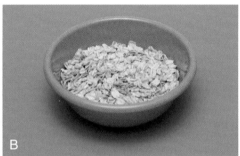

Fig. 20.1 (A) The amount of whole grain that equals a 1-oz slice of bread. (B) A 3-oz equivalent serving of whole grain.

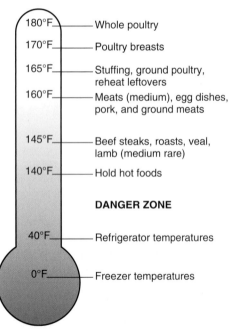

Fig. 20.2 Food temperature guide. *F*, Fahrenheit. (Redrawn from US Department of Health and Human Services and US Department of Agriculture: *Finding your way to a healthier you: based on the Dietary Guidelines for Americans, 2020-2025*.)

The *Dietary Guidelines* focus on:
- Consuming fewer calories.
- Making informed food choices.
- Being physically active.

MyPlate

The MyPlate symbol (Fig. 20.3) encourages healthy eating from five food groups. MyPlate, issued by the US Department of Agriculture (USDA), helps you make wise food choices by:
- Balancing calories:
  - Eating less
  - Avoiding oversized portions
- Increasing certain foods:
  - Making half of your plate fruits and vegetables
  - Making at least half of your grains whole grains
  - Drinking fat-free or low-fat (1%) milk
- Reducing certain foods:
  - Choosing low-sodium foods
  - Drinking water instead of sugary drinks

The amount needed from each food group depends on age, sex, and physical activity (Table 20.2).

Activity

Activity should be moderate or vigorous (Box 20.2). The US Department of Health and Human Services recommends that adults do at least one of the following:
- 150 to 300 minutes each week of moderate physical activity or
- 75 to 150 minutes each week of vigorous physical activity

Physical activity at least 3 days a week is best. Each activity should be for at least 10 minutes at a time. Adults should also do strengthening activities at least 2 days a week. Pushups, sit-ups, and weightlifting are examples. When older adults cannot do 150 minutes of moderate activity, they should try to be as

TABLE 20.1   Facts About Nutrition-Related Health Conditions in the United States

Health Conditions	Statistics
Overweight and Obesity	• About 74% of adults are overweight or have obesity. • Adults ages 40–59 have the highest rate of obesity (43%) of any age group with adults 60 years and older having a 41% rate of obesity. • About 40% of children and adolescents are overweight or have obesity; the rate of obesity increases throughout childhood and teen years.
Cardiovascular Disease (CVD) and Risk Factors: • Coronary artery disease • Hypertension • High low-density lipoprotein (LDL) and total blood cholesterol • Stroke	• Heart disease is the leading cause of death. • About 18.2 million adults have coronary artery disease, the most common type of heart disease. • Stroke is the fifth leading cause of death. • Hypertension, high LDL cholesterol, and high total cholesterol are major risk factors in heart disease and stroke. • Rates of hypertension and high total cholesterol are higher in adults with obesity than those who are at a healthy weight. • About 45% of adults have hypertension. • More Black adults (54%) than White adults (46%) have hypertension. • More adults ages 60 and older (75%) than adults ages 40 to 59 (55%) have hypertension. • Nearly 4% of adolescents have hypertension. • More than 11% of adults have high total cholesterol (≥240 mg/dL). • More women (12%) than men (10%) have high total cholesterol (≥240 mg/dL). • 7% of children and adolescents have high total cholesterol (≥200 mg/dL).
Diabetes	• Almost 11% of Americans have type 1 or type 2 diabetes. • Almost 35% of American adults have prediabetes, and people 65 years and older have the highest rate (48%) compared to other age groups. • Almost 90% of adults with diabetes also are overweight or have obesity. • About 210,000 children and adolescents have diabetes, including 187,000 with type 1 diabetes. • About 6–9% of pregnant women develop gestational diabetes
Cancer • Breast cancer • Colorectal cancer	• Colorectal cancer in men and breast cancer in women are among the most common types of cancer. • About 250,520 women will be diagnosed with breast cancer this year. • Close to 5% of men and women will be diagnosed with colorectal cancer at some point during their lifetime. • More than 1.3 million people are living with colorectal cancer. • The incidence and mortality rates are highest among those ages 65 and older for every cancer type.
Bone Health and Muscle Strength	• More women (17%) than men (5%) have osteoporosis. • 20% of older adults have reduced muscle strength. • Adults over 80 years, non-Hispanic Asians, and women are at the highest risk for reduced bone mass and muscle strength.

From Dietary Guidelines for Americans, 2020-2025

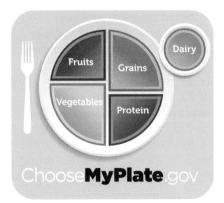

Fig. 20.3 The MyPlate symbol. (Courtesy US Department of Agriculture, Center for Nutrition and Policy Promotion, 2020-2025, www. ChooseMyplate.gov.)

physically active as their abilities allow. Many LTC centers offer exercise programs (Chapter 24) and have exercise equipment or a wellness center.

Grains Group

Food made from wheat, rice, oats, cornmeal, barley, or other cereal grain is a grain product. Bread, pasta, oatmeal, breakfast cereals, tortillas, and grits are examples. There are two types of grains.

- *Whole grains* contain the entire grain kernel. Whole-wheat flour, bulgur (cracked wheat), oatmeal, whole cornmeal, and brown rice are examples.
- *Refined grains* were processed to remove the grain kernel. These grains have a fine texture. White flour, white bread,

TABLE 20.2   MyPlate Serving Sizes

Group	Daily Servings	Serving Sizes
Grains	• Adult women: 5–6 oz; at least 3 oz from whole grains • Adult men: 6–8 oz; at least 3–4 oz from whole grains	1 oz = 1 slice of bread 1 oz = 1 cup of breakfast cereal 1 oz = ½ cup of cooked rice, cereal, or pasta
Vegetables	• Adult women: 2–2½ cups • Adult men: 2½–3 cups	1 cup = 1 cup of raw or cooked vegetables or vegetable juice 1 cup = 2 cups of raw leafy greens
Fruits	• Adult women: 1½–2 cups • Adult men: 2 cups	1 cup = 1 cup of fruit 1 cup = 1 cup of fruit juice 1 cup = ½ cup of dried fruit
Dairy	• Adult women: 3 cups • Adult men: 3 cups	1 cup = 1 cup of milk or yogurt 1 cup = 1½ oz of natural cheese 1 cup = 2 oz of processed cheese
Protein	• Adult women: 5–5½ oz • Adult men: 5½–6½ oz	1 oz = 1 oz of lean meat, poultry, or fish 1 oz = 1 egg 1 oz = 1 tablespoon of peanut butter 1 oz = ¼ cup of cooked dry beans 1 oz = ½ oz of nuts or seeds

Modified from US Department of Agriculture: *MyPlate,* Washington, DC, 2020, Author.

BOX 20.2   Moderate and Vigorous Physical Activities

Moderate Physical Activities
- Walking briskly (2.5 miles per hour or faster)
- Bicycling (less than 10 miles per hour)
- Gardening (raking, trimming bushes)
- Dancing
- Golf (walking and carrying clubs)
- Water aerobics
- Canoeing
- Tennis (doubles)

Vigorous Physical Activities
- Running and jogging
- Walking very fast (4½ miles per hour)
- Bicycling (more than 10 miles per hour)
- Heavy yard work (digging or shoveling)
- Swimming laps
- Aerobics
- Vigorous dancing
- Tennis (singles)

US Department of Health and Human Services: Physical activity guidelines for Americans, ed 2, Washington, DC, 2018, Author.

and white rice are examples. They have less dietary fiber than whole grains.

Grains have these health benefits:
- Reduce the risk of coronary artery disease
- May prevent constipation
- May help with weight management
- May prevent certain birth defects
- Contain these nutrients—dietary fiber, several B vitamins (thiamine, riboflavin, niacin, folate), and minerals (iron, magnesium, and selenium)

Vegetables Group

Vegetables can be eaten raw or cooked. They may be fresh, frozen, canned, dried, or juice. You can eat them whole, cut up, or mashed. The five vegetable subgroups are:
- *Dark green vegetables*—bok choy, broccoli, collard greens, dark green leafy lettuce, kale, mesclun, mustard greens, romaine lettuce, spinach, turnips, watercress
- *Red and orange vegetables*—acorn, butternut, and hubbard squashes; carrots; pumpkin; red peppers; sweet potatoes; tomatoes; tomato juice
- *Beans and peas*—black beans, black-eyed peas, garbanzo beans (chickpeas), kidney beans, lentils, navy beans, pinto beans, soybeans, split peas, white beans
- *Starchy vegetables*—corn, green bananas, green peas, green lima beans, plantains, potatoes, taro, water chestnuts
- *Other vegetables*—artichokes, asparagus, avocado, bean sprouts, beets, Brussels sprouts, cabbage, cauliflower, celery, cucumbers, eggplant, green beans, green peppers, iceberg (head) lettuce, mushrooms, okra, onions, parsnips, turnips, wax beans, zucchini

Vegetables have these health benefits:
- May reduce the risk for stroke, coronary artery disease, other cardiovascular diseases, and type 2 diabetes
- Protect against certain cancers (e.g., cancers of the mouth, stomach, colon-rectum)
- May reduce the risk of developing kidney stones
- May reduce the risk of bone loss
- May help lower calorie intake; most vegetables are naturally low in fat and calories
- Contain no cholesterol
- Contain these nutrients: potassium, dietary fiber, folate (folic acid), vitamins A and C

Fruits Group

Any fruit or 100% fruit juice counts as part of the fruit group. Fruit choices should vary. Fresh, frozen, canned, or dried fruits are best. Avoid fruits canned in syrup. Syrup contains added sugar. Choose fruits canned in 100% fruit juice or water.

Fruits have these health benefits:

- May reduce the risk for stroke, coronary artery disease, other cardiovascular diseases, and type 2 diabetes
- Protect against certain cancers (e.g., cancers of the mouth, stomach, and colon-rectum)
- May reduce the risk of developing kidney stones
- May reduce the risk of bone loss
- May help lower calorie intake; most fruits are naturally low in fat and calories
- Contain no cholesterol
- Are naturally low in sodium
- Contain these nutrients: potassium, dietary fiber, vitamin C, and folate (folic acid)

Dairy Group

All fluid milk products are part of the dairy group, as are many foods made from milk. Low-fat or fat-free choices are best. The milk group includes all fluid milk, yogurt, and cheese. (Cream, cream cheese, and butter are not part of the group.)

Milk has these health benefits:

- Helps build and maintain bone mass throughout the lifespan; this may reduce the risk of osteoporosis
- Improves the overall quality of the diet
- Contains these nutrients: calcium, potassium, and vitamin D

Protein Group

This group includes all foods made from meat, poultry, seafood, beans and peas, eggs, processed soy products, nuts, and seeds.

When selecting foods from this group, remember:

- To choose lean or low-fat meat and poultry. Higher-fat choices include regular ground beef (75% to 80% lean) and chicken with skin.
- Using fat for cooking increases the calories. Fried chicken and eggs fried in butter are examples.
- Salmon, trout, and herring are rich in substances that may reduce the risk of heart disease.
- Liver and other organ meats are high in cholesterol.
- Egg yolks are high in cholesterol. Egg whites are cholesterol free.
- Processed meats have added sodium (salt). They include ham, sausage, frankfurters, and luncheon and deli meats.

Many protein foods are high in fat and cholesterol. Heart disease is a major risk. However, this group provides nutrients needed for health and body maintenance:

- Protein
- B vitamins (niacin, thiamine, riboflavin, and B$_6$) and vitamin E
- Iron, zinc, and magnesium

Oils

Oils are fats that are liquid at room temperature. Vegetable oils for cooking are examples. They include canola oil, corn oil, and olive oil. Oils come from plants and fish. Because they have nutrients, the USDA includes oils in food patterns. However, *oils are not a food group*.

Adult women are allowed 5 to 6 teaspoons of oils daily. Adult men are allowed 6 to 7 teaspoons daily. Some foods are high in oil—nuts, olives, some fish, and avocados. When making oil choices, remember:

- Oils are high in calories.
- The best oil choices come from fish, nuts, and vegetable oils.
- Some foods are mainly oil. Mayonnaise, certain salad dressings, and soft margarine (tub or squeeze) are examples.
- Oils from plant sources do not contain cholesterol.
- *Solid fats* are solid at room temperature. Common solid fats include butter, beef fat (tallow, suet), chicken fat, pork fat (lard), stick margarine, and shortening.
- Oils contain some fatty acids that are essential for health. Oils also are a major source of vitamin E.

Nutrients

No food or food group has every essential nutrient. A well-balanced diet ensures an adequate intake of essential nutrients.

- *Protein* is the most important nutrient. It is needed for tissue growth and repair. Sources include meat, fish, poultry, eggs, milk and milk products, cereals, beans, peas, and nuts. Protein is needed for tissue growth and repair. The diets of some older persons may lack protein. High-protein foods are costly.
- *Carbohydrates* provide energy and fiber for bowel elimination. They are found in fruits, vegetables, breads, cereals, and sugar. Carbohydrates break down into sugars during digestion. The sugars are absorbed into the bloodstream. Fiber is not digested. It provides the bulky part of chyme for elimination.
- *Fats* provide energy. They add flavor to food and help the body use certain vitamins. Sources include meats, lard, butter, shortening, oils, milk, cheese, egg yolks, and nuts. Dietary fat not needed by the body is stored as body fat (*adipose tissue*).
- *Vitamins* are needed for certain body functions. They do not provide calories. The body stores vitamins A, D, E, and K. Vitamin C and the B complex vitamins are not stored. They must be ingested daily. The lack of a certain vitamin results in signs and symptoms of an illness (Table 20.3).
- *Minerals* are used for many body processes. Bone and tooth formation, nerve and muscle function, and fluid balance are examples. Foods containing calcium help prevent musculoskeletal changes (Table 20.4).
- *Water* is needed for all body processes (p. 314).

Food Labels

Most foods have labels (Fig. 20.4). They are used to make informed food choices for a healthy diet. In 2016 the Food and Drug Administration (FDA) announced the new Nutrition

TABLE 20.3 Functions and Sources of Common Vitamins

Vitamin	Major Functions	Sources
Vitamin A	Growth; vision; healthy hair, skin, and mucous membranes; resistance to infection	Liver, spinach, green leafy and yellow vegetables, yellow fruits, fish liver oils, egg yolks, butter, cream, whole milk
Vitamin B$_1$ (thiamine)	Muscle tone, nerve function, digestion, appetite, normal elimination, carbohydrate use	Pork, fish, poultry, eggs, liver, breads, pastas, cereals, oatmeal, potatoes, peas, beans, soybeans, peanuts
Vitamin B$_2$ (riboflavin)	Growth, healthy eyes, protein and carbohydrate metabolism, healthy skin and mucous membranes	Milk and milk products, liver, green leafy vegetables, eggs, breads, cereals
Vitamin B$_3$ (niacin)	Protein, fat, and carbohydrate metabolism; nervous system function; appetite; digestive system function	Meat, pork, liver, fish, peanuts, breads and cereals, green vegetables, dairy products
Vitamin B$_{12}$	Formation of red blood cells, protein metabolism, nervous system function	Liver, meats, poultry, fish, eggs, milk, cheese
Folate (folic acid)	Formation of red blood cells, intestinal function, protein metabolism	Liver, meats, fish, poultry, green leafy vegetables, whole grains
Vitamin C (ascorbic acid)	Formation of substances that hold tissues together; healthy blood vessels, skin, gums, bones, and teeth; wound healing; prevention of bleeding; resistance to infection	Citrus fruits, tomatoes, potatoes, cabbage, strawberries, green vegetables, melons
Vitamin D	Absorption and metabolism of calcium and phosphorus, healthy bones	Fish liver oils, milk, butter, liver, exposure to sunlight
Vitamin E	Normal reproduction, formation of red blood cells, muscle function	Vegetable oils, milk, eggs, meats, cereals, green leafy vegetables
Vitamin K	Blood clotting	Liver, green leafy vegetables, egg yolks, cheese

TABLE 20.4 Functions and Sources of Common Minerals

Mineral	Major Functions	Sources
Calcium	Formation of teeth and bones, blood clotting, muscle contraction, heart function, nerve function	Milk and milk products, green leafy vegetables, whole grains, egg yolks, dried peas and beans, nuts
Phosphorus	Formation of bones and teeth; use of proteins, fats, and carbohydrates; nerve and muscle function	Meat, fish, poultry, milk and milk products, nuts, egg yolks, dried peas and beans
Iron	Allows red blood cells to carry oxygen	Liver, meat, eggs, green leafy vegetables, breads and cereals, dried peas and beans, nuts
Iodine	Thyroid gland function, growth, metabolism	Iodized salt, seafood, shellfish
Sodium	Fluid balance, nerve and muscle function	Almost all foods
Potassium	Nerve function, muscle contraction, heart function	Fruits, vegetables, cereals, meats, dried peas and beans

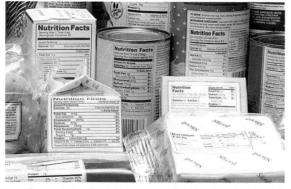

Fig. 20.4 Food labels. The labels are required by the Nutrition Labeling and Education Act of 1990.

- Serving size and the number of servings in each package.
- Calories and calories from fat. The number of servings eaten determines the number of calories of that food. For example: 1 cup of macaroni and cheese contains 250 calories with 110 of them from fat. If you eat 2 cups, you consume 500 calories (220 of which are from fat).
- Nutrients—total fat (saturated fat and trans fat), cholesterol, sodium, carbohydrate (dietary fibers and sugar), protein, vitamins A and C, calcium, and iron.

How a serving fits into the daily diet is called the Daily Value (DV). The DV is expressed in a percentage (%). The percentage is based on a daily diet of 2000 calories. The % DV helps you decide if a food is high or low in a nutrient. According to the FDA, a 5% DV is low. A DV of 20% or more is high.

Factors Affecting Eating and Nutrition

Poor nutrition is common in persons needing long-term care. They need good nutrition to correct or prevent health problems. A team approach is needed to meet a person's nutritional

Facts label for packaged foods to reflect new scientific information. This includes the link between diet and chronic diseases such as obesity and heart disease. It is believed that the new label will make it easier for people to make better food choices. Fig. 20.5 shows the new food label. Food labels contain information about:

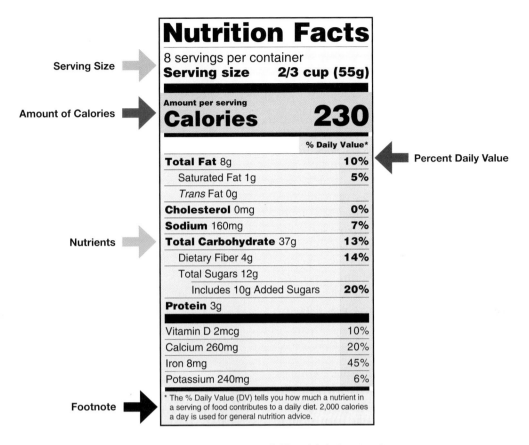

Fig. 20.5 Nutrition Facts label. (From US Food and Drug Administration. https://www.fda.gov/food/food-labeling-nutrition/nutrition-facts-label-images-download.)

needs. The nursing team, doctor, dietitian, speech-language pathologist, and occupational therapist are involved. The person is involved. So is the family if necessary. The person's likes, dislikes, and lifelong habits are part of the nutritional care plan.

Some of the following factors begin during infancy and continue throughout life. Others develop later.

Culture and Religion

Culture and religion influence dietary practices, food choices, and food preparation (Chapter 7). Frying, baking, smoking, or roasting food and eating raw food are cultural practices. So is the use of sauces, herbs, and spices.

Selecting, preparing, and eating food often involve religious or spiritual practices (Chapter 7). Persons may follow all, some, or none of the dietary practices of their chosen faith. You must respect each person's religious and spiritual practices.

Finances

People with limited incomes often buy the cheaper carbohydrate foods. Their diets often lack protein and certain vitamins and minerals.

Appetite

Appetite relates to the desire for food. When hungry, individuals seek food. They eat until the appetite is satisfied. Aromas and thoughts of food can stimulate the appetite. However, loss of appetite (anorexia) can occur. Causes include illness, medications, anxiety, pain, and depression. Unpleasant sights, thoughts, and smells are other causes.

Personal Choice

Food likes and dislikes are personal. They begin in childhood. They are influenced by foods served in the home. As children grow older, they try new foods at school and social events. Food choices depend on how food looks, how it is prepared, its smell, and ingredients. Usually food likes expand with age and social experiences.

Sometimes resident groups plan holiday and birthday meals. They may also plan picnics, pizza parties, ice cream socials, and other events. Remember, residents have the right to personal choice.

Body Reactions, Allergies, and Illness

People must avoid foods that cause allergic reactions. The person's medical record and diet card will note any food allergies. All workers who serve meals should be aware of these food allergies. Some people must avoid foods that cause nausea, vomiting, diarrhea, indigestion, gas, or headaches. People with celiac disease, for example, must avoid foods that contain the protein gluten. Gluten is found in many common grains such as wheat, barley, and rye. Cross-contamination with gluten can easily occur. An example would be toasting a slice of gluten-free bread in a toaster that is also used to toast wheat bread. Gluten-free foods should be stored in separate containers. Every effort must be made to prevent gluten products from coming in contact with gluten-free foods.

Appetite usually decreases during illness and recovery from injuries. However, nutritional needs are increased. The body must fight infection, heal tissue, and replace lost blood cells. Nutrients lost through vomiting and diarrhea need replacement.

Many medications can affect nutrition. They can cause loss of appetite, confusion, nausea, constipation, impaired taste, or changes in gastrointestinal (GI) function. They can cause inflammation of the mouth, throat, esophagus, and stomach. There are some foods that should not be given when a person takes a certain medication. This will be noted on the person's diet card. Some medications must be taken when the stomach is empty (before meals). Other medications are best tolerated when taken with food.

Chewing and Swallowing Problems

Mouth, teeth, and gum problems can affect chewing. Examples include oral pain, dry or sore mouth, gum disease (Chapter 18), and dentures that fit poorly. Broken, decayed, or missing teeth also affect chewing, especially protein foods (the meat group).

Foods providing soft bulk are often ordered for persons with chewing problems. These foods include whole-grain cereals and cooked fruits and vegetables.

Some people have to avoid high-fiber foods needed for bowel elimination. High-fiber foods are hard to chew and can irritate the intestines. Such foods include apricots, celery, and fruits and vegetables with skins and seeds.

Many health problems can affect swallowing. They include stroke, pain, confusion, dry mouth, and diseases of the mouth, throat, and esophagus. See "The Dysphagia Diet" on p. 311.

Disability

Disease or injury can affect the neck, hands, wrists, and arms. Assist devices let the person eat independently (Fig. 20.6). The speech-language pathologist and occupational therapist teach the person how to use them. Make sure each person has needed devices. Some examples of assist devices are eating utensils with special handles. A plate may have divisions or a rimmed edge (Fig. 20.7). A nonskid placemat may be placed under the plate. Special cups with handles or lids are often used. A nosey cup has a cutaway portion so the person does not have to put the head back to swallow liquids (Fig. 20.8). Special "safe straws" may be ordered. These limit the amount of liquid that flows into the mouth.

Impaired cognitive function may affect the person's ability to use eating utensils; and it may affect eating, chewing, and swallowing. Follow the care plan to assist the person.

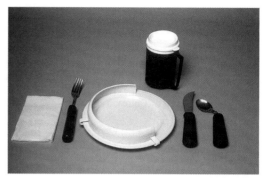

Fig. 20.6 Eating utensils for persons with special needs. (From Stromberg H: *Medical surgical nursing*, ed 5, St Louis, 2022, Saunders.)

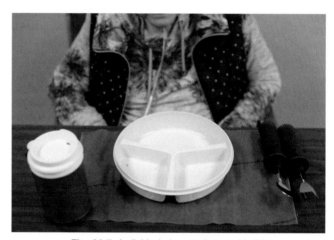

Fig. 20.7 A divided plate and cup with lid.

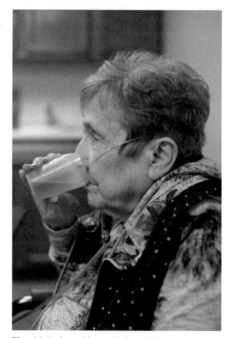

Fig. 20.8 A resident drinks with a nosey cup.

Age

With aging, changes occur in the GI system:

- Taste and smell dull. Good oral hygiene and denture care improve taste.
- Appetite decreases.
- Secretion of digestive juices decreases. Therefore, fried and fatty foods are hard to digest. They may cause indigestion. Dry, fried, and fatty foods are avoided. This helps digestion and swallowing problems (p. 310).

❖ OBRA DIETARY REQUIREMENTS

The Omnibus Budget Reconciliation Act of 1987 (OBRA) and the CMS have requirements for food served in nursing centers.

- *Each person*'s nutritional and dietary needs are met.
- The person's diet is well balanced. It is nourishing and tastes good. Food is well seasoned. It is not too salty or too sweet.
- Food is appetizing. It has an appealing aroma and is attractive.
- The foods served vary in color and texture.
- Food is served at the correct temperature. Hot food is served hot. Cold food is served cold. Food servers keep food at the correct temperature.
- Food is served promptly. Otherwise, hot food cools and cold food warms.
- Food is prepared to meet each person's needs. Some people need food cut, ground, or chopped. Others have special diets ordered by the doctor.
- Other foods are offered to residents who refuse the food served. Substituted food must have a similar nutritional value to the first foods served.
- Each person receives at least three meals a day.
- A bedtime snack is offered.
- The center provides assist devices and utensils (see Fig. 20.6).

SPECIAL DIETS

Health care providers may order special diets for a nutritional deficiency or a disease (Table 20.5). They also order them for weight control (gain or loss) or to eliminate or decrease certain substances in the diet. The doctor, nurses, and dietitian work together to meet the person's nutritional needs. They consider the need for dietary changes, personal choices, religion, culture, and eating problems. They also consider food allergies and sensitivities. The nurse and dietitian teach the person and family about the diet.

Regular diet, general diet, and *house diet* mean no dietary limits or restrictions. Persons with diseases of the heart, kidneys, gallbladder, liver, stomach, or intestines often need special diets. Persons with wounds, pressure injuries, or burns need high-protein diets for healing. Some persons may have bran added to their food. It provides fiber for bowel elimination. Allergies, excess weight, and other disorders also require special diets.

The sodium-controlled diet is often ordered. So is a diabetes meal plan. Persons with difficulty swallowing may need a dysphagia diet.

The Sodium-Controlled Diet

The average amount of sodium in the daily diet is 3000 to 5000 milligrams (mg). The body needs no more than 2400 mg a day. Healthy people excrete excess sodium in the urine.

Heart, liver, and kidney diseases and certain medications cause the body to retain extra sodium. A sodium-controlled diet is often needed. Sodium causes the body to retain water. If there is too much sodium, the body retains more water. Tissues swell with water (edema). There is excess fluid in the blood vessels. The heart has to work harder. That is, the workload of the heart increases. With heart disease, the extra workload can cause serious problems or death.

Sodium control decreases the amount of sodium in the body. The body retains less water. Less water in the tissues and blood vessels reduces the heart's workload.

The doctor orders the amount of sodium allowed. Sodium-controlled diets involve:

- Omitting high-sodium foods (Box 20.3).
- Not adding salt to food at the table.
- Limiting the amount of salt used in cooking.
- Diet planning.

Diabetes Meal Plan

Diabetes is a chronic illness in which the body cannot produce or use insulin properly (Chapter 37). The pancreas produces and secretes insulin. Insulin lets the body use sugar. Without enough insulin, sugar builds up in the bloodstream. It is not used by cells for energy. Diabetes is usually treated with insulin or other medications, diet, and exercise.

The dietitian and person develop a meal plan for healthy eating. Consistency is key. It involves:

- The person's food preferences (likes, eating habits, mealtimes, culture, and lifestyle). It may involve limiting the amount of food or changing how it is prepared.
- Calories needed. The same amounts of carbohydrates, protein, and fat are eaten each day.
- Eating meals and snacks at regular times. The person eats at the same time every day.

Serve meals and snacks on time. The person eats at regular times to maintain a certain blood sugar level.

Always check what was eaten. Report what the person did and did not eat. If all food was not eaten, a between-meal snack is needed (p. 323). The nurse tells you what to give the person. It makes up for what was not eaten at the meal. The amount of insulin given also depends on daily food intake. Report changes in the person's eating habits.

The Dysphagia Diet

Dysphagia means difficulty (*dys-*) swallowing (*-phagia*). Food thickness is changed to meet the person's needs. The doctor, speech-language pathologist, occupational therapist, dietitian,

TABLE 20.5 Special Diets

Diet	Use	Foods Allowed
Clear liquid—foods liquid at body temperature and that leave small amounts of residue; nonirritating and non–gas forming	Postoperatively, acute illness, infection, nausea and vomiting, and to prepare for gastrointestinal (GI) exams	Water, tea, and coffee (without milk or cream); carbonated drinks; gelatin; clear fruit juices (apple, grape, cranberry); fat-free clear broth; hard candy, sugar, and Popsicles
Full-liquid—foods liquid at room temperature or melt at body temperature	Advance from clear-liquid diet postoperatively; for stomach irritation, fever, nausea, and vomiting; for persons unable to chew, swallow, or digest solid foods	Foods on the clear-liquid diet; custard; eggnog; strained soups; strained fruit and vegetable juices; milk and milk shakes; strained, cooked cereals; plain ice cream and sherbet; pudding; yogurt
Mechanical soft—semisolid foods that are easily digested	Advance from full-liquid diet, chewing or swallowing problems, GI disorders, and infections	All liquids; eggs (not fried); broiled, baked, or roasted meat, fish, or poultry that is chopped or shredded; mild cheeses (American, Swiss, cheddar, cream, cottage); strained fruit juices; refined bread (no crust) and crackers; cooked cereal; cooked or pureed vegetables; cooked or canned fruit without skin or seeds; pudding; plain cakes and soft cookies without fruit or nuts
Fiber and residue restricted—food that leaves a small amount of residue in the colon	Diseases of the colon and diarrhea	Coffee, tea, milk, carbonated drinks, strained fruit juices; refined bread and crackers; creamed and refined cereal; rice; cottage and cream cheese; eggs (not fried); plain puddings and cakes; gelatin; custard; sherbet and ice cream; strained vegetable juices; canned or cooked fruit without skin or seeds; potatoes (not fried); strained cooked vegetables; plain pasta; *no raw fruits or vegetables*
High fiber—foods that increase the amount of residue and fiber in the colon to stimulate peristalsis	Constipation and GI disorders	All fruits and vegetables; whole-wheat bread; whole-grain cereals; fried foods; whole-grain rice; milk, cream, butter, and cheese; meats
Gluten free—foods that do not contain the protein gluten No wheat, barley, rye, or triticale	Celiac disease and gluten sensitivity conditions	Meat, milk, eggs, cheese, fish, fruits, vegetables, rice
Bland—foods that are mechanically and chemically nonirritating and low in roughage; foods served at moderate temperatures; no strong spices or condiments	Ulcers, gallbladder disorders, and some intestinal disorders; after abdominal surgery	Lean meats; white bread; creamed and refined cereals; cream or cottage cheese; gelatin; plain puddings, cakes, and cookies; eggs (not fried); butter and cream; canned fruits and vegetables without skin and seeds; strained fruit juices; potatoes (not fried); pastas and rice; strained or soft-cooked carrots, peas, beets, spinach, squash, and asparagus tips; creamed soups from allowed vegetables; no fried foods
High calorie—calorie intake is increased to about 3000–4000 daily; includes three full meals and between-meal snacks	Weight gain and some thyroid imbalances	Dietary increases in all foods; large portions of regular diet with three between-meal snacks
Calorie controlled—provides adequate nutrients while controlling calories to promote weight loss and reduce body fat	Weight reduction	Foods low in fats and carbohydrates and lean meats; avoid butter, cream, rice, gravies, salad oils, noodles, cakes, pastries, carbonated and alcoholic drinks, candy, potato chips, and similar foods
High iron—foods that are high in iron	Anemia, following blood loss, for women during the reproductive years	Liver and other organ meats, lean meats, egg yolks, shellfish, dried fruits, dried beans, green leafy vegetables, lima beans, peanut butter, enriched breads and cereals
Fat controlled (low cholesterol)—foods low in fat and prepared without adding fat	Heart disease, gallbladder disease, disorders of fat digestion, liver disease, diseases of the pancreas	Skim milk (fat-free) or buttermilk; cottage cheese (no other cheeses allowed); gelatin; sherbet; fruit; lean meat, poultry, and fish (baked, broiled, or roasted); fat-free broth; soups made with skim milk (fat-free); margarine; rice, pasta, breads, and cereals; vegetables; potatoes
High protein—aids and promotes tissue healing	For burns, high fever, infection, and some liver diseases	Meat, milk, eggs, cheese, fish, poultry; breads and cereals; green leafy vegetables
Sodium controlled—a certain amount of sodium is allowed	Heart disease, fluid retention, liver disease, and some kidney diseases	Fruits and vegetables and unsalted butter are allowed; adding salt at the table is not allowed; highly salted foods and foods high in sodium are not allowed; the use of salt during cooking may be restricted
Diabetes meal plan—the same amounts of carbohydrates, protein, and fat are eaten at the same time each day	Diabetes	Determined by nutritional and energy requirements

BOX 20.3 High-Sodium Foods

Grains Group
- Baked goods (biscuits, muffins, cakes, cookies, pies, pastries, sweet rolls, donuts)
- Breads and rolls
- Cereals (cold, instant hot)
- Noodle mixes
- Pancakes
- Salted snack foods (pretzels, corn chips, popcorn, crackers, chips)
- Stuffing mixes
- Waffles

Vegetables Group
- Canned vegetables
- Olives
- Pickles and other pickled vegetables
- Relish
- Sauerkraut
- Tomato sauce or paste
- Vegetable juices (tomato, V-8, bloody Mary mixes)
- Vegetables with sauces, creams, or seasonings

Fruits Group
- None—fruits are not high in sodium

Dairy Group
- Buttermilk
- Cheese
- Commercial dips made with sour cream

Protein Group
- Bacon
- Canadian bacon
- Canned meats and fish (chicken, tuna, salmon, anchovies, sardines)
- Caviar
- Chipped and corned beef
- Dried beef and other meats

- Dried fish
- Ham
- Herring
- Hot dogs (frankfurters)
- Liverwurst
- Lox
- Luncheon meats (turkey, ham, bologna, salami)
- Mackerel
- Pastrami
- Pepperoni
- Salt pork
- Sausages
- Scrapple
- Shellfish (shrimp, crab, clams, oysters, scallops, lobster)
- Smoked salmon

Other
- Asian foods (Chinese, Japanese, East Indian, Thai, Vietnamese)
- Baking soda and baking powder
- Catsup (ketchup)
- Cocoa mixes
- Commercially prepared dinners (frozen, canned, boxed)
- Mayonnaise
- Mexican foods
- Mustard
- Pasta dishes (lasagna, manicotti, ravioli)
- Peanut butter
- Pizzas
- Pot pies
- Salad dressings
- Salted nuts or seeds
- Sauces (soy, teriyaki, Worcestershire, steak, barbecue, pasta, chili, cocktail)
- Seasoning salts (garlic, onion, celery, meat tenderizers, monosodium glutamate [MSG])
- Soups (canned, packaged, instant, dried, bouillon)

and nurse collaborate to choose the right food texture and beverage thickness.

It is very important to be aware if the person is having difficulty swallowing. When food or liquid is not swallowed completely to enter into the esophagus, coughing or choking may occur. Coughing is the body's attempt to prevent matter from entering the airway. Choking is defined as severe obstruction of the airway. A person cannot "choke" when taking a drink of water. The person might cough while drinking water and the possibility of aspiration could occur. Aspiration is breathing fluid, food, vomitus, or an object into the lungs (Chapter 21). This can be serious and even life threatening (Chapter 11). Emergency care for choking is discussed in Chapter 44. A speech-language therapist evaluates the person for possible swallowing problems. A diet is then ordered to meet the person's needs. The food texture may be modified, and the thickness of the liquids will be adjusted (Fig. 20.9).

For many years, caregivers followed recommendations from the National Dysphagia Diet (NDD). This information was helpful, but the terminology was not always clear. An international group of volunteers was formed to help clarify the diet for those experiencing dysphagia. The International Dysphagia Diet Standardisation Initiative (IDDSI) committee was formed in 2013. According to IDDSI, "the goal is to develop international standardized terminology and descriptors for dysphagia diets. These would meet the needs of individuals with dysphagia across the age span, across all care settings, and across all cultures." The complete IDDSI Framework appears in Fig. 20.10. Colors and numbers are used to define the various levels. Notice how the colors and numbers are also labeled on the products in Fig. 20.9. The manufacturers of thickened products now use the labels, colors, and numbers from IDDSI to make it easier and more accurate to provide the prescribed consistency. Fig. 20.11 compares the NDD terminology with the new IDDSI framework. It is important to mix the thickener

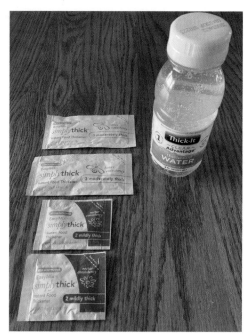

Fig. 20.9 Packages of thickener and bottle of prethickened water. Note the numbers and colors denoting consistency.

with the correct volume of liquid to get the prescribed consistency. Some states have recommended guidelines to follow. Always follow the person's diet order and the policies at your center.

You may need to feed a person with dysphagia. To promote safety and comfort, you must:

- Know the signs and symptoms of dysphagia (Box 20.4).
- Feed the person according to the care plan.
- Follow aspiration precautions (Box 20.5).
- Report changes in how the person eats.
- Observe for signs and symptoms of aspiration: choking, coughing, difficulty breathing during or after meals, and abnormal breathing or respiratory sounds; report these observations at once.

Fluid Balance

Water is needed to live. Death can result from too much or too little water. Water is ingested through fluids and foods. Water is lost through urine, feces, and vomit. It is also lost through the skin (perspiration) and the lungs (expiration).

Fluid balance is needed for health. The amount of fluid taken in (intake) and the amount of fluid lost (output) must be equal. If fluid intake exceeds fluid output, body tissues swell

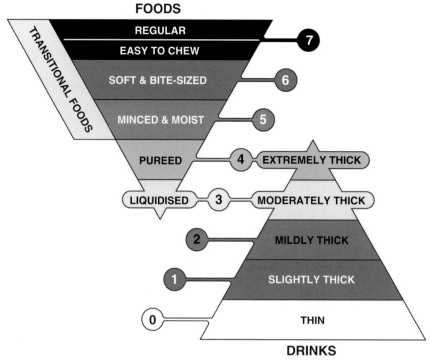

Fig. 20.10 International Dysphagia Diet Standardization Initiative (IDDSI) Framework. (From International Dysphagia Diet Standardization Initiative, https://iddsi.org/framework/.)

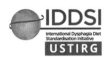

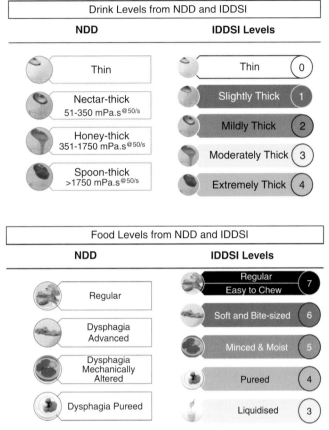

Fig. 20.11 Dysphagia diet comparing National Dysphagia Diet (NDD) to International Dysphagia Diet Standardisation Initiative (IDDSI). (From Common Ground between NDD and IDDSI, International Dysphagia Diet Standardization Initiative, 2021.)

with water. This is called edema. Edema is common in people with heart and kidney diseases. Dehydration is a decrease in the amount of water in body tissues. Fluid output exceeds intake. Common causes of dehydration are listed in Box 20.6.

BOX 20.4 Signs and Symptoms of Dysphagia

- The person avoids food that needs chewing.
- The person avoids food with certain textures and temperatures.
- The person tires during a meal or is short of breath.
- Food spills out of the person's mouth while eating.
- Food "pockets" or is "squirreled" in the person's cheeks. This means that food remains or is hidden in the mouth.
- The person eats slowly, especially solid foods.
- The person complains that food will not go down or that the food is stuck.
- The person frequently coughs or chokes before, during, or after swallowing.
- The person regurgitates food after eating.
- The person spits out food suddenly and almost violently.
- Food comes up through the person's nose.
- The person is hoarse—especially after eating.
- After swallowing, the person makes gargling sounds while talking or breathing.
- The person has a runny nose, sneezes, or has excessive drooling of saliva.
- The person complains of frequent heartburn or chest pressure.
- Appetite is decreased.
- There is a spike in temperature after meals.

BOX 20.5 Aspiration Precautions

- Help the person with meals and snacks. Follow the care plan.
- Position the person in Fowler position or upright in a chair for meals and snacks.
- Support the upper back, shoulders, and neck with a pillow. Follow the care plan.
- Observe for signs and symptoms of aspiration during meals and snacks.
- Check the person's mouth after eating for pocketing. Check inside the cheeks, under the tongue, and on the roof of the mouth. Remove any food.
- Position the person in a chair or in semi-Fowler position after eating. The person maintains this position for at least 1 hour after eating. Follow the care plan.
- Provide mouth care after eating.
- Report and record your observations.

BOX 20.6   Common Causes of Dehydration

- Bleeding
- Coma
- Dementia
- Diarrhea
- Fever
- Fluid intake: poor
- Fluid restriction
- Fluids: refusing
- Functional impairments: difficulty drinking, reaching fluids, communicating fluid needs
- Medication therapy
- Sweating: excess
- Urine production: increased
- Vomiting
- Excessive wound drainage

Normal Fluid Requirements

An adult needs 1500 milliliters (mL) of water daily to survive. About 2000 to 2500 mL are needed for normal fluid balance. The water requirement increases with hot weather, exercise, fever, illness, and excess fluid losses.

The amount of body water decreases with age. Older persons also are at risk for diseases that affect fluid balance. Examples include heart disease, kidney disease, cancer, and diabetes. Some medications cause the body to lose fluids. Others cause the body to retain water. The older person is at risk for dehydration and edema.

Older persons may have a decreased sense of thirst. Their bodies need water, but they may not feel thirsty. Offer water and other fluids often. Some persons have special fluid orders.

Special Fluid Orders

The doctor may order the amount of fluid a person can have during a 24-hour period. This is done to maintain fluid balance. Found in the care plan and in the Kardex, common orders are:

- *Encourage fluids.* The person drinks an increased amount of fluid. The order states the amount to ingest. Intake records are kept. The person is given a variety of fluids allowed on the diet. They are kept within the person's reach. They are served at the correct temperature. Fluids are offered regularly to persons who cannot feed themselves.
- *Restrict fluids.* Fluids are limited to a certain amount. They are offered in small amounts and in small containers. The water pitcher is removed from the room or kept out of sight. Intake records are kept. The person needs frequent oral hygiene. It helps keep mucous membranes of the mouth moist.

- *Nothing by mouth.* The person cannot eat or drink anything. *NPO* is the abbreviation for *non per os.* It means nothing *(non)* by *(per)* mouth *(os).* NPO often is ordered before and after surgery, before some laboratory tests and diagnostic procedures, and in treating certain illnesses. An NPO sign is posted above the bed. The water pitcher and glass are removed. Frequent oral hygiene is needed but the person must not swallow any fluid. The person is NPO for 6 to 8 hours before surgery and before some laboratory tests and diagnostic procedures.
- *Ice chips only. The person is usually NPO with the exception of ice chips to moisten the mouth.*
- *Thickened liquids.* All fluids are thickened, including water. The thickness depends on the person's ability to swallow. Thickener is added before fluids are served, or prethickened commercial fluids are used (see Fig. 20.9). When thickened liquids are consumed, a greater quantity of fluid may need to be taken in to prevent dehydration. Always refer to the care plan.

Intake and Output Records

The doctor or nurse may order intake and output (I&O) measurements. I&O records are kept. They are used to evaluate fluid balance and kidney function. They help in planning medical treatment. They also are kept when the person has special fluid orders.

All fluids taken by mouth are measured and recorded—water, milk, coffee, tea, juices, soups, and soft drinks. So are foods that melt at room temperature—ice cream, sherbet, custard, pudding, gelatin, and Popsicles. The nurse measures and records intravenous (IV) fluids and tube feedings (Chapter 21). Output includes urine, vomitus, diarrhea, and wound drainage.

Measuring Intake and Output

Intake and output are measured in milliliters (mL). You need to know these amounts:

- 1 ounce (oz) equals 30 mL
- 1 pint is about 500 mL
- 1 quart is about 1000 mL

You also need to know the serving sizes of bowls, dishes, cups, pitchers, glasses, and other containers. This information may be on the I&O record (Fig. 20.12). Ice chip intake is usually recorded at half the volume. For example, if the person was given an 8-oz cup of ice chips and consumed all, 4 oz or 120 mL would be recorded on the I&O record.

A measuring container for fluid is called a graduate. It is used to measure leftover fluids, urine, vomitus, and drainage from suction. Like a measuring cup, the graduate is marked in ounces and milliliters (Fig. 20.13). Plastic urinals and kidney

FLUID BALANCE CHART

OSF ST. JOSEPH MEDICAL CENTER
Bloomington, Illinois

DATE __6/15__

Water Glass	250mL		Ice Cream	120mL
Styrofoam Cup	180mL		Ice Chips	1/2 amt. of
Cup (coffee)	250mL			mL's in cup
Milk Carton	240mL		Pitcher	
Pop (1 can)	360mL		(Yellow)	1000mL
Broth-Soup	175mL			
Juice Carton	120mL			
Juice Glass	120mL			
Jello	120mL			

	INTAKE				OUTPUT					
					URINE		OTHER		CONT. IRRIGATION	
TIME	ORAL	Parenteral		Amt. mL Absbd.	Method Collected	Amt. (mL)	Method Collected	Amt. (mL)	In	Out
2400-0100		mL from previous shift			V	150				
0100-0200							Vom.	150		
0200-0300										
0300-0400										
0400-0500										
0500-0600	125				V	200				
0600-0700										
0700-0800										
	125	8 - hour Sub-total			8-hr T	350	8-hr T	150		
0800-0900	400	mL from previous shift			V	250				
0900-1000	100									
1000-1100										
1100-1200										
1200-1300	400				V	250				
1300-1400										
1400-1500	200									
1500-1600										
	1100	8 - hour Sub-total			8-hr T	500	8-hr T			
1600-1700		mL from previous shift			V	270				
1700-1800	350									
1800-1900	50									
1900-2000	200									
2000-2100					V	400				
2100-2200										
2200-2300										
2300-2400										
	600	8 - hour Sub-total			8-hr T	670	8-hr T			
	1825	24 - hour Sub-total			24-hr T	1520	24-hr T	150		

Source Key:
URINE
V - Voided
C - Catheter
INC - Incontinent
U.C. - Ureteral Catheter

Source Key:
OTHER
G.I.T. - Gastric Intestinal Tube
T.T. - T. Tube
Vom. - Vomitus
Liq S. - Liquid Stool
H.V. - Hemovac

310' *Marie Mills*

Form No. MF36722 (Rev. 5/97) **MFI**

Fig. 20.12 An intake and output record. (Modified from OSF St. Joseph Medical Center, Bloomington, IL.)

basins also have amounts marked. The measuring device is held at eye level to read the amount.

An I&O record is kept at the bedside (or other designated spot) or is recorded electronically. When intake or output is measured, the amount is recorded in the correct column (see Fig. 20.12). Amounts are totaled at the end of the shift. The totals are recorded in the person's chart. They also are shared during the end-of-shift report.

The purpose of measuring I&O and how to help are explained to the person. Some persons measure and record their intake. Family members may help. The urinal, commode, bedpan, or specimen pan is used for voiding. Remind the person not to void in the toilet. Also remind the person not to put toilet tissue into the receptacle.

See *Delegation Guidelines: Intake and Output*.
See *Promoting Safety and Comfort: Intake and Output*.

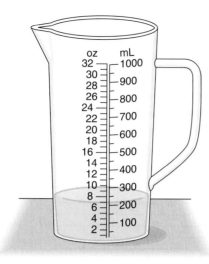

Fig. 20.13 A graduate marked in ounces (oz) and milliliters (mL).

 DELEGATION GUIDELINES

Intake and Output
When measuring I&O, you need this information from the nurse and the care plan:

- If the person has a special fluid order—encourage fluids, restrict fluids, NPO, or thickened fluids
- When to report measurements—hourly or end of shift
- What the person uses for voiding—urinal, bedpan, commode, or specimen pan (Chapter 22)
- If the person has a catheter
- What specific resident concerns to report at once

PROMOTING SAFETY AND COMFORT

Intake and Output
Safety
Urine may contain microbes or blood. Microbes can grow in urinals, commodes, bedpans, specimen pans, and drainage systems. Follow Standard Precautions and the Bloodborne Pathogen Standard when handling such equipment. Thoroughly clean the item after it is used. Use a disinfectant for cleaning.

Comfort
Promptly measure the contents of urinals, bedpans, commodes, and specimen pans. This helps prevent or reduce odors, which can be disturbing to residents.

MEETING FOOD AND FLUID NEEDS

Weakness, illness, and confusion can affect appetite and ability to eat. So can unpleasant odors, sights, and sounds. An uncomfortable position, the need for oral hygiene, the need to eliminate, and pain also affect appetite.

See *Focus on Communication: Meeting Food and Fluid Needs.*

FOCUS ON COMMUNICATION

Meeting Food and Fluid Needs
The person may not eat or drink all the food and fluids served. You need to find out why and tell the nurse. Politely ask the person to explain the reason.

- "I see you didn't eat anything today. How are you feeling?"
- "How can we make the food better next time?"
- "Did your food taste okay?"
- "Was there something you didn't like?"
- "Was your food too hot or too cold?"
- "Would you like something else? What small snack can I get you?"
- "Could you try to eat a small amount?"

❊ MEASURING INTAKE AND OUTPUT (NATCEP)

Quality of Life
Remember to:

- Knock before entering the person's room.
- Address the person by name.
- Introduce yourself by name and title.
- Explain the procedure to the person before beginning and during the procedure.
- Protect the person's rights during the procedure.
- Handle the person gently during the procedure.

Preprocedure
1. Follow *Delegation Guidelines: Intake and Output.* See *Promoting Safety and Comfort: Intake and Output.*
2. Practice hand hygiene.
3. Collect the following:
   - I&O record
   - Graduates
   - Gloves

Procedure
4. Put on gloves.
5. Measure intake as follows:
   a. Pour liquid remaining in the container into the graduate.
   b. Measure the amount at eye level or on a flat surface. Keep the container level.

c. Check the serving amount on the I&O record.
d. Subtract the remaining amount from the full serving amount. Note the amount.
e. Pour fluid in the graduate back into the container.
f. Repeat steps 5a–e for each liquid.
g. Add the amounts from each liquid together.
h. Record the time and amount on the I&O record.
▶ 6. Measure output as follows:
   a. Pour the fluid into the graduate used to measure output.
   b. Measure the amount at eye level or on a flat surface. Keep the container level.
   c. Dispose of fluid in the toilet. Avoid splashes.
7. Clean and rinse the graduates. Dispose of rinse into the toilet. Return the graduates to their proper place.
8. Clean and rinse the voiding receptacle or drainage container. Dispose of rinse in the toilet. Return the item to its proper place.
9. Remove the gloves. Practice hand hygiene.
10. Record the output amount on the I&O record.

Postprocedure
11. Provide for comfort. (See the inside of the front cover.)
12. Make sure the call light is within reach.
13. Complete a safety check of the room. (See the inside of the front cover.)
14. Report and record your observations.

This skill is also covered in *Clinical Skills: Nurse Assisting.*

Dining Programs

Most people enjoy going to a restaurant for a delicious meal. The combination of enjoyable conversation and good food is something that many people treasure. The staff in long-term care centers should try very hard to make dining the most pleasurable experience possible. Loud noises should be avoided. Residents should be attended in a courteous and friendly manner. Many residents are alert and oriented. They enjoy being together for meals. Others like eating in their rooms. Others are confused and noisy at mealtime. Some persons are incontinent or have odor problems. Some are too weak or ill to leave their rooms for meals.

The following dining programs are common in nursing centers:

- *Social dining.* Four to six residents are seated at a dining room table (Fig. 20.14). Food is served as in a restaurant. This program is for persons who are oriented and can feed themselves. Sometimes quietly confused persons are included. They must be able to feed themselves and not disrupt others.
- *Family dining.* This is like social dining. However, food is served in bowls and on platters. Residents serve themselves as at home.
- *Low-stimulation dining.* Mealtime distractions are prevented. The health team decides on the best place for each person to sit.
- *Restaurant-style menus.* The person selects food from a menu. This program allows more food choices. The person is served as in a restaurant.
- *Open dining.* A buffet is open for several hours. A breakfast buffet is an example. Residents can eat any time while the buffet is open.

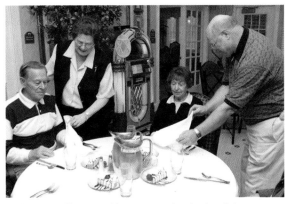

Fig. 20.14 These residents are eating in the dining room.

Some centers have areas where residents can dine privately with guests. The person can have a meal with a partner, children, and other family or friends. They can celebrate holidays, birthdays, anniversaries, or other events. Food is provided by guests or the dietary department. To avoid conflicts, arrangements are often made in advance to reserve a private dining area.

Preparing for Meals

Preparing residents for meals promotes their comfort. To promote comfort:

- Assist with elimination needs.
- Provide oral hygiene. Make sure dentures are in place.
- Make sure eyeglasses and hearing aids are in place.
- Make sure incontinent persons are clean and dry.
- Position the person in a comfortable position.
- Assist the person with hand washing.
  See *Delegation Guidelines: Preparing for Meals.*
  See *Promoting Safety and Comfort: Preparing for Meals.*

DELEGATION GUIDELINES

Preparing for Meals

To prepare a person for a meal, you need this information from the nurse and the care plan:

- How much help the person needs
- Where the person will eat—the person's room or the dining room
- What the person uses for elimination—bathroom, commode, bedpan, urinal, or specimen pan
- What type of oral hygiene the person needs
- If the person wears dentures
- If the person wears eyeglasses or hearing aids
- How to position the person—in bed, a chair, or a wheelchair
- How the person gets to the dining room—by self or with help
- If the person uses a wheelchair, walker, or cane
- When to report observations
- What specific resident concerns to report at once

PROMOTING SAFETY AND COMFORT

Preparing for Meals

Safety

Before meals, the person needs to eliminate and have oral hygiene. Follow Standard Precautions and the Bloodborne Pathogen Standard. Also follow them when cleaning equipment and the room.

Comfort

The meal setting must be free of unpleasant sights, sounds, and odors. Remove unpleasant equipment from the room.

PREPARING THE PERSON FOR A MEAL

Quality of Life

Remember to:

- Knock before entering the person's room.
- Address the person by name.
- Introduce yourself by name and title.
- Explain the procedure to the person before beginning and during the procedure.
- Protect the person's rights during the procedure.
- Handle the person gently during the procedure.

Preprocedure

1. Follow *Delegation Guidelines: Preparing for Meals.* See *Promoting Safety and Comfort: Preparing for Meals.*
2. Practice hand hygiene.
3. Collect the following:
   - Equipment for oral hygiene
   - Bedpan and cover, urinal, commode, or specimen pan
   - Toilet tissue
   - Wash basin
   - Soap
   - Washcloth
   - Towel
   - Gloves
4. Provide for privacy.

Procedure

5. Make sure eyeglasses and hearing aids are in place.
6. Assist with oral hygiene. Make sure dentures are in place. Wear gloves and decontaminate your hands after removing them.

7. Assist with elimination. Make sure the incontinent person is clean and dry. Wear gloves and practice hand hygiene after removing them.
8. Assist with hand washing. Wear gloves and practice hand hygiene after removing them.
9. Do the following if the person will eat in bed:
   a. Raise the head of the bed to a comfortable position. Fowler position is preferred.
   b. Remove items from the overbed table. Clean the overbed table.
   c. Adjust the overbed table in front of the person.
10. Do the following if the person will sit in a chair:
    a. Position the person in a chair with arms or wheelchair.
    b. Remove items from the overbed table. Clean the table.
    c. Adjust the overbed table in front of the person.
11. Assist the person to the dining area. (This step is for the person who eats in a dining area.) It is best if the person can sit in a chair with arms. The feet should rest on the floor. It may be necessary to place a pillow behind the person's back for good alignment (Fig. 20.15). In some cases, the person remains in the wheelchair.

Postprocedure

12. Provide for comfort. (See the inside of the front cover.)
13. Place the call light within reach.
14. Empty, clean, and disinfect equipment. Return equipment to its proper place. Wear gloves and practice hand hygiene after removing them.
15. Straighten the room. Eliminate unpleasant noise, odors, or equipment.
16. Unscreen the person.
17. Complete a safety check of the room. (See the inside of the front cover.)
18. Decontaminate your hands.

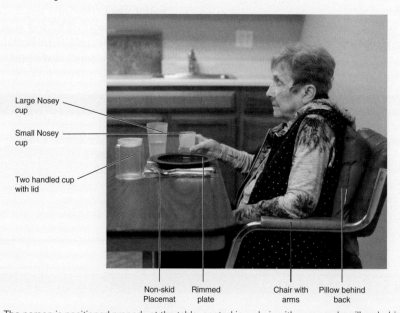

Large Nosey cup

Small Nosey cup

Two handled cup with lid

Non-skid Placemat

Rimmed plate

Chair with arms

Pillow behind back

Fig. 20.15 The person is positioned properly at the table, seated in a chair with arms and a pillow behind the back.

Serving Meals

❖ Food is served in containers that keep foods at the correct temperature. Hot food is kept hot. Cold food is kept cold. OBRA requires that food be at the correct temperature when ◆ the person receives it.

You serve meals after preparing residents for meals. You can serve meals promptly if residents are ready to eat. Prompt serving keeps food at the correct temperature.

📄 DELEGATION GUIDELINES

Serving Meals

Before serving meal trays, you need this information from the nurse and the care plan:
- What assist devices the person uses
- If the person needs help opening cartons, cutting food, buttering bread, and so on
- If the person's intake is measured (p. 316)
- If calorie counts are done (p. 323)
- When to report observations
- What specific resident concerns to report at once

👤 PROMOTING SAFETY AND COMFORT

Serving Meals
Safety
Always check food temperature after reheating. Food that is too hot can cause burns.

Comfort
The preferred position is to have the person sitting in a chair with arms. The feet should rest on the floor. There are occasions when this is not possible. The person may be brought to the table in a wheelchair. Still other situations may require the person to remain in bed. Check the person's position when serving a meal. The position may have changed after the person was prepared to eat. Provide other comfort measures as needed. See the inside of the front cover for comfort measures.

🧩 TEAMWORK AND TIME MANAGEMENT

Serving Meals

Meal trays are served in the order set by the health team. You will serve trays to your residents and to those assigned to other nursing assistants. Your coworkers will do the same. The goal is to serve trays as fast as possible. This keeps food at the desired temperature. Every attempt is made to serve all the individuals sitting at the same table at the same time.

Serve meals in the assigned order. Residents seated at tables are served at the same time.

If food is not served within 15 minutes, recheck food temperatures. Follow center policy. If not at the correct temperature, get fresh food. Temperature guides and food thermometers are in dining rooms and in nursing unit kitchens. Some centers allow reheating in microwave ovens.

See *Delegation Guidelines: Serving Meals.*
See *Promoting Safety and Comfort: Serving Meals.*
See *Teamwork and Time Management: Serving Meals.*

✳ SERVING MEAL TRAYS

Quality of Life
Remember to:
- Knock before entering the person's room.
- Address the person by name.
- Introduce yourself by name and title.
- Explain the procedure to the person before beginning and during the procedure.
- Protect the person's rights during the procedure.
- Handle the person gently during the procedure.

Preprocedure
1. Follow *Delegation Guidelines: Serving Meals.* See *Promoting Safety and Comfort: Serving Meals.*
2. Practice hand hygiene.

Procedure
3. Make sure the tray is complete. Check items on the tray with the dietary card. Be aware of any allergies. Make sure assist devices are included.
4. Identify the person. Check the ID (identification) bracelet against the dietary card. Also call the person by name.
5. Place the tray within the person's reach. Adjust the overbed table as needed.
6. Remove food covers. Open cartons, cut food into bite-sized pieces, butter bread, and so on as needed (Fig. 20.16). Season food as the person prefers and is allowed on the care plan.
7. Place the napkin, clothes protector, assist devices, and eating utensils within reach.
8. Place the call light within reach.
9. Do the following when the person is done eating:
   a. Measure and record intake if ordered (p. 316).
   b. Note the amount and type of foods eaten. (See "Calorie Counts" on p. 323.)
   c. Check for and remove any food in the person's mouth (pocketing). Wear gloves. Decontaminate your hands after removing them.

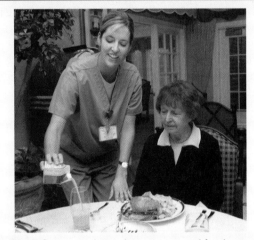
Fig. 20.16 Cartons and containers are opened for the person.

d. Remove the tray.
e. Clean up spills. Change soiled linen and clothing.
f. Help the person return to bed if needed.
g. Assist with oral hygiene and hand washing. Wear gloves. Decontaminate your hands after removing the gloves.

Postprocedure
10. Provide for comfort. (See the inside of the front cover.)
11. Place the call light within reach.
12. Raise or lower bed rails. Follow the care plan.
13. Complete a safety check of the room. (See the inside of the front cover.)
14. Follow center policy for soiled linen.
15. Decontaminate your hands.
16. Report and record your observations.

This skill is also covered in *Clinical Skills: Nurse Assisting.*

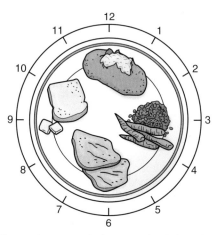

Fig. 20.17 The numbers on a clock are used to help a visually impaired person locate food.

✳ Feeding the Person

Weakness, paralysis, casts, confusion, and other limits may make self-feeding impossible. These persons are fed.

Serve food and fluids in the order the person prefers. Offer fluids during the meal. Fluids help the person chew and swallow.

Use teaspoons to feed the person. They are less likely to cause injury than forks. The teaspoon should only be one-third full. This portion is chewed and swallowed easily. Some people need smaller portions. Follow the care plan.

Persons who need to be fed are often angry, humiliated, and embarrassed. Some are depressed or resentful or refuse to eat. Let them do as much as possible. Some can manage "finger foods" (bread, cookies, crackers). If strong enough, let them hold milk or juice cups (never hot drinks). Do not exceed activity limits ordered by the doctor. Provide support. Encourage them to try, even if food is spilled.

Visually impaired persons are often very aware of food aromas. They may know the food served. Always tell the person what is on the tray. When feeding visually impaired persons, describe what you are offering. For persons who feed themselves, describe foods and fluids and their place on the tray. Use the numbers on a clock for the location of foods (Fig. 20.17).

Many people pray before eating. Allow time and privacy for prayer (Chapter 7). This shows respect and caring.

Meals provide social contact with others. Engage the person in pleasant conversation. However, allow time for chewing and swallowing. Do not ask a question while the person has food in the mouth. Also, sit facing the person. Sitting is more relaxing. It shows that you have time for the person. By facing the person, you can see how well the person is eating. You can also see if the person has problems swallowing.

See *Residents with Dementia: Feeding the Person.*
See *Delegation Guidelines: Feeding the Person.*
See *Promoting Safety and Comfort: Feeding the Person.*

🐭 RESIDENTS WITH DEMENTIA

Feeding the Person

Residents with dementia may become distracted during meals. Some persons cannot sit long enough for a meal. Others forget how to use eating utensils. Some persons resist your efforts to assist them with eating. A confused person may throw or spit food.

The Alzheimer's Disease Education and Referral Center (ADEAR) recommends the following. The measures may be part of the person's care plan.

- Provide a calm, quiet setting for eating. Limit noise and other distractions. This helps the person focus on the meal.
- Limit the number of food choices.
- Offer several small meals throughout the day instead of larger ones.
- Use straws or cups with lids. These make drinking easier.
- Provide finger foods if the person has problems with utensils. A bowl may be easier to use than a plate.
- Provide healthy snacks. Keep snacks where the person can see them.

You must be patient. Talk to the nurse if you feel upset or impatient. Remember, the person has the right to be treated with dignity and respect.

📄 DELEGATION GUIDELINES

Feeding the Person

Before feeding a person, you need this information from the nurse and the care plan:

- Why the person needs help
- How much help the person needs
- If the person needs any assist devices
- If the person can manage finger foods
- What the person's activity limits are
- What the person's dietary restrictions are
- What size portion to feed the person—$\frac{1}{3}$ teaspoonful or less
- What safety measures are needed if the person has dysphagia
- If the person can use a straw
- What observations to report and record:
  - The amount and kind of food eaten
  - Complaints of nausea or dysphagia
  - Signs and symptoms of dysphagia
  - Signs and symptoms of aspiration
- When to report observations
- What specific resident concerns to report at once

📋 FOCUS ON COMMUNICATION

Feeding the Person

The person must be treated with dignity at all times. Do not make statements aloud that refer to the person's dietary restrictions. For example, in the dining room, don't say, "Mrs. Miller needs to have pureed vegetables and she needs to wear a bib. She can't have pudding because she is diabetic." Statements like this are degrading. They can cause hurt feelings. Visit with the person you are assisting, but do not ask a question after putting food in the person's mouth. Do not make negative comments about the appearance of food. Focus on the resident and refrain from conversations with coworkers.

PROMOTING SAFETY AND COMFORT

Feeding the Person

Safety

Check food temperature. Very hot foods can burn the person.

Prevent aspiration. Check the person's mouth before offering more food or fluids. The person's mouth must be empty between bites and swallows.

Comfort

The person will eat better if not rushed. Sit to show the person that you have time for the meal. Standing communicates that you are in a hurry.

Wipe the person's hands, face, and mouth as needed during the meal. Use the napkin. If necessary, use a wet washcloth. Then dry the person with a towel.

Between-Meal Snacks

Many special diets involve between-meal snacks. Common snacks are crackers, milk, juice, a milkshake, cake, wafers, a sandwich, gelatin, and custard.

Snacks are served upon arrival on the nursing unit. Provide needed utensils, a straw, and a napkin. Follow the same considerations and procedures for serving meals and feeding persons.

Calorie Counts

Calorie records are kept for some people. On a flow sheet, note what the person ate and how much. For example, a chicken breast, rice, beans, a roll, pudding, and two pats of butter were served. The person ate all the chicken, half the rice, and the roll. One pat of butter was used. The beans and pudding were not eaten. Note these on the flow sheet. A nurse or dietitian

FEEDING THE PERSON (NATCEP)

Quality of Life

Remember to:
- Knock before entering the person's room.
- Address the person by name.
- Introduce yourself by name and title.
- Explain the procedure to the person before beginning and during the procedure.
- Protect the person's rights during the procedure.
- Handle the person gently during the procedure.

Preprocedure

1. Follow *Delegation Guidelines: Feeding the Person*. See *Promoting Safety and Comfort: Feeding the Person*.
2. Practice hand hygiene.
3. Position the person in a comfortable position for eating—usually sitting or Fowler.
4. Get the tray. Place it on the overbed table or dining table. Gather any assist devices.

Procedure

5. Identify the person. Check the ID bracelet against the dietary card. Also call the person by name.
6. Drape a napkin or clothes protector across the person's chest and underneath the chin. Always refer to this as a napkin or clothes protector. To protect the person's dignity do not call it a "bib."
7. Tell the person what foods and fluids are on the tray.
8. Prepare food for eating. Cut food into bite-sized pieces. Season foods as the person prefers and is allowed on the care plan.
9. Place the chair where you can sit comfortably. Sit facing the person.
10. Serve foods in the order the person prefers. Identify foods as you serve them. If the person has a dry mouth, it may be best to begin by offering a drink of water and then alternate between solid and liquid foods. Use a spoon for safety (Fig. 20.18). Allow enough time for chewing and swallowing. Do not rush the person. Also offer water, coffee, tea, or other beverages on the tray.
11. Check the person's mouth before offering more food or fluids. Make sure the person's mouth is empty between bites and swallows.
12. Use straws for liquids if the person cannot drink out of a glass or cup. Have one straw for each liquid. Some residents have an order for a "safe straw." This allows only small amounts of liquid to enter the mouth at one time. Straws are *not* used for some residents. Follow the care plan.
13. Wipe the person's hands, face, and mouth as needed during the meal. Use the napkin.

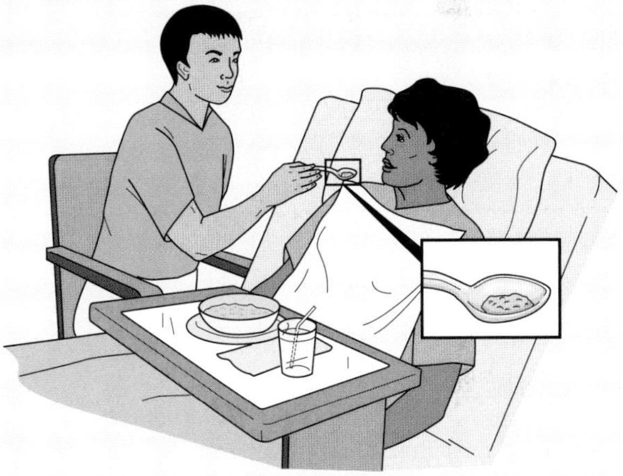

Fig. 20.18 A spoon is used to feed the person. The spoon is one-third full.

14. Follow the care plan if the person has dysphagia. Give thickened liquid with a spoon.
15. Converse with the person in a pleasant manner, however, do not ask a resident a question immediately after placing a bit of food in the mouth.
16. Encourage the person to eat as much as possible.
17. Wipe the person's mouth with a napkin. Discard the napkin.
18. Note how much and which foods were eaten. See "Calorie Counts."
19. Measure and record intake if ordered (p. 316).
20. Remove the tray.
21. Take the person back to his or her room (if in a dining area).
22. Assist with oral hygiene and hand washing. Wear gloves. Provide for privacy. Decontaminate your hands after removing the gloves.

Postprocedure

23. Provide for comfort. (See the inside of the front cover.)
24. Place the call light within reach.
25. Raise or lower bed rails. Follow the care plan.
26. Complete a safety check of the room. (See the inside of the front cover.)
27. Return the food tray to the food cart.
28. Decontaminate your hands.
29. Report and record your observations.

This skill is also covered in *Clinical Skills: Nurse Assisting.*

converts these portions into calories. The nurse tells you which persons need calorie counts.

 Providing Drinking Water

Residents need fresh drinking water each shift. They also need water whenever the pitcher is empty.

Some centers do not use the procedure that follows. Each person's pitcher may be filled as needed. Many centers have a schedule for collecting and sanitizing water pitchers on a daily basis. The resident's used pitcher should never be taken to the ice machine and filled directly from the machine. This could transmit microorganisms from the resident to the ice machine. When filling water pitchers, fill with ice first, then add water. Follow the center's procedure for providing fresh drinking water.

See *Delegation Guidelines: Providing Drinking Water.*
See *Promoting Safety and Comfort: Providing Drinking Water.*

DELEGATION GUIDELINES

Providing Drinking Water
Before providing water, you need this information from the nurse and the care plan:
- The person's fluid orders
- If the person can have ice
- If the person uses a straw

PROMOTING SAFETY AND COMFORT

Providing Drinking Water
Safety
Water cups and pitchers can spread microbes. To prevent the spread of microbes:
- Make sure the pitcher is labeled with the person's name and room and bed number.
- Do not touch the rim or inside of the cup or pitcher.
- Do not let the ice scoop touch the rim or inside of the cup or pitcher.

PROVIDING DRINKING WATER

Quality of Life
Remember to:
- Knock before entering the person's room.
- Address the person by name.
- Introduce yourself by name and title.
- Explain the procedure to the person before beginning and during the procedure.
- Protect the person's rights during the procedure.
- Handle the person gently during the procedure.

Preprocedure
1. Follow *Delegation Guidelines: Providing Drinking Water.* See *Promoting Safety and Comfort: Providing Drinking Water.*
2. Obtain a list of persons who have special fluid orders from the nurse, or use your assignment sheet.
3. Practice hand hygiene.
4. Collect the following:
   - Cart
   - Ice chest filled with ice
   - Cover for the ice chest
   - Scoop
   - Water cups
   - Straws
   - Paper towels
   - Water pitchers for resident use
   - Large water pitcher filled with cold water (optional, depending on center procedure)
   - Towel for the scoop
5. Cover the cart with paper towels. Arrange equipment on top of the paper towels.

Procedure
6. Take the cart to the person's room door. Do not take the cart into the room.
7. Check the person's fluid orders. Use the list from the nurse.
8. Identify the person. Check the ID bracelet against the fluid orders sheet or your assignment sheet. Also call the person by name.
9. Take the pitcher from the person's overbed table. Empty it into the bathroom sink.
10. Determine if a new pitcher is needed.

11. Use the scoop to fill the pitcher with ice (Fig. 20.19). Do not let the scoop touch the rim or inside of the pitcher. Do not place the person's pitcher on the cart.

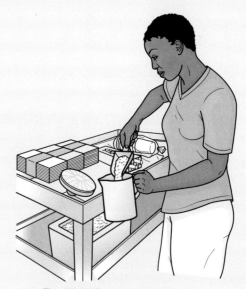

Fig. 20.19 Providing drinking water.

12. Place the ice scoop on the towel.
13. Fill the pitcher with water. Get water from the bathroom or use the larger water pitcher on the cart.
14. Place the pitcher, cup, and straw (if used) on the overbed table. Fill the cup with water. Do not let the water pitcher touch the rim or inside of the cup.
15. Make sure the pitcher, cup, and straw (if used) are within the person's reach.

Postprocedure
16. Provide for comfort. (See the inside of the front cover.)
17. Place the call light within reach.
18. Complete a safety check of the room. (See the inside of the front cover.)
19. Decontaminate your hands.
20. Repeat steps 6 through 19 for each person.

PROMOTING SAFETY AND COMFORT—CONT'D

- Do not put the ice scoop in the ice container or dispenser. Place it in the scoop holder or on a towel for the scoop.
- Make sure the person's pitcher and cup are clean. Also check for cracks and chips. Provide a new pitcher or cup as needed.
- Do not take the person's used water pitcher to the clean ice machine. This could transmit pathogens.

FOODBORNE ILLNESSES

A foodborne illness (food poisoning) is caused by pathogens in food and fluids. Report the signs and symptoms listed in Box 20.7 to the nurse at once.

Food is not sterile. Therefore pathogens are present in food. Cooked and ready-to-eat foods can become contaminated from other food. For example, meat juices can spill or splash onto other food. Food handlers with poor hygiene can contaminate the food.

Pathogens grow rapidly between 40°F (Fahrenheit) and 140°F. This range is called the "danger zone" by the USDA. You must keep food out of this zone of harm. To do so, keep cold food cold and hot food hot.

To keep food safe, the USDA recommends these four safety tips:

- *Clean.* Wash hands, utensils, and countertops often.

BOX 20.7 Signs and Symptoms of Foodborne Illnesses

- Abdominal cramps or pain
- Backache
- Breathing problems
- Chills
- Diarrhea (may be bloody)
- Eyelids: droopy
- Fever
- Headache
- Muscle pain
- Nausea
- Speaking problems
- Swallowing problems
- Vision: double
- Vomiting

- *Separate.* Avoid cross contamination. Do not let raw meat, poultry, or their juices touch other foods that will not be cooked.
- *Cook.* Cook food to a safe internal temperature (see Fig. 20.2). Use a food thermometer to check the internal temperature. When reheating cooked food, reheat to 165°F.
- *Chill.* Refrigerate or freeze food within 2 hours. If the air is 90°F or above, chill food within 1 hour.

QUALITY OF LIFE

OBRA serves to promote the person's quality of life. Nutrition and fluid balance are important for quality of life.

The right to personal choice is important in meeting food and fluid needs. Everyone has a lifetime of likes and dislikes. These do not change when in a nursing center. Cultural, social, religious, medical, and personal factors affect food choices. Persons often express their food likes and dislikes. A person may say that the food is too cold. Or it is too bland. Or the food tastes bad.

Residents have the right to express their preferences. Do not become angry or upset. Do not make the person feel like a complainer or picky eater. Learning the person's likes and dislikes can improve nutrition. It also shows interest and concern for the person. Respect the person's right to express personal choices. Some residents prefer to wear a clothing protector. Others may wish to use a cloth napkin. With time, you will learn the person's preferences. Share this information with the staff. With the person's help, the dietitian plans healthy meals that include personal choices.

Persons with dementia may require special measures to meet their nutritional needs (Chapter 40). Be patient. Provide a quiet and calm mealtime. They may become overwhelmed when many food items are placed before them. Try placing one or two items on the table at a time. Gradually add other items. Treat the person with dignity and respect.

Sometimes families and friends bring food from home. This helps meet love and belonging needs. Sometimes the center cannot provide everything the person likes. Residents are usually pleased to receive homemade food. Holidays have food traditions. Holidays mean more when lifelong traditions are shared. Gifts of food are common. Tell the nurse when the person receives food. The food must not interfere with the person's diet.

OBRA requires that food be served correctly. Hot food must be hot. Cold food must be cold. Cold mashed potatoes are not very good. You would not eat them. The person should not have to. Serve meals promptly. If a meal is delayed, tell the person why. Then get fresh food. Provide needed help with eating. This includes providing eating devices and utensils.

TIME TO REFLECT

You are assisting residents in the dining room for breakfast. Mrs. O'Malley has celiac disease and requires a gluten-free diet. She asks for some toast to eat with her scrambled eggs. Can her request be granted? What are some considerations of this special diet?

REVIEW QUESTIONS

Circle the BEST answer.

1. Nutrition is
   a. Fats, proteins, carbohydrates, vitamins, and minerals
   b. The many processes involved in the ingestion, digestion, absorption, and use of food and fluids by the body
   c. The MyPlate symbol
   d. The balance between calories taken in and used by the body

2. MyPlate encourages the following *except*
   a. The same diet for everyone
   b. Balancing calories
   c. Increasing the amount of fruits and vegetables
   d. Choosing low-sodium foods

3. On a 2000-calorie-a-day diet, what is the amount of grains needed for an adult woman?
   a. 6 oz
   b. 4 to 5 oz
   c. 2 to 4 oz
   d. 3 oz

4. On a 2000-calorie-a-day diet, what is the amount of protein foods needed by an adult man?
   a. 2½ oz
   b. 3 to 4 oz
   c. 4 to 5 oz
   d. 5½ to 6½ oz

5. Which food group contains the *most* fat?
   a. Grains
   b. Vegetables
   c. Milk
   d. Meat and beans

6. These statements are about oils. Which is *false*?
   a. Oils are high in calories.
   b. The best oil choices come from fish, nuts, and vegetable oils.
   c. Oils from plant sources contain cholesterol.
   d. Mayonnaise, certain salad dressings, and soft margarine are mainly oil.

7. Protein is needed for
   a. Tissue growth and repair
   b. Energy and the fiber for bowel elimination
   c. Body heat and to protect organs from injury
   d. Improving the taste of food

8. Which foods provide the *most* protein?
   a. Butter and cream
   b. Tomatoes and potatoes
   c. Meats and fish
   d. Corn and lettuce

9. The sodium-controlled diet involves
   a. Omitting high-sodium foods
   b. Adding salt to food at the table
   c. Using 2400 mg of salt in cooking
   d. A sodium-intake flow sheet

10. A person on a sodium-controlled diet wants a salt shaker. You should
    a. Provide the salt
    b. Salt the person's food
    c. Explain that added salt is not allowed on the diet
    d. Ignore the request

11. Diabetes meal planning involves the following *except*
    a. Food the person likes
    b. Eating the same amount of carbohydrates, protein, and fat each day
    c. Eating at regular times
    d. Sodium control

12. OBRA requires the following *except*
    a. Offering 24-hour meal service
    b. Serving hot food hot; serving cold food cold
    c. Providing needed eating devices
    d. Serving food promptly

13. OBRA requires
    a. Two regular meals
    b. Three regular meals
    c. Four regular meals and a bedtime snack
    d. Meals every 6 hours

14. Which of the following special diets would a person with celiac disease need?
    a. Full liquid
    b. High fiber
    c. Gluten free
    d. Sodium controlled

15. A person is NPO. You should
    a. Provide a variety of fluids
    b. Offer fluids in small amounts and in small containers
    c. Remove the water pitcher and cup from the room
    d. Remove oral hygiene equipment from the room

16. Which are *not* counted as liquids on the I&O record?
    a. Coffee, tea, juices, soft drinks
    b. Butter, mashed potatoes, applesauce
    c. Ice cream, sherbet, custard, pudding
    d. Gelatin, popsicles, ice chips

17. Residents are eating in the dining room. They serve themselves from bowls and platters on their tables. This is a(n)
    a. Social dining program
    b. Family dining program
    c. Low-stimulation feeding program
    d. Open-dining program

18. Persons with dysphagia
    a. Use straws for all liquids
    b. Have a regular diet
    c. Are fed according to the care plan
    d. Eat alone in their rooms

19. Which is *not* a sign of a swallowing problem?
    a. Drooling
    b. Coughing while eating
    c. Pocketing
    d. Edema
20. You are feeding a person. Which action is *not* correct?
    a. Allow the person time to pray before eating
    b. Use a fork to feed the person
    c. Ask the person the order in which to serve food and fluids
    d. Engage the person in a pleasant conversation
21. Before providing fresh drinking water, you need to know the person's
    a. I&O
    b. Diet
    c. Fluid orders
    d. Preferred beverages
22. You are reheating cooked food. The food temperature should be
    a. 40°F
    b. 90°F
    c. 140°F
    d. 165°F
23. The drinking glasses and mugs at your center each hold 8 oz. You are recording Mr. Denner's fluid intake after he finished dinner. He consumed the following: a cup of coffee, half a glass of milk, and a 3-oz dish of pudding. What would you record?
    a. 15 oz
    b. 12 oz
    c. 480 mL
    d. 450 mL
24. Mrs. Miller is unable to feed herself. Which is *incorrect*?
    a. Assist with elimination needs before the meal
    b. Stand near her weak side while feeding
    c. Cover her clothing with a napkin or clothes protector
    d. Use a spoon to feed her

See Appendix A for answers to these questions.

21

Nutritional Support and Intravenous Therapy

OBJECTIVES

- Define the key terms and key abbreviations listed in this chapter.
- Identify the reasons for nutritional support and intravenous (IV) therapy.
- Explain how tube feedings are given.
- Describe scheduled and continuous feedings.
- Explain how to prevent aspiration.
- Describe the comfort measures for the person with a feeding tube.
- Describe parenteral nutrition.

- Describe the IV therapy sites.
- Identify the equipment used in IV therapy.
- Describe how to assist with the IV flow rate.
- Identify the safety measures for IV therapy.
- Identify the observations to report when a person has nutritional support or IV therapy.
- Explain how to assist with nutritional support and IV therapy.
- Explain how to promote quality of life.

KEY TERMS

aspiration Breathing fluid, food, vomitus, or an object into the lungs

enteral nutrition Giving nutrients into the gastrointestinal (GI) tract (enteral) through a feeding tube

flow rate The number of drops per minute (gtt/min)

gastrostomy tube A tube inserted through a surgically created opening (-stomy) in the stomach (gastro-); stomach tube

gavage The process of giving a tube feeding

intravenous (IV) therapy Giving fluids through a needle or catheter inserted into a vein; IV and IV infusion

jejunostomy tube A feeding tube inserted into a surgically created opening (-stomy) in the jejunum of the small intestine

nasoenteral tube A feeding tube inserted through the nose (naso-) into the small bowel (-enteral)

nasogastric (NG) tube A feeding tube inserted through the nose (naso-) into the stomach (-gastro)

parenteral nutrition Giving nutrients through a catheter inserted into a vein; para means "beyond"; enteral relates to the bowel

percutaneous endoscopic gastrostomy (PEG) tube A feeding tube inserted into the stomach (gastro-) through a small incision (-stomy) made through (per) the skin (cutaneous); a lighted instrument (scope) is used to see inside a body cavity or organ (endo-)

regurgitation The backward flow of stomach contents into the mouth

KEY ABBREVIATIONS

GI	Gastrointestinal
gtt	Drops
gtt/min	Drops per minute
IV	Intravenous
mL	Milliliter
NG	Nasogastric

NPO	Nothing by mouth
oz	Ounce
PEG	Percutaneous endoscopic gastrostomy
PICC	Peripherally inserted central catheter
TPN	Total parenteral nutrition

Many persons cannot eat or drink because of illness, surgery, or injury. They may have chewing or swallowing problems. Aspiration is a risk. Aspiration is breathing fluid, food, vomitus, or an object into the lungs. Some persons have problems eating or refuse to eat or drink. Others cannot eat enough to meet their nutritional needs. The doctor may order nutritional support or intravenous (IV) therapy to meet food and fluid needs.

ENTERAL NUTRITION

Some persons cannot or will not ingest, chew, or swallow food. Or food cannot pass from the mouth into the esophagus and into the stomach or small intestine, resulting in poor nutrition. Common causes include the following:

- Cancer, especially cancers of the head, neck, and esophagus
- Trauma to the face, mouth, head, or neck

- Coma
- Dysphagia
- Dementia
- Eating disorders
- Nervous system disorders (Chapter 35)
- Prolonged vomiting
- Major trauma or surgery
- Acquired immunodeficiency syndrome (AIDS)
- Illnesses and disorders affecting eating and nutrition

  Enteral nutrition is giving nutrients into the gastrointestinal (GI) tract *(enteral)* through a feeding tube. Gavage is the process of giving a tube feeding. Tube feedings replace or supplement normal nutrition.

Types of Feeding Tubes

These feeding tubes are common:

- Nasogastric (NG) tube. A feeding tube is inserted through the nose *(naso)* into the stomach *(gastro)* (Fig. 21.1). A doctor or registered nurse (RN) inserts the tube.
- Nasoenteral tube. A feeding tube is inserted through the nose *(naso)* into the small bowel *(enteral)* (Fig. 21.2). A doctor or RN inserts the tube.
- Gastrostomy tube. Also called a *stomach tube,* it is inserted into the stomach (Fig. 21.3). A doctor surgically creates an opening *(stomy)* in the stomach *(gastro)*.
- Jejunostomy tube. A feeding tube inserted into a surgically created opening *(stomy)* in the *jejunum* of the small intestine (Fig. 21.4).
- Percutaneous endoscopic gastrostomy (PEG) tube. The doctor inserts the feeding tube with an endoscope. An endoscope is a lighted instrument *(scope)* used to see inside a body cavity or organ *(endo)*. The tube is inserted through the mouth and esophagus and into the stomach. The doctor makes a small incision *(stomy)* through *(per)* the skin *(cutaneous)* and into the stomach *(gastro)*. A tube is inserted into

the stomach through the incision (Fig. 21.5). The endoscope allows the doctor to see correct tube placement in the stomach.

NG and nasoenteral tubes are used for short-term nutritional support—usually less than 6 weeks. Gastrostomy, jejunostomy, and PEG tubes are used for long-term nutritional support—usually longer than 6 weeks.

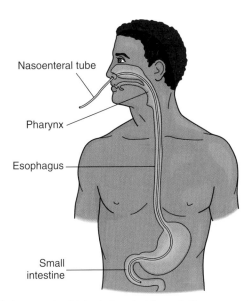

Fig. 21.2 A nasoenteral tube is inserted through the nose and into the small intestine.

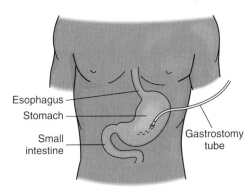

Fig. 21.3 A gastrostomy tube.

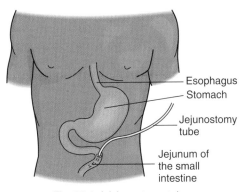

Fig. 21.4 A jejunostomy tube.

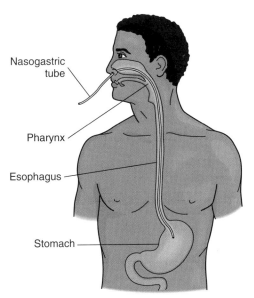

Fig. 21.1 A nasogastric (NG) tube is inserted through the nose and esophagus and into the stomach.

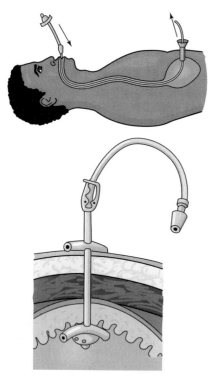

Fig. 21.5 A percutaneous endoscopic gastrostomy (PEG) tube.

Formulas

The doctor orders the type of formula, the amount to give, and when to give tube feedings. Most formulas contain protein, carbohydrates, fat, vitamins, and minerals. Commercial formulas are common.

A nurse gives formula through the feeding tube. Formula is given at room temperature. Cold fluids can cause cramping.

Opened formula can remain at room temperature for about 8 hours. Microbes can grow in warm formula.

See *Teamwork and Time Management: Formulas.*

TEAMWORK AND TIME MANAGEMENT

Formulas

Refrigerated formula needs to warm to room temperature. The nurse may ask you to warm the formula. To do so, place the container in a wash basin filled with warm water. If warmed in the sink, other staff cannot use the sink. They need to go elsewhere. This wastes their time and energy. Or someone may remove the container to use the sink. The container does not warm in a timely manner. That affects you, the nurse, and the resident.

The nurse and manufacturer instructions tell you how long formula can hang. Check the time that the feeding started. Remind the nurse when the time limit is near. For example, a feeding started at 0800. The formula can hang for 8 hours. At 1530 or 1545, tell the nurse how much time is left. Also report the amount of formula left.

Feeding Times

Tube feedings are given at certain times (scheduled feedings). Or they are given over a 24-hour period (continuous feedings).

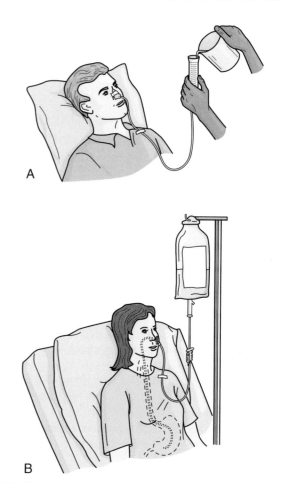

Fig. 21.6 (A) A tube feeding is given with a syringe. (B) Formula drips from a feeding bag into the feeding tube.

Scheduled Feedings

Such feedings also are called intermittent feedings. (*Intermittent* means "to start, stop, and then start again.") Feeding times are scheduled. Four or more feedings are given each day. Usually 8 to 12 ounces (oz) (240 to 360 milliliters [mL]) are given over about 30 minutes. The frequency, amount, and time are like a normal eating pattern.

The nurse uses a syringe or a feeding bag (Fig. 21.6). The syringe attaches to the feeding tube. Connecting tubing connects the feeding bag to the tube. Formula is added to the syringe or to the feeding bag. Then it slowly flows through the feeding tube into the stomach.

The nurse removes the syringe or connecting tubing after the feeding. Then the nurse clamps and covers the end of the feeding tube with a cap or gauze. Gauze is secured in place with a rubber band. Clamping prevents air from entering the tube. It also prevents fluid from leaking out of the tube. Covering the end of the tube also prevents leaking.

Continuous Feedings

These feedings are usually given over 24 hours. A feeding pump is used (Fig. 21.7). Formula drips into the feeding tube at a

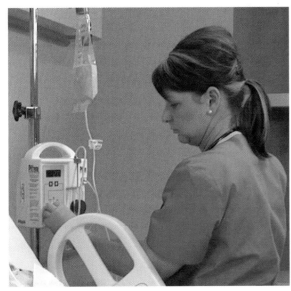

Fig. 21.7 Feeding pump. (Copyright Mosby's Clinical Skills: Essentials Collection.)

certain rate per minute. The person receives a certain amount every hour.

A pump alarm sounds if something is wrong. When you hear an alarm, tell the nurse.

Observations

Diarrhea, constipation, delayed stomach emptying, and aspiration are risks. Report the following at once:

- Nausea
- Discomfort during the feeding
- Vomiting
- Distended (enlarged and swollen) abdomen
- Coughing
- Complaints of indigestion or heartburn
- Redness, swelling, drainage, odor, or pain at the ostomy site
- Fever
- Signs and symptoms of respiratory distress (Chapter 26)
- Increased pulse rate (Chapter 27)
- Complaints of flatulence (Chapter 23)
- Diarrhea (Chapter 23)

Preventing Aspiration

Aspiration is a major risk from tube feedings. It can cause pneumonia and death. Aspiration can occur:

- *During insertion.* NG tubes and nasoenteral tubes are passed through the esophagus and then into the stomach or small intestine. The tube can slip into the airway. An x-ray is taken after insertion to check tube placement.
- *From tube movement out of place.* Coughing, sneezing, vomiting, suctioning, and poor positioning are common causes. A tube can move from the stomach or intestines into the esophagus and then into the airway. The RN checks tube placement before every scheduled tube feeding. With

continuous feedings, the RN checks tube placement every 4 hours. To do so, the RN attaches a syringe to the tube. GI secretions are withdrawn through the syringe. Then the pH of the secretions is measured. *You never check feeding tube placement.*

- *From regurgitation.* Regurgitation is the backward flow of stomach contents into the mouth. Delayed stomach emptying and overfeeding are common causes.
- To help prevent regurgitation and aspiration:
- Position the person in Fowler or semi-Fowler position before the feeding. Follow the care plan and the nurse's directions.
- Maintain Fowler or semi-Fowler position after the feeding. It allows formula to move through the GI tract. The position is required for 1 to 2 hours after the feeding or at all times. Follow the care plan and the nurse's directions.
- Avoid the left side-lying position. When the person lies on the left side, the stomach cannot empty into the small intestine.

Persons with NG or gastrostomy tubes are at great risk for regurgitation. The risk is less with intestinal tubes. Formula passes directly into the small intestine. Also, formula is given at a slow rate. During digestion, food slowly passes from the stomach into the small intestine. The stomach handles larger amounts of food at one time than does the small intestine.

Digestion slows with aging. Stomach emptying also slows. Older persons are at risk for regurgitation and aspiration. Less formula and longer feeding times prevent overfeeding.

Comfort Measures

Persons with feeding tubes usually are not allowed to eat or drink. They are NPO—nothing by mouth (Chapter 20). Dry mouth, dry lips, and sore throat cause discomfort. Sometimes hard candy or gum is allowed. These measures are common:

- Oral hygiene every 2 hours while the person is awake
- Lubricant for the lips every 2 hours while the person is awake
- Mouth rinses every 2 hours while the person is awake

Feeding tubes can irritate and cause pressure on the nose. Tubes can change the shape of the nostrils or cause pressure injuries. These measures are common:

- Clean the nose and nostrils every 4 to 8 hours.
- Secure the tube to the nose (Fig. 21.8). Use tape or a tube holder. Tube holders have foam cushions that prevent pressure on the nose. Retaping is not needed, as it irritates the nose. Do not use safety pins.
- Secure the tube to the person's garment at the shoulder area. This prevents the tube from pulling or dangling. Both can cause pressure on the nose. These methods are common. Follow center policy.
- Loop a rubber band around the tube. Then pin the rubber band to the garment with a safety pin.
- Tape the tube to the garment.

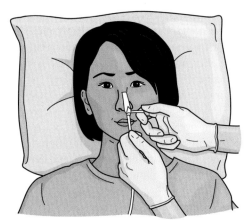

Fig. 21.8 The feeding tube is secured to the nose.

Giving Tube Feedings

You assist the nurse with tube feedings. In some states and centers, nursing assistants give tube feedings and remove NG tubes. *Remember, you never insert feeding tubes or check their placement. They are the RN's responsibility.*

See *Delegation Guidelines: Giving Tube Feedings.*
See *Promoting Safety and Comfort: Giving Tube Feedings.*

DELEGATION GUIDELINES

Giving Tube Feedings

Before giving tube feedings or removing an NG tube, make sure that:

- Your state allows you to perform the procedure.
- The procedure is in your job description.
- You have had the necessary education and training.
- You know how to use the center's equipment and supplies.
- You review the procedure in the center's procedure manual.
- You review the procedure with the nurse.
- A nurse is available to answer questions and to supervise you.
- An RN has identified and labeled all other tubes, catheters, and needles.
- An RN checks tube placement.

If the above mentioned conditions are met, you need this information from the nurse and the care plan:

- The type of tube—NG, nasoenteral, gastrostomy, PEG, or jejunostomy
- What feeding method to use—syringe, feeding bag, or feeding pump
- What size syringe to use—usually 30 or 60 mL for an adult
- How to position the person for the feeding—Fowler or semi-Fowler
- How to position the person after the feeding—Fowler or semi-Fowler
- What formula to use
- How much formula to give
- How high to raise the syringe or hang the feeding bag (usually 18 inches above the stomach or intestines)
- The amount of flushing solution to use—usually 30 to 60 mL (1 to 2 oz) of water for an adult
- How fast to give the feeding if using a syringe—usually over 30 minutes
- The flow rate if a feeding bag is used (Flow rate is the number of drops per minute [see p. 335].)
- The flow rate if a feeding pump is used
- If ice is kept around the bag for a continuous feeding
- If you are to remove an NG tube, when to remove the tube
- What observations to report and record (see p. 333)
- When to report observations
- What specific resident concerns to report at once

PROMOTING SAFETY AND COMFORT

Giving Tube Feedings
Safety

The person may have an IV line, a breathing tube (Chapter 26), and drainage tubes (Chapter 31). You must know the purpose of each tube. Ask the nurse to label each tube to identify its purpose. *Formula must enter only the feeding tube.* Otherwise, the person can die.

Before giving a tube feeding, always:

- Turn on the light if the room is dark. Do so even if the person is sleeping.
- Check and inspect the feeding tube and label with the nurse.
- Make sure an RN checks for tube placement.
- Make sure every tube, catheter, or needle is labeled.
- Trace the feeding tube back to the insertion site. Start at the end of the feeding tube. Trace the tube backward. For example, if the person has an NG tube, you will end at the nose. If the person has a gastrostomy tube, you will end at the abdomen. *If you do not end at the correct place, do not give the tube feeding.* Call for the nurse.

Nasal secretions may contain blood or microbes. So can drainage at an ostomy site. Wear gloves. Follow Standard Precautions and the Bloodborne Pathogen Standard.

Remind visitors to call for a nurse if any tube becomes disconnected. They could connect the wrong tubes together.

Confusion and disorientation can cause a person to pull out the feeding tube. Tell the nurse at once if this happens. At times, the person may need to have limb restraints (Chapter 13) applied to prevent removal of tubes or IVs.

PARENTERAL NUTRITION

Parenteral nutrition is giving nutrients through a catheter inserted into a vein (Fig. 21.9). (*Para-* means "beyond"; *enteral* relates to the bowel.) A nutrient solution is given directly into the bloodstream. Nutrients do not enter the GI tract. Parenteral nutrition is often called *total parenteral nutrition (TPN)* or *hyperalimentation.* (*Hyper-* means "high or excessive"; *alimentation* means "nourishment.")

The solution contains water, proteins, carbohydrates, vitamins, and minerals. It drips through a catheter inserted into a large vein. TPN is used when the person cannot receive oral or

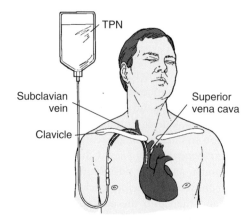

Fig. 21.9 Parenteral nutrition. *TPN,* Total parenteral nutrition. (From *Mosby's dictionary of medicine, nursing, and health professions,* ed 11, St Louis, 2022, Mosby.)

enteral feedings. Or it is used when oral or enteral feedings are not enough to meet the person's needs.

Common reasons for TPN:

- Disease, injury, or surgery to the GI tract
- Severe trauma, infection, or burns
- Being NPO for more than 5 to 7 days
- GI side effects from cancer treatments (Chapter 34)
- Prolonged coma
- Prolonged anorexia (loss of appetite)

Observations

TPN risks include infection, fluid imbalances, and blood sugar imbalances. Report these signs and symptoms to the nurse at once:

- Fever, chills, and other signs and symptoms of infection (Chapter 14)
- Signs and symptoms of sugar imbalances (see "Diabetes" in Chapter 37)
- Chest pain
- Difficulty breathing or shortness of breath
- Cough
- Nausea and vomiting
- Diarrhea
- Thirst
- Rapid heart rate or an irregular heartbeat
- Weakness or fatigue
- Sweating
- Pallor (pale skin)
- Trembling
- Confusion or behavior changes

Assisting with TPN

The nurse is responsible for all aspects of TPN. You assist by carefully observing the person. You also assist with the person's basic needs and activities of daily living. Persons receiving TPN may be NPO. Provide frequent oral hygiene, lubricant to the lips, and mouth rinses as the nurse and care plan direct. Also follow other aspects of the person's care plan.

Many aspects of IV therapy apply to TPN.

IV THERAPY

Intravenous (IV) therapy is giving fluids through a needle or catheter inserted into a vein (Fig. 21.10). Fluid flows directly into the bloodstream. *IV* and *IV infusion* also refer to IV therapy. Doctors order IV therapy to:

- Provide fluids when they cannot be taken by mouth.
- Replace minerals and vitamins lost because of illness or injury.
- Provide sugar for energy.
- Give medications and blood.

RNs are responsible for IV therapy. They start and maintain the infusion according to the doctor's orders. RNs also give IV medications and administer blood. State laws vary about the role of licensed practical nurses/licensed vocational nurses (LPNs/LVNs) and nursing assistants in IV therapy.

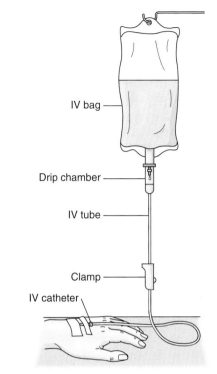

Fig. 21.10 Equipment for intravenous *(IV)* therapy.

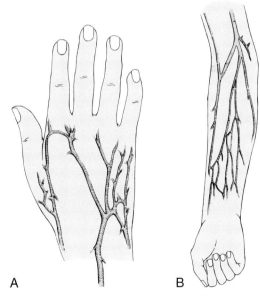

Fig. 21.11 Peripheral intravenous sites. (A) Back of the hand. (B) Inner forearm. (From Potter PA, Perry AG: *Fundamentals of nursing*, ed 10, St Louis, 2021, Mosby.)

IV Sites

Peripheral and central venous sites are used. Peripheral means "around *(peri-)* a boundary *(-pheral)*." The boundary is the center of the body near the heart. *Peripheral IV sites* are away from the center of the body. For adults, the back of the hand and inner forearm are useful sites (Fig. 21.11).

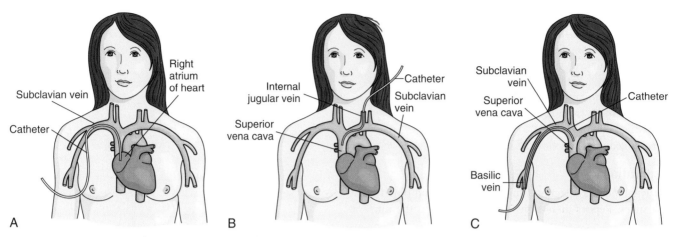

Fig. 21.12 Central venous sites. (A) Subclavian vein. The catheter tip is in the right atrium. (B) Internal jugular vein. The catheter tip is in the superior vena cava. (C) Basilic vein. This is a peripherally inserted central catheter.

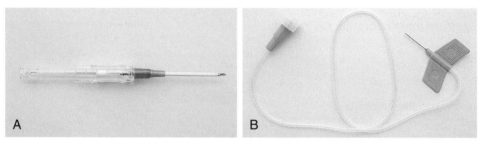

Fig. 21.13 (A) Intravenous catheter. (B) Butterfly needle.

The subclavian vein and the internal jugular vein are *central venous sites.* They are close to the heart. A catheter is threaded into the right atrium or superior vena cava (Fig. 21.12A and B). The catheter is called a *central venous catheter* or a *central line.* The cephalic and basilic veins in the arm also are used. A catheter inserted into one of these sites is called a *peripherally inserted central catheter (PICC).* The catheter is threaded into the subclavian vein or the superior vena cava (see Fig. 21.12C). At times it may be necessary for the doctor to implant a venous port. This is often used for persons receiving chemotherapy for cancer treatment (Chapter 34).

Central venous sites are used:
- For parenteral nutrition.
- To give large amounts of fluid.
- For long-term IV therapy.
- To give medications that irritate peripheral veins.

IV Equipment

The basic equipment used in IV therapy is shown in Fig. 21.10:
- The solution container is a plastic bag. It is called the *IV bag.*
- A *catheter* or *needle* is inserted into a vein (Fig. 21.13).
- The *IV tube* or *infusion tubing* connects the IV bag to the catheter or needle. Fluid drips from the bag into the *drip chamber.* The *clamp* is used to regulate the flow rate. Some IV fluids are given continuously. Intermittent administration allows the tubing to be disconnected from the catheter for a

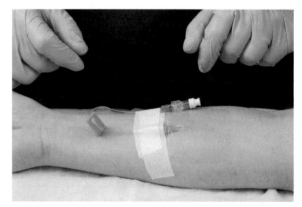

Fig. 21.14 A short-peripheral intravenous device. (From Potter PA, Perry AG, Stockert Pe, et al: *Fundamentals of nursing*, ed 10, St Louis, 2022, Elsevier.)

time. These are called short peripheral IV devices (Fig. 21.14). This allows the person to be more mobile. For example, Mr. Brown receives an antibiotic through his IV every 12 hours. After the medication is given, the nurse infuses a small amount of solution that prevents the vein from closing. The IV is still inserted but the tubing is disconnected, and he can be up and about.
- The IV bag hangs from an IV pole (IV standard) or ceiling hook.

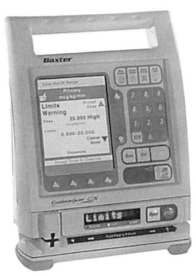

Fig. 21.15 Electronic intravenous pump. (Courtesy Baxter Healthcare Corp., Round Lake, IL.)

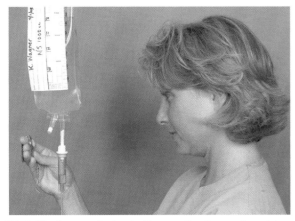

Fig. 21.16 The flow rate is checked by counting the number of drops per minute.

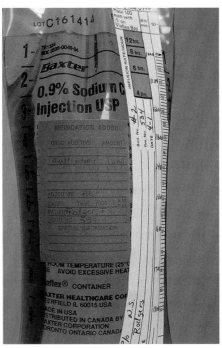

Fig. 21.17 Time tape applied to an intravenous bag. (From Elkin MK, Perry AG, Potter PA: *Nursing interventions and clinical skills,* ed 4, St Louis, 2007, Mosby.)

The time tape shows how much fluid to give over a period of time (Fig. 21.17). For example, the doctor orders 1000 mL of fluid over 8 hours. The RN marks the tape in eight 1-hour intervals. To check if the infusion is on time, compare the fluid line with the time line on the tape. If the fluid line is above or below the time line, the flow rate is too slow or too fast. Tell the RN at once if too much or too little fluid was given.

See *Promoting Safety and Comfort: Flow Rate.*

> **PROMOTING SAFETY AND COMFORT**
>
> **Flow Rate**
> *Safety*
> The person can suffer serious harm if the flow rate is too fast or too slow. The flow rate can change from position changes. Kinked tubes and lying on the tube also affect the flow rate.
>
> Never change the position of the clamp or adjust any controls on infusion pumps. Tell the nurse at once if there is a problem with the flow rate. An electronic pump can be unplugged from the wall outlet and used on battery power. This may be necessary when the person needs to walk to the bathroom. Always remember to plug the cord into the electrical source when returning the person to bed.

Flow Rate

The doctor orders the amount of fluid to give *(infuse)* and the amount of time to give it in. With this information, the RN figures the flow rate. The flow rate is the number of drops per minute *(gtt/min).* The Latin word *guttae (gtt)* means "drops."

The fluid may infuse by gravity. The RN sets the clamp for the flow rate. Or an electronic pump is used to control the flow rate (Fig. 21.15). An alarm sounds if something is wrong. Tell the nurse at once if you hear an alarm. *Never change the position of the clamp or adjust any controls on IV pumps.*

You can check the flow rate. The RN tells you the number of drops per minute (gtt/min). To check the flow rate, count the number of drops in 1 minute (Fig. 21.16). Tell the RN at once if:

• No fluid is dripping.
• The rate is too fast.
• The rate is too slow.

Assisting with IV Therapy

You help meet the safety, hygiene, and activity needs of persons with IVs. Follow the safety measures in Box 21.1. Report any of the signs and symptoms listed in Box 21.2 at once.

Your state and center may allow you to change dressings at peripheral IV sites. They also may let you discontinue a peripheral IV.

BOX 21.1 Safety Measures for Intravenous Therapy

- Follow Standard Precautions and the Bloodborne Pathogen Standard.
- Do not move the needle or catheter. Needle or catheter position must be maintained. If the needle or catheter is moved, it may come out of the vein. Then fluid flows into tissues (*infiltration*) or the flow stops.
- Follow the safety measures for restraints (Chapter 13). The nurse may splint or restrain the extremity to prevent movement (Fig. 21.18). The nurse may apply a protective device (Fig. 21.19). This helps prevent the needle or catheter from moving.
- Protect the IV bag, tubing, and needle or catheter when the person walks. Portable IV standards are rolled along next to the person (Fig. 21.20). Portable IV pumps can operate on battery power. Always plug them back into the wall electrical outlet when returning the person to bed.
- Assist the person with turning and repositioning. Move the IV bag to the side of the bed on which the person is lying. Always allow enough slack in the tubing. The needle or catheter can move from pressure on the tube.
- Always follow the person's care plan for bathing and hygiene needs. For example, can Mr. Jenkins shower with his IV? Always ask the nurse if in doubt.
- It is best to use the opposite arm for blood pressures (the arm that the IV is *not* in). If the person has a PICC line, *never* measure blood pressure in that arm.
- Tell the nurse at once if bleeding occurs from the insertion site. Follow Standard Precautions and the Bloodborne Pathogen Standard.
- Tell the nurse at once of any signs and symptoms listed in Box 21.2.

BOX 21.2 Signs and Symptoms of Intravenous Therapy Complications

Local—At the IV Site
- Bleeding
- Puffiness, swelling, or leaking fluid
- Pale or reddened skin
- Complaints of pain at or above the IV site
- Hot or cold skin near the site

Systemic—Involving the Whole Body
- Fever
- Itching
- Drop in blood pressure
- Pulse rate greater than 100 beats per minute
- Irregular pulse
- Cyanosis
- Confusion or changes in mental function
- Loss of consciousness
- Difficulty breathing
- Shortness of breath
- Decreasing or no urine output
- Chest pain
- Nausea

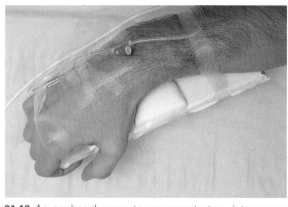

Fig. 21.18 An armboard prevents movement at an intravenous site. (From Elkin MK, Perry AG, Potter PA: *Nursing interventions and clinical skills,* ed 4, St Louis, 2007, Mosby.)

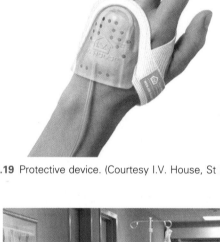

Fig. 21.19 Protective device. (Courtesy I.V. House, St Louis, MO.)

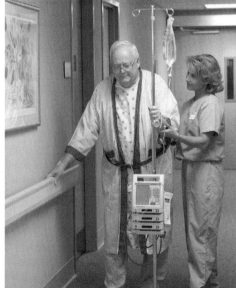

Fig. 21.20 A person walking with an intravenous line in place.

You never start or maintain IV therapy. Nor do you regulate the flow rate or change IV bags. You never give blood or IV medications.

See *Teamwork and Time Management: Assisting with IV Therapy.*

See *Delegation Guidelines: Assisting with IV Therapy.*

TEAMWORK AND TIME MANAGEMENT

Assisting with IV Therapy

If a person's care is part of your assignment, you must know the IV flow rate. When you are with the person, always check the flow rate. Report any problems to the nurse at once.

Also check the amount of fluid in the bag. Tell the nurse at once if the bag is empty or almost empty.

Residents cared for by other staff may have IVs. When you are near the person or walking past the person's room, always make sure the IV is dripping. Also check the amount of fluid in the bag. Report any problems to a nurse at once.

DELEGATION GUIDELINES

Assisting with IV Therapy

Before changing a peripheral IV dressing or discontinuing a peripheral IV, make sure:

- Your state lets nursing assistants perform the procedure.
- The procedure is in your job description.
- You have the necessary education and training.
- You know how to use the center's supplies and equipment.
- You review the procedure in the center's procedure manual.
- You review the procedure with the nurse.
- A nurse is available to answer questions and to supervise you.
- An RN has identified and labeled all other tubes, catheters, and needles.

If the abovementioned conditions are met, you need this information from the nurse and the care plan:

- When to change the IV dressing
- If the person has an IV needle or catheter
- When to discontinue the IV
- If the person has more than one IV, which IV to discontinue
- What supplies to use
- What observations to report and record (see Box 21.2)
- When to report observations
- What specific resident concerns to report at once

QUALITY OF LIFE

Persons who need nutritional support or IV therapy are often very ill. Their care needs may be great and take a lot of time. Do not take shortcuts or omit care. Doing so is unethical. It could also cause great harm. At all times, you must give quality care and protect the person's rights.

Sometimes decisions are made to stop nutritional support or IV therapy. The person is allowed to die. The person may make the decision. Or the family does so after talking to the doctor (Chapter 45). You may agree or disagree with such choices. The choice may or may not be within your religious or cultural beliefs and values. The person's or family's wishes and doctor's orders must be followed. The person must receive quality care. Talk to the nurse if you have problems with the decision. The nurse may need to change your assignment.

TIME TO REFLECT

Mr. Lee has an IV inserted into a vein in his left hand. He is allowed to go to the bathroom without help. He is in the bathroom when he catches the tubing on the grab bar and the IV catheter is pulled out. He signals by pulling the call light.

You are the first to arrive. When you open the bathroom door you see blood everywhere. What should you do first? How will you assist Mr. Lee with getting cleaned up? What special precautions must you take?

REVIEW QUESTIONS

Circle the BEST answer.

1. Enteral nutrition
   a. Requires an NG tube
   b. Is given into a central venous site
   c. Is given into the GI tract
   d. Requires an IV
2. The process of giving a tube feeding is called
   a. Gavage
   b. Parenteral nutrition
   c. Aspiration
   d. Regurgitation
3. For a tube feeding, the person is positioned in
   a. Fowler or semi-Fowler position
   b. The left side-lying position
   c. The right side-lying position
   d. The supine position

4. Formula for a tube feeding is given
   a. At body temperature
   b. At room temperature
   c. Hot
   d. Cold
5. Continuous feedings are given with a
   a. Syringe
   b. Feeding bag
   c. PEG tube
   d. Feeding pump
6. The nurse checks feeding tube placement to prevent
   a. Aspiration
   b. Regurgitation
   c. Overfeeding
   d. Cramping

7. Which position prevents regurgitation after a tube feeding?
   a. Left or right side-lying position
   b. Supine position
   c. Fowler or semi-Fowler position
   d. Prone position
8. The risk of regurgitation is the greatest with
   a. NG and gastrostomy tubes
   b. PEG tube
   c. Nasoenteral tube
   d. Jejunostomy tube
9. A person with a feeding tube is NPO. You should do the following *except*
   a. Give the person hard candy or gum
   b. Provide oral hygiene
   c. Provide mouth rinses
   d. Apply lubricant to the lips
10. A person has an NG tube. The care plan includes the following measures to prevent nasal irritation. Which measure should you question?
    a. Clean the nose and nostrils every 4 hours
    b. Tape the tube to the nose
    c. Remove the tube every 4 hours
    d. Secure the tube to the person's gown
11. A nurse asks you to give a tube feeding. The procedure is not in your job description. What should you do?
    a. Refuse to perform the task
    b. Give the tube feeding
    c. Tell the director of nursing
    d. Ask another nurse what you should do
12. A person is receiving TPN. The person complains of chest pain and difficulty breathing. What should you do?
    a. Position the person in Fowler position
    b. Call for the nurse
    c. Stop the TPN
    d. Provide oral hygiene

13. A person is receiving TPN. You know that TPN
    a. Involves a nutrient solution
    b. Is given through a feeding tube
    c. Can cause pressure injuries on the nose
    d. Requires that the person be NPO
14. Which is a peripheral IV site?
    a. Subclavian vein
    b. Superior vena cava
    c. Jugular vein
    d. A vein on the back of the hand
15. The IV flow rate is
    a. The number of gtt/mL
    b. The number of gtt/min
    c. The amount of fluid given in 1 hour
    d. The amount of fluid in the IV bag
16. You note that an IV bag is almost empty. What should you do?
    a. Clamp the IV tubing
    b. Tell the nurse
    c. Discontinue the IV
    d. Adjust the flow rate
17. You note bleeding from an IV insertion site. What should you do?
    a. Tell the nurse
    b. Move the needle or catheter
    c. Discontinue the IV
    d. Clamp the IV tubing
18. Mrs. Ross has a PICC line in her right arm. You need to check her blood pressure. How should you proceed?
    a. Measure the blood pressure in her left arm
    b. Measure the blood pressure in her right arm
    c. Use either arm to measure her blood pressure
    d. Ask the nurse to check her blood pressure

See Appendix A for answers to these questions.

22

Urinary Elimination

OBJECTIVES

- Define the key terms and key abbreviations listed in this chapter.
- Describe normal urine.
- Describe the rules for normal urinary elimination.
- Identify the observations to report to the nurse.
- Describe urinary incontinence and the care required.
- Describe straight, indwelling, external, and condom catheters.
- Explain why catheters are used.
- Explain how to care for persons with catheters.
- Describe two methods of bladder training.
- Perform the procedures described in this chapter.
- Explain how to promote quality of life.

KEY TERMS

catheter A tube used to drain or inject fluid through a body opening

catheterization The process of inserting a catheter

dysuria Painful or difficult (*dys-*) urination (*-uria*)

external catheter A catheter placed on the outside of the body (male or female) and drains urine to a collection container

Foley catheter See "indwelling catheter"

functional incontinence The person has bladder control but cannot use the toilet in time

hematuria Blood (*hemat-*) in the urine (*-uria*)

incontinence The inability to control urination or defecation

indwelling catheter A catheter left in the bladder so urine drains constantly into a drainage bag; retention catheter or Foley catheter

micturition See "urination"

mixed incontinence The combination of stress incontinence and urge incontinence

nocturia Frequent urination (*-uria*) at night (*noct-*)

oliguria Scant amount (*olig-*) of urine (*-uria*); less than 500 mL in 24 hours

overflow incontinence Small amounts of urine leak from a full bladder

polyuria Abnormally large amounts (*poly-*) of urine (*-uria*)

reflex incontinence Urine is lost at predictable intervals when the bladder is full

retention catheter See "indwelling catheter"

straight catheter A catheter that drains the bladder and then is removed

stress incontinence When urine leaks during exercise and certain movements that cause pressure on the bladder

transient incontinence Temporary or occasional incontinence that is reversed when the cause is treated

urge incontinence The loss of urine in response to a sudden, urgent need to void; the person cannot get to a toilet in time

urinary frequency Voiding at frequent intervals

urinary incontinence The involuntary loss or leakage of urine

urinary urgency The need to void at once

urination The process of emptying urine from the bladder; micturition or voiding

voiding See "urination"

KEY ABBREVIATIONS

C Centigrade
CAUTI Catheter-associated urinary tract infection
CMS Centers for Medicare & Medicaid Services
F Fahrenheit
ID Identification
I&O Intake and output
IV Intravenous
mL Milliliter
UTI Urinary tract infection

Eliminating waste is a physical need. The respiratory, digestive, integumentary, and urinary systems remove body wastes. The digestive system rids the body of solid wastes. The lungs remove carbon dioxide. Sweat contains water and other substances. Blood contains waste products from body cells burning food for energy. The urinary system removes waste products from the blood. It also maintains the body's water balance.

NORMAL URINATION

The healthy adult produces about 1500 milliliters (mL) or 3 pints of urine a day. Many factors affect urine production: age, disease, the amount and kinds of fluid ingested, dietary salt, body temperature, perspiration, and medications. Some substances increase urine production: coffee, tea, alcohol, and some medications. A diet high in salt causes the body to retain water. When water is retained, less urine is produced.

FOCUS ON COMMUNICATION

Normal Urination

Residents may not use "voiding" or "urinating" terms. The person may not understand what you are saying. Instead you can ask these questions:
- "Do you need to use the bathroom?"
- "Do you need to use the bedpan?"
- "Do you need to pass urine?"
- "Do you need to pee?"

TEAMWORK AND TIME MANAGEMENT

Normal Urination

The need to void may be urgent. Answer call lights promptly. Also answer call lights for coworkers. Otherwise incontinence may result. **Incontinence** means the inability to control urination or defecation. The person is wet and embarrassed. The person is at risk for skin breakdown and infection. Your coworker has extra work—changing linens and garments. You appreciate help when you are busy, and so do your coworkers.

Urination, micturition, and *voiding* mean the process of emptying urine from the bladder. The amount of fluid intake, habits, and available toilet facilities affect frequency. So do activity, work, and illness. People usually void at bedtime, after sleep, and before meals. Some people void every 2 to 3 hours. The need to void at night disturbs sleep.

Some persons need help getting to the bathroom. Others use bedpans, urinals, or commodes. Follow the rules in Box 22.1 and the person's care plan.

See *Focus on Communication: Normal Urination.*

See *Teamwork and Time Management: Normal Urination.*

Observations

Normal urine is pale yellow, straw colored, or amber (Fig. 22.1). It is clear with no particles. A faint odor is normal. Observe urine for color, clarity, odor, amount, and particles.

Some foods affect urine color. Red food dyes, beets, blackberries, and rhubarb cause red urine. Carrots and sweet potatoes cause bright yellow urine. Certain medications change urine color. Asparagus causes a urine odor.

Ask the nurse to observe urine that looks or smells abnormal. Report complaints of urgency, burning on urination, or painful or difficult urination. Also report the problems in Table 22.1. The nurse uses the information for the nursing process.

Bedpans

Bedpans are used by persons who cannot be out of bed. Women use bedpans for voiding and bowel movements. Men use them for bowel movements.

The *standard bedpan* is shown in Fig. 22.2. A *fracture pan* has a thin rim. It is only about ½-inch deep at one end (see

BOX 22.1 Rules for Normal Urination

- Practice medical asepsis.
- Follow Standard Precautions and the Bloodborne Pathogen Standard.
- Provide fluids as the nurse and care plan direct.
- Follow the person's voiding routines and habits. Check with the nurse and the care plan.
- Help the person to the bathroom when the request is made. Or provide the commode, bedpan, or urinal. The need to void may be urgent.
- Help the person assume a normal position for voiding if possible. Women sit or squat. Men stand.
- Warm the bedpan or urinal.
- Cover the person for warmth and privacy.
- Provide for privacy. Pull the curtain around the bed, close room and bathroom doors, and close window coverings. Leave the room if the person can be alone.
- Tell the person that running water, flushing the toilet, or playing music can mask voiding sounds. Voiding with others close by embarrasses some people.
- Stay nearby if the person is weak or unsteady.
- Place the call light and toilet tissue within reach.
- Allow enough time. Do not rush the person.
- Promote relaxation. Some people like to read.
- Run water in a sink if the person cannot start the stream. Or place the person's fingers in warm water.
- Provide perineal care as needed (Chapter 18).
- Assist with hand washing after voiding. Provide a wash basin, soap, washcloth, and towel.
- Assist the person to the bathroom or offer the bedpan, urinal, or commode at regular times. Some people are embarrassed or are too weak to ask for help.

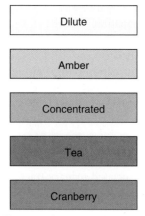

Fig. 22.1 Color chart for urine.

Fig. 22.2). The smaller end is placed under the buttocks (Fig. 22.3). Fracture pans are used:
- By persons with casts.
- By persons in traction.
- By persons with limited back motion.
- After spinal cord injury or surgery.
- After a hip fracture.
- After hip replacement surgery.

TABLE 22.1   Urinary Elimination Problems

Problem	Definition	Causes
Dysuria	Painful or difficult *(dys)* urination *(uria)*	Urinary tract infection (UTI), trauma, urinary tract obstruction
Hematuria	Blood *(hemat)* in the urine *(uria)*	Kidney disease, UTI, trauma
Nocturia	Frequent urination *(uria)* at night *(noct)*	Excess fluid intake, kidney disease, prostate disease
Oliguria	Scant amount *(olig)* of urine *(uria)*; less than 500 mL in 24 hours	Poor fluid intake, shock, burns, kidney disease, heart failure
Polyuria	Abnormally large amounts *(poly)* of urine *(uria)*	Medications, excess fluid intake, diabetes, hormone imbalance
Urinary frequency	Voiding at frequent intervals	Excess fluid intake, UTI, pressure on the bladder, medications
Urinary incontinence	The involuntary loss or leakage of urine	Trauma, disease, UTI, reproductive or urinary tract surgeries, aging, fecal impaction, constipation, not getting to the bathroom in time
Urinary urgency	The need to void at once	UTI, fear of incontinence, full bladder, stress

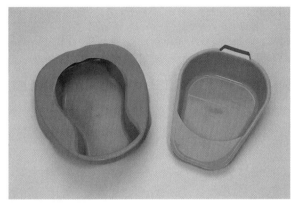

Fig. 22.2 Standard bedpan *(left)* and the fracture pan *(right)*.

See *Delegation Guidelines: Bedpans.*
See *Promoting Safety and Comfort: Bedpans.*

📄 DELEGATION GUIDELINES

Bedpans

Before assisting with a bedpan, you need this information from the nurse and the care plan:

- What bedpan to use—standard bedpan or fracture pan
- Position or activity limits
- If you can leave the room or if you need to stay with the person
- If the nurse needs to observe the results before disposing of the contents
- What observations to report and record:
  - Urine color, clarity, and odor
  - Amount
  - Presence of particles

- Blood in the urine
- Cloudy urine
- Complaints of urgency, burning, dysuria, or other problems (see Table 22.1)
- For bowel movements (Chapter 23)
- When to report observations
- What specific resident concerns to report at once

👤 PROMOTING SAFETY AND COMFORT

Bedpans

Safety

Urine and bowel movements may contain blood and microbes. Microbes can live and grow in dirty bedpans. Follow Standard Precautions and the Bloodborne Pathogen Standard when handling bedpans and their contents. Thoroughly clean and disinfect bedpans after use.

Remember to raise the bed as needed for good body mechanics. Lower the bed before leaving the room. Raise or lower the bed rails according to the care plan.

Comfort

Some older persons have fragile bones from osteoporosis or painful joints from arthritis (Chapter 35). Fracture pans provide more comfort for them than standard bedpans.

Most bedpans are made of plastic. Some are made of metal. Metal bedpans are often cold. Warm them with warm water and then dry them before use.

The person must not sit on a bedpan for a long time. Bedpans are uncomfortable, and they can lead to pressure injuries from prolonged pressure (Chapter 32).

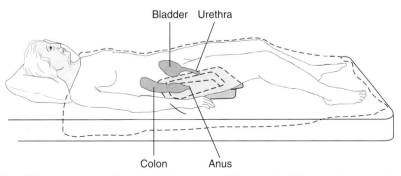

Fig. 22.3 A person positioned on a fracture pan. The small end is under the buttocks.

✳ GIVING THE BEDPAN (NATCEP)

Quality of Life

Remember to:

- Knock before entering the person's room.
- Address the person by name.
- Introduce yourself by name and title.
- Explain the procedure to the person before beginning and during the procedure.
- Protect the person's rights during the procedure.
- Handle the person gently during the procedure.

Preprocedure

1. Follow Delegation Guidelines: Bedpans. See *Promoting Safety and Comfort: Bedpans* (p. 341).
2. Provide for privacy.
3. Practice hand hygiene.
4. Put on gloves.
5. Collect the following:
   - Bedpan
   - Bedpan cover
   - Toilet tissue
   - Waterproof pad (if required by the center)
6. Arrange equipment on the chair or bed.

Procedure

7. Lower the bed rail near you if up.
8. Position the person supine. Raise the head of the bed slightly.
9. Fold the top linens and gown out of the way. Keep the lower body covered.
10. Ask the person to flex the knees and raise the buttocks by pushing against the mattress with the feet.
11. Slide your hand under the lower back. Help raise the buttocks. If using a waterproof pad, place it under the person's buttocks.
12. Slide the bedpan under the person (Fig. 22.4).
13. If the person cannot assist in getting on the bedpan:
    a. Place the waterproof pad under the person's buttocks if using one.
    b. Turn the person onto the side away from you.
    c. Place the bedpan firmly against the buttocks (Fig. 22.5A).
    d. Push the bedpan down and toward the person (see Fig. 22.5B).

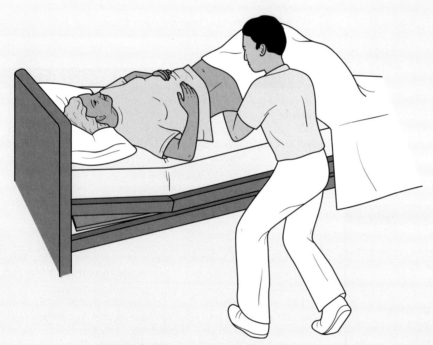
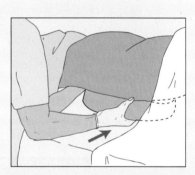

Fig. 22.4 The person raises the buttocks off the bed with help. The bedpan is slid under the person.

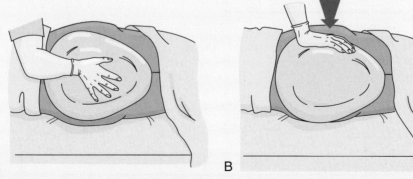

A

B

Fig. 22.5 Giving a bedpan. (A) Position the person on one side. Place the bedpan firmly against the buttocks. (B) Push downward on the bedpan and toward the person.

✲ GIVING THE BEDPAN (NATCEP)—cont'd

e. Hold the bedpan securely. Turn the person onto the back.

f. Make sure the bedpan is centered under the person.

14. Cover the person.

15. Raise the head of the bed so the person is in a sitting (Fowler) position if using a standard bedpan. (*NOTE:* Some state competency tests require that you remove gloves and wash your hands before raising the head of the bed.)

16. Make sure the person is correctly positioned on the bedpan (Fig. 22.6).

17. Raise the bed rail if used.

18. Place the toilet tissue and call light within reach.

19. Ask the person to signal when done or when help is needed.

20. Remove the gloves. Practice hand hygiene.

21. Leave the room; close the door.

22. Return when the person signals. Or check on the person every 5 minutes. Knock before entering.

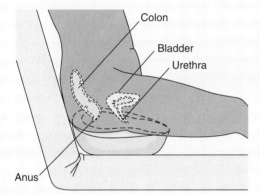

Fig. 22.6 The person is positioned on the bedpan so the urethra and anus are directly over the opening.

This skill is also covered in Clinical Skills: Nurse Assisting.

23. Practice hand hygiene. Put on gloves.

24. Raise the bed for body mechanics. Lower the bed rail (if used) and lower the head of the bed.

25. Ask the person to raise the buttocks. Remove the bedpan. Or hold the bedpan and turn the person onto the side away from you.

26. Clean the genital area if the person cannot do so. Clean from front (urethra) to back (anus) with toilet tissue. Use fresh tissue for each wipe. Provide perineal care if needed. Remove and discard the waterproof pad if using one.

27. Cover the bedpan. Take it to the bathroom. Raise the bed rail (if used) before leaving the bedside.

28. Note the color, amount, and character of urine or feces.

29. Empty the bedpan contents into the toilet and flush.

30. Rinse the bedpan. Pour the rinse into the toilet and flush.

31. Clean the bedpan with a disinfectant.

32. Remove soiled gloves. Practice hand hygiene and put on clean gloves.

33. Return the bedpan and clean cover to the bedside stand.

34. Help the person with hand washing. (Wear gloves for this step.)

35. Remove the gloves. Practice hand hygiene.

Postprocedure

36. Provide for comfort. (See the inside of the front cover.)

37. Place the call light within reach.

38. Lower the bed to its lowest position.

39. Raise or lower bed rails. Follow the care plan.

40. Unscreen the person.

41. Complete a safety check of the room. (See the inside of the front cover.)

42. Follow center policy for soiled linens.

43. Practice hand hygiene.

44. Report and record your observations.

✲ Urinals

Most urinals are used by men to void (Fig. 22.7A). There are specially designed urinals for women (see Fig. 22.7B). The female urinal has a larger opening at the top. Most women prefer to use a bedpan to void. Plastic urinals have caps and hook-type handles. The urinal hooks to the bed rail within the person's reach. The person stands to use the urinal if possible. Or the person sits on the side of the bed or lies in bed to use it. Some persons need support when standing. You may have to place and hold the urinal for some persons.

After voiding, the urinal cap is closed. This prevents urine spills. Remind the person to hang urinals on bed rails and to use the call light after using them. Remind them not to place urinals on overbed tables and bedside stands. The overbed table is used for eating and as a work surface. Bedside stands are used for supplies. These surfaces must not be contaminated with urine.

Some beds may not have bed rails. Follow center policy for where to place urinals.

See *Focus on Communication: Urinals.*

See *Delegation Guidelines: Urinals.*

See *Promoting Safety and Comfort: Urinals.*

📋 FOCUS ON COMMUNICATION

Urinals

Some people cannot use a urinal on their own. You may need to assist them and/or stay with them. For their comfort, explain why you must help them. You can say:

- "Mrs. Turner, I'll help you use your urinal. I need to stay with you to make sure you don't fall."
- "Mr. Gomez, I'll help you place and remove your urinal so it doesn't spill."

📄 DELEGATION GUIDELINES

Urinals

Before assisting with urinals, you need this information from the nurse and the care plan:

- How the urinal is used—standing, sitting, or lying in bed
- If help is needed with placing or holding the urinal
- If the person needs support to stand (If yes, how many staff members are needed?)
- If you can leave the room or if you need to stay with the person
- If the nurse needs to observe the urine before its disposal
- What observations to report and record (see *Delegation Guidelines: Bedpans,* p. 341)
- When to report observations
- What specific resident concerns to report at once

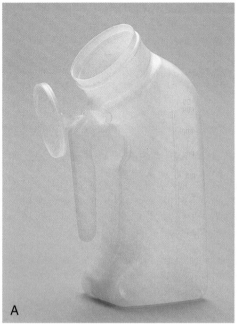
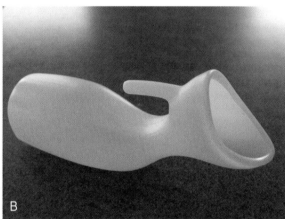

Fig. 22.7 Types of male (A) and female (B) urinals.

PROMOTING SAFETY AND COMFORT

Urinals

Safety

Urine may contain microbes and blood. Follow Standard Precautions and the Bloodborne Pathogen Standard when handling urinals and their contents. Empty them promptly to prevent odors and the spread of microbes. A filled urinal spills easily, causing safety hazards. Also, it is an unpleasant sight and a source of odor. Urinals are cleaned and disinfected like bedpans.

Comfort

You may have to place the urinal for some men. This means that you have to place the penis in the urinal. This may embarrass both the person and you. Act in a professional manner at all times.

GIVING THE URINAL

Quality of Life

Remember to:

- Knock before entering the person's room.
- Address the person by name.
- Introduce yourself by name and title.
- Explain the procedure to the person before beginning and during the procedure.
- Protect the person's rights during the procedure.
- Handle the person gently during the procedure.

Preprocedure

1. Follow Delegation Guidelines: Urinals. See *Promoting Safety and Comfort: Urinals*.
2. Provide for privacy.
3. Determine if the man will stand, sit, or lie in bed.
4. Practice hand hygiene.
5. Put on gloves.
6. Collect the following:
   - Urinal
   - Nonskid footwear if the person will stand to void

Procedure

7. Give the person the urinal if in bed. Remind the person to tilt the bottom down to prevent spills.

8. If the person is going to stand:
   a. Help to sit on the side of the bed.
   b. Put on the person nonskid footwear.
   c. Help the person stand. Provide support if the person is unsteady.
   d. Give the person the urinal.
9. Position the urinal if necessary. For a male, position his penis in the urinal if he cannot do so. For a female, position the urinal closely against her genitalia.
10. Place the call light within reach. Ask the person to signal when done or needs help.
11. Provide for privacy.
12. Remove the gloves. Practice hand hygiene.
13. Leave the room and close the door.
14. Return when the person signals for you. Or check on them every 5 minutes. Knock before entering.
15. Practice hand hygiene. Put on gloves.
16. Provide perineal care if needed.
17. Close the cap on the urinal. Take it to the bathroom.
18. Note the color and clarity of urine. Note the amount of urine in milliliters.
19. Empty the urinal into the toilet and flush.
20. Rinse the urinal with cold water. Pour rinse into the toilet and flush.
21. Clean the urinal with a disinfectant.
22. Return the urinal to its proper place.

✳ GIVING THE URINAL—cont'd

23. Remove soiled gloves. Practice hand hygiene and put on clean gloves.
24. Assist with hand washing.
25. Remove the gloves. Practice hand hygiene.

Postprocedure
26. Provide for comfort. (See the inside of the front cover.)
27. Place the call light within reach.

28. Raise or lower bed rails. Follow the care plan.
29. Unscreen the person.
30. Complete a safety check of the room. (See the inside of the front cover.)
31. Follow center policy for soiled linens.
32. Practice hand hygiene.
33. Report and record your observations. Record on the intake and output (I&O) record if necessary.

This skill is also covered in *Clinical Skills: Nurse Assisting.*

✳ Commodes

A commode is a chair or wheelchair with an opening for a container (Fig. 22.8A). Persons unable to walk to the bathroom often use commodes. The commode allows a normal position for elimination. The commode arms and back provide support and help prevent falls.

Some commodes are wheeled into bathrooms and placed over toilets (Fig. 22.8B). They are useful for persons who need support when sitting. The container is removed if the commode is used with the toilet. Wheels are locked after the commode is positioned over the toilet.

See *Delegation Guidelines: Commodes.*
See *Promoting Safety and Comfort: Commodes.*

📄 DELEGATION GUIDELINES

Commodes
You need this information from the nurse and care plan when assisting with commodes:
- If the commode is used at the bedside or over the toilet
- How much help the person needs
- If you can leave the room or if you need to stay with the person

- If the nurse needs to observe urine or bowel movements
- What observations to report and record (see *Delegation Guidelines: Bedpans*, p. 341)
- When to report observations
- What specific resident concerns to report at once

👤 PROMOTING SAFETY AND COMFORT

Commodes
Safety
For commode use, transfer the person from the bed, chair, or wheelchair to the commode. Practice safe transfer procedures (Chapter 15). Use the transfer belt and lock the wheels. Remember to remove the transfer belt after the transfer. See "Transfer/Gait Belts" in Chapter 12.

Urine and feces may contain blood and microbes. Follow Standard Precautions and the Bloodborne Pathogen Standard. Thoroughly clean and disinfect the

commode container after use. Clean and disinfect the seat and other commode parts if necessary.

Comfort
After the person transfers to the commode, cover the lap and legs with a bath blanket. This provides warmth and promotes privacy.

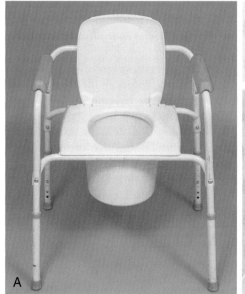
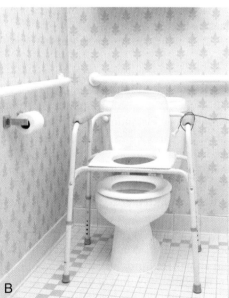

Fig. 22.8 (A) The commode has a toilet seat with a container. The container slides out from under the seat for emptying. (B) The container is removed. The commode chair is placed over the toilet.

✳ HELPING THE PERSON TO THE COMMODE

Quality of Life

Remember to:

- Knock before entering the person's room.
- Address the person by name.
- Introduce yourself by name and title.
- Explain the procedure to the person before beginning and during the procedure.
- Protect the person's rights during the procedure.
- Handle the person gently during the procedure.

Preprocedure

1. Follow Delegation Guidelines: Commodes. See *Promoting Safety and Comfort: Commodes.*
2. Provide for privacy.
3. Practice hand hygiene.
4. Put on gloves.
5. Collect the following:
   - Commode
   - Toilet tissue
   - Bath blanket
   - Transfer belt
   - Robe and nonskid footwear

Procedure

6. Bring the commode next to the bed. Remove the chair seat and container lid.
7. Help the person sit on the side of the bed. Lower the bed rail if used.
8. Help the person put on a robe and nonskid footwear.
9. Assist the person to the commode. Use the transfer belt.
10. Remove the transfer belt. Cover the person with a bath blanket for warmth.
11. Place the toilet tissue and call light within reach.
12. Ask them to signal when done or when help is needed. (Stay with the person if necessary. Be respectful. Provide as much privacy as possible.)
13. Remove the gloves. Practice hand hygiene.

14. Leave the room. Close the door.
15. Return when the person signals. Or check on the person every 5 minutes. Knock before entering.
16. Decontaminate your hands. Put on the gloves.
17. Help the person clean the genital area as needed. Remove the gloves and practice hand hygiene.
18. Apply the transfer belt. Help the person back to bed using the transfer belt. Remove the transfer belt, robe, and footwear. Raise the bed rail if used.
19. Put on clean gloves. Remove and cover the commode container. Clean the commode.
20. Take the container to the bathroom.
21. Observe urine and feces for color, amount, and character.
22. Pour into graduate container if the person's output is to be measured.
23. Empty the container contents into the toilet and flush.
24. Rinse the container. Pour the rinse into the toilet and flush.
25. Clean and disinfect the container.
26. Return the container to the commode. Return other supplies to their proper place.
27. Remove soiled gloves. Practice hand hygiene and put on clean gloves.
28. Assist with hand washing.
29. Remove the gloves. Practice hand hygiene.

Postprocedure

30. Provide for comfort. (See the inside of the front cover.)
31. Place the call light within reach.
32. Raise or lower bed rails. Follow the care plan.
33. Unscreen the person.
34. Complete a safety check of the room. (See the inside of the front cover.)
35. Follow center policy for dirty linens.
36. Practice hand hygiene.
37. Report and record your observations. Record on I&O sheet if necessary.

This skill is also covered in *Clinical Skills: Nurse Assisting.*

✳ URINARY INCONTINENCE

Urinary incontinence is the involuntary loss or leakage of urine. While it occurs in some older persons, it is not a normal part of aging. However, older persons are at risk for incontinence because of changes in the urinary tract, medical and surgical conditions, and medication therapy.

Incontinence may be temporary or permanent. The basic types of incontinence are:

- **Stress incontinence.** Urine leaks during exercise and certain movements that cause pressure on the bladder. Urine loss is small (less than 50 mL). Often called dribbling, it occurs with laughing, sneezing, coughing, lifting, or other activities. Obesity and late pregnancy also are causes. The problem is common in women and may begin during menopause. Pelvic muscles weaken from pregnancies and with aging.
- **Urge incontinence.** Urine is lost in response to a sudden, urgent need to void. The person cannot get to a toilet in time. Urinary frequency, urinary urgency, and nighttime voiding are common. Causes include urinary tract infections (UTIs), Alzheimer disease, nervous system disorders, bladder cancer, and an enlarged prostate.
- **Overflow incontinence.** Small amounts of urine leak from a full bladder. The person feels like the bladder is not empty. The person only dribbles or has a weak urine stream.

Diabetes, enlarged prostate, and spinal cord injuries are causes. Some medications may also cause this type of incontinence.

- **Functional incontinence.** The person has bladder control but cannot use the toilet in time. Immobility, restraints, unanswered call lights, no call light within reach, and not knowing where to find the bathroom are causes. Confusion, disorientation, and difficulty removing clothing are other causes.
- **Reflex incontinence.** Urine is lost at predictable intervals when the bladder is full. The person does not feel the need to void. Nervous system disorders and injuries are common causes.
- **Mixed incontinence.** The person has a combination of stress incontinence and urge incontinence. Many older women have this type.
- **Transient incontinence.** *Transient* means "for a short time." Transient incontinence refers to temporary or occasional incontinence that is reversed when the cause is treated. Common causes are delirium (Chapter 40), UTIs, some medications, increased urine production, restricted mobility, and fecal impaction (Chapter 23).

Sometimes incontinence results from intestinal, rectal, and reproductive system surgeries. Incontinence may result from a physical illness or medications. Some causes of incontinence can be reversed. Others cannot. If incontinence is a new problem, tell the nurse at once.

❖ *The Centers for Medicare & Medicaid Services (CMS) require appropriate treatment and services for persons who are incontinent. The goals are to:*
- *Prevent UTIs.*
◆ - *Restore as much normal bladder function as possible.*

Incontinence is embarrassing. Garments get wet and odors develop. The person is uncomfortable. Skin irritation, infection, and pressure injuries are risks. Falling is a risk when trying to get to the bathroom quickly. Pride, dignity, and self-esteem are affected. Social isolation, loss of independence, and depression are common. Quality of life suffers.

The person's care plan may include some of the measures listed in Box 22.2. *Good skin care and dry garments and linens are essential.* Promoting normal urinary elimination prevents incontinence in some people (see Box 22.1). Others need bladder training (p. 358). Sometimes catheters are needed (p. 350).

Incontinence products help keep the person dry (Fig. 22.9). They have several layers and a waterproof back. Fluid passes through the first layer. It is absorbed by the lower layers. The nurse suggests products that best meet the person's needs. Follow the manufacturer instructions and center procedures when using them.

Incontinence is linked to abuse, mistreatment, and neglect. Persons who are incontinent need frequent care. They may wet again right after skin care and changing wet garments and linens. Remember, incontinence is beyond the person's control. It is not something the person chooses to do. The person is often embarrassed. Be patient. The person's needs are great. If you are becoming short-tempered and impatient, talk to the nurse at once. The person has the right to be free from abuse, mistreatment, and neglect. Kindness, empathy, understanding, and patience are needed.

See *Residents with Dementia: Urinary Incontinence.*

BOX 22.2 Nursing Measures for Persons with Urinary Incontinence

- Record the person's voidings. This includes incontinent times and successful use of the toilet, commode, bedpan, or urinal.
- Answer call lights promptly. The need to void may be urgent.
- Promote normal urinary elimination (see Box 22.1).
- Promote normal bowel elimination (Chapter 23).
- Assist with elimination after sleep, before and after meals, and at bedtime.
- Follow the person's bladder training program (p. 358).
- Make sure the person has a clear pathway to the bathroom.
- Have the person wear easy-to-remove clothing. Incontinence can occur while trying to deal with buttons, zippers, other closures, and undergarments.
- Encourage the person to do pelvic muscle exercises as instructed by the nurse.
- Check the person often for cleanliness and dryness.
- Help prevent UTIs.
  - Promote fluid intake as the nurse directs.
  - Have the person wear cotton underwear.
  - Keep the perineal area clean and dry.
- Decrease fluid intake at bedtime.
- Provide good skin care.
- Apply a barrier cream or moisturizer (cream, lotion, paste) as directed by the nurse. The cream prevents irritation and skin damage.
- Provide dry garments and linens.
- Observe for signs of skin breakdown (Chapters 31 and 32).
- Use incontinence products as the nurse directs. Follow the manufacturer instructions.
- Do not leave urinals in place to catch urine in men who are incontinent.
- Keep the perineal area clean and dry (Chapter 18). Remember to:
  - Use soap and water or a no-rinse incontinence cleanser (perineal rinse). Follow the care plan. If using soap and water, remember to use a safe and comfortable water temperature and to rinse thoroughly.
  - Follow Standard Precautions and the Bloodborne Pathogen Standard.
  - Protect the person and dry garments and linens from the wet incontinence product.
  - Expose only the perineal area.
  - Dry the perineal area and buttocks.
  - Remove wet incontinence products, garments, and linen. Apply clean, dry ones.

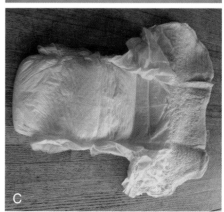
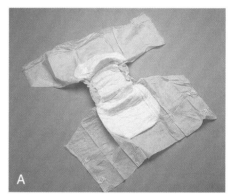
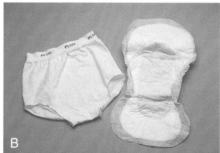

Fig. 22.9 Disposable garment protectors. (A) Complete incontinence brief. (B) Pant liner and undergarment. (C) Pull-on brief.

RESIDENTS WITH DEMENTIA

Urinary Incontinence

Persons with dementia may develop incontinence. They may void in the wrong places. Trash cans, planters, heating vents, and closets are examples. Some persons remove incontinence products and throw them on the floor or in the toilet. Other persons resist staff efforts to keep them clean and dry.

You must provide safe care for these persons. The care plan lists needed measures. The care plan may include these measures recommended by the Alzheimer's Disease Education and Referral Center (ADEAR):

- Follow the person's bathroom routine as closely as possible. For example, take the person to the bathroom every 2 to 3 hours during the day. Do not wait for the person to ask.
- Observe for signs that the person may need to void. Restlessness and pulling at clothes are examples. Respond quickly.

- Stay calm when the person is incontinent. Provide reassurance if the person becomes upset.
- Tell the nurse when the person is incontinent. Report the time, what the person was doing, and other observations. A pattern may emerge to the person's incontinence. If so, measures are planned to prevent the problem.
- Prevent episodes of incontinence during sleep. Limit the type and amount of fluids in the evening. Follow the care plan.
- Plan ahead if the person will leave the center. Have the person wear clothing that is easy to remove. Pack an extra set of clothing and incontinence products. Know where to find restrooms.

You may need a coworker's help to keep the person clean and dry. If you have questions, ask the nurse for help.

Remember, everyone has the right to safe care. They also have the right to be treated with dignity and privacy.

APPLYING AN INCONTINENCE BRIEF

Quality of Life

Remember to:

- Knock before entering the person's room.
- Address the person by name.
- Introduce yourself by name and title.
- Explain the procedure to the person before beginning and during the procedure.
- Protect the person's rights during the procedure.
- Handle the person gently during the procedure.

Preprocedure

1. Follow Delegation Guidelines Perineal Care (Chapter 18); see Promoting Safety and Comfort Perineal Care (Chapter 18).
2. Provide for privacy.
3. Practice hand hygiene.
4. Put on gloves.
5. Collect the following:
   - Correct type and size of brief for resident
   - Gloves
   - Supplies for perineal care (basin of warm water, soap, wash cloth, towel) or disposable periwipes
   - Waterproof pad
   - Bath blanket
   - Plastic trash bag

Procedure

6. Lower the head of the bed. The bed is as flat as possible.
7. Lower the bed rail near you if up.
8. Cover the person with a bath blanket. Lower top linens to the foot of the bed.
9. *To apply an incontinence brief with the person in bed:*
   a. Place a waterproof pad under the buttocks. Ask the person to raise the buttocks off the bed. Or turn the person from side to side.
   b. Loosen the tabs on each side of the soiled brief (Fig. 22.10A).
   c. Turn the person onto the side away from you.
   d. Remove the soiled brief from front to back. Observe the urine or feces as you roll the brief up (see Fig. 22.10B).
   e. Place the soiled brief in the trash bag. Set the bag aside.
   f. Remove gloves. Practice hand hygiene.
   g. Put on gloves.
   h. Perform perineal care (Chapter 18). Be sure to use facility-approved perineal cleanser and barrier cream if ordered.

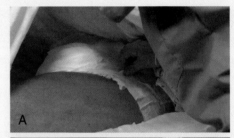
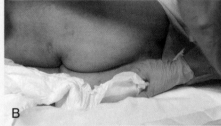
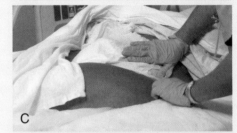
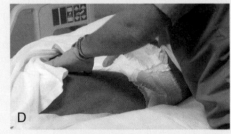

Fig. 22.10 Changing an incontinence product. (A) Loosen the tabs on each side of the soiled brief. (B) Remove the soiled brief from front to back. (C) Position the clean brief to fit the body. (D) Fasten the tape tabs. (From Mosby's Nursing Assistant Video Skills, 4.0, St. Louis, Elsevier.)

❋ APPLYING AN INCONTINENCE BRIEF—cont'd

i. Remove gloves. Practice hand hygiene.

j. Put on gloves.

k. Open the new brief. Fold it in half lengthwise along the center.

l. Insert the brief between the legs from front to back.

m. Unfold and spread the back panel.

n. Center the brief in the perineal area.

o. Turn the person onto the back.

p. Unfold and spread the front panel. Provide a "cup" shape in the perineal area. For a male, position the penis downward.

q. Make sure the brief is positioned high in the groin folds. This allows it to fit the shape of the body (see Fig. 22.10C).

r. Secure the brief by fastening the tape tabs. Pull the lower tab forward on the side near you. Attach it at a slightly upward angle. Do the same for the other side. Repeat for the upper tabs, attaching in a horizontal manner (see Fig. 22.10D).

s. Smooth out all wrinkles and folds.

t. Remove and discard gloves.

u. Practice hand hygiene.

10. *To apply a pad and undergarment with the person in bed:*

a. Place a waterproof pad under the buttocks. Ask the person to raise the buttocks off the bed. Or turn the person from side to side.

b. Turn the person onto the side away from you.

c. Pull the undergarment down. The waistband is over the knee.

d. Remove the pad from front to back. Observe the urine or feces as you roll the pad up.

e. Place the soiled pad in the trash bag. Remove gloves. Set the bag aside.

f. Perform hand hygiene.

g. Put on gloves.

h. Perform perineal care (Chapter 18). Be sure to use facility-approved perineal cleanser and barrier cream if ordered.

i. Remove gloves. Practice hand hygiene.

j. Put on gloves.

k. Fold the new pad in half lengthwise along the center.

l. Insert the pad between the legs from front to back.

m. Unfold and spread the back panel.

n. Center the pad in the perineal area (Fig. 22.11).

o. Pull the undergarment up at the back.

p. Check and adjust the pad and undergarment for a good fit.

11. *To apply pull-on underwear (briefs) with the person standing:*

a. Help the person put on nonskid footwear.

b. Help the person stand.

c. Tear the side seams to remove the soiled pull-on brief.

d. Remove the brief from front to back. Observe the urine or feces as you roll the brief up.

e. Place the brief in the trash bag. Remove your gloves. Set the bag aside.

f. Practice hand hygiene.

g. Perform perineal care (Chapter 18). Be sure to use facility-approved perineal cleanser and barrier cream if ordered.

h. Remove gloves. Practice hand hygiene.

i. Put on gloves. Place a waterproof pad on the bed.

j. Have the person sit on the side of the bed on a waterproof pad.

k. Slide the pull-on brief over the feet to past the knees (Fig. 22.12).

l. Help the person stand.

m. Pull the brief up.

n. Check for a good fit.

o. Discard waterproof pad. Remove and discard gloves.

p. Practice hand hygiene.

Postprocedure

12. Provide for comfort. (See the inside of the front cover.)

13. Place the call light within reach.

14. Lower the bed to its lowest position.

15. Raise or lower bed rails. Follow the care plan.

16. Clean, dry, and return equipment to its proper place. Discard disposable items. (Wear gloves for this step.) Never leave a trash bag with a soiled brief in the person's room. Tie up the plastic bag and take it to the proper place for disposal.

17. Unscreen the person.

18. Complete a safety check of the room. (See the inside of the front cover.)

19. Follow center policy for soiled linens.

20. Remove the gloves. Practice hand hygiene.

21. Report and record your observations

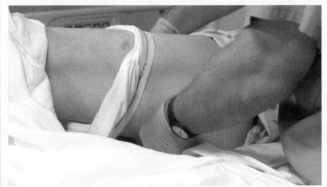

Fig. 22.11 Center the pad in the perineal area. (From Mosby's Nursing Assistant Video Skills, 4.0, St. Louis, Elsevier.)

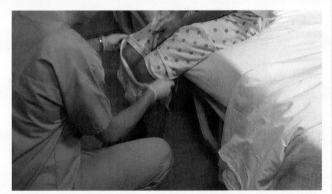

Fig. 22.12 Slide the pull-on brief over the feet past the knees. (From Mosby's Nursing Assistant Video Skills, 4.0, St. Louis, Elsevier.)

CATHETERS

A catheter is a tube used to drain or inject fluid through a body opening. Inserted through the urethra into the bladder, a urinary catheter drains urine.

- A straight catheter drains the bladder and then is removed.
- An indwelling catheter (retention catheter or Foley catheter) is left in the bladder. Urine drains constantly into a drainage bag. A balloon near the tip is inflated with sterile water after the catheter is inserted. The balloon prevents the catheter from slipping out of the bladder (Fig. 22.13). Tubing connects the catheter to the drainage bag.
- An external catheter is a catheter placed on the outside of the body to collect urine.

Catheterization is the process of inserting a catheter. It is done by a doctor, nurse, or other health care provider. With the proper education and supervision, some states and centers let nursing assistants insert or remove catheters.

Catheters often are used before, during, and after surgery. They keep the bladder empty. This reduces the risk of bladder injury during surgery. After surgery, a full bladder causes pressure on nearby organs. Such pressure can lead to pain or discomfort. A bladder scanner is a piece of equipment that can help tell the nurse the amount of urine that is in the bladder (Fig. 22.14). It is often used to determine whether the person will need a catheter to help empty the bladder.

Some people are too weak or disabled to use the bedpan, urinal, commode, or toilet. Dying persons are examples. For them, catheters can promote comfort and prevent incontinence. Catheters can protect wounds and pressure injuries from contact with urine. They also allow hourly urinary output measurements. However, they are a last resort for incontinence. Catheters do not treat the cause of incontinence.

Catheters also are used to:

- Collect sterile urine specimens.
- Measure the amount of urine left in the bladder after the person voids. This is called *residual urine.*

You will care for persons with indwelling catheters. The risk of CAUTI (catheter-associated urinary tract infection) is high. Follow the rules in Box 22.3 to promote safety and comfort.

CMS surveyors will determine if the person is receiving appropriate treatment and services. The surveyor may ask you questions about:

- Your understanding of the person's bladder management program.
- Your training related to handling catheters, catheter tubing, drainage bags, catheter care, CAUTIs, catheter-related injuries, dislodgement, and skin breakdown.
- What observations to report, when to report them, and to whom you should report them.

See *Delegation Guidelines: Catheters.*
See *Promoting Safety and Comfort: Catheters.*

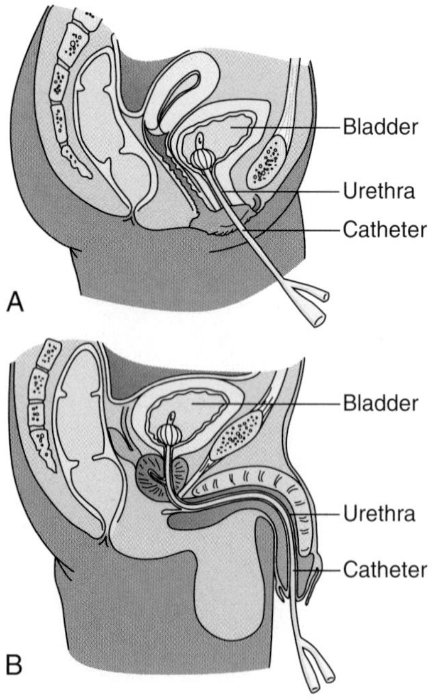

Fig. 22.13 Indwelling catheter. (A) Indwelling catheter in the female bladder. The inflated balloon at the tip prevents the catheter from slipping out through the urethra. (B) Indwelling catheter with the balloon inflated in the male bladder.

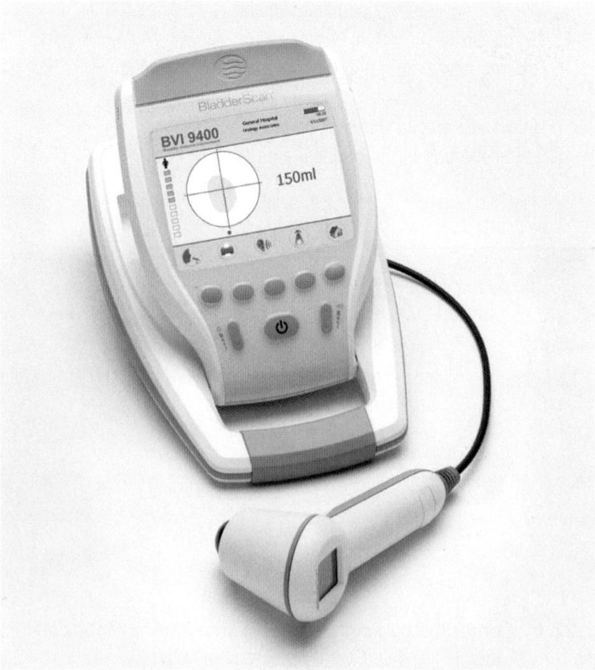

Fig. 22.14 A bladder scanner. (Courtesy Verathon Corporation, Bothell, WA.)

DELEGATION GUIDELINES

Catheters

The nurse may delegate catheter care to you. If so, you need this information from the nurse and the care plan:

- When to give catheter care—daily, twice a day, after bowel movements, or when vaginal discharge is present
- Where to secure the catheter—thigh or abdomen
- How to secure the catheter—tube holder, tape, or other device
- How to secure drainage tubing—clip, bed sheet clamp, tape, safety pin with rubber band, or other device
- What observations to report and record:

- Complaints of pain, burning, irritation, or the need to void (report at once)
- Crusting, abnormal drainage, or secretions
- The color, clarity, and odor of urine
- Particles in the urine
- Blood in the urine
- Cloudy urine
- Urine leaking at the insertion site
- Drainage system leaks
- When to report observations
- What specific resident concerns to report at once

PROMOTING SAFETY AND COMFORT

Catheters
Safety

Urine may contain microbes and blood. Follow Standard Precautions and the Bloodborne Pathogen Standard.

Be very careful when using a safety pin and rubber band to secure the drainage tubing to the bottom linens:

- Check the safety pin and rubber band.
- The safety pin must work properly. It must not be stretched out of shape.
- The rubber band must be intact. It should not be frayed or overstretched.

- Do not insert the pin through the catheter.
- Point the pin away from the person.

Comfort

The catheter must not pull at the insertion site. This causes discomfort and irritation. Hold the catheter securely during catheter care. Then properly secure the catheter. Make sure the tubing is not under the person. Besides obstructing urine flow, lying on the tubing is uncomfortable. It can also cause skin breakdown. To promote comfort, see Box 22.3.

BOX 22.3 Caring for Persons With Indwelling Catheters

- Follow the rules of medical asepsis.
- Follow Standard Precautions and the Bloodborne Pathogen Standard.
- Allow urine to flow freely through the catheter or tubing. Tubing should not have kinks. The person should not lie on the tubing.
- Keep the catheter connected to the drainage tubing. Follow the measures on p. 354 if the catheter and drainage tube are disconnected.
- Keep the drainage tube below the bladder. This prevents urine from flowing backward into the bladder.
- Move the bag to the other side of the bed when the person is turned and repositioned on the other side.
- Attach the drainage bag to the bed frame, back of the chair, or lower part of an intravenous (IV) pole. *Never attach the drainage bag to the bed rail.* Otherwise it is higher than the bladder when the bed rail is raised.
- Do not let the drainage bag rest on the floor. This can contaminate the system.
- Coil the drainage tubing on the bed. Secure it to the bottom linen (Fig. 22.15). Follow center policy. Use a clip, bed sheet clamp, tape, safety pin with rubber band, or other device as directed by the nurse. Tubing must not loop below the drainage bag.
- Secure the catheter to the inner thigh or secure it to the man's abdomen (see Fig. 22.15). This prevents excess catheter movement and friction at the insertion site. Secure the catheter with a tube holder (Fig. 22.16), tape, or other devices as the nurse directs.
- Check for leaks. Check the site where the catheter connects to the drainage bag. Report any leaks to the nurse at once.
- Provide catheter care according to the care plan—daily, twice a day, after bowel movements, or when vaginal discharge is present. (See procedure:

Giving Catheter Care, p. 352). Some centers consider perineal care to be sufficient. Follow the care plan.
- Provide perineal care daily or twice a day, after bowel movements, and when there is vaginal drainage. Follow the care plan.
- Empty the drainage bag at the end of the shift or as the nurse directs. Measure and record the amount of urine (see procedure: Emptying a Urinary Drainage Bag, p. 356). Report an increase or decrease in the amount of urine.
- When transporting the person in a wheelchair, place the drainage bag in a cover or holder (Fig. 22.17) to promote dignity.
- Use a separate measuring container for each person. This prevents the spread of microbes from one person to another.
- Do not let the drain on the drainage bag touch any surface.
- Encourage fluid intake as directed by the nurse and the care plan.
- Report complaints to the nurse at once—pain, burning, the need to void, or irritation. Also report the color, clarity, and odor of urine and the presence of particles.
- Observe for signs and symptoms of a CAUTI. Report the following at once:
  - Fever
  - Chills
  - Flank pain or tenderness (The flank area is in the back between the ribs and the hip.)
  - Change in the urine—blood, foul smell, particles, cloudiness, oliguria
  - Change in mental or functional status—confusion, decreased appetite, falls, decreased activity, tiredness, and so on
  - Urine leakage around the catheter

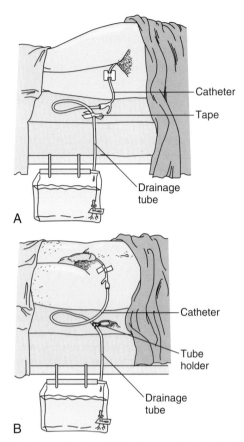

A

B

Fig. 22.15 Securing catheters. (A) The drainage tube is coiled on the bed and secured to the bottom linens. The catheter is secured to the inner thigh with a tube holder. Drainage tubing is secured to bottom linens with tape. (B) The catheter is secured to the man's abdomen with tape. Drainage tubing is secured to bottom linens with a clamp.

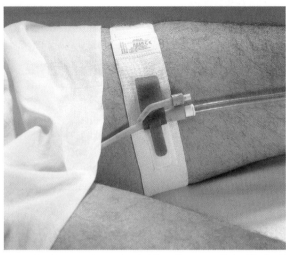

Fig. 22.16 A urinary catheter leg holder. (Courtesy Dale Medical Products, Inc, Planeville, MA.)

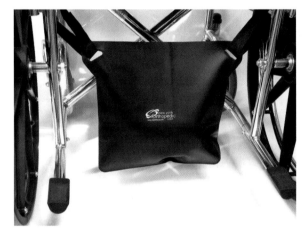

Fig. 22.17 A urine drainage bag holder for wheelchair. (Courtesy New York Orthopedic, New York, NY.)

✳ GIVING CATHETER CARE (NATCEP)

Quality of Life

Remember to:
- Knock before entering the person's room.
- Address the person by name.
- Introduce yourself by name and title.
- Explain the procedure to the person before beginning and during the procedure.
- Protect the person's rights during the procedure.
- Handle the person gently during the procedure.

Preprocedure

1. Follow Delegation Guidelines:
   a. *Perineal Care* (Chapter 18)
   b. *Catheters*
   See Promoting Safety and Comfort:
   a. *Perineal Care* (Chapter 18)
   b. *Catheters*
2. Practice hand hygiene.
3. Collect the following:
   - Items for perineal care (Chapter 18)
   - Gloves
   - Bath blanket

4. Cover the overbed table with paper towels. Arrange items on top of them.
5. Identify the person. Check the identification (ID) bracelet against the assignment sheet. Also call the person by name.
6. Provide for privacy.
7. Fill the wash basin. Water temperature is about 105°F (Fahrenheit) (40.5°C [Centigrade]). Measure water temperature according to center policy. Ask the person to check the water temperature. Adjust water temperature as needed.
8. Raise the bed for body mechanics. Bed rails are up if used.

Procedure

9. Lower the bed rail near you if up.
10. Decontaminate your hands. Put on the gloves.
11. Cover the person with a bath blanket. Fan-fold top linens to the foot of the bed.
12. Drape the person for perineal care (Chapter 18).
13. Fold back the bath blanket to expose the genital area.
14. Place the waterproof pad under the buttocks. Ask the person to flex the knees and raise the buttocks off the bed.
15. Separate the labia (female). In an uncircumcised male, retract the foreskin (Fig. 22.18). Check for crusts, abnormal drainage, or secretions.
16. Give perineal care (Chapter 18).

GIVING CATHETER CARE (NATCEP)—cont'd

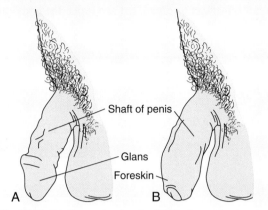

Fig. 22.18 (A) Circumcised male. (B) Uncircumcised male.

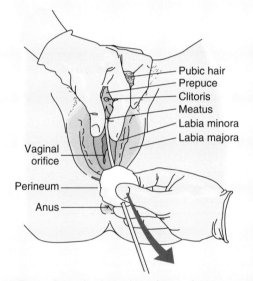

Fig. 22.19 The catheter is cleaned starting at the meatus. About 4 inches of the catheter are cleaned.

17. Apply soap to a clean, wet washcloth.
18. Hold the catheter near the meatus.
19. Clean the catheter from the meatus down the catheter about 4 inches (Fig. 22.19). Clean downward, away from the meatus with one stroke. Do not tug or pull on the catheter. Repeat as needed with a clean area of the washcloth. Use a clean washcloth if needed.
20. Rinse the catheter with a clean washcloth. Rinse from the meatus down the catheter about 4 inches. Rinse downward, away from the meatus with one stroke. Do not tug or pull on the catheter. Repeat as needed with a clean area of the washcloth. Use a clean washcloth if needed.
21. Dry the catheter with a towel. Dry from the meatus down the catheter about 4 inches. Do not tug or pull on the catheter.
22. Pat dry the perineal area. Dry from front to back.
23. Return the foreskin to its natural position.
24. Secure the catheter. Coil and secure tubing (see Fig. 22.15).
25. Remove the waterproof pad.
26. Cover the person. Remove the bath blanket.
27. Remove the gloves. Practice hand hygiene.

Postprocedure
28. Provide for comfort. (See the inside of the front cover.)
29. Place the call light within reach.
30. Lower the bed to its lowest position.
31. Raise or lower bed rails. Follow the care plan.
32. Clean, dry, and return equipment to its proper place. Discard disposable items. (Wear gloves for this step.)
33. Unscreen the person.
34. Complete a safety check of the room. (See the inside of the front cover.)
35. Follow center policy for soiled linens.
36. Remove the gloves. Practice hand hygiene.
37. Report and record your observations (Fig. 22.20).

Date	Time	Nursing Margin	Other Depts Margin
12/21	0900	Catheter care given. No drainage from around the catheter. Resident denies discomfort. Clear amber urine flowing freely. Catheter secured to abdomen with tape. Drainage tubing attached to bed with clip. Resident positioned on L side. Bed in low position. Call light within reach. Adam Aims, CNA ———	

Fig. 22.20 Charting sample.

This skill is also covered in *Clinical Skills: Nurse Assisting.*

Drainage Systems

A closed drainage system is used for indwelling catheters. Nothing can enter the system from the catheter to the drainage bag. The urinary system is sterile. Infection can occur if microbes enter the drainage system. The microbes travel up the tubing or catheter into the bladder and kidneys. A CAUTI can threaten health and life.

The drainage system has drainage tubing and a drainage bag (see Fig. 22.15). Tubing attaches at one end to the catheter. At the other end, it attaches to the drainage bag.

The bag hangs from the bed frame, chair, or wheelchair. It must not touch the floor. The bag is always kept lower than the person's bladder (see Fig. 22.15). Some people wear leg bags when up. The leg bag attaches to the thigh or calf (p. 356).

Microbes can grow in urine. If the drainage bag is higher than the bladder, urine can flow back into the bladder. A CAUTI can occur. *Therefore do not hang the drainage bag on a bed rail.* Otherwise when the bed rail is raised, the bag is higher than bladder level. When the person walks, the bag is held lower than the bladder.

Sometimes drainage systems are disconnected accidentally. If that happens, tell the nurse at once. Do not touch the ends of the catheter or tubing. Do the following:

- Practice hand hygiene. Put on gloves.
- Wipe the end of the tube with an antiseptic wipe.
- Wipe the end of the catheter with another antiseptic wipe.
- Do not put the ends down. Do not touch the ends after you clean them.
- Connect the tubing to the catheter.
- Discard the wipes into a biohazard bag.
- Remove the gloves. Practice hand hygiene.

Leg bags are changed to drainage bags when the person is in bed. This drainage bag stays lower than bladder level. You need to open the closed drainage system. You must prevent microbes from entering the system.

Drainage bags are emptied and urine is measured:

- At the end of every shift.
- When changing from a leg bag to a drainage bag.
- When changing from a drainage bag to a leg bag.
- When the bag is becoming full.
  See *Delegation Guidelines: Drainage Systems.*
  See *Promoting Safety and Comfort: Drainage Systems.*

📋 DELEGATION GUIDELINES

Drainage Systems

Your delegated tasks may involve urinary drainage systems. If so, you need this information from the nurse and the care plan:

- When to empty the drainage bag
- If the person uses a leg bag
- When to switch a drainage bag and leg bag
- If you should clean or discard the drainage bag
  - What observations to report and record:
  - The amount of urine measured

- The color, clarity, and odor of urine
- Particles in the urine
- Blood in the urine
- Cloudy urine
- Complaints of pain, burning, irritation, or the need to urinate
- Drainage system leaks
- When to report observations
- What specific resident concerns to report at once

👤 PROMOTING SAFETY AND COMFORT

Drainage Systems

Safety

Urine may contain microbes and blood. Follow Standard Precautions and the Bloodborne Pathogen Standard.

For the procedure: *Changing a Leg Bag to a Drainage Bag,* you will open sterile packages. You must keep sterile items free from contamination. Review "Surgical Asepsis" in Chapter 14.

A leg bag attaches to the thigh or calf (p. 356). Leg bags hold less than 1000 mL of urine. Most standard drainage bags hold at least 2000 mL of urine. Therefore leg bags fill faster than standard drainage bags. Check leg bags often. Empty the leg bag if it is becoming half full. Measure the contents.

Comfort

Having urine in a drainage bag embarrasses some people. Visitors can see the urine when they are with the person. To promote mental comfort, have visitors sit on the side away from the drainage bag. Sometimes you can empty the bag before visitors arrive. Make sure you measure, report, and record the amount of urine.

Some centers provide drainage bag holders (see Fig. 22.17). The drainage bag is placed inside the holder. Urine cannot be seen. This promotes dignity for the person.

✳️ CHANGING A LEG BAG TO A DRAINAGE BAG

Quality of Life

Remember to:

- Knock before entering the person's room.
- Address the person by name.
- Introduce yourself by name and title.
- Explain the procedure to the person before beginning and during the procedure.
- Protect the person's rights during the procedure.
- Handle the person gently during the procedure.

Preprocedure

1. Follow Delegation Guidelines: Drainage Systems. See *Promoting Safety and Comfort: Drainage Systems.*

2. Practice hand hygiene.
3. Collect the following:
   - Gloves
   - Drainage bag and tubing
   - Antiseptic wipes
   - Waterproof pad
   - Sterile cap and plug
   - Catheter clamp
   - Paper towels
   - Bedpan
   - Bath blanket
4. Arrange paper towels and equipment on the overbed table.

CHANGING A LEG BAG TO A DRAINAGE BAG—cont'd

5. Identify the person. Check the ID bracelet against the assignment sheet. Also call the person by name.
6. Provide for privacy.

Procedure

7. Have the person sit on the side of the bed.
8. Practice hand hygiene. Put on the gloves.
9. Expose the catheter and leg bag.
10. Clamp the catheter (Fig. 22.21). This prevents urine from draining from the catheter into the drainage tubing.
11. Let urine drain from below the clamp into the drainage tubing. This empties the lower end of the catheter.
12. Help the person lie down.
13. Raise the bed rails if used. Raise the bed for body mechanics.
14. Lower the bed rail near you if up.
15. Cover the person with a bath blanket. Fan-fold top linens to the foot of the bed. Expose the catheter and leg bag.
16. Place the waterproof pad under the person's leg.
17. Open the antiseptic wipes. Set them on the paper towels.
18. Open the package with the sterile cap and plug. Set the package on the paper towels. Do not let anything touch the sterile cap or plug (Fig. 22.22).
19. Open the package with the drainage bag and tubing.
20. Attach the drainage bag to the bed frame.
21. Disconnect the catheter from the drainage tubing. Do not let anything touch the ends.

22. Insert the sterile plug into the catheter end (Fig. 22.23). Touch only the end of the plug. Do not touch the part that goes inside the catheter. (If you contaminate the end of the catheter, wipe the end with an antiseptic wipe. Do so before you insert the sterile plug.)
23. Place the sterile cap on the end of the leg bag drainage tube (see Fig. 22.23). (If you contaminate the end of the tubing, wipe the end with an antiseptic wipe. Do so before you put on the sterile cap.)
24. Remove the cap from the new drainage tubing.
25. Remove the sterile plug from the catheter.
26. Insert the end of the drainage tubing into the catheter.
27. Remove the clamp from the catheter.
28. Loop the drainage tubing on the bed. Secure the tubing to the bottom linens.
29. Remove the leg bag. Place it in the bedpan.
30. Remove and discard the waterproof pad.
31. Cover the person. Remove the bath blanket.
32. Take the bedpan to the bathroom.
33. Remove the gloves. Practice hand hygiene.

Postprocedure

34. Provide for comfort. (See the inside of the front cover.)
35. Place the call light within reach.
36. Lower the bed to its lowest position.
37. Raise or lower bed rails. Follow the care plan.
38. Unscreen the person.
39. Put on clean gloves. Discard disposable items.
40. Empty the drainage bag. See procedure: *Emptying a Urinary Drainage Bag,* p. · ·.
41. Discard the drainage tubing and bag following center policy. Or clean the bag following center policy.
42. Clean and disinfect the bedpan. Place it in a clean cover.
43. Return the bedpan and other supplies to their proper place.
44. Remove the gloves. Practice hand hygiene.
45. Complete a safety check of the room. (See the inside of the front cover.)
46. Follow center policy for soiled linens.
47. Practice hand hygiene.
48. Report and record your observations.

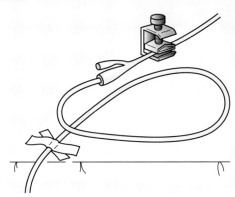

Fig. 22.21 The clamped catheter prevents urine from draining out of the bladder. The clamp is applied directly to the catheter—not to the drainage tube.

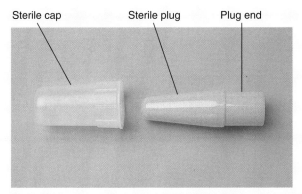

Fig. 22.22 Sterile cap and catheter plug. The inside of the cap is sterile. Touch only the end of the plug.

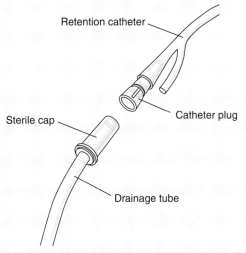

Fig. 22.23 Sterile plug inserted into the end of the catheter. The sterile cap is on the end of the drainage tube.

This skill is also covered in *Clinical Skills: Nurse Assisting.*

✳ EMPTYING A URINARY DRAINAGE BAG

Quality of Life

Remember to:

- Knock before entering the person's room.
- Address the person by name.
- Introduce yourself by name and title.
- Explain the procedure to the person before beginning and during the procedure.
- Protect the person's rights during the procedure.
- Handle the person gently during the procedure.

Preprocedure

1. Follow Delegation Guidelines: Drainage Systems, p. 354. See *Promoting Safety and Comfort: Drainage Systems,* p. 354.
2. Collect the following:
   - Graduate (measuring container)
   - Waterproof pad or plastic bag to place on floor under the graduate container
   - Gloves
   - Face shield (if required by your facility)
   - Paper towels
   - Antiseptic wipes (if required by your facility)
3. Practice hand hygiene.
4. Identify the person. Check the ID bracelet against the assignment sheet. Call the person by name.
5. Provide for privacy.

Procedure

6. Put on the gloves. (Some facilities may require wearing a face shield.)
7. Place a paper towel on the floor. Place the graduate on top of it.
8. Position the graduate under the collection bag and on a waterproof pad.
9. Open the clamp on the drain.
10. Let all urine drain into the graduate. Do not let the drain touch the graduate (Fig. 22.24).
11. Close and position the clamp.
12. Wipe the drain with an antiseptic wipe. (Not all facilities include this step.)
13. Measure urine.
14. Remove and discard the paper towel.
15. Empty the contents of the graduate into the toilet and flush.
16. Rinse the graduate. Empty the rinse into the toilet and flush.
17. Clean and disinfect the graduate.
18. Return the graduate to its proper place.

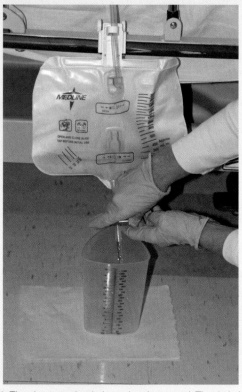

Fig. 22.24 The clamp on the drainage bag is opened. The drain is directed into the graduate. The drain must not touch the inside of the graduate. (From Cooper K: Foundations of nursing, ed 9, St Louis, 2023, Elsevier.)

19. Remove the gloves. Practice hand hygiene.
20. Record the time and amount on the I&O record (Chapter 20).

Postprocedure

21. Provide for comfort. (See the inside of the front cover.)
22. Place the call light within reach.
23. Unscreen the person.
24. Complete a safety check of the room. (See the inside of the front cover.)
25. Report and record the amount and other observations.

This skill is also covered in *Clinical Skills: Nurse Assisting.*

✳ Condom Catheters

Condom catheters are often used for incontinent men. They also are called *male external catheters, Texas catheters,* and *urinary sheaths.* A condom catheter is a soft sheath that slides over the penis. Tubing connects the condom catheter and the drainage bag. Many men prefer leg bags (Fig. 22.25).

Condom catheters are changed daily after perineal care. To apply a condom catheter, follow the manufacturer instruction. Thoroughly wash the penis with soap and water. Then dry it before applying the catheter.

Some condom catheters are self-adhering. Adhesive inside the catheter adheres to the penis. Other catheters are secured in place with elastic tape. Use the elastic tape packaged with the catheter. Elastic tape expands when the penis changes size. This allows blood flow to the penis. *Use only elastic tape. Never use*

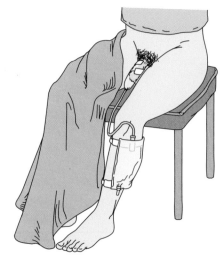

Fig. 22.25 Condom catheter attached to a leg bag.

adhesive or other tape to secure catheters. It does not expand. Blood flow to the penis is cut off, injuring the penis.

See *Delegation Guidelines: Condom Catheters.*
See *Promoting Safety and Comfort: Condom Catheters.*

📄 DELEGATION GUIDELINES

Condom Catheters

Before removing or applying a condom catheter, you need this information from the nurse and the care plan:

- What size to use—small, medium, or large
- When to remove the catheter and apply a new one
- If a leg bag or standard drainage system is used
- What observations to report and record:
  - Reddened or open areas on the penis
  - Swelling of the penis
  - Color, clarity, and odor of urine
  - Particles in the urine
  - Blood in the urine
  - Cloudy urine
- When to report observations
- What specific resident concerns to report at once

👤 PROMOTING SAFETY AND COMFORT

Condom Catheters

Safety

Do not apply a condom catheter if the penis is red, irritated, or shows signs of skin breakdown. Report your observations to the nurse at once.

If you do not know how to apply the condom catheters used by your center, ask the nurse to show you the correct application. Then ask the nurse to observe you applying the catheter.

Blood must flow to the penis. If tape is needed, use the elastic tape packaged with the catheter. Apply it in a spiral fashion.

Urine may contain microbes and blood. Follow Standard Precautions and the Bloodborne Pathogen Standard.

Comfort

To apply a condom catheter, you need to touch and handle the penis. This can embarrass the man. Some men become sexually aroused. Always act in a professional manner. If necessary, allow the man some privacy. Provide for his safety and place the urinal within reach. Tell him when you will return and then leave the room. Knock before entering the room again.

✴ APPLYING A CONDOM CATHETER

Quality of Life

Remember to:

- Knock before entering the person's room.
- Address the person by name.
- Introduce yourself by name and title.
- Explain the procedure to the person before beginning and during the procedure.
- Protect the person's rights during the procedure.
- Handle the person gently during the procedure.

Preprocedure

1. Follow *Delegation Guidelines:*
   a. *Perineal Care* (Chapter 18)
   b. *Condom Catheters*
   See *Promoting Safety and Comfort:*
   a. *Perineal Care* (Chapter 18)
   b. *Condom Catheters*
2. Practice hand hygiene.
3. Collect the following:
   - Condom catheter
   - Elastic tape
   - Drainage bag or leg bag
   - Cap for the drainage bag
   - Basin of warm water
   - Soap
   - Towel and washcloths
   - Bath blanket
   - Gloves
   - Waterproof pad
   - Paper towels

4. Cover the overbed table with paper towels. Arrange items on top of them.
5. Identify the person. Check the ID bracelet against the assignment sheet. Also call the person by name.
6. Provide for privacy.
7. Fill the wash basin. Water temperature is about 105°F (40.5°C). Measure water temperature according to center policy. Ask the person to check the water temperature. Adjust water temperature as needed.
8. Raise the bed for body mechanics. Bed rails are up if used.
   a. Procedure
9. Lower the bed rail near you if up.
10. Practice hand hygiene. Put on the gloves.
11. Cover the person with a bath blanket. Lower top linens to the knees.
12. Ask the person to raise his buttocks off the bed. Or turn him onto his side away from you.
13. Slide the waterproof pad under his buttocks.
14. Have the person lower his buttocks. Or turn him onto his back.
15. Secure the drainage bag to the bed frame. Or have a leg bag ready. Close the drain.
16. Expose the genital area.
17. Remove the condom catheter.
    1. Remove the tape. Roll the sheath off the penis.
    2. Disconnect the drainage tubing from the condom. Cap the drainage tube.
    3. Discard the tape and condom.
18. Provide perineal care (Chapter 18). Observe the penis for reddened areas, skin breakdown, and irritation.
19. Remove the gloves and practice hand hygiene. Put on clean gloves.
20. Remove the protective backing from the condom. This exposes the adhesive strip.
21. Hold the penis firmly. Roll the condom onto the penis. Leave a 1-inch space between the penis and the end of the catheter (Fig. 22.26).

Continued

✱ APPLYING A CONDOM CATHETER—cont'd

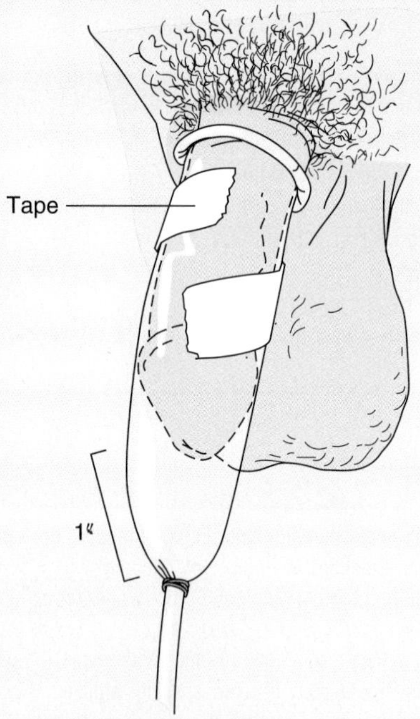

Tape

1"

Fig. 22.26 A condom catheter applied to the penis. A 1-inch space is between the penis and the end of the catheter. Elastic tape is applied in a spiral fashion to secure the condom catheter to the penis.

22. Secure the condom.
   a. For a self-adhering condom, press the condom to the penis.
   b. For a condom secured with elastic tape, apply elastic tape in a spiral fashion (see Fig. 22.26). Do not apply tape completely around the penis.
23. Make sure the penis tip does not touch the condom. Make sure the condom is not twisted.
24. Connect the condom to the drainage tubing. Coil and secure excess tubing on the bed. Or attach a leg bag.
25. Remove the waterproof pad and gloves. Discard them. Practice hand hygiene.
26. Cover the person. Remove the bath blanket.
   a. Postprocedure
27. Provide for comfort. (See the inside of the front cover.)
28. Place the call light within reach.
29. Lower the bed to its lowest position.
30. Raise or lower bed rails. Follow the care plan.
31. Unscreen the person.
32. Practice hand hygiene. Put on clean gloves.
33. Measure and record the amount of urine in the bag. Clean or discard the collection bag.
34. Clean, dry, and return the wash basin and other equipment. Return items to their proper place.
35. Remove the gloves. Practice hand hygiene.
36. Complete a safety check of the room. (See the inside of the front cover.)
37. Report and record your observations.

This skill is also covered in *Clinical Skills: Nurse Assisting*.

Female External Catheters

A recent product designed for females who experience incontinence is the female external catheter (Fig. 22.27). It is placed on the perineum of a woman (Fig. 22.28). The tubing is connected to a suction drainage container. A soft, flexible wick draws urine away from the body into a sealed collection canister. This wick is replaced every 8 to 12 hours. It is designed to be used when the woman is supine in bed. For this reason, some women may only have this applied at night. Perineal care is provided before application of the wick and after it is removed. In many centers the nurse applies the wick. The wick is always discarded after each use. Manufacturer's instructions are followed.

BLADDER TRAINING

Bladder training helps some persons with urinary incontinence. Some persons need bladder training after indwelling catheter removal. Control of urination is the goal. Bladder control

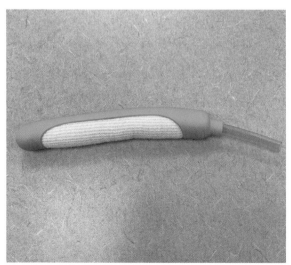

Fig 22.27 A female external catheter.

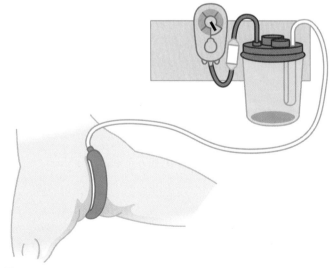

Fig. 22.28 Placement of female external catheter. (Courtesy and Copyright Becton, Dickinson and Company.)

promotes comfort and quality of life. It also increases self-esteem. You assist with bladder training as directed by the nurse and the care plan. Successful bladder training may take several weeks.

The rules for normal elimination are followed. The normal position for urination is assumed if possible. Privacy is important. The person's care plan may include one of the following:

- *Bladder retraining (bladder rehabilitation).* This requires that the person:
- Resist or ignore the strong desire to urinate.
- Postpone or delay voiding.
- Urinate following a schedule rather than the urge to void.
- The time between voidings may be increased as bladder retraining progresses.
- *Prompted voiding.* The person uses the toilet, commode, bedpan, or urinal at scheduled times. The person is taught to:

- Recognize when the bladder is full.
- Recognize the need to void.
- Ask for help.
- Respond when prompted to void.
- *Habit training/scheduled voiding.* Voiding is scheduled at regular times to match the person's voiding habits. This is usually every 3 to 4 hours while awake. The person does not delay or resist voiding. Timed voiding is based on the person's usual voiding pattern.
- *Catheter clamping.* The catheter is clamped to prevent urine flow from the bladder (see Fig. 22.21). It is usually clamped for 1 hour at first. Over time, it is clamped for 3 to 4 hours. Urine drains when the catheter is unclamped. When the catheter is removed, voiding is encouraged every 3 to 4 hours or as directed by the nurse and the care plan.

QUALITY OF LIFE

People do not usually void in front of others. Illness, disease, and aging can affect this private act. Residents often depend on the nursing staff to assist with elimination needs. Some are very weak and disabled. They cannot use the bathroom, commode, bedpan, or urinal alone.

You must protect the person's privacy. Pull privacy curtains and close doors and window coverings. If you must stay in the room, allow as much privacy as possible. Stand just outside the bathroom door in case the person needs you. Or stand on the other side of the privacy curtain if safe to do so. The nurse helps you with ways to protect the person's privacy.

Some persons can place bedpans and urinals themselves. Some can get on and off bedside commodes themselves. Other persons need some help but can be left alone to void. Allow persons to do as much as safely possible.

To safely promote independence, keep devices within reach for persons who use them without help. For persons who need some help, check on them often.

Do not leave a person sitting on a bedpan or commode for a long time. Discomfort, odors, and skin breakdown are likely. Also, the person may feel forgotten, and so try to get off the bedpan or commode alone. The person may be harmed. Make sure the call light is within reach. Respond promptly when a person calls for help.

Empty urinals, bedpans, and commodes promptly. Leaving urine-filled devices in the person's room does not respect the person's right to a neat and clean setting. It also may cause embarrassment. Do your best to promote comfort, dignity, and respect when assisting with elimination needs.

Privacy and confidentiality are important for persons who are incontinent. Incontinence is embarrassing. It affects the person's pride, dignity, and self-esteem. Only those involved in the person's care need to know about incontinence. Patience and understanding are important. Incontinence is not something the person wants or chooses.

TIME TO REFLECT

Mrs. Palmer has a urinary catheter attached to a drainage bag. During the change-of-shift report, Carol, the nursing assistant going off duty, tells you that she performed catheter care and that Mrs. Palmer's urinary output was 400 mL for her shift. Shortly after getting the report, Mrs. Palmer signals and asks if you could transport her by wheelchair to the activity room for bingo. You are glad to help Mrs. Palmer to the activity. Ten minutes later, the activity assistant calls to say that there is a pool of urine under Mrs. Palmer's wheelchair in the activity room. Mrs. Palmer is very upset and embarrassed. What could have happened to cause this accident? How should it be dealt with now? What precautions should take place so that there are no future occurrences of this type?

REVIEW QUESTIONS

Circle the BEST answer.

1. Which is *false?*
   a. Urine is normally clear and yellow or amber in color
   b. Urine normally has an ammonia odor
   c. Micturition usually occurs before going to bed and upon awakening
   d. A person normally voids 1500 mL a day
2. Which is *not* a rule for normal elimination?
   a. Help the person assume a normal position for voiding
   b. Provide for privacy
   c. Help the person to the bathroom or commode. Or provide the bedpan or urinal as soon as requested
   d. Stay with the person who uses the bedpan

3. The person using a standard bedpan is in the
   a. Fowler position
   b. Supine position
   c. Prone position
   d. Side-lying position
4. After using the urinal, the man should
   a. Put it on the bedside stand
   b. Use the call light
   c. Put it on the overbed table
   d. Empty it

5. After a person uses a commode, you should
   a. Clean and disinfect the container, seat, and commode parts
   b. Return the commode to the supply area
   c. Get a new container
   d. Get a new commode

6. Urinary incontinence
   a. Is always permanent
   b. Requires good skin care
   c. Is treated with a catheter
   d. Requires bladder training

7. Which is *not* a cause of functional incontinence?
   a. Unanswered call light
   b. No call light within reach
   c. Problems removing clothing
   d. UTI

8. A person has an indwelling catheter. Which is *not* correct?
   a. Keep the drainage bag above the level of the bladder
   b. Keep drainage tubing free of kinks
   c. Coil the drainage tubing on the bed
   d. Secure the catheter according to center policy

9. A person has an indwelling catheter. Which is *not* correct?
   a. Tape any leaks at the connection site
   b. Follow Standard Precautions and the Bloodborne Pathogen Standard
   c. Empty the drainage bag at the end of your shift
   d. Report complaints of pain, burning, the need to void, or irritation at once

10. A person has an indwelling catheter. You are going to turn the person from the left side to the right side. What should you do with the drainage bag?
    a. Hang it from an IV pole
    b. Keep it on the left side
    c. Move it to the right side
    d. Remove the catheter and the drainage bag

11. When giving catheter care, you clean the catheter
    a. From the meatus down the catheter about 4 inches
    b. From the meatus down the entire catheter
    c. From the drainage tube connection up the catheter to the meatus
    d. From the drainage tube connection up the catheter about 4 inches

12. Mr. Cooper has a condom catheter. You apply elastic tape
    a. Completely around the penis
    b. To the inner thigh
    c. To the abdomen
    d. In a spiral fashion

13. The goal of bladder training is to
    a. Remove the catheter
    b. Clamp the catheter
    c. Allow the person to walk to the bathroom
    d. Gain control of urination

14. A person is taught to ignore the urge to void. This type of bladder training is called
    a. Bladder retraining
    b. Prompted voiding
    c. Habit training
    d. Scheduled voiding

15. When applying an incontinence product, what part should you place in the person's perineal area?
    a. The front
    b. The back
    c. The center
    d. The plastic backing

See Appendix A for answers to these questions.

23

Bowel Elimination

OBJECTIVES

- Define the key terms and key abbreviations listed in this chapter.
- Describe normal defecation.
- List the observations to make about defecation.
- Identify the factors that affect bowel elimination.
- Describe the common bowel elimination problems.
- Explain how to promote comfort and safety during defecation.
- Describe bowel training.
- Explain why enemas are given.
- Describe the common enema solutions.
- Describe the rules for giving enemas.
- Describe how to care for a person with an ostomy.
- Perform the procedures described in this chapter.
- Explain how to promote quality of life.

KEY TERMS

colostomy A surgically created opening (*-stomy*) between the colon (*colo-*) and abdominal wall

constipation The passage of a hard, dry stool

defecation The process of excreting feces from the rectum through the anus; bowel movement

dehydration The excessive loss of water from tissues

diarrhea The frequent passage of liquid stools

enema The introduction of fluid into the rectum and lower colon

fecal impaction The prolonged retention and buildup of feces in the rectum

fecal incontinence The inability to control the passage of feces and gas through the anus

feces The semisolid mass of waste products in the colon that is expelled through the anus

flatulence The excessive formation of gas or air in the stomach and intestines

flatus Gas or air passed through the anus

ileostomy A surgically created opening (*-stomy*) between the ileum (small intestine [*ileo-*]) and the abdominal wall

melena Black, tarry stools caused by gastrointestinal bleeding

ostomy A surgically created opening for the elimination of body wastes; see "colostomy" and "ileostomy"

peristalsis The alternating contraction and relaxation of intestinal muscles

stoma An opening that can be seen through the abdominal wall; see "colostomy" and "ileostomy"

stool Excreted feces

suppository A cone-shaped, solid medication that is inserted into a body opening; it melts at body temperature

KEY ABBREVIATIONS

BM Bowel movement
C Centigrade
F Fahrenheit
GI Gastrointestinal
ID Identification

IV Intravenous
mL Milliliter
oz Ounce
SSE Soapsuds enema
TWE Tapwater enema

Bowel elimination is a basic physical need. It is the excretion of wastes from the gastrointestinal (GI) system (Chapter 8). Many factors affect bowel elimination. They include privacy, habits, age, diet, exercise and activity, fluids, and medications. Problems easily occur. Promoting normal bowel elimination is important. You assist residents in meeting elimination needs.

NORMAL BOWEL ELIMINATION

Foods and fluids are partially digested in the stomach. The partially digested food and fluids are called *chyme*. Chyme passes from the stomach into the small intestine. It enters the large intestine (large bowel or colon) where fluid is absorbed. Chyme becomes less fluid and more solid in consistency. Feces refers to the semisolid mass of waste products in the colon that is expelled through the anus.

Feces move through the intestines by peristalsis. Peristalsis is the alternating contraction and relaxation of intestinal muscles. The feces move through the large intestine to the rectum. Feces are stored in the rectum until excreted from the body. Defecation (bowel movement [BM]) is the process of excreting feces from the rectum through the anus. Stool refers to excreted feces.

Some people have a BM every day. Others have one every 2 to 3 days. Some people have two or three BMs a day. Many people have a BM after breakfast. Others do so in the evening. Many older persons expect to have a BM every day. They are very concerned if they do not have one. The nurse teaches them about normal elimination.

Stools are normally brown. Bleeding in the stomach and small intestine causes black or tarry stools (melena). Bleeding in the lower colon and rectum causes red stools, as do beets, tomato juice or soup, red gelatin, and foods with red food coloring. A diet high in green vegetables can cause green stools. Diseases and infection can cause clay-colored or white, pale, orange, or green stools.

Stools are normally soft, formed, moist, and shaped like the rectum. They have a normal odor caused by bacterial action in the intestines. Certain foods and medications also cause odors.

Observations

Your observations are used for the nursing process. Carefully observe stools before disposing of them. Ask the nurse to observe abnormal stools. Observe and report the following to the nurse. If allowed to chart, also record the following:

- Color
- Amount
- Consistency
- Presence of blood or mucus
- Odor
- Shape
- Frequency of BMs
- Complaints of pain or discomfort
  See *Focus on Communication: Observations*.

FOCUS ON COMMUNICATION

Observations

Many residents tend to their own bowel elimination needs. However, information is still needed for the person's record and the nursing process. You may need to ask these questions:

- "Did you have a bowel movement today?"
- "Please tell me about your bowel movement."
- "When did you have a bowel movement?"
- "What was the amount?"
- "Were the stools formed or loose?"
- "What was the color?"
- "Did you have any bleeding, pain, or problems having a bowel movement?"
- "Did you pass any gas?"
- "How much gas did you pass?"
- "Do you need to pass more gas?"
- "Do you need help cleaning yourself?"

FACTORS AFFECTING BOWEL ELIMINATION

These factors affect stool frequency, consistency, color, and odor. The nurse considers them when using the nursing process to meet the person's elimination needs. Normal, regular elimination is the goal.

- *Privacy.* Bowel elimination is a private act. Odors and sounds are embarrassing. Lack of privacy can prevent a BM despite having the urge. Some people ignore the urge when others are present.
- *Habits.* Many people have a BM after breakfast. Some drink a hot beverage, read, or take a walk. These activities are relaxing. A BM is easier when a person is relaxed, not tense.
- *Diet—high-fiber foods.* High-fiber foods leave a residue for needed bulk. Fruits, vegetables, and whole-grain cereals and breads are high in fiber. Many people do not eat enough fruits and vegetables. Some cannot chew these foods. They may not have teeth, or dentures may fit poorly. Some people think they cannot digest fruits and vegetables so they refuse to eat them. In nursing centers, bran may be added to cereal, prunes, or prune juice. These foods provide fiber and prevent constipation.
- *Diet—other foods.* Milk and milk products can cause constipation or diarrhea. Chocolate and other foods cause similar reactions. Spicy foods can irritate the intestines. Frequent stools or diarrhea can result. Gas-forming foods stimulate peristalsis, which aids a BM. Such foods include onions, beans, cabbage, cauliflower, radishes, and cucumbers.
- *Fluids.* Feces contain water. Stool consistency depends on the amount of water absorbed in the colon. The amount of fluid intake, urine output, and vomiting are factors. Feces harden and dry when large amounts of water are absorbed or when fluid intake is poor. Hard, dry feces move slowly through the colon. Constipation can occur. Drinking 6 to 8 glasses of water daily promotes normal bowel elimination. Warm fluids—coffee, tea, hot cider, warm water—increase peristalsis.
- *Activity.* Exercise and activity maintain muscle tone and stimulate peristalsis. Irregular elimination and constipation often occur from inactivity and bedrest. Inactivity may result from disease, surgery, injury, and aging.
- *Medications.* Medications can prevent constipation or control diarrhea. Other medications have diarrhea or constipation as side effects. Medications for pain relief often cause constipation. Antibiotics (used to fight or prevent infections) often cause diarrhea. Diarrhea occurs when the antibiotics kill normal flora in the colon. Normal flora is needed to form feces.
- *Disability.* Some people cannot control bowel movements. They have a BM whenever feces enter the rectum. A bowel training program is needed (pp. 364-365).
- *Aging.* Aging causes changes in the GI tract. Feces pass through the intestines at a slower rate. Constipation is a risk. Some older persons lose bowel control. Older persons may not completely empty the rectum. They often need to have another BM about 30 to 45 minutes after the first BM. Older persons are at risk for intestinal tumors and disorders.

Safety and Comfort

The care plan includes measures to meet the person's elimination needs. It may involve diet, fluids, and exercise. Follow the measures in Box 23.1 to promote safety and comfort.

BOX 23.1 Safety and Comfort During Bowel Elimination

- Follow Standard Precautions and the Bloodborne Pathogen Standard.
- Provide for privacy. Ask visitors to leave the room. Close doors, privacy curtains, and window coverings.
- Help the person to the toilet or commode. Or provide the bedpan as soon as requested.
- Wheel the person into the bathroom on the commode if possible. Place the commode over the toilet. This provides privacy. Remember to lock the commode wheels.
- Make sure the bedpan is warm.
- Position the person in a normal sitting or squatting position.
- Cover the person for warmth and privacy.
- Allow enough time for a BM.
- Place the call light and toilet tissue within reach.
- Leave the room if the person can be alone. Check on the person every 5 minutes.
- Stay nearby if the person is weak or unsteady.
- Provide perineal care.
- Dispose of stools promptly, to reduce odors and prevent the spread of microbes.
- Assist the person with hand washing after elimination.
- Follow the care plan if the person has fecal incontinence. The care plan tells you when to assist with elimination.

See *Teamwork and Time Management: Safety and Comfort.*

TEAMWORK AND TIME MANAGEMENT

Safety and Comfort

The need to have a BM may be urgent. Answer call lights promptly. Also help coworkers answer call lights. Residents must not be left sitting on toilets, commodes, or bedpans. They must not be left sitting or lying in stools.

COMMON PROBLEMS

Common problems include constipation, fecal impaction, diarrhea, fecal incontinence, and flatulence.

Constipation

Constipation is the passage of a hard, dry stool. The person usually strains to have a BM. Stools are large or marble sized. Large stools cause pain as they pass through the anus. Constipation occurs when feces move slowly through the bowel. This allows more time for water absorption. Common causes of constipation include the following:

- A low-fiber diet
- Ignoring the urge to have a BM
- Decreased fluid intake
- Inactivity
- Medications
- Aging
- Certain diseases

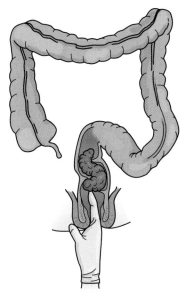

Fig. 23.1 A gloved index finger is used to check for a fecal impaction.

Dietary changes, fluids, and activity prevent or relieve constipation, as do medications and enemas.

Fecal Impaction

A fecal impaction is the prolonged retention and buildup of feces in the rectum. Feces are hard or puttylike. Fecal impaction results if constipation is not relieved. The person cannot defecate. More water is absorbed from the already hard feces. Liquid feces pass around the hardened fecal mass in the rectum. The liquid feces seep from the anus.

The person tries many times to have a BM. Abdominal discomfort, abdominal distention (swelling), nausea, cramping, and rectal pain are common. Older persons may have poor appetite or confusion. Some persons may have a fever. Report these signs and symptoms to the nurse.

The nurse does a digital (finger) exam to check for an impaction. A lubricated, gloved finger is inserted into the rectum to feel for a hard mass (Fig. 23.1). The mass is felt in the lower rectum. Sometimes it is higher in the colon and out of reach. The digital exam often causes the urge to have a BM. The doctor may order medications and enemas to remove the impaction.

Sometimes the nurse removes the fecal mass with a gloved finger. This is called *digital removal of an impaction.*

Diarrhea

Diarrhea is the frequent passage of liquid stools. Feces move through the intestines rapidly. This reduces the time for fluid absorption. The need for a BM is urgent. Some people cannot get to a bathroom in time. Abdominal cramping, nausea, and vomiting may occur.

Causes of diarrhea include infections, some medications, irritating foods, and microbes in food and water. Diet and medications are ordered to reduce peristalsis. You need to:

- Assist with elimination needs promptly.

- Dispose of stools promptly, to prevent odors and the spread of microbes.
- Give good skin care. Liquid stools irritate the skin, as does frequent wiping with toilet tissue. Skin breakdown and pressure injuries are risks.

Fluid lost through diarrhea is replaced. Otherwise, dehydration occurs. Dehydration is the excessive loss of water from tissues. The person has pale or flushed skin, dry skin, and a coated tongue. The urine is dark and scant in amount (*oliguria*). Thirst, weakness, dizziness, and confusion also occur. Falling blood pressure and increased pulse and respirations are serious signs. Death can occur. The nursing process is used to meet the person's fluid needs. The doctor may order intravenous (IV) fluids in severe cases (Chapter 21).

Microbes can cause diarrhea. Preventing the spread of infection is important. Always follow Standard Precautions and the Bloodborne Pathogen Standard when in contact with stools.

See *Promoting Safety and Comfort: Diarrhea.*

PROMOTING SAFETY AND COMFORT

Diarrhea

Safety

Death is a risk when dehydration is not recognized and treated. Older persons are at risk for dehydration. The amount of body water decreases with aging. Therefore, diarrhea is very serious in older persons. Report signs of diarrhea at once. Ask the nurse to observe the stool.

Clostridium difficile

Clostridium difficile (*C. diff*) is a microbe that causes diarrhea and intestinal infections. It can also cause death. Persons at risk include those who are older, ill, or need the prolonged use of antibiotics. Signs and symptoms include:

- Watery diarrhea with a foul odor.
- Fever.
- Loss of appetite.
- Nausea.
- Abdominal pain or tenderness.

The microbe is found in feces. A person becomes infected by touching items or surfaces contaminated with feces and then touching the mouth or mucous membranes. You can spread the microbe if your contaminated hands or gloves:

- Touch a person.
- Contaminate surfaces.

You must practice good hand hygiene. Alcohol-based hand rubs are not effective against *C. diff*. You must wash your hands with soap and water. Also follow Standard Precautions.

Fecal Incontinence

Fecal incontinence is the inability to control the passage of feces and gas through the anus. Causes include the following:

- Intestinal diseases
- Nervous system diseases and injuries
- Fecal impaction
- Diarrhea
- Some medications
- Chronic illness
- Aging

- Mental health disorders or dementia (Chapters 39 and 40)—the person may not recognize the need for or act of having a BM
- Not answering call lights when help is needed with elimination
- Not getting to the bathroom in time
- Not finding the bathroom when in a new setting

Fecal incontinence affects the person emotionally. Frustration, embarrassment, anger, and humiliation are common. The person may need:

- Bowel training.
- Help with elimination after meals and every 2 to 3 hours.
- Incontinence products to keep garments and linens clean (see "Applying Incontinence Products," Chapter 22).
- Good skin care.

See *Residents with Dementia: Fecal Incontinence.*

RESIDENTS WITH DEMENTIA

Fecal Incontinence

Persons with dementia may smear stools on themselves, furniture, and walls. Some are not aware of having BMs. Some resist care. Follow the person's care plan. The measures for urinary incontinence (Chapter 22) may be part of the care plan. Be patient. Ask for help from coworkers. Talk to the nurse if you have problems keeping the person clean.

Flatulence

Gas and air are normally in the stomach and intestines. They are expelled through the mouth (burping, belching, eructating) and anus. Gas or air passed through the anus is called flatus. Flatulence is the excessive formation of gas or air in the stomach and intestines. Causes include the following:

- Swallowing air while eating and drinking. This includes chewing gum, eating fast, drinking through a straw, and drinking carbonated beverages. Tense or anxious people may swallow large amounts of air when drinking.
- Bacterial action in the intestines
- Gas-forming foods (onions, beans, cabbage, cauliflower, radishes, and cucumbers)
- Constipation
- Bowel and abdominal surgeries
- Medications that decrease peristalsis

If flatus is not expelled, the intestines distend. That is, they swell or enlarge from the pressure of gases. Abdominal cramping or pain, shortness of breath, and a swollen abdomen occur. "Bloating" is a common complaint. Exercise, walking, moving in bed, and the left side-lying position often produce flatus. Doctors may order enemas and medications to relieve flatulence.

BOWEL TRAINING

Bowel training has two goals:

- To gain control of bowel movements
- To develop a regular pattern of elimination, thus preventing fecal impaction, constipation, and fecal incontinence

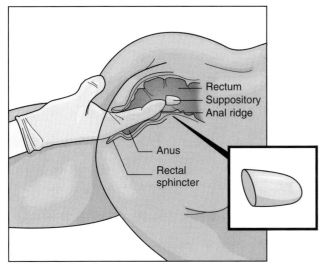

Fig. 23.2 The suppository *(inset)* is inserted into the rectum.

Meals, especially breakfast, stimulate the urge for a BM. The person's usual time of day for a BM is noted on the care plan. So is toilet, commode, or bedpan use. Offer help with elimination at the times noted. Factors that promote elimination are part of the care plan and bowel training program. These include a high-fiber diet, increased fluids, warm fluids, activity, and privacy. The nurse tells you about a person's bowel training program.

The doctor may order a suppository to stimulate a BM. A *suppository* is a cone-shaped, solid medication that is inserted into a body opening. It melts at body temperature. A nurse inserts a rectal suppository into the rectum (Fig. 23.2). A BM occurs about 30 minutes later.

ENEMAS

An *enema* is the introduction of fluid into the rectum and lower colon. Doctors order enemas to:
- Remove feces.
- Relieve constipation, fecal impaction, or flatulence.
- Clean the bowel of feces before certain surgeries and diagnostic procedures.

Safety and comfort measures for bowel elimination are practiced when giving an enema (see Box 23.1), as are the rules in Box 23.2.

The doctor orders the enema solution. The solution depends on the enema's purpose:
- *Tapwater enema (TWE)*—is obtained from a faucet.
- *Saline enema*—is a solution of salt and water. For adults, add 1 to 2 teaspoons of table salt to 500 to 1000 milliliters (mL) of tapwater.
- *Soapsuds enema (SSE)*—for adults, add 3 to 5 mL of castile soap to 500 to 1000 mL of tapwater.
- *Small-volume enema*—the adult size contains about 120 mL (4 ounces [oz]) of solution. The commercially prepared enema is ready to use.
- *Oil-retention enema*—has mineral, olive, or cottonseed oil. The adult size contains about 120 mL (4 oz) of solution. The commercially prepared enema is ready to use.

Other enema solutions may be ordered. Consult with the nurse and use the center's procedure manual to safely prepare and give enemas. You do not give enemas that contain medications. Nurses give them.

See *Delegation Guidelines: Enemas.*
See *Promoting Safety and Comfort: Enemas.*

DELEGATION GUIDELINES

Enemas

Some states and centers let nursing assistants give enemas. Others do not. Before giving an enema, make sure that:
- Your state allows you to perform the procedure.
- The procedure is in your job description.
- You have the necessary education and training.
- You review the procedure with the nurse.
- A nurse is available to answer questions and to supervise you.
- If the abovementioned conditions are met, you need this information from the nurse:
- What type of enema to give—cleansing, small volume, or oil retention
- What size enema tube to use
- When to give the enema
- How many times to repeat the enema
- The amount of solution ordered by the doctor—usually 500 to 1000 mL for a cleansing enema (for adults)
- How much castile soap to use for an SSE
- How much salt to use for a saline enema

- What the solution temperature should be—usually body temperature (98.6°F [Fahrenheit] or 37°C [Centigrade]); sometimes warmer temperatures (105°F [40.5°C]) are used for adults
- How to position the person—the left side-lying position
- How far to insert the enema tubing—usually 2 to 4 inches for adults
- How high to hold the solution container—usually 12 inches above the anus
- How fast to give the solution—750 to 1000 mL are usually given over 10 to 15 minutes
- How long the person should try to retain the solution
- What to report and record:
  - The amount of solution given
  - If you noted bleeding or resistance when inserting the tube
  - How long the person retained the enema solution
  - Color, amount, consistency, shape, and odor of stools
  - Complaints of cramping, pain, or discomfort
  - Complaints of nausea or weakness
  - How the person tolerated the procedure
- When to report observations
- What specific resident concerns to report at once

BOX 23.2 Safety and Comfort Measures for Giving Enemas

- Have the person void first. This increases the person's comfort during the enema procedure.
- Cover the person with a bath blanket.
- Measure solution temperature with a bath thermometer. See *Delegation Guidelines: Enemas*.
- Give the amount of solution ordered.
- Position the person as the nurse directs. The left side-lying position is preferred.
- Ask the nurse and check the procedure manual for how far to insert the enema tubing. It is usually inserted 2 to 4 inches in adults.
- Lubricate the enema tip before inserting it.
- Stop tube insertion if you feel resistance, the person complains of pain, or bleeding occurs.

- Ask the nurse how high to raise the enema bag. For adults, it is usually held 12 inches above the anus.
- Give the solution slowly. Usually it takes 10 to 15 minutes to give 750 to 1000 mL.
- Hold the enema tube in place while giving the solution.
- Ask the nurse how long the person should retain the solution. The length of time depends on the amount and type of solution.
- Make sure the bathroom will be vacant when the person needs to defecate. Make sure that another person will not use the bathroom. If the person uses the commode, have the commode ready. Always have a bedpan handy in case the person cannot get to the bathroom or commode in time.
- Ask the nurse to observe the enema results.

PROMOTING SAFETY AND COMFORT

Enemas

Safety

Enemas are usually safe procedures. Many people give themselves enemas at home. However, enemas are dangerous for older persons and those with certain heart and kidney diseases.

Contact with stools is likely when giving enemas. They contain microbes and may contain blood. Follow Standard Precautions and the Bloodborne Pathogen Standard.

Comfort

Before starting the procedure, ensure that the bathroom is ready for the person's use. If the person will use the commode or bedpan, make sure the device is ready. Always keep a bedpan nearby in case the person starts to expel the enema solution and stools. Mental comfort is promoted when the person knows that the bathroom, commode, or bedpan is ready for use.

Make sure the person is comfortable in the left semiprone side position. When comfortable, it is easier for the person to tolerate the procedure.

To prevent cramping:
- Use the correct water temperature. Cool water causes cramping.
- Give the solution slowly.

✳ The Cleansing Enema

Cleansing enemas clean the bowel of feces and flatus. They relieve constipation and fecal impaction. They are needed before certain surgeries and diagnostic procedures. Cleansing enemas take effect in 10 to 20 minutes.

The doctor orders a tap water, saline, or soapsuds enema. The doctor may order *enemas until clear*. This means that enemas are given until the return solution is clear and free of stools. Ask the nurse how many enemas to give. Center policy may allow repeating enemas two or three times.

Tapwater enemas can be dangerous. The colon may absorb some of the water into the bloodstream. This creates a fluid imbalance. *Only one tapwater enema is given. Do not repeat the enema.* Repeated enemas increase the risk of excessive fluid absorption.

The *saline enema* solution is similar to body fluid. However, some of the salt solution may be absorbed. This too can cause a fluid imbalance. When excess salt is in the body, the body retains water.

SSEs irritate the bowel's mucous lining. Repeated enemas can damage the bowel. So can using more than 3 to 5 mL of castile soap or stronger soaps.

✳ GIVING A CLEANSING ENEMA

Quality of Life

Remember to:
- Knock before entering the person's room.
- Address the person by name.
- Introduce yourself by name and title.
- Explain the procedure to the person before beginning and during the procedure.
- Protect the person's rights during the procedure.
- Handle the person gently during the procedure.

Preprocedure

1. Follow *Delegation Guidelines: Enemas*, p. 365. See *Promoting Safety and Comfort: Enemas*.
2. Practice hand hygiene.

3. Collect the following before going to the person's room:
   - Disposable enema kit as directed by the nurse (enema bag, tube, clamp, and waterproof pad)
   - Bath thermometer
   - Waterproof pad (if not in the enema kit)
   - Water-soluble lubricant
   - 3 to 5 mL (1 teaspoon) of castile soap or 1 to 2 teaspoons of salt
   - IV pole
   - Gloves
4. Arrange items in the person's room and bathroom.
5. Decontaminate your hands.
6. Identify the person. Check the identification (ID) bracelet against the assignment sheet. Also call the person by name.

✳ GIVING A CLEANSING ENEMA—cont'd

7. Put on gloves.
8. Collect the following:
   - Commode or bedpan and cover
   - Toilet tissue
   - Bath blanket
   - Robe and nonskid footwear
   - Paper towels
9. Provide for privacy.
10. Raise the bed for body mechanics. Bed rails are up if used.

Procedure

11. Remove the gloves and decontaminate your hands. Put on clean gloves.
12. Lower the bed rail near you if up.
13. Cover the person with a bath blanket. Fan-fold top linens to the foot of the bed.
14. Position the IV pole so the enema bag is 12 inches above the anus. Or it is at the height directed by the nurse.
15. Raise the bed rail if used.
16. Prepare the enema.
    a. Close the clamp on the tube.
    b. Adjust water flow until it is lukewarm.
    c. Fill the enema bag for the amount ordered.
    d. Measure water temperature with the bath thermometer. The nurse tells you what temperature to use.
    e. Prepare the solution as directed by the nurse.
       (1) TWE: add nothing
       (2) Saline enema: add salt as directed
       (3) SSE: add castile soap as directed
    f. Stir the solution with the bath thermometer. Scoop off any suds (SSE).
    g. Seal the bag.
    h. Hang the bag on the IV pole.
17. Lower the bed rail near you if up.
18. Position the person in a left side-lying position.
19. Place a waterproof pad under the buttocks.
20. Expose the anal area.
21. Place the bedpan behind the person.
22. Position the enema tube in the bedpan. Remove the cap from the tubing.
23. Open the clamp. Let solution flow through the tube to remove air. Clamp the tube.
24. Lubricate the tube 2 to 4 inches from the tip.
25. Separate the buttocks to see the anus.
26. Ask the person to take a deep breath through the mouth.

27. Insert the tube gently 2 to 4 inches into the adult's rectum (Fig. 23.3). Do this when the person is exhaling. Stop if the person complains of pain, you feel resistance, or bleeding occurs.
28. Check the amount of solution in the bag.
29. Unclamp the tube. Give the solution slowly (Fig. 23.4).
30. Ask the person to take slow, deep breaths. This helps the person relax.
31. Clamp the tube if the person needs to have a BM, has cramping, or starts to expel solution. Also clamp the tube if the person is sweating or complains of nausea or weakness. Unclamp when symptoms subside.
32. Give the amount of solution ordered. Stop if the person cannot tolerate the procedure.
33. Clamp the tube before it is empty. This prevents air from entering the bowel.
34. Hold toilet tissue around the tube and against the anus. Remove the tube.
35. Discard toilet tissue in the bedpan.
36. Wrap the tubing tip with paper towels. Place it inside the enema bag.
37. Assist the person to the bathroom or commode. The person wears a robe and nonskid footwear when up. The bed is in the lowest position. Or help the person onto the bedpan. Raise the head of the bed. Raise or lower bed rails according to the care plan.
38. Place the call light and toilet tissue within reach. Remind the person not to flush the toilet.
39. Discard disposable items.
40. Remove the gloves. Practice hand hygiene.
41. Leave the room if the person can be left alone.
42. Return when the person signals. Or check on the person every 5 minutes. Knock before entering the room or bathroom.
43. Decontaminate your hands and put on gloves. Lower the bed rail if up.
44. Observe enema results for amount, color, consistency, shape, and odor. Call the nurse to observe the results.
45. Provide perineal care as needed.
46. Remove the waterproof pad.
47. Empty, clean, and disinfect equipment. Flush the toilet after the nurse observes the results.
48. Return equipment to its proper place.
49. Remove the gloves and practice hand hygiene.
50. Assist with hand washing. Wear gloves for this step.

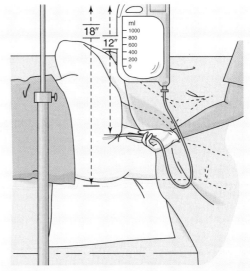

Fig. 23.4 Giving an enema. The person is in left side-lying position. The enema bag hangs from an intravenous pole. The bag is 12 inches above the anus and 18 inches above the mattress.

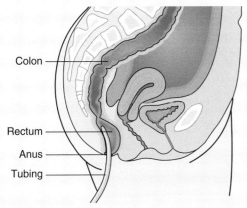

Fig. 23.3 Enema tubing inserted into the adult rectum.

Continued

✴ **GIVING A CLEANSING ENEMA—cont'd**

Date	Time	Nursing Margin	Other Depts Margin
7/8	1700	750 mL tap water enema given with the resident in the L side-lying position.	
		The resident was asked to retain the enema for at least 15 minutes. Bed in low	
		position. Call light within reach. No resident complaints at this time. Resident	
		informed that I would check on her in 5 minutes or when the call light was used.	
		Angie Martinez, CNA ————————————	
	1715	Assisted resident to the bedside commode. Privacy curtain pulled. Call light and	
		toilet tissue within reach. Resident reminded to signal when finished expelling the	
		enema or if she needs assistance. Angie Martinez, CNA ————————	

Fig. 23.5 Charting sample.

51. Cover the person. Remove the bath blanket.
    a. Postprocedure
52. Provide for comfort. (See the inside of the front cover.)
53. Place the call light within reach.
54. Lower the bed to its lowest position.
55. Raise or lower bed rails. Follow the care plan.
56. Unscreen the person.
57. Complete a safety check of the room. (See the inside of the front cover.)
58. Follow center policy for dirty linens and used supplies.
59. Practice hand hygiene.
60. Report and record your observations (Fig. 23.5).

This skill also covered in *Clinical Skills: Nurse Assisting.*

✴ The Small-Volume Enema

Small-volume enemas irritate and distend the rectum, which causes a BM. They are often ordered for constipation or when the bowel does not need complete cleansing.

These enemas are ready to give. The solution is usually given at room temperature. To give the enema, squeeze and roll up the plastic bottle from the bottom. Do not release pressure on the bottle. Otherwise, solution is drawn from the rectum back into the bottle.

Urge the person to retain the solution until there is a need to have a BM. This usually takes about 5 to 10 minutes. Staying in the Sims or left side-lying position helps retain the enema.

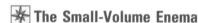

✴ GIVING A SMALL-VOLUME ENEMA

Quality of Life

Remember to:
- Knock before entering the person's room.
- Address the person by name.
- Introduce yourself by name and title.
- Explain the procedure to the person before beginning and during the procedure.
- Protect the person's rights during the procedure.
- Handle the person gently during the procedure.

Preprocedure

1. Follow *Delegation Guidelines: Enemas*, p. 365. See *Promoting Safety and Comfort: Enemas*, p. 366.
2. Practice hand hygiene.
3. Collect the following before going to the person's room:
   - Small-volume enema
   - Waterproof pad
   - Gloves
4. Arrange items in the person's room.
5. Practice hand hygiene.
6. Identify the person. Check the ID bracelet against the assignment sheet. Also call the person by name.
7. Put on gloves.
8. Collect the following:
   - Commode or bedpan
   - Waterproof pad
   - Toilet tissue
   - Robe and nonskid footwear
   - Bath blanket
9. Provide for privacy.
10. Raise the bed for body mechanics. Bed rails are up if used.

Procedure

11. Remove the gloves and practice hand hygiene. Put on clean gloves.
12. Lower the bed rail near you if up.
13. Cover the person with a bath blanket. Fan-fold top linens to the foot of the bed.
14. Position the person in the left side-lying position.

✳ GIVING A SMALL-VOLUME ENEMA—cont'd

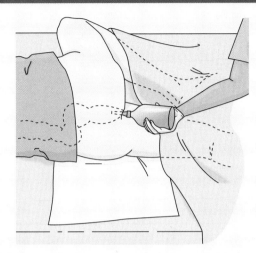

Fig. 23.6 The small-volume enema tip is inserted 2 inches into the rectum.

15. Place the waterproof pad under the buttocks.
16. Expose the anal area.
17. Position the bedpan near the person.
18. Remove the cap from the enema tip.
19. Separate the buttocks to see the anus.
20. Ask the person to take a deep breath through the mouth.
21. Insert the enema tip 2 inches into the adult's rectum (Fig. 23.6). Do this when the person is exhaling. Insert the tip gently. Stop if the person complains of pain, you feel resistance, or bleeding occurs.
22. Squeeze and roll the bottle gently. Release pressure on the bottle after you remove the tip from the rectum.
23. Put the bottle into the box, tip first.
24. Assist the person to the bathroom or commode when there is the urge to have a BM. The person wears a robe and nonskid footwear when up. The bed

is in the lowest position. Or help the person onto the bedpan and raise the head of the bed. Raise or lower bed rails according to the care plan.
25. Place the call light and toilet tissue within reach. Remind the person not to flush the toilet.
26. Discard disposable items.
27. Remove the gloves. Practice hand hygiene.
28. Leave the room if the person can be left alone.
29. Return when the person signals. Or check on the person every 5 minutes. Knock before entering the room or bathroom.
30. Practice hand hygiene. Put on gloves.
31. Lower the bed rail if up.
32. Observe enema results for amount, color, consistency, shape, and odor. Call the nurse to observe the results.
33. Provide perineal care as needed.
34. Remove the waterproof pad.
35. Empty, clean, and disinfect equipment. Flush the toilet after the nurse observes the results.
36. Return equipment to its proper place.
37. Remove the gloves and practice hand hygiene.
38. Assist with hand washing. Wear gloves for this step.
39. Cover the person. Remove the bath blanket.

Postprocedure
40. Provide for comfort. (See the inside of the front cover.)
41. Place the call light within reach.
42. Lower the bed to its lowest position.
43. Raise or lower bed rails. Follow the care plan.
44. Unscreen the person.
45. Complete a safety check of the room. (See the inside of the front cover.)
46. Follow center policy for dirty linens and used supplies.
47. Practice hand hygiene.
48. Report and record your observations.

This skill also covered in *Clinical Skills: Nurse Assisting.*

✳ The Oil-Retention Enema

Oil-retention enemas relieve constipation and fecal impactions. The oil is retained for 30 to 60 minutes or longer (1 to 3 hours). Retaining oil softens feces and lubricates the rectum. This lets feces pass with ease. Most oil-retention enemas are commercially prepared.

See *Promoting Safety and Comfort: The Oil-Retention Enema.*

👤 PROMOTING SAFETY AND COMFORT

The Oil-Retention Enema
Safety
The oil-retention enema is retained for at least 30 to 60 minutes. Leave the room after giving the enema. Make sure you check on the person often. After checking, tell the person when you will return. Remind the person to signal for you if help is needed.

✳ GIVING AN OIL-RETENTION ENEMA

Quality of Life
Remember to:
- Knock before entering the person's room.
- Address the person by name.
- Introduce yourself by name and title.
- Explain the procedure to the person before beginning and during the procedure.
- Protect the person's rights during the procedure.
- Handle the person gently during the procedure.

Preprocedure
1. Follow *Delegation Guidelines: Enemas,* p. 365. See *Promoting Safety and Comfort:*
   a. *Enemas,* p. 366
   b. *The Oil-Retention Enema*
2. Practice hand hygiene.
3. Collect the following before going to the person's room:
   - Oil-retention enema
   - Waterproof pads

Continued

✳ GIVING AN OIL-RETENTION ENEMA—cont'd

4. Arrange items in the person's room.
5. Practice hand hygiene.
6. Identify the person. Check the ID bracelet against the assignment sheet. Also call the person by name.
7. Put on gloves.
8. Collect the following:
   • Gloves
   • Bath blanket
9. Provide for privacy.
10. Raise the bed for body mechanics. Bed rails are up if used.

Procedure
11. Follow steps 11 through 23 in procedure: *Giving a Small-Volume Enema*, pp. 368-369.
12. Cover the person. Leave the person in the left side-lying position.

13. Encourage the person to retain the enema for the time ordered.
14. Place more waterproof pads on the bed if needed.
15. Remove the gloves. Practice hand hygiene.

Postprocedure
16. Provide for comfort. (See the inside of the front cover.)
17. Place the call light within reach.
18. Lower the bed to its lowest position.
19. Raise or lower bed rails. Follow the care plan.
20. Unscreen the person.
21. Complete a safety check of the room. (See the inside of the front cover.)
22. Follow center policy for dirty linen and used supplies.
23. Practice hand hygiene.
24. Report and record your observations.
25. Check the person often.

This skill also covered in *Clinical Skills: Nurse Assisting*.

THE PERSON WITH AN OSTOMY

Sometimes part of the intestines is removed surgically. Cancer, bowel disease, and trauma (stab or bullet wounds) are common reasons. An ostomy is sometimes necessary. An **ostomy** is a surgically created opening for the elimination of body wastes. The opening that can be seen through the abdominal wall is called a **stoma**. The person wears a pouch over the stoma to collect stools and flatus.

Colostomy

A **colostomy** is a surgically created opening *(stomy)* between the colon *(colo)* and abdominal wall. Part of the colon is brought out onto the abdominal wall and a stoma is made. Feces and flatus pass through the stoma instead of the anus.

Colostomies are temporary or permanent. If permanent, the diseased part of the colon is removed. A temporary colostomy gives the diseased or injured bowel time to heal. After healing, surgery is done to reconnect the bowel.

The colostomy site depends on the site of disease or injury (Fig. 23.7). Stool consistency—liquid to formed—depends on the colostomy site. The more colon remaining to absorb water, the more solid and formed the stool. If the colostomy is near the start of the colon, stools are liquid. A colostomy near the end of the colon results in formed stools.

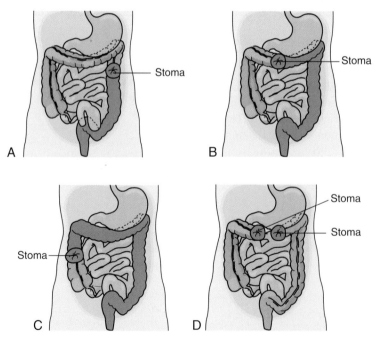

Fig. 23.7 Colostomy sites. Shading in A, B, and C shows the part of the bowel surgically removed. (A) Sigmoid or descending colostomy. (B) Transverse colostomy. (C) Ascending colostomy. (D) Double-barrel colostomy has two stomas. One allows for the excretion of feces. The other is for the introduction of medications to help the bowel heal. This type of colostomy is usually temporary.

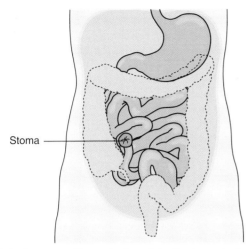

Fig. 23.8 An ileostomy. The entire large intestine is surgically removed.

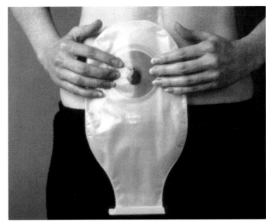

Fig. 23.9 A one-piece ostomy pouch. (From Potter PA, Perry AG: *Fundamentals of nursing*, ed. 8, St. Louis, 2013, Elsevier.)

Stools irritate the skin. Skin care prevents skin breakdown around the stoma. The skin is washed and dried. Then a skin barrier is applied around the stoma. It prevents stools from having contact with the skin. The skin barrier is part of the pouch or a separate device.

Ileostomy

An ileostomy is a surgically created opening *(stomy)* between the ileum (small intestine *[ileo]*) and the abdominal wall. Part of the ileum is brought out onto the abdominal wall and a stoma is made. The entire colon is removed (Fig. 23.8).

Liquid stools drain constantly from an ileostomy. Water is not absorbed because the colon was removed. Feces in the small intestine contain digestive juices that are very irritating to the skin. The ileostomy pouch must fit well. Stools must not touch the skin. Good skin care is required.

✳ Ostomy Pouches

The pouch has an adhesive backing that is applied to the skin (Fig. 23.9). Sometimes pouches are secured to ostomy belts.

Many pouches have a drain at the bottom that closes with a clip, clamp, Velcro, or wire closure. The drain is opened to empty the pouch. The pouch is emptied when stools are present. It is opened when it balloons or bulges with flatus. The drain is wiped with toilet tissue before it is closed.

The pouch is changed every 3 to 7 days and when it leaks. Frequent pouch changes can damage the skin.

Odors are prevented by:
- Good hygiene.
- Emptying the pouch.
- Avoiding gas-forming foods.
- Putting deodorants into the pouch. (The nurse tells you what to use.)

The person wears normal clothes. However, tight garments can prevent feces from entering the pouch. Also, bulging from stools and flatus can be seen with tight clothes.

Peristalsis increases after eating and drinking. Therefore, stomas are usually quiet after sleep. That is, expelling feces is less likely at this time. If the person showers or bathes with the pouch off, it is best done before breakfast. Showers and baths are delayed for 1 to 2 hours after applying a new pouch. This gives the adhesive time to seal to the skin.

Do not flush pouches down the toilet. Follow center policy for disposing of them.

See *Delegation Guidelines: Ostomy Pouches.*

See *Promoting Safety and Comfort: Ostomy Pouches.*

📄 DELEGATION GUIDELINES

Ostomy Pouches

Many people manage their own ostomies. Others need help. When the nurse delegates changing an ostomy pouch to you, make sure that:
- Your state allows you to perform the procedure.
- The procedure is in your job description.
- You have the necessary education and training.
- You review the procedure with the nurse.
- The nurse is available to answer questions and to supervise you.

If the abovementioned conditions are met, you need this information from the nurse and the care plan:
- If the person has a colostomy or ileostomy
- When to change the pouch
- What equipment and supplies to use
- What soap or cleaning agent to use
- Drying time for the skin barrier (usually 1 to 2 minutes)
- What pouch deodorant to use
- What observations to report and record:
  - Signs of skin breakdown (the normal stoma is red, like a mucous membrane)
  - Color, amount, consistency, and odor of stools
  - Complaints of pain or discomfort
- When to report observations
- What specific resident concerns to report at once

👤 PROMOTING SAFETY AND COMFORT

Ostomy Pouches

Safety

When changing an ostomy pouch, contact with stools and the stoma is likely. Stools contain microbes and may contain blood. The stoma may bleed slightly when washed. Follow Standard Precautions and the Bloodborne Pathogen Standard.

Comfort

The stoma does not have sensation. Touching the stoma does not cause pain or discomfort.

✴ CHANGING AN OSTOMY POUCH

Quality of Life

Remember to:

- Knock before entering the person's room.
- Address the person by name.
- Introduce yourself by name and title.
- Explain the procedure to the person before beginning and during the procedure.
- Protect the person's rights during the procedure.
- Handle the person gently during the procedure.

Preprocedure

1. Follow *Delegation Guidelines: Ostomy Pouches*, p. 371. See *Promoting Safety and Comfort: Ostomy Pouches*.
2. Practice hand hygiene.
3. Collect the following before going to the person's room:
   - Clean pouch with skin barrier
   - Pouch clamp, clip, or wire closure
   - Clean ostomy belt (if used)
   - Gauze pads or washcloths
   - Adhesive remover wipes
   - Skin paste (optional)
   - Pouch deodorant
   - Disposable bag
4. Arrange your work area.
5. Practice hand hygiene.
6. Identify the person. Check the ID bracelet against the assignment sheet. Also call the person by name.
7. Put on gloves.
8. Collect the following:
   - Bedpan with cover
   - Waterproof pad
   - Bath blanket
   - Wash basin with warm water
   - Paper towels
   - Gloves
9. Provide for privacy.
10. Raise the bed for body mechanics. Bed rails are up if used.

Procedure

11. Remove the gloves and practice hand hygiene. Put on clean gloves.
12. Lower the bed rail near you if up.
13. Cover the person with a bath blanket. Fan-fold linens to the foot of the bed.
14. Place the waterproof pad under the buttocks.
15. Disconnect the pouch from the belt if one is worn. Remove the belt.
16. Remove and place the pouch and skin barrier in the bedpan. Gently push the skin down and lift up on the barrier. Use the adhesive remover wipes if necessary.

17. Wipe the stoma and around it with a gauze pad. This removes excess stool and mucus. Discard the gauze pad into the disposable bag.
18. Wet the gauze pads or the washcloth.
19. Wash the stoma and the skin around it with a gauze pad or washcloth. Wash gently. Do not scrub or rub the skin.
20. Pat dry with a gauze pad or the towel.
21. Observe the stoma and the skin around the stoma. Report bleeding, skin irritation, or skin breakdown to the nurse.
22. Remove the backing from the new pouch.
23. Apply a thin layer of paste around the pouch opening. Let it dry following the manufacturer instructions.
24. Pull the skin around the stoma taut. The skin must be wrinkle free.
25. Center the pouch over the stoma. The drain points downward.
26. Press around the pouch and skin barrier so it seals to the skin. Apply gentle pressure with your fingers. Start at the bottom and work up around the sides to the top.
27. Maintain the pressure for 1 to 2 minutes. Follow the manufacturer instructions.
28. Tug downward on the pouch gently. Make sure the pouch is secure.
29. Add deodorant to the pouch.
30. Close the pouch at the bottom. Use a clamp, clip, or wire closure.
31. Attach the ostomy belt if used. The belt should not be too tight. You should be able to slide two fingers under the belt.
32. Remove the waterproof pad.
33. Discard disposable supplies into the disposable bag.
34. Remove the gloves. Practice hand hygiene.
35. Cover the person. Remove the bath blanket.

Postprocedure

36. Provide for comfort. (See the inside of the front cover.)
37. Place the call light within reach.
38. Lower the bed to its lowest position.
39. Raise or lower bed rails. Follow the care plan.
40. Unscreen the person.
41. Practice hand hygiene. Put on gloves.
42. Take the bedpan and disposable bag into the bathroom.
43. Empty the pouch and bedpan into the toilet. Observe the color, amount, consistency, and odor of stools. Flush the toilet.
44. Discard the pouch into the disposable bag. Discard the disposable bag.
45. Empty, clean, and disinfect equipment. Return equipment to its proper place.
46. Remove the gloves. Practice hand hygiene.
47. Complete a safety check of the room. (See the inside of the front cover.)
48. Follow center policy for dirty linens.
49. Practice hand hygiene.
50. Report and record your observations.

This skill also covered in *Clinical Skills: Nurse Assisting*.

👥 QUALITY OF LIFE

The "Quality of Life" described for urinary elimination (Chapter 22) applies for bowel elimination as well. As always, protect the person's rights. Assist with bowel elimination as directed by the nurse and the care plan.

Bowel elimination is a very private act. People want and need privacy. Do all you can to protect the person's right to privacy. Otherwise, normal bowel elimination can be affected. Constipation and fecal impaction can result.

Odors and sounds often occur with BMs. You must control your verbal and nonverbal responses. Act in a professional manner at all times. Do not laugh at or make fun of another person. Such reactions are unprofessional. They lessen the person's dignity and self-esteem.

Bowel control is important to people. Physical and mental well-being are related to normal bowel function. Personal BM habits also affect well-being. Good hygiene is needed after BMs.

Normal bowel elimination is not always possible. Constipation, fecal impaction, diarrhea, fecal incontinence, and flatulence are common problems. The doctor may order diet changes, medications, or enemas to relieve the problem. The nurse may ask you to give an enema. You must completely understand the nurse's instructions and the procedure.

Residents have the right to personal choice. Persons with ostomies manage their own care if able. Some have had ostomies for a long time. They have their own routines and care measures. Their choices in ostomy care are followed.

⚡ TIME TO REFLECT

Mr. Sanchez had colon cancer. The doctor needed to remove his colon and perform a colostomy. He is having a hard time adjusting to this change in his body image. He refuses to learn how to care for the colostomy and will not look at the stoma. When you care for Mr. Sanchez, what will you keep in mind when you interact with him? How will you and the nursing team help Mr. Sanchez adjust to this change in his life?

■ REVIEW QUESTIONS

Circle the BEST answer.

1. Which is *false*?
   a. A person must have a BM every day
   b. Stools are normally brown, soft, and formed
   c. Diarrhea occurs when feces move rapidly through the bowels
   d. Constipation results when feces move slowly through the colon

2. The prolonged retention and accumulation of feces in the rectum is called
   a. Constipation
   b. Fecal impaction
   c. Diarrhea
   d. Fecal incontinence

3. Which does *not* promote comfort and safety for bowel elimination?
   a. Asking visitors to leave the room
   b. Helping the person to a sitting position
   c. Offering the bedpan after meals
   d. Telling the person you will return very soon

4. Bowel training is aimed at
   a. Bowel control and regular elimination
   b. Ostomy control
   c. Preventing fecal impaction, constipation, and fecal incontinence
   d. Preventing bleeding

5. Which of the following is *not a common cause of constipation*?
   a. Inactivity
   b. High-fiber diet
   c. Decreased fluid intake
   d. Medications

6. Which is *not* used for a cleansing enema?
   a. Castile soap
   b. Salt
   c. Oil
   d. Tapwater

7. These statements are about enemas. Which is *false*?
   a. The solution should be cool
   b. The left side-lying position is used
   c. The enema bag is held 12 inches above the anus
   d. The solution is given slowly

8. In adults, the enema tube is inserted
   a. 2 to 4 inches
   b. 4 to 6 inches
   c. 6 to 8 inches
   d. 8 to 10 inches

9. The oil-retention enema is retained for at least
   a. 10 to 15 minutes
   b. 15 to 30 minutes
   c. 30 to 60 minutes
   d. 60 to 90 minutes

10. These statements are about ostomies. Which is *false*?
    a. Good skin care around the stoma is needed
    b. Deodorants can control odors
    c. The person wears a pouch
    d. Stools are liquid

11. An ostomy pouch is usually emptied
    a. Every 4 to 6 hours
    b. Every shift
    c. Every 3 to 7 days
    d. When stools are present

12. Melena is
    a. clay-colored stool
    b. green stool
    c. black, tarry stool
    d. bright red stool

See Appendix A for answers to these questions.

24

Exercise and Activity

OBJECTIVES

- Define the key terms and key abbreviations listed in this chapter.
- Describe bedrest.
- Explain how to prevent the complications from bedrest.
- Describe the devices used to support and maintain body alignment.

- Explain the purpose of a trapeze.
- Describe range-of-motion exercises.
- Describe four walking aids.
- Perform the procedures described in this chapter.
- Explain how to promote quality of life.

KEY TERMS

abduction Moving a body part away from the midline of the body

adduction Moving a body part toward the midline of the body

ambulation The act of walking

atrophy The decrease in size or the wasting away of tissue

contracture The lack of joint mobility caused by abnormal shortening of a muscle

deconditioning The loss of muscle strength from inactivity

dorsiflexion Bending the toes and foot up at the ankle

extension Straightening a body part

external rotation Turning the joint outward

flexion Bending a body part

footdrop The foot falls down at the ankle; permanent plantar flexion

hyperextension Excessive straightening of a body part

internal rotation Turning the joint inward

orthostatic hypotension Abnormally low *(hypo-)* blood pressure when the person suddenly stands up *(ortho* and *static)*; postural hypotension

plantar flexion The foot *(plantar)* is bent *(flexion)*; bending the foot down at the ankle

postural hypotension See "orthostatic hypotension"

pronation Turning the joint downward

range of motion (ROM) The movement of a joint to the extent possible without causing pain

rotation Turning the joint

supination Turning the joint upward

syncope A brief loss of consciousness; fainting

KEY ABBREVIATIONS

ADL Activities of daily living
CMS Centers for Medicare & Medicaid Services
ID Identification

OBRA Omnibus Budget Reconciliation Act of 1987
PT Physical therapist
ROM Range of motion

Being active is important for physical and mental well-being. Most people move about and function without help. Illness, surgery, injury, pain, and aging cause weakness and some activity limits. Some people are in bed for a long time. Some are paralyzed. Some disorders worsen over time. They cause decreases in activity. Examples include arthritis and nervous system and muscular disorders (Chapter 35). Inactivity, whether mild or severe, affects every body system. It also affects mental well-being.

Deconditioning is the loss of muscle strength from inactivity. When not active, older persons become deconditioned quickly. Nurses use the nursing process to promote exercise and activity in all persons to the extent possible. The care plan and your assignment sheet include the person's activity level and needed exercises.

See *Residents with Dementia: Exercise and Activity.*

🧑 RESIDENTS WITH DEMENTIA

Exercise and Activity
Persons with dementia may resist exercise and activity. They do not understand what is happening and may fear harm. They may become agitated and combative. Some cry out for help. Do not force the person to exercise or take part in activities. Stay calm and ask the nurse for help. Follow the care plan.

BEDREST

The doctor orders bedrest to treat a health problem. It may be a nursing measure if the person's condition changes. Generally bedrest is ordered to:

- Reduce physical activity.
- Reduce pain.
- Encourage rest.
- Regain strength.
- Promote healing.
    These types of bedrest are common:
- *Strict bedrest.* Everything is done for the person. No activities of daily living (ADLs) are allowed.
- *Bedrest.* Some ADLs are allowed. Self-feeding, oral hygiene, bathing, shaving, and hair care are often allowed.
- *Bedrest with commode privileges.* The person uses the commode for elimination.
- *Bedrest with bathroom privileges (bedrest with BRP).* The person uses the bathroom for elimination.

The person's care plan and your assignment sheet tell you the activities allowed. Always ask the nurse what bedrest means for each person. Check with the nurse if you have questions about a person's activity limits.

Complications from Bedrest

Bedrest and lack of exercise and activity can cause serious complications. Every system is affected. Pressure injuries, constipation, and fecal impaction can result. Urinary tract infections and renal calculi (kidney stones) can occur. So can blood clots (thrombi) and pneumonia (inflammation and infection of the lung).

The musculoskeletal system is affected by lack of exercise and activity. These complications must be prevented to maintain normal movement:

- A contracture is the lack of joint mobility caused by abnormal shortening of a muscle. The contracted muscle is fixed into position, is deformed, and cannot stretch (Fig. 24.1). Common sites are the fingers, wrists, elbows, toes, ankles, knees, and hips. They can also occur in the neck and spine. The person is permanently deformed and disabled.
- Atrophy is the decrease in size or the wasting away of tissue. Tissues shrink in size. Muscle atrophy is a decrease in size or a wasting away of muscle (Fig. 24.2).

Orthostatic hypotension and blood clots occur in the circulatory system. Orthostatic hypotension is abnormally low *(hypo)* blood pressure when the person suddenly stands up *(ortho* and *static).* When a person moves from lying or sitting to a standing position, the blood pressure drops. The person is dizzy and weak and has spots before the eyes. Syncope can occur. Syncope (fainting) is a brief loss of consciousness. (Syncope comes from the Greek word *synkoptein,* meaning "to cut short.") Orthostatic hypotension also is called postural hypotension. *(Postural* relates to posture or standing.) Box 24.1 lists the measures that prevent orthostatic hypotension. Slowly changing positions is key.

See *Focus on Communication: Complications of Bedrest.*

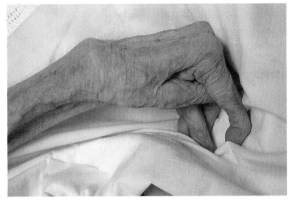

Fig. 24.1 A contracture.

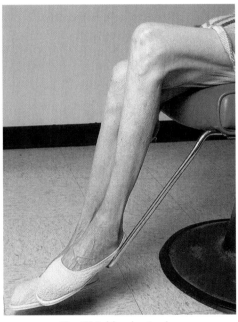

Fig. 24.2 Muscle atrophy.

📋 FOCUS ON COMMUNICATION

Complications of Bedrest
Orthostatic hypotension can occur when the person moves from lying to sitting or standing. Fainting is a risk. To check for orthostatic hypotension, ask these questions:

- "Do you feel weak?"
- "Do you feel dizzy?"
- "Do you see spots before your eyes?"
- "Do you feel like fainting?"

Positioning

Body alignment and positioning were discussed in Chapter 15. Supportive devices are often used to support and maintain the person in a certain position.

- *Bedboards*—are placed under the mattress. They prevent the mattress from sagging (Fig. 24.3). Usually made of plywood, they are covered with canvas or other material. There are

BOX 24.1 Preventing Orthostatic Hypotension

- Measure blood pressure, pulse, and respirations with the person supine.
- Position the person in Fowler position. Raise the head of the bed slowly.
  - Ask the person about weakness, dizziness, or spots before the eyes. Lower the head of the bed if symptoms occur.
  - Measure blood pressure, pulse, and respirations.
  - Keep the person in Fowler position for a short while. Ask about weakness, dizziness, or spots before the eyes.
- Help the person sit on the side of the bed (Chapter 15).
  - Ask about weakness, dizziness, or spots before the eyes. Help the person to Fowler position if symptoms occur.
  - Measure blood pressure, pulse, and respirations.
  - Have the person sit on the side of the bed for a short while.
- Help the person stand.
  - Ask about weakness, dizziness, or spots before the eyes. Help the person sit on the side of the bed if any symptoms occur.
  - Measure blood pressure, pulse, and respirations.
- Help the person sit in a chair or walk as directed by the nurse.
  - Ask about weakness, dizziness, or spots before the eyes. If the person is walking, help the person to sit if symptoms occur.
  - Measure blood pressure, pulse, and respirations.
- Report blood pressure, pulse, and respirations to the nurse. Also report other symptoms or complaints.

Good nursing care prevents complications from bedrest. Good alignment, range-of-motion exercises (p. ··), and frequent position changes are important measures. These are part of the care plan.

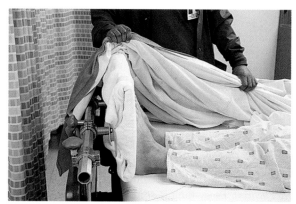

Fig. 24.4 A footboard. Feet are flush with the board to keep them in normal alignment.

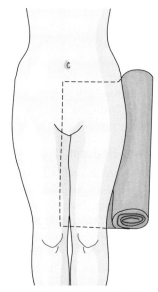

Fig. 24.5 A trochanter roll is made from a bath blanket. It extends from the hip to the knee.

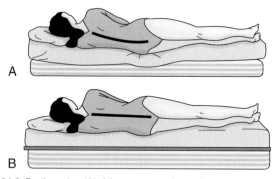

Fig. 24.3 Bedboards. (A) Mattress sagging without bedboards. (B) Bedboards are under the mattress. No sagging occurs.

two sections so the head of the bed can be raised. One section is for the head of the bed. The other is for the foot of the bed.

- *Footboards*—are placed at the foot of mattresses (Fig. 24.4). They prevent plantar flexion that can lead to footdrop. In plantar flexion, the foot (*plantar*) is bent (*flexion*). Footdrop is when the foot falls down at the ankle (permanent plantar flexion). The footboard is placed so the soles of the feet are flush against it. The feet are in good alignment as when standing. Footboards also serve as bed cradles. They prevent pressure ulcers by keeping top linens off the feet and toes.
- *Trochanter rolls*—prevent the hips and legs from turning outward (external rotation) (Fig. 24.5). A bath blanket is folded to the desired length and rolled up. The loose end is placed under the person from the hip to the knee. Then the roll is tucked alongside the body. Pillows or sandbags also keep the hips and knees in alignment.

- *Hip abduction wedges*—keep the hips abducted (apart) (Fig. 24.6). The wedge is placed between the person's legs. These are common after hip replacement surgery.
- *Hand rolls or hand grips*—prevent contractures of the thumb, fingers, and wrist (Fig. 24.7). Foam rubber sponges, rubber balls, and finger cushions (Fig. 24.8) also are used. These are often ordered by the doctor or therapist.
- *Splints*—keep the elbows, wrists, thumbs, fingers, ankles, and knees in normal position. They are usually secured in place with Velcro (Fig. 24.9).
- *Bed cradles*—keep the weight of top linens off the feet and toes (Fig. 24.10). The weight of top linens can cause footdrop and pressure injuries.

Exercise

Exercise helps prevent contractures, muscle atrophy, and other complications from bedrest. Some exercise occurs with ADL and when turning and moving in bed without help. Other exercises are needed for muscles and joints. (See "Range-of-Motion Exercises" [p. ··] and "Ambulation" [p. ··]).

Some centers may have a therapy pool (Fig 24.11) where a therapist can work with residents and help them exercise.

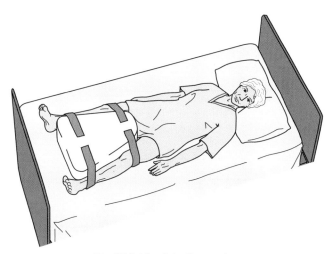

Fig. 24.6 Hip abduction wedge.

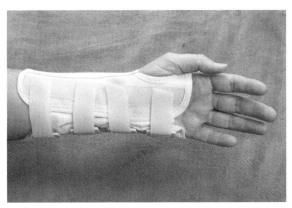

Fig. 24.9 A splint.

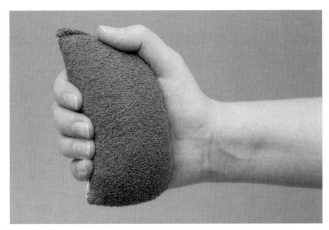

Fig. 24.7 Hand grip. (From Sorrentino SA, Remmert LN: *Mosby's textbook for long-term care nursing assistants*, ed. 10, St. Louis, 2021, Elsevier.)

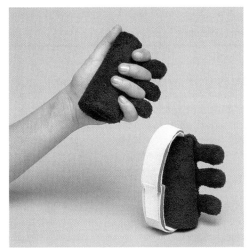

Fig. 24.8 Finger cushion. (From Scott K: *Long-term caring: residential, home and community aged care*, ed. 2, St. Louis, 2010, Elsevier.)

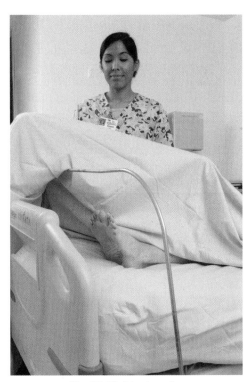

Fig. 24.10 A bed cradle.

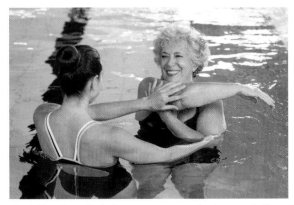

Fig. 24.11 The therapist helps a person exercise in a pool. (From Leonard PC: *Quick & easy medical terminology*, ed. 8, St. Louis, 2017, Elsevier.)

Hydrotherapy (water therapy) is usually less painful, and the warm water increases joint mobility. Some therapy pools have underwater treadmills. These help obese people to lose weight and build muscle mass. Water aerobic exercises may also take place.

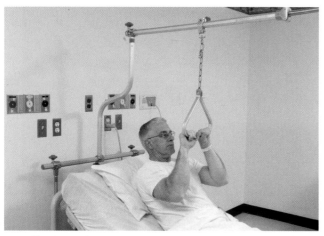

Fig. 24.12 A trapeze is used to strengthen arm muscles.

BOX 24.2 **Joint Movements**

Abduction—moving a body part away from the midline of the body
Adduction—moving a body part toward the midline of the body
Extension—straightening a body part
Flexion—bending a body part
Hyperextension—excessive straightening of a body part
Dorsiflexion—bending the toes and foot up at the ankle
Rotation—turning the joint
Internal rotation—turning the joint inward
External rotation—turning the joint outward
Plantar flexion—bending the foot down at the ankle
Pronation—turning the joint downward
Supination—turning the joint upward

A trapeze is used for exercises to strengthen arm muscles. The trapeze hangs from an overbed frame (Fig. 24.12). The person grasps the bar with both hands to lift the trunk off the bed. The trapeze is also used to move up and turn in bed.

See *Focus on Rehabilitation: Exercise.*

FOCUS ON REHABILITATION

Exercise
The person works closely with physical and occupational therapists to improve strength and endurance. Care plan goals for exercise and ambulation (p. ··) may change daily. The goal may be to improve the person's independence enough to go home. Or the goal may be to attain the highest level of function possible. The health team works with the person to meet rehabilitation goals. Follow the care plan carefully.

✴ RANGE-OF-MOTION EXERCISES

The movement of a joint to the extent possible without causing pain is the range of motion (ROM) of that joint. Range-of-motion exercises involve moving the joints through their complete ROM (Box 24.2). They are usually done at least two times a day.

• *Active* ROM exercises—are done by the person alone.
• *Passive* ROM exercises—you move the joints through their ROM.
• *Active-assistive* ROM exercises—the person does the exercises with some help.

Bathing, hair care, eating, reaching, dressing and undressing, and walking all involve joint movements. Persons on bedrest need more frequent ROM exercises. So do those who cannot walk, turn, or transfer themselves because of illness or injury. The doctor or nurse may order ROM exercises.

 The Omnibus Budget Reconciliation Act of 1987 (OBRA) and the Centers for Medicare & Medicaid Services (CMS) require an assessment and care planning process focused on a person's ROM. The intent is to have the person reach or maintain one's own highest level of ROM. Or the focus is on preventing a decline in ROM. The goal may be one of the following:

• Prevent loss in ROM
• Increase ROM
• Prevent further decrease in ROM

During a survey, CMS surveyors may observe you performing ROM exercises.

See *Focus on Communication: Range-of-Motion Exercises.*
See *Delegation Guidelines: Range-of-Motion Exercises.*
See *Promoting Safety and Comfort: Range-of-Motion Exercises.*

FOCUS ON COMMUNICATION

Range-of-Motion Exercises
You must not force a joint beyond its present ROM or to the point of pain. Ask persons to tell you if they:
• Feel that the joint cannot move any farther.
• Feel pain or discomfort in the joint.

DELEGATION GUIDELINES

Range-of-Motion Exercises
When delegated ROM exercises, you need this information from the nurse and the care plan:
• The kind of ROM ordered—active, passive, active-assistive
• Which joints to exercise
• How often the exercises are done
• How many times to repeat each exercise
• What observations to report and record:
  • The time the exercises were performed
  • The joints exercised
  • The number of times the exercises were performed on each joint
  • Complaints of pain or signs of stiffness or spasm
  • The degree to which the person took part in the exercises
• When to report observations
• What specific resident concerns to report at once

BOX 24.3 Performing Range-of-Motion Exercises

- Exercise only the joints the nurse tells you to exercise.
- Expose only the body part being exercised.
- Use good body mechanics.
- Support the part being exercised.
- Move the joint slowly, smoothly, and gently.
- Do not force a joint beyond its present range of motion.

- Do not force a joint to the point of pain.
- Ask the person about pain or discomfort.
- *Perform range-of-motion exercises to the neck only if allowed by center policy.* In some centers, only physical or occupational therapists do neck exercises. This is because of the danger of neck injuries.

👤 PROMOTING SAFETY AND COMFORT

Range-of-Motion Exercises

Safety

ROM exercises can cause injury if not done properly. Muscle strain, joint injury, and pain are possible. Practice the rules in Box 24.3 when performing or assisting with ROM exercises.

ROM exercises to the neck can cause serious injury if not done properly. Some centers require that nursing assistants have special training before doing such exercises. Other centers do not let nursing assistants do them. Know your center's policy. *Perform ROM exercises to the neck only if allowed by your center and if the nurse instructs you to do so.*

Comfort

To promote physical comfort during ROM exercises, follow the rules in Box 24.3. Also cover the person with a bath blanket. Expose only the part being exercised. Providing for privacy promotes physical and mental comfort.

✳ PERFORMING RANGE-OF-MOTION EXERCISES (NATCEP)

Quality of Life

Remember to:

- Knock before entering the person's room.
- Address the person by name.
- Introduce yourself by name and title.
- Explain the procedure to the person before beginning and during the procedure.
- Protect the person's rights during the procedure.
- Handle the person gently during the procedure.

Preprocedure

1. Follow *Delegation Guidelines: Range-of-Motion Exercises.* See *Promoting Safety and Comfort: Range-of-Motion Exercises.*
2. Practice hand hygiene.
3. Identify the person. Check the identification (ID) bracelet against the assignment sheet. Also call the person by name.
4. Obtain a bath blanket.
5. Provide for privacy.
6. Raise the bed for body mechanics. Bed rails are up if used.

Procedure

7. Lower the bed rail near you if up.
8. Position the person supine.
9. Cover the person with a bath blanket. Fan-fold top linens to the foot of the bed.
10. Exercise the neck *if allowed by your center and if the nurse instructs you to do so* (Fig. 24.13).
    a. Place your hands over the person's ears to support the head. Support the jaws with your fingers.

    b. Flexion—bring the head forward. The chin touches the chest.
    c. Extension—straighten the head.
    d. Hyperextension—bring the head backward until the chin points up.
    e. Rotation—turn the head from side to side.
    f. Lateral flexion—move the head to the right and to the left.
    g. Repeat flexion, extension, hyperextension, rotation, and lateral flexion five times—or the number of times stated on the care plan.
11. Exercise the shoulder (Fig. 24.14).
    a. Grasp the wrist with one hand. Grasp the elbow with the other hand.
    b. Flexion—raise the arm straight in front and over the head.
    c. Extension—bring the arm down to the side.
    d. Hyperextension—move the arm behind the body. (Do this if the person sits in a straight-backed chair or is standing.)
    e. Abduction—move the straight arm away from the side of the body.
    f. Adduction—move the straight arm to the side of the body.
    g. Internal rotation—bend the elbow. Place it at the same level as the shoulder. Move the forearm down toward the body.
    h. External rotation—move the forearm toward the head.
    i. Repeat flexion, extension, hyperextension, abduction, adduction, and internal and external rotation five times—or the number of times stated on the care plan.

Flexion   Extension   Hyperextension   Rotation   Lateral flexion

Fig. 24.13 Range-of-motion exercises for the neck.

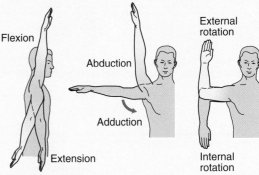

Fig. 24.14 Range-of-motion exercises for the shoulder.

✳ PERFORMING RANGE-OF-MOTION EXERCISES (NATCEP)—cont'd

12. Exercise the elbow (Fig. 24.15).
    a. Grasp the person's wrist with one hand. Grasp the elbow with your other hand.
    b. Flexion—bend the arm so the same-side shoulder is touched.
    c. Extension—straighten the arm.
    d. Repeat flexion and extension five times—or the number of times stated on the care plan.
13. Exercise the forearm (Fig. 24.16).
    a. Continue to support the wrist and elbow.
    b. Pronation—turn the hand so the palm is down.
    c. Supination—turn the hand so the palm is up.
    d. Repeat pronation and supination five times—or the number of times stated on the care plan.
14. Exercise the wrist (Fig. 24.17).
    a. Hold the wrist with both of your hands.
    b. Flexion—bend the hand down.
    c. Extension—straighten the hand.
    d. Hyperextension—bend the hand back.
    e. Radial flexion—turn the hand toward the thumb.
    f. Ulnar flexion—turn the hand toward the little finger.
    g. Repeat flexion, extension, hyperextension, radial flexion, and ulnar flexion five times—or the number of times stated on the care plan.

15. Exercise the thumb (Fig. 24.18).
    a. Hold the person's hand with one hand. Hold the thumb with your other hand.
    b. Abduction—move the thumb out from the inner part of the index finger.
    c. Adduction—move the thumb back next to the index finger.
    d. Opposition—touch each fingertip with the thumb.
    e. Flexion—bend the thumb into the hand.
    f. Extension—move the thumb out to the side of the fingers.
    g. Repeat abduction, adduction, opposition, flexion, and extension five times—or the number of times stated on the care plan.
16. Exercise the fingers (Fig. 24.19).
    a. Abduction—spread the fingers and the thumb apart.
    b. Adduction—bring the fingers and thumb together.
    c. Flexion—make a fist.
    d. Extension—straighten the fingers so the fingers, hand, and arm are straight.
    e. Repeat abduction, adduction, flexion, and extension five times—or the number of times stated on the care plan.

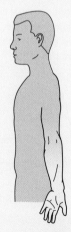
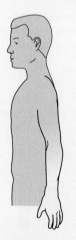

Fig. 24.15 Range-of-motion exercises for the elbow.

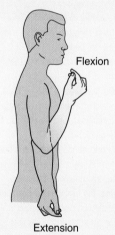

Fig. 24.16 Range-of-motion exercises for the forearm.

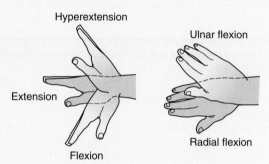

Fig. 24.17 Range-of-motion exercises for the wrist.

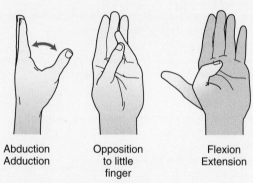

Fig. 24.18 Range-of-motion exercises for the thumb.

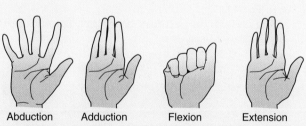

Fig. 24.19 Range-of-motion exercises for the fingers.

Continued

✳ PERFORMING RANGE-OF-MOTION EXERCISES (NATCEP)—cont'd

17. Exercise the hip (Fig. 24.20).
    a. Support the leg. Place one hand under the knee. Place your other hand under the ankle.
    b. Flexion—raise the leg.
    c. Extension—straighten the leg.
    d. Abduction—move the leg away from the body.
    e. Adduction—move the leg toward the other leg.
    f. Internal rotation—turn the leg inward.
    g. External rotation—turn the leg outward.
    h. Repeat flexion, extension, abduction, adduction, and internal and external rotation five times—or the number of times stated on the care plan.
18. Exercise the knee (Fig. 24.21).
    a. Support the knee. Place one hand under the knee. Place your other hand under the ankle.
    b. Flexion—bend the knee.
    c. Extension—straighten the knee.
    d. Repeat flexion and extension of the knee five times—or the number of times stated on the care plan.

19. Exercise the ankle (Fig. 24.22).
    a. Support the foot and ankle. Place one hand under the foot. Place your other hand under the ankle.
    b. Dorsiflexion—pull the foot upward. Push down on the heel at the same time.
    c. Plantar flexion—turn the foot down. Or point the toes.
    d. Repeat dorsiflexion and plantar flexion five times—or the number of times stated on the care plan.
20. Exercise the foot (Fig. 24.23).
    a. Continue to support the foot and ankle.
    b. Pronation—turn the outside of the foot up and the inside down.
    c. Supination—turn the inside of the foot up and the outside down.
    d. Repeat pronation and supination five times—or the number of times stated on the care plan.
21. Exercise the toes (Fig. 24.24).
    a. Flexion—curl the toes.
    b. Extension—straighten the toes.
    c. Abduction—spread the toes apart.
    d. Adduction—pull the toes together.
    e. Repeat flexion, extension, abduction, and adduction five times—or the number of times stated on the care plan.

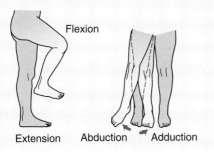

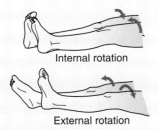

Fig. 24.20 Range-of-motion exercises for the hip.

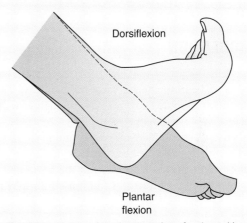

Fig. 24.22 Range-of-motion exercises for the ankle.

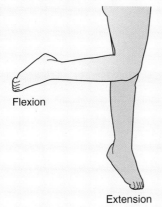

Fig. 24.21 Range-of-motion exercises for the knee.

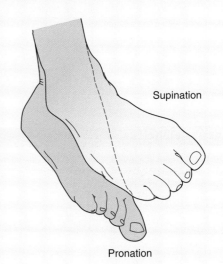

Fig. 24.23 Range-of-motion exercises for the foot.

Continued

✴ PERFORMING RANGE-OF-MOTION EXERCISES (NATCEP)—cont'd

Flexion	Extension	Abduction	Adduction
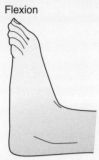	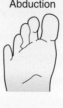	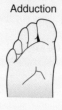	

Fig. 24.24 Range-of-motion exercises for the toes.

22. Cover the leg. Raise the bed rail if used.
23. Go to the other side. Lower the bed rail near you if up.
24. Repeat steps 11 through 21.

Postprocedure
25. Provide for comfort. (See the inside of the front cover.)
26. Remove the bath blanket.
27. Place the call light within reach.

28. Lower the bed to its lowest level.
29. Raise or lower bed rails. Follow the care plan.
30. Fold and return the bath blanket to its proper place.
31. Unscreen the person.
32. Complete a safety check of the room. (See the inside of the front cover.)
33. Decontaminate your hands.
34. Report and record your observations.

This skill also covered in *Clinical Skills: Nurse Assisting.*

✴ AMBULATION

Ambulation is the act of walking. Some people are weak and unsteady from bedrest, illness, surgery, or injury. They may need help walking. Some become strong enough to walk alone. Others will always need help.

After bedrest, activity increases slowly and in steps. First, the person sits on the side of the bed (dangles). Sitting in a bedside chair follows. Next, the person walks in the room and then in the hallway. To walk, contractures and muscle atrophy must be prevented. Proper positioning and exercises are needed during bedrest.

Regular walking helps prevent deconditioning. Some persons who use wheelchairs can walk with help. Follow the care plan when helping a person walk. Use a gait (transfer) belt if the person is weak or unsteady. The person also uses handrails along the wall. Always check for orthostatic hypotension (p. ··).

See *Focus on Communication: Ambulation.*
See *Delegation Guidelines: Ambulation.*
See *Promoting Safety and Comfort: Ambulation.*

📋 FOCUS ON COMMUNICATION

Ambulation
Before ambulating, talk with the person about the activity. Doing so promotes comfort and reduces fear. Explain to the person:
- How far to walk
- What assist devices are used
- How you will assist
- What the person is to report to you

- How you will help if the person begins to fall

For example, you can say: "Mr. Owens, I am going to help you walk from your bed to the doorway and back. This belt helps support you while you walk. I will be at your side and hold the belt at all times. Tell me right away if you feel unsteady, dizzy, or weak. Also tell me if you feel any pain or discomfort. If you begin to fall, I will use the belt to pull you close to me and gently lower you to the floor. Do you have any questions?"

📄 DELEGATION GUIDELINES

Ambulation
Before helping with ambulation, you need this information from the nurse and the care plan:
- How much help the person needs
- If the person uses a cane, walker, crutches, or a brace
- Areas of weakness—right arm or leg, left arm or leg
- How far to walk the person
- What observations to report and record:

- How well the person tolerated the activity
- Shuffling, sliding, limping, or walking on tiptoes
- Complaints of pain or discomfort
- Complaints of orthostatic hypotension—weakness, dizziness, spots before the eyes, feeling faint
- The distance walked
- When to report observations
- What specific resident concerns to report at once

👤 PROMOTING SAFETY AND COMFORT

Ambulation

Safety

Practice the safety measures to prevent falls (Chapter 12). Use a gait belt to help the person stand. Also use it during ambulation. If there is a question about how strong the person is, the nurse or therapist may require another assistant to follow behind with an empty wheelchair. If the person begins to become weak, then have the person sit down in the wheelchair to prevent a fall.

Comfort

The fear of falling affects mental comfort. Explain the purpose of the gait belt. Also explain how you will help if the person starts to fall (Chapter 12).

✳️ HELPING THE PERSON WALK

Quality of Life

Remember to:

- Knock before entering the person's room.
- Address the person by name.
- Introduce yourself by name and title.
- Explain the procedure to the person before beginning and during the procedure.
- Protect the person's rights during the procedure.
- Handle the person gently during the procedure.

Preprocedure

1. Follow *Delegation Guidelines: Ambulation.* See *Promoting Safety and Comfort: Ambulation.*
2. Practice hand hygiene.
3. Collect the following:
   - Robe, socks, and nonskid shoes
   - Paper or sheet to protect bottom linens
   - Gait (transfer) belt
4. Identify the person. Check the ID bracelet against the assignment sheet. Also call the person by name.
5. Provide for privacy.

Procedure

6. Lower the bed to its lowest position. Lock the bed wheels. Lower the bed rail if up.
7. Fan-fold top linens to the foot of the bed.
8. Place the paper or sheet under the person's feet. Put the socks and shoes on the person. Fasten the shoes.
9. Help the person sit on the side of the bed. (See procedure: *Sitting on the Side of the Bed [Dangling]*, Chapter 15.)
10. Help the person put on the robe.
11. Make sure the person's feet are flat on the floor.
12. Apply the gait belt. (See procedure: *Applying a Transfer/Gait Belt*, Chapter 12.)
13. Help the person stand. (See procedure: *Transferring the Person to a Chair or Wheelchair*, Chapter 15.) Grasp the gait belt at each side. If no gait belt, place your arms under the person's arms around to the shoulder blades.
14. Stand at the person's weak side while the person gains balance. Hold the belt at the side and back. If not using a gait belt, have one arm around the back and the other at the elbow to support the person.
15. Encourage the person to stand erect with the head up and back straight.
16. Help the person walk. Walk to the side and slightly behind the person on the person's weak side. Provide support with the gait belt (Fig. 24.25). If not using a gait belt, have one arm around the back and the other at the elbow to support the person. Encourage the person to use the handrail on the strong side.
17. Encourage the person to walk normally. The heel strikes the floor first. Discourage shuffling, sliding, or walking on tiptoes.

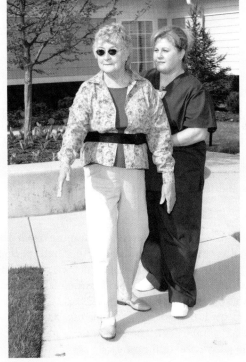

Fig. 24.25 The nursing assistant walks at the person's side and slightly behind her.

18. Walk the required distance if the person tolerates the activity. Do not rush the person.
19. Help the person return to bed. Remove the gait belt. (See procedure: *Transferring the Person from a Chair or Wheelchair to Bed*, Chapter 15.)
20. Lower the head of the bed. Help the person to the center of the bed.
21. Remove the shoes. Remove and discard the paper or sheet over the bottom sheet.

Postprocedure

22. Provide for comfort. (See the inside of the front cover.)
23. Place the call light within reach.
24. Raise or lower bed rails. Follow the care plan.
25. Return the robe and shoes to their proper place.
26. Unscreen the person.
27. Complete a safety check of the room. (See the inside of the front cover.)
28. Decontaminate your hands.
29. Report and record your observations (Fig. 24.26).

✳ **HELPING THE PERSON WALK—cont'd**

Date	Time	Nursing Margin	Other Depts Margin
10/10	1400	Ambulated 25 feet in the hallway c̄ assist of one and use of a gait belt.	
		Reminded not to shuffle her feet. Showed no signs of distress or discomfort.	
		Denied feeling dizzy, light-headed, or weak. No c/o pain. Assisted to her recliner	
		chair and elevated her feet after ambulating. BP-132/84 L arm sitting. P-76	
		regular rate and rhythm. R-20 and unlabored. Over-bed table c̄ water pitcher	
		and glass within reach. Call light within reach. Adam Aims, CNA —————	

Fig. 24.26 Charting sample. *BP,* Blood pressure; *c/o,* complaints of; *L,* left; *P,* pulse; *R,* respirations.

This skill also covered in *Clinical Skills: Nurse Assisting.*

Walking Aids

Walking aids support the body. The doctor, nurse, or physical therapist (PT) orders them. The need may be temporary or permanent. The type ordered depends on the person's condition, the amount of support needed, and the type of disability. Older persons often need walkers or canes for safety. The PT measures and teaches the person to use the device.

Crutches

Crutches are used when the person cannot use one leg or when one or both legs need to gain strength. Some persons with permanent leg weakness can use crutches. They often use forearm crutches (Fig. 24.27). Underarm crutches extend from the underarm to the ground (Fig. 24.28).

The person learns to crutch walk, use stairs, and sit and stand. Safety is important. The person on crutches is at risk for falls. Follow these safety measures:

- Check the crutch tips. They must not be worn down, torn, or wet. Replace worn or torn crutch tips. Dry wet tips with a towel or paper towels.
- Check crutches for flaws. Check wooden crutches for cracks and metal crutches for bends.
- Tighten all bolts.
- Have the person wear street shoes. They must be flat and have nonskid soles.
- Make sure clothes fit well. Loose clothes may get caught between the crutches and underarms. Loose clothes and long skirts can hang forward and block the person's view of the feet and crutch tips.
- Practice safety rules to prevent falls (Chapter 12).
- Keep crutches within the person's reach. Put them by the person's chair or against a wall.
- Know which crutch gait the person uses:
  - Four-point gait (Fig. 24.29)
  - Three-point gait (Fig. 24.30)
  - Two-point gait (Fig. 24.31)

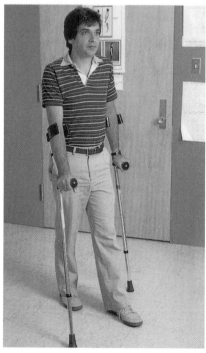

Fig. 24.27 Forearm crutches. (From Elkin MK, Perry AG, Potter PA: *Nursing interventions & clinical skills,* ed. 2, St. Louis, 2000, Mosby.)

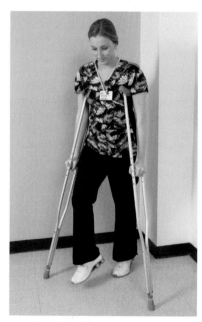

Fig. 24.28 Underarm crutches.

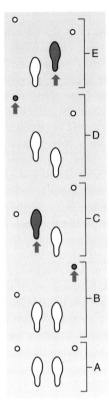

Fig. 24.29 The four-point gait. The person uses both legs. The right crutch is moved forward and then the left foot. Then the left crutch is moved forward followed by the right foot.

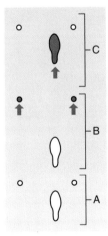

Fig. 24.30 The three-point gait. One leg is used. Both crutches are moved forward. Then the good foot is moved forward.

- Swing-to gait (Fig. 24.32)
- Swing-through gait (Fig. 24.33)

Canes

Canes are used for weakness on one side of the body. They help provide balance and support. Single-tip and four-point *(quad)* canes are common (Fig. 24.34). A cane is held on the *strong side* of the body. (If the left leg is weak, the cane is held in the right hand.) Four-point canes give more support than single-tip canes. However, they are harder to move.

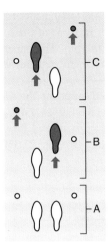

Fig. 24.31 The two-point gait. The person bears some weight on each foot. The left crutch and right foot are moved forward at the same time. Then the right crutch and left foot are moved forward.

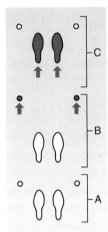

Fig. 24.32 Swing-to gait. The person bears some weight on each leg. Both crutches are moved forward. Then the person lifts both legs and swings to the crutches.

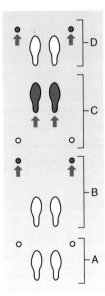

Fig. 24.33 Swing-through gait. The person bears some weight on each leg. Both crutches are moved forward. Then the person lifts both legs and swings through the crutches.

The cane tip is about 6 to 10 inches to the side of the foot. It is about 6 to 10 inches in front of the foot on the strong side. The grip is level with the hip. The person walks as follows:

- *Step A:* The cane is moved forward 6 to 10 inches (Fig. 24.35A).
- *Step B:* The weak leg (opposite the cane) is moved forward even with the cane (see Fig. 24.35B).
- *Step C:* The strong leg is moved forward and ahead of the cane and the weak leg (see Fig. 24.35C).

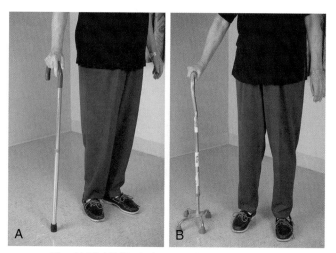

Fig. 24.34 (A) Single-tip cane. (B) Four-point cane.

Walkers

A walker gives more support than a cane. There are different types of walkers to fit the needs of the person. The physical therapist decides which type will be best for the person. A standard walker (Fig. 24.36A) offers the most support. The person grasps it by the hand grips, picks it up, and places it squarely on the floor about 10 inches in front of the body. All four legs of the walker should be in contact with the floor when the person steps into the frame. Wheeled walkers are another type (see Fig. 24.36B). They have wheels on the front legs and rubber tips, tennis balls, or plastic glides on the back legs. The person pushes the walker about 6 to 8 inches in front of the feet. Rubber tips or tennis balls on the back legs prevent the walker from moving while the person is standing. Some have a braking action when weight is applied to the walker's back legs. Some walkers have wheels in the front and back and may have handbrakes. This type of walker allows a person to walk faster, but the person needs to be stable on the feet. A walker may have a built-in seat for the person to rest (see Fig 24.36C). This seat is not meant to be used when the walker is moving. Never push a person while the person is sitting on the seat of a walker. A wheelchair should be used instead. An additional type of walker is a hemiwalker (Fig. 24.37). A hemiwalker may be used for a person who has the use of only one arm or hand. For example, someone who has suffered a stroke and has a weak side.

Baskets, pouches, and trays attach to the walker. They are used for needed items. This allows more independence. They also free the hands to grip the walker.

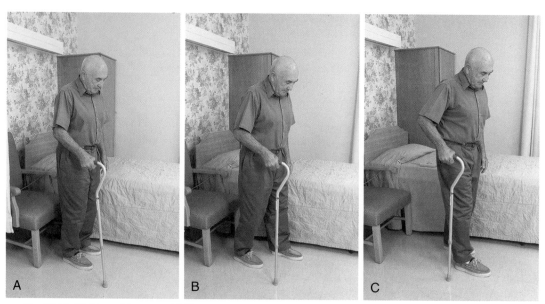

Fig. 24.35 Walking with a cane. (A) The cane is moved forward about 6 to 10 inches. (B) The leg opposite the cane (weak leg) is brought forward even with the cane. (C) The leg on the cane side (strong side) is moved ahead of the cane and the weak leg.

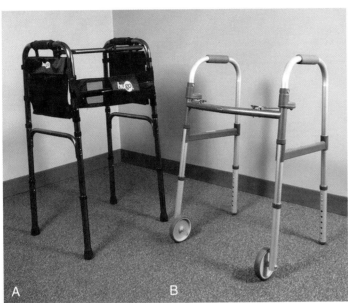

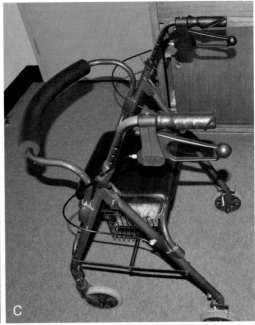

Fig. 24.36 (A) Standard walker. (B) Two-wheel rolling walker. (C) Four-wheel rolling (rollator) walker. ((A and B) From Bonewit-West, 2012Bonewit-West K: *Clinical procedures for medical assistants*, ed. 8, St. Louis, 2012, Saunders. (C) From Talley NJ, O'Connor S: *Clinical Examination: A Systematic Guide to Physical Diagnosis*, ed. 7, Australia, 2013, Churchill Livingstone.)

PROMOTING SAFETY AND COMFORT

Using a Walker

Safety

The walker should be fitted to the person by the physical or occupational therapist, who will also suggest the best type of walker. The person should be taught to never hold onto the walker when getting up. Instead, the person should grasp the arms of a chair or push off of a mattress with the hands. When sitting, the person should back up to the chair and touch the chair with the legs. Next, the person should reach back for the arms of the chair. Finally, the person should lower into the chair using the arms for support. Walkers should not be used on stairs.

Comfort

Some walkers have built-in seats (see Fig 24.35C). These offer a resting place for the person to sit down. The person should never be pushed while sitting on the seat. Many people attach baskets, bags, or cup holders to their walkers. This allows them to transport objects with them. Their hands are free to hold onto the hand grips.

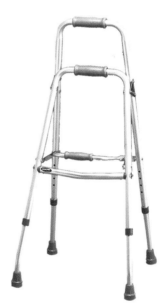

Fig. 24.37 Hemiwalker. (Courtesy Invacare Corporation. Used with permission.)

Braces

Braces support weak body parts. They also prevent or correct deformities or prevent joint movement. Metal, plastic, or leather is used for braces. A brace is applied over the ankle, knee, or back (Fig. 24.38). An ankle-foot orthosis (AFO) is placed in the shoe (Fig. 24.39). Then the foot is inserted. The AFO is secured in place with a Velcro strap. This type of brace is common after a stroke.

Keep skin and bony points under braces clean and dry. This prevents skin breakdown. Report redness or signs of skin breakdown at once. Also report complaints of pain or discomfort. The nurse assesses the skin under braces every shift. The care plan tells you when to apply and remove a brace.

RECREATIONAL ACTIVITIES

OBRA requires activity programs for residents.

Recreational activities are important for an older person's physical and mental well-being. Joints and muscles are exercised. Circulation is stimulated. Recreational activities also are social events and are mentally stimulating. A good activity

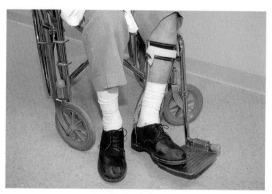

Fig. 24.38 Leg brace.

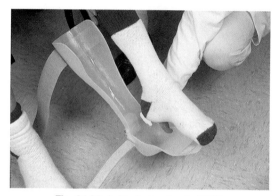

Fig. 24.39 Ankle-foot orthosis (AFO).

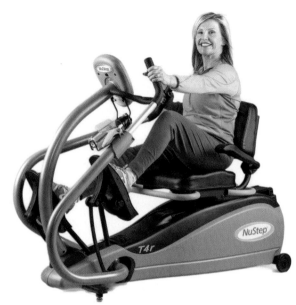

Fig. 24.40 Exercise machine. (Courtesy NuStep, Inc., Ann Arbor, MI.)

resident group that plans activities. *Remember, OBRA also re-quires that persons be allowed to take part in resident group activities.*

See *Teamwork and Time Management: Recreational Activities.*

program improves a person's quality of life. Some centers plan activities that encourage physical activity while having fun. An example might be offering prizes for a level of physical activity that is achieved. A walking club and logging time spent on a treadmill or exercise machine are examples (Fig. 24.40).

❖ *Activities must meet each person's interests and physical, mental, spiritual, and psychosocial needs. When residents are first admitted to the center, their personal interests are documented. The social worker, activity director, and other staff consider their interests when planning events. Small groups may be arranged with residents who share common interests.*

Bingo, movies, dances, exercise groups, shopping trips, museum trips, concerts, guest speakers, crafts, book discussions, and gardening activities are common.

❖ The right to personal choice is protected. Well-being is promoted when the person attends activities of personal choice. The person is not forced to do things that are not of interest.

TEAMWORK AND TIME MANAGEMENT

Recreational Activities

Some persons need help getting to activity programs. Some also need help with activities. When you can, help coworkers assist residents to and from and with activity programs. For example, you have one or two persons who need help. A coworker has four or five persons who need help.

Some persons need help getting to an activity. Some also need help taking part in them. You must assist as needed.

Activity ideas are always welcome. Residents may share ideas with you or tell you about favorite pastimes. Or you may have ideas. Share these with the health team. They are given to the

---

QUALITY OF LIFE

You assist residents with exercise and activity. You must protect their rights to privacy and personal choice. Privacy is protected. During ROM, cover the person with a bath blanket. Expose only the body part being exercised. The person is properly clothed when walking. The person's body is not exposed. Remember, privacy promotes dignity and mental comfort.

Personal choice in walking is encouraged. The person may want to walk outside. The person may prefer to walk in the morning, afternoon, or evening. Or the person may want to wait until a visitor arrives or leaves. Such choices are allowed whenever safe and possible. Be sure to get the nurse's approval.

Disease, injury, pain, and aging affect a person's activities. Even with such limits, you can promote activity, exercise, and well-being. You can:

- Encourage the person to be as active as possible.
- Resist the urge to do things for the person that can be safely done alone or with some help.
- Focus on the person's abilities.
- Encourage the person when doing well or making progress.
- Tell the person you are proud of the efforts.

TIME TO REFLECT

Mrs. Turner had knee surgery 6 months ago. She now uses a wheeled walker to ambulate. Her doctor and physical therapist have encouraged her to walk as much as possible. She usually walks a certain distance in the center's halls on a regular basis. One day, as she neared an entrance at the end of the hall, she looked out the doorway and saw what a pleasant, sunny day it was. She went out the door without notifying staff and walked around the block before returning to the center. A concerned passerby called the center to report an elderly lady walking with a walker on the sidewalk. What do you think about this situation? Is it safe for Mrs. Turner to walk outside unattended? Would her rights be restricted if she was told she could not do this? Is there a compromise that would allow her to exercise yet promote her safety?

REVIEW QUESTIONS

Circle the BEST answer.

1. Deconditioning is
   a. The loss of muscle strength from inactivity
   b. Bending a body part
   c. The lack of joint mobility
   d. The act of walking

2. Moving a body part away from the midline is
   a. Rotation
   b. Abduction
   c. Adduction
   d. Pronation

3. Which of the following is *incorrect* when performing ROM?
   a. Cover the person with a bath blanket
   b. Follow your center's policy for ROM
   c. Ask the person to tell you if there is pain
   d. Force the joint beyond its present ROM

4. Which is true about the use of walkers?
   a. A person can be pushed while seated on a wheeled walker
   b. The nursing assistant decides which type of walker the person will use
   c. The person pushes a wheeled walker about 12 inches in front of the feet
   d. A walker gives more support than a cane

5. The purpose of bedrest is to
   a. Prevent orthostatic hypotension
   b. Reduce pain and promote healing
   c. Prevent pressure injuries, constipation, and blood clots
   d. Cause contractures and muscle atrophy

6. Which helps prevent plantar flexion?
   a. Bedboards
   b. A footboard
   c. A trochanter roll
   d. Hand rolls

7. Which prevents the hip from turning outward?
   a. Bedboards
   b. A footboard
   c. A trochanter roll
   d. A leg brace

8. A contracture is
   a. The loss of muscle strength from inactivity
   b. The lack of joint mobility from shortening of a muscle
   c. A decrease in the size of a muscle
   d. A blood clot in the muscle

9. A trapeze is used to
   a. Prevent footdrop
   b. Prevent contractures
   c. Strengthen arm muscles
   d. Strengthen leg muscles

10. Passive ROM exercises are performed by
    a. The person
    b. Someone else
    c. The person with the help of another
    d. The person with the use of a trapeze

11. ROM exercises are ordered. You do the following *except*
    a. Support the part being exercised
    b. Move the joint slowly, smoothly, and gently
    c. Force the joint through its full ROM
    d. Exercise only the joints indicated by the nurse

12. Flexion involves
    a. Bending the body part
    b. Straightening the body part
    c. Moving the body part toward the body
    d. Moving the body part away from the body

13. When ambulating a person
    a. A gait belt is used if the person is weak or unsteady
    b. The person can shuffle or slide when walking after bedrest
    c. Have the person walk on tiptoes
    d. You walk on the person's strong side

14. You are getting a person ready to crutch walk. You should do the following *except*
    a. Check the crutch tips
    b. Have the person wear nonskid shoes
    c. Get a pair of crutches from physical therapy
    d. Tighten the bolts on the crutches

15. A single-tip cane is used
    a. At waist level
    b. On the strong side
    c. On the weak side
    d. On either side

See Appendix A for answers to these questions.

25

Comfort, Rest, and Sleep

OBJECTIVES

- Define the key terms and key abbreviations listed in this chapter.
- Explain why comfort, rest, and sleep are important.
- List the OBRA room requirements for comfort, rest, and sleep.
- Describe four types of pain and the factors affecting pain.
- Explain why pain is personal.
- List the signs and symptoms of pain.
- List the nursing measures that relieve pain.
- Explain why meeting basic needs is important for rest.

- Identify when rest is needed.
- Explain how circadian rhythm affects sleep.
- Describe the stages of sleep.
- Know the sleep requirements for each age group.
- Describe the factors that affect sleep.
- Describe the common sleep disorders.
- List the nursing measures that promote rest and sleep.
- Explain how dementia affects sleep.
- Explain how to promote quality of life.

KEY TERMS

acute pain Pain that is felt suddenly from injury, disease, trauma, or surgery

chronic pain Pain that continues for a long time (months or years) or occurs off and on; persistent pain

circadian rhythm Daily rhythm based on a 24-hour cycle; the day-night cycle or body rhythm

comfort A state of well-being; the person has no physical or emotional pain and is calm and at peace

discomfort See "pain"

distraction To change the person's center of attention

enuresis Urinary incontinence in bed at night

guided imagery Creating and focusing on an image

insomnia A chronic condition in which the person cannot sleep or stay asleep all night

NREM sleep The phase of sleep when there is no rapid eye movement; non-REM sleep

pain To ache, hurt, or be sore; discomfort

persistent pain See "chronic pain"

phantom pain Pain felt in a body part that is no longer there

radiating pain Pain felt at the site of tissue damage and in nearby areas

relaxation To be free from mental and physical stress

REM sleep The phase of sleep when there is rapid eye movement

rest To be calm, at ease, and relaxed; no anxiety or stress

sleep A state of unconsciousness, reduced voluntary muscle activity, and lowered metabolism

KEY ABBREVIATIONS

CMS Centers for Medicare & Medicaid Services	**NREM** Nonrapid eye movement
CPAP Continuous positive airway pressure	**OBRA** Omnibus Budget Reconciliation Act of 1987
F Fahrenheit	**REM** Rapid eye movement
HS Hour of sleep	**TENS** Transcutaneous electrical nerve stimulation
NPO Nothing by mouth	

Comfort, rest, and sleep are needed for well-being. The total person—the physical, emotional, social, and spiritual—is affected by comfort, rest, and sleep problems. Discomfort and pain can be physical or emotional. Whatever the cause, they affect rest and sleep. They also decrease function and quality of life.

Rest and sleep restore energy and well-being. Illness and injury increase the need for rest and sleep. The body needs more energy for healing and repair. And more energy is needed for daily functions.

COMFORT

Comfort is a state of well-being. The person has no physical or emotional pain. The person is calm and at peace. Age, illness, and activity affect comfort. So do temperature, ventilation, noise, odors, and lighting. Such factors are controlled to meet the person's needs (Chapter 16).

See *Focus on Communication: Comfort.*

📋 FOCUS ON COMMUNICATION

Comfort

Do not assume that a person is comfortable. Ask the following:
- "Are you comfortable?"
- "How can I help you be more comfortable?"
- "Are you warm enough?"
- "Do you need another blanket?"
- "Do you need another pillow?"
- "Should I adjust your pillow?"

❖ OBRA Requirements

The Omnibus Budget Reconciliation Act of 1987 (OBRA) and the Centers for Medicare & Medicaid Services (CMS) require care that promotes well-being. Comfort, rest, and sleep are needed for physical, emotional, and mental well-being. Rooms are designed and equipped for comfort.

- No more than four persons in a room
- A suspended curtain that goes around the bed for privacy
- A bed of proper height and size for the person
- A clean, comfortable mattress
- Linens (sheets, blankets, spreads) that suit the weather and climate
- A clean and orderly room
- An odor-free room
- A room temperature between 71°F (Fahrenheit) and 81°F
- A comfortable sound level
- Adequate ventilation and room humidity
- Adequate and comfortable lighting

PAIN

Pain or *discomfort* means to ache, hurt, or be sore. It is unpleasant. Comfort and discomfort are subjective (Chapter 4). That is, you cannot see, hear, touch, or smell pain or discomfort. You must rely on what the person says. A common complaint of long-term care residents is that they don't feel they are believed when they state they are experiencing pain. Report complaints to the nurse for the nursing process.

Pain differs for each person. What *hurts* to one person may *ache* to another. What one person calls *sore*, another may call *aching*. If a person complains of pain or discomfort, the person *has* pain or discomfort. Believe the person. You cannot see, hear, feel, or smell the person's pain or discomfort.

Pain is a warning from the body. Often called the fifth vital sign (Chapter 27), pain signals tissue damage. Pain often causes the person to seek health care.

See *Focus on Communication: Pain.*

Types of Pain

There are different types of pain.

- *Acute pain* is felt suddenly from injury, disease, trauma, or surgery. It may signal a new injury or a life-threatening event. There is tissue damage. Acute pain lasts a short time. It lessens with healing.
- *Chronic pain (persistent pain)* continues for a long time (months or years) or occurs off and on. There is no longer tissue damage. Chronic pain remains long after healing. Arthritis is a common cause.

📋 FOCUS ON COMMUNICATION

Pain

Communicating with persons about pain promotes comfort. You can say:
- "I want you to be comfortable. Please tell me if you are having any pain."
- "I will tell the nurse about your pain."

If a person complains of pain, then it is real. You must rely on what the person tells you. Promptly report any complaints of pain to the nurse.

- *Radiating pain* is felt at the site of tissue damage and in nearby areas. Pain from a heart attack is often felt in the left chest, left jaw, left shoulder, and left arm. Gallbladder disease can cause pain in the right upper abdomen, the back, and the right shoulder (Fig. 25.1).
- *Phantom pain* is felt in a body part that is no longer there. A person with an amputated leg may still sense leg pain.

Factors Affecting Pain

A person may handle pain well one time and poorly the next time. Many factors affect reactions to pain.

Past Experience

We learn from past experiences. They help us know what to do or what to expect. Whether it is going to school, driving, taking a test, shopping, having a baby, or caring for children, the past prepares us for similar events at another time. We also learn from the experiences of family and friends.

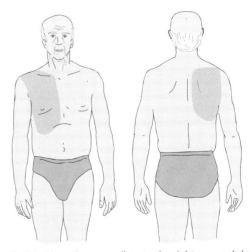

Fig. 25.1 Gallbladder pain may radiate to the right upper abdomen, the back, and the right shoulder.

A person may have had pain before. The severity of pain, its cause, how long it lasted, and if relief occurred all affect the current response to pain. Knowing what to expect can help or hinder how the person handles pain.

Some people have not had pain. When it occurs, pain can cause fear and anxiety. They can make pain worse.

Anxiety

Anxiety relates to feelings of fear, dread, worry, and concern. The person is uneasy and tense. The person may feel troubled or threatened. Or the person may sense danger. Something is wrong but the person does not know what or why.

Pain and anxiety are related. Pain can cause anxiety. Anxiety increases how much pain is felt. Reducing anxiety helps lessen pain. For example, the nurse explains to Mr. Smith about pain after surgery. The nurse also explains that medications are given for pain relief. Mr. Smith knows the cause of pain and what to expect. This helps lessen anxiety and therefore the amount of pain felt.

Rest and Sleep

Rest and sleep restore energy. They reduce body demands. The body repairs itself. Lack of needed rest and sleep affects thinking and coping with daily life. Sleep and rest needs increase with illness and injury. Pain seems worse when tired or restless. Also, the person tends to focus on pain when tired and unable to rest or sleep.

Attention

The more a person thinks about the pain, the worse it seems. Sometimes severe pain is all the person thinks about. Even mild pain can seem worse if the person thinks about it all the time.

Pain often seems worse at night. Activity is less and it is quiet. There are no visitors. The radio or TV is off. Others are asleep. When unable to sleep, the person has time to think about the pain.

Personal and Family Duties

Personal and family duties affect pain responses. Often pain is ignored when there are children to care for. Some people go to work with pain. Others deny pain if a serious illness is feared. The illness can interfere with a job, going to school, or caring for children, a partner, or ill parents.

The Value or Meaning of Pain

To some people, pain is a sign of weakness. It may mean a serious illness and the need for painful tests and treatments. Therefore pain is ignored or denied. Sometimes pain gives pleasure. The pain of childbirth is one example.

For some persons, pain means not having to work or assume daily routines. Pain is used to avoid certain people or things.

The pain is useful. Some people like doting and pampering by others. The person values and wants such attention.

Support from Others

Dealing with pain is often easier when family and friends offer comfort and support. The pain of childbirth is easier when a loving father gives support and encouragement. A child bears pain much better when comforted by a caring parent or family member. The use of touch by a valued person is very comforting. Just being nearby also helps.

Some people do not have caring family or friends. They deal with pain alone. Being alone can increase anxiety. The person has more time to think about the pain. Facing pain alone is hard for everyone, especially children and older persons.

Culture

Culture affects pain responses (Chapter 7). In some cultures, the person in pain is *stoic*. To be stoic means to show no reaction to joy, sorrow, pleasure, or pain. Strong verbal and nonverbal reactions to pain are seen in other cultures.

OBRA requires that the care planning process reflect the person's culture. Non–English-speaking persons may have problems describing pain. The center must be aware of these people. Someone must be available to interpret their needs. All persons have the right to be comfortable and as pain free as possible.

Illness

Some diseases cause decreased pain sensations. Central nervous system disorders are examples. The person may not feel pain, or the pain may not feel severe. The person is at risk for undetected disease or injury. Pain occurs with tissue damage. The pain signals illness or injury. If pain is not felt, the person does not know to seek health care.

Age

Some older persons have many painful health problems. Chronic pain may mask new pain. Older persons may ignore or deny new pain. They may think it relates to a known health problem. Older persons often deny or ignore pain because of what it may mean.

Older persons may have decreased pain sensations. They may not feel pain, or the pain may not feel severe. The person is at risk for undetected disease or injury. Pain occurs with tissue damage. The pain signals illness or injury. If pain is not felt, the person does not know to seek health care.

Thinking and reasoning are affected in some older persons. Some cannot verbally communicate pain. Increased confusion, grimacing, or restlessness may signal pain. So may changes in usual behavior. You must be alert for the signs of pain. Always report changes in the person's behavior.

See *Residents with Dementia: Factors Affecting Pain—Age.*

🔵 RESIDENTS WITH DEMENTIA

Factors Affecting Pain—Age

Persons with dementia may not be able to tell you about their pain. Changes in usual behavior may signal pain. A person who normally moans and groans may become quiet and withdrawn. A person who is friendly and outgoing may become agitated and aggressive. One who is nonverbal and quiet may become restless and cry easily. Loss of appetite also signals pain.

Report any changes in a person's usual behavior to the nurse. All persons have the right to correct pain management. The nurse does a pain assessment when behavior changes.

Signs and Symptoms

You cannot see, hear, feel, or smell the person's pain. You must rely on what the person tells you. Promptly report any information you collect about pain. Write down what the person says. Use the person's exact words when reporting and recording. The nurse needs this information to assess the person's pain:

- *Location.* Where is the pain? Ask the person to point to the area of pain (Fig. 25.2). Pain can radiate. Ask the person if the pain is anywhere else and to point to those areas.

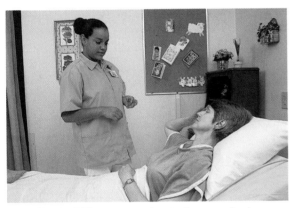

Fig. 25.2 The person points to the area of pain.

PAIN: Ask patient to rate pain on scale of 0-10										
No pain									Worst pain imaginable	
0	1	2	3	4	5	6	7	8	9	10

Fig. 25.3 Pain rating scale. (From deWit SC, O'Neil P: *Fundamental concepts and skills for nursing,* ed 6, St Louis, 2022, Elsevier.)

- *Onset and duration.* When did the pain start? How long has it lasted?
- *Intensity.* Is the pain mild, moderate, or severe? Ask the person to rate the pain on a scale of 0 to 10, with 10 as the most severe (Fig. 25.3). Or use the Wong-Baker Faces Pain Rating Scale (Fig. 25.4). Designed for children, the scale is useful for persons of all ages. To use the scale, tell the person that each face shows how a person is feeling. Read the description for each face. Then ask the person to choose the face that best describes the feelings.
- *Description.* Ask the person to describe the pain. If the person cannot describe the pain, offer some of the words listed in Box 25.1.
- *Factors causing pain.* These are called *precipitating* factors. To precipitate means "to cause." Such factors include moving or turning in bed, coughing or deep breathing, and exercise. Ask what the person was doing before the pain started and when it started.
- *Factors affecting pain.* Ask the person what makes the pain better. Also ask what makes it worse.
- *Vital signs.* Measure the person's pulse, respirations, and blood pressure (Chapter 27). Increases in these vital signs often occur with acute pain. Vital signs may be normal with chronic pain.
- *Other signs and symptoms.* Does the person have other symptoms? Box 25.2 lists the signs and symptoms that often occur with pain.

Nursing Measures

The nurse uses the nursing process to promote comfort and relieve pain. The care plan may include the measures in Box 25.3 and in Fig. 25.5.

Other measures are often needed. They include distraction, relaxation, and guided imagery. If asked to assist, the nurse tells you what to do.

Distraction means to change the person's center of attention. Attention is moved away from the pain. Music, games, singing, praying, TV, and needlework can distract attention (Fig. 25.6).

Relaxation means to be free from mental and physical stress. This state reduces pain and anxiety. The person is taught relaxation methods. The person is taught to breathe deeply and slowly and to contract and relax muscle groups. A comfortable position is important, as is a quiet room.

Guided imagery is creating and focusing on an image. The person is asked to create a pleasant scene. This is noted on the

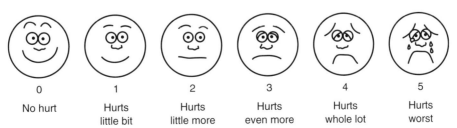

Fig. 25.4 Wong-Baker Faces Pain Rating Scale. (From Hockenberry MJ et al: *Wong's essentials of pediatric nursing,* ed 10, St Louis, 2015, Mosby.)

BOX 25.1 Words Used to Describe Pain

- Aching
- Burning
- Cramping
- Crushing
- Discomfort
- Dull
- Gnawing
- Heaviness
- Hurting
- Knifelike
- Numbness
- Piercing
- Pins and needles
- Pressure
- Radiating
- Ripping
- Sharp
- Shooting
- Soreness
- Spasms
- Squeezing
- Stabbing
- Tearing
- Tenderness
- Throbbing
- Tingling
- Viselike

BOX 25.2 Signs and Symptoms of Pain

Body Responses
- Appetite: changes in
- Dizziness
- Nausea
- Numbness
- Pulse, respirations, and blood pressure: increased
- Skin: pale (pallor)
- Sleep: difficulty with
- Sweating (diaphoresis)
- Tingling
- Vomiting
- Weakness
- Weight loss

Behaviors
- Clenching of the jaw
- Crying
- Frowning
- Gait: changes in; limping
- Gasping
- Grimacing
- Groaning
- Grunting
- Holding the affected body part (splinting; guarding)
- Irritability
- Moaning
- Mood: changes in; depressed
- Pacing
- Positioning: maintaining one position; refusing to move
- Quietness
- Resisting care
- Restlessness
- Rubbing a body part or area
- Screaming
- Speech: slow or rapid; loud or quiet
- Whimpering

---

care plan so all staff members use the same image with the person. A calm, soft voice is used to help the person focus on the image. Soft music, a blanket for warmth, and a darkened room may help. The person is coached to focus on the image and then to practice relaxation exercises.

Medications

Doctors often order medications to control or relieve pain. Nurses give these medications. For many people over-the-counter pain medications, such as aspirin or acetaminophen, may relieve their pain. For more severe pain, stronger medications or narcotics may be needed. Medications may be given by mouth, as injections (shots), or through patches worn on the skin. Only nurses may apply or remove pain medication patches. If a pain patch falls off or has been removed by anyone other than the nurse, report this at once. If a person requests a pain pill, report this to the nurse immediately. Some medications can cause orthostatic hypotension (Chapter 24). They also can cause drowsiness, dizziness, and coordination problems. Protect the person from injury, falls, and fractures. The nurse and care plan alert you to needed safety measures.

Other Therapy Measures

Transcutaneous electrical nerve stimulation (TENS) (Fig. 25.7) may be ordered by the doctor. Electrodes are placed on the skin near the painful area. They are connected to a device that sends electrical impulses. These block pain signals. The person may

be taught to apply the TENS unit. Or a member of the health care team applies the electrodes for the person.

Ice and heat applications are often effective in relieving pain (Chapter 31). Always follow the care plan and ask the nurse if there are questions about these applications.

Ultrasound therapy may be used by a physical therapist to transmit sound waves to a painful area. This may cause the muscles or tissue to relax and lessen the pain.

Exercise and massage therapy may also be used by a physical therapist to reduce pain and stiffness associated with musculoskeletal disorders.

REST

Rest means to be calm, at ease, and relaxed. The person has no anxiety or stress. Rest may involve inactivity. Or the person does things that are calming and relaxing. Examples include reading, music, TV, needlework, and prayer. Some people garden, bake, golf, walk, or do woodworking.

BOX 25.3 Nursing Measures to Promote Comfort and Relieve Pain

- Position the person in good alignment. Use pillows for support.
- Keep bed linens tight and wrinkle free.
- Make sure the person is not lying on tubes.
- Assist with elimination needs.
- Adjust the room temperature to meet the person's needs.
- Provide blankets for warmth and to prevent chilling.
- Use correct handling, moving, and turning procedures.
- Wait 30 minutes after pain medications are given before giving care or starting activities.
- Give a back massage.
- Provide soft music to distract the person.
- Talk softly and gently.
- Use touch to provide comfort.
- Allow family and friends at the bedside as requested by the person.
- Avoid sudden or jarring movements of the bed or chair.
- Handle the person gently.
- Practice safety measures if the person takes strong pain medications or sedatives.
- Keep the bed in the low position.
- Raise bed rails as directed. Follow the care plan.
- Check on the person every 10 to 15 minutes.
- Provide help when the person needs to get up and while up and about.
- Apply warm or cold applications as directed by the nurse (Chapter 31).
- Provide a calm, quiet, darkened setting.

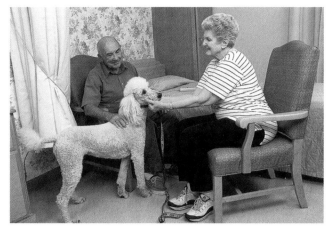

Fig. 25.6 A comforting pet can distract attention away from pain.

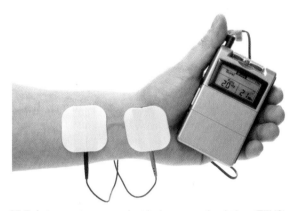

Fig. 25.7 A transcutaneous electrical nerve stimulation (TENS) unit. (Robert Byron/Getty Images.)

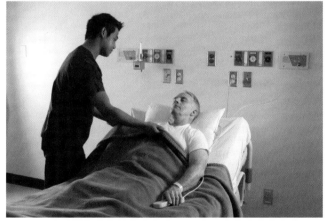

Fig. 25.5 Measures are implemented to relieve pain. The person is positioned in good alignment with pillows used for comfort. The room is darkened. Blankets provide warmth.

Promote rest by meeting physical needs. Thirst, hunger, and elimination needs can affect rest, as can pain or discomfort. A comfortable position and good alignment are important. A quiet setting promotes rest, as does a clean, dry, and wrinkle-free bed. Some people rest easier in a clean, neat, and uncluttered room.

Meet safety and security needs. The person must feel safe from falling or other injuries. The person is secure with the call light within reach. Understanding the reasons for care also helps the person feel safe, as does knowing how care is given. That is why you always explain procedures before doing them.

Many people have rituals or routines before resting. These may include going to the bathroom, brushing teeth, and washing the face and hands. Some people meditate or pray. Some may listen to soft music. Some have a snack or beverage, lock doors, or make sure loved ones are safe at home. The person may want a certain blanket or afghan. Follow routines and rituals whenever possible. Some centers may refer to this as *hour of sleep (HS)* care.

Love and belonging promote rest. Visits or calls from family and friends may relax the person. The person knows that others care and are concerned. Reading cards and letters may also help the person relax and rest (Fig. 25.8).

Self-esteem needs relate to feeling good about oneself. Some people find hospital gowns embarrassing. Others fear exposure. Many persons rest better in their own sleepwear. Hygiene and grooming also affect self-esteem. This includes hair care and being clean and odor free. Hygiene and grooming measures help people feel good about themselves. If esteem needs are met, they may rest easier.

Some people are refreshed after a 15- or 20-minute rest. Others need more time. Health care routines usually allow time

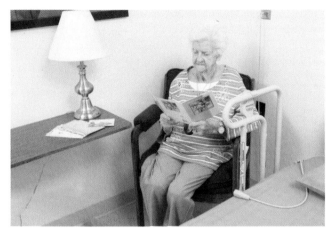

Fig. 25.8 The resident reads cards and letters from family and friends.

for afternoon rest. Some centers will dim the hallway lights and remind staff and visitors to keep noise levels to a minimum to promote a restful environment.

Ill or injured persons need to rest more often. Some rest during or after a procedure. For example, a bath tires a person, as does getting dressed. The person needs to rest before you make the bed. Some people need a few hours for hygiene and grooming. Others need to rest after meals. Do not push the person beyond limits. Allow rest when needed. Do not rush the person.

Distraction, relaxation, and guided imagery also promote rest, as does a back massage. Plan and organize care to allow uninterrupted rest.

The doctor may order bedrest for a person.

SLEEP

Sleep is a state of unconsciousness, reduced voluntary muscle activity, and lowered metabolism. Unconscious persons are not aware of their own settings and cannot respond to people and things. There are no voluntary arm or leg movements. *Metabolism* is the burning of food to produce energy for the body. Less energy is needed during sleep. Thus metabolism is reduced during sleep. The sleep state is temporary. People wake up from sleep.

Sleep is a basic need. It lets the mind and body rest. The body saves energy. Body functions slow. Vital signs are lower than when awake. Tissue healing and repair occur. Sleep lowers stress, tension, and anxiety. It refreshes and renews the person. The person regains energy and mental alertness. The person thinks and functions better after sleep.

Circadian Rhythm

Sleep is part of circadian rhythm. (*Circa* means "about"; *dies* means "day.") Circadian rhythm is a daily rhythm based on a 24-hour cycle. It is called the *day-night cycle* or *body rhythm*. It affects functioning. Some people function better in the morning. They are more alert and active. They think and react better. Others do better in the evening.

Circadian rhythm includes a sleep-wake cycle. The person's *biologic clock* signals when to sleep and when to wake up. You sleep and wake up at certain times. You may awaken before the alarm clock goes off. That is part of your biologic clock. Health care often interferes with a person's circadian rhythm and the sleep-wake cycle. Sleep problems easily occur.

Many people work evening and night shifts. Their bodies must adjust to changes in the sleep-wake cycle.

Sleep Cycle

There are two phases of sleep (Box 25.4). NREM sleep (*non-REM sleep*) is the phase of sleep where there is *no rapid eye*

BOX 25.4 Sleep Cycle

Stage 1: NREM Sleep
- Lightest sleep level
- Lasts a few minutes
- Gradual decrease in vital signs
- Gradual lowering of metabolism
- Person feels drowsy and relaxed
- Person is easily aroused
- Daydreaming feeling after being aroused

Stage 2: NREM Sleep
- Sound sleep
- Relaxation increases
- Still easy to arouse
- Lasts 10 to 20 minutes
- Body functions continue to slow

Stage 3: NREM Sleep
- First stage of deep sleep
- Hard to arouse the person
- Person rarely moves
- Muscles relax completely
- Vital signs decrease
- Lasts 15 to 30 minutes

Stage 4: NREM Sleep
- Deepest stage of sleep
- Hard to arouse the person
- Body rests and is restored
- Vital signs much lower than when awake
- Lasts about 15 to 30 minutes
- Sleepwalking may occur
- Enuresis (urinary incontinence in bed at night) may occur

REM Sleep
- Vivid, full-color dreaming
- Usually starts 50 to 90 minutes after sleep has begun
- Rapid eye movements
- Blood pressure, pulse, and respirations may fluctuate
- Voluntary muscles are relaxed
- Mental restoration occurs
- Hard to arouse the person
- Lasts about 20 minutes

Modified from Potter PA, Perry AG: *Fundamentals of nursing*, ed 9, St Louis, 2017, Mosby.

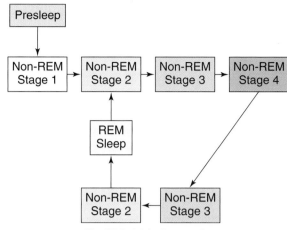

Fig. 25.9 Adult sleep cycle.

TABLE 25.1 Average Sleep Requirements	
Age Group	**Hours per Day**
Newborns (birth to 4 weeks)	14 to 18
Infants (4 weeks to 1 year)	12 to 14
Toddlers (1 to 3 years)	11 to 12
Preschoolers (3 to 6 years)	11 to 12
Middle and late childhood (6 to 12 years)	10 to 11
Adolescents (12 to 18 years)	8 to 9
Young adults (18 to 40 years)	7 to 8
Middle-age adults (40 to 65 years)	7
Older adults (65 years and older)	5 to 7

movement. NREM sleep has four stages. Sleep goes from light to deep as the person moves through the four stages.

The *rapid eye movement* phase is called REM sleep. The person is hard to arouse. Mental restoration occurs. Events and problems of the day are thought to be reviewed. The person prepares for the next day.

There are usually four to six cycles of NREM and REM sleep during 7 to 8 hours of sleep. Stage 1 of NREM is usually not repeated (Fig. 25.9).

Sleep Requirements

Sleep needs vary for each age group. The amount needed decreases with age (Table 25.1). Infants need more sleep than toddlers. Toddlers need more than preschool children. School-age children need more than teenagers. Older persons need less sleep than middle-age adults.

Factors Affecting Sleep

Many factors affect the amount and quality of sleep. Quality relates to how well the person slept. It also involves getting needed amounts of NREM and REM sleep.

- *Illness.* Illness increases the need for sleep. However, signs and symptoms of illness can interfere with sleep. They include pain, nausea, vomiting, coughing, difficulty breathing, diarrhea, frequent voiding, and itching. Treatments and therapies can also interfere with sleep. Often residents

are awakened for treatments or medications. Care devices can cause uncomfortable positions. The emotional effects of illness can affect sleep. These include fear, anxiety, and worry.

- *Nutrition.* Sleep needs increase with weight gain. They decrease with weight loss. Some foods affect sleep. Those with caffeine (chocolate, coffee, tea, or colas) prevent sleep. The protein *tryptophan* tends to help sleep. It is found in protein sources—milk, cheese, red meat, fish, poultry, and peanuts.
- *Exercise.* Exercise improves health and fitness. Exercise requires energy. People usually feel good after exercising. Eventually they tire. Being tired helps them sleep well. Exercise before bedtime interferes with sleep. Exercise causes the release of substances into the bloodstream that stimulate the body. Exercise is avoided 2 hours before bedtime.
- *Environment.* People adjust to their usual sleep settings. They get used to such things as the bed, pillows, noises, lighting, and a sleeping partner. Any change in the usual setting can affect the amount and quality of sleep.
- *Medications and other substances.* Sleeping pills promote sleep. Medications for anxiety, depression, and pain may cause the person to sleep. However, these medications and sleeping pills reduce the length of REM sleep. Mental restoration occurs during REM sleep. Behavior problems and sleep deprivation can occur. Alcohol is a drug. It causes drowsiness and sleep. However, it interferes with REM sleep. Those under the influence of alcohol may awaken during sleep. Difficulty returning to sleep is common. Some medications contain caffeine. Caffeine is a stimulant and prevents sleep. Besides medications, caffeine is found in coffee, tea, chocolate, and colas. The side effects of some medications may cause frequent voiding and nightmares.
- *Lifestyle changes.* Lifestyle relates to a person's daily routines and way of living. Work, school, play, and social events are all part of lifestyle. Lifestyle changes can affect sleep. Travel, vacation, and social events often affect usual sleep and wake times. If work hours change, sleep hours may change. Such changes affect normal sleep-wake cycles and the circadian rhythm.
- *Emotional problems.* Fear, worry, depression, and anxiety affect sleep. Causes include work, personal, or family problems. Loss of a loved one or friend is another cause. Money problems are stressful. People may have problems falling asleep or they awaken often. Some have problems getting back to sleep.

Sleep Disorders

Sleep disorders involve repeated sleep problems. The amount and quality of sleep are affected. Sleep disorders affect lifestyle. Box 25.5 lists the signs and symptoms that occur.

Insomnia

Insomnia is a chronic condition in which the person cannot sleep or stay asleep all night. There are three forms of insomnia:

BOX 25.5 Signs and Symptoms of Sleep Disorders

- Agitation
- Attention: decreased
- Coordination: problems with
- Disorientation
- Eyes: red, puffy, dark circles under the eyes
- Fatigue
- Hallucinations (Chapters 39 and 40)
- Irritability
- Memory: reduced word memory; problems finding the right word
- Mood: moodiness; mood swings
- Pulse: irregular
- Respirations: irregular, apnea, snoring
- Reasoning and judgment: decreased
- Responses to questions, conversations, or situations: slowed
- Restlessness
- Sleepiness
- Speech: slurred
- Tremors: in the hands

- Cannot fall asleep
- Cannot stay asleep
- Early awakening and cannot fall back asleep

Emotional problems are common causes of insomnia. The fear of dying during sleep is another cause. Some people are afraid of not waking up. This may occur with heart disease or when told of a terminal illness. The fear of not being able to sleep is another cause. The physical and emotional discomforts of illness can also cause insomnia.

The nurse plans certain measures to promote sleep. However, the emotional or physical problems causing the insomnia also are treated.

Sleep Deprivation

With sleep deprivation, the amount and quality of sleep are decreased. Sleep is interrupted. NREM and REM sleep stages are not completed. Illness, pain, and hospital care are common causes. Factors that affect sleep can also lead to sleep deprivation. The signs and symptoms in Box 25.5 may occur.

Sleepwalking

The person leaves the bed and walks about. The person is not aware of sleepwalking and has no memory of the event on awakening. Children sleepwalk more than adults. The event may last 3 to 4 minutes or longer.

Stress, fatigue, and some medications are common causes. Protect the person from injury. Falling is a risk. Care tubings (IV, catheters, nasogastric) can cause injury. They can be pulled out of the body when the person gets out of bed. Guide sleepwalkers back to bed. They startle easily. Awaken them gently.

TEAMWORK AND TIME MANAGEMENT

Sleepwalking

You may find a person sleepwalking. Help the person back to bed even if you are not assigned to provide the person's care. Provide for the person's comfort. Then tell the nurse what happened and what you did.

See *Teamwork and Time Management: Sleepwalking.*

Sleep Apnea

A person with sleep apnea may temporarily stop breathing for short periods of time throughout the night. Sleep apnea has different causes. Some people do not know they have sleep apnea. They may report being sleepy and tired during the day. A sleep study is performed to observe the person while sleeping. One way of treating sleep apnea is to have the person wear a continuous positive airway pressure (CPAP) mask while sleeping (Fig. 25.10). The mask forms a tight seal over the person's nose or over both the nose and mouth. A tube connects the mask to a machine that keeps air flowing through the person's airway. A doctor orders the CPAP therapy. Some people can apply their own mask at night. Others may need help. Follow the policy at your center for assisting with a CPAP mask. Always report to the nurse if the person takes off the mask or refuses to wear it.

Promoting Sleep

The nurse assesses the person's sleep patterns. Report any of the signs and symptoms listed in Box 25.5. Measures are planned to promote sleep (Box 25.6). Follow the care plan. Also report your observations about how the person slept. This helps the nurse evaluate if the person has a regular sleep pattern.

Many people have rituals and routines before bedtime. They are important to the person. They are allowed if safe. The

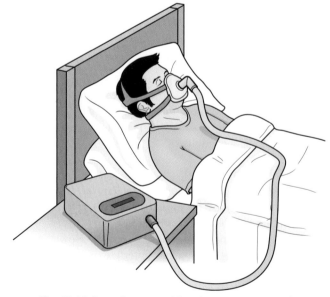

Fig. 25.10 A continuous positive airway pressure mask.

BOX 25.6 Nursing Measures to Promote Sleep

- Plan care for uninterrupted rest.
- Avoid physical activity before bedtime.
- Encourage the person to avoid business or family matters before bedtime.
- Allow a flexible bedtime. Bedtime is when the person is tired, not a certain time.
- Provide a comfortable room temperature.
- Let the person take a warm bath or shower.
- Provide a bedtime snack.
- Avoid caffeine (coffee, tea, colas, chocolate).
- Avoid alcoholic beverages.
- Have the person void before going to bed.
- Make sure incontinent persons are clean and dry.
- Follow bedtime routines.
- Have the person wear loose-fitting sleepwear.
- Provide for warmth (blankets, socks) for those who tend to be cold.
- Weighted blankets may be beneficial for some. They are not used for some persons with respiratory or circulatory conditions. Always check with the nurse and the person's care plan.
- Reduce noise.
- Darken the room—close window coverings and the privacy curtain. Shut off or dim lights.
- Dim lights in hallways and the nursing unit.
- Make sure linens are clean, dry, and wrinkle free.
- Position the person in good alignment and in a comfortable position.
- Support body parts as ordered.
- Give a back massage.
- Provide measures to relieve pain.
- Let the person read, or read to the person if asked to do so.
- Let the person listen to music or watch TV.
- There are videos, CDs, DVDs, and computer applications devoted to soothing music and peaceful images of nature. The center may have access to these, or the family might bring these for the resident.
- Assist with relaxation exercises as ordered.
- Sit and talk with the person.

person may perform personal hygiene in a certain order. A bedtime snack may be important. Some persons watch certain TV shows in bed. Others read religious or spiritual writings, meditate, pray, or say a rosary before going to sleep. Some benefit from listening to peaceful music.

Older persons have less energy than younger people. They may nap during the day. Let the person sleep. Plan the person's care to allow uninterrupted naps.

The person is involved in planning care. The person chooses when to nap or go to bed. The person chooses the measures that promote comfort, rest, and sleep. Follow the care plan and the person's wishes.

See *Residents with Dementia: Promoting Sleep.*

RESIDENTS WITH DEMENTIA

Promoting Sleep
Sleep problems are common in persons with Alzheimer disease and other dementias. Night wandering is common. Restlessness and confusion often increase at night. This increases the risk of falls. It may help to quietly and calmly direct the person to bed. Nighttime wandering in a safe and supervised setting is the best approach for some persons. The measures listed in Box 25.6 are tried. Follow the care plan.

QUALITY OF LIFE

Comfort, rest, and sleep are needed for quality of life and well-being. OBRA and the CMS require measures that promote comfort, rest, and sleep. They relate to the bed, mattress, room temperature, noise level, lighting, linens, odors, and the number of persons in each room. The right to personal choice and taking part in planning care also promote comfort, rest, and sleep.

Comfort involves more than physical needs alone. Emotional, spiritual, and social needs must also be met. Time spent with friends and family provides comfort for residents. For some, religious ceremonies or rituals promote peace and healing. Allow time and privacy for these needs.

Residents have the right to have pain assessed and managed. Untreated pain decreases quality of life. You must report signs and symptoms of pain. This helps the nurse meet the person's needs.

TIME TO REFLECT

Mr. Lansing had surgery for colon cancer 3 years ago. Recently he has had lower abdominal pain, nausea, and vomiting. Tomorrow he is scheduled for diagnostic tests at the hospital. He will be NPO (nothing by mouth) after midnight. You help him get ready for bed. He tells you he is afraid of what the doctors may find. He also admits he will find it hard to sleep tonight. What will you report to the nurse? What are some measures that can be tried to help Mr. Lansing in this difficult situation?

REVIEW QUESTIONS

Circle the BEST answer.
1. Which is not an OBRA requirement for physical comfort?
   a. An odor-free room
   b. Adequate ventilation and room humidity
   c. No more than four persons in a room
   d. A room temperature between 82°F and 92°F

2. Mr. Lang had his right foot amputated. Which type of pain might he experience?
   a. Phantom pain
   b. Radiating pain
   c. Chronic pain
   d. Persistent pain

3. To change the person's center of attention when they have pain is
   a. Guided imagery
   b. Distraction
   c. Relaxation
   d. Intensity

4. These statements are about pain. Which is *false*?
   a. Pain can be seen, heard, smelled, or felt
   b. Pain is a warning from the body
   c. Pain differs for each person
   d. Pain is used to make diagnoses

5. A person has pain in the left chest, the left jaw, and the left shoulder and arm. This is
   a. Acute pain
   b. Chronic pain
   c. Radiating pain
   d. Phantom pain

6. A person complains of pain. You should ask the person to do the following *except*
   a. Point to where the pain is felt
   b. Tell you when the pain started
   c. Describe the pain
   d. Let you look at the pain

7. The nurse gives a person a medication for pain relief. When should you give scheduled care?
   a. Before the medication is given
   b. Right after the medication is given
   c. 30 minutes after the medication is given
   d. The next day

8. A medication was given for pain relief. To promote safety, you should do the following *except*
   a. Keep the bed in the high position
   b. Raise bed rails as directed
   c. Check on the person every 10 to 15 minutes
   d. Provide help if the person needs to get up

9. Which measure will *not* help relieve pain?
   a. Providing blankets as needed
   b. Keeping lights on in the room
   c. Providing soft music
   d. Giving a back massage

10. A person's care plan has these measures. Which will *not* promote rest or sleep?
    a. Voiding before rest or sleep
    b. Positioning in a comfortable position
    c. Having the person walk before rest or sleep
    d. Letting the person choose sleepwear

11. A person tires easily. Morning care includes a bath, hair care, getting dressed, and making the bed. When should the person rest?
    a. After you complete morning care
    b. After the bath and before hair care
    c. After you make the bed
    d. When the person needs to

12. These statements are about sleep. Which is *false*?
    a. Tissue healing and repair occur during sleep
    b. Voluntary muscle activity increases during sleep
    c. Sleep refreshes and renews the person
    d. Sleep lowers stress, tension, and anxiety

13. A person was awake several nights. Which is *false*?
    a. Circadian rhythm may be affected
    b. NREM and REM sleep are affected
    c. The person's biologic clock still tells when to sleep and wake up
    d. Functioning may be affected

14. A healthy 70-year-old person needs about
    a. 12 to 14 hours of sleep per day
    b. 8 to 9 hours of sleep per day
    c. 7 to 8 hours of sleep per day
    d. 5 to 7 hours of sleep per day

15. Which prevents sleep?
    a. Chocolate
    b. Cheese
    c. Milk
    d. Beef

16. These measures for sleep are in the person's care plan. Which should you question?
    a. Let the person choose the bedtime
    b. Provide hot cocoa and a cheese sandwich at bedtime
    c. Position the person in good alignment
    d. Follow the person's bedtime rituals

See Appendix A for answers to these questions.

26

Oxygen Needs and Respiratory Therapies

OBJECTIVES

- Define the key terms and key abbreviations listed in this chapter.
- Describe the factors affecting oxygen needs.
- List the signs and symptoms of hypoxia and altered respiratory function.
- Describe the tests used to diagnose respiratory problems.
- Explain the measures that promote oxygenation.
- Describe the devices used to give oxygen.
- Explain how to safely assist with oxygen therapy.
- Explain how to assist in the care of persons with artificial airways.
- Describe the principles and safety measures for suctioning.
- Explain how to assist in the care of persons on mechanical ventilation.
- Perform the procedures described in this chapter.
- Explain how to promote quality of life.

KEY TERMS

allergy A sensitivity to a substance that causes the body to react with signs and symptoms

apnea The lack or absence (a-) of breathing (-pnea)

Biot respirations Rapid and deep respirations followed by 10 to 30 seconds of apnea

bradypnea Slow (brady-) breathing (-pnea); respirations are fewer than 12 per minute

Cheyne-Stokes respirations Respirations gradually increase in rate and depth and then become shallow and slow; breathing may stop (apnea) for 10 to 20 seconds

cyanosis Bluish color to the skin, lips, mucous membranes, and nail beds

dyspnea Difficult, labored, or painful (dys-) breathing (-pnea)

hemoptysis Bloody (hemo-) sputum (ptysis means "to spit")

hemothorax Blood (hemo-) in the pleural space (thorax)

hyperventilation Respirations (ventilation) are rapid (hyper-) and deeper than normal

hypoventilation Respirations (ventilation) are slow (hypo-), shallow, and sometimes irregular

hypoxemia A reduced amount (hypo-) of oxygen (ox) in the blood (-emia)

hypoxia Cells do not have enough (hypo-) oxygen (-oxia)

intubation Inserting an artificial airway

Kussmaul respirations Very deep and rapid respirations

mechanical ventilation Using a machine to move air into and out of the lungs

orthopnea Breathing (-pnea) deeply and comfortably only when sitting (ortho-)

orthopneic position Sitting up (ortho-) and leaning over a table to breathe (pneic)

oxygen concentration The amount (percentage) of hemoglobin containing oxygen

patent Open and unblocked

pleural effusion The escape and collection of fluid (effusion) in the pleural space

pneumothorax Air (pneum-) in the pleural space (thorax)

pollutant A harmful chemical or substance in the air or water

respiratory arrest When breathing stops

respiratory depression Slow, weak respirations at a rate of fewer than 12 per minute

sputum Mucus from the respiratory system that is expectorated (expelled) through the mouth

suction The process of withdrawing or sucking up fluid (secretions)

tachypnea Rapid (tachy-) breathing (-pnea); respirations are more than 20 per minute

tracheostomy A surgically created opening (-stomy) into the trachea (trachea-)

KEY ABBREVIATIONS

CO_2 Carbon dioxide	NPO Nothing by mouth
ET Endotracheal	O_2 Oxygen
ID Identification	RBC Red blood cell
L/min Liters per minute	SpO_2 Saturation of peripheral oxygen (pulse oximetry)

Oxygen (O_2) is a gas. It has no taste, odor, or color. It is a basic need required for life. Death occurs within minutes if breathing stops. Brain damage and serious illness can occur without enough oxygen. Illness, surgery, and injuries affect the amount of oxygen in the blood and cells.

You assist in the care of persons with oxygen needs. You must give safe and effective care.

FACTORS AFFECTING OXYGEN NEEDS

The respiratory and circulatory systems must function properly for cells to get enough oxygen. Any disease, injury, or surgery involving these systems affects the intake and use of oxygen. Body systems depend on each other. Altered function of any system (for example, the nervous, musculoskeletal, or urinary system) affects oxygen needs. Oxygen needs are affected by:

- *Respiratory system.* Structures must be intact and function properly. An open *(patent)* airway is needed. Alveoli (air sacs) must exchange O_2 and carbon dioxide (CO_2).
- *Circulatory system.* Blood must flow to and from the heart. Narrowed vessels affect blood flow. Capillaries and cells must exchange O_2 and CO_2.
- *Red blood cell (RBC) count.* RBCs contain hemoglobin. Hemoglobin picks up O_2 in the lungs and carries it to the cells. The bone marrow must produce enough RBCs. Poor diet, chemotherapy, and leukemia affect bone marrow function. Blood loss also reduces the number of RBCs.
- *Nervous system.* Nervous system diseases and injuries can affect respiratory muscles. Breathing may be difficult or impossible. Brain damage affects respiratory rate, rhythm, and depth. Narcotics and depressant medications affect the brain. They slow respirations. O_2 and CO_2 blood levels also affect brain function. Respirations increase to bring in more O_2. They also increase to rid the body of excess CO_2.
- *Aging.* Respiratory muscles weaken. Lung tissue is less elastic. Strength for coughing decreases. The person must cough and remove secretions from the upper airway. Otherwise, *pneumonia* (inflammation and infection of the lung) can develop. Respiratory complications are risks after surgery.
- *Exercise.* O_2 needs increase with exercise. Respiratory rate and depth increase to bring in O_2. Persons with heart and respiratory diseases may have enough oxygen at rest. However, even slight activity can increase O_2 needs. Their bodies may not be able to bring in O_2 and carry it to the cells.
- *Fever.* O_2 needs increase. Respiratory rate and depth increase to meet the body's needs.
- *Pain.* O_2 needs increase. Respirations increase to meet this need. Chest and abdominal injuries and surgeries often involve respiratory muscles. It hurts to breathe in and out.
- *Medications.* Some medications depress the respiratory center in the brain. Respiratory depression means slow, weak respirations at a rate of fewer than 12 per minute. Respirations are too shallow to bring enough O_2 into the lungs. Respiratory arrest is when breathing stops. Narcotics

(morphine, Demerol, and others) can have these effects. (*Narcotic* comes from the Greek word *narkoun*, which means "stupor" or "to be numb.") In safe amounts, these medications relieve severe pain. Substance abusers are at risk for respiratory depression and respiratory arrest from medication overdoses.

- *Smoking.* Smoking causes lung cancer and chronic obstructive pulmonary disease (COPD). It is a risk factor for coronary artery disease.
- *Allergies.* An allergy is a sensitivity to a substance that causes the body to react with signs and symptoms. Runny nose, wheezing, and congestion are common. Mucous membranes in the upper airway swell. With severe swelling, the airway closes. Shock and death are risks. Pollens, dust, foods, medications, insect bites, and cigarette smoke often cause allergies. Chronic bronchitis and asthma are risks.
- *Pollutant exposure.* A pollutant is a harmful chemical or substance in the air or water. Examples are dust, fumes, toxins, asbestos, coal dust, and sawdust. They damage the lungs. Pollutant exposure occurs in home, work, and public settings.
- *Nutrition.* The body needs iron and vitamins (vitamin B_{12}, vitamin C, and folate) to produce RBCs.
- *Alcohol.* Alcohol depresses the brain. Excessive amounts reduce the cough reflex and increase the risk of aspiration. Obstructed airway and pneumonia are risks from aspiration.

ALTERED RESPIRATORY FUNCTION

Respiratory function involves three processes. Respiratory function is altered if even one process is affected.

- Air moves into and out of the lungs.
- O_2 and CO_2 are exchanged at the alveoli.
- The blood carries O_2 to the cells and removes CO_2 from them.

Hypoxia

Hypoxia means that cells do not have enough *(hypo)* oxygen *(oxia)*. Without enough oxygen, cells cannot function properly. Anything affecting respiratory function can cause hypoxia. The brain is very sensitive to inadequate O_2. Restlessness is an early sign. So are dizziness and disorientation. Report the signs and symptoms in Box 26.1 at once.

Hypoxia threatens life. All organs need oxygen to function. Oxygen is given. The cause of hypoxia is treated.

Abnormal Respirations

Normal adult respirations are 12 to 20 per minute. They are quiet, effortless, and regular. Both sides of the chest rise and fall equally. These breathing patterns are abnormal (Fig. 26.1):

- Tachypnea—rapid *(tachy)* breathing *(pnea)*. Respirations are more than 20 per minute. Fever, exercise, pain, pregnancy, airway obstruction, and hypoxemia are common causes. Hypoxemia is a reduced amount *(hypo)* of oxygen *(ox)* in the blood *(emia)*.

BOX 26.1 Signs and Symptoms of Hypoxia

- Restlessness
- Dizziness
- Disorientation
- Confusion
- Behavior and personality changes
- Concentrating and following directions: problems with
- Apprehension
- Anxiety
- Fatigue
- Agitation
- Pulse rate: increased
- Respirations: increased rate and depth
- Sitting position: often leaning forward
- Cyanosis (bluish color to the skin, lips, mucous membranes, and nail beds)
- Dyspnea

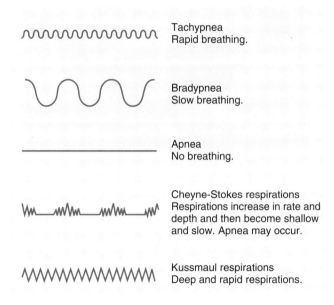

Tachypnea
Rapid breathing.

Bradypnea
Slow breathing.

Apnea
No breathing.

Cheyne-Stokes respirations
Respirations increase in rate and depth and then become shallow and slow. Apnea may occur.

Kussmaul respirations
Deep and rapid respirations.

Fig. 26.1 Some abnormal breathing patterns. (Modified from Talbot L, Meyers-Marquardt M: *Pocket guide to critical care assessment*, ed. 3, St. Louis, 1997, Mosby.)

- Bradypnea—slow *(brady)* breathing *(pnea)*. Respirations are fewer than 12 per minute. Medication overdose and nervous system disorders are common causes.
- Apnea—lack or absence *(a)* of breathing *(pnea)*. It occurs in sudden cardiac arrest and respiratory arrest. Sleep apnea is another type of apnea.
- Hypoventilation—respirations *(ventilation)* are slow *(hypo)*, shallow, and sometimes irregular. Lung disorders affecting the alveoli are common causes. Pneumonia is an example. Other causes include obesity, airway obstruction, and medication side effects. Nervous system and musculoskeletal disorders affecting the respiratory muscles also are causes.
- Hyperventilation—respirations *(ventilation)* are rapid *(hyper)* and deeper than normal. Causes include asthma,

emphysema, infection, fever, nervous system disorders, hypoxia, anxiety, pain, and some medications.
- Dyspnea—difficult, labored, or painful *(dys)* breathing *(pnea)*. Heart disease and anxiety are common causes.
- Cheyne-Stokes respirations—respirations gradually increase in rate and depth. Then they become shallow and slow. Breathing may stop *(apnea)* for 10 to 20 seconds. Medication overdose, heart failure, renal failure, and brain disorders are common causes. Cheyne-Stokes are common when death is near.
- Orthopnea—breathing *(pnea)* deeply and comfortably only when sitting *(ortho)*. Common causes are emphysema, asthma, pneumonia, angina, and other heart and respiratory disorders.
- Biot respirations—rapid and deep respirations followed by 10 to 30 seconds of apnea. They occur with nervous system disorders.
- Kussmaul respirations—very deep and rapid respirations. They signal diabetic coma.

ASSISTING WITH ASSESSMENT AND DIAGNOSTIC TESTS

Altered respiratory function may be an acute or chronic problem. Report your observations promptly and accurately (Box 26.2). Quick action is needed to meet the person's oxygen needs. Measures are taken to correct the problem and to prevent it from becoming worse.

See *Focus on Communication: Assisting with Assessment and Diagnostic Tests.*

FOCUS ON COMMUNICATION

Assisting with Assessment and Diagnostic Tests
The questions you ask the person aid the nurse in the assessment step of the nursing process. For example:
- "Do you need more pillows?"
- "Do you want the head of your bed raised more?"
- "How often are you coughing?"
- "Are you coughing anything up?"
- "Please use a tissue when you cough up mucus, then put on your call light. The nurse needs to observe the mucus."

The doctor orders tests to find the cause of the problem. These tests are commonly done in hospitals.
- *Chest x-ray (CXR).* An x-ray is taken of the chest to study lung changes.
- *Lung scan.* The lungs are scanned to see what areas are not getting air or blood. The person inhales radioactive gas. *Radioactive* means to give off radiation. A radioisotope is injected into a vein. A *radioisotope* is a substance that gives off radiation. Lung tissue getting air and blood flow "take up" the substance.
- *Bronchoscopy.* A scope *(scopy)* is passed into the trachea and bronchi *(broncho)*. Airway structures are checked for bleeding and tumors. Tissue samples *(biopsies)* are taken.

BOX 26.2 Signs and Symptoms of Altered Respiratory Function

- Hypoxia: signs and symptoms of (see Box 26.1)
- Breathing pattern: abnormal
- Shortness of breath or complaints of being "winded" or "short-winded"
- Cough (note frequency and time of day)
  - Dry and hacking
  - Harsh and barking
  - Productive (produces sputum) or nonproductive
- Sputum (mucus from the respiratory system)
  - Color: clear, white, yellow, green, brown, or red
  - Odor: none or foul odor
  - Consistency: thick, watery, or frothy (with bubbles or foam)
  - Hemoptysis: bloody *(hemo)* sputum *(ptysis* means "to spit"); note if the sputum is bright red, dark red, blood-tinged, or streaked with blood
- Respirations: noisy
  - Wheezing
  - Wet-sounding
  - Crowing sounds
- Chest pain (note location)
  - Constant or comes and goes
  - Person's description (stabbing, knifelike, aching)
  - What makes it worse (movement, coughing, yawning, sneezing, sighing, deep breathing)
- Cyanosis (bluish color)
  - Skin
  - Mucous membranes
  - Lips
  - Nail beds
- Vital signs: changes in
- Position
  - Sitting upright
  - Leaning forward or hunched over a table

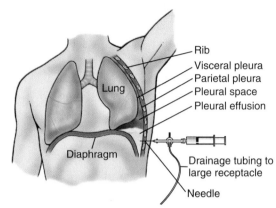

Fig. 26.2 Thoracentesis. (Modified from Monahan FD, Neighbors M: *Foundations for clinical practice*, ed. 2, Philadelphia, 1998, Saunders.)

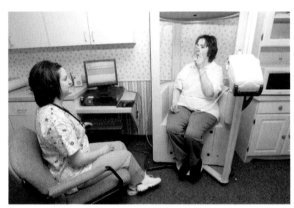

Fig. 26.3 Pulmonary function testing.

Or mucous plugs and foreign objects are removed. The person is NPO (*non per os*; nothing by mouth) for 6 to 8 hours before the procedure. This reduces the risks of vomiting and aspiration. An anesthetic is given. After the procedure, the person is NPO and observed carefully until the gag and swallow reflexes return. This can take about 2 hours.

- *Thoracentesis.* The pleura *(thora)* is punctured. Air or fluid is removed *(centesis)* from it. The doctor inserts a needle through the chest wall into the pleural sac (Fig. 26.2). Injury or disease can cause the sac to fill with air, blood, or fluid. Anticancer medications can be injected into the pleural sac. The procedure takes a few minutes. Vital signs are taken. Then a local anesthetic is given. The person sits up and leans forward. The person must not talk, cough, or move suddenly. Afterward, a dressing is applied to the puncture site. Vital signs are taken. A chest x-ray is taken to detect lung damage. The person is observed for shortness of breath, dyspnea, cough, sputum, chest pain, cyanosis, vital sign changes, and other respiratory signs and symptoms.
- *Pulmonary function tests.* These measure the amount of air moving into and out of the lungs *(volume).* They also measure how much air the lungs can hold *(capacity).* The person takes as deep a breath as possible. Using a mouthpiece, the person blows into a machine (Fig. 26.3). The tests help assess the risk for lung diseases or postoperative lung complications. They also measure the progress of lung disease and its treatment. Fatigue is common after the tests. The person needs to rest.
- *Arterial blood gases (ABGs).* A radial, femoral, or brachial artery is punctured to obtain arterial blood. Laboratory tests measure the amount of O_2 in the blood. Bleeding from the artery must be prevented. Pressure is applied to the artery for at least 5 minutes after the procedure. Pressure is applied longer if there are blood-clotting problems.

✳ Pulse Oximetry

Pulse oximetry measures *(metry)* the oxygen *(oxi)* concentration in arterial blood. Oxygen concentration is the amount (percentage) of hemoglobin containing O_2. Measurements are used to prevent and treat hypoxia. The normal range is 95% to 100%. For example, if 97% of all hemoglobin (100%) carries O_2, tissues get enough oxygen. If only 90% contains O_2, tissues do not get enough oxygen. As low as 85% may be normal for persons with some chronic diseases.

A sensor attaches to a finger, toe, earlobe, nose, or forehead (Fig. 26.4). Light beams on one side of the sensor pass through the tissues. A detector on the other side measures the amount

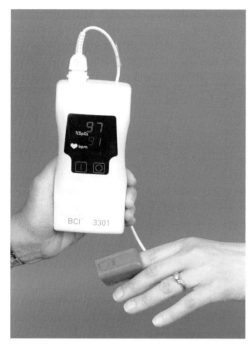

Fig. 26.4 A pulse oximetry sensor is attached to a finger.

of light passing through the tissues. With this information, the oximeter measures the O_2 concentration. The value and pulse rate are shown. Oximeter alarms are set when continuous monitoring is needed. An alarm sounds if:

- O_2 concentration is low.
- The pulse is too fast or slow.
- Other problems occur.

A good sensor site is needed. Avoid swollen sites and sites with skin breaks. It is good to rotate the sensor to different sites. Aging and vascular disease often cause poor circulation. Sometimes blood flow to the fingers or toes is poor. Then the earlobe, nose, and forehead sites are used.

Bright light, nail polish, fake nails, and movements affect measurements. Place a towel over the sensor to block bright light. Remove nail polish or use another site. Do not use a finger site if the person has fake nails. Movements from shivering, seizures, or tremors affect finger sensors. The earlobe is a better site for such problems. Blood pressure cuffs affect blood flow. If using a finger site, do not measure blood pressure on that side.

Report and record oxygen concentration accurately according to center policy. A center may use:

- Pulse oximetry (pulse ox).
- O_2 saturation (O_2 sat).
- Saturation of peripheral oxygen (SpO_2).
  See *Promoting Safety and Comfort: Pulse Oximetry.*
  See *Delegation Guidelines: Pulse Oximetry.*

PROMOTING SAFETY AND COMFORT

Pulse Oximetry

Safety

The person's condition can change rapidly. Pulse oximetry does not lessen the need for good observations. Observe for signs and symptoms of hypoxia (see Box 26.1) and altered respiratory system function (see Box 26.2).

Comfort

A clip-on sensor feels like a clothespin when applied. It should not hurt or cause discomfort. Ask the person to tell you at once if it causes pain, discomfort, or too much pressure. Change the sensor site when the nurse tells you to do so.

DELEGATION GUIDELINES

Pulse Oximetry

When assisting with pulse oximetry, you need this information from the nurse and the care plan:

- What site to use
- How to use the equipment
- What sensor to use
- What type of tape to use
- The normal saturation of peripheral oxygen (pulse ox; SpO_2) range for the person
- Alarm limits for SpO_2 and pulse rate for continuous monitoring
  - Tell the nurse at once if the SpO_2 goes below the alarm limit (usually 95%)
  - Tell the nurse at once if the pulse rate goes above or below the alarm limit
- When to do the measurement
- What pulse site to use: apical or radial
- How often to check the sensor site (usually every 2 hours)
- What observations to report and record:
  - The date and time
  - The SpO_2 and display pulse rate
  - Apical or radial pulse rate
  - What the person was doing at the time
  - Oxygen flow rate (p. ··) and the device used (p. ··)
  - Reason for the measurement: routine or condition change
- When to report observations
- What specific resident concerns to report at once

USING A PULSE OXIMETER

Quality of Life

Remember to:

- Knock before entering the person's room.
- Address the person by name.
- Introduce yourself by name and title.
- Explain the procedure to the person before beginning and during the procedure.
- Protect the person's rights during the procedure.
- Handle the person gently during the procedure.

Preprocedure

1. Follow *Delegation Guidelines: Pulse Oximetry.* See *Promoting Safety and Comfort: Pulse Oximetry.*
2. Practice hand hygiene.
3. Collect the following before going to the person's room:
   - Oximeter and sensor
   - Tape
   - Towel
4. Arrange your work area.

Continued

✳ USING A PULSE OXIMETER—cont'd

5. Decontaminate your hands.
6. Identify the person. Check the identification (ID) bracelet against your assignment sheet. Also call the person by name.
7. Provide for privacy.

Procedure

8. Provide for comfort.
9. Dry the site with a towel.
10. Clip or tape the sensor to the site.
11. Turn on the oximeter.
12. Set the high and low alarm limits for SpO_2 and pulse rate. Turn on audio and visual alarms. (This step is for continuous monitoring.)
13. Check the person's pulse (apical or radial) with the pulse on the display. The pulses should be about the same. Note both pulse rates on your assignment sheet.

14. Read the SpO_2 on the display. Note the value on the flow sheet and your assignment sheet. Also record if the person is receiving supplemental oxygen and the flow rate.
15. Leave the sensor in place for continuous monitoring. Otherwise, turn off the device and remove the sensor. For continuous monitoring, the site of the sensor should be changed at least every 2 hours.

Postprocedure

16. Provide for comfort. (See the inside of the front cover.)
17. Place the call light within reach.
18. Unscreen the person.
19. Complete a safety check of the room. (See the inside of the front cover.)
20. Return the device to its proper place (unless monitoring is continuous).
21. Decontaminate your hands.
22. Report and record the SpO_2, the pulse rates, and your other observations.

This skill is also covered in *Clinical Skills: Nurse Assisting.*

Sputum Specimens

Respiratory disorders cause the lungs, bronchi, and trachea to secrete mucus. Mucus from the respiratory system is called sputum when expectorated *(expelled)* through the mouth. Sputum specimens are studied for blood, microbes, and abnormal cells (Chapter 29).

PROMOTING OXYGENATION

To get enough oxygen, air must move deep into the lungs. Air must reach the alveoli where O_2 and CO_2 are exchanged. Disease and injury can prevent air from reaching the alveoli. Pain and immobility interfere with deep breathing and coughing, as do narcotics. Therefore, secretions collect in the airway and lungs. They interfere with air movement and lung function. Secretions also provide a place for microbes to grow and multiply. Infection is a threat.

Oxygen needs must be met. The following measures are common in care plans.

Positioning

Breathing is usually easier in semi-Fowler and Fowler positions. Persons with difficulty breathing often prefer sitting up and leaning over a table to breathe. This is called the orthopneic position. (*Ortho* means "sitting or standing"; *pneic* means "breathing.") Place a pillow on the table to increase the person's comfort (Fig. 26.5).

Frequent position changes are needed. Unless the doctor limits positioning, the person must not lie on one side for a long time. Secretions pool. The lungs cannot expand on that side. Position changes are needed at least every 2 hours. Follow the care plan.

✳ Deep Breathing and Coughing

Deep breathing moves air into most parts of the lungs. Coughing removes mucus. Deep-breathing and coughing exercises promote oxygenation. They are done after surgery or injury and during bedrest. The exercises are painful after surgery or injury. Breaking an incision open while coughing is a fear.

Deep breathing and coughing help prevent pneumonia and atelectasis. *Atelectasis* is the collapse of a portion of the lung. It occurs when mucus collects in the airway. Air cannot get to a part of the lung. The lung collapses. Atelectasis is a risk after surgery. Bedrest, lung diseases, and paralysis are other risk factors.

Deep breathing and coughing are usually done every 2 hours while the person is awake. Sometimes they are done every hour while the person is awake.

See *Focus on Communication: Deep Breathing and Coughing.*

See *Delegation Guidelines: Deep Breathing and Coughing.*

See *Promoting Safety and Comfort: Deep Breathing and Coughing.*

📋 FOCUS ON COMMUNICATION

Deep Breathing and Coughing

To encourage cough etiquette (Chapter 14), you can say, "Please remember to cover your nose and mouth when coughing. I'll put these tissues where you can reach them. Here is a waste container to dispose of your tissues. Where would you like me to place it? Also, please remember to disinfect or wash your hands often. Let me know if you need help."

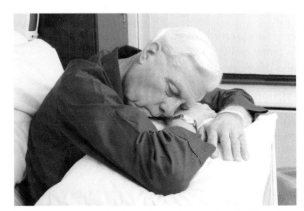

Fig. 26.5 The person is in the orthopneic position. A pillow is on the overbed table for the person's comfort.

DELEGATION GUIDELINES

Deep Breathing and Coughing

When delegated deep-breathing and coughing exercises, you need this information from the nurse and the care plan:

- When to do them
- How many deep breaths and coughs the person needs to do

- What observations to report and record:
  - The number of deep breaths and coughs
  - How the person tolerated the procedure
- When to report observations
- What specific resident concerns to report at once

PROMOTING SAFETY AND COMFORT

Deep Breathing and Coughing
Safety

Respiratory hygiene and cough etiquette are needed if the person has a productive cough (Chapter 14). The person needs to:

- Cover the nose and mouth when coughing or sneezing.
- Use tissues to contain respiratory secretions.
- Dispose of tissues in the nearest waste container after use.
- Wash hands after coughing or contact with respiratory secretions.

ASSISTING WITH DEEP-BREATHING AND COUGHING EXERCISES

Quality of Life

Remember to:

- Knock before entering the person's room.
- Address the person by name.
- Introduce yourself by name and title.
- Explain the procedure to the person before beginning and during the procedure.
- Protect the person's rights during the procedure.
- Handle the person gently during the procedure.

Preprocedure

1. Follow *Delegation Guidelines: Deep Breathing and Coughing*. See *Promoting Safety and Comfort: Deep Breathing and Coughing*.
2. Practice hand hygiene.
3. Collect the following before going to the person's room:
   - Box of tissues
   - Gloves
   - Mask (may be needed for persons with respiratory infections)
4. Identify the person. Check the ID bracelet against the assignment sheet. Also call the person by name.
5. Provide for privacy.

Procedure

6. Lower the bed rail if up.
7. Help the person to a comfortable sitting position: sitting on the side of the bed, semi-Fowler, or Fowler.

8. Put on gloves and mask if required.
9. Have the person deep breathe.
   a. Have the person place the hands over the rib cage (Fig. 26.6).
   b. Have the person take a deep breath. It should be as deep as possible. Remind the person to inhale through the nose.
   c. Ask the person to hold the breath for 2 to 3 seconds.
   d. Ask the person to exhale slowly through pursed lips (Fig. 26.7). Ask the person to exhale until the ribs move as far down as possible.
   e. Repeat this step four more times.
10. Ask the person to cough.
    a. Have the person place both hands over the incision. One hand is on top of the other (Fig. 26.8A). The person can hold a pillow or folded towel over the incision (see Fig. 26.8B).
    b. Have the person take a deep breath as in step 9.
    c. Ask the person to cough strongly twice with the mouth open.
    d. Have a box of tissues within the person's reach for productive cough.

Postprocedure

11. Provide for comfort. (See the inside of the front cover.)
12. Place the call light within reach.
13. Raise or lower bed rails. Follow the care plan.
14. Unscreen the person.
15. Complete a safety check of the room. (See the inside of the front cover.)
16. Remove gloves and decontaminate your hands.
17. Report and record your observations (Fig. 26.9).

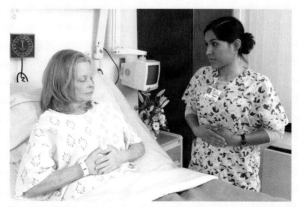

Fig. 26.6 The hands are over the rib cage for deep breathing.

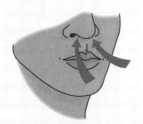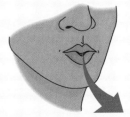

Fig. 26.7 The person inhales through the nose and exhales through pursed lips during the deep-breathing exercise.

Continued

✳ ASSISTING WITH DEEP-BREATHING AND COUGHING EXERCISES—cont'd

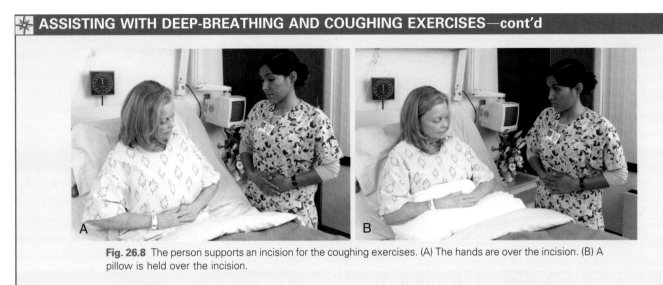

Fig. 26.8 The person supports an incision for the coughing exercises. (A) The hands are over the incision. (B) A pillow is held over the incision.

Date	Time	Nursing Margin	Other Depts Margin
3/15	0830	Assisted resident with deep-breathing and coughing exercises.	
		Resident performed exercises x2. He states "It is getting easier every	
		day." Denied pain or discomfort. Requested to sit in his chair after	
		the exercises. Tray table with water pitcher and glass, tissues, and	
		a book within reach. Call light within reach. Jean Hein, CNA	

Fig. 26.9 Charting sample.

This skill is also covered in *Clinical Skills: Nurse Assisting.*

✳ Incentive Spirometry

Incentive means "to encourage." A *spirometer* is a machine that measures the amount *(volume)* of air inhaled. With incentive spirometry, the person is encouraged to inhale until reaching a preset volume of air. Balls or bars in the machine let the person see air movement when inhaling (Fig. 26.10).

Incentive spirometry also is called *sustained maximal inspiration (SMI)*. (*Sustained* means "constant"; *maximal* means "the most" or "the greatest"; and *inspiration* relates to breathing in.) SMI means inhaling as deeply as possible and holding the breath for a certain time. The breath is usually held for at least 3 seconds.

The goal is to improve lung function. Atelectasis is prevented or treated. Like yawning or sighing, breathing is long, slow, and deep. This moves air deep into the lungs. Secretions loosen. O_2 and CO_2 exchange occurs between the alveoli and the capillaries.

See *Delegation Guidelines: Incentive Spirometry.*

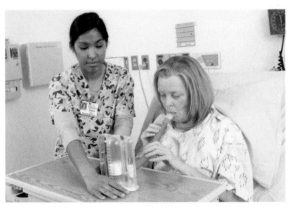

Fig. 26.10 The person uses a spirometer.

DELEGATION GUIDELINES

Incentive Spirometry

Before assisting a person with incentive spirometry, you need this information from the nurse and the care plan:

- How often the person needs incentive spirometry
- If the person needs to have pain medication before performing incentive spirometry
- How many breaths the person needs to take
- The desired height of the floating balls
- How to clean the mouthpiece

- When to replace the mouthpiece
- What observations to report and record:
  - How many breaths the person took
  - The height of the floating balls
  - If the person coughed after using the spirometer
  - How the person tolerated the incentive spirometry
- When to report observations
- What specific resident concerns to report at once

ASSISTING WITH INCENTIVE SPIROMETRY

Quality of Life

Remember to:

- Knock before entering the person's room.
- Address the person by name.
- Introduce yourself by name and title.
- Explain the procedure to the person before beginning and during the procedure.
- Protect the person's rights during the procedure.
- Handle the person gently during the procedure.

Preprocedure

1. Follow *Delegation Guidelines: Incentive Spirometry.*
2. Practice hand hygiene.
3. Collect the following before going to the person's room:
   - Box of tissues
   - Gloves
   - Spirometer
4. Identify the person. Check the ID bracelet against the assignment sheet. Also call the person by name.
5. Provide for privacy.

Procedure

6. Lower the bed rail if up.
7. Help the person to a comfortable sitting position: sitting on the side of the bed, semi-Fowler, or Fowler.

8. Have the person hold the spirometer upright.
9. Ask the person to exhale normally.
10. Have the person seal the lips around the mouthpiece of the spirometer (see Fig. 26.10).
11. Ask the person to take a slow, deep breath until the balls rise to the desired height.
12. Ask the person to hold the breath for 3 to 6 seconds to keep the balls floating.
13. Have the person remove the mouthpiece and exhale slowly. The person may cough at this time.
14. Ask the person to take some normal breaths. Then the device is used again.
15. Have the person repeat steps 8 through 13. The nurse or the care plan will direct how many times the person should repeat the breaths with the spirometer (often 10 times).

Postprocedure

16. Provide for comfort. (See the inside of the front cover.)
17. Place the call light within reach.
18. Raise or lower bed rails. Follow the care plan.
19. Unscreen the person.
20. Complete a safety check of the room. (See the inside of the front cover.)
21. Decontaminate your hands.
22. Report and record your observations.

This skill is also covered in *Clinical Skills: Nurse Assisting.*

ASSISTING WITH OXYGEN THERAPY

Disease, injury, and surgery often interfere with breathing. The amount of O_2 in the blood may be less than normal *(hypoxemia).* If so, the doctor orders oxygen therapy.

Oxygen is treated as a medication. The doctor orders the amount of oxygen to give, the device to use, and when to give it. Some people need oxygen constantly. Others need it for symptom relief—chest pain or shortness of breath. Oxygen helps relieve chest pain. Persons with respiratory diseases may have enough oxygen at rest. With mild exercise or activity, they become short of breath. Oxygen helps relieve shortness of breath.

You do not give oxygen. The nurse and respiratory therapist start and maintain oxygen therapy. You assist the nurse in providing safe care.

Oxygen Sources

Oxygen is supplied as follows:

- *Wall outlet.* O_2 is piped into each person's unit (Fig. 26.11).

- *Oxygen tank.* The oxygen tank is placed at the bedside. Small tanks are used during emergencies and transfers. They also are used by persons who walk or use wheelchairs (Fig. 26.12). A gauge tells how much oxygen is left (Fig. 26.13).
- *Oxygen concentrator.* The machine removes oxygen from the air (Fig. 26.14). A power source is needed. If the machine is not portable, the person stays near it. A portable oxygen tank is needed for power failures and mobility.
- *Liquid oxygen system.* A portable unit is filled from a stationary unit. The portable unit has enough oxygen for about 8 hours of use. A dial shows the amount of oxygen in the unit. The portable unit can be worn over the shoulder (Fig. 26.15). This allows the person to be mobile.

See *Promoting Safety and Comfort: Oxygen Sources.*
See *Teamwork and Time Management: Oxygen Sources.*

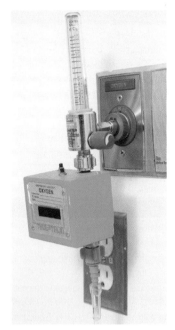

Fig. 26.11 Wall oxygen outlet.

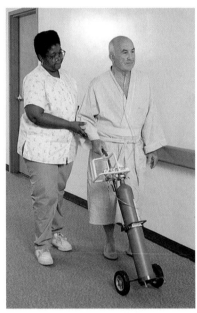

Fig. 26.12 A portable oxygen tank is used when walking.

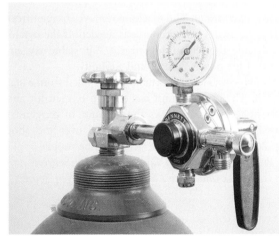

Fig. 26.13 The gauge shows the amount of oxygen in the tank.

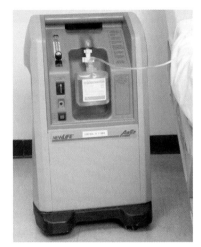

Fig. 26.14 Oxygen concentrator.

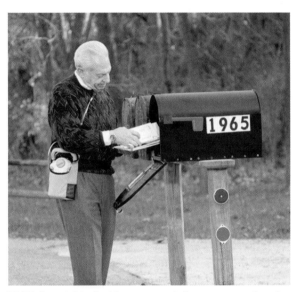

Fig. 26.15 A portable liquid oxygen unit is worn over the shoulder. (Image used by permission from Nellcor Puritan Bennet LLC, Boulder, CO; part of Covidien.)

PROMOTING SAFETY AND COMFORT

Oxygen Sources

Safety

Liquid oxygen is very cold. If touched, it can freeze the skin. Never tamper with the equipment. Doing so is unsafe and could damage the equipment. Follow center procedures and the manufacturer instructions when working with liquid oxygen.

TEAMWORK AND TIME MANAGEMENT

Oxygen Sources

Oxygen tanks and liquid oxygen systems contain a certain amount of oxygen. When the oxygen level is low, another tank is needed or the liquid oxygen system is refilled. Always check the oxygen level when you are with or near persons using these oxygen sources. Report a low oxygen level at once.

Oxygen Devices

The doctor orders the device for giving oxygen. These devices are common:

- *Nasal cannula* (Fig. 26.16). The prongs are inserted into the nostrils. A band goes behind the ears and under the chin to keep the device in place. A cannula allows eating and drinking. Tight prongs can irritate the nose. Pressure on the ears and cheekbones is possible.
- *Simple face mask* (Fig. 26.17). It covers the nose and mouth. The mask has small holes in the sides; CO_2 escapes when exhaling.
- *Partial-rebreather mask* (Fig. 26.18). A bag is added to the simple face mask. The bag is for exhaled air. When breathing in, the person inhales oxygen and some exhaled air. Some room air also is inhaled. The bag should not totally deflate when inhaling.

- *Nonrebreather mask* (Fig. 26.19). Exhaled air and room air cannot enter the bag. Exhaled air leaves through holes in the mask. When inhaling, only oxygen from the bag is inhaled. The bag must not totally collapse during inhalation.
- *Venturi mask* (Fig. 26.20). Precise amounts of oxygen are given. Color-coded adapters show the amount of oxygen given.

Talking and eating are hard to do with a mask. Listen carefully. Moisture can build up under the mask. Keep the face clean and dry. This helps prevent irritation from the mask. Masks are removed for eating. Usually oxygen is given by cannula during meals.

Oxygen Flow Rates

The *flow rate* is the amount of oxygen given. It is measured in liters per minute (L/min). The doctor orders 2 to 15 L of O_2 per minute. The nurse or respiratory therapist sets the flow rate according to the doctor's orders (Fig. 26.21).

The nurse and care plan tell you the person's flow rate. When giving care and checking the person, always check the flow rate. Tell the nurse at once if it is too high or too low. A nurse or respiratory therapist will adjust the flow rate. Some states and centers let nursing assistants adjust O_2 flow rates. Know your center's policy.

✦ Oxygen Administration Setup

Oxygen is a dry gas. If not humidified (made moist), oxygen dries the airway's mucous membranes. Distilled water is added

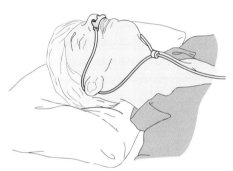

Fig. 26.16 Nasal cannula.

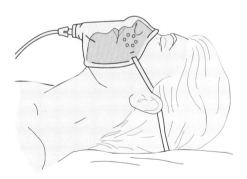

Fig. 26.17 Simple face mask.

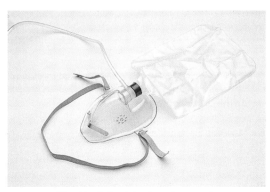

Fig. 26.18 Partial-rebreather mask.

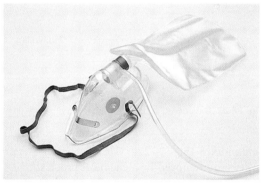

Fig. 26.19 Nonrebreather mask.

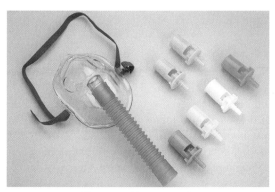

Fig. 26.20 Venturi mask.

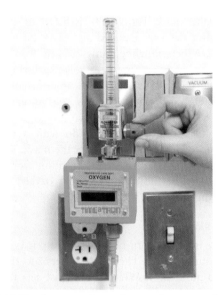

Fig. 26.21 The flowmeter is used to set the oxygen flow rate.

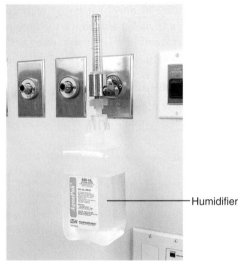
Humidifier

Fig. 26.22 Oxygen administration system with humidifier.

to the humidifier (Fig. 26.22). (Distilled water is pure. Dissolved salts were removed by a chemical process.)

When added to the humidifier, the distilled water creates water vapor. Oxygen picks up the water vapor as it flows into the system. Bubbling in the humidifier means that water vapor is being produced. Low flow rates (1 to 2 L/min) by cannula are not usually humidified.

Oxygen Safety

You assist the nurse with oxygen therapy. You do not give oxygen. You do not adjust the flow rate unless allowed by your state and center. However, you must give safe care. Follow the rules in Box 26.3. Also follow the rules for fire and the use of oxygen (Chapter 11).

See *Delegation Guidelines: Oxygen Administration Setup.*

See *Promoting Safety and Comfort: Oxygen Administration Setup.*

BOX 26.3 Safety Rules for Oxygen Therapy

- Never remove the oxygen device.
- A sign should be posted on the door stating that oxygen is in use.
- Remove all flammable substances from the area.
- Make sure the oxygen device is secure but not tight.
- Check for signs of irritation from the device. Check behind the ears, under the nose (cannula), and around the face (mask). Also check the cheekbones.
- If the person complains of dry lips, do not use petroleum jelly. Use a water-based lubricant instead.
- Keep the face clean and dry when a mask is used.
- Never shut off the oxygen flow.
- Do not adjust the flow rate unless allowed by your state and center.
- Tell the nurse at once if the flow rate is too high or too low.
- Tell the nurse at once if the humidifier is not bubbling.
- Secure tubing in place. Tape or pin it to the person's garment following center policy.
- Make sure there are no kinks in the tubing.
- Make sure the person does not lie on any part of the tubing.
- Make sure the oxygen tank is secure in its holder.
- Report signs and symptoms of hypoxia, respiratory distress, or abnormal breathing patterns to the nurse at once (see Boxes 26.1 and 26.2).
- Give oral hygiene as directed. Follow the care plan.
- Make sure the oxygen device is clean and free of mucus.
- Maintain an adequate water level in the humidifier.

See *Teamwork and Time Management: Oxygen Administration Setup.*

📄 DELEGATION GUIDELINES

Oxygen Administration Setup

If setting up oxygen is delegated to you, you need this information from the nurse:

- The person's name and room and bed number
- What oxygen device was ordered
- If humidification was ordered

👤 PROMOTING SAFETY AND COMFORT

Oxygen Administration Setup
Safety
You do not give oxygen. Tell the nurse when the oxygen administration system is set up. The nurse turns on the oxygen, sets the flow rate, and applies the oxygen device.

Practice medical asepsis. Do not let the connecting tubing hang on the floor.

👥 TEAMWORK AND TIME MANAGEMENT

Oxygen Administration Setup

As you walk past the room of any person receiving oxygen, always check the humidifier. Make sure the humidifier is bubbling. Also make sure it has enough water. Tell the nurse if:

- There is no bubbling.
- The water level is low.

✳ SETTING UP FOR OXYGEN ADMINISTRATION

Quality of Life

Remember to:
- Knock before entering the person's room.
- Address the person by name.
- Introduce yourself by name and title.
- Explain the procedure to the person before beginning and during the procedure.
- Protect the person's rights during the procedure.
- Handle the person gently during the procedure.

Preprocedure

1. Follow *Delegation Guidelines: Oxygen Administration Setup.* See *Promoting Safety and Comfort: Oxygen Administration Setup.*
2. Practice hand hygiene.
3. Collect the following before going to the person's room:
   - Oxygen device with connecting tubing
   - Flowmeter
   - Humidifier (if ordered)
   - Distilled water (if using a humidifier)
4. Arrange your work area.
5. Decontaminate your hands.
6. Identify the person. Check the ID bracelet against the assignment sheet. Also call the person by name.

Procedure

7. Make sure the flowmeter is in the *OFF* position.
8. Attach the flowmeter to the wall outlet or to the tank.
9. Fill the humidifier with distilled water.
10. Attach the humidifier to the bottom of the flowmeter.
11. Attach the oxygen device and connecting tubing to the humidifier. *Do not set the flowmeter. Do not apply the oxygen device on the person.*
12. Place the cap securely on the distilled water. Store the water according to center policy.
13. Discard the packaging from the oxygen device and connecting tubing.

Postprocedure

14. Provide for comfort. (See the inside of the front cover.)
15. Place the call light within reach.
16. Decontaminate your hands.
17. Complete a safety check of the room. (See the inside of the front cover.)
18. Tell the nurse when you are done. *The nurse will:*
    a. *Turn on the oxygen and set the flow rate.*
    b. *Apply the oxygen device on the person.*

Some persons need inhalers, nebulizer treatments, artificial airways, suctioning, mechanical ventilation, and chest tubes. Persons who need respiratory rehabilitation are often very ill. They need to recover from problems affecting the airway and lungs. They need complex procedures and equipment.

The nurse may ask you to assist in their care. The center must teach and train you to provide needed care. The goals of care are to help persons:
- Reach their highest level of function.
- Live as independently as possible.
- Return home.

TYPES OF RESPIRATORY THERAPIES

Inhalers

Some persons need medication to help keep their air passages open. Asthma, bronchitis, and emphysema (Chapter 36) are examples of conditions that may have obstruction that needs to be cleared. Inhalers (Fig. 26.23) help open the air passages quickly. An acute asthma attack can be frightening for people. They cannot catch their breath, and often wheezing can be heard. They may need to have an inhaler immediately. Notify the nurse quickly, stay with the person, and offer reassurance.

Nebulizer Treatments

Another type of breathing treatment uses a machine called a *nebulizer.* A nebulizer (Fig. 26.24) gives the person medication that is inhaled in the form of a mist. The medication can be inhaled into the lungs through a mouthpiece or mask. The nurse gives the nebulizer treatment. Know your center's policy about caring for people who are receiving nebulizer treatments.

After the treatment, it is helpful to give the person a drink of water or assist with oral care (Chapter 18).

Artificial Airways

Artificial airways keep the airway patent (open and unblocked). They are needed:
- When disease, injury, secretions, or aspiration obstructs the airway.
- For mechanical ventilation (p. ⋯).
- By some persons who are semiconscious or unconscious.

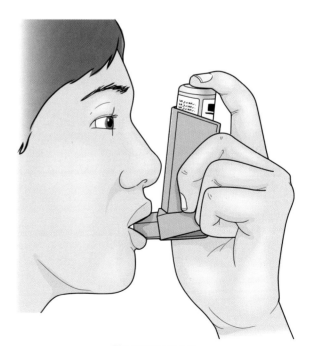

Fig. 26.23 Inhaler.

Intubation means inserting an artificial airway. They are usually plastic and disposable. They come in various sizes. These airways are common:

- *Oropharyngeal airway*—inserted through the mouth and into the pharynx (Fig. 26.25A). A nurse or respiratory therapist inserts the airway.
- *Endotracheal (ET) tube*—inserted through the mouth or nose and into the trachea (see Fig. 26.25B). A doctor inserts it using a lighted scope. Some registered nurses (RNs) and respiratory therapists are trained to insert ET tubes. A cuff is inflated to keep the airway in place.
- *Tracheostomy tube*—inserted through a surgically created opening *(stomy)* into the trachea *(tracheo)* (see Fig. 26.25C). Cuffed tubes are common. The cuff is inflated to keep the tube in place. Doctors perform tracheostomies.

Vital signs are checked often. Observe for hypoxia and other signs and symptoms. If an airway comes out or is dislodged, tell the nurse at once. Frequent oral hygiene is needed. Follow the care plan.

Gagging and choking feelings are common. Imagine something in your mouth, nose, or throat. Comfort and reassure the person. Remind the person that the airway helps breathing. Use touch to show you care.

Persons with ET tubes cannot speak. Some tracheostomy tubes allow speech. Paper and pencils, Magic Slates, and communication boards are ways to communicate. Hand signals, nodding the head, and hand squeezes are common for simple "yes" and "no" questions. Follow the care plan. *Always keep the call light within reach.*

Tracheostomies

A **tracheostomy** is a surgically created opening *(stomy)* into the trachea *(tracheo)*. Tracheostomies are temporary or permanent for mechanical ventilation (p. ··). They are permanent when airway structures are surgically removed. Cancer, severe airway trauma, or brain damage may require a permanent tracheostomy.

A tracheostomy tube is made of plastic, silicone, or metal. It has three parts (Fig. 26.26):

- The *obturator* has a round end. It is used to guide the insertion of the outer cannula (tube). Then it is removed. The obturator is placed within easy reach in case the tracheostomy tube falls out and needs reinsertion. It is taped to the wall or bedside stand.
- The *inner cannula* is inserted and locked in place. It fits inside the outer cannula. It is removed for cleaning and mucus removal. This keeps the airway patent. Some inner cannulas are disposable. Other tracheostomy tubes do not have inner cannulas.
- The *outer cannula* is secured in place with ties around the neck or a Velcro collar. The outer cannula is not removed. It keeps the tracheostomy patent.

The cuffed tracheostomy tube provides a seal between the cannula and the trachea (see Fig. 26.25C). This prevents air from leaking around the tube. It also prevents aspiration. A nurse or respiratory therapist inflates and deflates the cuff.

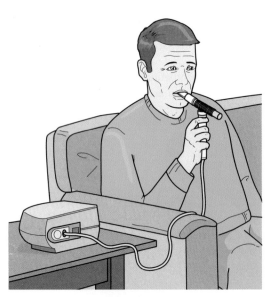

Fig. 26.24 Nebulizer.

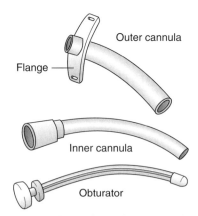

Fig. 26.26 Parts of a tracheostomy tube.

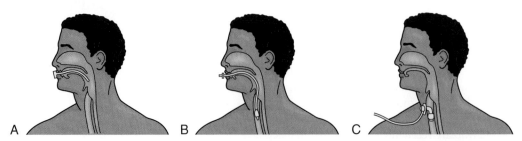

Fig. 26.25 Artificial airways. (A) Oropharyngeal airway. (B) Endotracheal tube. (C) Tracheostomy tube.

The tube must not come out *(extubation)*. If not secure, it could come out with coughing or if pulled on. A loose tube moves up and down. It can damage the trachea. *Call the nurse if the outer cannula comes out.*

The tube must remain patent. If able, the person coughs up secretions. Otherwise, suctioning is needed. *Call for the nurse if you note signs and symptoms of hypoxia or respiratory distress.*

Nothing must enter the stoma. Otherwise, the person can aspirate. These safety measures are needed:
- Dressings do not have loose gauze or lint.
- The stoma or tube is covered when outdoors. The person wears a stoma cover, scarf, or shirt or blouse that buttons at the neck. The cover prevents dust, insects, and other small particles from entering the stoma.
- The stoma is not covered with plastic, leather, or similar materials. They prevent air from entering the stoma. The person cannot breathe.
- Tub baths are taken. If showers are taken, a shower guard is worn. A handheld nozzle is used to direct water away from the stoma.
- The person is assisted with shampooing. Water must not enter the stoma.
- The stoma is covered when shaving.
- Swimming is not allowed. Water will enter the tube or stoma.
- Medical-alert jewelry is worn. The person carries a medical-alert ID card.

The nurse may ask you to assist with tracheostomy care. The care is done daily or every 8 to 12 hours. It also is done as needed for excess secretions, soiled ties or collar, or soiled or moist dressings. The care involves:
- Cleaning the inner cannula to remove mucus and keep the airway patent. Disposable inner cannulas are discarded after one use. A new cannula is inserted. Reusable inner cannulas are cleaned with a small bottle brush or a pipe cleaner. The nurse tells you what cleaning agent to use—usually hydrogen peroxide or a mild soap.
- Cleaning the stoma to prevent infection and skin breakdown.
- Applying clean ties or a Velcro collar to prevent infection. Clean ties are applied before removing the dirty ones. Hold the outer cannula in place when the nurse changes the ties or collar. Continue to do so until the nurse secures the new ties or collar. The ties or collar must be secure but not tight. For an adult, a finger should slide under the ties or collar (Fig. 26.27).

See *Promoting Safety and Comfort: Tracheostomies.*

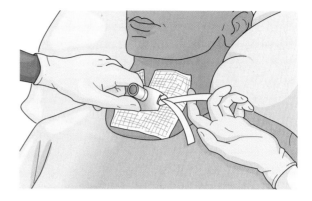
Fig. 26.27 For an adult, a finger is inserted under the ties.

SUCTIONING THE AIRWAY

Secretions can collect in the airway. Retained secretions:
- Obstruct air flow into and out of the airway.
- Provide an environment for microbes.
- Interfere with oxygen (O_2) and carbon dioxide (CO_2) exchange.

Hypoxia can occur. Usually coughing removes secretions. Some persons cannot cough, or the cough is too weak to remove secretions. They need suctioning.

Suction is the process of withdrawing or sucking up fluid *(secretions)*. A suction source is needed—wall outlet or suction machine. A tube connects to a suction source at one end and to a suction catheter at the other end. The catheter is inserted into the airway. Secretions are withdrawn through the catheter.

The nose, mouth, and pharynx make up the upper airway. The trachea and bronchi make up the lower airway. These routes are used to suction the airway:
- *Oropharyngeal.* The mouth *(oro)* and pharynx *(pharyngeal)* are suctioned. A suction catheter is passed through the mouth and into the pharynx. The Yankauer suction catheter is often used for thick secretions (Fig. 26.28).

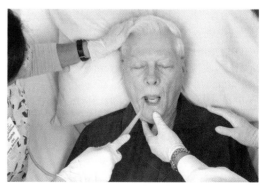
Fig. 26.28 The Yankauer suction catheter is often used when there are large amounts of thick secretions.

👤 PROMOTING SAFETY AND COMFORT

Tracheostomies
Safety
Mucus may contain microbes or blood. Follow Standard Precautions and the Bloodborne Pathogen Standard.

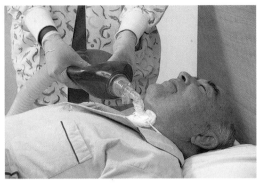

Fig. 26.29 The Ambu bag is squeezed with two hands.

- *Nasopharyngeal.* The nose *(naso)* and pharynx *(pharyngeal)* are suctioned. The suction catheter is passed through the nose into the pharynx.
- *Lower airway.* The suction catheter is passed through an ET or tracheostomy tube.

The person's lungs are hyperventilated before suctioning an ET or a tracheostomy tube. *Hyperventilate* means to give extra *(hyper)* breaths *(ventilate).* An Ambu bag is used (Fig. 26.29). The Ambu bag is attached to an oxygen source. Then the oxygen delivery device is removed from the ET or tracheostomy tube. The Ambu bag is attached to the ET or tracheostomy tube. To give a breath, the bag is squeezed with both hands. The nurse or respiratory therapist gives three to five breaths.

PROMOTING SAFETY AND COMFORT

Suctioning

Safety

If not done correctly, suctioning can cause serious harm. Suctioning removes oxygen from the airway. The person does not get oxygen during suctioning. Hypoxia and life-threatening problems can occur. They arise from the respiratory, cardiovascular, and nervous systems. Cardiac arrest can occur. Infection and airway injury are possible.

You can *assist* the nurse with suctioning (Box 26.4). However, you do not perform the suctioning procedure.

Always keep needed suction equipment and supplies at the bedside. When suctioning is needed, you do not have time to collect items from the supply area.

Mucus may contain microbes or blood. Follow Standard Precautions and the Bloodborne Pathogen Standard.

Oxygen is treated like a medication. You do not give medications. Check if your state and center allow you to use an Ambu bag attached to an oxygen source.

See *Promoting Safety and Comfort: Suctioning.*

MECHANICAL VENTILATION

Weak muscle effort, obstructed airway, and damaged lung tissue cause hypoxia. Nervous system diseases and injuries can affect the respiratory center in the brain. Nerve damage interferes with messages between the lungs and the brain. Medication overdose depresses the brain. With severe

---

BOX 26.4 Assisting with Suctioning: Safety Measures

- Review the procedure with the nurse. Know what the nurse wants you to do.
- Report coughing and the signs and symptoms of respiratory distress. They signal the need for suctioning. Suctioning is done as needed, not on a schedule.
- Standard Precautions and the Bloodborne Pathogen Standard are followed. Secretions may contain blood and are potentially infectious.
- Sterile technique is used (Chapter 14). This helps prevent microbes from entering the airway.
- The nurse tells you the catheter type and size needed. If too large, it can injure the airway.
- Needed suction supplies and equipment are kept at the bedside. They are ready when the person needs suctioning.
- Suction is *not* applied while inserting the catheter. When suction is applied, air is sucked out of the airway.
- The catheter is inserted smoothly. This helps prevent injury to mucous membranes.
- A suction cycle for adults takes no more than 10 to 15 seconds. A suction cycle involves:
  - Inserting the catheter.
  - Suctioning.
  - Removing the catheter.
- The catheter is cleared with sterile water or saline between suction cycles.
- The nurse waits 20 to 30 seconds between each suction cycle. Some centers require waiting 60 seconds.
- The suction catheter is passed (inserted) no more than three times. Injury and hypoxia are risks each time the suction catheter is passed.
- Check the person's pulse, respirations, and pulse oximeter measurements before, during, and after the procedure. Also observe the person's level of consciousness. Tell the nurse at once if any of these occur:
  - A drop in pulse rate or a pulse rate less than 60 beats per minute
  - Irregular pulse rhythms
  - A drop or rise in blood pressure
  - Respiratory distress
  - A drop in oxygen saturation (normal range is 95% to 100%)

---

problems, the person cannot breathe. Or normal blood oxygen levels are not maintained. Often, mechanical ventilation is needed.

Mechanical ventilation is using a machine to move air into and out of the lungs (Fig. 26.30). Oxygen enters the lungs. Carbon dioxide leaves them. An ET or tracheostomy tube is needed.

Mechanical ventilation is started in the hospital. Some people need it for a few hours or days. Others need it longer. They may require long-term care. Often, the person needs *weaning* from the ventilator. That is, the person needs to breathe without the machine. The respiratory therapist and RN plan the weaning process. Weaning can take many weeks.

Alarms sound when something is wrong. One alarm means the person is disconnected from the ventilator. The nurse shows you how to reconnect the ET or tracheostomy tube. *When any alarm sounds, first check to see if the tube is attached to the ventilator. If not, attach it to the ventilator. The person can die if*

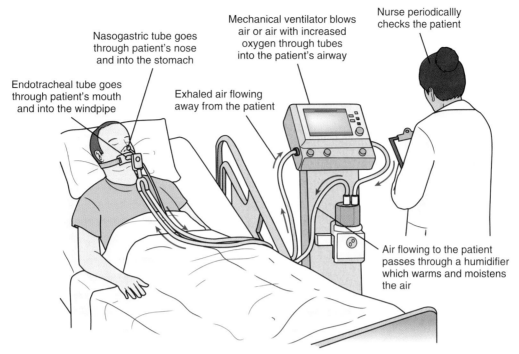

Fig. 26.30 A mechanical ventilator. (Redrawn from National Heart, Lung, and Blood Institute, National Institute of Health [NHLBI, NIH]: *What to expect while on a ventilator*, Bethesda, MD, 2011, Author.)

not attached to the ventilator. Then tell the nurse at once about the alarm. Do not reset alarms.

Persons needing mechanical ventilation are often very ill. Other problems and injuries are common. Some persons are confused, disoriented, or cannot think clearly. The machine and fear of dying frighten many. Some are relieved to get enough oxygen. Many fear needing the machine for life. Mechanical ventilation can be painful for those with chest injuries or chest surgery. Tubes and hoses restrict movement. This causes more discomfort.

The nurse may ask you to assist with the person's care (Box 26.5).

CHEST TUBES

Air, blood, or fluid can collect in the pleural space (sac or cavity). This occurs when the chest is entered because of injury or surgery.

- Pneumothorax is air *(pneumo)* in the pleural space *(thorax)*.
- Hemothorax is blood *(hemo)* in the pleural space *(thorax)*.
- Pleural effusion is the escape and collection of fluid *(effusion)* in the pleural space.

Pressure occurs when air, blood, or fluid collects in the pleural space. The pressure collapses the lung. Air cannot reach affected alveoli. O_2 and CO_2 are not exchanged. Respiratory distress and hypoxia result. Pressure on the heart affects the heart's ability to pump blood.

Hospital care is required. The doctor inserts chest tubes to remove the air, blood, or fluid (Fig. 26.31). The sterile procedure is done in surgery, in the emergency room, or at the bedside. A nurse assists.

Chest tubes attach to a drainage system (Fig. 26.32). The system must be airtight so air does not enter the pleural space. Water-seal drainage keeps the system airtight.

Box 26.6 indicates care of the person with chest tubes.

BOX 26.5 Care of Persons on Mechanical Ventilation

- Keep the call light within reach.
- Make sure hoses and connecting tubing have slack. They must not pull on the artificial airway.
- Answer call lights promptly. The person depends on others for basic needs.
- Explain who you are and what you are going to do. Do this whenever you enter the room.
- Give the day, date, and time every time you give care.
- Report signs of respiratory distress or discomfort at once.
- Do not change settings on the machine or reset alarms.
- Follow the care plan for communication. The person cannot talk. Use agreed-upon hand or eye signals for "yes" and "no." For effective communication, everyone must use the same signals. Some persons can use paper and pencils, Magic Slates, communication boards, and hand signals.
- Ask questions that have simple answers. It may be hard to write long responses.
- Watch what you say and do. This includes when you are near and away from the person and family. They pay close attention to your verbal and nonverbal communication. Do not say or do anything that could upset the person.
- Use touch to comfort and reassure the person. Also tell the person about the weather, pleasant news events, and gifts and cards.
- Meet basic needs. Follow the care plan.
- Tell the person when you are leaving the room and when you will return.
- Complete a safety check before leaving the room. (See the inside of the front cover.)

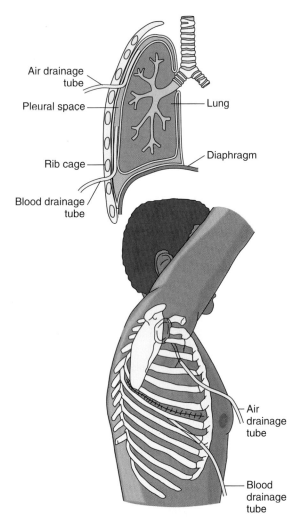

Fig. 26.31 Chest tubes inserted into the pleural space. (From Potter PA et al.: *Fundamentals of nursing*, ed. 9, St. Louis, 2017, Mosby.)

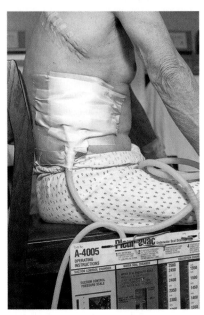

Fig. 26.32 Chest tubes attached to a disposable water-seal drainage system. Chest tubes are inserted into the pleural space. (From Perry AG, Potter PA, Ostendorf WR: *Clinical nursing skills and techniques*, ed. 8, St. Louis, 2014, Mosby.)

BOX 26.6 Care of the Person with Chest Tubes

- Keep the drainage system below the chest.
- Measure vital signs as directed. Report vital sign changes at once.
- Report signs and symptoms of hypoxia and respiratory distress at once. Also report complaints of pain or difficulty breathing.
- Keep connecting tubing coiled on the bed. Allow enough slack so the chest tubes are not dislodged when the person moves. If tubing hangs in loops, drainage collects in the loops.
- Prevent tubing kinks. Kinks obstruct the chest tube. Air, blood, or fluid collects in the pleural space.
- Observe chest drainage. Report any change in chest drainage at once. This includes increases in drainage or the appearance of bright red drainage.
- Record chest drainage according to agency policy.
- Turn and position the person as directed. When ambulating a person with a chest tube, always keep the drainage container below the insertion site. Be careful and gentle to prevent the chest tubes from dislodging.
- Assist with deep-breathing and coughing exercises as directed.
- Assist with incentive spirometry as directed.
- Note bubbling in the drainage system. Tell the nurse at once if bubbling increases, decreases, or stops.
- Tell the nurse at once if any part of the system is loose or disconnected.
- Keep sterile petrolatum gauze at the bedside. It is needed if a chest tube comes out.
- Call for help at once if a chest tube comes out. Cover the insertion site with sterile petrolatum gauze. Stay with the person. Follow the nurse's directions.
- Complete a safety check before leaving the room. (See the inside of the front cover.)

QUALITY OF LIFE

Residents have the right to safe care. Perform only procedures that you understand. Do not perform unfamiliar procedures.

You do not give oxygen. You assist in providing safe care to persons receiving oxygen. You need to understand oxygen therapy and its safety rules. Careful observation is needed. Promptly report observations and complaints. Some treatments and procedures have severe side effects and complications. Every sign, symptom, or complaint is important.

Protect the right to privacy. Do all you can to provide privacy. Screening with the privacy curtain is not enough. If possible, provide care when the roommate is out of the room. Close doors and window coverings.

Respiratory support and therapies involve complex care. Serious problems can occur from the wrong care. Know your limits. Follow the nurse's directions when assisting with care measures. Remember your legal and ethical responsibilities. You have the right to refuse a function or task. Do not function beyond your legal scope, preparation, and skill level.

TIME TO REFLECT

Mr. Watkins has chronic obstructive pulmonary disease (COPD). He has an oxygen concentrator in his room and receives oxygen through a nasal cannula at 2 L/min. Today, after returning from the bathroom, he is having trouble breathing. He becomes very anxious and presses his call light. When you arrive at his room, you find him sitting on the edge of the bed and barely able to catch his breath. His respirations are rapid and labored. His color is dusky. What would you do in this situation?

REVIEW QUESTIONS

Circle the BEST answer.

1. Alcohol and narcotics affect oxygen needs because they
   a. Depress the brain
   b. Are pollutants
   c. Cause allergies
   d. Cause infection

2. Hypoxia is
   a. Not enough oxygen in the blood
   b. The amount of hemoglobin that affects oxygen
   c. Not enough oxygen in the cells
   d. The lack of carbon dioxide

3. An early sign of hypoxia is
   a. Cyanosis
   b. Increased pulse and respiratory rates
   c. Restlessness
   d. Dyspnea

4. A person can breathe deeply and comfortably only while sitting. This is called
   a. Biot respirations
   b. Orthopnea
   c. Bradypnea
   d. Kussmaul respirations

5. The nurse tells you that a person has tachypnea. The person's respirations are
   a. Slow
   b. Rapid
   c. Absent
   d. Difficult or painful

6. The person needs to rest after
   a. A chest x-ray
   b. A lung scan
   c. Arterial blood gases
   d. Pulmonary function tests

7. A person's pulse oximeter measurement is 98%. Which is *true*?
   a. The pulse oximeter is wrong
   b. The pulse is 98 beats per minute
   c. The measurement is within normal range
   d. The person has respiratory depression

8. Which is *not* a site for a pulse oximetry sensor?
   a. Toe
   b. Finger
   c. Earlobe
   d. Upper arm

9. You are assisting with deep breathing and coughing. Which is *false*?
   a. The person inhales through pursed lips
   b. The person sits in a comfortable sitting position
   c. The person inhales deeply through the nose
   d. The person holds a pillow over an incision

10. Deep-breathing and coughing exercises are ordered. The person has a productive cough. You need to remind the person to
    a. Cover the nose and mouth when coughing
    b. Use a face mask
    c. Provide a sputum specimen
    d. Inhale through the mouth

11. A person has a tracheostomy. Which is *false*?
    a. The person must not cough
    b. The obturator is taped to the wall or bedside stand
    c. The nurse removes the inner cannula for cleaning
    d. The outer cannula must be secured in place

12. A person with a tracheostomy *cannot*
    a. Shampoo
    b. Shave
    c. Shower with a handheld nozzle
    d. Swim

13. The nurse is changing tracheostomy ties. You must
    a. Remove the inner cannula
    b. Clean the stoma
    c. Remove the dressing
    d. Hold the outer cannula in place

14. A person has a tracheostomy. You cannot slide a finger under the ties. This means that the ties
    a. Are secure
    b. Are too tight
    c. Need to be replaced
    d. Need to be removed

15. Which signals the need for suctioning?
    a. A pulse rate of 90 beats per minute
    b. Signs and symptoms of respiratory distress
    c. The orthopneic position
    d. Being unable to speak

16. Tracheostomy suctioning requires
    a. Sterile technique
    b. Mechanical ventilation
    c. An artificial airway
    d. Chest tubes

17. You note the following while assisting with suctioning. Which should you report at once?
    a. A pulse rate of 82 beats per minute
    b. A regular heart rhythm
    c. O_2 saturation of 92%
    d. Thick secretions

18. A person requires mechanical ventilation. Which is *false*?
    a. The person has an ET or tracheostomy tube
    b. The call light must always be within reach
    c. Touch provides comfort and reassurance
    d. You can reset alarms on the ventilator

19. An alarm sounds on a person's ventilator. What should you do *first*?
    a. Reset the alarm
    b. Check to see if the airway is attached to the machine
    c. Call the nurse at once
    d. Ask the person what is wrong

20. A person has a pneumothorax. This is
    a. Fluid in the pleural space
    b. Blood in the pleural space
    c. Air in the pleural space
    d. Secretions in the pleural space

See Appendix A for answers to these questions.

27

Measuring Vital Signs

OBJECTIVES

- Define the key terms and key abbreviations listed in this chapter.
- Explain why vital signs are measured.
- List the factors affecting vital signs.
- Identify the normal ranges for each temperature site.
- Explain when to use each temperature site.
- Describe the different types of thermometers.
- Identify the pulse sites.
- Describe a normal pulse and normal respirations.
- Describe the practices to follow when measuring blood pressure.
- Perform the procedures described in this chapter.
- Explain how to promote quality of life.

KEY TERMS

apical-radial pulse Taking the apical and radial pulses at the same time

blood pressure (BP) The amount of force exerted against the walls of an artery by the blood

body temperature The amount of heat in the body that is a balance between the amount of heat produced and the amount lost by the body

bradycardia A slow (*brady-*) heart rate (*cardia*); less than 60 beats per minute

diastole The period of heart muscle relaxation; the heart is at rest

diastolic pressure The pressure in the arteries when the heart is at rest

fever Elevated body temperature

hypertension Blood pressure measurements remaining above (*hyper-*) a systolic pressure of 120 mm Hg or a diastolic pressure of 80 mm Hg

hypotension When the systolic blood pressure is below (*hypo-*) 90 mm Hg and the diastolic pressure is below 60 mm Hg

pulse The beat of the heart felt at an artery as a wave of blood passes through the artery

pulse deficit The difference between the apical and radial pulse rates

pulse rate The number of heartbeats or pulses felt in 1 minute

respiration Breathing air into (inhalation) and out of (exhalation) the lungs

sphygmomanometer A cuff and measuring device used to measure blood pressure

stethoscope An instrument used to listen to sounds produced by the heart, lungs, and other body organs

systole The period of heart muscle contraction; the heart is pumping blood

systolic pressure The pressure in the arteries when the heart contracts

tachycardia A rapid (*tachy-*) heart rate (*cardia*); more than 100 beats per minute

vital signs Temperature, pulse, respirations, and blood pressure

KEY ABBREVIATIONS

AHA American Heart Association	ID Identification
BP Blood pressure	IV Intravenous
C Centigrade	mm Millimeter
F Fahrenheit	mm Hg Millimeters of mercury
Hg Mercury	TPR Temperature, pulse, and respiration

Vital signs reflect the function of three body processes essential for life: regulation of body temperature, breathing, and heart function. There are four vital signs of body function:

- Temperature
- Pulse
- Respirations
- Blood pressure

Vital signs are often called TPR (temperature, pulse, and respiration) and BP (blood pressure). This is the commonly accepted order of recording vital signs. Many facilities check pulse oximetry readings in addition to TPR and BP. This procedure was discussed in Chapter 26. Follow the policies of your nursing center.

MEASURING AND REPORTING VITAL SIGNS

A person's vital signs vary within certain limits. They are affected by sleep, activity, eating, weather, noise, exercise, medications, anger, fear, anxiety, pain, and illness.

Vital signs are measured to detect changes in normal body function. They tell about treatment response. They often signal life-threatening events. Vital signs are part of the assessment step in the nursing process. Vital signs are measured:

- During physical exams.
- When the person is admitted to the center.
- As often as the person's condition requires.
- Before and after surgery, complex procedures, and diagnostic tests.
- After some care measures, such as ambulation.
- After a fall or other injury.
- When medications affect the respiratory or circulatory system.
- When the person complains of pain, dizziness, lightheadedness, feeling faint, shortness of breath, a rapid heart rate, or not feeling well.
- When there is increased risk for the spread of infection.
- As stated on the care plan (usually daily, twice a day, or weekly in nursing centers).

Vital signs show even minor changes in the person's condition. Accuracy is essential when you measure, record, and report vital signs. If unsure of your measurements, promptly ask the nurse to take them again. Unless otherwise ordered, take vital signs with the person at rest—lying or sitting. Report the following at once:

- Any vital sign that is changed from a prior measurement
- Vital signs above the normal range
- Vital signs below the normal range

Vital signs are recorded in the person's medical record. If measured often, a flow sheet is used. The doctor or nurse compares current and previous measurements.

See *Residents with Dementia: Measuring and Reporting Vital Signs.*

See *Focus on Communication: Measuring and Reporting Vital Signs.*

🧑 RESIDENTS WITH DEMENTIA

Measuring and Reporting Vital Signs

Measuring vital signs on persons with dementia may be difficult. The person may move about, hit at you, and grab equipment. This is not safe for the person or for you. Two workers may be needed. One uses touch and a soothing voice to calm and distract the person. The other measures the vital signs.

You may need to try the procedure when the person is calmer. Or take the pulse and respirations at one time. Then take the temperature and blood pressure at another time.

Always approach the person calmly. Use a soothing voice. Tell the person what you are going to do. Do not rush the person. Follow the care plan. If you cannot measure vital signs, tell the nurse right away.

📋 FOCUS ON COMMUNICATION

Measuring and Reporting Vital Signs

Residents like to know their measurements. If center policy allows, tell the person the measurements. Remember, this information is private and confidential. Roommates and visitors must not hear what you are saying.

A measurement may be abnormal. Or you may not be able to feel a pulse or hear a blood pressure. Do not alarm the person. You can say:

- "I'm not sure that I counted your pulse correctly. I'll ask the nurse to take it."
- "I'm not sure that I heard your blood pressure correctly. I'll ask the nurse to take it again."
- "Your pulse is a little slow (or fast). I'll ask the nurse to check it."
- "Your temperature is higher than normal. I'm going to use another thermometer. I'll also ask the nurse to check you."

BODY TEMPERATURE

Body temperature is the amount of heat in the body. It is a balance between the amount of heat produced and the amount lost by the body. Heat is produced as cells use food for energy. It is lost through the skin, breathing, urine, and feces. Body temperature stays fairly stable. It is lower in the morning and higher in the afternoon and evening. See p. ·· for the factors affecting vital signs. Pregnancy and the menstrual cycle are other factors affecting body temperature.

You use thermometers to measure temperature. It is measured using the Fahrenheit (F) and Centigrade (C) scales.

Temperature Sites

Temperature sites are the mouth, rectum, axilla (underarm), tympanic membrane (ear), and temporal artery (forehead) (Box 27.1). Each site has a normal range (Table 27.1). **Fever** means an elevated body temperature.

Older persons have lower body temperatures than younger persons. An oral temperature of 98.6°F may signal fever in an older person. Always report temperatures that are above or below the normal range.

See *Promoting Safety and Comfort: Temperature Sites.*
See *Delegation Guidelines: Taking Temperatures.*
See *Promoting Safety and Comfort: Taking Temperatures.*

🧑 PROMOTING SAFETY AND COMFORT

Temperature Sites
Safety
Rectal temperatures are dangerous for persons with heart disease. The thermometer can stimulate the vagus nerve in the rectum. This nerve also affects the heart. Stimulation of the vagus nerve slows the heart rate. The heart rate can slow to dangerous levels in some persons.

BOX 27.1 Temperature Sites

Oral Site

Oral temperatures are *not* taken if the person:
- Is under 4 or 5 years of age.
- Is unconscious.
- Has had surgery or an injury to the face, neck, nose, or mouth.
- Is receiving oxygen.
- Breathes through the mouth.
- Has a nasogastric tube.
- Is delirious, restless, confused, or disoriented.
- Is paralyzed on one side of the body.
- Has a sore mouth.
- Has a convulsive (seizure) disorder.

Rectal Site

Rectal temperatures are taken when the other sites cannot be used. Rectal temperatures are *not* taken if the person:
- Has diarrhea.

- Has a rectal disorder or injury.
- Has heart disease.
- Had rectal surgery.
- Is confused or agitated.

Tympanic Membrane Site

The site has fewer microbes than the mouth or rectum. The risk of spreading infection is reduced. This site is *not* used if the person has:
- An ear disorder.
- Ear drainage.

Temporal Artery Site

Measures body temperature at the temporal artery in the forehead. The site is noninvasive.

Axillary Site

Less reliable than the other sites. It is used when the other sites cannot be used.

DELEGATION GUIDELINES

Taking Temperatures

Before taking temperatures, you need this information from the nurse and the care plan:
- What site to use for each person—oral, rectal, axillary, tympanic membrane, or temporal artery
- What thermometer to use for each person—electronic or other type (p. 427)
- When to take temperatures
- Which persons are at risk for elevated temperatures
- What observations to report and record:
  - A temperature that is changed from a prior measurement
  - A temperature above or below the normal range for the site used
- When to report observations
- What specific resident concerns to report at once

TABLE 27.1 Normal Body Temperatures

Site	Baseline	Normal Range
Oral	98.6°F (37°C)	97.6°F to 99.6°F (36.5°C to 37.5°C)
Rectal	99.6°F (37.5°C)	98.6°F to 100.6°F (37.0°C to 38.1°C)
Axillary	97.6°F (36.5°C)	96.6°F to 98.6°F (35.9°C to 37.0°C)
Tympanic membrane	98.6°F (37°C)	97.6°F to 99.6°F (36.5°C to 37.5°C)
Temporal artery	98.6°F (37°C)	97.6°F to 99.6°F (36.5°C to 37.5°C)

PROMOTING SAFETY AND COMFORT

Taking Temperatures

Safety

Thermometers are inserted into the mouth, rectum, axilla, and ear. Each area has many microbes. The area may contain blood. Follow Standard Precautions and the Bloodborne Pathogen Standard when taking temperatures.

With rectal temperatures, your gloved hands may have contact with feces. If so, remove gloves and practice hand hygiene. Then note the temperature on your note pad or assignment sheet. Put on clean gloves to complete the procedure.

Electronic Thermometers

Electronic thermometers are battery operated. They measure temperature in a few seconds. The temperature is shown on the front of the device. Some have batteries. Others are larger and kept in battery chargers when not in use (Fig. 27.1). Most electronic thermometers are designed to measure temperature at the oral (Fig. 27.2) and axillary (Fig. 27.3) sites. Rectal temperatures require a separate rectal thermometer or a special rectal probe (Fig. 27.4). Rectal thermometers and probes are always color-coded red. A disposable cover (sheath) protects the probe. You discard the probe cover after use. This helps prevent the spread of infection.

Types of Thermometers

Currently the two most common types of thermometers used are electronic and disposable. Glass thermometers have been eliminated from health care settings because of the environmental hazards of mercury and the risk of injury from broken glass. There are several variations of electronic thermometers.

Tympanic Membrane Thermometers

Tympanic membrane thermometers measure temperature at the tympanic membrane in the ear (Figs. 27.5 and 27.6). The covered probe is gently inserted into the ear. The temperature is measured in 1 to 3 seconds.

Tympanic membrane thermometers are comfortable. They are not invasive like rectal thermometers and probes. There are

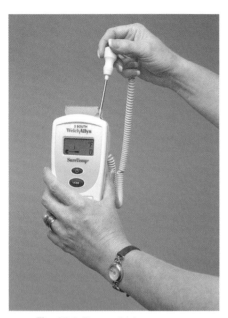

Fig. 27.1 Electronic thermometer.

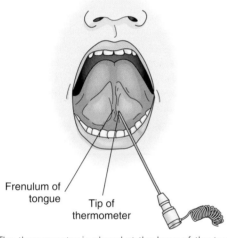

Frenulum of tongue

Tip of thermometer

Fig. 27.2 The thermometer is placed at the base of the tongue and to one side.

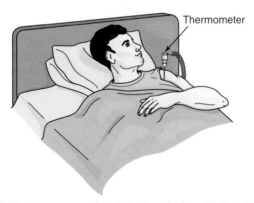

Thermometer

Fig. 27.3 The thermometer is held in place in the axilla by bringing the person's arm over the chest.

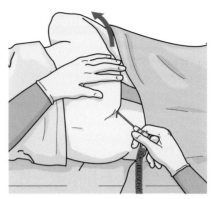

Fig. 27.4 The rectal temperature is taken with the person in the left side-lying position. The buttock is raised to expose the anus.

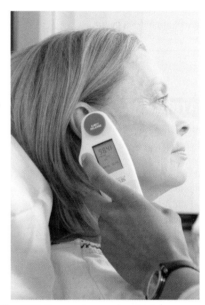

Fig. 27.5 Tympanic membrane thermometer.

fewer microbes in the ear than in the mouth or rectum. The risk of spreading infection is reduced. These devices are not used if there is ear drainage or if the person complains of an earache. If the person wears hearing aids in both ears, ask the person to remove one hearing aid. Wait 5 minutes and then insert the covered probe into the ear.

Temporal Artery Thermometers

Body temperature is measured at the temporal artery in the forehead (Fig. 27.7). You gently stroke the device across the forehead and across the temporal artery. It measures the temperature of the blood in the temporal artery—the same temperature of the blood coming from the heart.

These noninvasive devices measure body temperature in 3 to 4 seconds. Follow the manufacturer instructions to use, clean, and store the device. Some devices have probe covers. To measure temperature:

- Use the side of the head that is exposed. Do not use the side covered by hair, a dressing, a hat, or other covering. Do not use the side that was on a pillow.

- Place the device at the side of the forehead between the hairline and eyebrows.
- Slide the device across the forehead.
- Read the temperature display.

Infrared or Noncontact Thermometers

Noncontact thermometers are safe and easy to use, as nothing comes in contact with the person's body (Fig. 27.8).

- The test area of the forehead must be clean, dry, and unblocked during measurement.
- The person's forehead test area has not been increased or decreased by wearing head covers (for example, headbands, bandanas).
- The thermometer sensing area should be held perpendicular to the forehead.
- The person remains stationary.
- Consult the manufacturer's instructions for measurement distances.
- Do not touch the sensing area. Keep it clean and dry.
  See *Residents with Dementia: Electronic Thermometers.*

See *Teamwork and Time Management: Electronic Thermometers.*

RESIDENTS WITH DEMENTIA

Electronic Thermometers

Tympanic membrane, temporal artery, and infrared thermometers are used for persons who are confused and resist care. They are fast and comfortable. Oral and rectal thermometers are unsafe because an electronic thermometer can injure the mouth and teeth if the person bites down on it. It also can cause injury if the person moves quickly and without warning.

TEAMWORK AND TIME MANAGEMENT

Electronic Thermometers

Electronic, tympanic membrane, infrared, and temporal artery thermometers are shared with your coworkers. When using these devices, tell your coworkers what thermometer you have. Work quickly but carefully. Return the device to the charging unit in a timely manner. Check to see that there is an adequate supply of disposable probe covers if the thermometer needs these.

TAKING A TEMPERATURE WITH AN ELECTRONIC THERMOMETER (NATCEP)

Quality of Life

Remember to:

- Knock before entering the person's room.
- Address the person by name.
- Introduce yourself by name and title.
- Explain the procedure to the person before beginning and during the procedure.
- Protect the person's rights during the procedure.
- Handle the person gently during the procedure.

Preprocedure

1. Follow *Delegation Guidelines: Taking Temperatures,* p. 423. See *Promoting Safety and Comfort: Taking Temperatures,* p. 423.
2. For an oral temperature, ask the person not to eat, drink, smoke, or chew gum for at least 15 to 20 minutes before the measurement or as required by center policy.
3. Practice hand hygiene.
4. Collect the following:
   - Thermometer—electronic, tympanic membrane, or temporal
   - Probe (blue for an oral or axillary temperature; red for a rectal temperature)
   - Probe covers
   - Toilet tissue (rectal temperature)
   - Water-soluble lubricant (rectal temperature)
   - Gloves
   - Towel (axillary temperature)
5. Plug the probe into the thermometer, if using an electronic thermometer.
6. Decontaminate your hands.
7. Identify the person. Check the identification (ID) bracelet against the assignment sheet. Also call the person by name.

Procedure

8. Provide for privacy. Position the person for an oral, rectal, axillary, or tympanic membrane temperature.
9. Put on gloves if contact with blood, body fluids, secretions, or excretions is likely.

10. Insert the probe into a probe cover.
11. For an *oral temperature:*
    a. Ask the person to open the mouth and raise the tongue.
    b. Place the covered probe at the base of the tongue and to one side (see Fig. 27.2).
    c. Ask the person to lower the tongue and close the mouth.
12. For a *rectal temperature:*
    a. Place some lubricant on toilet tissue.
    b. Lubricate the end of the covered probe.
    c. Expose the anal area.
    d. Raise the upper buttock.
    e. Insert the probe ½ inch into the rectum (see Fig. 27.4).
    f. Hold the probe in place.
13. For an *axillary temperature:*
    a. Help the person remove an arm from the gown. Do not expose the person.
    b. Dry the axilla with the towel.
    c. Place the covered probe in the center of the axilla (see Fig. 27.3).
    d. Place the person's arm over the chest.
    e. Hold the probe in place.
14. For a *tympanic membrane temperature:*
    a. Ask the person to turn the head so the ear is in front of you (see Fig. 27.5).
    b. Pull up and back on the adult's ear to straighten the ear canal (Fig. 27.6).
    c. Insert the covered probe gently.
15. Start the thermometer.
16. Hold the probe in place until you hear a tone or see a flashing or steady light.
17. Read the temperature on the display.
18. Remove the probe. Press the eject button to discard the cover.
19. For a *temporal artery temperature:*
    a. Ask the person to look (turn the face) toward you (see Fig. 27.7).
    b. Place the device near the center of the forehead. Press the button.
    c. While keeping the button depressed, slide the device across the forehead and over the temporal artery, ending in front of the ear. (If the person has perspiration on the forehead, continue sliding the device to the back of the ear.) Always follow manufacturer instructions.

Continued

✳ TAKING A TEMPERATURE WITH AN ELECTRONIC THERMOMETER (NATCEP)—cont'd

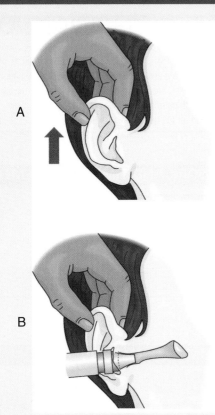

Fig. 27.6 Using a tympanic membrane thermometer. (A) The ear is pulled up and back. (B) The probe is inserted into the ear canal.

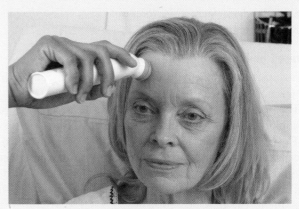

Fig. 27.7 Temporal artery thermometer.

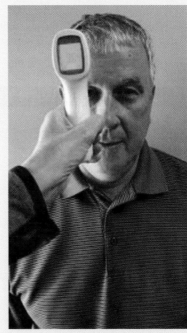

Fig. 27.8 A noncontact infrared thermometer. (From Fairchild SL, O'Shea RK: *Pierson and Fairchild's principles & techniques of patient care*, ed. 7, St. Louis, 2023, Elsevier.)

20. Note the person's name and temperature on your note pad or assignment sheet. Note the temperature site.
21. Return the probe to the holder.
22. Help the person put the gown back on (axillary temperature). For a *rectal temperature:*
    a. Wipe the anal area with toilet tissue to remove lubricant.
    b. Cover the person.
    c. Dispose of used toilet tissue.
    d. Remove the gloves. Practice hand hygiene.
23. For a noncontact infrared thermometer:
    a. Ask the person to pull back any hair from forehead.
    b. Hold thermometer the recommended distance from the person's forehead (see Fig. 27.8)
    c. Press the button on the thermometer.
    d. Note the reading.

Postprocedure
24. Provide for comfort. (See the inside of the front cover.)
25. Place the call light within reach.

26. Unscreen the person.
27. Complete a safety check of the room. (See the inside of the front cover.)
28. Return the thermometer to the charging unit.
29. Decontaminate your hands.
30. Report and record the temperature. Note the temperature site when reporting and recording. A rectal temperature should always be noted with "R" after the value. An axillary temperature should always be recorded with "Ax" after the value. Report an abnormal temperature at once.

This skill is also covered in *Clinical Skills: Nurse Assisting.*

Other Thermometers

Other thermometers are used. Follow the manufacturer instructions.

- *Digital thermometers*—show the temperature on the front of the thermometer (Fig. 27.9). Depending on the type, the temperature is measured in 6 to 60 seconds. Some of these thermometers have disposable sheath covers (Fig. 27.10). A rectal version will be color-coded red (see Fig. 27.10).
- *Disposable oral thermometers*—have small chemical dots (Fig. 27.11). The dots change color when heated. Each dot is heated to a certain temperature before it changes color. These thermometers are used once. They measure temperatures in 45 to 60 seconds.

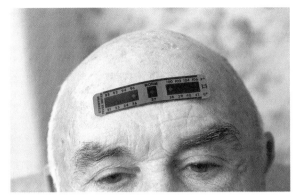

Fig. 27.12 Temperature-sensitive tape.

- *Temperature-sensitive tape*—changes color in response to body heat (Fig. 27.12). The tape is applied to the forehead. The measurement takes about 15 seconds.

PULSE

The **pulse** is the beat of the heart felt at an artery as a wave of blood passes through the artery. A pulse is felt every time the heart beats.

Pulse Sites

The temporal, carotid, brachial, radial, femoral, popliteal, posterior tibial, and dorsalis pedis (pedal) pulses are on each side of the body (Fig. 27.13). The arteries are close to the body surface and lie over a bone; therefore, they are easy to feel.

The radial pulse is used most often. It is easy to reach and find. You can take a radial pulse without disturbing or exposing

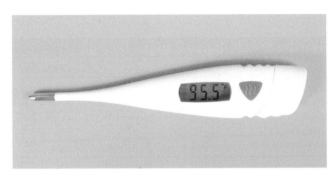

Fig. 27.9 Digital thermometer.

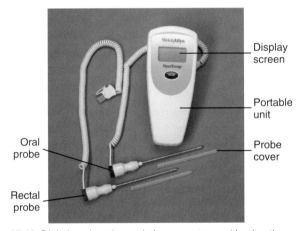

Display screen

Portable unit

Oral probe

Probe cover

Rectal probe

Fig. 27.10 Digital oral and rectal thermometers with sheath covers. (From Bonewit-West K: *Clinical procedures for medical assistants*, ed. 9, St. Louis, 2015, Saunders.)

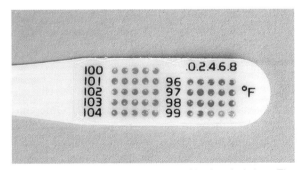

Fig. 27.11 Disposable oral thermometer with chemical dots. The dots change color when heated by the body.

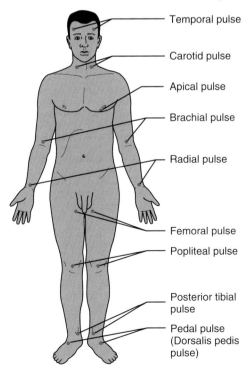

Temporal pulse

Carotid pulse

Apical pulse

Brachial pulse

Radial pulse

Femoral pulse

Popliteal pulse

Posterior tibial pulse

Pedal pulse (Dorsalis pedis pulse)

Fig. 27.13 The pulse sites.

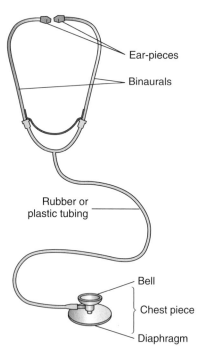

Ear-pieces

Binaurals

Rubber or plastic tubing

Bell

Chest piece

Diaphragm

Fig. 27.14 Parts of a stethoscope.

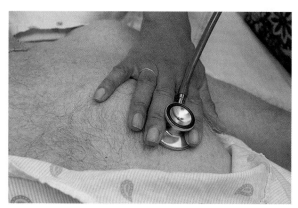

Fig. 27.15 The stethoscope is held in place with the fingertips of the index and middle fingers.

TABLE 27.2	**Pulse Ranges by Age**
Age	**Pulse Rate per Minute**
Birth to 1 year	80—190
2 years	80—160
6 years	75—120
10 years	70—110
12 years and older	60—100

the person. The carotid pulse is taken during cardiopulmonary resuscitation (CPR) and other emergencies (Chapter 44).

The apical pulse is heard over the heart. The apex *(apical)* of the heart is at the tip of the heart, just below the left nipple (see Fig. 27.15, later). This pulse is taken with a stethoscope.

Using a Stethoscope

A stethoscope is an instrument used to listen to the sounds produced by the heart, lungs, and other body organs (Fig. 27.14). It is used to take apical pulses and blood pressures. The device makes sounds louder for easy hearing.

To use a stethoscope:

- Wipe the earpieces and diaphragm with antiseptic wipes before and after use.
- Place the earpiece tips in your ears. The bend of the tips points forward. Earpieces should fit snugly to block out noises. They should not cause pain or ear discomfort.
- Tap the diaphragm gently. You should hear the tapping. If not, turn the chest piece at the tubing. Gently tap the diaphragm again. Proceed if you hear the tapping sound. Check with the nurse if you do not hear the tapping.
- Place the diaphragm over the artery. Hold it in place (Fig. 27.15).
- Prevent noise. Do not let anything touch the tubing. Ask the person to be silent. Mute the TV or radio.

See *Focus on Communication: Using a Stethoscope.*
See *Promoting Safety and Comfort: Using a Stethoscope.*

Pulse Rate

The pulse rate is the number of heartbeats or pulses felt in 1 minute. The rate varies for each age group (Table 27.2). The pulse rate is affected by many factors (p. 422).

> 📋 **FOCUS ON COMMUNICATION**
>
> **Using a Stethoscope**
> Hearing through the stethoscope is hard if the person is talking. Politely ask the person to be silent. Explain the procedure. Tell the person when and for how long to remain silent. You can say: "Mr. Bradley, I am going to check your pulse with a stethoscope. It is hard for me to hear your heartbeat when you talk. Please do not talk when my stethoscope is on your chest. It will take about 1 minute."
>
> The person may forget and begin talking. You can politely say: "I am almost finished. Please stay quiet for just a little longer." Thank the person when you are done.

> 👤 **PROMOTING SAFETY AND COMFORT**
>
> **Using a Stethoscope**
> *Safety*
> Stethoscopes are in contact with many persons and staff. You must prevent infection. Wipe the earpieces and diaphragm with antiseptic wipes before and after use.
>
> *Comfort*
> Stethoscope diaphragms tend to be cold. Warm the diaphragm in your hand before applying it to the person (Fig. 27.16). Cold diaphragms can startle the person.

Some medications increase the pulse rate. Other medications slow down the pulse.

The adult pulse rate is between 60 and 100 beats per minute. A rate of less than 60 or more than 100 is considered abnormal. Report abnormal pulses to the nurse at once.

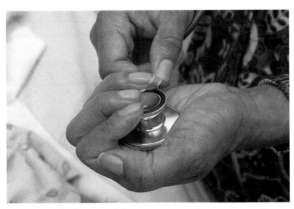

Fig. 27.16 The diaphragm of the stethoscope is warmed in the palm of the hand.

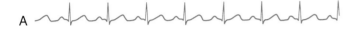

A

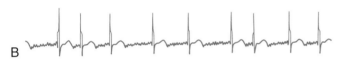

B

Fig. 27.17 (A) The electrocardiogram shows a regular pulse. The beats occur at regular intervals. (B) These beats are at irregular intervals.

- Tachycardia is a rapid *(tachy)* heart rate *(cardia)*. The heart rate is more than 100 beats per minute.
- Bradycardia is a slow *(brady)* heart rate *(cardia)*. The heart rate is less than 60 beats per minute.

Rhythm and Force of the Pulse

The pulse *rhythm* should be regular. That is, pulses are felt in a pattern. The same interval occurs between beats. An irregular pulse occurs when the beats are not evenly spaced or beats are skipped (Fig. 27.17).

Force relates to pulse strength. A forceful pulse is easy to feel. It is described as *strong*, *full*, or *bounding*. Hard-to-feel pulses are described as *weak*, *thready*, or *feeble*.

Electronic blood pressure equipment (p. 434) can also count pulses. The pulse rate and blood pressures are shown.

Some show if the pulse is regular or irregular. However, you need to feel the pulse to determine its force.

Taking Pulses

You will take radial, apical, and apical-radial pulses. You must count, report, and record accurately.

See *Delegation Guidelines: Taking Pulses.*
See *Promoting Safety and Comfort: Taking Pulses.*

DELEGATION GUIDELINES

Taking Pulses
Before taking a pulse, you need this information from the nurse and the care plan:
- What pulse to take for each person—radial, apical, or apical-radial (p. 431)
- When to take the pulse
- What other vital signs to measure
- How long to count the pulse—30 seconds or 1 minute
- If the nurse has concerns about certain residents
- What observations to report and record:
  - The pulse site
  - The pulse rate—report a pulse rate less than 60 (bradycardia) or more than 100 beats (tachycardia) per minute at once
  - Pulse deficit for an apical-radial pulse (p. 431)
  - If the pulse is regular or irregular
  - Pulse force—strong, full, bounding, weak, thready, or feeble
- When to report the pulse rate
- What specific resident concerns to report at once

PROMOTING SAFETY AND COMFORT

Taking Pulses
Safety
Use your first two or three middle fingertips to take a pulse. Do not use your thumb. The thumb has a pulse. You could mistake the pulse in your thumb for the person's pulse. Reporting and recording the wrong pulse rate can harm the person.

Taking a Radial Pulse

The radial pulse is used for routine vital signs. Place the first two or three fingertips of one hand against the radial artery. The radial artery is on the thumb side of the wrist (Fig. 27.18). Count the pulse for 30 seconds, then multiply the number by 2. This gives the number of beats per minute. If the pulse is irregular, count it for 1 minute.

In some centers, all radial pulses are taken for 1 minute. Follow center policy.

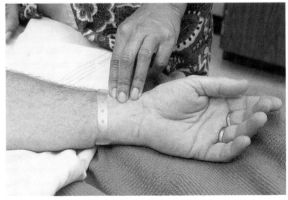

Fig. 27.18 The middle three fingertips are used to take the radial pulse.

✳ TAKING A RADIAL PULSE (NATCEP)

Quality of Life

Remember to:

- Knock before entering the person's room.
- Address the person by name.
- Introduce yourself by name and title.
- Explain the procedure to the person before beginning and during the procedure.
- Protect the person's rights during the procedure.
- Handle the person gently during the procedure.

Preprocedure

1. Follow *Delegation Guidelines: Taking Pulses.* See *Promoting Safety and Comfort: Taking Pulses.*
2. Practice hand hygiene.
3. Identify the person. Check the ID bracelet against the assignment sheet. Also call the person by name.
4. Provide for privacy.

Procedure

5. Have the person sit or lie down.

6. Locate the radial pulse on the thumb side of the person's wrist. Use your first two or three middle fingertips (see Fig. 27.18).
7. Note if the pulse is strong or weak and regular or irregular.
8. Count the pulse for 30 seconds, then multiply the number of beats by 2. Or count the pulse for 1 minute if:
   a. Directed by the nurse and care plan.
   b. Required by center policy.
   c. The pulse was irregular.
   d. Required for your state competency test.
9. Note the person's name and pulse on your note pad or assignment sheet. Note the strength of the pulse. Note if it was regular or irregular.

Postprocedure

10. Provide for comfort. (See the inside of the front cover.)
11. Place the call light within reach.
12. Unscreen the person.
13. Complete a safety check of the room. (See the inside of the front cover.)
14. Decontaminate your hands.
15. Report and record the pulse rate and your observations. Report an abnormal pulse at once.

This skill is also covered in *Clinical Skills: Nurse Assisting.*

✳ Taking an Apical Pulse

The apical pulse is on the left side of the chest slightly below the nipple (Fig. 27.19). It is taken with a stethoscope. Apical pulses are taken on persons who:

- Have heart disease.
- Have irregular heart rhythms.
- Take medications that affect the heart.

Count the apical pulse for 1 minute. The heartbeat normally sounds like a *lub-dub*. Count each *lub-dub* as one beat. Do not count the *lub* as one beat and the *dub* as another.

✳ TAKING AN APICAL PULSE

Quality of Life

Remember to:

- Knock before entering the person's room.
- Address the person by name.
- Introduce yourself by name and title.
- Explain the procedure to the person before beginning and during the procedure.
- Protect the person's rights during the procedure.
- Handle the person gently during the procedure.

Preprocedure

1. Follow *Delegation Guidelines: Taking Pulses*, p. 429. See *Promoting Safety and Comfort: Using a Stethoscope*, p. 428.
2. Practice hand hygiene.
3. Collect a stethoscope and antiseptic wipes.
4. Decontaminate your hands.
5. Identify the person. Check the ID bracelet against the assignment sheet. Also call the person by name.
6. Provide for privacy.

Procedure

7. Clean the earpieces and diaphragm with the wipes.
8. Have the person sit or lie down.
9. Expose the nipple area of the left chest. Expose a woman's breasts to the extent necessary.
10. Warm the diaphragm in your palm.
11. Place the earpieces in your ears.
12. Find the apical pulse. Place the diaphragm 2 to 3 inches to the left of the breastbone and below the left nipple (see Fig. 27.19).
13. Count the pulse for 1 minute. Note if it was regular or irregular.
14. Cover the person. Remove the earpieces.

15. Note the person's name and pulse on your note pad or assignment sheet. Note if the pulse was regular or irregular.

Postprocedure

16. Provide for comfort. (See the inside of the front cover.)
17. Place the call light within reach.
18. Unscreen the person.
19. Complete a safety check of the room. (See the inside of the front cover.)
20. Clean the earpieces and diaphragm with the wipes.
21. Return the stethoscope to its proper place.
22. Decontaminate your hands.
23. Report and record your observations. Record the pulse rate with *Ap* for apical. Report an abnormal pulse rate at once.

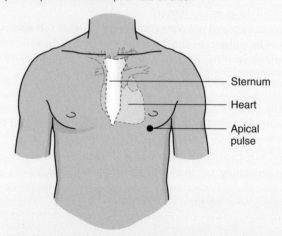

Fig. 27.19 The apical pulse is located 2 to 3 inches to the left of the sternum (breastbone) and below the left nipple.

This skill is also covered in *Clinical Skills: Nurse Assisting.*

Taking an Apical-Radial Pulse

The apical and radial pulse rates should be the same. Sometimes heart contractions are not strong enough to create pulses in the radial artery. Then the radial rate is less than the apical rate. Heart disease is a common cause.

To see if the apical and radial pulses are equal, two staff members are needed. One takes the radial pulse; the other takes the apical pulse. Taking the apical and radial pulses at the same time is called the apical-radial pulse.

The pulse deficit is the difference between the apical and radial pulse rates. That is, you subtract the radial rate from the apical rate. (The radial rate is never greater than the apical rate.) For example:

- The apical rate is 84 beats per minute. The radial rate is 84 beats per minute. The pulse deficit is zero (0).
- The apical rate is 90 beats per minute. The radial rate is 86 beats per minute. The pulse deficit is 4.

TAKING AN APICAL-RADIAL PULSE

Quality of Life

Remember to:

- Knock before entering the person's room.
- Address the person by name.
- Introduce yourself by name and title.
- Explain the procedure to the person before beginning and during the procedure.
- Protect the person's rights during the procedure.
- Handle the person gently during the procedure.

Preprocedure

1. Follow *Delegation Guidelines: Taking Pulses*, p. 429. See *Promoting Safety and Comfort:*
   a. *Using a Stethoscope*, p. 428
   b. *Taking Pulses*, p. 429
2. Ask a coworker to help you.
3. Practice hand hygiene.
4. Collect a stethoscope and antiseptic wipes.
5. Decontaminate your hands.
6. Identify the person. Check the ID bracelet against the assignment sheet. Also call the person by name.
7. Provide for privacy.

Procedure

8. Clean the earpieces and diaphragm with the wipes.
9. Have the person sit or lie down.
10. Expose the nipple area of the left chest. Expose a woman's breasts only to the extent necessary.
11. Warm the diaphragm in your palm.
12. Place the earpieces in your ears.
13. Find the apical pulse. Your helper finds the radial pulse (Fig. 27.20).
14. Give the signal to begin counting at the same time.
15. Count the pulse for 1 minute.
16. Give the signal to stop counting.

17. Cover the person. Remove the stethoscope earpieces.
18. Note the person's name and the apical and radial pulses on your note pad or assignment sheet. Subtract the radial pulse from the apical pulse for the pulse deficit. Note whether the pulse was regular or irregular.

Postprocedure

19. Provide for comfort. (See the inside of the front cover.)
20. Place the call light within reach.
21. Unscreen the person.
22. Complete a safety check of the room. (See the inside of the front cover.)
23. Clean the earpieces and diaphragm with the wipes.
24. Return the stethoscope to its proper place.
25. Decontaminate your hands.
26. Report and record your observations. (Report an abnormal pulse at once.) Include the:
    a. Apical and radial pulse rates.
    b. Pulse deficit.

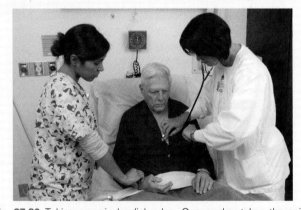

Fig. 27.20 Taking an apical-radial pulse. One worker takes the apical pulse. The other takes the radial pulse.

This skill is also covered in *Clinical Nursing Skills: Nurse Assisting.*

RESPIRATIONS

Respiration means breathing air into *(inhalation)* and out of *(exhalation)* the lungs. Oxygen enters the lungs during inhalation. Carbon dioxide leaves the lungs during exhalation. Each respiration involves one inhalation and one exhalation. The chest rises during inhalation. It falls during exhalation.

The healthy adult has 12 to 20 respirations per minute. See p. 422 for the factors affecting vital signs. Heart and respiratory diseases often increase the respiratory rate.

Respirations are normally quiet, effortless, and regular. Both sides of the chest rise and fall equally. See Chapter 26 for abnormal respiratory patterns.

Count respirations when the person is at rest. Position the person so you can see the chest rise and fall. To some extent, a person can control the rate and depth of breathing. People tend to change their breathing patterns when they know their respirations are being counted. Therefore, do not tell the person that you are counting them.

Count respirations right after taking a pulse. Keep your fingers or stethoscope over the pulse site. (The person assumes you are taking the pulse.) To count respirations, watch the chest rise and fall. Count them for 30 seconds. Multiply the number by 2 for the number of respirations in 1 minute. If you note an abnormal pattern, count the respirations for 1 minute.

In nursing centers, respirations may be counted for 1 minute. Follow center policy.

See *Delegation Guidelines: Respirations.*

📄 DELEGATION GUIDELINES

Respirations

Before counting respirations, you need this information from the nurse and the care plan:

- How long to count respirations for each person—30 seconds or 1 minute
- When to count respirations
- If the nurse has concerns about certain residents
- What other vital signs to measure
- What observations to report and record:
  - The respiratory rate
  - Equality and depth of respirations
  - If the respirations were regular or irregular
  - If the person has pain or difficulty breathing
  - Any respiratory noises
  - An abnormal respiratory pattern (Chapter 26)
- When to report observations
- What specific resident concerns to report at once

✴ COUNTING RESPIRATIONS (NATCEP)

Procedure

1. Follow *Delegation Guidelines: Respirations.*
2. Keep your fingers or stethoscope over the pulse site.
3. Do not tell the person you are counting respirations.
4. Begin counting when the chest rises. Count each rise and fall of the chest as one respiration.
5. Note the following:
   a. If respirations are regular
   b. If both sides of the chest rise equally
   c. The depth of respirations
   d. If the person has any pain or difficulty breathing
   e. An abnormal respiratory pattern
6. Count respirations for 30 seconds, then multiply the number by 2. Count respirations for 1 minute if:
   a. Directed by the nurse and care plan.
   b. Required by center policy.
   c. They are abnormal or irregular.
   d. Required for your state competency test.
7. Note the person's name, respiratory rate, and other observations on your note pad or assignment sheet.

Postprocedure

8. Provide for comfort. (See the inside of the front cover.)
9. Place the call light within reach.
10. Unscreen the person.
11. Complete a safety check of the room. (See the inside of the front cover.)
12. Decontaminate your hands.
13. Report and record the respiratory rate and your observations. Report abnormal respirations at once.

This skill is also covered in *Clinical Skills: Nurse Assisting.*

Blood Pressure

Blood pressure (BP) is the amount of force exerted against the walls of an artery by the blood. BP is controlled by:

- The force of heart contractions.
- The amount of blood pumped with each heartbeat.
- How easily the blood flows through the blood vessels.

Systole is the period of heart muscle contraction. The heart is pumping blood. **Diastole** is the period of heart muscle relaxation. The heart is at rest.

You measure systolic and diastolic pressures. The **systolic pressure** is the pressure in the arteries when the heart contracts. It is the higher pressure. The **diastolic pressure** is the pressure in the arteries when the heart is at rest. It is the lower pressure.

Blood pressure is measured in millimeters (mm) of mercury (Hg). The systolic pressure is recorded over the diastolic pressure. A systolic pressure of 120 mm Hg and a diastolic pressure of 80 mm Hg is written as 120/80 mm Hg.

Normal and Abnormal Blood Pressures

Blood pressure can change from minute to minute. Factors affecting blood pressure are listed in Box 27.2.

In 2017 the American College of Cardiology and the American Heart Association (AHA) revised the guidelines for the detection and treatment of high BP (hypertension). The new categories for blood pressure are shown in Table 27.3.

Blood pressure has normal ranges:

- *Systolic pressure*—less than 120 mm Hg
- *Diastolic pressure*—less than 80 mm Hg

BOX 27.2 Factors Affecting Blood Pressure

- *Age.* BP increases with age. It is lowest in infancy and childhood. It is highest in adulthood.
- *Gender (male or female).* Women usually have lower blood pressures than men. Blood pressures may rise in women after menopause.
- *Blood volume.* This is the amount of blood in the system. Severe bleeding lowers the blood volume; therefore, BP lowers. Giving intravenous (IV) fluids rapidly increases the blood volume, and the BP rises.
- *Stress.* Stress includes anxiety, fear, and emotions. BP increases as the body responds to stress.
- *Pain.* Pain generally increases BP. However, severe pain can cause shock. BP is seriously low in the state of shock (Chapter 44).
- *Exercise.* BP increases. Do not measure BP right after exercise.
- *Weight.* BP is higher in overweight persons. It lowers with weight loss.
- *Race.* Blacks generally have higher BPs than Whites.
- *Diet.* A high-sodium diet increases the amount of water in the body. The extra fluid volume increases BP.
- *Medications.* Medications can be given to raise or lower BP. Other medications have the side effects of high or low BP.
- *Position.* BP is higher when lying down. It is lower in the standing position. Sudden changes in position can cause a sudden drop in BP (orthostatic hypotension). When standing suddenly, the person may have a sudden drop in BP. Dizziness and fainting can occur.
- *Smoking.* BP increases. Nicotine in cigarettes causes blood vessels to narrow. The heart must work harder to pump blood through narrowed vessels.
- *Alcohol.* Excessive alcohol intake can raise BP.

TABLE 27.3 Blood Pressure Categories

Blood Pressure Category	Systolic (mm Hg)		Diastolic (mm Hg)
Normal	Less than 120	and	Less than 80
Elevated	120–129	and	Less than 80
Hypertension stage 1	130–139	or	80–89
Hypertension stage 2	140 or higher	or	90 or higher
Hypertensive crisis	Higher than 180	and/or	Higher than 120

- Hypertension—Can be classified as elevated, stage 1, stage 2, or hypertensive crisis (see Table 27.3). Some persons may be treated for hypertension based on their medical history. If untreated, hypertension can lead to stroke or heart attack (Chapters 35 and 36). Always report elevated BP readings to the nurse.

- Hypotension—when the systolic blood pressure is below *(hypo)* 90 mm Hg and the diastolic pressure is below 60 mm Hg. Report a systolic pressure below 90 mm Hg. Also report a diastolic pressure below 60 mm Hg. Some people normally have low blood pressures. Older persons are at risk for orthostatic hypotension (Chapter 24). However, hypotension can signal a life-threatening problem.

Equipment

You use a stethoscope and a sphygmomanometer to measure blood pressure. The sphygmomanometer has a cuff and a measuring device.

- The *aneroid type* has a round dial and a needle that points to the numbers (Fig. 27.21A and B).

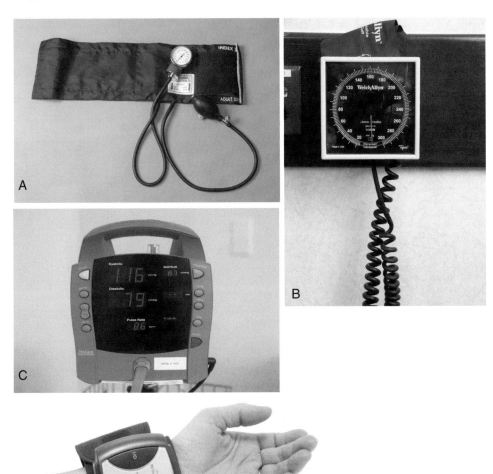

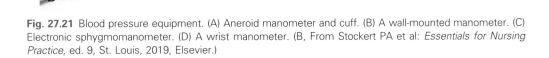

Fig. 27.21 Blood pressure equipment. (A) Aneroid manometer and cuff. (B) A wall-mounted manometer. (C) Electronic sphygmomanometer. (D) A wrist manometer. (B, From Stockert PA et al: *Essentials for Nursing Practice*, ed. 9, St. Louis, 2019, Elsevier.)

- The *electronic type* shows the systolic and diastolic blood pressures on the front of the device (see Fig. 27.21C). Small wrist manometers (Fig. 27.21D) use the radial pulse to detect BP. These are convenient for a person who monitors their BP at home. They can also be useful when the brachial site is difficult to access. Some vital sign machines may be mounted on wheels. This makes them mobile so they can easily be transported to multiple rooms. Often, they have thermometers and pulse oximeters attached (Fig. 27.22). To use the devices, follow the manufacturer instructions. When not in use, these machines are usually plugged into an electric wall outlet so they are charged when needed.

You wrap the blood pressure cuff around the upper arm. Tubing connects the cuff to the manometer. Another tube connects the cuff to a small, handheld bulb. To inflate the cuff, turn the valve on the bulb clockwise to close the valve and then squeeze the bulb. The inflated cuff causes pressure over the brachial artery. Turn the valve counterclockwise to open the valve to deflate the cuff. Measure BP as the cuff deflates.

Blood flowing through the arteries produces sounds. Use the stethoscope to listen to the sounds in the brachial artery as you deflate the cuff. You do not need a stethoscope for an electronic manometer.

Measuring Blood Pressure

You measure blood pressure in the brachial artery. Box 27.3 lists the guidelines for measuring blood pressure.

See *Delegation Guidelines: Measuring Blood Pressure.*

DELEGATION GUIDELINES

Measuring Blood Pressure

Before measuring BP, you need this information from the nurse and the care plan:

- When to measure BP
- What arm to use
- The person's normal BP range
- If the nurse has concerns about certain residents
- If neither arm can be used, the nurse will instruct you with an alternate site. (At times the leg may be used.)
- If the person needs to be lying down, sitting, or standing or if measurements need to be taken in each of these positions (orthostatic vital signs) (see Box 27.3)
- What size cuff to use—regular, child-sized, or extra large
- What observations to report and record
- When to report the BP measurement
- What specific resident concerns to report at once

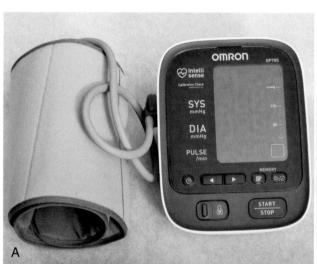
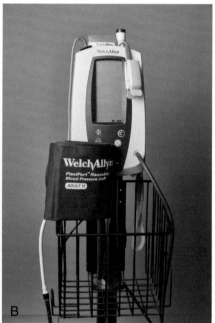

Fig. 27.22 An automatic blood pressure monitor. (A) Automatic monitor. (B) Mobile floor stand with monitor electronic thermometer and pulse oximeter. (A, From Bonewit-West K: *Today's medical assistant: clinical administrative procedures*, ed. 5, St. Louis, 2021, Elsevier; B, From Potter P et al: *Fundamentals of Nursing*, ed. 11, St. Louis, 2023, Elsevier.)

BOX 27.3 **Guidelines for Measuring Blood Pressure**

- Do not take BP on an arm with an IV infusion, a cast, or a dialysis access site. If a person had breast surgery, do not take BP on that side. Avoid taking BP on an injured arm.
- If neither arm can be used, ask the nurse to show you how to measure the person's BP. (The leg may be used for some persons.)
- Let the person rest for 10 to 20 minutes before measuring BP.
- Measure BP with the person sitting or lying. Sometimes the doctor orders BP measured in the standing position.
- If sitting in a chair, ask the person not to cross the legs. Have the person place both feet on the floor.
- If orthostatic vital signs are ordered, follow the center's policy. Often, this means measuring BP and pulse after the person has been supine for at least 5 minutes. Next, have the person sit at the bedside and repeat the BP and pulse measurements. Finally, have the person stand, repeating the BP and pulse measurements. If the person complains of feeling dizzy or faint, immediately put the person in the supine position. Notify the nurse of your observations.
- Apply the cuff to the bare upper arm. Clothing can affect the measurement.
- Make sure the cuff is snug. Loose cuffs can cause inaccurate readings.

- Use a larger cuff if the person is obese or has a large arm. Use a small cuff if the person has a very small arm. Ask the nurse what size to use. Also check the care plan.
- Place the diaphragm of the stethoscope firmly over the brachial artery. The entire diaphragm must have contact with the skin. The person's arm must not be bent.
- Make sure the room is quiet. Talking, TV, radio, and sounds from the hallway can affect an accurate measurement.
- Have the sphygmomanometer where you can clearly see it.
- Measure the systolic and diastolic pressures.
  - Expect to hear the first BP sound at the point where you last felt the radial or brachial pulse. The first sound is the systolic pressure.
  - The point where the sound disappears is the diastolic pressure.
- Take the BP again if you are not sure of an accurate measurement. Wait 30 to 60 seconds before repeating the measurement. Ask the nurse to take the BP if you are unsure of the measurement.
- Record the systolic and diastolic measurements in even numbers for manual blood pressures. Automatic (electronic) blood pressure machines record readings in both even and odd numbers.
- Tell the nurse at once if you cannot hear the BP.

✴ MEASURING BLOOD PRESSURE (NATCEP)

Quality of Life
Remember to:
- Knock before entering the person's room.
- Address the person by name.
- Introduce yourself by name and title.
- Explain the procedure to the person before beginning and during the procedure.
- Protect the person's rights during the procedure.
- Handle the person gently during the procedure.

Preprocedure
1. Follow *Delegation Guidelines: Measuring Blood Pressure.* See *Promoting Safety and Comfort: Using a Stethoscope*, p. 428.
2. Practice hand hygiene.
3. Collect the following:
   - Sphygmomanometer
   - Stethoscope
   - Antiseptic wipes
4. Decontaminate your hands.
5. Identify the person. Check the ID bracelet against the assignment sheet. Also call the person by name.
6. Provide for privacy.

Procedure
7. Wipe the stethoscope earpieces and diaphragm with the wipes. Warm the diaphragm in your palm.
8. Have the person sit or lie down. If sitting, ask the person to place both feet on the floor.
9. Position the person's arm level with the heart. The palm is up.
10. Stand no more than 3 feet away from the manometer. The aneroid type is directly in front of you or mounted on the wall (see Fig. 27.21B).
11. Expose the upper arm.
12. Squeeze the cuff to expel any remaining air. Close the valve on the bulb.

13. Find the brachial artery at the inner aspect of the elbow. (The brachial artery is on the little finger side of the arm.) Use your fingertips.
14. Locate the arrow on the cuff (Fig. 27.23A). Place the arrow on the cuff over the brachial artery (see Fig. 27.23B). Wrap the cuff around the upper arm at least 1 inch above the elbow. It is even and snug.
15. Place the stethoscope earpieces in your ears.
16. Place the diaphragm of the stethoscope over the brachial artery (see Fig. 27.23C). Do not place it under the cuff.
17. Inflate the cuff between 160 and 180 mm Hg.
18. Deflate the cuff at an even rate of 2 to 4 mm per second. Turn the valve counterclockwise to deflate the cuff.
19. If a beat is heard immediately upon deflation, completely deflate the cuff. Wait 30 to 60 seconds. Reinflate the cuff to no more than 200 mm Hg.
20. Note the point where you hear the first sound. This is the systolic reading.
21. Continue to deflate the cuff. Note the point where the sound disappears. This is the diastolic reading.
22. Deflate the cuff completely. Remove it from the person's arm. Remove the stethoscope earpieces from your ears.
23. Note the person's name and blood pressure on your note pad or assignment sheet.
24. Return the cuff to the case or wall holder.

Postprocedure
25. Provide for comfort. (See the inside of the front cover.)
26. Place the call light within reach.
27. Unscreen the person.
28. Complete a safety check of the room. (See the inside of the front cover.)
29. Clean the earpieces and diaphragm with the wipes.
30. Return the equipment to its proper place.
31. Decontaminate your hands.
32. Report and record the BP (Fig. 27.24). Note which arm was used. Report an abnormal blood pressure at once.

Continued

✦ MEASURING BLOOD PRESSURE (NATCEP)—cont'd

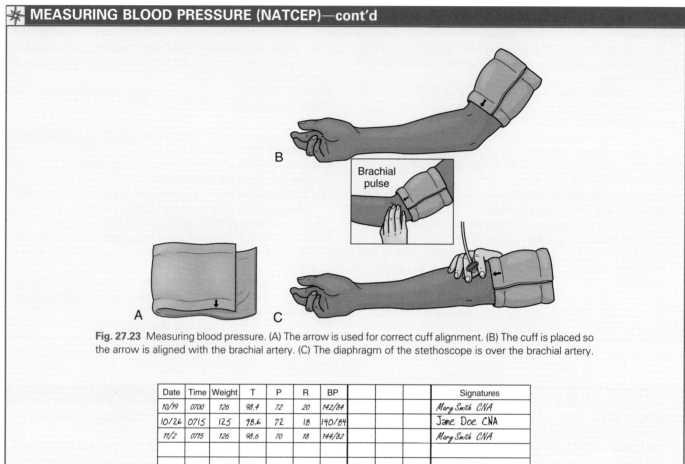

Fig. 27.23 Measuring blood pressure. (A) The arrow is used for correct cuff alignment. (B) The cuff is placed so the arrow is aligned with the brachial artery. (C) The diaphragm of the stethoscope is over the brachial artery.

Date	Time	Weight	T	P	R	BP				Signatures
10/19	0700	126	98.4	72	20	142/84				Mary Smith CNA
10/26	0715	125	98.6	72	18	140/84				Jane Doe CNA
11/2	0715	126	98.6	70	18	144/82				Mary Smith CNA

Fig. 27.24 Charting sample.

This skill is also covered in *Clinical Skills: Nurse Assisting.*

👥 QUALITY OF LIFE

Protect the right to privacy when measuring vital signs. This is very important when taking axillary or rectal temperatures and apical and apical-radial pulses. Expose the person only to the extent needed.

Always keep resident information confidential. Vital signs are just as private as other information. Do not share the information with family, visitors, or roommates.

The right to personal choice is important. Unless directed otherwise, vital signs are measured with the person sitting or lying down. Let the person choose the position. The person may also prefer that you use the right or left arm for pulses and blood pressure. If safe to do so, use the arm the person prefers.

👤 TIME TO REFLECT

Mrs. Zigler was transferred to your care center last week from the hospital. She suffered a stroke 3 years ago. She has contractures of both upper extremities. She receives oxygen by nasal cannula. When measuring her vital signs, what considerations do you need to keep in mind? What are possible methods for checking her temperature? How will her BP be measured?

REVIEW QUESTIONS

Circle the BEST answer.

1. Which statement is *false*?
   a. The vital signs are temperature, pulse, respirations, and blood pressure
   b. Vital signs detect changes in body function
   c. Vital signs change only during illness
   d. Sleep, exercise, medications, emotions, and noise affect vital signs

2. Which should you report at once?
   a. An oral temperature of 98.4°F
   b. A rectal temperature of 101.6°F
   c. An axillary temperature of 97.6°F
   d. An oral temperature of 99.0°F

3. A rectal temperature is taken when the person
   a. Is unconscious
   b. Has heart disease
   c. Is confused
   d. Has diarrhea

4. Which gives the *least* accurate measurement of body temperature?
   a. Oral site
   b. Rectal site
   c. Axillary site
   d. Tympanic membrane site

5. Your center uses tympanic membrane thermometers. Mrs. Yee wears a hearing aid in her left ear. How should you proceed?
   a. Ask the nurse to take her temperature
   b. Ask Mrs. Yee if she can remove her hearing aid
   c. Take her temperature in her right ear
   d. Write unavailable on the vital sign sheet

6. As you enter Mr. Cooper's room to check his temperature, he is drinking a cup of ice water. You have an oral electronic thermometer. What should you do?
   a. Go ahead and check his temperature
   b. Come back in 5 minutes
   c. Tell him you will come back in 15 to 20 minutes and ask him to refrain from drinking until you return
   d. Ask another nursing assistant to take his temperature

7. Which is usually used to take an adult's pulse?
   a. Radial pulse
   b. Apical pulse
   c. Apical-radial pulse
   d. Brachial pulse

8. Which is reported to the nurse at once?
   a. An adult has a pulse of 124 beats per minute
   b. An adult has a pulse of 90 beats per minute
   c. An adult has a pulse of 86 beats per minute
   d. An adult has a pulse of 64 beats per minute

9. Which statement about the apical-radial pulse is *true*?
   a. The radial pulse can be greater than the apical pulse.
   b. The apical pulse can be greater than the radial pulse.
   c. The apical and radial pulses are always equal.
   d. The pulse deficit is always 0.

10. In an adult, normal respirations are
    a. 10 to 18 per minute
    b. 12 to 20 per minute
    c. Less than 20 per minute
    d. More than 20 per minute

11. Normal respirations
    a. Are heard as the person inhales
    b. Are heard as the person exhales
    c. Are quiet
    d. Sound like wheezing with inhalation and exhalation

12. Respirations are usually counted
    a. After taking the temperature
    b. After taking the pulse
    c. Before taking the pulse
    d. After taking the blood pressure

13. Which blood pressure is normal for an adult?
    a. 88/54 mm Hg
    b. 140/90 mm Hg
    c. 100/48 mm Hg
    d. 112/78 mm Hg

14. When measuring BP, you should do the following *except*
    a. Use the arm with an intravenous infusion
    b. Apply the cuff to a bare upper arm
    c. Turn off the TV
    d. Locate the brachial artery

15. The systolic pressure is the point
    a. Where the pulse is no longer felt
    b. Where the first sound is heard
    c. Where the last sound is heard
    d. 30 mm Hg above where the pulse was felt

16. You are not sure of hearing an accurate BP measurement. What should you do?
    a. Record what you think you heard
    b. Measure the BP again after 60 seconds
    c. Use the bell part of the stethoscope
    d. Ask another nursing assistant to take the BP

17. Which of the following does *not* cause an increase in the person's BP?
    a. Smoking
    b. High sodium intake
    c. Excessive alcohol intake
    d. Sudden change from lying position to standing

18. You are measuring a person's blood pressure while they are sitting in a chair? Which is *false*?
    a. The person can rest the arm on a table
    b. The person can cross the legs
    c. You may mute the person's TV temporarily while measuring the BP
    d. You may tell the person the BP reading
19. Where should the person's arm be positioned when measuring BP?
    a. Resting on the bed or table at the level of the heart
    b. Above the head
    c. Hanging at the side
    d. Any position will work

20. What is the correct order for recording vital signs?
    a. BP-P-T-R
    b. R-P-T-BP
    c. T-P-R-BP
    d. P-T-R-BP

See Appendix A for answers to these questions.

28

Assisting with the Physical Examination

OBJECTIVES

- Define the key terms listed in this chapter.
- Explain what to do before, during, and after an examination (exam).
- Identify the rules for measuring weight and height.
- Identify the equipment used for an exam.

- Describe how to prepare and drape a person for an exam.
- Explain the rules for assisting with an exam.
- Perform the procedures described in this chapter.
- Explain how to promote quality of life.

KEY TERMS

dorsal recumbent position The supine position with the legs together; horizontal recumbent position

genupectoral position See "knee-chest position"

horizontal recumbent position See "dorsal recumbent position"

knee-chest position The person kneels and rests the body on the knees and chest; the head is turned to one side, the arms are above the head or flexed at the elbows, the back is straight, and the body is flexed about 90 degrees at the hips; genupectoral position

laryngeal mirror An instrument used to examine the mouth, teeth, and throat

lithotomy position The woman lies on her back with her hips at the edge of the exam table; her knees are flexed, her hips are externally rotated, and her feet are in stirrups

nasal speculum An instrument used to examine the inside of the nose

ophthalmoscope A lighted instrument used to examine the internal eye structures

otoscope A lighted instrument used to examine the external ear and the eardrum (tympanic membrane)

percussion hammer An instrument used to tap body parts to test reflexes; reflex hammer

tuning fork An instrument vibrated to test hearing

vaginal speculum An instrument used to open the vagina to examine it and the cervix

KEY ABBREVIATIONS

cm Centimeter
ID Identification
kg Kilogram

lb Pound
oz Ounce
RN Registered nurse

Doctors and many registered nurses (RNs) perform physical examinations (exams). Exams are done to:

- Promote health.
- Determine fitness for work.
- Diagnose disease.

YOUR ROLE

Your role depends on center policies and procedures. It also depends on what the examiner prefers. You may do some or all of the following:

- Collect needed linens
- Collect equipment and supplies
- Prepare the room for the exam
- Provide lighting
- Transport the person to and from the exam room
- Measure vital signs, weight, and height

- Position and drape the person
- Hand equipment and supplies to the examiner
- Label specimen containers
- Discard used supplies
- Clean equipment
- Help the person dress or move to a comfortable position after the exam
- Follow center policy for soiled linens

EQUIPMENT

The instruments in Fig. 28.1 may be used in the exam.

- Laryngeal mirror—used to examine the mouth, teeth, and throat.
- Nasal speculum—used to examine the inside of the nose.
- Ophthalmoscope—a lighted instrument used to examine the internal eye structures.

- **Otoscope**—a lighted instrument used to examine the external ear and the eardrum (tympanic membrane). Some scopes can be changed into an ophthalmoscope.
- **Percussion hammer** (reflex hammer)—used to tap body parts to test reflexes.

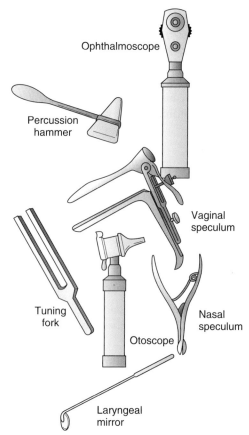

Ophthalmoscope

Percussion hammer

Vaginal speculum

Tuning fork

Otoscope

Nasal speculum

Laryngeal mirror

Fig. 28.1 Instruments used for a physical exam.

- **Tuning fork**—vibrated to test hearing.
- **Vaginal speculum**—used to open the vagina to examine it and the cervix.

Some centers have exam trays in the supply department. If not, collect the items listed in the procedure: *Preparing the Person for an Examination,* p. 444. Arrange them on a tray or table. A tray prepared and arranged with supplies and common instruments is shown in Fig. 28.2.

Measure vital signs before the exam (Chapter 27). Measure the person's height and weight. Record the measurements on the exam form.

✳ WEIGHT AND HEIGHT

Weight and height are measured prior to a physical exam. They are also measured on admission to the center. Then the person is weighed daily, weekly, or monthly. This is done to measure weight gain or loss.

Standing, chair, bed, lift, and wheelchair scales are used (Fig. 28.3). These types of scales are used for persons who cannot stand. Follow the manufacturer instructions and center procedures. Know the center's policy for recording weight and height. For example: Is weight recorded in pounds or kilograms? Is height recorded in inches or centimeters? Some measuring equipment can measure in both inches and centimeters. Likewise, some scales can measure in pounds and ounces or kilograms. If you need to do the conversion, use the formula noted in Box 28.1.

When measuring weight and height, follow these guidelines:
- The person wears only a gown or pajamas. Clothes add weight. No footwear is worn. Footwear adds to the weight and height measurements.
- The person voids before being weighed. A full bladder adds weight.

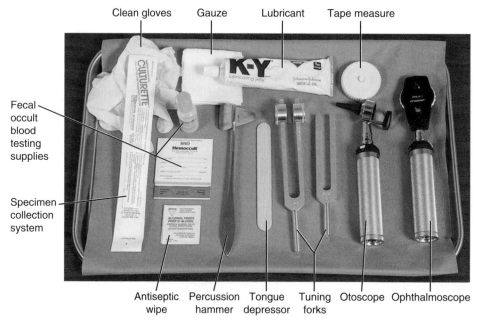

Clean gloves   Gauze   Lubricant   Tape measure

Fecal occult blood testing supplies

Specimen collection system

Antiseptic wipe   Percussion hammer   Tongue depressor   Tuning forks   Otoscope   Ophthalmoscope

Fig. 28.2 A tray of common instruments and supplies arranged for a physical exam. (From Bonewit-West K, Hunt SA, Applegate E: *Today's medical assistant: clinical & administrative procedures,* ed. 3, St. Louis, 2016, Elsevier.)

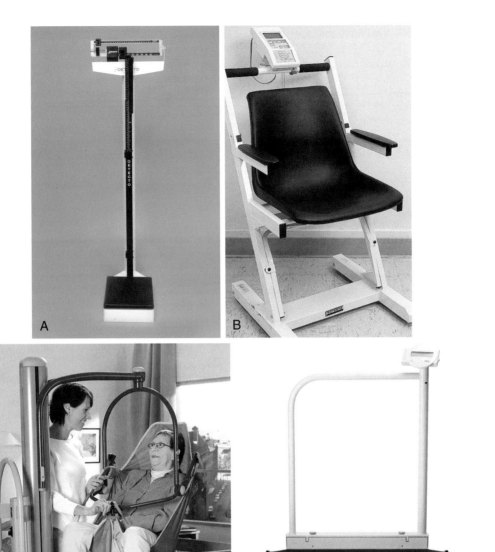

Fig. 28.3 Types of scales. (A) Standing scale. (B) Chair scale. (C) Lift scale. (D) Wheelchair scale. (C, Courtesy ARJO, Morton Grove, IL; D, courtesy Seca Corp., Chino, CA.)

BOX 28.1 Conversions

Weight
- 1 pound = 16 ounces
- 1 kilogram = 2.2 pounds

Height
- 1 foot = 12 inches
- 1 inch = 2.54 centimeters

- Weigh the person at the same time of day. Before breakfast is the best time. Food and fluids add weight.
- Use the same scale for daily, weekly, and monthly weights. Scales weigh differently.

- Balance the scale at zero (0) before weighing the person. For balance scales, move the weights to zero. A digital scale should read at zero.

  See *Teamwork and Time Management: Weight and Height.*
  See *Delegation Guidelines: Weight and Height.*
  See *Promoting Safety and Comfort: Weight and Height.*

TEAMWORK AND TIME MANAGEMENT

Weight and Height

Nursing units usually have just one standing scale. In some centers, chair, wheelchair, and lift scales are shared with other nursing units. Return the device to the storage area as quickly as possible. Do not have your coworkers wait or look for the scale.

DELEGATION GUIDELINES

Weight and Height

Before measuring weight and height, you need this information from the nurse and the care plan:

- When to measure weight and height

- What scale to use
- If height is measured with the person in bed
- When to report the measurements
- What specific resident concerns to report at once

PROMOTING SAFETY AND COMFORT

Weight and Height

Safety

Follow the manufacturer instructions when using chair, bed, wheelchair, or lift scales. Also follow the center's procedures. Practice safety measures to prevent falls.

Comfort

The person wears only a gown or pajamas for the weight measurement. Prevent chilling and drafts.

MEASURING WEIGHT AND HEIGHT (NATCEP)

Quality of Life

Remember to:

- Knock before entering the person's room.
- Address the person by name.
- Introduce yourself by name and title.
- Explain the procedure to the person before beginning and during the procedure.
- Protect the person's rights during the procedure.
- Handle the person gently during the procedure.

Preprocedure

1. Follow *Delegation Guidelines: Weight and Height,* p. 442. See *Promoting Safety and Comfort: Weight and Height,* p. 442.
2. Ask the person to void.
3. Practice hand hygiene.

4. Bring the scale and paper towels (for a standing scale) to the person's room or transport the person by wheelchair to the wheelchair platform scale.
5. Decontaminate your hands.
6. Identify the person. Check the identification (ID) bracelet against the assignment sheet. Also call the person by name.
7. Provide for privacy.

Procedure

8. Place the paper towels on the scale platform.
9. Raise the height rod.
10. Move the weights to zero (0). The pointer is in the middle.
11. Have the person remove the robe and footwear. Assist as needed.
12. Help the person stand on the scale. The person stands in the center of the scale. Arms are at the sides.
13. Move the weights until the balance pointer is in the middle (Fig. 28.4).

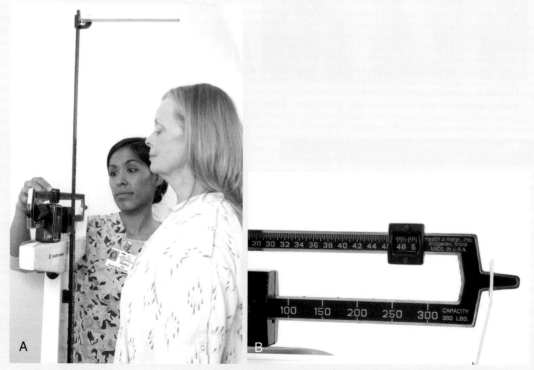

Fig. 28.4 (A) The person is weighed. (B) The weight is read when the balance pointer is in the middle.

✳ MEASURING WEIGHT AND HEIGHT (NATCEP)—cont'd

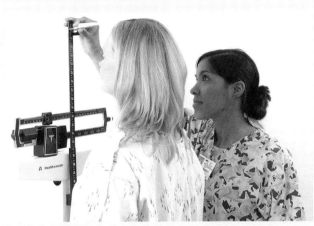

Fig. 28.5 The person's height is measured.

14. If using a wheelchair scale, push the person sitting in the wheelchair onto the scale. Note the weight. Safely move the person in the wheelchair off the platform. Subtract the weight of the wheelchair from the total weight. This will be the value to record.

15. Note the weight on your note pad or assignment sheet. Record in pounds or kilograms according to your center's policy.
16. Ask the person to stand very straight.
17. Lower the height rod until it rests on the person's head (Fig. 28.5).
18. Note the height on your note pad or assignment sheet. Record in inches or centimeters according to your center's policy.
19. Raise the height rod. Help the person step off the scale.
20. Help the person put on a robe and nonskid footwear if the person will be up. Or help the person back to bed.
21. Lower the height rod. Adjust the weights to zero (0) if this is your center's policy.

Postprocedure
22. Provide for comfort. (See the inside of the front cover.)
23. Place the call light within reach.
24. Raise or lower bed rails. Follow the care plan.
25. Unscreen the person.
26. Complete a safety check of the room. (See the inside of the front cover.)
27. Discard the paper towels.
28. Return the scale to its proper place.
29. Decontaminate your hands.
30. Report and record the measurements.

This skill is also covered in *Clinical Skills: Nurse Assisting.*

✳ MEASURING HEIGHT—THE PERSON IS IN BED

Quality of Life

Remember to:
- Knock before entering the person's room.
- Address the person by name.
- Introduce yourself by name and title.
- Explain the procedure to the person before beginning and during the procedure.
- Protect the person's rights during the procedure.
- Handle the person gently during the procedure.

Preprocedure
1. Follow *Delegation Guidelines: Weight and Height*, p. 442. See *Promoting Safety and Comfort: Weight and Height*, p. 442.
2. Practice hand hygiene.
3. Ask a coworker to help you.
4. Collect a measuring tape and ruler.
5. Decontaminate your hands.
6. Identify the person. Check the ID bracelet against the assignment sheet. Also call the person by name.
7. Provide for privacy.
8. Raise the bed for body mechanics. Bed rails are up if used.

Procedure
9. Lower the bed rails if up.
10. Position the person supine if the position is allowed.
11. Have your coworker hold the end of the measuring tape so it extends to the person's heel.
12. Pull the measuring tape along the person's body. Pull until it extends past the head (Fig. 28.6).
13. Place the ruler flat across the top of the person's head. It extends from the person's head to the measuring tape. Make sure the ruler is level.
14. Note the height on your note pad or assignment sheet. Record in either inches or centimeters according to your center's policy.

Postprocedure
15. Provide for comfort. (See the inside of the front cover.)
16. Place the call light within reach.

17. Lower the bed to its lowest position.
18. Raise or lower bed rails. Follow the care plan.
19. Complete a safety check of the room. (See the inside of the front cover.)
20. Return equipment to its proper place.
21. Decontaminate your hands.
22. Report and record the height.

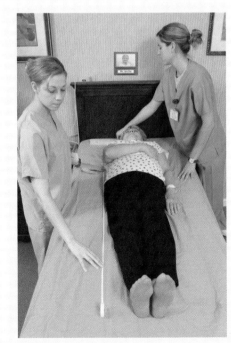

Fig. 28.6 The person's height is measured in bed. The tape measure extends from the top of the head to the heel. The ruler is flat across the top of the person's head.

✴ PREPARING THE PERSON

The physical exam is a concern to many persons. They worry about the findings. Some are confused or fearful about the procedure. Discomfort, embarrassment, fearing exposure, and not knowing the procedure cause anxiety. You must respect the person's feelings and concerns. To prepare the person physically and mentally, the nurse explains the exam's purpose and what to expect. The person must give informed consent for the exam.

Privacy is protected. The person is screened and the room door closed. All clothes are removed for a complete exam. A patient gown is worn. It reduces the naked feeling and the fear of exposure. So does covering the person with a drape—paper drape, bath blanket, sheet, or drawsheet. Explain that only the part being examined is exposed.

The person voids before the exam to empty the bladder. This lets the examiner feel the abdominal organs. A full bladder can change the normal position and shape of organs. It also causes discomfort, especially when feeling the abdominal organs. If a urine specimen is needed, obtain it at this time. Explain how to collect the specimen (Chapter 29). Label the container.

Nursing center residents have an exam at least once a year. The person is told who will do the exam and when it will be done. The person may want a different examiner. Or the person may want a family member present during the exam and when the results are explained.

See *Delegation Guidelines: Preparing the Person.*
See *Promoting Safety and Comfort: Preparing the Person.*

📄 DELEGATION GUIDELINES

Preparing the Person

To prepare a person for an exam, you need this information from the nurse and the care plan:

- When to prepare the person
- Where it will be done—an exam room or the person's room
- How to position the person
- What equipment and supplies are needed
- If a urine specimen is needed
- What specific resident concerns to report at once

👤 PROMOTING SAFETY AND COMFORT

Preparing the Person

Safety

Protect the person from falls and injury. Do not leave the person unattended.

Comfort

Warmth is a major concern during an exam. Protect the person from chilling. Have an extra bath blanket nearby. Also take measures to prevent drafts.

✴ PREPARING THE PERSON FOR AN EXAMINATION

Quality of Life

Remember to:

- Knock before entering the person's room.
- Address the person by name.
- Introduce yourself by name and title.
- Explain the procedure to the person before beginning and during the procedure.
- Protect the person's rights during the procedure.
- Handle the person gently during the procedure.

Preprocedure

1. Follow *Delegation Guidelines: Preparing the Person.* See *Promoting Safety and Comfort: Preparing the Person.*
2. Practice hand hygiene.
3. Collect the following:
   - Flashlight
   - Sphygmomanometer
   - Stethoscope
   - Thermometer
   - Tongue depressors (blades)
   - Laryngeal mirror
   - Ophthalmoscope
   - Otoscope
   - Nasal speculum
   - Percussion (reflex) hammer
   - Tuning fork
   - Tape measure
   - Gloves
   - Water-soluble lubricant
   - Vaginal speculum
   - Cotton-tipped applicators
   - Occult blood slides and developer (Chapter 29)
   - Specimen containers and labels
   - Disposable bag
   - Kidney basin
   - Towel
   - Bath blanket
   - Tissues
   - Drape (sheet, bath blanket, drawsheet, or paper drape)
   - Paper towels
   - Cotton balls
   - Waterproof pad
   - Eye chart (Snellen chart)
   - Slides
   - Gown
   - Alcohol wipes
   - Exam gloves (size for the examiner)
   - Wastebasket
   - Container for soiled instruments
   - Marking pencils or pens
4. Decontaminate your hands.
5. Identify the person. Check the ID bracelet against the assignment sheet. Also call the person by name.
6. Provide for privacy.

Procedure

7. Ask the person to remove all clothes. Have the person put on the gown. Assist as needed.
8. Ask the person to void. Collect a urine specimen if needed. Provide for privacy.

✳ PREPARING THE PERSON FOR AN EXAMINATION—cont'd

9. Transport the person to the exam room. (This is not done for an exam in the person's room.)
10. Measure weight and height. Record the measurements on the exam form.
11. Help the person onto the exam table. Provide a step stool if necessary. (Omit this step for an exam in the person's room.)
12. Raise the far bed rail (if used). Raise the bed to its highest level. (This step is not done if an exam table is used.)
13. Measure vital signs. Record them on the exam form.
14. Position the person as directed.
15. Drape the person.
16. Place a waterproof pad under the buttocks.
17. Raise the bed rail near you (if used).
18. Provide adequate lighting.
19. Put on the call light for the examiner. Do not leave the person alone.

Postprocedure
20. Assist the examiner as needed.
21. If any specimens were taken, process them according to directions (Chapter 29).
22. Perform hand hygiene.
23. Assist the person to get dressed if necessary.
24. Assist the person off the exam table or, if in bed, help the person to a comfortable position.
25. After the person has left the exam room, clean the area and put away all equipment and supplies.
26. Complete a safety check of the room. (See inside of the front cover.)

POSITIONING AND DRAPING

The examiner tells you how to position the person. Some positions are uncomfortable and embarrassing. Before helping the person assume and maintain the position, explain:

- Why the position is needed.
- How to assume the position.
- How the body is draped for warmth and privacy.
- How long to expect to stay in the position.

The dorsal recumbent position (horizontal recumbent position) is used to examine the abdomen, chest, and breasts. The person is supine with the legs together. To examine the perineal area, the knees are flexed and hips externally rotated. Drape the person as in Fig. 28.7A.

The lithotomy position (see Fig. 28.7B) is used to examine the vagina and cervix. The woman lies on her back. Hips are at the edge of the exam table. Knees are flexed and the hips are externally rotated. Feet are in stirrups. Drape the woman as for perineal care (Chapter 18). Some centers provide socks for the feet and calves. Some women cannot assume this position. If so, the examiner tells you how to position the woman. It is helpful to have an adjustable floor lamp available for the exam.

The knee-chest position (see Fig. 28.7C) is used to examine the rectum. It also is called the genupectoral position. (*Genu* means "knee"; *pectoral* relates to the breast.) The person kneels and rests the body on the knees and chest. The head is turned to one side. The arms are above the head or flexed at the elbows. The back is straight. The body is flexed about 90 degrees at the hips. Apply the drape in a diamond shape to cover the back, buttocks, and thighs. This position is rarely used for older persons. For them, the side-lying position is used to examine the rectum.

The *left side-lying position* (see Fig. 28.7D) is sometimes used to examine the rectum or vagina (Chapter 15). Apply the drape in a diamond shape. The examiner folds back the near corner to expose the rectum or vagina.

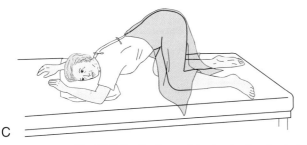
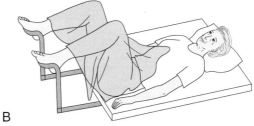
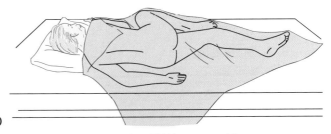
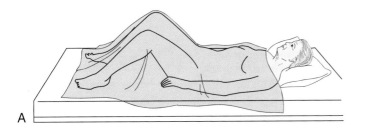

Fig. 28.7 Positioning and draping for the physical exam. (A) Dorsal recumbent position. (B) Lithotomy position. (C) Knee-chest position. (D) Left side-lying position.

ASSISTING WITH THE EXAM

You may be asked to prepare, position, and drape the person. If assisting with the exam, follow the rules in Box 28.2.

See *Residents with Dementia: Assisting with the Exam.*
See *Focus on Communication: Assisting with the Exam.*

RESIDENTS WITH DEMENTIA

Assisting with the Exam

Persons with dementia may resist the examiner's efforts. The person may be agitated and aggressive because of confusion and fear. Do not restrain or force the person to have the exam. The exam is tried another time. Sometimes a family member can calm the person. The doctor may order medications to help the person relax. The person's rights are always respected.

FOCUS ON COMMUNICATION

Assisting with the Exam

Each examiner has a routine and does things in a certain order. To better assist, ask the examiner to explain the routine to you. Also ask the examiner to tell you what equipment and supplies are needed. For example:

- "Dr. Weaver, I want to help in the best way that I can. Please tell me how you will start the exam and how you will proceed."
- "Ms. Carrigan, please ask for equipment and supplies as you need them. That way I can hand you the correct item."

After the Exam

After the exam, the person dresses or returns to bed. Lubricant is used to examine the vagina or rectum. The area is wiped or cleaned before the person dresses or returns to the room. Assist as needed. You also need to:

BOX 28.2 Rules for Assisting with the Physical Exam

- Practice hand hygiene before and after the exam.
- Provide for privacy.
  - Close doors and window coverings.
  - Screen and drape the person.
  - Expose only the body part being examined.
- Position the person as directed by the examiner.
- Place instruments and equipment near the examiner.
- Adjust lighting for the examiner.
- Stay in the room when a female is examined (unless you are a male). When a man examines a female, another female is in the room. This is for the legal protection of the female and the male examiner. A female attendant also adds to the woman's mental comfort. A female examiner may want a male attendant present when examining a male. This also is for legal protection.
- Protect the person from falling.
- Reassure the person throughout the exam.
- Anticipate the examiner's need for equipment and supplies.
- Place paper or paper towels on the floor if the person is asked to stand.
- Follow Standard Precautions and the Bloodborne Pathogen Standard.

- Discard disposable items.
- Replace supplies so the tray is ready for the next exam.
- Clean reusable items according to center policy. Return them to the tray or storage area. This includes the otoscope and ophthalmoscope tips and stethoscope.
- Send a reusable speculum to the supply area. It needs to be sterilized.
- Cover the exam table with a clean drawsheet or paper.
- Label specimens. Take them to the designated area with a requisition slip.
- Clean and straighten the person's unit or exam room.
- Follow center policy for soiled linens.
  See *Teamwork and Time Management: After the Exam.*

TEAMWORK AND TIME MANAGEMENT

After the Exam

Make sure that the exam room is clean and that supplies and equipment are ready for the next exam. Otherwise, you delay the resident, examiner, and the staff member assisting.

You may find an exam room that is not clean. Or you may find that equipment and supplies are not ready for an exam. Call for the nurse before you start to prepare the room and ready supplies and equipment. The nurse needs to see the problem. The nurse can find out who last used the room or tray. The nurse can then talk to the staff members involved.

QUALITY OF LIFE

Resident care is given in a way that promotes dignity; self-esteem; and physical, mental, and social well-being. Often, only a gown is worn for an exam. Sometimes an uncomfortable position is required. Often, private body parts (breasts, vagina, penis, rectum) are examined.

Fears about the exam affect the person's dignity, self-esteem, and well-being. These fears are common:
- Who will perform the exam?
- How will the exam be done?
- Why is the exam needed?
- Is the person dying?
- Will cancer be found?
- Will surgery be needed?
- Will more medications be needed?
- Will an illness be found?

The person has the right to personal choice. The person also has the right to privacy and confidentiality. Protect the person from exposure. Only the examiner and the person assisting have the right to see the person's body. The person must consent for others to be present. Proper draping and screening are needed. Expose only the body part being examined. Remember to keep the person covered.

Only staff involved in the person's care need to know the reason for the exam and its results. If the person consents, the doctor tells the family. The person can share the information with others by choice.

The person needs to feel safe and secure. Protect the person from falls and other injuries. Keep the person covered to provide warmth and protect from chills and drafts. The person must feel covered and protected from exposure.

Safety and security affect mental well-being. The person should know the reasons for the exam and how it will be done. The person should feel comfortable with the examiner and the person assisting. Touch and comforting words also help the person feel safe and secure.

TIME TO REFLECT

The doctor has come to do Ms. Groves's annual exam. The nurse explains to Ms. Groves that the doctor wants to perform a pelvic exam. The nurse asks you to transport Ms. Groves to the center's exam room and prepare her for the examination. You have just finished measuring her vital signs when Ms. Groves begins to cry. She asks you if the pelvic exam will hurt and tells you she is too afraid to continue. How would you react in this situation?

REVIEW QUESTIONS

Circle the BEST answer.

1. The otoscope is used to examine
   a. Internal eye structures
   b. The external ear and the eardrum
   c. Reflexes
   d. The vagina

2. You are preparing a person for an exam. You should do the following *except*
   a. Ask the person to void
   b. Ask the person to undress
   c. Drape the person
   d. Leave the person and go get the nurse

3. Which part of an exam can you do?
   a. Test reflexes
   b. Inspect the mouth, teeth, and throat
   c. Measure weight, height, and vital signs
   d. Observe the perineum and rectum

4. A person is supine. The hips are flexed and externally rotated. The feet are supported in stirrups. The person is in the
   a. Dorsal recumbent position
   b. Lithotomy position
   c. Knee-chest position
   d. Side-lying position

5. You will assist with Mrs. Janz's exam. Which is *false*?
   a. Hand hygiene is practiced before and after the exam
   b. Instruments are placed near the examiner
   c. A male nursing team member stays in the room
   d. Provide for privacy by screening, closing the door, and proper draping

6. You are preparing Mrs. Janz for the physical exam. Which is *false*?
   a. She will wear only a gown
   b. The doctor or nurse tells you what position to place Mrs. Janz
   c. Her vital signs are measured before the exam
   d. She will void after the exam

7. The health care provider needs to do a rectal exam on Mr. Angelo. In what position will he most likely be placed?
   a. Supine position
   b. Left side-lying position
   c. Lithotomy position
   d. Fowler's position

8. A person is weighed daily. Which of the following does *not* need to be the same each day?
   a. The same nursing assistant needs to do the weighing
   b. The weight should be measured the same time each day
   c. The same amount of clothing should be worn
   d. The same scale should be used

9. A person is weighed on a wheelchair scale. Which is *true*?
   a. The person can have a pillow or cushion in the wheelchair
   b. The wheelchair weight must be subtracted from the total weight that the scale reads
   c. The person does not need to void before being weighed
   d. It makes no difference if the footrests are on or off

10. Mrs. Janz's height is 5 feet 2 inches. What is her height in centimeters?
    a. 25 cm
    b. 62 cm
    c. 132.56 cm
    d. 157.48 cm

11. Mr. Angelo's height is 188 centimeters. What is his height in inches?
    a. 25 inches
    b. 62 inches
    c. 74 inches
    d. 160 inches

12. Mrs. Janz's weight is 62 kilograms. She asks you to tell her the weight in pounds. Your answer to her would be approximately
    a. 125 pounds
    b. 137 pounds
    c. 150 pounds
    d. 168 pounds

13. Mr. Angelo's weight is 176 pounds. What is his weight in kilograms?
    a. Approximately 80 kg
    b. Approximately 120 kg
    c. Approximately 250 kg
    d. Approximately 387 kg

14. Mr. Sanchez cannot stand. The nurse asks you to measure his height. Which is *false*?
    a. It is helpful to have another person assist you
    b. His height can be measured in bed
    c. Use a tape measure and ruler
    d. Position him in the prone position

See Appendix A for answers to these questions.

29

Collecting and Testing Specimens

OBJECTIVES

- Define the key terms and key abbreviations listed in this chapter.
- Explain why urine, stool, sputum, and blood specimens are collected.
- Explain the rules for collecting specimens.
- Describe the different types of urine specimens.
- Describe the equipment used for blood glucose testing.
- Identify the sites used for skin punctures.
- Perform the procedures described in this chapter.
- Explain how to promote quality of life.

KEY TERMS

acetone See "ketone"
glucosuria Sugar (*glucose-*) in the urine (*-uria*); glycosuria
glycosuria Sugar (*glycos-*) in the urine (*-uria*); glucosuria
hematoma A swelling (*-oma*) that contains blood (*hemat-*)
hematuria Blood (*hemat-*) in the urine (*-uria*)
hemoptysis Bloody (*hemo-*) sputum (*ptysis* means "to spit")

ketone A substance that appears in urine from the rapid breakdown of fat for energy; acetone, ketone body
ketone body See "ketone"
melena A black, tarry stool
sputum Mucus from the respiratory system that is expectorated (expelled) through the mouth

KEY ABBREVIATIONS

BM Bowel movement
ID Identification
I&O Intake and output

mL Milliliter
oz Ounce

Ordered by doctors, specimens (samples) are collected and tested to prevent, detect, and treat disease. Most specimens are tested in the laboratory. All specimens sent to the laboratory require requisition slips. The slip has the person's identifying information and the test ordered. And the specimen container is labeled according to center policy. Some tests are done at the bedside. When collecting specimens, follow the rules in Box 29.1.

See *Teamwork and Time Management: Collecting and Testing Specimens*.

URINE SPECIMENS

Urine specimens are collected for urine tests. Follow the rules in Box 29.1.

See *Delegation Guidelines: Urine Specimens*.
See *Promoting Safety and Comfort: Urine Specimens*.

TEAMWORK AND TIME MANAGEMENT

Collecting and Testing Specimens
Nursing centers send specimens to a laboratory for study or analysis. The center has a storage area for specimens. A driver picks up specimens at a certain time and transports them to the laboratory.

Have ordered specimens collected and in the storage area by the pickup time. If the specimen is not collected, the results are delayed at least 1 day.

This can cause the person harm. If the specimen was not collected in time, it may need to be discarded. If discarded, another specimen is collected the next day. This also causes a delay in the results and can harm the person. Using more supplies and equipment also costs more money.

DELEGATION GUIDELINES

Urine Specimens
Before collecting a urine specimen, you need this information from the nurse and the care plan:

- If the person uses the toilet, bedpan, urinal, or commode for voiding
- The type of specimen needed
- What time to collect the specimen
- What special measures are needed
- If you need to test the specimen (p. 452)
- If measuring intake and output (I&O) is ordered
- What observations to report and record:
  - Problems obtaining the specimen
  - Color, clarity, and odor of urine
  - Blood in the urine
  - Particles in the urine
  - Complaints of pain, burning, urgency, difficulty voiding, or other problems
- When to report observations
- What specific resident concerns to report at once

BOX 29.1 Rules for Collecting Specimens

- Follow the rules of medical asepsis.
- Follow Standard Precautions and the Bloodborne Pathogen Standard.
- Use a clean container for each specimen.
- Use the correct container.
- Do not touch the inside of the container or lid.
- Identify the person. Check the ID bracelet against the laboratory requisition slip or assignment sheet. Compare *all* information.
- Label the container in the person's presence. Provide accurate information.
- Collect the specimen at the correct time.
- Ask the person not to have a BM when collecting a urine specimen. The specimen must not contain stools.

- Ask the person to void before collecting a stool specimen. The specimen must not contain urine.
- Ask the person to put toilet tissue in the toilet or wastebasket. Urine and stool specimens must not contain tissue.
- Place the specimen container in a labeled BIOHAZARD plastic bag. Do not let the container touch the outside of the bag. If your center's policy requires placing the specimen in a second plastic bag, make sure to follow this. Seal the bag(s).
- Take the specimen and requisition slip to the storage area.
- Know whether the specimen needs to be stored in a refrigerator or at room temperature. Some specimens must be transported immediately to the laboratory.

PROMOTING SAFETY AND COMFORT

Urine Specimens

Safety

Microbes can grow in urine. Urine also may contain blood. Follow Standard Precautions and the Bloodborne Pathogen Standard.

Comfort

Urine specimens may embarrass some people. They do not like clear specimen containers that show urine. Placing the urine specimen container in a paper bag is often helpful.

The Random Urine Specimen

The random urine specimen is collected for a routine urinalysis. No special measures are needed. It is collected any time during a 24-hour period. Many people can collect the specimen themselves. Weak and very ill persons need help.

COLLECTING A RANDOM URINE SPECIMEN

Quality of Life

Remember to:

- Knock before entering the person's room.
- Address the person by name.
- Introduce yourself by name and title.
- Explain the procedure to the person before beginning and during the procedure.
- Protect the person's rights during the procedure.
- Handle the person gently during the procedure.

Preprocedure

1. Follow *Delegation Guidelines: Urine Specimens*, p. 448. See *Promoting Safety and Comfort: Urine Specimens.*
2. Practice hand hygiene.
3. Collect the following before going to the person's room:
   - Laboratory requisition slip
   - Specimen container and lid
   - Specimen label
   - Plastic bag(s)
   - BIOHAZARD label (if needed)
   - Gloves
4. Arrange collected items in the person's bathroom.
5. Decontaminate your hands.
6. Identify the person. Check the identification (ID) bracelet against the requisition slip. Also call the person by name.
7. Label the container in the person's presence.
8. Put on gloves.
9. Collect the following:
   - Voiding receptacle—bedpan and cover, urinal, commode, or specimen pan (Fig. 29.1)
   - Graduate to measure output
10. Provide for privacy.

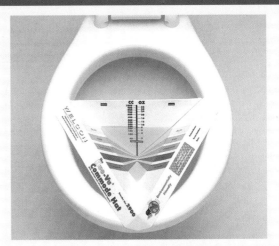

Fig. 29.1 The specimen pan is placed at the front of the toilet on the toilet rim. This pan has a color chart for urine. (Courtesy Welcon, Inc., Fort Worth, TX.)

Procedure

11. Ask the person to void into the receptacle. Remind the person to put toilet tissue in the wastebasket or toilet. Toilet tissue is not put in the bedpan or specimen pan.
12. Take the receptacle to the bathroom.
13. Pour about 120 milliliters (mL) (4 ounces [oz]) into the specimen container.
14. Place the lid on the specimen container. Put the container in the plastic bag. Do not let the container touch the outside of the bag. Some facilities require double-bagging of the specimen. Apply a BIOHAZARD label according to center policy.
15. Measure urine if I&O are ordered. Include the amount in the specimen container.
16. Empty, clean, and disinfect equipment. Return equipment to its proper place.

❊ COLLECTING A RANDOM URINE SPECIMEN—cont'd

17. Remove the gloves and practice hand hygiene. Put on clean gloves.
18. Assist with hand washing.
19. Remove the gloves. Practice hand hygiene.

Postprocedure
20. Provide for comfort. (See the inside of the front cover.)
21. Place the call light within reach.

22. Raise or lower bed rails. Follow the care plan.
23. Unscreen the person.
24. Complete a safety check of the room. (See the inside of the front cover.)
25. Decontaminate your hands.
26. Take specimen and requisition slip to the storage area. Follow center policy. Wear gloves.
27. Report and record your observations.

❊ The Midstream Specimen

The midstream specimen is also called a *clean-voided specimen* or *clean-catch specimen*. The perineal area is cleaned before collecting the specimen. This reduces the number of microbes in the urethral area. The person starts to void into a receptacle. Then the person stops the stream of urine, and a sterile specimen container is positioned. The person voids into the container until the specimen is obtained.

Stopping the stream of urine is hard for many people. You may need to position and hold the specimen container in place after the person starts to void (Fig. 29.2).

See *Focus on Communication: The Midstream Specimen.*

▤ FOCUS ON COMMUNICATION

The Midstream Specimen
Some persons can collect the midstream specimen on their own. You may need to explain the procedure. Use words the person understands. Show what supplies to use. Also, ask if the person has any questions. For example: "Ms. Jacobs, I need to collect a midstream urine specimen from you. This means I need urine that comes from the middle of your urine stream. First, wipe well with this towelette (show the towelette). Wipe from front to back. The specimen will go in this cup (show the specimen cup). Please do not touch the inside of the cup. Start your urine stream and then stop. Position the cup to catch urine and begin your stream again. If you cannot stop your stream, just position the cup during the middle of the stream. I need at least this much urine in the cup if possible (point to the 30 mL measure on the cup). Remove the cup when it is about that full. Finish urinating. Secure the lid on top of the cup. I will take the specimen when you are done. Do you have any questions?"

❊ COLLECTING A MIDSTREAM SPECIMEN

Quality of Life
Remember to:
- Knock before entering the person's room.
- Address the person by name.
- Introduce yourself by name and title.
- Explain the procedure to the person before beginning and during the procedure.
- Protect the person's rights during the procedure.
- Handle the person gently during the procedure.

Preprocedure
1. Follow *Delegation Guidelines: Urine Specimens,* p. 448. See *Promoting Safety and Comfort: Urine Specimens,* p. 449.
2. Practice hand hygiene.
3. Collect the following before going to the person's room:
   - Laboratory requisition slip
   - Midstream specimen kit—includes specimen container, label, and towelettes; may include sterile gloves
   - Plastic bag(s)
   - Sterile gloves (if not part of the kit)
   - Disposable gloves
   - BIOHAZARD label (if needed)
4. Arrange your work area.
5. Decontaminate your hands.
6. Identify the person. Check the ID bracelet against the requisition slip. Also call the person by name.
7. Put on disposable gloves.

8. Collect the following:
   - Voiding receptacle—bedpan and cover, urinal, commode, or specimen pan if needed
   - Supplies for perineal care
   - Graduate to measure output
   - Paper towel
9. Provide for privacy.
10. Provide perineal care. (Wear gloves for this step. Decontaminate your hands after removing them.)
11. Open the sterile kit.
12. Put on the sterile gloves.
13. Open the packet of towelettes inside the kit.
14. Open the sterile specimen container. Do not touch the inside of the container or lid. Set the lid down so the inside is up.
15. *For a female*—clean the perineal area with the towelettes.
    a. Spread the labia with your thumb and index finger. Use your nondominant hand. (This hand is now contaminated. It must not touch anything sterile.)
    b. Clean the urethral area from front to back. Use a clean towelette for each stroke.
    c. Keep the labia separated to collect the urine specimen (steps 17 through 20).
16. *For a male*—clean the penis with the towelettes.
    a. Hold the penis with your nondominant hand. (This hand is now contaminated. It must not touch anything sterile.)
    b. Clean the penis starting at the meatus. Clean in a circular motion. Start at the center and work outward.
    c. Keep holding the penis until the specimen is collected (steps 17 through 20).

Continued

✳ COLLECTING A MIDSTREAM SPECIMEN—cont'd

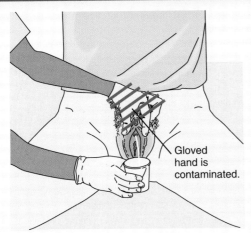

Fig. 29.2 The labia are separated to collect a midstream specimen.

17. Ask the person to void into a receptacle.
18. Pass the specimen container into the stream of urine. Keep the labia separated (see Fig. 29.2).
19. Collect about 30 to 60 mL (1 to 2 oz) of urine.
20. Remove the specimen container before the person stops voiding.
21. Release the labia or penis. Let the person finish voiding into the receptacle.
22. Put the lid on the specimen container. Touch only the outside of the container and lid. Wipe the outside of the container. Set the container on a paper towel.

23. Provide toilet tissue after the person is done voiding.
24. Take the receptacle to the bathroom.
25. Measure urine if I&O are ordered. Include the amount in the specimen container.
26. Empty, clean, and disinfect equipment. Return equipment to its proper place.
27. Remove the gloves and practice hand hygiene. Put on clean disposable gloves.
28. Label the specimen container in the person's presence. Place the container in the plastic bag. Do not let the container touch the outside of the bag. (Some facilities require double-bagging of the specimen.) Apply a BIOHAZARD label according to center policy.
29. Assist with hand washing.
30. Remove the gloves. Practice hand hygiene.

Postprocedure
31. Provide for comfort. (See the inside of the front cover.)
32. Place the call light within reach.
33. Raise or lower bed rails. Follow the care plan.
34. Unscreen the person.
35. Complete a safety check of the room. (See the inside of the front cover.)
36. Decontaminate your hands.
37. Take the specimen and requisition slip to the storage area. Follow center policy. Wear gloves.
38. Report and record your observations.

This skill is also covered in *Clinical Skills: Nurse Assisting.*

✳ The 24-Hour Urine Specimen

All urine voided during a 24-hour period is collected for a 24-hour urine specimen. Urine is chilled on ice or refrigerated during this time. This prevents the growth of microbes. A preservative is added to the collection container for some tests.

The person voids to begin the test with an empty bladder. Discard this voiding. Save *all voidings* for the next 24 hours. The person and nursing staff must clearly understand the procedure and the test period. The test is restarted if:

- A voiding was not saved.
- Toilet tissue was discarded into the specimen.
- The specimen contains feces.

See *Promoting Safety and Comfort: The 24-Hour Urine Specimen.*

🛈 PROMOTING SAFETY AND COMFORT

The 24-Hour Urine Specimen
Safety
The collection container or preservative may contain an acid. Do not get the preservative or urine from the container on your skin or in your eyes. If you do, flush your skin or eyes with a large amount of water. Tell the nurse what happened and check the Safety Data Sheet (SDS) (Chapter 11). Also complete an incident report.

Keep the specimen chilled to prevent the growth of microbes. If not refrigerated, place the urine collection container in a bucket with ice. Add ice to the bucket as needed.

Assist the person with hand washing after every voiding. This prevents the spread of microbes that may be in the urine.

✳ COLLECTING A 24-HOUR URINE SPECIMEN

Quality of Life
Remember to:
- Knock before entering the person's room.
- Address the person by name.
- Introduce yourself by name and title.
- Explain the procedure to the person before beginning and during the procedure.

- Protect the person's rights during the procedure.
- Handle the person gently during the procedure.

Preprocedure
1. Follow *Delegation Guidelines: Urine Specimens*, p. 448. See Promoting Safety and Comfort:
   a. *Urine Specimens*, p. 449
   b. *The 24-Hour Urine Specimen*

✳ COLLECTING A 24-HOUR URINE SPECIMEN—cont'd

2. Practice hand hygiene.
3. Collect the following before going to the person's room:
   - Laboratory requisition slip
   - Urine container for a 24-hour collection
   - Specimen label
   - Preservative if needed
   - Bucket with ice if needed
   - Two 24-HOUR URINE labels
   - Funnel
   - BIOHAZARD LABEL
4. Arrange collected items in the person's bathroom.
5. Place one 24-HOUR URINE label in the bathroom. Place the other near the bed.
6. Decontaminate your hands.
7. Identify the person. Check the ID bracelet against the requisition slip. Also call the person by name.
8. Label the urine container in the person's presence. Apply the BIOHAZARD label.
9. Put on gloves.
10. Collect the following:
    - Voiding receptacle—bedpan and cover, urinal, commode, or specimen pan
    - Gloves
    - Graduate to measure output
11. Provide for privacy.

Procedure

12. Ask the person to void. Provide a voiding receptacle.
13. Measure and discard the urine. Note the time. This starts the 24-hour collection period.
14. Mark the time on the collection container.
15. Empty, clean, and disinfect equipment. Return equipment to its proper place.
16. Remove the gloves and practice hand hygiene. Put on clean gloves.
17. Assist with hand washing.
18. Remove the gloves. Practice hand hygiene.

19. Mark the time the test began and the time it ends on the room and bathroom labels.
20. Remind the person to:
    a. Use the voiding receptacle when voiding during the next 24 hours.
    b. Not have a bowel movement (BM) when voiding.
    c. Put toilet tissue in the toilet or wastebasket.
    d. Put on the call light after voiding.
21. Return to the room when the person signals for you. Knock before entering the room.
22. Do the following after every voiding:
    a. Decontaminate your hands. Put on gloves.
    b. Measure urine if I&O are ordered.
    c. Pour urine into the container using the funnel. Do not spill any urine. Restart the test if you spill or discard the urine.
    d. Empty, clean, and disinfect equipment. Return equipment to its proper place.
    e. Remove the gloves and practice hand hygiene. Put on clean gloves.
    f. Assist with hand washing.
    g. Remove the gloves. Practice hand hygiene.
    h. Follow "Postprocedure" steps *except* for steps 28 and 33.
23. Ask the person to void at the end of the 24-hour period. Follow steps 22a–g.

Postprocedure

24. Provide for comfort. (See the inside of the front cover.)
25. Place the call light within reach.
26. Raise or lower bed rails. Follow the care plan.
27. Put on gloves.
28. Remove the labels from the room and bathroom.
29. Clean and return equipment to its proper place. Discard disposable items.
30. Remove the gloves. Practice hand hygiene.
31. Unscreen the person.
32. Complete a safety check of the room. (See the inside of the front cover.)
33. Take the specimen and requisition slip to the storage area. Wear gloves.
34. Report and record your observations.

This skill is also covered in *Clinical Skills: Nurse Assisting.*

Testing Urine

The nurse may ask you to do simple urine tests. You can test for pH, glucose, and blood using reagent strips (dipsticks). The doctor orders the type and frequency of urine tests. Random urine specimens are needed.

- *Testing for pH*—Urine pH measures if urine is acidic or alkaline. Changes in normal pH (4.6 to 8.0) occur from illness, food, and medications.
- *Testing for glucose and ketones*—In diabetes, the pancreas does not secrete enough insulin (Chapter 37). The body needs insulin to use sugar for energy. If not used, sugar builds up in the blood. Some sugar appears in the urine. Glucosuria or glycosuria means "sugar" (*glucos, glycos*) in the urine (*uria*). The diabetic person may also have ketones (ketone bodies, acetone) in the urine. These substances appear in urine from the rapid breakdown of fat for energy. The body uses fat for energy if it cannot use sugar. Urine is also tested for ketones. These tests are

usually done four times a day—30 minutes before each meal and at bedtime. The doctor uses the test to make medication and diet decisions.

- *Testing for blood*—Injury and disease can cause hematuria. It means blood (*hemat*) in the urine (*uria*). Sometimes blood is seen in the urine. At other times it is unseen (*occult*).

See *Teamwork and Time Management: Testing Urine.*
See *Delegation Guidelines: Testing Urine.*
See *Promoting Safety and Comfort: Testing Urine.*

✳✳ TEAMWORK AND TIME MANAGEMENT

Testing Urine

Blood glucose testing is usually used for persons with diabetes (p. 459). However, the nurse may want urine tested for glucose and ketones. Perform the tests when directed by the nurse and care plan. The nurse uses the test results to decide about giving the person diabetic medications. The medications are given at a certain time. The nurse needs the results before giving the medications.

📄 DELEGATION GUIDELINES

Testing Urine

When testing urine is delegated to you, you need this information from the nurse and the care plan:

- What test is needed
- What equipment to use
- When to test urine
- Instructions for the test ordered
- If the nurse wants to observe the results of each test
- What observations to report and record:
  - The time you collected and tested the specimen
  - Test results
  - Problems obtaining the specimen
  - Color, clarity, and odor of urine
  - Blood in the urine
  - Particles in the urine
  - Complaints of pain, burning, urgency, difficulty voiding, or other problems
- When to report test results and observations
- What specific resident concerns to report at once

✳ Using Reagent Strips

Reagent strips (dipsticks) have sections that change color when they react with urine. To use a reagent strip:

- Do not touch the test area on the strip.
- Dip the strip into urine.

- Compare the strip with the color chart on the bottle (Fig. 29.3).

See *Promoting Safety and Comfort: Using Reagent Strips.*

👤 PROMOTING SAFETY AND COMFORT

Testing Urine

Safety

You must be accurate when testing urine. Promptly report the results to the nurse. Ordered medications may depend on the results.

Urine may contain microbes and blood. Follow Standard Precautions and the Bloodborne Pathogen Standard.

Comfort

The person may want to know the test results. If allowed by center policy, you can tell the person the results. Remember, this information is private and confidential. Make sure only the person hears what you are saying.

👤 PROMOTING SAFETY AND COMFORT

Using Reagent Strips

Safety

When using reagent strips, follow the manufacturer instructions. Otherwise, you could get the wrong result. The doctor uses the test results in diagnosing and treating the person. A wrong result could lead to serious harm.

✳ TESTING URINE WITH REAGENT STRIPS

Quality of Life

Remember to:

- Knock before entering the person's room.
- Address the person by name.
- Introduce yourself by name and title.
- Explain the procedure to the person before beginning and during the procedure.
- Protect the person's rights during the procedure.
- Handle the person gently during the procedure.

Preprocedure

1. Follow *Delegation Guidelines: Testing Urine.* See *Promoting Safety and Comfort:*
   a. *Testing Urine*
   b. *Using Reagent Strips*
2. Practice hand hygiene.
3. Collect gloves and the reagent strips ordered.
4. Decontaminate your hands.
5. Identify the person. Check the ID bracelet against the assignment sheet. Also call the person by name.
6. Put on gloves.
7. Collect equipment for the urine specimen. (See procedure: *Collecting a Random Urine Specimen,* pp. 449-450.)
8. Provide for privacy.

Procedure

9. Collect the urine specimen. (See procedure: *Collecting a Random Urine Specimen,* pp. 449-450.)
10. Remove the strip from the bottle. Put the cap on the bottle at once. It must be on tight.
11. Dip the strip test areas into the urine.
12. Remove the strip after the correct amount of time. See the manufacturer instructions.

13. Tap the strip gently against the container. This removes excess urine.
14. Wait the required amount of time. See the manufacturer instructions.
15. Compare the strip with the color chart on the bottle (see Fig. 29.3). Read the results.
16. Discard disposable items and the specimen.
17. Empty, clean, and disinfect equipment. Return equipment to its proper place.
18. Remove the gloves. Practice hand hygiene.

Postprocedure

19. Provide for comfort. (See the inside of the front cover.)
20. Place the call light within reach.
21. Raise or lower bed rails. Follow the care plan.
22. Unscreen the person.
23. Complete a safety check of the room. (See the inside of the front cover.)
24. Decontaminate your hands.
25. Report and record the test results and other observations.

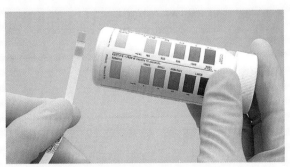

Fig. 29.3 Reagent strip for sugar and ketones.

✳ Straining Urine

A stone *(calculus)* can develop in the kidney, ureter, or bladder. Stones *(calculi)* vary in size (Chapter 38). They can be as small as grains of sand, pearl-sized, or larger. Stones causing severe pain and urinary system damage may require surgical removal.

Some stones pass through urine; therefore, all urine is strained. Passed stones are sent to the laboratory.

The person drinks 8 to 12 glasses of water a day to help pass the stone. Expect the person to void in large amounts.

✳ STRAINING URINE

Quality of Life

Remember to:

- Knock before entering the person's room.
- Address the person by name.
- Introduce yourself by name and title.
- Explain the procedure to the person before beginning and during the procedure.
- Protect the person's rights during the procedure.
- Handle the person gently during the procedure.

Preprocedure

1. Follow *Delegation Guidelines: Testing Urine*, p. 448. See *Promoting Safety and Comfort: Testing Urine*, p. 449.
2. Practice hand hygiene.
3. Collect the following before going to the person's room:
   - Laboratory requisition slip
   - Gauze or strainer
   - Specimen container
   - Specimen label
   - Two STRAIN ALL URINE labels
   - Plastic bag
   - BIOHAZARD label (if needed)
   - Gloves
4. Arrange collected items in the person's bathroom.
5. Place one STRAIN ALL URINE label in the bathroom. Place the other near the bed.
6. Decontaminate your hands.
7. Identify the person. Check the ID bracelet against the assignment sheet. Call the person by name.
8. Label the specimen container in the person's presence.
9. Put on gloves.
10. Collect the following:
    - Voiding receptacle—bedpan and cover, urinal, commode, or specimen pan
    - Graduate
    - Gloves
11. Provide for privacy.

Procedure

12. Ask the person to use the voiding receptacle for urinating. Ask the person to put on the call light after voiding.
13. Remove the gloves. Practice hand hygiene.
14. Return to the room when the person signals for you. Knock before entering the room.
15. Decontaminate your hands. Put on clean gloves.
16. Place the gauze or strainer into the graduate.
17. Pour urine into the graduate. Urine passes through the gauze or strainer (Fig. 29.4).

18. Place the gauze or strainer in the specimen container if any crystals, stones, or particles appear.
19. Place the specimen container in the plastic bag. Do not let the container touch the outside of the bag. Apply a BIOHAZARD label according to center policy.
20. Measure urine if I&O were ordered.
21. Empty, clean, and disinfect equipment. Return equipment to its proper place.
22. Remove the gloves and practice hand hygiene. Put on clean gloves.
23. Assist with hand washing.
24. Remove the gloves. Practice hand hygiene.

Postprocedure

25. Provide for comfort. (See the inside of the front cover.)
26. Place the call light within reach.
27. Raise or lower bed rails. Follow the care plan.
28. Unscreen the person.
29. Complete a safety check of the room. (See the inside of the front cover.)
30. Decontaminate your hands.
31. Take the specimen container and requisition slip to the laboratory or storage area. Wear gloves.
32. Report and record your observations.

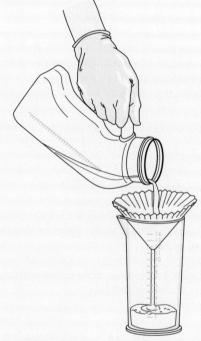

Fig. 29.4 A strainer is placed in the graduate. Urine is poured through the strainer into the graduate.

✳ STOOL SPECIMENS

When internal bleeding is suspected, stools are checked for blood. Stools also are studied for fat, microbes, worms, and other abnormal contents.

Urine must not contaminate the stool specimen. The person uses one receptacle for voiding and another for a BM. Some tests require a warm stool. The specimen is taken at once to the storage area for transport to the laboratory. Follow the rules in Box 29.1.

See *Focus on Communication: Stool Specimens.*

See *Delegation Guidelines: Stool Specimens.*

See *Promoting Safety and Comfort: Stool Specimens.*

📋 FOCUS ON COMMUNICATION

Stool Specimens

Always explain the procedure before you begin. Explain what the person needs to do and what you will do. Also show what equipment and supplies you will use. For example: "The doctor wants your stools tested. Meaning, we need a specimen from a bowel movement. I'm going to place this specimen pan (show the specimen pan) at the back of the toilet seat. You will urinate into the toilet. Your bowel movement will collect in the specimen pan rather than in the toilet. Please put toilet tissue in the toilet, not in the specimen pan. After you have a bowel movement, put your call light on right away. I'll use a tongue blade (show the tongue blade) to take some stool from the specimen pan to put in this specimen container (show the specimen container)."

After explaining the procedure, ask if person has any questions. If you do not know the answer, refer questions to the nurse.

Also make sure the person understands what to do. You can say: "Mrs. Clark, please help me make sure that you understand what I said. To collect a stool specimen, please tell me what you're going to do."

📄 DELEGATION GUIDELINES

Stool Specimens

Before collecting a stool specimen, you need this information from the nurse:
- What time to collect the specimen
- What special measures are needed
- What observations to report and record:
  - Problems obtaining the specimen
  - Color, amount, consistency, and odor of stools
  - Blood in the stool
  - Complaints of pain or discomfort
  - The time when the specimen was collected
- When to report observations
- What specific resident concerns to report at once

🧍 PROMOTING SAFETY AND COMFORT

Stool Specimens

Safety

Stools contain microbes, and they may contain blood. Follow Standard Precautions and the Bloodborne Pathogen Standard.

Comfort

Stools normally have an odor. A person may be embarrassed that you need to collect a specimen. Complete the task quickly and carefully. Also act in a professional manner.

✳ COLLECTING A STOOL SPECIMEN

Quality of Life

Remember to:
- Knock before entering the person's room.
- Address the person by name.
- Introduce yourself by name and title.
- Explain the procedure to the person before beginning and during the procedure.
- Protect the person's rights during the procedure.
- Handle the person gently during the procedure.

Preprocedure

1. Follow *Delegation Guidelines: Stool Specimens.* See *Promoting Safety and Comfort: Stool Specimens.*
2. Practice hand hygiene.
3. Collect the following before going to the person's room:
   - Laboratory requisition slip
   - Specimen pan for the toilet
   - Specimen container and lid
   - Specimen label
   - Tongue blade
   - Disposable bag
   - Plastic bag(s)
   - BIOHAZARD label (if needed)
   - Gloves
4. Arrange collected items in the person's bathroom.
5. Decontaminate your hands.

6. Identify the person. Check the ID bracelet against the requisition slip. Also call the person by name.
7. Label the specimen container in the person's presence.
8. Put on gloves.
9. Collect the following:
   - Receptacle for voiding—bedpan and cover, urinal, commode, or specimen pan
   - Toilet tissue
10. Provide for privacy.

Procedure

11. Ask the person to void. Provide the receptacle for voiding if the person does not use the bathroom. Empty, clean, and disinfect the device. Return it to its proper place.
12. Put the specimen pan on the toilet if the person will use the bathroom. Place it at the back of the toilet (Fig. 29.5). Or provide a bedpan or commode.
13. Ask the person not to put toilet tissue into the bedpan, commode, or specimen pan. Provide a bag for toilet tissue.
14. Place the call light and toilet tissue within reach. Raise or lower bed rails. Follow the care plan.
15. Remove the gloves. Decontaminate your hands. Leave the room.
16. Return when the person signals. Or check on the person every 5 minutes. Knock before entering.
17. Decontaminate your hands. Put on clean gloves.
18. Lower the bed rail near you if up.

✴ COLLECTING A STOOL SPECIMEN—cont'd

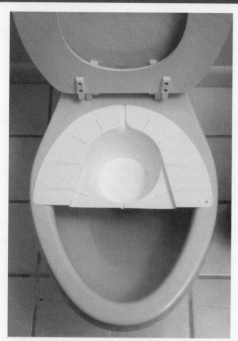

Fig. 29.5 The specimen pan is placed at the back of the toilet for a stool specimen.

19. Remove the bedpan (if used). Note the color, amount, consistency, and odor of stools.
20. Provide perineal care if needed.
21. Collect the specimen:
    a. Use a tongue blade to take about 2 tablespoons of stool to the specimen container (Fig. 29.6). Take the sample from the middle of a formed stool.
    b. Include pus, mucus, or blood present in the stool.
    c. Take stool from two different places in the BM if required by center policy.
    d. Put the lid on the specimen container.
    e. Place the container in the plastic bag. Do not let the container touch the outside of the bag. (Some facilities require double-bagging.) Apply a biohazard label according to center policy.

This skill is also covered in *Clinical Skills: Nurse Assisting*.

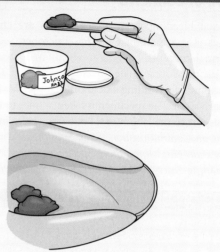

Fig. 29.6 A tongue blade is used to transfer a small amount of stool from the bedpan to the specimen container.

22. Wrap the tongue blade in toilet tissue. Discard it in the disposable bag.
23. Empty, clean, and disinfect equipment. Return equipment to its proper place.
24. Remove the gloves and practice hand hygiene. Put on clean gloves.
25. Assist with hand washing.
26. Remove the gloves. Practice hand hygiene.

Postprocedure
27. Provide for comfort. (See the inside of the front cover.)
28. Place the call light within reach.
29. Raise or lower bed rails. Follow the care plan.
30. Unscreen the person.
31. Complete a safety check of the room. (See the inside of the front cover.)
32. Deliver the specimen and requisition slip to the storage area. Follow center policy. Wear gloves.
33. Report and record your observations.

✴ Testing Stools for Blood

Stools may contain blood. Ulcers, colon cancer, and hemorrhoids are common causes. Often, blood is seen if bleeding is low in the bowels. Stools are black and tarry from bleeding in the stomach or upper gastrointestinal tract. Melena is a black, tarry stool.

Sometimes bleeding occurs in very small amounts. Then stools are tested for *occult blood*. *Occult* means "hidden" or "not seen." The test is done to screen for colon cancer and other digestive disorders.

Occult blood test kits vary. Follow the manufacturer instructions. The following procedure is presented as a guide.

See *Delegation Guidelines: Testing Stools for Blood*.
See *Promoting Safety and Comfort: Testing Stools for Blood*.

📄 DELEGATION GUIDELINES

Testing Stools for Blood
Before testing a stool specimen for blood, you need this information from the nurse:
- What test is needed
- What equipment to use
- When to test the stool
- Instructions for the test ordered
- If the nurse wants to observe the results of each test
- What observations to report and record:

- The time you collected and tested the specimen
- Test results
- Problems obtaining the specimen
- Color, amount, consistency, and odor of feces
- Blood in the stool
- Complaints of pain or discomfort
- When to report observations
- What specific resident concerns to report at once

PROMOTING SAFETY AND COMFORT

Testing Stools for Blood
Safety
You must be accurate when testing stools. Follow the manufacturer instructions for the test used. Promptly report the results to the nurse.

Stools contain microbes and may contain blood. Follow Standard Precautions and the Bloodborne Pathogen Standard.

TESTING A STOOL SPECIMEN FOR BLOOD

Quality of Life
Remember to:
- Knock before entering the person's room.
- Address the person by name.
- Introduce yourself by name and title.
- Explain the procedure to the person before beginning and during the procedure.
- Protect the person's rights during the procedure.
- Handle the person gently during the procedure.

Preprocedure
1. *Follow Delegation Guidelines: Testing Stools for Blood.* See *Promoting Safety and Comfort:*
   a. *Stool Specimens,* p. 456
   b. *Testing Stools for Blood*
2. Practice hand hygiene.
3. Collect the following before going to the person's room:
   - Occult blood test kit
   - Tongue blades (if needed)
   - Gloves
4. Arrange collected items in the person's bathroom.
5. Decontaminate your hands.
6. Identify the person. Check the ID bracelet against the assignment sheet. Also call the person by name.
7. Put on gloves.
8. Collect the following:
   - Equipment for a stool specimen (see procedure: *Collecting a Stool Specimen,* pp. 455-456)
   - Paper towels
9. Provide for privacy.

Procedure
10. Collect a stool specimen. See procedure: *Collecting a Stool Specimen,* pp. 455-456.
11. Practice hand hygiene. Put on clean gloves.
12. Open the test kit.
13. Use a tongue blade to obtain a small amount of stool.
14. Apply a thin smear of stool on *box A* on the test paper (Fig. 29.7A).
15. Use another tongue blade to obtain stool from another part of the specimen.
16. Apply a thin smear of stool on *box B* on the test paper (see Fig. 29.7B).
17. Close the packet.
18. Turn the test packet to the other side. Open the flap. Apply developer (from the kit) to *boxes A* and *B*. Follow the manufacturer instructions (see Fig. 29.7C).
19. Wait 10 to 60 seconds as required by the manufacturer.
20. Note the color changes on your assignment sheet (see Fig. 29.7D).
21. Dispose of the test packet.
22. Wrap the tongue blades with toilet tissue, then discard them.
23. Empty, clean, and disinfect equipment. Return equipment to its proper place.
24. Remove the gloves. Practice hand hygiene.

Postprocedure
25. Provide for comfort. (See the inside of the front cover.)
26. Place the call light within reach.
27. Raise or lower bed rails. Follow the care plan.
28. Complete a safety check of the room. (See the inside of the front cover.)
29. Decontaminate your hands.
30. Report and record the test results and your observations.

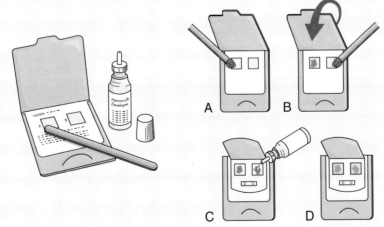

Fig. 29.7 Testing for occult blood. (A) Stool is smeared on *box A*. (B) Stool is smeared on *box B* and then the flap is closed. (C) Developer is applied to *boxes A* and *B* on the back side of the test packet. (D) Color changes are noted.

This skill is also covered in *Clinical Skills: Nurse Assisting.*

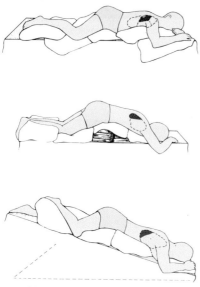

Fig. 29.8 Some positions for postural drainage. (From Potter PA, Perry AG: *Fundamentals of nursing*, ed. 10, St. Louis, 2021, Mosby.)

✳ SPUTUM SPECIMENS

Respiratory disorders cause the lungs, bronchi, and trachea to secrete mucus. Mucus from the respiratory system is called sputum when expectorated *(expelled)* through the mouth. Sputum is not saliva. Saliva ("spit") is a thin, clear liquid produced by the salivary glands in the mouth.

Sputum specimens are studied for blood, microbes, and abnormal cells. The person coughs up sputum from the bronchi and trachea. This is often painful and hard to do. It is easier to collect a specimen in the morning. Secretions collect in the trachea and bronchi during sleep. They are coughed up on awakening.

To collect a specimen, follow the rules in Box 29.1. Also have the person rinse the mouth with water. Rinsing decreases saliva and removes food particles. Mouthwash is not used. It destroys some of the microbes in the mouth.

Older persons may lack the strength to cough up sputum. Coughing is easier after postural drainage. It drains secretions by gravity. Gravity causes fluids to flow down. The person is positioned so a lung part is higher than the airway (Fig. 29.8). The nurse or respiratory therapist does postural drainage.

See *Delegation Guidelines: Sputum Specimens.*
See *Promoting Safety and Comfort: Sputum Specimens.*

📋 DELEGATION GUIDELINES

Sputum Specimens

Before collecting a sputum specimen, you need this information from the nurse:

- When to collect the specimen
- How much sputum is needed—usually 1 to 2 teaspoons
- If the person uses the bathroom
- If the person can hold the specimen container
- What observations to report and record:
  - The time the specimen was collected
  - The amount of sputum collected
  - How easily the person raised the sputum
  - Sputum color—clear, white, yellow, green, brown, or red
  - Sputum odor—none or foul odor
  - Sputum consistency—thick, watery, or frothy (with bubbles or foam)
  - Hemoptysis—bloody *(hemo)* sputum *(ptysis* means "to spit")
  - If the person was not able to produce sputum
  - Any other observations
- When to report observations
- What specific resident concerns to report at once

👤 PROMOTING SAFETY AND COMFORT

Sputum Specimens

Safety

Follow Standard Precautions and the Bloodborne Pathogen Standard to prevent contact with mucus. It may contain blood or microbes.

The person may have tuberculosis (TB) (Chapter 36). Follow isolation precautions and protect yourself by wearing a TB respirator (Chapter 14).

Comfort

The procedure can embarrass the person. Coughing and expectorating sounds can disturb others. Also, sputum is not pleasant to look at. For these reasons, privacy is important. Cover the specimen container and place it in a bag. Some sputum specimen containers are cloudy in color to hide the contents.

✳ COLLECTING A SPUTUM SPECIMEN

Quality of Life

Remember to:

- Knock before entering the person's room.
- Address the person by name.
- Introduce yourself by name and title.
- Explain the procedure to the person before beginning and during the procedure.
- Protect the person's rights during the procedure.
- Handle the person gently during the procedure.

Preprocedure

1. Follow *Delegation Guidelines: Sputum Specimens*, p. 458. See *Promoting Safety and Comfort: Sputum Specimens.*
2. Practice hand hygiene.

3. Collect the following before going to the person's room:
   - Laboratory requisition slip
   - Sputum specimen container and lid
   - Specimen label
   - Plastic bag(s)
   - BIOHAZARD label (if needed)
4. Arrange collected items in the person's bathroom.
5. Decontaminate your hands.
6. Identify the person. Check the ID bracelet against the requisition slip. Also call the person by name.
7. Label the specimen container in the person's presence.
8. Collect mask, gloves, and tissues.
9. Provide for privacy. If able, the person uses the bathroom for the procedure.

Continued

✳ COLLECTING A SPUTUM SPECIMEN—cont'd

Procedure

10. Put on mask and gloves.
11. Ask the person to rinse the mouth out with clear water. Do not have the person use mouthwash.
12. Have the person hold the container. Only the outside is touched.
13. Ask the person to cover the mouth and nose with tissues when coughing. Follow center policy for used tissues.
14. Ask the person to take two or three deep breaths and cough up the sputum.
15. Have the person expectorate directly into the container (Fig. 29.9). Sputum should not touch the outside of the container.
16. Collect 1 to 2 teaspoons of sputum unless told to collect more.
17. Put the lid on the container.
18. Place the container in the plastic bag. Do not let the container touch the outside of the bag. (Some facilities require double-bagging.) Apply a BIOHAZARD label according to center policy.
19. Remove the gloves and decontaminate your hands. Put on clean gloves.
20. Assist with hand washing.
21. Remove the gloves. Remove the mask. Decontaminate your hands.

Postprocedure

22. Provide for comfort. (See the inside of the front cover.)
23. Place the call light within reach.
24. Raise or lower bed rails. Follow the care plan.

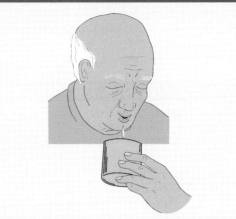

Fig. 29.9 The person expectorates into the center of the specimen container.

25. Unscreen the person.
26. Complete a safety check of the room. (See the inside of the front cover.)
27. Decontaminate your hands.
28. Deliver the specimen and the requisition slip to the storage area. Follow center policy. Wear gloves.
29. Report and record your observations.

This skill is also covered in *Clinical Skills: Nurse Assisting*.

✳ BLOOD GLUCOSE TESTING

Blood glucose testing is used for persons with diabetes. The doctor uses the results to regulate the person's medications and diet. In some states or centers, nursing assistants do not perform blood glucose testing. Follow the policies of your nursing center.

Capillary blood is obtained through a skin puncture. A drop of blood is collected. A fingertip is the most common site for skin punctures. This provides easy access and clothing is not removed.

Inspect the puncture site for signs of trauma and skin breaks. Do not use swollen, bruised, cyanotic (bluish color), scarred, or callused sites. Such areas have poor blood flow. A *callus* is a thick, hardened area on the skin. Calluses often form over frequently used areas, such as the tips of the thumbs and index fingers. Therefore, thumbs, index fingers, and fifth (pinkie) fingers are not good skin puncture sites.

Use the side toward the tip of the middle or ring finger (Fig. 29.10). Do not use the center, fleshy part of the fingertip. This site has many nerve endings, making punctures painful.

You use a sterile, disposable lancet to puncture the skin (Fig. 29.11). The person feels a brief, sharp pinch. A *lancet* is a short, pointed blade. It punctures but does not cut the skin. The lancet is inside a protective cover. You do not touch the blade. Discard it in the sharps container after use.

A *glucose meter (glucometer)* measures blood glucose. You apply a drop of blood to a reagent strip. Then you insert the strip in the glucose meter. The blood glucose level appears on

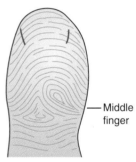

Middle finger

Fig. 29.10 Site for skin punctures. (From Bonewit-West K: *Clinical procedures for medical assistants*, ed. 7, St. Louis, 2008, Saunders.)

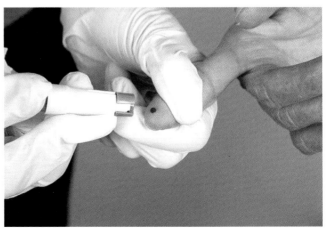

Fig. 29.11 A lancet. (From iStock/aabejon/173917280.)

the screen. Many types of glucose meters are available. How fast results are displayed varies. Some take 5 seconds.

You will learn to use your center's device. Always follow the manufacturer instructions.

See *Teamwork and Time Management: Blood Glucose Testing.*
See *Delegation Guidelines: Blood Glucose Testing.*
See *Promoting Safety and Comfort: Blood Glucose Testing.*

TEAMWORK AND TIME MANAGEMENT

Blood Glucose Testing
Perform blood glucose testing at times directed by the nurse and the care plan. The nurse uses the results to make decisions about the person's diet and medication dosages. The medications are given at a certain time. The nurse needs the blood glucose results before giving the medications.

Glucose meters are shared with other staff. Tell your coworkers when you have one. Work quickly but carefully. Return the device to the storage area in a timely manner.

DELEGATION GUIDELINES

Blood Glucose Testing
If testing blood glucose is delegated to you, make sure that:
- Your state and center allow you to perform the procedure.
- The procedure is in your job description.
- You have the necessary training.
- You know how to use the center's equipment.
- You review the procedure with a nurse.
- The nurse is available to answer questions and to supervise you.

If the abovementioned conditions are met, you need the following information from the nurse and the care plan:
- What sites to avoid for a skin puncture
- When to collect and test the specimen—usually before meals

- If the person receives medications that affect blood clotting (Note: If yes, it may take a longer time to stop bleeding. Apply pressure until bleeding stops.)
- What to report and record:
  - The time the specimen was collected
  - The blood glucose test results
  - The site used for the skin puncture
  - The amount of bleeding at the skin puncture site
  - Any signs of a **hematoma** (a swelling *[oma]* that contains blood *[hemat]*)
  - How the person tolerated the procedure
  - Complaints of pain at the skin puncture site
  - Other observations or resident complaints
- When to report observations and the test result
- What specific resident concerns to report at once

PROMOTING SAFETY AND COMFORT

Blood Glucose Testing
Safety
Accurate results are important. Inaccurate results can harm the person. Follow the rules in Box 29.2.

You must know how to use the equipment. Use only the type of reagent strip specified by the manufacturer. Otherwise, you will get inaccurate results.

Contact with blood is likely. Follow Standard Precautions and the Bloodborne Pathogen Standard.

Comfort
Older persons often have poor circulation in their fingers. To increase blood flow, apply a warm washcloth or wash the hands in warm water.

BOX 29.2 Rules for Blood Glucose Testing

- Follow the manufacturer instructions for the glucose meter.
- Know how to use the equipment. Request any necessary training.
- Make sure the glucose meter was tested for accuracy. Check the testing log.
- Enter a code or username if required by the glucose meter. This is provided by the center. Do not share your username with others.
- Make sure you have the correct reagent strips for the glucose meter you are using. Compare the code number on the strip with the code number on the glucose meter. The code numbers should be the same.

- Scan the bar code on the bottle of reagent strips if needed (see Fig. 29.12).
- Check the color of reagent strips. Do not use discolored strips.
- Check the expiration date of the reagent strips. Do not use them if the date has passed.
- Report the result to the nurse at once.
- Record the result following center policy.

✳ MEASURING BLOOD GLUCOSE

Quality of Life

Remember to:

- Knock before entering the person's room.
- Address the person by name.
- Introduce yourself by name and title.
- Explain the procedure to the person before beginning and during the procedure.
- Protect the person's rights during the procedure.
- Handle the person gently during the procedure.

Preprocedure

1. Follow *Delegation Guidelines: Blood Glucose Testing*, p. 460. See *Promoting Safety and Comfort: Blood Glucose Testing*, p. 460.
2. Practice hand hygiene.
3. Collect the following:
   - Sterile lancet
   - Antiseptic wipes
   - Gloves
   - Cotton balls
   - Bandage
   - Glucose meter
   - Reagent strips (Use the correct ones for the meter. Check the expiration date.)
   - Paper towels
   - Warm washcloth
4. Read the manufacturer instructions for the lancet and glucose meter.
5. Arrange your work area.
6. Identify the person. Check the ID bracelet against the assignment sheet. Also call the person by name.
7. Provide for privacy.
8. Raise the bed for body mechanics. The far bed rail is up if used.

Procedure

9. Help the person to a comfortable position.
10. Put on the gloves.
11. Prepare the supplies.
    a. Open the antiseptic wipes.
    b. Remove a reagent strip from the bottle. Place it on the paper towel. Place the cap securely on the bottle.
    c. Prepare the lancet.
    d. Turn on the glucose meter.
    e. Follow the prompts. You may need to enter a username and the person's ID number. Scan the bar code on the bottle of reagent strips if needed (Fig. 29.12).
    f. Insert a reagent strip into the glucose meter (Fig. 29.13).
12. Perform a skin puncture to obtain a drop of blood.
    a. Inspect the person's fingers. Select a puncture site.
    b. Warm the finger. Rub it gently or apply a warm washcloth.
    c. Lightly massage twice only the hand and finger toward the puncture site. And lower the finger below the person's waist. These actions increase blood flow to the site.
    d. Hold the finger with your thumb and forefinger. Use your nondominant hand. Hold the finger until step 13c.
    e. Clean the site with an antiseptic wipe. *Do not touch the site after cleaning.*
    f. Let the site dry.
    g. Pick up the sterile lancet.
    h. Place the lancet against the puncture site.
    i. Push the button on the lancet to puncture the skin. (Follow the manufacturer instructions.)
    j. Wipe away the first blood drop. Use a cotton ball.
    k. Apply gentle pressure below the puncture site.
    l. Let a large drop of blood form.
13. Collect and test the specimen. Follow the manufacturer instructions and center procedures for the glucose meter used.
    a. Hold the test area of the reagent strip close to the drop of blood.
    b. Lightly touch the reagent strip to the blood drop (Fig. 29.14). Do not smear the blood. The meter will test the sample when enough blood is applied.
    c. Apply pressure to the puncture site until bleeding stops. Use a cotton ball or gauze. If able, let the person apply pressure to the site.
    d. Read the result on the display (Fig. 29.15). Note the result on your note pad or assignment sheet. Tell the person the result.
    e. Turn off the glucose meter.
    f. Apply a bandage to the area. Tell the person it may be removed after 15 minutes.

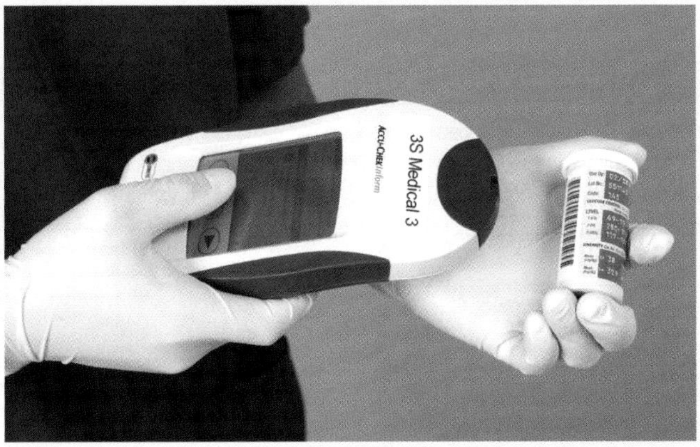

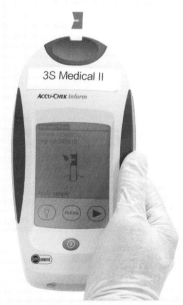

Fig. 29.12 The bar code on the bottle of reagent strips is scanned.

Fig. 29.13 A reagent strip is in the glucose meter.

Continued

✳ MEASURING BLOOD GLUCOSE—cont'd

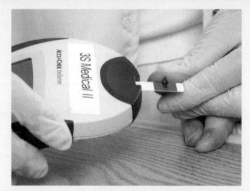

Fig. 29.14 A drop of blood is applied to the reagent strip.

14. Discard the lancet in the sharps container.
15. Discard the cotton balls and reagent strip following center policy.
16. Remove and discard the gloves. Decontaminate your hands.

Postprocedure

17. Provide for comfort. (See the inside of the front cover.)
18. Place the call light within reach.
19. Lower the bed to its lowest position.
20. Raise or lower bed rails. Follow the care plan.
21. Unscreen the person.
22. Discard used supplies.
23. Complete a safety check of the room. (See the inside of the front cover.)

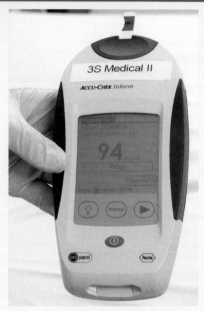

Fig. 29.15 The result is displayed on the glucose meter.

24. Follow center policy for soiled linens.
25. Decontaminate your hands.
26. Report and record the test result and your observations.

This skill is also covered in *Clinical Skills: Nurse Assisting.*

👥 QUALITY OF LIFE

You must collect and test specimens on the right person. Otherwise, one or more persons could suffer harm. Before collecting or testing a specimen, carefully identify the person. Check the ID bracelet against the laboratory requisition slip or assignment sheet. Compare all information, not just the person's name.

Some centers require you to place the collection date, collection time, and your name or initials on the container. This promotes safety. Follow center policy for labeling specimens.

Specimen collection embarrasses many people. To promote comfort and privacy:

- Politely ask visitors to leave the room.
- Close doors, the privacy curtain, and window coverings.

- Leave the room if it is safe to do so. If you cannot leave, explain this to the person.
- Place the specimen container in a paper bag or wrap it in a paper towel or washcloth. Then others will not see the specimen.
- Always act professionally. Do not say things that may embarrass the person.

Some people can collect their own urine and sputum specimens. Doing so promotes independence. It also helps reduce embarrassment. Explain the procedure to the person. This helps the person know how to collect the specimen correctly. Show the person the specimen container and how it is used. Also ask the person where to place the container. When ready to collect the specimen, the person knows where to find the container.

❓ TIME TO REFLECT

The doctor has ordered a 24-hour urine test for Mr. Lightfoot. The nurse has instructed Mr. Lightfoot and you will be caring for him today. As you make your first rounds of the morning, you see that all of the equipment is in his bathroom. You visit with Mr. Lightfoot and remind him to put on his call light after he uses the urinal. He nods and appears to understand. After lunch you check on Mr. Lightfoot. He is napping in bed and his wife has come to visit. She tells you that her husband used the urinal and she emptied it in the toilet because she did not want there to be an odor in the room. What has this done to the procedure of the 24-hour urine test? What has to happen next? How could this have been prevented?

REVIEW QUESTIONS

Circle the BEST answer.

1. A random urine specimen is collected
   a. After sleep
   b. Before meals
   c. After meals
   d. Any time

2. Perineal care is given before collecting a
   a. Random specimen
   b. Midstream specimen
   c. 24-hour urine specimen
   d. Stool specimen

3. A 24-hour urine specimen involves
   a. Collecting all urine voided during a 24-hour period
   b. Collecting a random specimen every hour for 24 hours
   c. Testing urine for ketones every day
   d. Measuring output every hour for 24 hours

4. Urine is tested for ketones
   a. At bedtime
   b. 30 minutes after meals and at bedtime
   c. 30 minutes before meals and at bedtime
   d. Before breakfast

5. You need to strain a person's urine. Straining is done to find
   a. Blood
   b. Stones
   c. Ketones
   d. Acetone

6. You note a black, tarry stool. This is called
   a. Melena
   b. Feces
   c. Hemostool
   d. Occult blood

7. A stool specimen must be kept warm. After collecting the specimen
   a. Put it in an oven
   b. Put it in a paper bag
   c. Cover it with a towel
   d. Take it to the storage area

8. The best time to collect a sputum specimen is
   a. On awakening
   b. After meals
   c. At bedtime
   d. After oral hygiene

9. A sputum specimen is needed. You should ask the person to
   a. Use mouthwash
   b. Rinse the mouth with clear water
   c. Brush the teeth
   d. Remove dentures

10. Which is the best site for a skin puncture?
    a. Thumb
    b. Index finger
    c. Ring finger
    d. Little finger

11. Which is used to measure blood glucose?
    a. Glucose meter
    b. Lancet
    c. Reagent strip
    d. Sphygmomanometer

12. Before using reagent strips for blood glucose testing, you need to
    a. Check the expiration date
    b. Make sure they are discolored
    c. Label each strip with the person's name
    d. Check the size of the test area

See Appendix A for answers to these questions.

30

Admissions, Transfers, and Discharges

OBJECTIVES

- Define the key terms listed in this chapter.
- Describe your role during admissions, transfers, discharges, and when moving the person to a new room.
- Explain how you can help the resident and family feel comfortable in the nursing center.
- Identify the rules for measuring weight and height.
- Explain the reasons for moving a resident to a new room.
- Perform the procedures described in this chapter.
- Explain how to promote quality of life.

KEY TERMS

admission Official entry of a person into a nursing center

discharge Official departure of a person from a nursing center

transfer Moving the person to another health care setting; moving the person to a new room within the center

KEY ABBREVIATIONS

CMS Centers for Medicare & Medicaid Services

ID Identification

IV Intravenous

OBRA Omnibus Budget Reconciliation Act of 1987

Admission is the official entry of a person into a nursing center. It causes anxiety and fear in residents and families. They are in a new, strange setting. They may have concerns and fears about:

- Where to go, what to do, and what to expect.
- Never returning home.
- Who gives care, how care is given, and if the correct care is given.
- Getting meals.
- Finding the bathroom.
- How to get help.
- Being abused.
- Strange sights and sounds.
- Being apart from family and friends.
- Making new friends.
- Leaving homes and possessions behind.
- How care will be paid for.

Moving to another room may cause similar concerns. So may transfer to another health care setting—hospital or nursing center. Discharge to a home setting is usually a happy time. However, the person may need home care. Discharge and transfer are defined as follows:

- **Discharge** is the official departure of a person from a nursing center.
- **Transfer** is moving the person to another health care setting. In some centers it also means moving the person to a new room or level of care within the center.

Admission, transfer, and discharge are critical events. So is moving the person to a new room. Sometimes the new room is on another nursing unit. These events involve the following:

- Privacy and confidentiality
- Reporting and recording
- Understanding and communicating with the person
- Communicating with the health team
- Respect for the person and the person's property
- Being kind, courteous, and respectful

See *Teamwork and Time Management: Admissions, Transfers, and Discharges.*

See *Delegation Guidelines: Admissions, Transfers, and Discharges.*

See *Promoting Safety and Comfort: Admissions, Transfers, and Discharges.*

TEAMWORK AND TIME MANAGEMENT

Admissions, Transfers, and Discharges

Transfers and discharges are easier if a coworker helps you. So is moving the person to a new room. When asking for help, politely tell your coworker:

- The procedure you need help with.
- When you plan to do the procedure.
- What you need the person to do.
- How much time it will take.

Remember to thank the person for helping you.

🖹 DELEGATION GUIDELINES

Admissions, Transfers, and Discharges
When admitting, transferring, or discharging a person, you need this information from the nurse. You also need the same information when moving a person to a new room.
- If you need to admit, transfer, or discharge the person or move the person to a new room
- If moving to a new room, the person's new room and bed number
- The person's method of transportation to or from the center—car, ambulance, or wheelchair van
- How the person will move about within the center—walking, wheelchair, stretcher, or bed
- The person's room and bed number
- What equipment and supplies are needed
- If the person stays dressed or needs to wear a gown or sleepwear
- If the person stays in bed or can be in a chair
- When to report observations
- What specific resident concerns to report at once

👤 PROMOTING SAFETY AND COMFORT

Admissions, Transfers, and Discharges
Safety
The person may develop pain or become distressed during admission, transfer, discharge, or when moving to a new room. If so, call for the nurse at once. Stay with the person. When the nurse arrives, assist as needed.

Comfort
Admission, transfer, or discharge may be stressful for the person. Moving to a new room may cause some to worry. Some persons are happy. Others are sad and fearful. Some anxiety is normal. To provide for the person's mental comfort:
- Explain what you are doing and why.
- Do not rush the person.
- Be sensitive to the person's needs and feelings.

✴ ADMISSIONS

An admission coordinator starts the process. The goal is to make it simple and easy. Often, the process starts 2 or 3 days before the person enters the center.

The person's identifying information is obtained. This includes the person's:
- Full name.
- Age and birth date.
- Doctor's name.
- Medicare number.
- Religion.

A nurse or social worker explains the resident's rights to the person and family. They also receive the rights in writing.

Admitting papers and a consent for treatment are signed. The person signs them or the person's legal representative does so. The nurse or admission coordinator obtains needed signatures.

The person's photo is taken. Then the person may receive an identification (ID) bracelet. The photo or ID bracelet is used to identify the person (Chapter 11).

Admission is often a hard time for the person and family. They do not part until ready to do so. Allow privacy and as much time as needed. Answer any questions they have or refer their questions to the nurse or social worker.

See *Residents with Dementia: Admissions.*
See *Focus on Rehabilitation: Admissions.*

👤 RESIDENTS WITH DEMENTIA

Admissions
Persons with dementia and their families may need extra help during the admission process. Often, confusion increases in a new setting. Fear, agitation, and wanting to leave are common. The family also is fearful. Many feel guilty about the need for nursing center care. The health team helps the person and family feel safe and welcome.

Patients are admitted to rehabilitation units from hospitals. Often, they arrive with special equipment and supplies.

🌿 FOCUS ON REHABILITATION

Admissions
A nurse usually greets the person and starts the admission process. Assist as needed. The nurse may ask you to complete parts of the admission process if:
- The person's condition is stable.
- The person has no serious discomfort or distress.

Preparing the Room

You prepare the room before the person arrives. Fig. 30.1 shows a room ready for a new resident.

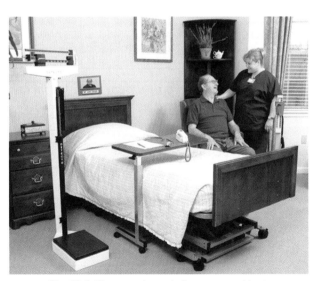

Fig. 30.1 The room is ready for a new resident.

✴ PREPARING THE PERSON'S ROOM

Procedure

1. Follow *Delegation Guidelines: Admissions, Transfers, and Discharges.*
2. Practice hand hygiene.
3. Collect the following:
   - Admission kit—wash basin, soap, toothpaste, toothbrush, water pitcher and cup, and so on
   - Bedpan and urinal (for a man)
   - Admission form (Fig. 30.2)

- Thermometer
- Sphygmomanometer
- Stethoscope
- Gown or pajamas (if needed)
- Towels and washcloth
- Intravenous (IV) pole (if needed)
- Other items requested by the nurse

ADMISSION NURSING ASSESSMENT

STATUS UPON ADMISSION

Admission Notes

Date of admission ___/___/___   Time _____ a.m. p.m.

Transported by _____

Accompanied by _____

Age _____ Sex _____ Weight _____ Height: _____ Ft. _____ In.

Vitals: T _____ P _____ (☐ Reg ☐ Irreg) R _____ B/P _____/_____

Attending physician notified? ☐ No ☐ Yes, date/time ___/___/___ a.m. p.m.

Diagnosis: _____ Date last chest x-ray or PPD ___/___/___

Allergies

Meds _____

Food _____

Other _____

Skin Condition

Using the diagrams provided, indicate all body marks such as old/recent scars (surgical and other), bruises, discolorations, abrasions, pressure ulcers, or questionable markings. Indicate size, depth (in cms), color and drainage.

COMMENTS: _____

SPECIAL TREATMENTS & PROCEDURES: _____

PAIN
(As described by resident/representative)

Frequency:
☐ No pain   ☐ Daily, but not
☐ Less than daily   constant
                   ☐ Constant

Location: _____

Intensity:
☐ No pain   ☐ Severe pain
☐ Mild pain   ☐ Horrible pain
☐ Distressing pain ☐ Excruciating
                      pain

Pain on admission:
☐ No ☐ Yes, describe _____

RIGHT   LEFT

CURRENT STATUS

General Skin Condition	**Physical Status** (describe if applicable otherwise indicate NA)
Check all that apply.	Paralysis/paresis-site, degree _____
☐ Reddened ☐ Pale ☐ Jaundiced	Contracture(s)-site, degree _____
☐ Cyanotic ☐ Ashen	Congenital anomalies _____
☐ Dry ☐ Moist ☐ Oily ☐ Warm ☐ Cold	Prosthesis: _____
☐ Edema, site _____	Other _____

Functional Status

TRANSFERS-ABLE TO TRANSFER
☐ Independently
☐ 1 person assist
☐ 2 person assist
☐ Total assist

WEIGHT BEARING-ABLE TO BEAR
☐ Full weight
☐ Partial weight
☐ Non-weight bearing

AMBULATION-ABLE TO AMBULATE
☐ Independently
☐ 1 person assist
☐ 2 person assist
☐ With device
   Type _____
☐ Wheelchair only
☐ Wheelchair/propels self
☐ Bedrest

SUPPORTIVE DEVICES USED:
☐ Elastic hose   ☐ Footboard
☐ Bed cradle   ☐ Air mattress
☐ Sheepskin   ☐ Eggcrate
☐ Hand rolls ☐ Sling ☐ Trapeze
☐ Other _____
☐ Other _____

Drug Therapy

DRUG	DOSE/FREQUENCY	DRUG	DOSE/FREQUENCY
1		**6**	
2		**7**	
3		**8**	
4		**9**	
5		**10**	

NAME–Last	First	Middle	Attending Physician	Record No.	Room/Bed

CFS 5-3HH   © 1992 Briggs Corporation, Des Moines, IA 50305 (800) 247-2343
R1001   PRINTED IN U.S.A.

ADMISSION NURSING ASSESSMENT
☐ Continued on Reverse

Fig. 30.2 Admission form. (Courtesy Briggs Corp., Des Moines, IA.)

PREPARING THE PERSON'S ROOM—cont'd

4. Place the following on the overbed table:
   - Thermometer
   - Sphygmomanometer
   - Stethoscope
   - Admission form
5. Place the water pitcher and cup on the bedside stand or overbed table.
6. Place the following in the bedside stand:
   - Admission kit
   - Bedpan and urinal

- Gown or pajamas
- Towels and washcloth
7. *If the person arrives by stretcher:*
   a. Make a surgical bed (Chapter 17).
   b. Raise the bed to its highest level.
8. *If the person is ambulatory or arrives by wheelchair:*
   a. Leave the bed closed.
   b. Lower the bed to its lowest position.
9. Attach the call light to the bed linens.
10. Decontaminate your hands.

CURRENT STATUS - CONTINUED

Hearing	Right	Left	R & L	Vision	Right	Left	R & L	Communication
Adequate				Adequate				❑ Clear
Adequate w/aid				Adequate w/glasses				❑ Aphasic ❑ Dysphasic
Poor				Poor				Language(s) Spoken:
Deaf				Blind				_____

Oral Assessment | **Eating/Nutrition**

Complete oral cavity exam: ❑ Yes ❑ No
If yes, condition _____
_____

Own teeth: ❑ Yes ❑ No
If yes, condition _____

Dentures: Upper ❑ Comp ❑ Part
Lower ❑ Comp ❑ Part
Do dentures fit? ❑ Yes ❑ No

❑ Dependent ❑ Independent ❑ Needs assist
❑ Dysphagic; reason _____
❑ Adaptive equipment (specify) _____
Type/consistency of diet _____
_____

Food likes _____
Food dislikes _____
Bev. preference _____
HS snack preferred: ❑ Yes ❑ No

Sleep Patterns	Bathing/Oral Hyg.	Indep.	Assist	Dep.	General Grooming	Indep.	Assist	Dep.
Usual bed time _____ a.m./p.m.	Tub				Shave			
Usual arising time _____ a.m./p.m.	Shower				Grooming			
Usual nap time _____ a.m./p.m.	Bed bath				Dressing			
Other _____	Oral hygiene				Shampoo			

Psychosocial Functioning

FAMILY RELATIONSHIPS:
Members visit (frequency) _____
_____
Closest relationship with _____

WHICH WORDS BEST DESCRIBE RESIDENT? ❑ Alert ❑ Angry ❑ Fearful
❑ Noisy ❑ Friendly ❑ Cooperative ❑ Lethargic ❑ _____
❑ Non-questioning ❑ Combative
ANSWERS QUESTIONS: ❑ Readily ❑ Reluctantly ❑ Inappropriately
MOOD: ❑ Passive ❑ Depressed ❑ Elated ❑ Quiet ❑ Secure
❑ Questioning ❑ Talkative ❑ Homesick ❑ Wanders mentally
❑ Hyperactive ❑ _____

ORIENTED: ❑ Yes ❑ No, if No, _____
DISORIENTED TO: ❑ Time ❑ Place
❑ Person
COMPREHENSION: ❑ Slow ❑ Quick ❑ Unable to understand
MOTIVATION: ❑ Good ❑ Fair ❑ Poor
PERSONAL HABITS: Smokes? ❑ Yes ❑ No Uses alcohol? ❑ Yes ❑ No
RESIDENT GIVEN EXPLANATION OF/OR INVOLVED IN PLAN OF CARE? ❑ Yes ❑ No
RESIDENT ORIENTED TO FACILITY? ❑ Call light ❑ Bathroom ❑ Mealtime ❑ Activities

Bowel and Bladder Evaluation

Uses: ❑ Toilet ❑ Urinal ❑ Bedpan ❑ Bedside commode
BOWEL HABITS: Continent? ❑ Yes ❑ No Constipated? ❑ Yes ❑ No Laxative used? ❑ Yes ❑ No
Enemas used? ❑ Yes ❑ No Last bowel movement _____ a.m./p.m.
BLADDER HABITS: Continent? ❑ Yes ❑ No Dribbles? ❑ Yes ❑ No Catheter? ❑ Yes, type _____ ❑ No
Urine color _____ Consistency _____ Time last voiding _____ a.m./p.m.

Restorative Programs Indicated | Therapy Indicated

Based on the foregoing assessment, check all that apply.
❑ ROM
❑ Splint or brace assistance
❑ Bed mobility training & skill practice
❑ Transfer training & skill practice
❑ Walking training & skill practice
❑ Dressing/grooming training & skill practice
❑ Eating/swallowing training & skill practice
❑ Appliance/prosthesis training & skill practice
❑ Communication training & skill practice
❑ Scheduled toileting
❑ Bladder retraining

Comments: _____
_____

❑ Physical
❑ Occupational
❑ Speech
Comments: _____
_____
_____
_____
_____

Completed by:
Signature/Title _____ Date _____

NAME–Last	First	Middle	Attending Physician	Record No.	Room/Bed

ADMISSION NURSING ASSESSMENT

Fig. 30.2 cont'd

✳ Admitting the Person

The room assignment is made before the person arrives. Some residents arrive by ambulance or wheelchair van. Attendants take them to their rooms. Some arrive by car. A nurse usually greets and escorts the person to the room. The nurse may ask you to do so if the person has no discomfort or distress.

Admission is your first chance to make a good impression. You must:

- Greet the person by name and title; use the admission form to find out the person's name.
- Introduce yourself by name and title to the person, family, and friends (Fig. 30.3).
- Make roommate introductions.
- Act in a professional manner.
- Treat the person with dignity and respect.

Safety and Security

Physical and mental comfort are important. So is feeling safe and secure. Do not rush the admission procedures. Rather, treat the person and family as guests in your home. Offer them a beverage. Visit with them. Tell them some of the good things about the center.

Introduce residents in nearby rooms. This way the person knows other residents. They can provide comfort and support. Some centers may appoint another resident as a "buddy" to help acquaint the new person during the first few days. They understand, better than anyone else, what a nursing center is like.

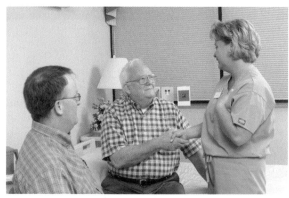

Fig. 30.3 The nursing assistant introduces herself to the person and family member.

The center is the person's home. Help make the room as homelike as possible. Also help the person unpack. Perhaps the person needs help putting clothes away. The person may want to hang pictures or display photos. Show care and compassion. Help the person feel safe, comfortable, and secure.

The Admission Procedure

During the admission procedure the nurse may ask you to:

- Collect some information for the admission form.
- Measure the person's weight and height.
- Measure the person's vital signs.
- Complete a clothing and personal belongings list.
- Orient the person to the room, the nursing unit, and the center.

✳ ADMITTING THE PERSON

Quality of Life

Remember to:
- Knock before entering the person's room.
- Address the person by name.
- Introduce yourself by name and title.
- Explain the procedure to the person before beginning and during the procedure.
- Protect the person's rights during the procedure.
- Handle the person gently during the procedure.

Preprocedure

1. Follow *Delegation Guidelines: Admissions, Transfers, and Discharges*, p. 465. See *Promoting Safety and Comfort: Admissions, Transfers, and Discharges*, p. 465.
2. Practice hand hygiene.
3. Prepare the room. See procedure: Preparing the Person's Room, pp. 466-467.

Procedure

4. Check the person's name on the admission form.
5. Greet the person by name. Ask if the person prefers a certain name.
6. Introduce yourself to the person and others present. Give your name and title. Explain that you assist the nurses in giving care.
7. Introduce the roommate.
8. Provide for privacy. Ask family or friends to leave the room. Tell them how much time you need and direct them to the waiting area. Let a family member or friend stay if the person prefers.
9. Let the person stay dressed if physical condition permits. Or help the person change into a gown or pajamas.

10. Provide for comfort. The person is in bed or in a chair as directed by the nurse.
11. Assist the nurse with assessment.
    a. Measure vital signs (Chapter 27) and pulse oximetry (Chapter 26) if required by your facility.
    b. Measure weight and height (Chapter 28).
    c. Collect information for the admission form as requested by the nurse.
12. Complete a clothing and personal belongings list (Chapter 11).
13. Help the person put away clothes and personal items. Put them in the closet, drawers, and bedside stand. (The family may wish to help with this step.)
14. Explain ordered activity limits.
15. Orient the person and family to the area.
    a. Give names of the nurses and nursing assistants.
    b. Identify items in the bedside stand. Explain the purpose of each.
    c. Explain how to use the overbed table.
    d. Show how to use the call light.
    e. Show how to use the bed, TV, and light controls.
    f. Explain how to make phone calls. Place the phone within reach.
    g. Show the person the bathroom. Also show how to use the call light in the bathroom.
    h. Explain visiting hours and policies.
    i. Explain where to find the nurses' station, lounge, chapel, dining room, and other areas.
    j. Identify staff—housekeeping, dietary, physical therapy, and others. Also identify students who may be in the center.
    k. Explain when meals and snacks are served.

✶ ADMITTING THE PERSON—cont'd

16. Fill the water pitcher and cup if oral fluids are allowed.
17. Place the call light within reach.
18. Place other controls and needed items within reach.
19. Provide a denture container if needed. Label it with the person's name and room and bed number.
20. Label the personal property and care items with the resident's name (if not done so by the family).

Postprocedure
21. Provide for comfort. (See the inside of the front cover.)
22. Lower the bed to its lowest position.
23. Raise or lower bed rails. Follow the care plan.
24. Answer any questions that the person or family may have. If needed, ask the nurse to offer more information.
25. Complete a safety check of the room. (See the inside of the front cover.)
26. Decontaminate your hands.
27. Report and record your observations.

✶ MOVING THE PERSON TO A NEW ROOM

Sometimes a person is moved to a new room. Reasons include the following:

- A change in condition
- The person requests a room change
- Roommates do not get along
- Changes in care needs
- The need for closer supervision

The doctor, nurse, or social worker explains the reasons for the move. The family and business office are told. You assist with the move or perform the entire procedure. The person is transported by wheelchair, stretcher, or the bed.

Support and reassure the person. If the new room is on another nursing unit, the person does not know the staff. Use good communication skills.

- Avoid pat answers, such as "It will be okay."
- Use touch to provide comfort.
- Introduce the person to the staff and roommate.
- Wish the person well as you leave the room.

✶ MOVING THE PERSON TO A NEW ROOM

Quality of Life

Remember to:
- Knock before entering the person's room.
- Address the person by name.
- Introduce yourself by name and title.
- Explain the procedure to the person before beginning and during the procedure.
- Protect the person's rights during the procedure.
- Handle the person gently during the procedure.

Preprocedure
1. Follow *Delegation Guidelines: Admissions, Transfers, and Discharges,* p. 465. See *Promoting Safety and Comfort: Admissions, Transfers, and Discharges,* p. 465.
2. Confirm that the new room is ready for the person. Make sure that the staff of the new unit are expecting the person. It is helpful if you can give them an approximate time of arrival.
3. Ask a coworker to help you.
4. Practice hand hygiene.
5. Collect the following:
   - Wheelchair or stretcher
   - Utility cart
   - Bath blanket
6. Decontaminate your hands.
7. Identify the person. Check the ID bracelet against the assignment sheet. Call the person by name.
8. Provide for privacy.

Procedure
9. Collect the person's belongings and care equipment. Place them on the cart.

10. Transfer the person to a wheelchair or stretcher (Chapter 15). Cover the person with the bath blanket.
11. Transport the person to the new room. Your coworker brings the cart.
12. Help transfer the person to the bed or chair. Help position the person (Chapter 15).
13. Help arrange the person's belongings and equipment.
14. Report the following to the receiving nurse:
   a. How the person tolerated the transfer
   b. Any observations made during the transfer
   c. That the nurse will bring the medical record, care plan, Kardex, and medications

Postprocedure
15. Return the wheelchair or stretcher and the cart to the storage area.
16. Decontaminate your hands.
17. Report and record the following:
   - The time of the transfer
   - Who helped you with the transfer
   - Where the person was taken
   - How the person was transferred (bed, wheelchair, or stretcher)
   - How the person tolerated the transfer
   - Who received the person
   - Any other observations
18. Strip the bed and clean the unit. Decontaminate your hands and put on gloves for this step. (The housekeeping staff may do this step.)
19. Remove the gloves. Decontaminate your hands.
20. Follow center policy for dirty linen.
21. Make a closed bed.
22. Decontaminate your hands.

TRANSFERS AND DISCHARGES

When transferred or discharged, the person leaves the center and goes home or to another health care setting. The Omnibus Budget and Reconciliation Act of 1987 (OBRA) and the Centers for Medicare & Medicaid Services (CMS) have standards for transfers and discharges. The person's rights are protected. Reasons for the transfer or discharge are part of the person's medical record. The person and family are informed in advance of the transfer or discharge plans. A procedure is followed if the person objects. An ombudsman protects the person's interests.

According to OBRA and the CMS, reasons for a transfer or discharge are the following:

- The measure is necessary to meet the person's welfare. The person's welfare cannot be met in the center.
- The person's health has improved to the extent that the center's services are no longer needed.
- The health or safety of other people in the nursing center is in danger.
- The person has failed to pay for the stay in the nursing center.
- The nursing center closes.

The person and family are told of the date and time of the transfer or discharge. And they are given the name and location of the hospital or nursing center where the person will be going.

Transfers and discharges are usually planned in advance. When transferred, the person goes to a hospital or another nursing center. Discharge is a happy time if the person is going home.

The health team plans the transfer or discharge. If being discharged, they teach the person and family about diet, exercise, and medications. They also teach about procedures and treatments. They arrange for home care, equipment, and therapies as needed. A doctor's appointment is given.

The nurse tells you when to start the transfer or discharge procedure. The doctor must give the order before the person can

TRANSFERRING OR DISCHARGING THE PERSON

Quality of Life

Remember to:

- Knock before entering the person's room.
- Address the person by name.
- Introduce yourself by name and title.
- Explain the procedure to the person before beginning and during the procedure.
- Protect the person's rights during the procedure.
- Handle the person gently during the procedure.

Preprocedure

1. Follow *Delegation Guidelines: Admissions, Transfers, and Discharges,* p. 465. See *Promoting Safety and Comfort: Admissions, Transfers, and Discharges,* p. 465.
2. Ask a coworker to help you.
3. Practice hand hygiene.
4. Identify the person. Check the ID bracelet against the assignment sheet. Also call the person by name.
5. Provide for privacy.

Procedure

6. Help the person dress as needed.
7. Help the person pack. Check all drawers and closets. Check the bathroom. Make sure all items are collected. If the person needs plastic bags to place belongings in, gather these from the supply room. Some may have a suitcase or bag for clothing.
8. Check off the clothing list and personal belongings list. Make sure the person has eyeglasses, hearing aids, and dentures. Give the list to the nurse.
9. Tell the nurse that the person is ready for the final visit. The nurse:
   a. Gives prescriptions written by the doctor.
   b. Provides discharge instructions.
   c. Gets valuables from the safe.
   d. Has the person sign the clothing and personal belongings list.
10. If the person will leave by wheelchair:
    a. Get a wheelchair and a utility cart for the person's items. Ask a coworker to help you.
    b. Help the person into the wheelchair.
    c. Take the person to the exit area.
    d. Lock the wheelchair wheels.
    e. Help the person out of the wheelchair and into the car (Fig. 30.4).
    f. Help put the person's items into the car.

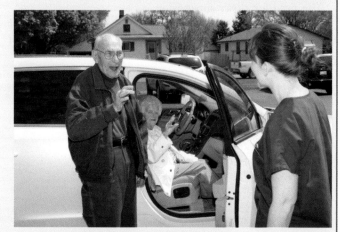

Fig. 30.4 This resident is going home with her husband.

11. *If the person will leave by ambulance:*
    a. Raise the bed rails.
    b. Raise the bed to its highest level.
    c. Place the call light within reach.
    d. Wait for the ambulance attendants.

Postprocedure

12. Return the wheelchair and cart to the storage area.
13. Decontaminate your hands.
14. Report and record the following:
    - The time of the discharge
    - Who helped you with the procedure
    - How the person was transported
    - Who was with the person
    - The person's destination
    - Any other observations
15. Strip the bed and clean the unit. Decontaminate your hands and put on gloves for this step. (The housekeeping staff may do this step.)
16. Remove the gloves. Decontaminate your hands.
17. Follow center policy for dirty linens.
18. Make a closed bed.
19. Decontaminate your hands.

leave. The nurse tells you when the person is ready to leave. Usually a wheelchair is used. If leaving by ambulance, a stretcher is used.

Use good communication skills when assisting with a transfer or discharge. Wish the person and family well as they leave the center.

A person may want to leave the center without the doctor's permission. Tell the nurse at once. The nurse or social worker handles the matter.

Use the procedure that follows for discharges and transfers.

QUALITY OF LIFE

Admission to a nursing center usually is a hard time for the person and family. Transfers and discharges also can cause fear and worry. Discharge often is a happy and pleasant event. However, it may cause worries and concerns if more care and treatment are needed. To help the person and family:

- Be courteous, caring, efficient, and competent.
- Be sensitive to fears and concerns.
- Handle the person's property and valuables carefully and with respect. Protect them from loss or damage.
- Treat the person and family like you want your loved ones treated.

The first hours and days in the center are often very lonely. Visit new residents often. Introduce them to other residents. Encourage them to take part in activities.

Explain all procedures and what the various sounds mean. Repeat information as needed. The new resident is in a new place. There is much new information. It may take time to remember things. Knowing what is happening and why helps the person feel safer and more secure. Remember to always protect the person's rights and to promote quality of life.

TIME TO REFLECT

Mrs. Ellwood has lived with her daughter and son-in-law since her husband died 8 years ago. She is 92 years old, uses a walker, and has osteoporosis. Recently she fell in her bathroom at home and broke her hip. After surgery at the hospital, she is admitted to your care center for physical therapy and rehabilitation. Mrs. Ellwood is very hard-of-hearing and has mild confusion. She misses her family and her cat, Smokey. She is not happy about being in the care center. You are caring for her on the second day after being admitted. You come to her room and find her packing her clothing into a suitcase. She tells you: "I need to get out of this place and go home!" How do you respond? What are some measures that can be taken to help Mrs. Ellwood adjust to her stay in the center for rehabilitation?

REVIEW QUESTIONS

Circle the BEST answer.

1. The nurse asks you to assist with the admission procedure. Which is *incorrect*?
   a. Greet the person by name and title
   b. Introduce yourself by name and title
   c. Introduce any roommates
   d. Rush the admission procedure so you can get back to your other residents

2. You are preparing the room for a new resident. The nurse tells you that the person will be arriving by stretcher. Which is *correct*?
   a. Make a closed bed
   b. Lower the bed to the lowest position
   c. Make a surgical bed
   d. Wait until the person arrives before collecting the admission kit

3. Which of the following does *not* promote comfort and support for the new resident?
   a. Help make the room as homelike as possible
   b. Help the person unpack
   c. Let the person find own way to the dining room
   d. Appoint another resident as a "buddy"

4. Which is *false* concerning residents' rights?
   a. The nurse or social worker explains the residents' rights
   b. The nursing assistant explains the residents' rights
   c. Residents' rights are given in writing
   d. Residents' rights are posted in the center

5. Which of the following is *not* a valid reason to transfer a person to another unit?
   a. The person's condition changes
   b. Roommates do not get along
   c. There is a need for closer supervision
   d. The staff do not get along with the resident

6. Which is *not* the nursing assistant's role in the discharge of the resident?
   a. Giving the resident prescriptions written by the doctor
   b. Helping the resident dress
   c. Helping the resident pack
   d. Making sure all items are collected from drawers and closets

7. A person wants to leave the center without the doctor's permission. What should the nursing assistant do?
   a. Help the person pack the belongings
   b. Tell the nurse at once
   c. Call the person's family
   d. Call the doctor

8. Mrs. Wilson is being discharged and is returning to her home. She will be leaving by wheelchair and has many belongings. Which is *incorrect*?
   a. Ask a coworker to help you
   b. Use a utility cart for her belongings
   c. Help put items into the car
   d. Let Mrs. Wilson get into the car by herself

See Appendix A for answers to these questions.

31

Wound Care

OBJECTIVES

- Define the key terms and key abbreviations listed in this chapter.
- Describe skin tears, circulatory ulcers, and diabetic foot ulcers; the persons at risk; and how to prevent them.
- Describe the process and complications of wound healing.
- Describe what to observe about wounds.
- Explain how to secure dressings.
- Explain the rules for applying dressings.
- Explain the purpose of binders and how to apply them.
- Explain the purpose, effects, and complications of heat and cold applications.
- Describe the rules for applying heat and cold.
- Describe how to meet the basic needs of persons with wounds.
- Perform the procedures described in this chapter.
- Explain how to promote quality of life.

KEY TERMS

abrasion A partial-thickness wound caused by the scraping away or rubbing of the skin

arterial ulcer An open wound on the lower legs or feet caused by poor arterial blood flow

chronic wound A wound that does not heal easily

clean-contaminated wound A wound that occurs from the surgical entry of the reproductive, urinary, respiratory, or gastrointestinal system

clean wound A wound that is not infected

closed wound Tissues are injured but the skin is not broken

compress A soft pad applied over a body area

constrict To narrow

contaminated wound A wound with a high risk of infection

contusion A closed wound caused by a blow to the body; a bruise

dehiscence The separation of wound layers

diabetic foot ulcer An open wound on the foot caused by complications from diabetes

dilate To expand or open wider

dirty wound See "infected wound"

edema Swelling caused by fluid collecting in tissues

embolus A blood clot (or other foreign matter) that travels through the vascular system until it lodges in a vessel

evisceration The separation of the wound along with the protrusion of abdominal organs

full-thickness wound The dermis, epidermis, and subcutaneous tissue are penetrated; muscle and bone may be involved

gangrene A condition in which there is death of tissue

hyperthermia A body temperature *(thermia)* that is much higher *(hyper-)* than the person's normal range

hypothermia A very low *(hypo-)* body temperature *(thermia)*

incision A cut produced surgically by a sharp instrument; it creates an opening into an organ or body space

infected wound A wound containing large amounts of microbes that shows signs of infection; dirty wound

intentional wound A wound created for therapy

laceration An open wound with torn tissues and jagged edges

open wound The skin or mucous membrane is broken

pack Wrapping a body part with a wet or dry application

partial-thickness wound The dermis and epidermis of the skin are broken

penetrating wound An open wound that breaks the skin and enters a body area, organ, or cavity

phlebitis Inflammation *(-itis)* of a vein *(phleb-)*

puncture wound An open wound made by a sharp object

purulent drainage Thick green, yellow, or brown drainage

sanguineous drainage Bloody *(sanguis)* drainage

serosanguineous drainage Thin, watery drainage *(sero-)* that is blood-tinged *(sanguineous)*

serous drainage Clear, watery fluid *(serum)*

skin tear A break or rip in the outer layers of the skin; the epidermis (top skin layer) separates from the underlying tissues

stasis ulcer See "venous ulcer"

thrombus A blood clot

trauma An accident or violent act that injures the skin, mucous membranes, bones, and organs

ulcer A shallow or deep craterlike sore of the skin or a mucous membrane

unintentional wound A wound resulting from trauma

vascular ulcer An open sore on the lower legs or feet caused by decreased blood flow through the arteries or veins

venous ulcer An open sore on the lower legs or feet caused by poor venous blood flow; stasis ulcer

wound A break in the skin or mucous membrane

KEY ABBREVIATIONS

C Centigrade
F Fahrenheit
GI Gastrointestinal

ID Identification
PPE Personal protective equipment

A wound is a break in the skin or mucous membrane. Common causes are the following:

- Surgery
- Trauma—an accident or violent act that injures the skin, mucous membranes, bones, and organs; falls, vehicle crashes, gun shots, stabbings, human and animal bites, burns, and frostbite are examples
- Pressure injuries from unrelieved pressure (Chapter 32)
- Decreased blood flow through the arteries or veins
- Nerve damage

Infection is a major threat. Wound care involves preventing infection and further injury to the wound and nearby tissues. Blood loss and pain also are prevented.

The nurse uses the nursing process to keep the person's skin healthy. Some centers have a skin care team to manage all skin problems. The team includes a registered nurse (RN), physical therapist, dietitian, and often a wound, ostomy, continence nurse (WOCN).

See *Focus on Rehabilitation: Wound Care.*

TYPES OF WOUNDS

Types of wounds are described in Box 31.1. Wounds also are described by their cause.

- Abrasion—a partial-thickness wound caused by the scraping away or rubbing of the skin (Fig. 31.1)
- Contusion—a closed wound caused by a blow to the body (a bruise); also called a deep tissue injury (Fig. 31.2)
- Incision—a cut produced surgically by a sharp instrument that creates an opening into an organ or body space (Fig. 31.3)

- Laceration—an open wound with torn tissues and jagged edges (Fig. 31.4)

FOCUS ON REHABILITATION

Wound Care
Some persons have poor or delayed wound healing. Others have complications from wound healing. Rehabilitation and subacute care units often provide special wound care.

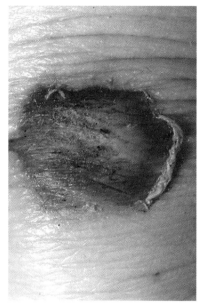

Fig. 31.1 An abrasion. (From Lynch VA, Duval JB: *Forensic nursing science*, ed. 2, St. Louis, 2011, Mosby.)

BOX 31.1 Types of Wounds

Intentional and Unintentional Wounds
- Intentional wound—is created for therapy. Surgical incisions are examples, as are venipunctures for starting intravenous therapy and for drawing blood specimens.
- Unintentional wound—results from trauma.

Open and Closed Wounds
- Open wound—when the skin or mucous membrane is broken. Intentional and most unintentional wounds are open.
- Closed wound—tissues are injured but the skin is not broken. Bruises, twists, and sprains are examples.

Clean and Dirty Wounds
- Clean wound—is not infected. Microbes have not entered the wound. Closed wounds are usually clean. So are intentional wounds created under surgical asepsis. The reproductive, urinary, respiratory, and gastrointestinal (GI) systems are not entered.

- Clean-contaminated wound—occurs from the surgical entry of the reproductive, urinary, respiratory, or GI system. Some or all parts of these systems are not sterile and contain normal flora.
- Contaminated wound—has a high risk of infection. Unintentional wounds are generally contaminated. Wound contamination occurs from breaks in surgical asepsis and spillage of intestinal contents. Tissues may show signs of inflammation.
- Infected wound (dirty wound)—contains large amounts of microbes and shows signs of infection. Examples include old wounds, surgical incisions into infected areas, and traumatic injuries that rupture the bowel.
- Chronic wound—does not heal easily. Pressure ulcers and circulatory ulcers are examples.

Partial- and Full-Thickness Wounds (Describe Wound Depth)
- Partial-thickness wound—the dermis and epidermis of the skin are broken.
- Full-thickness wound—the dermis, epidermis, and subcutaneous tissue are penetrated. Muscle and bone may be involved.

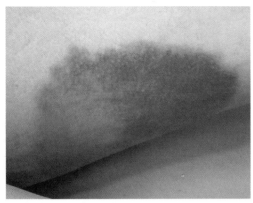

Fig. 31.2 Contusion. (From Finkbeiner W, Ursell P, Davis R: *Autopsy pathology: a manual and atlas*, ed. 2, Philadelphia, 2009, Saunders.)

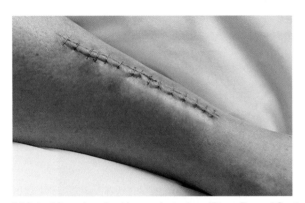

Fig. 31.3 Incision closed with metal staples. (From Perry AG et al.: *Fundamentals of nursing*, ed. 10, St. Louis, 2021, Mosby.)

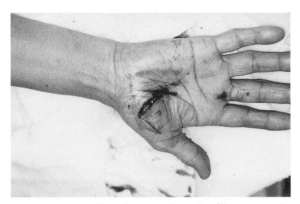

Fig. 31.4 Laceration. (From Roberts JR et al.: *Clinical procedures in emergency medicine*, ed. 6, Philadelphia, 2014, Saunders.)

- Penetrating wound—an open wound that breaks the skin and enters a body area, organ, or cavity (Fig. 31.5)
- Puncture wound—an open wound made by a sharp object (knife, nail, metal, wood, glass); entry of the skin and underlying tissues may be intentional or unintentional (Fig. 31.6)
- Ulcer—a shallow or deep craterlike sore of the skin or a mucous membrane (p. 475)

SKIN TEARS

A skin tear is a break or rip in the outer layers of the skin (Fig. 31.7). The epidermis (top skin layer) separates from the

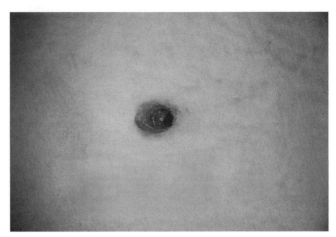

Fig. 31.5 Penetrating wound. (From McCance KL, Huether SE: *Pathophysiology: the biologic basis for disease in adults and children*, ed. 6, St. Louis, 2010, Mosby.)

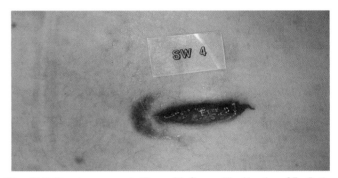

Fig. 31.6 Puncture wound. (From McCance KL, Huether SE: *Pathophysiology: the biologic basis for disease in adults and children*, ed. 6, St. Louis, 2010, Mosby.)

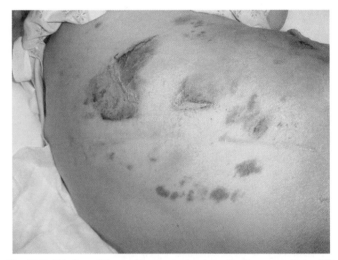

Fig. 31.7 Skin tear. (Used with permission from Dr. Rosemary Kohr, RN, PhD, ACNP [cert], www.lhsc.on.ca/wound.)

underlying tissues (Chapter 8). The skin is "peeled back." The hands, arms, and lower legs are common sites for skin tears. Very thin and fragile skin is common in older persons. Slight pressure can cause a skin tear.

Causes

Skin tears are caused by the following:

- Friction, shearing (Chapter 15), pulling, or pressure on the skin
- Falls or bumping a hand, arm, or leg on any hard surface; beds, bed rails, chairs, wheelchair footplates, mechanical lifts, and tables are dangers
- Holding the person's arm or leg too tightly
- Removing tape or adhesives
- Bathing, dressing, and other tasks
- Pulling buttons and zippers across fragile skin
- Jewelry—yours or the person's; rings, watches, and bracelets are examples

Skin tears are painful. They are portals of entry for microbes. Infection is a risk. Tell the nurse at once if you cause or find a skin tear.

Persons at Risk

Persons at risk for skin tears:

- Need some to total help in moving.
- Have poor nutrition.
- Have poor hydration.
- Have altered mental awareness.
- Are very thin.

See *Residents with Dementia: Persons at Risk (Skin Tears).*

Prevention and Treatment

Careful and safe care helps prevent skin tears and further injury. Follow the measures in Box 31.2. Also follow the care plan and the nurse's directions. They may include dressings that

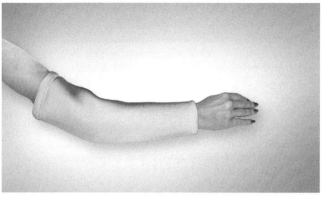

Fig. 31.8 Limb protector. (Courtesy DermaSaver.)

prevent taping of fragile skin and protective arm or leg sleeves (Fig. 31.8). Persons who have contusions, deep tissue injury, and areas of bruising should be protected with arm or leg sleeves. The skin should be examined daily. Elastic bandages also may be used to protect the skin and promote healing if ordered by the doctor or wound specialist (p. 478).

RESIDENTS WITH DEMENTIA

Persons at Risk (Skin Tears)

Some persons are confused and may resist care. They often move quickly and without warning, or they pull away from you during care. Some try to hit or kick. These sudden movements can cause skin tears.

Never force care on a person. Chapter 40 describes how to care for persons who are confused and resist care. Always follow the care plan.

VASCULAR ULCERS

Some diseases affect blood flow to and from the legs and feet. Such poor circulation can lead to pain, open wounds, and edema. Edema is swelling caused by fluid collecting in tissues. Infection and gangrene can result from the open wound and poor circulation. Gangrene is a condition in which there is death of tissue.

Vascular ulcers are open sores on the lower legs or feet. They are caused by decreased blood flow through the arteries or veins. Persons with diseases affecting the blood vessels are at risk. These wounds are painful and hard to heal.

The doctor orders medications and treatments as needed. The nurse uses the nursing process to meet the person's needs (Box 31.3). You must help prevent skin breakdown on the legs and feet.

Venous Ulcers

Venous ulcers (stasis ulcers) are open sores on the lower legs or feet. *Stasis* means "stopped or slowed fluid flow." These ulcers are caused by poor venous blood flow (Fig. 31.9).

Venous ulcers can develop when valves in the leg's veins do not close well. The veins do not pump blood back to the heart in a normal way. Blood and fluid collect in the legs and feet. Small skin veins rupture. This allows hemoglobin to enter the tissue, causing the skin to turn brown. (Hemoglobin gives

---

BOX 31.2 Measures to Prevent Skin Tears

- Keep your fingernails short and smoothly filed.
- Keep the person's fingernails short and smoothly filed. Report long and tough toenails.
- Do not wear rings with large or raised stones. Do not wear bracelets.
- Be patient and calm when the person is confused or agitated or resists care.
- Follow the care plan and safety rules to handle, move, turn, position, or transfer the person.
  - Prevent shearing and friction.
  - Use an assist device to move and turn the person in bed.
  - Use pillows to support arms and legs. Follow the care plan.
- Pad bed rails and wheelchair arms, footplates, and leg supports. Follow the care plan.
- Follow the care plan and safety rules to bathe the person.
- Dress and undress the person carefully.
- Dress the person in soft clothes with long sleeves and long pants.
- Provide good lighting so the person can see. The person needs to avoid bumping into furniture, walls, and equipment.
- Provide a safe area for wandering (Chapter 40).
- Keep the skin moisturized. Apply lotion according to the care plan.
- Offer fluids. Follow the care plan.
- Remove tape carefully (p. 487).
- Do not apply adhesive tape (p. 485).

BOX 31.3 Measures to Prevent Vascular Ulcers

- Remind the person not to sit with the legs crossed.
- Reposition the person according to the care plan—at least every 2 hours.
- Do not use elastic or rubber band-type garters to hold socks or hose in place.
- Do not dress the person in tight clothes.
- Provide good skin care daily. Keep the feet clean and dry. Clean and dry between the toes.
- Do not scrub or rub the skin during bathing and drying.
- Keep linens clean, dry, and wrinkle free.
- Avoid injury to the legs and feet.
- Make sure shoes fit well.
- Keep pressure off the heels and other bony areas. Use pillows or other devices as the nurse and care plan direct.
- Check the person's legs and feet. Report skin breaks or changes in skin color.
- Do not massage over pressure points (Chapter 32). *Never rub or massage reddened areas.*
- Use protective devices as the nurse directs. Follow the care plan.
- Follow the care plan for walking and exercise.

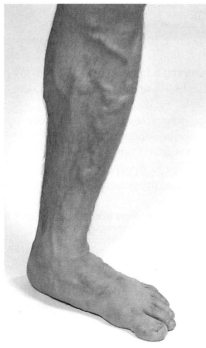

Fig. 31.10 Varicose veins. Veins under the skin are dilated (wide) and bulging. (From Belch J et al.: *Color atlas of peripheral vascular diseases,* ed. 2, London, 1996, Wolfe Medical Publishers.)

- Surgery on the bones and joints
- Phlebitis (inflammation *[itis]* of a vein *[phleb]*)

Prevention and Treatment

To prevent venous ulcers:
- Follow the care plan to prevent skin breakdown. See the measures in Box 31.3.
- Prevent injury. Do not bump the legs and feet.
- Elevate the extremities. Do not put pressure on the heels or calves.
- Handle, move, and transfer the person carefully and gently. Persons at risk need professional foot care. Attention is given to toenails, corns, calluses, and other toe and foot problems. *You do not cut the toenails of persons with diseases affecting the circulation.*

Venous ulcers are hard to heal. The doctor may order medications for infection and to decrease swelling. Medicated bandages and other wound care products are often ordered. The doctor may order compression stockings or elastic bandages to:
- Promote comfort.
- Promote circulation by providing support and pressure to the veins.
- Promote healing.
- Prevent injury.

✷ Compression (Antiembolism) Stockings

Compression stockings exert pressure on the veins. The pressure promotes venous blood return to the heart. The stockings help prevent venous ulcers and blood clots in leg veins.

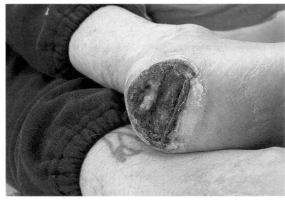

Fig. 31.9 Venous ulcer.

blood its red color.) The skin is dry, leathery, flaky, and hard. Itching is common. The person will sometimes have serous drainage due to the edema.

The lower legs and inner part of the ankles are common sites for venous ulcers. They can occur from skin injury. Venous ulcers are painful, and walking is difficult. Pain may be relieved by elevating the legs. Fluid may seep from the wound. Infection is a risk. Healing is slow.

Risk Factors

Risk factors for venous ulcers include the following:
- History of blood clots
- History of varicose veins (Fig. 31.10)
- Decreased mobility
- Obesity
- Heredity
- Leg or foot surgery
- Advanced age

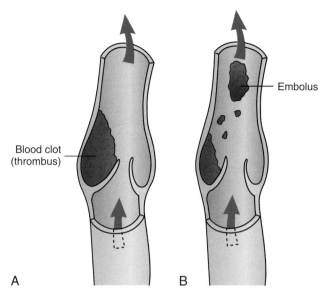

Fig. 31.11 (A) A blood clot is attached to the wall of a vein. The *arrow* shows the direction of blood flow. (B) Part of the thrombus breaks off and becomes an embolus. The embolus travels in the bloodstream until it lodges in a distant vessel.

A blood clot is called a thrombus. If blood flow is sluggish, blood clots may form. They can form in the deep leg veins in the lower leg or thigh (Fig. 31.11A). A thrombus can break loose and travel through the bloodstream. It then becomes an embolus. An embolus is a blood clot (or other foreign matter) that travels through the vascular system until it lodges in a vessel (see Fig. 31.11B). An embolus from a vein lodges in the lungs *(pulmonary embolism)*. A pulmonary embolus can cause severe respiratory problems and death. Report chest pain or shortness of breath at once.

Other terms for compression stockings are AE stockings (AE means *antiembolism* or *antiembolic*), TED hose (TED means *thromboembolic disease*), or elastic stockings. Persons at risk for thrombi include those who:

- Have heart and circulatory disorders.
- Are on bedrest.
- Have had surgery.
- Are older.
- Are pregnant.
- Have legs in a dependent position.

The person usually has two pairs of stockings. Wash one pair while the other pair is worn. Wash them by hand with a mild soap. Rinse them well. Roll them up in a towel and then hang them to dry. Do *not* send them to the laundry to be washed in machines.

See *Delegation Guidelines: Compression Stockings.*
See *Promoting Safety and Comfort: Compression Stockings.*

DELEGATION GUIDELINES

Compression Stockings

Before applying compression stockings, you need this information from the nurse and the care plan:

- What size to use—small, medium, or large
- What length to use—thigh-high or knee-high
- When to remove them and for how long—usually every 8 hours for 30 minutes
- What observations to report and record:
  - The size and length of stockings applied
  - When you applied the stockings
  - Skin color and temperature
  - Leg and foot swelling
  - Skin tears, wounds, or signs of skin breakdown
  - Complaints of pain, tingling, or numbness
  - When you removed the stockings and for how long
  - When you reapplied the stockings
  - When you washed the stockings
- When to report observations
- What specific resident concerns to report at once

PROMOTING SAFETY AND COMFORT

Compression Stockings
Safety

Stockings should not have twists, creases, or wrinkles after you apply them. Twists can affect circulation. Creases and wrinkles can cause skin breakdown.

Loose stockings do not promote venous blood return to the heart. Never fold over the top of the stocking. Stockings that are too tight can affect circulation. Tell the nurse if the stockings are too loose or too tight.

Comfort

Apply stockings before the person gets out of bed. Otherwise, the person's legs can swell from sitting or standing. Stockings are hard to put on when the legs are swollen. The person lies in bed while they are off. This prevents the legs from swelling.

Gently handle and move the person's foot and leg. Do not force the joints (toes, foot, ankle, knee, and hip) beyond their range of motion or to the point of pain.

✳ APPLYING COMPRESSION STOCKINGS (NATCEP)

Quality of Life
Remember to:

- Knock before entering the person's room.
- Address the person by name.
- Introduce yourself by name and title.
- Explain the procedure to the person before beginning and during the procedure.
- Protect the person's rights during the procedure.
- Handle the person gently during the procedure.

Preprocedure

1. Follow *Delegation Guidelines: Compression Stockings.* See *Promoting Safety and Comfort: Compression Stockings.*
2. Practice hand hygiene.
3. Obtain compression stockings in the correct size and length. (Often, the nurse measures the leg.)
4. Identify the person. Check the identification (ID) bracelet against the assignment sheet. Also call the person by name.

✳ APPLYING COMPRESSION STOCKINGS (NATCEP)—cont'd

A   B   C

Fig. 31.12 Applying antiembolism compression stockings. (A) The stocking is slipped over the toes. (B) The heel is in place. (C) The stocking turns right side out as it is pulled up over the leg. (From Potter PA et al.: *Fundamentals of nursing*, ed. 10, St. Louis, 2021, Mosby.)

5. Provide for privacy.
6. Raise the bed for body mechanics. Bed rails are up if used.

Procedure

7. Lower the bed rail near you if up.
8. Position the person supine.
9. Expose the legs. Fan-fold top linens toward the thighs.
10. Turn the stocking inside out down to the heel.
11. Slip the foot of the stocking over the toes, foot, and heel (Fig. 31.12A). Make sure the stocking heel is properly positioned on the person's heel.
12. Grasp the stocking top. Pull the stocking up the leg (see Fig. 31.12B). It turns right side out as it is pulled up. The stocking is even and snug (see Fig. 31.12C).

13. Remove twists, creases, or wrinkles.
14. Repeat steps 10 through 13 for the other leg.

Postprocedure

15. Cover the person.
16. Provide for comfort. (See the inside of the front cover.)
17. Place the call light within reach.
18. Lower the bed to its lowest position.
19. Raise or lower bed rails. Follow the care plan.
20. Unscreen the person.
21. Complete a safety check of the room. (See the inside of the front cover.)
22. Decontaminate your hands.
23. Report and record your observations.

This skill is also covered in *Clinical Skills: Nurse Assisting.*

✳ Elastic Bandages

Elastic bandages have the same purposes as compression stockings. They provide support and reduce swelling from injuries. Sometimes they are used to hold dressings in place. They are applied to arms and legs. Some centers do not allow nursing assistants to apply elastic bandages. Know your center's policy. When applying bandages:

- Use the correct size—length and width—to bandage the extremity.
- Position the person in good alignment.
- Face the person during the procedure.
- Start at the lower (*distal*) part of the extremity; work upward to the top (*proximal*) part.
- Expose fingers or toes if possible; this allows circulation checks.
- Apply the bandage with firm, even pressure with a 50% overlay.

- Check the color and temperature of the extremity every hour.
- Reapply a loose or wrinkled bandage.
- Replace a moist or soiled bandage.
  See *Focus on Communication: Elastic Bandages.*
  See *Delegation Guidelines: Elastic Bandages.*
  See *Promoting Safety and Comfort: Elastic Bandages.*

📋 FOCUS ON COMMUNICATION

Elastic Bandages

Elastic bandages should promote comfort. To check for comfort, you can ask:
- "Does the bandage feel too tight?"
- "Do you feel pain, itching, tingling, or numbness?" If yes: "What do you feel?" "Where do you feel it?"

📄 DELEGATION GUIDELINES

Elastic Bandages

Before applying elastic bandages, you need this information from the nurse and the care plan:
- Where to apply the bandage
- What width and length to use
- When to remove the bandage and for how long—usually every 8 hours for 30 minutes
- What to do if the bandage is wet or soiled
- What observations to report and record:
  - The width and length applied

- When you applied the bandage
- Skin color and temperature
- Swelling of the part
- Skin tears, wounds, or signs of skin breakdown
- Complaints of pain, itching, tingling, or numbness
- When you removed the bandage and for how long
- When you reapplied the bandage
- When to report observations
- What specific resident concerns to report at once

PROMOTING SAFETY AND COMFORT

Elastic Bandages

Safety

Elastic bandages must be firm and snug but not tight. A tight bandage can affect circulation.

Bandages are secured in place with clips, tape, or Velcro. Clips are made of metal or plastic. Clips can injure the skin if they become loose, fall off, or cause pressure. Use clips only if the nurse tells you to. Check the bandage often to make sure the clips are correctly in place.

Some centers do not allow you to apply elastic bandages. Know your center's policy.

Comfort

A tight bandage can cause pain and discomfort. Apply it with firm, even pressure. If the person complains of pain, tingling, or numbness, remove the bandage. Tell the nurse at once.

APPLYING ELASTIC BANDAGES

Quality of Life

Remember to:

- Knock before entering the person's room.
- Address the person by name.
- Introduce yourself by name and title.
- Explain the procedure to the person before beginning and during the procedure.
- Protect the person's rights during the procedure.
- Handle the person gently during the procedure.

Preprocedure

1. Follow Delegation Guidelines: Elastic Bandages, p. 478. See *Promoting Safety and Comfort: Elastic Bandages.*
2. Practice hand hygiene.
3. Collect the following:
   - Elastic bandage as directed by the nurse
   - Tape or clips (unless the bandage has Velcro)
4. Identify the person. Check the ID bracelet against the assignment sheet. Also call the person by name.
5. Provide for privacy.
6. Raise the bed for body mechanics. Bed rails are up if used.

Procedure

7. Lower the bed rail near you if up.
8. Help the person to a comfortable position. Expose the part you will bandage.

9. Make sure the area is clean and dry.
10. Hold the bandage so the roll is up. The loose end is on the bottom (Fig. 31.13A).
11. Apply the bandage to the smallest part of the wrist, foot, ankle, or knee.
12. Make two circular turns around the part (see Fig. 31.13B).
13. Make overlapping spiral turns in an upward direction. Each turn overlaps about ½ to ⅔ of the previous turn (see Fig. 31.13C). Each overlap is equal.
14. Apply the bandage smoothly with firm, even pressure. It is not tight.
15. End the bandage with two circular turns.
16. Secure the bandage in place with Velcro, tape, or clips. Clips are not under the body part.
17. Check the fingers or toes for coldness or cyanosis (bluish color). Ask about pain, itching, numbness, or tingling. Remove the bandage if any are noted. Report your observations.

Postprocedure

18. Provide for comfort. (See the inside of the front cover.)
19. Place the call light within reach.
20. Lower the bed to its lowest position.
21. Raise or lower bed rails. Follow the care plan.
22. Unscreen the person.
23. Complete a safety check of the room. (See the inside of the front cover.)
24. Decontaminate your hands.
25. Report and record your observations.

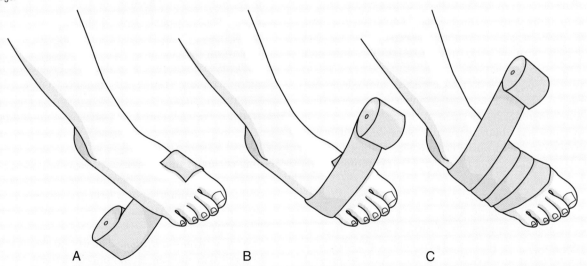

A   B   C

Fig. 31.13 Applying an elastic bandage. (A) The roll of the bandage is up. The loose end is at the bottom. (B) The bandage is applied to the smallest part with two circular turns. (C) The bandage is applied with spiral turns in an upward direction.

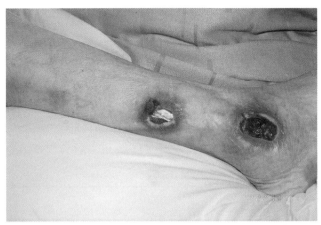

Fig. 31.14 Arterial ulcer. (From Black JM, Hawks JH: *Medical-surgical nursing: clinical management for positive outcomes*, ed. 7, St. Louis, 2005, WB Saunders.)

Arterial Ulcers

Arterial ulcers are open wounds on the lower legs or feet caused by poor arterial blood flow. They are found between the toes, on top of the toes, and on the outer side of the ankle (Fig. 31.14). The leg and foot may feel cold and look blue or shiny. The ulcer is very painful, especially at night.

These ulcers are caused by diseases or injuries that decrease arterial blood flow to the legs and feet. High blood pressure and diabetes are common causes. So are narrowed arteries from aging. Smoking is a risk factor.

The doctor treats the disease causing the ulcer. Medications, wound care, and a walking and exercise program are ordered. Professional foot care is important. Follow the care plan (see Box 31.3) and prevent further injury.

Diabetic Foot Ulcers

A diabetic foot ulcer is an open wound on the foot caused by complications from diabetes. Diabetes (Chapter 37) can affect the nerves and blood vessels.

- *Nerves.* The person can lose sensation in a foot or leg. Loss of sensation can be complete or partial. The person may not feel pain, heat, or cold. Therefore, the person may not feel a cut, blister, burn, or other trauma to the foot. Infection and a large sore can develop.
- *Blood vessels.* Blood flow decreases. Tissues and cells do not get needed oxygen and nutrients. Wounds heal poorly. Tissue death (gangrene) can occur.

Some persons have both nerve and blood vessel damage. Both problems can lead to diabetic foot ulcers. Infection and gangrene are risks. Sometimes the affected part is amputated to prevent the spread of gangrene.

Check the person's feet every day. Check the person's shoes to make sure they fit properly. Tight shoes and shoes that are too big can cause ulcerations and blisters. Look for the foot problems described in Box 31.4. Report any sign of a foot problem to the nurse at once. Follow the care plan to prevent and treat diabetic foot ulcers.

BOX 31.4 Foot Problems Common in Persons with Diabetes

- *Corns and calluses* (Fig. 31.15A). These are thick layers of the skin caused by too much rubbing or pressure on the same spot. They occur over bony areas or the soles of the feet. Infection is a risk.
- *Blisters* (see Fig. 31.15B). These form when shoes rub on the same spot. Shoes that do not fit well and wearing shoes without socks are causes. Infection is a risk.
- *In-grown toenails* (see Fig. 31.15C). An edge of a toenail grows into the skin. This occurs when the skin is cut while trimming toenails or from tight shoes. The skin becomes red and infected.
- *Bunions* (see Fig. 31.15D). The big toe slants toward the small toes. The space between the bones near the base of the big toe grows larger. Bunions can occur on one or both feet. Heredity is a factor. Shoes that fit poorly and pointy shoes are causes. Bunions are removed by surgery.
- *Plantar warts* (see Fig. 31.15E). *Plantar* means "sole." Plantar warts occur on the soles (bottoms) of the feet. Caused by a virus, plantar warts are painful.
- *Hammer toes* (see Fig. 31.15F). One or more toes are permanently flexed. They form when a foot muscle weakens. Diabetic nerve damage can weaken foot muscles. The second toe is commonly affected. Because of deformed toes, the person has problems walking. Shoes do not fit well. Sores can develop on the tops of the toes and on the bottoms of the feet.
- *Dry and cracked skin* (see Fig. 31.15G). Dry skin can occur from nerve damage in the legs and feet. These areas do not receive messages from the brain to keep the skin soft and moist. The dry skin can crack, causing portals of entry for microbes. Infection can occur.
- *Athlete's foot* (see Fig. 31.15H). This is a fungus causing redness and cracked skin between the toes and on the bottoms of the feet. The cracks are portals of entry for microbes. The fungus can spread to the toenails. The toenails become thick, yellow, and hard to cut.

WOUND HEALING

The healing process has three phases.

- *Inflammatory phase* (3 days). Bleeding stops. A scab forms over the wound. The scab protects against microbes entering the wound. Blood supply to the wound increases. The blood brings nutrients and healing substances. Because blood supply increases, signs and symptoms of inflammation appear—redness, swelling, heat or warmth, and pain. Loss of function may occur.
- *Proliferative phase* (day 3 to day 21). Proliferate means "to multiply rapidly." Tissue cells multiply to repair the wound.
- *Maturation phase* (day 21 to 2 years). The scar gains strength. The red, raised scar becomes thin and pale.

Types of Wound Healing

Healing occurs in three ways.

- *Primary (first) intention:* Wound edges are brought together to close the wound. Sutures (stitches), staples, clips, special glue, or adhesive strips hold the wound edges together (Fig. 31.16A).
- *Secondary (second) intention:* The wound extends through all layers of skin and can extend into underlying tissues. This is for contaminated and infected wounds. Wounds are cleaned

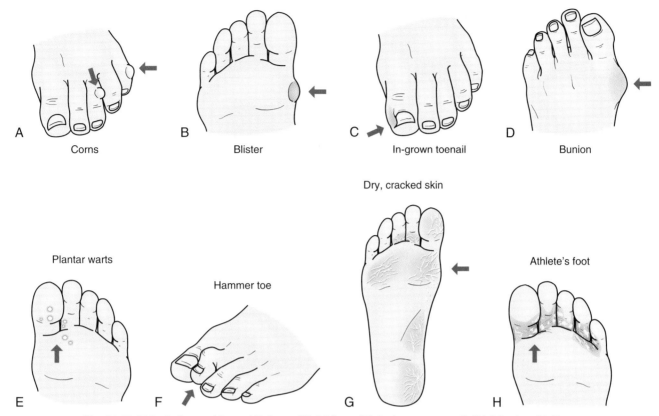

Fig. 31.15 Diabetic foot problems. (A) Corns. (B) A blister. (C) An in-grown toenail. (D) A bunion. (E) Plantar warts. (F) Hammer toe. (G) Dry and cracked skin. (H) Athlete's foot. (Redrawn from National Diabetes Information Clearinghouse [NDIC]: *Prevent diabetes problems: keep your feet and skin healthy*, NIH Publication No. 08-4282, Bethesda, MD, 2008, Author.)

and dead tissue is removed. Wound edges are not brought together. Healing takes longer and leaves a larger scar. Infection is a great risk (see Fig. 31.16B).

- *Tertiary (third) intention:* The wound is left open and closed later. It combines first and second intention. Infection and poor circulation are common reasons for tertiary intention (see Fig. 31.16C).

Complications of Wound Healing

Many factors affect healing and increase the risk of complications. They include wound type and the person's age, general health, nutrition, and lifestyle.

Good circulation is needed. Age, smoking, circulatory disease, and diabetes all affect circulation. Certain medications (Coumadin and heparin) prolong bleeding.

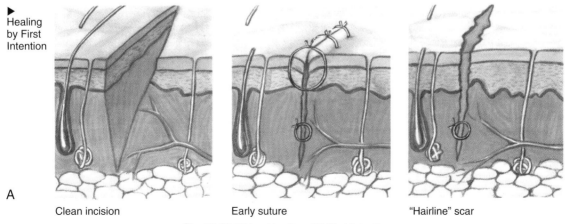

▶ Healing by First Intention

Clean incision   Early suture   "Hairline" scar

Fig. 31.16 Wound healing. (A) First intention.

▶ Healing by Second Intention (Granulation and Contraction)

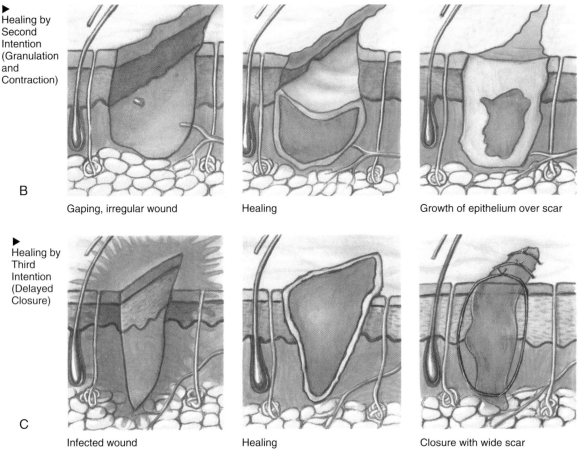

B

Gaping, irregular wound   Healing   Growth of epithelium over scar

▶ Healing by Third Intention (Delayed Closure)

C

Infected wound   Healing   Closure with wide scar

Fig. 31.16, cont'd (B) Second intention. (C) Third intention. (Modified from Ignatavicius DD, Workman ML: *Medical-surgical nursing: critical thinking for collaborative care,* ed. 7, St. Louis, 2013, Saunders.)

Good nutrition is needed. Protein is needed for tissue growth and repair.

Infection is a risk for persons with immune system changes and for those taking antibiotics. Antibiotics kill pathogens. Specific antibiotics kill specific pathogens. In doing so, other pathogens may be allowed to grow and multiply.

See *Focus on Rehabilitation: Complications of Wound Healing.*

FOCUS ON REHABILITATION

Complications of Wound Healing

Some persons need rehabilitation or subacute care because of:

- *Infection.* Contamination can occur during or after the injury. Trauma is a common cause. Surgical wounds can be contaminated during or after surgery. An infected wound appears inflamed (reddened) and has drainage that may have an odor. The wound is painful and tender. The person may have a fever.
- *Dehiscence.* **Dehiscence** is the separation of wound layers (Fig. 31.17). It may involve the skin layer or underlying tissues. Abdominal wounds are commonly affected. Coughing, vomiting, and abdominal distention place stress on the wound. The person often describes the sensation of the wound "popping open."
- *Evisceration.* **Evisceration** is the separation of the wound along with the protrusion of abdominal organs (Fig. 31.18). Causes are the same as for dehiscence.

Dehiscence and evisceration are surgical emergencies. Tell the nurse at once. The nurse covers the wound with large sterile dressings saturated with saline. Help prepare the person for surgery as directed.

Wound Appearance

Doctors and nurses observe the wound and its drainage. They observe for healing and complications. See Box 31.5 for the observations to make when assisting with wound care. Report and record your observations according to center policy.

Wound Drainage

During injury and the inflammatory phase of wound healing, fluid and cells escape from the tissues. Drainage amounts may be large or small. This depends on wound size and site. Bleeding and infection also affect the amount and kind of drainage. Wound drainage is observed and measured (Fig. 31.19).

- **Serous drainage**—clear, watery fluid (Fig. 31.20A). Serous comes from the word *serum.* The fluid in a blister is serous. Serum is the clear, thin, fluid portion of blood. Serum does not contain blood cells or platelets.
- **Sanguineous drainage**—bloody drainage (see Fig. 30.20B). The Latin word *sanguis* means "blood." The amount and color of sanguineous drainage is important. Hemorrhage is suspected when large amounts are present. Bright drainage means fresh bleeding. Older bleeding is darker.
- **Serosanguineous drainage**—thin, watery drainage *(sero)* that is blood-tinged *(sanguineous)* (see Fig. 31.20C).
- **Purulent drainage**—thick green, yellow, or brown drainage (see Fig. 31.20D).

Drainage must leave the wound for healing. Trapped drainage causes swelling of underlying tissues. The wound may heal at the skin level, but underlying tissues do not close. Infection and complications can occur.

When large amounts of drainage are expected, the doctor inserts a drain. A *Penrose drain* is a rubber tube that drains onto a dressing (Fig. 31.21). It opens

FOCUS ON REHABILITATION—cont'd

onto the dressing. Therefore, it is an open drain. Microbes can enter the drain and wound.

Closed drainage systems prevent microbes from entering the wound. A drain is attached to suction. The *Hemovac* (Fig. 31.22) and *Jackson-Pratt* (Fig. 31.23) systems are examples. Recently, another type of closed drainage system has become helpful for persons with wounds. Negative-pressure wound therapy uses suction applied over a foam dressing that is secured with a transparent film (Fig. 31.24). The nurse or wound specialist is responsible for the care. However, it may be your responsibility to change the drainage canister when necessary and record the output. Other systems are used depending on wound type, size, and site.

Drainage is measured in two ways:

- Noting the number and size of dressings with drainage. What is the amount and kind of drainage? Are dressings saturated? Is drainage on just part of the dressing? If so, which part? Is drainage through some or all layers?
- Measuring the amount of drainage in the collection container. This is done for closed drainage. Always follow the policy at your center. Some drainage systems are emptied only by the nurse.

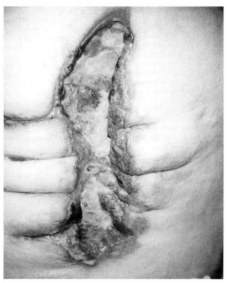

Fig. 31.17 Wound dehiscence. (Courtesy KCI Licensing, Inc., San Antonio, TX.)

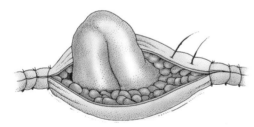

Fig. 31.18 Wound evisceration. (From Ignatavicius DD, Workman ML: *Medical-surgical nursing: critical thinking for collaborative care*, ed. 5, St. Louis, 2006, Saunders.)

BOX 31.5   Wound Observations

- Wound site
  - The person may have multiple wounds from surgery or trauma.
- Wound size and depth (measure in centimeters)
  - Size: Measure from top to bottom and side to side (Fig. 31.19).
  - Depth. To measure depth, the nurse:
    - Inserts a swab inside the deepest part of the wound.
    - Removes the swab.
    - Measures the distance on the swab.
    - Use a disposable ruler.
- Wound appearance
  - Is the wound red and swollen?
  - Is the area around the wound warm to touch?
  - Are sutures, staples, or clips intact or broken?
  - Are wound edges closed or separated?
  - Did the wound break open?
- Drainage
  - Is the drainage serous, sanguineous, serosanguineous, or purulent?
  - What is the amount of drainage?
- Odor
  - Does the wound or drainage have an odor?
- Surrounding skin
  - Is surrounding skin intact?
  - What is the color of surrounding skin?
  - Are surrounding tissues swollen?

DRESSINGS

Wound dressings have the following functions:
- Protect wounds from injury and microbes
- Absorb drainage
- Remove dead tissue
- Promote comfort
- Cover unsightly wounds

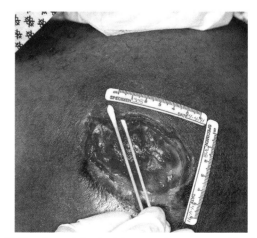

Fig. 31.19 The size and depth of the wound are measured by the nurse. (From Potter PA et al.: *Fundamentals of nursing*, ed. 8, St. Louis, 2013, Mosby.)

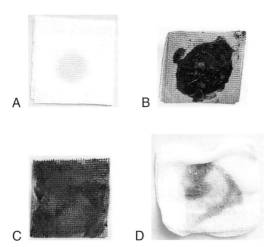

Fig. 31.20 Wound drainage. (A) Serous drainage. (B) Sanguineous drainage. (C) Serosanguineous drainage. (D) Purulent drainage. (Modified from Potter PA et al.: *Fundamentals of nursing*, ed. 10, St. Louis, 2021, Mosby.)

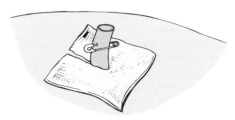

Fig. 31.21 Penrose drain. (From Potter PA et al.: *Fundamentals of nursing*, ed. 10, St. Louis, 2021, Mosby.)

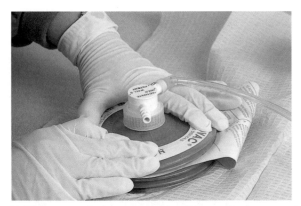

Fig. 31.22 Hemovac. Drains are sutured to the wound and connected to a reservoir. (From Potter PA et al.: *Fundamentals of nursing*, ed. 10, St. Louis, 2021, Mosby.)

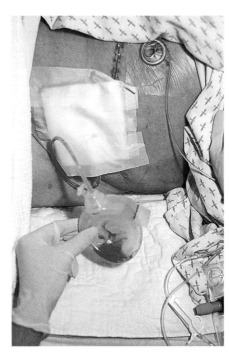

Fig. 31.23 Jackson-Pratt drainage system. (From Potter PA et al.: *Fundamentals of nursing*, ed. 10, St. Louis, 2021, Mosby.)

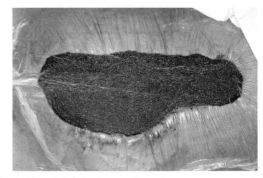

Fig. 31.24 Wound V.A.C. therapy (negative-pressure wound therapy). (Courtesy Kinetic Concepts, Inc. [KCI], San Antonio, TX.)

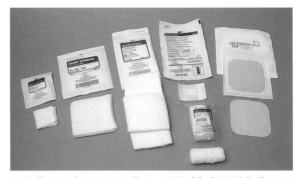

Fig. 31.25 Types of dressings. (From deWit SC, O' Neill P: *Fundamental concepts and skills for nursing*, ed. 5, St. Louis, 2018, Saunders.)

Types of Dressings

Dressings are described by the material used and how it is applied. There are many dressing products (Fig. 31.25). The following are common:

- *Gauze.* It comes in squares, rectangles, pads, and rolls. Gauze dressings absorb drainage and moisture.

- Provide a moist environment for wound healing
- Apply pressure (pressure dressings) to help control bleeding

Dressing type and size depend on many factors. These include the type of wound, its size and site, and amount of drainage. Infection is a factor. The dressing's function and the frequency of dressing changes are other factors. The doctor and nurse choose the dressing for each wound.

- *Nonadherent gauze.* It is a gauze dressing with a nonstick surface. It does not absorb drainage. It does not stick to the wound. It removes easily without injuring tissue.
- *Transparent adhesive film.* Air can reach the wound, but fluids and microbes cannot. The wound is kept moist. Drainage is not absorbed. The transparent film allows wound observation.
- *Hydrocolloids* (DuoDERM, Coloplast). An adhesive dressing that interacts with the wound drainage to form a gel. These cannot get wet with bathing.
- *Hydrogels.* A glycerin or water-based dressing that is commonly used to hydrate a wound. These dressings may be lifted to assess the wound and replaced. The doctor's order may allow removal of the dressing for bathing. Follow the care plan and the nurse's directions.
- *Negative-pressure dressings.* A type of wound therapy dressing that speeds up healing by using a controlled negative-pressure device (see Fig. 31.24). A foam or gauze dressing is placed in the wound. Then a clear adhesive drape is applied to form a seal. Finally, a tube is placed. It connects to a pump that applies negative pressure to the wound. The pump is at the person's bedside and must stay on at all times. It can be unplugged from the electrical outlet and the battery will take over. The machine signals when the canister is full. The canister is changed. The full canister is disposed of as biohazardous waste. Follow the Bloodborne Pathogen Standard.

Some dressings contain special agents to promote wound healing. If you assist with a dressing change, the nurse explains its use to you.

Dressings are wet or dry.

- *Dry dressing.* A dry gauze dressing is placed over the wound. More dressings are placed on top of the first dressing as needed. The dressings absorb drainage. The drainage is removed with the dressing. A dry dressing can stick to the wound. The dressing is removed carefully to prevent tissue injury and discomfort.
- *Wet-to-dry dressing.* This is used to remove dead tissue from the wound. Gauze dressings are saturated with a solution. These "wet" dressings are applied to the wound. The solution softens dead tissue. The dressing absorbs the dead tissue, which is removed when the dressings are dry.
- *Wet-to-wet dressing.* Gauze dressings saturated with solution are placed in the wound. The dressing is kept moist. It is not allowed to dry.

Securing Dressings

Dressings must be secured over wounds. Microbes can enter the wound and drainage can escape if the dressing is dislodged. Tape and adherent wraps are used to secure dressings. Binders may hold dressings in place.

Tape

Adhesive, paper, plastic, cloth, and elastic tapes are common. Adhesive tape sticks well to the skin. However, adhesive remaining on the skin is hard to remove. It can irritate the skin. An abrasion occurs if skin is removed with tape. Many people are allergic to adhesive tape. Paper, plastic, and cloth tapes usually do not cause allergic reactions. Elastic tape allows movement of the body part.

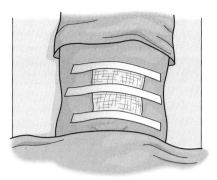

Fig. 31.26 Tape is applied at the top, middle, and bottom of the dressing. The tape extends several inches beyond both sides of the dressing.

Tape comes in different sizes—widths of ½, ¾, 1, 2, and 3 inches. Tape is applied to the top, middle, and bottom parts of the dressing. The tape extends several inches beyond each side of the dressing (Fig. 31.26). Sometimes a dressing is taped on all four sides (like a picture frame). *Do not apply tape to circle the entire body part. If swelling occurs, circulation to the part is impaired.*

See *Focus on Communication: Tape.*

FOCUS ON COMMUNICATION

Tape

Before applying tape, ask if the person has an allergy to tape. You can ask:
- "Do any types of tape irritate your skin?"
- "Do you have an allergy to tape?"

Applying Dressings

The nurse may ask you to assist with dressing changes. Some centers let you apply simple, dry, nonsterile dressings to simple wounds. Follow the rules in Box 31.6.

See *Focus on Communication: Applying Dressings.*

See *Teamwork and Time Management: Applying Dressings.*

BOX 31.6 Rules for Applying Dressings

- Let pain medications take effect, usually 30 minutes. The dressing change may cause discomfort. The nurse gives the medication and tells you how long to wait.
- Meet the person's fluid and elimination needs before you begin.
- Collect equipment and supplies before you begin.
- Do not bend or reach over your work area.
- Control your nonverbal communication. Wound odors, appearance, and drainage may be unpleasant. Do not communicate your thoughts or reactions to the person.
- Remove soiled dressings so the person cannot see the soiled side. The drainage and its odor may upset the person.
- Do not force the person to look at the wound. A wound can affect body image and self-esteem. The nurse helps the person deal with the wound.
- Remove tape by pulling it toward the wound.
- Remove dressings gently. They may stick to the wound, drain, or surrounding skin. If the dry dressing sticks, the nurse may have you wet the dressing with a saline solution. A wet dressing is easier to remove.
- Touch only the outer edges of old and new dressings (Chapter 14).
- Report and record your observations. *See Delegation Guidelines: Applying Dressings,* p. 486.

See *Delegation Guidelines: Applying Dressings.*
See *Promoting Safety and Comfort: Applying Dressings.*

FOCUS ON COMMUNICATION

Applying Dressings
The person may not report discomfort from a dressing. You should ask:
• "Is the dressing comfortable?"
• "Does the tape cause pain or itching?"

TEAMWORK AND TIME MANAGEMENT

Applying Dressings
Collect all needed items before starting the procedure. Have extra dressings, tape, and other supplies on hand. Leave unused items in the room for the next dressing change. Wound contamination can occur if you need to leave the room during the procedure.

DELEGATION GUIDELINES

Applying Dressings
When applying a dressing is delegated to you, make sure that:
• Your state allows you to perform the procedure.
• The procedure is in your job description.
• You have the necessary training.
• You know how to use the equipment.
• You review the procedure with the nurse.
• A nurse is available to answer questions and to supervise you.

If the abovementioned conditions are met, you need this information from the nurse:
• When to change the dressing
• When the person received a pain-relief medication and when it will take effect
• What to do if the dressing sticks to the wound
• How to clean the wound
• What dressings to use
• How to secure the dressing—where to apply the tape
• What kind of tape to use—adhesive, paper, plastic, cloth, or elastic
• What size tape to use—width of ½, ¾, 1, 2, or 3 inches

• What observations to report and record:
  • What you used to dress the wound and secure the dressing
  • A red or swollen wound
  • An area around the wound that is warm to touch
  • If wound edges are closed or separated
  • A wound that has broken open
  • Drainage appearance—clear, bloody, or watery and blood-tinged; thick and green, yellow, or brown
  • The amount of drainage
  • Wound or drainage odor
  • Intactness and color of surrounding tissues
  • Swelling of surrounding tissues
  • Possible dressing contamination—urine, feces; other body fluids, secretions, or excretions; dislodged dressing
  • Pain
  • Fever
• When to report observations
• What specific resident concerns to report at once

PROMOTING SAFETY AND COMFORT

Applying Dressings
Safety
Contact with blood, body fluids, secretions, or excretions is likely. Follow Standard Precautions and the Bloodborne Pathogen Standard. Wear personal protective equipment (PPE) as needed.

Do not apply tape to irritated, injured, or nonintact skin. Tape can further damage the skin.

Older persons have thin, fragile skin. Prevent skin tears. Use extreme care when removing tape.

Comfort
Wounds and dressing changes can cause discomfort or pain. If so, the nurse gives a pain-relief medication before the dressing change. Allow time for the medication to take effect. Be gentle when applying and removing tape and dressings.

APPLYING A DRY, NONSTERILE DRESSING

Quality of Life
Remember to:
• Knock before entering the person's room.
• Address the person by name.
• Introduce yourself by name and title.
• Explain the procedure to the person before beginning and during the procedure.
• Protect the person's rights during the procedure.
• Handle the person gently during the procedure.

Preprocedure
1. Follow *Delegation Guidelines: Applying Dressings.* See *Promoting Safety and Comfort: Applying Dressings.*
2. Practice hand hygiene.
3. Collect the following:
  • Gloves
  • PPE as needed
  • Tape
  • Dressings as directed by the nurse

Continued

✳ APPLYING A DRY, NONSTERILE DRESSING—cont'd

- Saline solution as directed by the nurse
- Cleansing solution as directed by the nurse
- Adhesive remover
- Dressing set with scissors and forceps
- Plastic bag
- Bath blanket

4. Decontaminate your hands.
5. Identify the person. Check the ID bracelet against the assignment sheet. Also call the person by name.
6. Provide for privacy.
7. Arrange your work area. You should not have to reach over or turn your back on your work area.
8. Raise the bed for body mechanics. Bed rails are up if used.

Procedure

9. Lower the bed rail near you if up.
10. Help the person to a comfortable position.
11. Cover the person with a bath blanket. Fan-fold top linens to the foot of the bed.
12. Expose the affected body part.
13. Make a cuff on the plastic bag. Place it within reach.
14. Decontaminate your hands.
15. Put on needed PPE. Put on gloves.
16. Remove tape. Hold the skin down. Gently pull the tape toward the wound.
17. Remove any adhesive from the skin. Wet a 4 × 4 gauze dressing with adhesive remover. Clean away from the wound.
18. Remove gauze dressings. Start with the top dressing and remove each layer. Keep the soiled side away from the person's sight. Put dressings in the plastic bag. They must not touch the outside of the bag.

19. Remove the dressing over the wound very gently. It may stick to the wound or drain site. Moisten the dressing with saline if it sticks to the wound.
20. Observe the wound, drain site, and wound drainage.
21. Remove the gloves and discard in the plastic bag. Decontaminate your hands.
22. Open the new dressings.
23. Cut the length of tape needed.
24. Put on clean gloves.
25. Clean the wound with saline or as directed by the nurse.
26. Apply dressings as directed by the nurse.
27. Secure the dressings in place with tape.
28. Remove the gloves. Put them in the bag.
29. Remove and discard PPE.
30. Decontaminate your hands.
31. Cover the person. Remove the bath blanket.

Postprocedure

32. Provide for comfort. (See the inside of the front cover.)
33. Place the call light within reach.
34. Lower the bed to its lowest position.
35. Raise or lower bed rails. Follow the care plan.
36. Return equipment and supplies to the proper place. Leave extra dressings and tape in the room.
37. Discard used supplies in the bag. Tie the bag closed. Discard the bag following center policy. (Wear gloves for this step.)
38. Clean your work area. Follow the Bloodborne Pathogen Standard.
39. Unscreen the person.
40. Complete a safety check of the room. (See the inside of the front cover.)
41. Decontaminate your hands.
42. Report and record your observations.

This skill is also covered in *Clinical Skills: Nurse Assisting.*

BINDERS

Binders are wide bands of elastic fabric. They are applied to the abdomen, chest, or perineal areas. Binders promote healing because they support wounds and hold dressings in place. They also prevent or reduce swelling, promote comfort, and prevent injury. Box 31.7 lists the rules for applying binders.

BOX 31.7 Rules for Applying Binders

- Follow the manufacturer instructions.
- Apply the binder so there is firm, even pressure over the area.
- Apply the binder so it is snug. It must not interfere with breathing or circulation.
- Position the person in good alignment.
- Reapply the binder if it is loose or wrinkled.
- Reapply the binder if it is out of position or causes discomfort.
- Secure safety pins so they point away from the wound (if used).
- Change binders that are moist or soiled. This prevents the growth of microbes.
- Tell the nurse at once if there is a change in the person's breathing.
- Check the person's skin under and around the binder. Tell the nurse at once if there is redness, irritation, or other signs of a skin problem.

Abdominal binders provide abdominal support and hold dressings in place (Fig. 31.27). The top part is at the person's waist. The lower part is over the hips. Binders are usually secured in place with Velcro.

See *Focus on Communication: Binders.*

See *Promoting Safety and Comfort: Binders.*

📋 FOCUS ON COMMUNICATION

Binders

The person may not tell you about pain or discomfort. Therefore, you need to ask these questions:
- "Is the binder too tight or too loose?"
- "Does the binder cause pain?"
- "Do you feel pressure from the binder?" If yes: "Where? Please show me."

WARM AND COLD APPLICATIONS

Warm and cold applications promote healing and comfort. They also reduce tissue swelling. Warm and cold have opposite effects on body function. Severe injuries and changes in body function can occur. The risks are great.

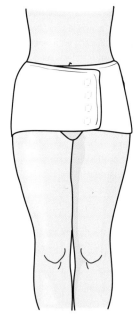

Fig. 31.27 Abdominal binder.

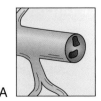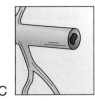

A	B	C
Normal	Dilated	Constricted

Fig. 31.28 (A) Blood vessel under normal conditions. (B) Dilated blood vessel. (C) Constricted blood vessel.

Also observe for pale skin. When heat is applied for too long, blood vessels constrict (narrow) (see Fig. 31.28). Blood flow decreases. Tissues receive less blood. Tissue damage occurs and the skin is pale.

Older and fair-skinned persons have fragile skin that is easily burned. Persons with problems sensing heat and pain are also at risk. Nervous system damage, loss of consciousness, and circulatory disorders affect sensation. So do confusion and some medications.

Metal implants pose risks. Metal conducts heat. Deep tissues can be burned. Pacemakers (cardiac devices) and joint replacements are made of metal. Do not apply heat to an implant area.

See *Residents with Dementia: Complications.*

Moist and Dry Warm Applications

With a *moist heat application*, water is in contact with the skin. Water conducts heat. Moist heat has greater and faster effects than dry heat. Heat penetrates deeper with a moist application. To prevent injury, moist heat applications have lower (cooler) temperatures than dry heat applications. Moist heat applications include:

- *Warm compresses* (Fig. 31.29A)—a compress is a soft pad applied over a body area. It is usually made of cloth. Sometimes an aquathermia pad is applied over the compress. It maintains the temperature of the compress.
- *Warm soaks* (see Fig. 31.29B)—a body part is put into water. This is usually used for small parts—a hand, lower arm, foot, or lower leg. A tub is used for larger areas.
- *Sitz baths* (see Fig. 31.29C)—the perineal and rectal areas are immersed in warm water. (*Sitz* means "seat" in German.) Sitz baths are common for hemorrhoids and after rectal or pelvic surgeries. They are used to:
  - Clean perineal and anal wounds.
  - Promote healing.
  - Relieve pain and soreness.
  - Increase circulation.
  - Stimulate voiding.
- *Warm packs* (see Fig. 31.29D)—a pack involves wrapping a body part with a wet or dry application. There are single-use and reusable packs. Some can be used for heat or cold. Follow the manufacturer instructions to activate the heat or cold. Clean reusable packs after use. To clean them, follow center policy and the manufacturer instructions.

With *dry heat applications*, water is not in contact with the skin. A dry heat application stays at the desired temperature longer. Dry heat does not penetrate as deeply as moist heat. Because water is

---

PROMOTING SAFETY AND COMFORT

Binders

Safety

Apply binders properly. Otherwise, severe discomfort, skin irritation, and circulatory and respiratory problems can occur. Correct application is needed for safety and for the binder to work effectively.

Comfort

A binder should promote comfort. Reapply the binder if it causes pain or discomfort.

RESIDENTS WITH DEMENTIA

Complications

Confused persons and those with dementia may not recognize pain. Look for changes in the person's behavior. Behavior changes can signal pain.

Warm Applications

Warm applications are often used for musculoskeletal injuries or problems (arthritis). Warmth:

- Relieves pain.
- Relaxes muscles.
- Decreases joint stiffness.
- Promotes healing.
- Reduces tissue swelling.

When heat is applied to the skin, blood vessels in the area dilate. Dilate means "to expand or open wider" (Fig. 31.28). Blood flow increases. Tissues have more oxygen and nutrients for healing. Excess fluid is removed from the area faster. The skin is red and warm.

Complications

High temperatures can cause burns. Report pain, excessive redness, and blisters at once.

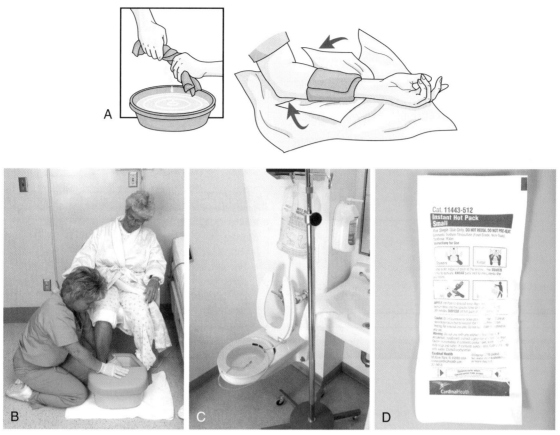

Fig. 31.29 Wet warm applications. (A) Compress. (B) Warm soak. (C) Disposable sitz bath. (D) Warm pack.

not used, dry heat needs higher (warmer) temperatures to achieve the desired effect. Therefore, burns are still a risk.

Some *warm packs* and the *aquathermia pad* are dry heat applications. The aquathermia pad is an electric device (Fig. 31.30). Tubes inside the pad are filled with distilled water. Heated water flows to the pad through a hose. Another hose returns water to the heating unit. The water is reheated and returned back into the pad.

Cold Applications

Cold applications reduce pain, prevent swelling, and decrease circulation and bleeding. Cold cools the body when fever is present.

Cold has the opposite effect of heat. When cold is applied to the skin, blood vessels constrict (see Fig. 31.28). Blood flow decreases. Tissues receive less oxygen and nutrients.

Cold applications are useful right after an injury. Decreased blood flow reduces the amount of bleeding. Less fluid collects in the tissues. Cold has a numbing effect on the skin. This helps reduce or relieve pain in the part.

Complications

Complications include pain, burns, blisters, and poor circulation. Burns and blisters occur from intense cold. They also occur when dry cold is in direct contact with the skin.

When cold is applied for a long time, blood vessels dilate. Blood flow increases. The prolonged application of cold has the same effect as heat applications.

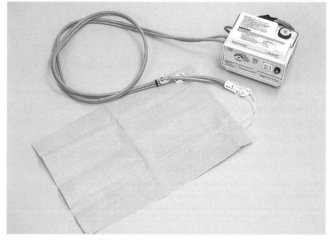

Fig. 31.30 The aquathermia pad.

Older and fair-skinned persons have fragile skin. They are at great risk for complications. So are persons with sensory impairments.

See *Residents with Dementia: Complications.*

Moist and Dry Cold Applications

Moist cold applications penetrate deeper than dry ones. Therefore, moist applications are not as cold as dry applications.

The cold compress is a moist cold application (see Fig. 31.29A). Dry cold applications include ice bags, ice collars, and ice gloves. Cold packs can be moist or dry applications.

✳ Applying Warm and Cold

Protect the person from injury during heat and cold applications. Follow the rules listed in Box 31.8.

See *Focus on Communication: Applying Warm and Cold.*
See *Teamwork and Time Management: Applying Warm and Cold.*
See *Delegation Guidelines: Applying Warm and Cold.*
See *Promoting Safety and Comfort: Applying Warm and Cold.*

TEAMWORK AND TIME MANAGEMENT

Applying Warm and Cold

After applying warm or cold, check the person and the application every 5 minutes. Plan your work so that you can stay in or near the person's room. For example, during the application:

- Make the bed and straighten the person's unit.
- Provide care to the roommate if you are assigned to this person.
- Help the person complete a daily or weekly menu.
- Read cards and letters to the person, with consent.
- Address envelopes and other correspondence for the person.
- Take time to visit with the person.

DELEGATION GUIDELINES

Applying Warm and Cold

Before applying warm or cold, you need this information from the nurse and the care plan:

- The type of application—warm compress or pack, commercial compress, warm soak, sitz bath, aquathermia pad; ice bag, ice collar, ice glove, cold pack, or cold compress
- How to cover the application
- What temperature to use
- The application site
- How long to leave the application in place
- What observations to report and record:
  - Complaints of pain or discomfort, numbness, or burning
  - Excessive redness
  - Blisters
  - Pale, white, or gray skin
  - *Cyanosis* (bluish color)
  - Shivering
  - Rapid pulse, weakness, faintness, and drowsiness (sitz bath)
  - Time, site, and length of application
- When to report observations
- What specific resident concerns to report at once

FOCUS ON COMMUNICATION

Applying Warm and Cold

The person may not tell you about pain or discomfort. The person may not know what symptoms to report. For heat and cold applications, you need to ask:

- "Does the application feel too hot or too cold?"
- "Do you feel any pain, numbness, or burning?"
- "Are you warm enough?"
- "Do you feel weak, faint, or drowsy?" If yes: "Tell me how you feel."

PROMOTING SAFETY AND COMFORT

Applying Warm and Cold
Safety

Check the person every 5 minutes. Also follow these safety measures:

- *Sitz bath.* Blood flow increases to the perineum and rectum. Therefore, less blood flows to other body parts. The person may become weak or feel faint. Drowsiness can occur from the bath's relaxing effect. Observe for signs of weakness, fainting, or fatigue. Also protect the person from injury. Keep the call light within reach and prevent chills and burns.
- *Commercial hot and cold packs.* Read warning labels and follow the manufacturer instructions.
- *Aquathermia pad:*
  - Follow electrical safety precautions (Chapter 11).
  - Check the device for damage or flaws.
  - Follow the manufacturer instructions.
  - Place the heating unit on an even, uncluttered surface. This prevents it from being knocked over or knocked off the surface.
  - Make sure the hoses do not have kinks or bubbles.
  - Use a flannel cover to insulate the pad. It absorbs perspiration at the application site. (Some centers use towels or pillowcases.)
  - Secure the pad in place with ties, tape, or rolled gauze. Do not use pins. They can puncture the pad and cause leaks.
  - Do not place the pad under the person or under a body part. This prevents the escape of heat. Burns can result if heat cannot escape.
  - Give the key used to set the temperature to the nurse. This prevents anyone from changing the temperature.

Some persons have medicated patches or ointments applied to the skin. Do not apply heat over such areas.

Comfort

Cold applications can cause chills and shivering. Provide for warmth. Use bath blankets or other blankets as needed.

BOX 31.8 **Rules for Applying Warm and Cold**

- Know how to use the equipment. Follow the manufacturer instructions for commercial devices.
- Measure the temperature of moist applications. Use a bath thermometer or follow center policy for measuring temperature.
- Follow center policies for safe temperature ranges.
- Do not apply *very hot* (above 106°F [46.1°C]) applications. Tissue damage can occur.
- Ask the nurse what the temperature should be.
  - Warm—cooler temperatures are needed for persons at risk.
  - Cold—warmer temperatures are needed for persons at risk.
- Know the exact site of the application. Ask the nurse to show you the site.
- Cover dry warm or cold applications before applying them. Use a flannel cover, towel, or other cover as directed by the nurse.
- Provide for privacy. Properly screen and drape the person. Expose only the body part involved. Avoid unnecessary exposure.
- Maintain comfort and body alignment during the procedure.
- Observe the skin every 5 minutes for signs of complications. See *Delegation Guidelines: Applying Warm and Cold.*
- Do not let the person change the temperature of the application.
- Know how long to leave the application in place. See *Delegation Guidelines: Applying Warm and Cold.* Carefully watch the time. Warm and cold are applied no longer than 15 to 20 minutes.
- Follow the rules of electrical safety when using electrical appliances to apply heat.
- Place the call light within the person's reach.
- Complete a safety check before leaving the room. (See the inside of the front cover.)

APPLYING WARM AND COLD APPLICATIONS

Quality of Life

Remember to:

- Knock before entering the person's room.
- Address the person by name.
- Introduce yourself by name and title.
- Explain the procedure to the person before beginning and during the procedure.
- Protect the person's rights during the procedure.
- Handle the person gently during the procedure.

Preprocedure

1. Follow *Delegation Guidelines: Applying Warm and Cold*, p. 490. See *Promoting Safety and Comfort: Applying Warm and Cold*, p. 490.
2. Practice hand hygiene.
3. Collect needed equipment.
   a. For a warm compress:
      - Basin
      - Bath thermometer
      - Small towel, washcloth, or gauze squares
      - Plastic wrap or aquathermia pad
      - Ties, tape, or rolled gauze
      - Bath towel
      - Waterproof pad
   b. For a warm soak:
      - Water basin or arm or foot bath
      - Bath thermometer
      - Waterproof pad
      - Bath blanket
      - Towel
   c. For a sitz bath:
      - Disposable sitz bath
      - Bath thermometer
      - Two bath blankets, bath towels, and a clean gown
   d. For a warm or cold pack:
      - Commercial pack
      - Pack cover
      - Ties, tape, or rolled gauze (if needed)
      - Waterproof pad
   e. For an aquathermia pad:
      - Aquathermia pad and heating unit
      - Distilled water
      - Flannel cover or other cover as directed by the nurse
      - Ties, tape, or rolled gauze
   f. For an ice bag, ice collar, ice glove, or dry cold pack:
      - Ice bag, collar, glove, or cold pack
      - Crushed ice (except for a cold pack)
      - Flannel cover or other cover as directed by the nurse
      - Paper towels
   g. For a cold compress:
      - Large basin with ice
      - Small basin with cold water
      - Gauze squares, washcloths, or small towels
      - Waterproof pad
4. Identify the person. Check the ID bracelet against the assignment sheet. Also call the person by name.
5. Provide for privacy.

Procedure

6. Position the person for the procedure.
7. Place the waterproof pad (if needed) under the body part.
8. For a *warm compress:*
   a. Fill the basin ½ to ⅔ full with warm water as directed by the nurse. Measure water temperature.
   b. Place the compress in the water.
   c. Wring out the compress.
   d. Apply the compress over the area. Note the time.
   e. Cover the compress quickly. Use one of the following as directed by the nurse:
      - Apply plastic wrap and then a bath towel. Secure the towel in place with ties, tape, or rolled gauze, or
      - Apply an aquathermia pad.
9. For a *warm soak:*
   a. Fill the container ½ full with warm water as directed by the nurse. Measure water temperature.
   b. Place the body part into the water. Pad the edge of the container with a towel. Note the time.
   c. Cover the person with a bath blanket for warmth.
10. For a *sitz bath:*
    a. Place the disposable sitz bath on the toilet seat.
    b. Fill the sitz bath ⅔ full with water as directed by the nurse. Measure water temperature.
    c. Secure the gown above the waist.
    d. Help the person sit on the sitz bath. Note the time.
    e. Provide for warmth. Place a bath blanket around the shoulders. Place another over the legs.
    f. Stay with the person if weak or unsteady.
11. For a warm or cold pack:
    a. Squeeze, knead, or strike the pack as directed by the manufacturer.
    b. Place the pack in the cover.
    c. Apply the pack. Note the time.
    d. Secure the pack in place with ties, tape, or rolled gauze. Some packs are secured with Velcro straps.
12. For an *aquathermia pad:*
    a. Fill the heating unit to the fill line with distilled water.
    b. Remove the bubbles. Place the pad and tubing below the heating unit. Tilt the heating unit from side to side.
    c. Set the temperature as the nurse directs (usually 105°F [40.5°C]). Remove the key.
    d. Place the pad in the cover.
    e. Plug in the unit. Let water warm to the desired temperature.
    f. Set the heating unit on the bedside stand. Keep the pad and connecting hoses level with the unit. Hoses must not have kinks.
    g. Apply the pad to the part. Note the time.
    h. Secure the pad in place with ties, tape, or rolled gauze. Do not use pins.
13. For an ice bag, collar, or glove:
    a. Fill the device with water. Put in the stopper. Turn the device upside down to check for leaks.
    b. Empty the device.
    c. Fill the device ½ to ⅔ full with crushed ice or ice chips (Fig. 31.31).
    d. Remove excess air. Bend, twist, or squeeze the device, or press it against a firm surface.
    e. Place the cap or stopper on securely.

✴ APPLYING WARM AND COLD APPLICATIONS—cont'd

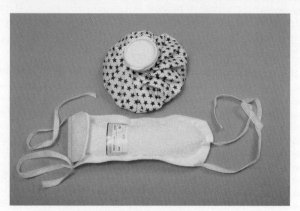

Fig. 31.31 Ice bags.

f. Dry the device with paper towels.
g. Place the device in the cover.
▶ h. Apply the device. Note the time.
i. Secure the device in place with ties, tape, or rolled gauze.
14. For a cold compress:
   a. Place the small basin with cold water into the large basin with ice.
   b. Place the compresses into the cold water.

c. Wring out a compress.
d. Apply the compress to the body part. Note the time.
15. Place the call light within reach. Unscreen the person.
16. Raise or lower bed rails. Follow the care plan.
17. Check the person every 5 minutes. Check for signs and symptoms of complications (see *Delegation Guidelines: Applying Warm and Cold*, p. 490). Remove the application if any occur. Tell the nurse at once.
18. Check the application every 5 minutes. Change the application if cooling (warm applications) or warming (cold applications) occurs.
▶ 19. Remove the application at the specified time. Warm and cold applications are usually left on for 15 to 20 minutes. (If bed rails are up, lower the near one for this step.)

Postprocedure
20. Provide for comfort. (See the inside of the front cover.)
21. Place the call light within reach.
22. Raise or lower bed rails. Follow the care plan.
23. Unscreen the person.
24. Clean and return reusable items to their proper place. Follow center policy for soiled linens. Wear gloves for this step.
25. Complete a safety check of the room. (See the inside of the front cover.)
26. Remove and discard the gloves. Decontaminate your hands.
27. Report and record your observations (Fig. 31.32).

Date	Time	Nursing Margin	Other Depts Margin
3/6	1000	Aquathermia heating unit set at 105° F. The pad was placed in a flannel	
		cover and applied to the anterior R thigh. Secured in place with tape.	
		Resident positioned in semi-Fowler's position. States she is comfortable.	
		States the pad does not feel too hot. Over-bed table with water pitcher and	
		water glass within reach. Bed in the low position. Call light within	
		reach. Adam Aims, CNA ⟵	
3/6	1005	Aquathermia pad checked. Resident states she feels comfortable. States the	
		pad is not too hot. Denies pain or discomfort. There is no redness, swelling,	
		or blistering of the skin under the pad. Pad re-secured with tape. Over-bed	
		table with water pitcher and glass within reach. Bed in the low position.	
		Call light within reach. Adam Aims, CNA ⟵	

Fig. 31.32 Charting sample.

This skill is also covered in *Clinical Skills: Nurse Assisting*.

Cooling and Warming Blanket

Hyperthermia is a body temperature *(thermia)* that is much higher *(hyper)* than the person's normal range. Body temperature is usually greater than 103°F (39.4°C). It is often called *heat stroke* when caused by hot weather. Other causes include illness, dehydration, and not being able to perspire. Lowering the body temperature is necessary. Otherwise, death can occur. The doctor orders ice packs applied to the head, neck, underarms, and groin. Sometimes cooling blankets are used alone or with ice packs.

A cooling blanket is an electrical device. Made of rubber or plastic, the device has tubes filled with fluid. The fluid flows through the tubes. The blanket is placed on the bed and covered with a sheet. The blanket is turned on the cool setting and allowed to cool. The person lies on the blanket.

Hypothermia is a very low (hypo) body temperature (thermia). Body temperature is less than 95°F (35°C). Cold weather is a common cause. The person is warmed to prevent death. Treatment may include a warming blanket. A warming blanket is like a cooling blanket except warm settings are used.

When used for cooling, the device is called a *hypothermia blanket.* When used for warming, it is called a *hyperthermia blanket.* The device has warm and cool settings. Vital signs are measured often. Rapid and excess cooling or warming is prevented.

MEETING BASIC NEEDS

The wound can affect basic needs. However, it is only one part of the person's care. Remember, the *person* has the wound.

The person is recovering from surgery or trauma. The wound causes pain and discomfort. These may affect breathing and moving. Turning, repositioning, and walking may be painful. Handle the person gently. Allow pain medications to take effect before giving care.

Good nutrition is needed for healing. However, pain and discomfort can affect appetite. So can odors from wound drainage. Promptly remove soiled dressings from the room. Use room deodorizers as directed. Also keep drainage containers out of the person's sight. Tell the nurse if the person wants certain foods or drinks.

Infection is always a threat. Follow Standard Precautions and the Bloodborne Pathogen Standard. Carefully observe the wound for signs and symptoms of infection.

Delayed healing is a risk for persons who are older, obese, or have poor nutrition. Protein is needed for tissue growth and repair. Poor circulation and diabetes also affect healing. These conditions are risk factors for infection.

Many factors affect safety and security needs. The person fears scarring, disfigurement, delayed healing, and infection. Fears about the wound "popping open" are common. Medical bills are other concerns. The person may need care for a long time.

Victims of violence have many other concerns. Future attacks, finding and convicting the attacker, and fear for family members are common concerns. Victims of domestic, child, and elder abuse often hide the source of their injuries.

Wounds may be large or small. Others can see wounds on the face, arms, or legs. Clothing can hide some wounds. Wound drainage may have odors. Some wounds are disfiguring. They can affect sexual performance or feelings of sexual attraction. Amputation of a finger, hand, arm, toe, foot, or leg can affect function, everyday activities, and jobs. Eye injuries can affect vision. Abdominal trauma and surgery can affect eating and elimination.

Whatever the wound site or size, it affects function and body image. Love and belonging and self-esteem needs are affected. The person may be sad and tearful or angry and hostile. Adjustment may be hard and rehabilitation necessary. Be gentle and kind, give thoughtful care, and practice good communication. Other health team members—therapists, social workers, psychiatrists, and the clergy—may be involved in the person's care.

QUALITY OF LIFE

Wounds result from surgery, trauma, pressure (Chapter 32), and circulatory problems. Many factors affect wound healing. They include wound type and site. The person's age, general health, nutrition, and lifestyle are other factors. Wounds cause pain and discomfort. Basic needs are affected. Treat the person with dignity and respect.

Many persons have poor arterial or venous circulation. They are at risk for open wounds on the lower legs and feet. Persons with diabetes are at risk for foot ulcers. Follow the person's care plan. Be very careful not to injure the skin during care.

Warm and cold applications promote healing and comfort. They also reduce tissue swelling. A person may worry about the need for a warm or cold application. Be kind, caring, and patient. Refer questions to the nurse. Remember the right to personal choice. The person has the right to be involved in planning care. To do so, the person must know the reason for the application.

Remember to explain procedures to residents. They can plan if they know what will happen. A person may want to make a phone call or finish an activity first. Or a person may want the procedure done by a certain time—before visitors arrive, before a TV program, or before an activity. You protect the right to personal choice when the person helps plan procedure times.

Protect the right to privacy. It shows respect and protects the person's dignity. Expose only the body part involved in the procedure. Unnecessary exposure violates the person's right to privacy. It also affects comfort and chilling.

Warm and cold are usually applied for 15 to 20 minutes. The person cannot move about during this time. To promote comfort and safety:
- Meet elimination needs before the procedure.
- Keep the room free of unpleasant equipment and odors.
- Place needed items within the person's reach. These include the call light, water pitcher and cup, reading material, needlework, phone, and other items requested by the person.
- Check the person often.

TIME TO REFLECT

You are assisting Mr. Tyson with a morning shower. He is a new resident who was recently discharged from the hospital. As you help him remove his pajama top in the shower room, you notice that he has a dressing over his spine in the middle of his back. The nurse did not mention the purpose of this dressing and you did not see any information in the care plan. Mr. Tyson is slightly confused and cannot offer any information about the dressing. What would be the best way to proceed at this point?

REVIEW QUESTIONS

Circle the BEST answer.

1. A person has a laceration on the right leg from a fall. The wound is
   a. Open, unintentional, and contaminated
   b. Open, unintentional, and infected
   c. Closed, intentional, and clean
   d. Closed, intentional, and chronic
2. A person had rectal surgery. The person has a
   a. Clean wound
   b. Dirty wound
   c. Clean-contaminated wound
   d. Contaminated wound
3. The skin and underlying tissues are pierced. This is a(n)
   a. Penetrating wound
   b. Incision
   c. Contusion
   d. Abrasion
4. Which can cause skin tears?
   a. Keeping your nails trimmed and smooth
   b. Dressing the person in soft clothing
   c. Wearing rings
   d. Padding wheelchair footplates
5. A person has a vascular ulcer. Which measure should you question?
   a. Hold socks in place with elastic garters
   b. Do not cut or trim toenails
   c. Apply compression (antiembolism) stockings
   d. Reposition the person every hour
6. Compression (antiembolism) stockings
   a. Hold dressings in place
   b. Prevent blood clots
   c. Increase swelling after injury
   d. Prevent venous blood flow
7. Compression (antiembolism) stockings are applied
   a. Before the person gets out of bed
   b. When the person is standing
   c. After the person's shower or bath
   d. For 30 minutes and then removed
8. When applying an elastic bandage
   a. Position the part in good alignment
   b. Cover the fingers or toes if possible
   c. Apply it from the largest to smallest part of the extremity
   d. Apply it from the upper to lower part of the extremity
9. Persons with diabetes are at risk for diabetic foot ulcers because of
   a. Gangrene
   b. Amputation
   c. Infection
   d. Nerve and blood vessel damage

10. A person has diabetes. You should check the person's feet every
    a. 2 hours
    b. Day
    c. Week
    d. Month
11. A person with diabetes needs to wear socks with shoes to prevent
    a. Corns
    b. Bunions
    c. Plantar warts
    d. Blisters
12. A wound is separating. This is called
    a. Primary intention
    b. Third intention
    c. Dehiscence
    d. Evisceration
13. Clear, watery drainage from a wound is called
    a. Purulent drainage
    b. Serous drainage
    c. Seropurulent drainage
    d. Serosanguineous drainage
14. A dressing does the following except
    a. Protect the wound from injury
    b. Absorb drainage
    c. Provide moisture for wound healing
    d. Support the wound and reduce swelling
15. A person receives a pain-relief medication before a dressing change. How long should you wait for the medication to take effect?
    a. 5 minutes
    b. 10 minutes
    c. 15 minutes
    d. 30 minutes
16. To remove tape
    a. Pull it toward the wound
    b. Pull it away from the wound
    c. Use an alcohol swab
    d. Use a saline solution
17. An abdominal binder is used to
    a. Prevent blood clots
    b. Prevent wound infection
    c. Provide support and hold dressings in place
    d. Decrease swelling and circulation
18. Warm applications have these effects except
    a. Pain relief
    b. Muscle relaxation
    c. Healing
    d. Decreased blood flow

19. The *greatest* threat from warm applications is
    a. Infection
    b. Burns
    c. Chilling
    d. Venous ulcers
20. These statements are about moist warm applications. Which is *false*?
    a. Water is in contact with the skin
    b. The effects from moist heat are less than from a dry heat application
    c. Moist heat penetrates deeper than dry heat
    d. A moist warm application has a lower temperature than a dry heat application
21. These statements are about sitz baths. Which is *false*?
    a. The perineal and rectal areas are immersed in warm water.
    b. Sitz baths last 25 to 30 minutes.
    c. They clean the perineum, relieve pain, increase circulation, or stimulate voiding.
    d. Weakness and fainting can occur.

22. A person uses an aquathermia pad. Which is *false*?
    a. It is a dry heat application
    b. A cover is used
    c. Electrical safety precautions are practiced
    d. Pins secure the pad in place
23. Cold applications
    a. Reduce pain, prevent swelling, and decrease circulation
    b. Dilate blood vessels
    c. Prevent the spread of microbes
    d. Prevent infection
24. Which is *not* a complication of cold applications?
    a. Pain
    b. Burns
    c. Blisters
    d. Infection

See Appendix A for answers to these questions.

32

Pressure Injuries

OBJECTIVES

- Define the key terms and key abbreviations listed in this chapter.
- Describe the causes and risk factors for pressure injuries.
- Identify the persons at risk for pressure injuries.
- Describe the stages of pressure injuries.
- Identify the sites for pressure injuries.
- Explain how to prevent pressure injuries.
- Identify the complications from pressure injuries.
- Explain how to promote quality of life.

KEY TERMS

avoidable pressure injury A pressure injury that develops from the improper use of the nursing process

bony prominence An area where the bone sticks out or projects from the flat surface of the body

chairfast Confined to a chair

colonized The presence of bacteria on the wound surface or in wound tissue; the person does not have signs and symptoms of an infection

erythema Redness of the skin

eschar Thick, leathery dead tissue that may be loose or adhered to the skin; it is often black or brown

friction The rubbing of one surface against another

intact skin Normal skin without openings or damage

pressure injury Localized damage to the skin and/or underlying soft tissue, usually over a bony prominence or related to a medical or other device. The injury can present as intact skin or an open ulcer and may be painful. Injury occurs as a result of intense and/or prolonged pressure or pressure in combination with shear.

shear When layers of the skin rub against each other; when the skin remains in place and underlying tissues move and stretch and tear underlying capillaries and blood vessels, causing tissue damage

slough Dead tissue that is soft and often moist and appears white, yellow, green, or tan; tissue may be firmly attached or loose and stringy

unavoidable pressure injury A pressure injury that occurs despite efforts to prevent one through proper use of the nursing process

KEY ABBREVIATIONS

CMS Centers for Medicare & Medicaid Services
MDRPI Medical device-related pressure injuries
NPIAP National Pressure Injury Advisory Panel

OBRA Omnibus Budget Reconciliation Act of 1987
TJC The Joint Commission

In 2016 the National Pressure Ulcer Advisory Panel replaced the term *pressure ulcer* with pressure injury. A pressure injury is localized damage to the skin and underlying tissue, usually over a bony prominence (Fig. 32.1). It is the result of pressure or pressure in combination with shear. *Prominence* means "to stick out." A bony prominence is an area where the bone sticks out or projects from the flat surface of the body. The back of the head, shoulder blades, elbows, hips, spine, sacrum, knees, ankles, heels, and toes are bony prominences (Fig. 32.2). *Decubitus ulcer, bed sore, pressure sore,* and *pressure ulcer* are other terms for pressure injury. The preferred term for health care providers is *pressure injury.*

❖ The Centers for Medicare & Medicaid Services (CMS) defines a pressure injury as any lesion caused by unrelieved pressure that results in damage to underlying tissues. According to the CMS, friction and shear are not the main causes of pressure injuries. However, friction and shear are important contributing factors. Shear is when layers of the skin rub against each other. Or shear is when the skin remains in place and underlying tissues move and stretch and tear underlying capillaries and blood vessels. Tissue damage occurs. Friction is the rubbing of one surface against another. The skin is dragged across a surface. Friction is always present with shearing.

The CMS has standards focusing on pressure injuries. Some persons are admitted to the center with pressure injuries. They come from hospitals or from home. According to the CMS, nursing centers must ensure that:

- A person does not develop a pressure injury after entering the center. However, sometimes developing a pressure injury cannot be avoided. A pressure injury occurs despite efforts

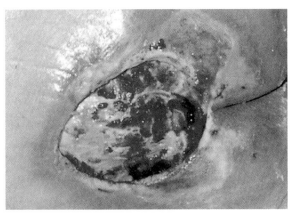

Fig. 32.1 A pressure injury. (From Proceedings from the November National V.A.C.: HMP communications, *Ostomy Wound Manage* 51:S7, 2005.)

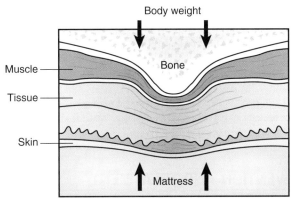

Fig. 32.2 Tissue under pressure. The skin is squeezed between two hard surfaces: the bone and the mattress. (Redrawn from U.S. Department of Health & Human Services, Agency for Healthcare Research and Quality: *Understanding your body: what are pressure ulcers?* Washington, D.C., 2009, Author.)

to prevent one through proper use of the nursing process. This is called an unavoidable pressure injury. An avoidable pressure injury is one that develops from the improper use of the nursing process. The center must:

- Evaluate the person's condition and pressure injury risk factors.
- Identify and implement measures that meet the resident's needs and goals.
- Monitor and evaluate the effect of such measures.
- Revise the measures as needed.
- A person with a pressure injury receives the necessary treatment and services to promote healing, prevent infection, and prevent new sores.

Centers must identify persons at risk for developing pressure injuries. The nurse does a thorough examination of the person's skin upon admission. Some persons are at greater risk than others, and their risk may increase during an illness (cold, flu) or when their condition changes. Many pressure injuries occur within the first 4 weeks of admission to a nursing center. A person at risk can develop a pressure injury within 2 to 6 hours after the onset of pressure. The center must develop a comprehensive care plan to meet the person's needs. The care plan must include measures to reduce or remove the person's risk factors.

BOX 32.1 Skin Breakdown: Common Causes

- Age-related changes in the skin
- Dryness
- Fragile and weak capillaries
- General thinning of the skin
- Loss of the fatty layer under the skin
- Decreased sensation to touch, heat, and cold
- Decreased mobility
- Sitting in a chair or lying in bed most or all of the day
- Chronic diseases (diabetes, high blood pressure)
- Diseases that decrease circulation
- Poor nutrition
- Poor hydration
- Incontinence (urinary, fecal)
- Moisture in dark body areas (skin folds, under breasts, perineal area)
- Pressure on bony parts
- Poor fingernail and toenail care
- Friction and shearing
- Edema

RISK FACTORS

Pressure is the major cause of pressure injuries. Shearing and friction are important factors. They also cause skin breakdown (Box 32.1) that can lead to a pressure injury. Risk factors include immobility, breaks in the skin, poor circulation to an area, moisture, dry skin, and irritation by urine and feces. Older and disabled persons are at great risk for pressure injuries. Their skin is easily injured. Causes include age-related skin changes, chronic disease, and general debility.

Unrelieved pressure squeezes tiny blood vessels. The skin does not receive oxygen and nutrients. Tissues die and a pressure ulcer forms when the skin is starved of oxygen and nutrients for too long. For example, pressure occurs when the skin over a bony area is squeezed between hard surfaces (see Fig. 32.2). The bone is one hard surface. The other is usually the mattress or chair seat. Squeezing or pressure prevents blood flow to the skin and underlying tissues. Oxygen and nutrients cannot get to the cells. Involved skin and tissues die.

Friction scrapes the skin, causing an open area. The open area needs to heal. A good blood supply is needed. A poor blood supply or an infection can lead to a pressure injury.

Shear occurs when the person slides down in the bed or chair. Blood vessels and tissues are damaged. Blood flow to the area is reduced.

PERSONS AT RISK

Persons at risk for pressure injuries are those who:

- Are bedfast (confined to a bed) or chairfast (confined to a chair). Pressure occurs from lying or sitting in the same position for too long.
- Need some or total help in moving. Coma, paralysis, or a hip fracture increases the risk for pressure injuries.

- Are agitated or have involuntary muscle movements. The person's movements cause rubbing (friction) against linens and other surfaces.
- Have urinary or fecal incontinence. Urine and feces contain substances that irritate the skin and lead to skin breakdown. They are also sources of moisture.
- Are exposed to moisture. Urine, feces, wound drainage, sweat, and saliva expose the person to moisture. Moisture irritates the skin. It also increases the risk of damage from friction and shearing during repositioning.
- Have poor nutrition. A balanced diet is needed to properly nourish the skin. The risk for pressure injuries increases when the skin is not healthy.
- Have poor fluid balance. Fluid balance is needed for healthy skin.
- Have lowered mental awareness. The person cannot act (move, change positions) to prevent pressure injuries. Medications and health problems affect mental awareness.
- Have problems sensing pain or pressure. These are symptoms of tissue damage. If unable to sense pain or pressure, the person does not know to alert the staff to the symptoms.
- Have circulatory problems. Good blood flow is needed to bring oxygen and nutrients to the cells. Cells and tissues die when starved of oxygen and nutrients.
- Are older. Older persons have thin and fragile skin. Such skin is easily injured. They may have chronic diseases that affect mobility, nutrition, circulation, and mental awareness.
- Are obese or very thin. Friction can damage the skin.
- Refuse care. The person needs proper care to prevent pressure injuries. The CMS requires that the person make informed choices. The center and resident must discuss the person's condition, treatment options, expected outcomes, and problems from refusing treatment. The center must address the person's concerns and offer options if a certain treatment is refused. The presence of a "Do Not Resuscitate" order (Chapter 45) does not mean the person is refusing measures to prevent or treat a pressure injury. It only means that the person will not be resuscitated in the event of a cardiac or respiratory arrest.

- Have a healed pressure injury. According to the CMS, areas of healed Stage 3 or Stage 4 pressure injury are more likely to recur. See "Pressure Injury Stages."

PRESSURE INJURY STAGES

In persons with light skin, a reddened bony area is the first sign of a pressure injury. In persons with dark skin, skin color may differ from surrounding areas. The color change remains after the pressure is relieved. The area may feel warm or cool. The person may complain of pain, burning, tingling, or itching in the area. Some persons do not feel anything unusual. Box 32.2 describes pressure injury stages.

See *Focus on Communication: Pressure Injury Stages.*

📋 FOCUS ON COMMUNICATION

Pressure Injury Stages

Tell the nurse if you see areas of redness, skin color changes, blisters, or skin or tissue loss. Describe what you observed as best as you can. Tell the nurse the site. The nurse needs to assess the area. For example, you can say:

- "I saw a reddened area on Mr. Drake's left heel. It was about the size of a quarter. The skin looked intact. Would you please take a look at it?"
- "I just gave Ms. Richards a bath. I noticed a reddened area with a blister on her left buttock. I didn't see any drainage. Would you please take a look at it? I can help you turn her."

PREVENTION AND TREATMENT

Preventing pressure injuries is much easier than trying to heal them. The Joint Commission (TJC) estimates that it costs up to $70,000 to treat a hospital-acquired pressure injury. In 2008 CMS announced it would no longer pay for additional costs incurred for hospital-acquired pressure ulcers. Pressure injuries also occur in long-term care and home settings. TJC estimates that it costs $11 billion a year to treat pressure injuries in the United States. Good nursing care, cleanliness, and skin care are essential. *TJC and the CMS require pressure injury prevention programs. The National Pressure Injury Advisory Panel (NPIAP) offers the information for preventing pressure injuries.*

BOX 32.2 **Pressure Injury Stages**

Stage 1 The skin is intact. There is usually redness (erythema) over a bony prominence. The color does not return to normal when the skin is relieved of pressure. In persons with dark skin, skin color may differ from surrounding areas. It may appear to be a persistent red, blue, or purple (Fig. 32.3).

Stage 2 Partial-thickness skin loss (see Fig. 32.3B). The wound may involve a blister or shallow ulcer. An ulcer may appear to be reddish pink. A blister may be intact or open.

Stage 3 Full-thickness skin loss (see Fig. 32.3C). The skin is gone. Subcutaneous fat may be exposed. Slough may be present. **Slough** is dead tissue that is soft and often moist and appears white, yellow, green, or tan. It may be firmly attached or loose and stringy.

Stage 4 Full-thickness skin and tissue loss with muscle, tendon, and bone exposure (see Fig. 32.3D). Slough and eschar may be present. **Eschar** is thick, leathery dead tissue that may be loose or adhered to the skin. It is often black or brown.

Unstageable Full-thickness tissue loss with the injury covered by slough and/or eschar (see Fig. 32.3E). Slough is yellow, tan, gray, green, or brown. Eschar is tan, brown, or black.

Deep Tissue Injury (see Fig. 32.3F) Purple or maroon localized area of discolored intact skin or blood-filled blister. Usually due to damage of underlying soft tissue from pressure and/or shear. The area may be preceded by tissue that is painful, firm, mushy, boggy, or warmer or cooler as compared to adjacent tissue. Deep tissue injury may be difficult to detect in individuals with dark skin tones.

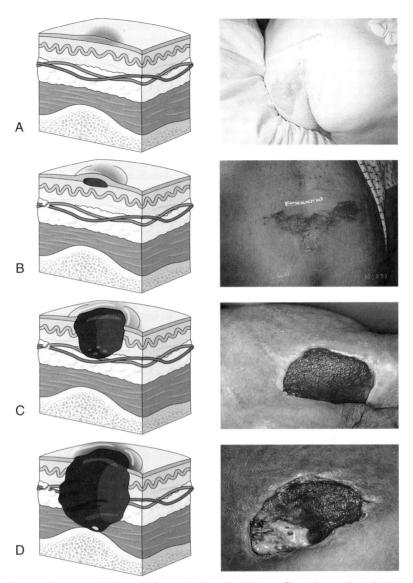

Fig. 32.3 Stages of pressure injuries. (A) Stage 1—the skin is intact. There is usually redness over a bony prominence. The color does not return to normal when the skin is relieved of pressure. In persons with dark skin, skin color may differ from surrounding areas. (B) Stage 2—partial-thickness skin loss with exposed dermis. The wound bed is pink or red and moist. A blister may be intact or open. (C) Stage 3—full-thickness skin loss. The skin is gone. Subcutaneous fat may be exposed. Tissue shedding (slough) may be present. (D) Stage 4—full-thickness skin and tissue loss with muscle, tendon, and bone exposure. Slough (tissue shedding) or eschar (a scab or dry crust) may be present. (Photos courtesy Laurel Wiersma, RN, MSN, Clinical Nurse Specialist, Barnes-Jewish Hospital, St. Louis. From Potter PA, Perry AG: Fundamentals of nursing, ed 7, St. Louis, 2009, Mosby.)

Pressure injury prevention involves:

- Identifying persons at risk. The nurse assesses the person when admitted to the center. The person's risk factors and skin condition are assessed. *The CMS requires that the nurse use the Minimum Data Set (MDS).* The Braden Scale for Predicting Pressure Sore Risk is a popular tool (Fig. 32.4). Existing pressure injuries are identified. Depending on the person's condition and risk factors, they are assessed daily or weekly.

- Implementing prevention measures for those at risk. Managing moisture, good nutrition, and fluid balance and relieving pressure are key measures. The daily care measures in Box 32.3 help prevent skin breakdown and pressure injuries. Follow the person's care plan.

Some centers use symbols or colored stickers as pressure injury alerts. They are placed on the person's door or chart. They remind the staff that the person is at risk for a pressure injury.

BRADEN SCALE FOR PREDICTING PRESSURE SORE RISK

Patient's name _____ Evaluator's name _____ Date of assessment

SENSORY PERCEPTION Ability to respond meaningfully to pressure-related discomfort	**1. Completely Limited** Unresponsive (does not moan, flinch, or grasp) to painful stimuli, due to diminished level of consciousness or sedation **OR** limited ability to feel pain over most of body	**2. Very Limited** Responds only to painful stimuli. Cannot communicate discomfort except by moaning or restlessness **OR** has a sensory impairment which limits the ability to feel pain or discomfort over 1/2 of body.	**3. Slightly Limited** Responds to verbal commands, but cannot always communicate discomfort or the need to be turned **OR** has some sensory impairment which limits ability to feel pain or discomfort in 1 or 2 extremities.	**4. No Impairment** Responds to verbal commands. Has no sensory deficit which would limit ability to feel or voice pain or discomfort.
MOISTURE Degree to which skin is exposed to moisture	**1. Constantly Moist** Skin is kept moist almost constantly by perspiration, urine, etc. Dampness is detected every time patient is moved or turned.	**2. Very Moist** Skin is often, but not always moist. Linen must be changed at least once a shift.	**3. Occasionally Moist** Skin is occasionally moist, requiring an extra linen change approximately once a day.	**4. Rarely Moist** Skin is usually dry, linen only requires changing at routine intervals.
ACTIVITY Degree of physical activity	**1. Bedfast** Confined to bed.	**2. Chairfast** Ability to walk severely limited or non-existent. Cannot bear own weight and/or must be assisted into chair or wheelchair.	**3. Walks Occasionally** Walks occasionally during day, but for very short distances, with or without assistance. Spends majority of each shift in bed or chair.	**4. Walks Frequently** Walks outside room at least twice a day and inside room at least once every two hours during waking hours.
MOBILITY Ability to change and control body position	**1. Completely Immobile** Does not make even slight changes in body or extremity position without assistance.	**2. Very Limited** Makes occasional slight changes in body or extremity position but unable to make frequent or significant changes independently.	**3. Slightly Limited** Makes frequent though slight changes in body or extremity position independently.	**4. No Limitation** Makes major and frequent changes in position without assistance.
NUTRITION Usual food intake pattern	**1. Very Poor** Never eats a complete meal. Rarely eats more than 1/3 of any food offered. Eats 2 servings or less of protein (meat or dairy products) per day. Takes fluids poorly. Does not take a liquid dietary supplement **OR** is NPO and/or maintained on clear liquids or IV's for more than 5 days.	**2. Probably Inadequate** Rarely eats a complete meal and generally eats only about 1/2 of any food offered. Protein intake includes only 3 servings of meat or dairy products per day. Occasionally will take a dietary supplement **OR** receives less than optimum amount of liquid diet or tube feeding.	**3. Adequate** Eats over half of most meals. Eats a total of 4 servings of protein (meat, dairy products) per day. Occasionally will refuse a meal, but will usually take a supplement when offered **OR** is on a tube feeding or TPN regimen which probably meets most of nutritional needs.	**4. Excellent** Eats most of every meal. Never refuses a meal. Usually eats a total of 4 or more servings of meat and dairy products. Occasionally eats between meals. Does not require supplementation.
FRICTION & SHEAR	**1. Problem** Requires moderate to maximum assistance in moving. Complete lifting without sliding against sheets is impossible. Frequently slides down in bed or chair, requiring frequent repositioning with maximum assistance. Spasticity, contractures or agitation leads to almost constant friction.	**2. Potential Problem** Moves feebly or requires minimum assistance. During a move skin probably slides to some extent against sheets, chair, restraints, or other devices. Maintains relatively good position in chair or bed most of the time, but occasionally slides down.	**3. No Apparent Problem** Moves in bed and in chair independently and has sufficient muscle strength to lift up completely during move. Maintains good position in bed or chair.	

© Copyright Barbara Braden and Nancy Bergstrom, 1988. All rights reserved. Total score

Fig. 32.4 Braden Scale for Predicting Pressure Sore Risk. *IV*, Intravenous; *NPO*, nothing by mouth. (Copyright 1988. Used with permission of Barbara Braden, PhD, RN, Professor, Creighton University School of Nursing, Omaha, NE; and Nancy Bergstrom, Professor, University of Texas-Houston, School of Nursing, Houston, TX.)

BOX 32.3 Daily Care to Prevent Skin Breakdown

Handling, Moving, and Positioning

- Follow the repositioning schedule in the person's care plan (Fig. 32.6). Reposition bedfast persons at least every 1 to 2 hours. Reposition chairfast persons every hour. Some persons are repositioned every 15 minutes. Some persons are allowed to sit in a chair three times a day for 60 minutes or less.
- Use assist devices (Chapter 15) according to the care plan.
- Position the person according to the care plan. Use pillows for support as instructed by the nurse. The 30-degree lateral position is recommended (Fig. 32.6).
- Do not position the person on a pressure injury.
- Do not position the person on a reddened area.
- Do not position the person on tubes or other medical devices.
- Do not leave a person on a bedpan longer than necessary.
- Prevent shearing and friction during handling, moving, and transfer procedures. Use assist devices as directed by the nurse and the care plan.
- Prevent friction in bed. Powder sheets lightly to prevent friction. Follow the care plan.
- Prevent shearing. Do not raise the head of the bed more than 30 degrees. Follow the care plan. The care plan tells you:
  - When to raise the head of the bed
  - How far to raise the head of the bed
  - How long (in minutes) to raise the head of the bed
- Use pillows, foam wedges, or other devices to prevent bony areas from contact with bony areas. The ankles, knees, hips, and sacrum are examples. Follow the care plan.
- Keep the heels and ankles off the bed. Use pillows or other devices as the nurse directs. Place the pillows or devices under the lower legs from midcalf to the ankles.
- Use protective devices as the nurse and care plan direct.
- Remind persons sitting in chairs to shift their positions every 15 minutes. This decreases pressure on bony points.
- Support the person's feet properly. Use a footrest if the person's feet do not touch the floor when sitting in a chair. The body slides forward when the person's feet do not touch the floor. If the person is in a wheelchair, position the feet on the footplates.

Skin Care

- Inspect the person's skin every time you provide care. This includes during or after transfers, repositioning, bathing, providing back massages, and elimination procedures. Report any concern at once.
- Follow the care plan for the person's bathing schedule. Some persons do not need a bath every day.
- Do not use hot water to bathe or clean the skin. Hot water can irritate the skin.
- Use a cleansing agent as directed by the nurse and the care plan. Soap can dry and irritate the skin.
- Provide good skin care. The skin is clean and dry after bathing. The skin is free of moisture from a bath, urine, stools, perspiration, wound drainage, and other secretions.
- Follow the care plan to prevent incontinence.
- Prevent skin exposure to moisture. Check persons who are incontinent of urine or feces often. Provide good skin care and change linens and garments at the time of soiling. Use incontinence products as directed by the nurse and the care plan.
- Apply an ointment or moisture barrier if the person is incontinent of urine or feces. Follow the care plan.
- Check persons often who perspire heavily or have wound drainage. Change linens and garments as needed. Provide good skin care.
- Apply moisturizer to dry areas—hands, elbows, legs, ankles, heels, and so on. The nurse tells you what to use and what areas need attention.
- Give a back massage when repositioning the person. *Do not massage bony areas.*
- Do not massage over pressure points. *Never rub or massage reddened areas.*
- Keep linens clean, dry, and wrinkle free.
- Do not irritate the skin. Avoid scrubbing or vigorous rubbing when bathing or drying the person.
- Use pillows and blankets to prevent skin from being in contact with skin. They also reduce moisture and friction.
- Make sure socks and shoes are in good repair. Inspect shoes for tightness. Poorly fitting shoes may cause pressure on bony prominences of the foot. Socks should not have wrinkles or creases. Socks or stockings should not be tight around the person's leg. Make sure there is nothing in the shoes before the person puts them on.
- Do not apply heat (Chapter 31) directly on a pressure injury.

Support surfaces are used to relieve or reduce pressure. Such surfaces include foam, air, alternating air, gel, or water mattresses. The best surface for the person is used.

SITES

Pressure injuries usually occur over bony areas. The bony areas are called *pressure points*. This is because they bear the weight of the body in a certain position (Fig. 32.7). Pressure from body weight can reduce the blood supply to the area. *According to the CMS, the sacrum is the most common site for a pressure injury.* However, pressure injuries on the heels often occur.

The ears also are sites for pressure injuries. This is from pressure of the ear on the mattress when in the side-lying position. Eyeglasses and oxygen tubing can also cause pressure on the ears (Fig. 32.8). A urinary catheter can cause pressure and friction on the meatus. Tubes, casts, braces, and other devices can cause pressure on arms, hands, legs, and feet. A pressure injury can develop where medical equipment is attached to the skin for a prolonged time. These are defined as medical device-related pressure injuries (MDRPIs) (Fig 32.9).

In obese people, pressure injuries can occur in areas where skin has contact with skin. Common sites are between abdominal folds, the legs, the buttocks, the thighs, and under the breasts. Friction occurs in these areas.

Protective Devices

The doctor orders wound care products, medications, treatments, and special equipment to promote healing. The nurse and care plan tell you what to do. Protective devices are often used to prevent and treat pressure injuries and skin breakdown. These devices are common:

- *Bed cradle*—A bed cradle is a metal frame placed on the bed and over the person (Chapter 24). Top linens are brought over the cradle to prevent pressure on the legs, feet, and

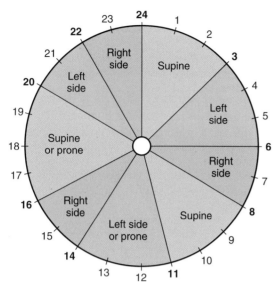

Fig. 32.5 Turn clock in 24-hour time. The clock shows the times to turn the person and to what position.

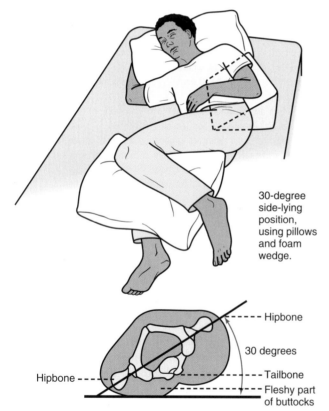

30-degree side-lying position, using pillows and foam wedge.

Fig. 32.6 The 30-degree lateral position. Pillows are placed under the head, shoulder, and leg. This position inclines (lifts up) the hip to avoid pressure on the hip. The person does not lie on the hip as in the side-lying position.

toes. Protect the person from drafts and chilling. To do so, tuck and miter linens at the bottom of the mattress. Also tuck them in under the mattress sides.

- *Heel and elbow protectors*—These devices are made of foam padding, pressure-relieving gel, sheepskin, and other cushion materials. They fit the shape of heels and elbows (Fig. 32.10). Some are inserted inside sleeves or mesh. Others are secured in place with straps. These devices promote comfort and reduce shear and friction.
- *Heel and foot elevators*—These raise the heels and feet off the bed (Fig. 32.11). They prevent pressure. Some also prevent footdrop (Chapter 24).
- *Gel or fluid-filled pads and cushions*—These devices involve a pressure-relieving gel or fluid (Fig. 32.12). They are used for chairs and wheelchairs to prevent pressure. The outer case is vinyl. The pad or cushion is placed in a fabric cover to protect the person's skin.
- *Alternating air mattress overlays*—Some beds may have a special air mattress overlay applied (Fig. 32.13).
- *Special beds*—Some beds have air flowing through the mattresses (Fig. 32.14). The person *floats* on the mattress. Body weight is distributed evenly. There is little pressure on body parts. Some beds allow repositioning without moving the person. The person is turned to the prone or supine position, or the bed is tilted various degrees. Alignment does not change. Pressure points change as the position changes. There is little friction. Some beds constantly rotate from side to side. They are useful for persons with spinal cord injuries.
- *Other equipment*—Pillows, trochanter rolls, footboards, and other positioning devices are used (Chapter 24). They help keep the person in good alignment.

See *Teamwork and Time Management: Prevention and Treatment.*

TEAMWORK AND TIME MANAGEMENT

Prevention and Treatment
The entire nursing team must prevent pressure injuries. As you walk down hallways, look into rooms to see if a person has slid down in bed or in a chair. Do the same when people are in dining and lounge areas. Help reposition the person. Ask a coworker to help you as needed. Report the repositioning to the nurse. Be aware of medical devices that can cause pressure. Even oxygen tubing or eyeglasses can cause a pressure injury.

Dressings

The nurse follows the orders of the treatment plan. At times, a multilayer foam dressing is applied as a preventative measure. This may prevent a pressure injury from occurring. For injuries that have already occurred, a special type of dressing is applied. A pressure injury may have drainage. A dressing that absorbs drainage is used. Wet-to-dry gauze dressings are sometimes used. The dressing absorbs slough. The slough is removed when the dressing is removed.

COMPLICATIONS

TJC estimates that about 60,000 people die each year from pressure injury complications. Infection is the most common complication. *According to the CMS, all Stage 2, 3, and 4*

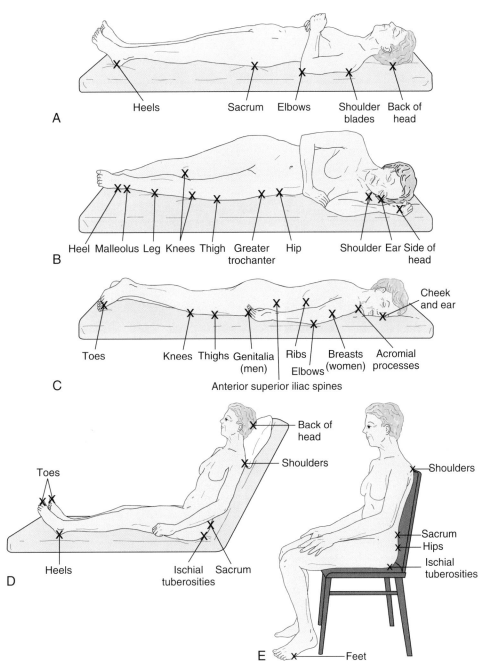

Fig. 32.7 Bony prominences (pressure points). (A) The supine position. (B) The lateral position. (C) The prone position. (D) Fowler position. (E) Sitting position.

pressure injuries are colonized with bacteria. Colonized refers to the presence of bacteria on the wound surface or in wound tissue. The person does not have signs and symptoms of an infection.

Wounds are infected if the person has signs and symptoms of infection (Chapter 14). For some persons, pain and delayed healing signal an infection. For the pressure injury to heal, infection must be diagnosed and treated.

Osteomyelitis is a risk if the pressure injury is over a bony prominence. The risk is great if the injury is not healing.

Osteomyelitis means "inflammation *(itis)* of the bone *(osteo)* and bone marrow *(myel)*." The person has severe pain. The person is treated with bedrest and antibiotics. Careful and gentle positioning is needed. Surgery may be needed to remove dead bone and tissue.

Pressure injuries can cause pain. Pain management is important (Chapter 25). Pain may interfere with movement and activity. The immobility is a risk factor for pressure injuries, and it may delay healing of an existing pressure injury.

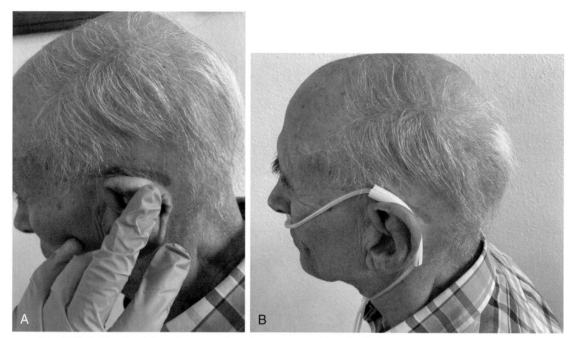

Fig. 32.8 A, Pressure injury above ear from from oxygen tubing. B, Cushion device on oxygen tubing for prevention of pressure injury.

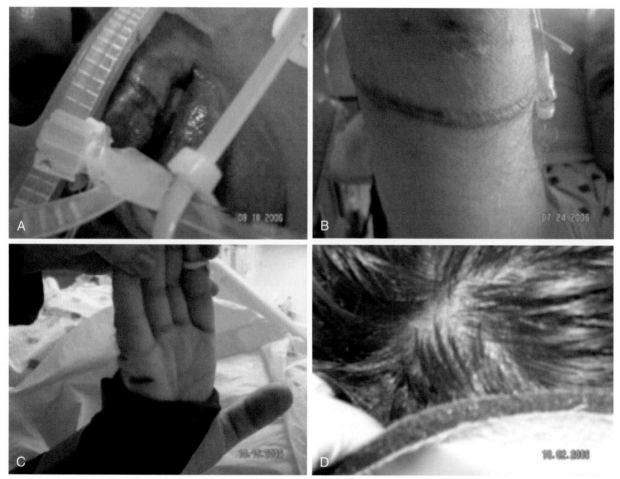

Fig. 32.9 Examples of medical device-related pressure injuries (MDRPI). (From Gefin A: Innovations and Emerging Technologies in Wound Care, ed 1, Elsevier, 2020, St. Louis)

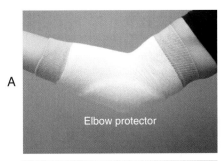

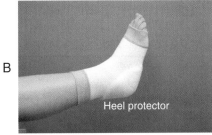

Fig. 32.10 (A) Elbow protector (B) Heel protector. (From Sorrentino SA, Remmert LN: *Mosby's textbook for nursing assistants*, ed. 10, St. Louis, 2021, Elsevier.)

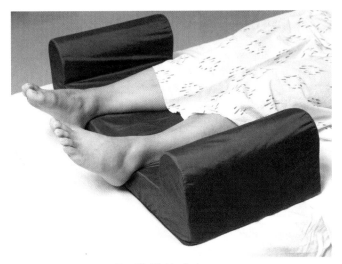

Fig. 32.11 Heel elevator.

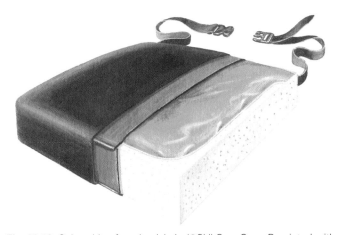

Fig. 32.12 Gel cushion for wheelchair. (©Skil-Care Corp. Reprinted with permission. All rights reserved.)

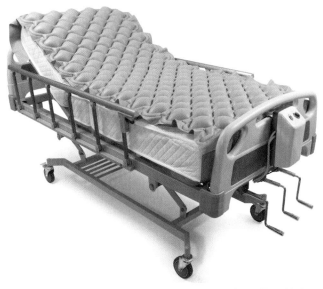

Fig. 32.13 An alternating air mattress. (From iStock/Recebin.)

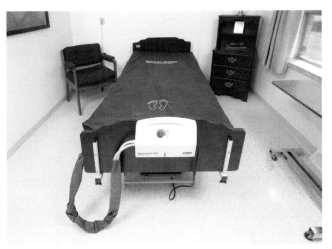

Fig. 32.14 Air flotation bed.

REPORTING AND RECORDING

Report and record any signs of skin breakdown or pressure injuries at once. See "Wound Appearance" in Chapter 31.

See *Focus on Communication: Reporting and Recording.*

📋 FOCUS ON COMMUNICATION

Reporting and Recording

During a site survey, CMS staff may interview you. They might ask questions about:

- How you are involved in the person's care.
- What measures the center uses to prevent and treat pressure injuries.
- What skin changes you should report and when.
- To whom you should report skin changes.
- Your knowledge of measures in a person's care plan.

Respond to the surveyor in a professional manner. Answer questions honestly and completely.

QUALITY OF LIFE

Residents have the right to care that promotes healthy skin and prevents skin breakdown and pressure injuries. The Omnibus Budget Reconciliation Act of 1987 (OBRA), the CMS, and TJC require a care plan for each person. It must address correct skin care. Use skin care products and protective devices as directed by the nurse and the care plan. Everyone must keep the person's skin healthy.

The skin is the body's first line of defense against changes in the environment. Keep the skin clean and intact. This promotes comfort and prevents infection. Giving good skin care is an important part of your job. Older persons require special skin care. Their skin is thin and fragile.

Preventing pressure injuries is easier than trying to heal them. Prolonged infection, pain, amputation, and longer hospital or nursing center stays are complications. The person's quality of life is reduced. Depression and death are risks.

TIME TO REFLECT

Mr. Michelson fell at home and fractured his right hip. He recently had surgery and was transferred from the hospital to your care center. He will have therapy and rehabilitation there. He has a urinary catheter inserted but is incontinent of feces. He cannot move independently in bed and cannot be positioned on his right side. He has now developed a Stage 2 pressure injury on his coccyx. What factors contributed to the formation of this pressure injury? What are some measures the nursing staff must take to help care for Mr. Michelson and to promote healing? Is he also at risk for a MDRPI?

REVIEW QUESTIONS

Circle the BEST answer.

1. A pressure injury is
   a. An open wound
   b. Localized damage to the skin and underlying soft tissue
   c. A bony prominence
   d. Dead tissue

2. Pressure injuries are the result of
   a. Unrelieved pressure
   b. Moisture
   c. Medical devices
   d. Aging

3. Which of the following contribute to the development of pressure injuries?
   a. Shear and friction
   b. Slough and eschar
   c. Bony prominences
   d. CMS and TJC

4. A pressure injury can develop within
   a. 2 to 6 hours
   b. 6 to 10 hours
   c. 10 to 14 hours
   d. 14 to 18 hours

5. The following are risk factors for pressure injuries *except*
   a. Urinary and fecal incontinence
   b. Lowered mental awareness
   c. Moisture
   d. Balanced diet

6. Which is the most common site for a pressure injury?
   a. Back of the head
   b. Hip
   c. Sacrum
   d. Heel

7. In a light-skinned person, the first sign of a pressure injury is
   a. A blister
   b. A reddened area
   c. Drainage
   d. Gangrene

8. A person's care plan includes the following. Which should you question?
   a. Reposition the person every 2 hours
   b. Scrub and rub the skin during bathing
   c. Apply lotion to dry areas
   d. Keep linens clean, dry, and wrinkle free

9. When positioning a person, you should position them
   a. On an existing pressure injury
   b. On a reddened area
   c. On tubes or other medical devices
   d. Using assist devices

10. What is the preferred position for preventing pressure injuries?
    a. 30-degree lateral position
    b. Semi-Fowler position
    c. Prone position
    d. Supine position

11. Besides heel and foot elevators, which are used to keep the heels and ankles off the bed?
    a. Bed cradles
    b. Pillows
    c. Heel protectors
    d. Sheepskin pads

12. Persons sitting in chairs should shift their positions every
    a. 15 minutes
    b. 30 minutes
    c. Hour
    d. 2 hours

13. A person is sitting in a chair. The feet do not touch the floor. What should you do?
    a. Have the person slide forward until the feet touch the floor
    b. Let the feet dangle
    c. Stack pillows under the person's feet
    d. Position the feet on a footrest

14. Which are *not* used to treat pressure injuries?
   a. Special beds
   b. Gel or fluid-filled pads and cushions
   c. Plastic drawsheets and waterproof pads
   d. Heel and elbow protectors

15. The following are sources of moisture *except*
   a. Urine and feces
   b. Wound drainage
   c. Perspiration
   d. Barrier ointment

16. You see a reddened area on the person's skin. What should you do?
   a. Rub or massage the area
   b. Apply a moisturizer
   c. Apply a moisture barrier
   d. Tell the nurse

17. The nurse tells you that the person's pressure injury is colonized. This means that
   a. The wound is infected
   b. Bacteria are present
   c. The person has osteomyelitis
   d. The person has a wet-to-dry gauze dressing

18. Inflammation of the bone and bone marrow is
   a. Osteoporosis
   b. Osteomyelitis
   c. Myositis
   d. Myalgia

19. Which of the following is *not* a prevention measure for pressure injuries?
   a. Reposition the person at least every 1 to 2 hours
   b. Keep the heels and ankles off the bed
   c. Massage bony areas
   d. Change linens and garments as needed

20. Which is correct for preventing or treating pressure injuries?
   a. Use hot water when bathing
   b. Allow the person to stay in one position during the night
   c. Keep the head of the bed raised as long as possible
   d. Make sure shoes fit properly

See Appendix A for answers to these questions.

33

Hearing, Speech, and Vision Problems

OBJECTIVES

- Define the key terms and key abbreviations listed in this chapter.
- Describe the common ear disorders.
- Describe how to communicate with persons who have hearing loss.
- Explain the purpose of a hearing aid.
- Describe how to care for hearing aids.
- Describe the common speech disorders.
- Explain how to communicate with speech-impaired persons.

- Describe the common eye disorders.
- Explain how to assist persons who are visually impaired or blind.
- Explain how to protect an ocular prosthesis from loss or damage.
- Perform the procedure described in this chapter.
- Explain how to promote quality of life.

KEY TERMS

aphasia The total or partial loss (*a-*) of the ability to use or understand language (*-phasia*); a language disorder resulting from damage to parts of the brain responsible for language

blindness The absence of sight

Braille A touch reading and writing system that uses raised dots for each letter of the alphabet; the first 10 letters also represent the numbers 0 through 9

Broca aphasia See "expressive aphasia"

cerumen Earwax

deafness Hearing loss in which it is impossible for the person to understand speech through hearing alone

expressive aphasia Difficulty expressing or sending out thoughts; Broca aphasia, motor aphasia

expressive-receptive aphasia Difficulty expressing or sending out thoughts and difficulty understanding language; global aphasia, mixed aphasia

global aphasia See "expressive-receptive aphasia"

hearing loss Not being able to hear the range of sounds associated with normal hearing

low vision Eyesight that cannot be corrected with eyeglasses, contact lenses, medications, or surgery

mixed aphasia See "expressive-receptive aphasia"

motor aphasia See "expressive aphasia"

receptive aphasia Difficulty understanding language; Wernicke aphasia

tinnitus A ringing, roaring, hissing, or buzzing sound in the ears or head

vertigo Dizziness

Wernicke aphasia See "receptive aphasia"

KEY ABBREVIATIONS

AFB American Foundation for the Blind
AMD Age-related macular degeneration

ASL American Sign Language
HOH Hard of hearing

Hearing, speech, and vision allow communication, learning, and moving about. They are important for self-care, work, and most activities. They also are important for safety and security needs. For example, you see dark clouds and hear tornado warning sirens. You know to seek shelter. With speech, you can alert others.

Many people have some degree of hearing or vision loss. Common causes are birth defects, accidents, infections, diseases, and aging.

EAR DISORDERS

The ear functions in hearing and balance. To review the structures and functions of the ear, see Chapter 8.

Otitis Media

Otitis media is infection (*itis*) of the middle (*media*) ear (*ot*). It often begins with infections that cause sore throats, colds, or other respiratory infections that spread to the middle ear. Viruses and bacteria are causes.

🧑 RESIDENTS WITH DEMENTIA

Otitis Media

Some persons with dementia cannot tell you about pain or when something is wrong. Be alert for behavior changes. Report the following to the nurse. They may signal otitis media.

- Unusual irritability
- Problems sleeping
- Tugging or pulling at one or both ears
- Fever
- Fluid draining from the ear
- Balance problems
- Signs of hearing problems

Otitis media is acute or chronic. Chronic otitis media can damage the tympanic membrane (eardrum) or the ossicles (Chapter 8). These structures are needed for hearing. Permanent hearing loss can occur.

Fluid builds up in the ear. Pain (earache) and hearing loss occur, as do fever and tinnitus. Tinnitus is a ringing, roaring, hissing, or buzzing sound in the ears or head. An untreated infection can travel to the brain and other structures in the head. The doctor orders antibiotics, medications for pain relief, or medications to relieve congestion.

See *Residents with Dementia: Otitis Media.*

Meniere Disease

Meniere disease involves the inner ear. It is a common cause of hearing loss. Usually, one ear is affected. Symptoms include the following:

- Vertigo (dizziness)
- Tinnitus
- Hearing loss
- Pain or pressure in the affected ear

With Meniere disease, there is increased fluid in the inner ear. The increased fluid causes swelling and pressure in the inner ear. Symptoms occur suddenly. They can occur daily or just once a year. An attack can last several hours.

An attack usually involves vertigo, tinnitus, and hearing loss. Vertigo causes whirling and spinning sensations. The dizziness causes severe nausea and vomiting.

Medications, fluid restriction, a low-salt diet, and no alcohol or caffeine decrease fluid in the inner ear. Safety is needed during vertigo. The person must lie down. Falls are prevented. Bed rails are used according to the care plan. The person's head is kept still. The person avoids turning the head. To talk to the person, stand directly in front of the person. When movement is necessary, move the person slowly. Sudden movements are avoided. So are bright or glaring lights. Assist with walking. The person should not walk alone in case vertigo occurs.

Hearing Loss

Hearing loss is not being able to hear the range of sounds associated with normal hearing. Losses are mild to severe. Sometimes the phrase "hard of hearing" (HOH) is used. Deafness is the most severe form. Deafness is hearing loss in which it is impossible for the person to understand speech through hearing alone.

📋 FOCUS ON COMMUNICATION

Hearing Loss

The National Association of the Deaf (NAD) uses the terms *deaf* and *hard-of-hearing* to describe persons with hearing loss. Do not use the terms *deaf and dumb*, *deaf-mute*, or *hearing-impaired*. Such terms offend persons who are deaf or hard-of-hearing.

👤 PROMOTING SAFETY AND COMFORT

Hearing Loss
Safety

Do not try to remove earwax. This is done by a health care provider. Do not insert anything, including cotton swabs, into the ear.

Hearing loss occurs in all age groups. According to the National Institute on Deafness and Other Communication Disorders (NIDCD), about one-third (33%) of Americans between ages 65 and 74 have hearing problems. About half (50%) of persons age 75 years and older have hearing loss. Hearing loss is more common in men than in women.

Common causes of hearing loss are the following:

- Damage to the outer, middle, or inner ear
- Damage to the auditory nerve
  Risk factors that can damage ear structures include:
- Aging
- Exposure to very loud sounds and noises—job-related noises, loud music, loud engines from vehicles, shooting firearms
- Medications—antibiotics, too much aspirin
- Infections
- Reduced blood flow to the ear caused by high blood pressure, heart and vascular diseases, and diabetes
- Stroke
- Head injuries
- Tumors
- Heredity
- Birth defects

Temporary hearing loss can occur from earwax (cerumen). Hearing improves after the earwax is removed.

Clear speech, responding to others, safety, and awareness of surroundings require hearing. Many people deny hearing problems. They relate hearing loss to aging.

See *Focus on Communication: Hearing Loss.*

See *Promoting Safety and Comfort: Hearing Loss.*

Effects on the Person

A person may not notice gradual hearing loss. Others may see changes in the person's behavior or attitude. They may not relate the changes to hearing loss. Obvious signs and symptoms of hearing loss include the following:

- Speaking too loudly
- Leaning forward to hear
- Turning and cupping the better ear toward the speaker
- Answering questions or responding inappropriately

- Asking for words to be repeated
- Asking others to speak louder or to speak more slowly and clearly
- Having trouble hearing over the phone
- Finding it hard to follow conversations when two or more people are talking
- Turning up the TV, radio, or music volume so loud that others complain
- Thinking that others are mumbling or slurring words
- Having problems understanding women and children

Psychologic and social changes are less obvious. People may give wrong answers or responses. Therefore, they tend to shun social events to avoid embarrassment. Often, they feel lonely, bored, and left out. Only parts of conversations are heard. They may become suspicious. They think others are talking about them or are talking softly on purpose. Some control conversations to avoid responding or being labeled "senile" because of poor answers. Straining and working hard to hear can cause fatigue, frustration, and irritability.

Hearing is needed for speech. How you pronounce words and voice volume depend on how you hear yourself. Hearing loss may result in slurred speech. Words may be pronounced incorrectly. Some have monotone speech or drop word endings. It may be hard to understand what the person says. Do not assume or pretend that you understand what the person says. Otherwise, serious problems can result. See "Speech Disorders" on p. ⋯.

Communication

Persons with hearing loss may wear hearing aids or lip-read (speech-read). They watch facial expressions, gestures, and body language. Some people learn American Sign Language (ASL) (Figs. 33.1 and 33.2). ASL uses signs made with the hands and other movements such as facial expressions, gestures, and postures. To promote communication, practice the measures in Box 33.1. (Different sign languages are used in different countries and regions. For example, British Sign Language is different from ASL.)

Some people have *hearing assistance dogs* (hearing dogs). The dog alerts the person to sounds. Phones, doorbells, smoke detectors, alarm clocks, sirens, and oncoming cars are examples.

❖ Hearing Aids

Hearing aids are electronic devices that fit inside or behind the ear (Figs. 33.3 and 33.4). They make sounds louder. They do not correct, restore, or cure hearing problems. Hearing ability does not improve. The person hears better because the device makes sounds louder. Background noise and speech are louder. The measures in Box 33.1 apply.

Hearing aids are battery operated. Sometimes they do not seem to work properly. Try these simple measures:

- Check if the hearing aid is *on*; it has an *on* and *off* switch.
- Check the battery position.
- Insert a new battery if needed.

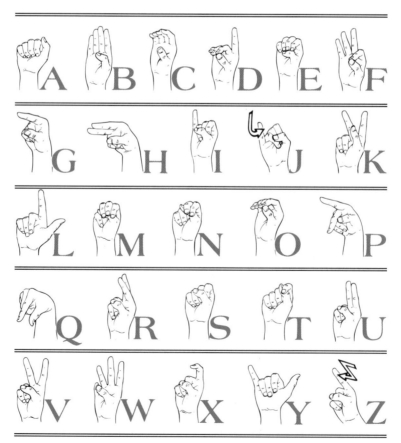

Fig. 33.1 Manual alphabet. (Courtesy National Association of the Deaf, Silver Spring, MD.)

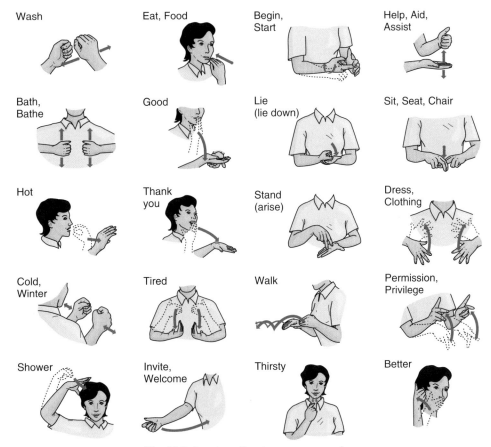

Fig. 33.2 American Sign Language examples.

BOX 33.1 Measures to Promote Hearing

The Environment
- Reduce or eliminate background noises. Turn off radios, stereos, music players, TVs, air conditioners, fans, and so on.
- Provide a quiet place to talk.
- Have the person sit in small groups or where the person can hear best.

The Person
- Have the person wear the hearing aid. It must be turned on and working.
- Have the person wear needed eyeglasses or contact lenses. The person needs to see your face for lip-reading (speech-reading).

You
- Gain attention. Alert the person to your presence. Raise an arm or hand or lightly touch the person's arm. Do not startle or approach the person from behind.
- Position yourself at the person's level. If the person is sitting, you sit. If the person is standing, you stand.
- Face the person when speaking. Do not turn or walk away while you are talking. Do not talk to the person from the doorway or another room.
- Stand or sit in good light. Shadows and glares affect the person's ability to see your face clearly.
- Speak clearly, distinctly, and slowly.
- Speak in a normal tone of voice. Do not shout.

- Adjust the pitch of your voice as needed. Ask if the person can hear you better.
- If the person does not wear a hearing aid, lower the pitch if you are a female. Women's voices are higher-pitched and harder to hear than lower-pitched male voices.
- If the person wears a hearing aid, raise the pitch slightly.
- Do not cover your mouth, smoke, eat, or chew gum while talking. Mouth movements are affected.
- Keep your hands away from your face. The person must be able to see your face clearly.
- Stand or sit on the side of the better ear.
- State the topic of conversation first.
- Tell the person when you are changing the subject. State the new subject of conversation.
- Use short sentences and simple words.
- Use gestures and facial expressions to give useful clues.
- Write out important names and words.
- Say things in another way if the person does not seem to understand.
- Keep conversations and discussions short. This avoids tiring the person.
- Repeat and rephrase statements as needed.
- Be alert to messages sent by your facial expressions, gestures, and body language.

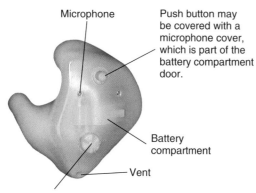

Microphone

Push button may be covered with a microphone cover, which is part of the battery compartment door.

Battery compartment

Vent

On/Off switch/Volume control

Fig. 33.3 A hearing aid. (Courtesy Siemens Hearing Instruments, Inc., Piscataway, NJ.)

- Clean the hearing aid; *follow the nurse's directions and the manufacturer instructions.*

Hearing aids are turned off when not in use, and the battery is removed. These measures help prolong battery life. The person should not use hair spray or other hair care products while wearing a hearing aid. They can damage the device.

Hearing aids are costly. Handle and care for them properly. When not in the person's ear, store a hearing aid in its case. Place the case in the top drawer of the bedside stand. Report lost or damaged hearing aids to the nurse at once.

 DELEGATION GUIDELINES

Hearing Aids

There are many different types of hearing aids. The nurse gives you instructions on specific ways to care for the hearing aid. Some residents are confused and would misplace their hearing aids. If the hearing aid cannot be stored in the bedside stand, the nurse will tell you where the hearing aid should be stored.

 PROMOTING SAFETY AND COMFORT

Hearing Aids
Safety

Hearing aids are costly. Protect them from loss or damage. When not worn, put them in their case. Place the case in the top drawer of the bedside stand. Never expose the hearing aid to water. Do not use a hair dryer with a hearing aid in place. Always remove before showering or shampooing the hair. Notify the nurse if the person complains of pain. Report any bleeding or drainage from the ear.

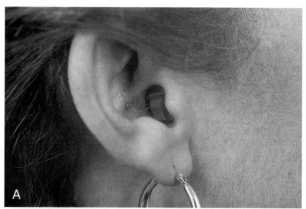

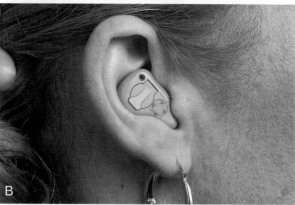

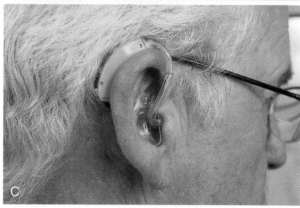

Fig. 33.4 Three common types of hearing aids. (A) In the canal (ITC). (B) In the ear (ITE). (C) Behind the ear (BTE). (From Potter PA et al.: *Fundamentals of nursing*, ed. 10, St. Louis, 2021, Mosby.)

✳ **CARING FOR HEARING AIDS**

Quality of Life

Remember to:
- Knock before entering the person's room.
- Address the person by name.
- Introduce yourself by name and title.
- Explain the procedure to the person before beginning and during the procedure.
- Protect the person's rights during the procedure.
- Handle the person gently during the procedure.

Preprocedure

1. Follow Delegation Guidelines: Hearing Aids. See *Promoting Safety and Comfort: Hearing Aids.*
2. Practice hand hygiene.
3. Collect the following:
   - Hearing aid case
   - Soft towel to place on work surface
   - Soft, dry cloth

Continued

✳️ CARING FOR HEARING AIDS—cont'd

Procedure

4. Place the towel over the surface where you are working.
5. Ask the resident to remove the hearing aid. If needed, carefully remove it for the person.
6. With a soft, dry cloth, carefully wipe the surfaces of the hearing aid.
   a. Wipe the hearing aid from top to bottom.
   b. Do not use water, alcohol, or any disinfectant unless told to do so.
7. Remove the battery and gently wipe the battery area. Replace the battery if needed.
8. *If the person wears the hearing aid:*
   a. Make sure the ear is clean and dry.
   b. Correctly place the hearing aid or have the resident place it.
   c. Make sure the hearing aid is on and adjusted properly.
   d. Ask if the resident is able to hear clearly.

If the person will not wear the hearing aid:
   a. Open the hearing aid case.
   b. Open the battery door and remove the battery.
   c. Put the hearing aid in the case.
   d. Place the case in the top drawer of the bedside stand.
   e. Do not expose the hearing aid to moisture or humidity.

Postprocedure

9. Provide for comfort. (See the inside of the front cover.)
10. Place the call light within reach.
11. Place the soiled cloth and towel in the proper place.
12. Complete a safety check of the room. (See the inside of the front cover.)
13. Decontaminate your hands.
14. Report and record your observations.

Cochlear Implants

A *cochlear implant* is a small, surgically implanted device that works by delivering impulses directly to the auditory nerve, which carries the signals to the brain (Chapter 8). A cochlear implant does not restore normal hearing. However, it can produce useful representation of sounds. Most people are able to understand speech in person or over the phone better than they can with a hearing aid. Some hear sounds in the environment better, such as telephones, doorbells, and alarms. Cochlear implants are used in very young children and elderly persons who have severe hearing loss. The implant is made up of several parts (Fig. 33.5). The implant package is secured inside the skull. The processor is worn outside the body. For the cochlear implant to work, the implant package and the sound processor must be aligned. Magnets are used to line up the internal and external parts (Fig. 33.6). If the implant package

and the sound processor are not aligned, the device does not work. Then the person cannot hear. *Follow the nurse's directions and the manufacturer instructions when caring for persons with cochlear implants. When not in use, the cochlear implant needs to be safely stored. Some have a special box that protects the processor from moisture and humidity.*

Other Hearing Devices

Other devices can help the person with hearing loss. They include the following:

- *Telephone amplifying devices.* Special telephone receivers make sounds louder. Some phones work with hearing aids.
- *TV and radio listening systems.* These can be used with or without hearing aids. The person does not have to turn the TV or radio volume up high.

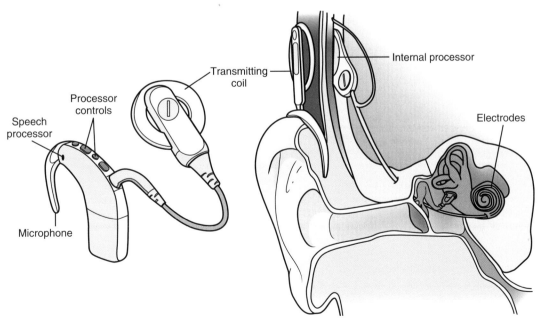

Fig. 33.5 Cochlear implants.

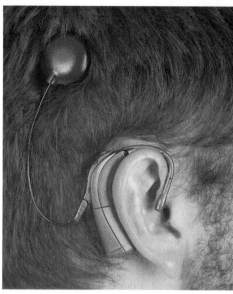

Fig. 33.6 External components of a cochlear implant hearing system. (Elizabeth Hoffmann/iStock.)

SPEECH DISORDERS

Speech is used to communicate with others. Speech disorders result in impaired or ineffective oral communication. Hearing loss, developmental disabilities (Chapter 41), and brain injury are common causes. The following are common problems.

- *Aphasia.* See "Aphasia."
- *Apraxia* means "not *(a)* to act, do, or perform *(praxia)*." The person with *apraxia of speech* cannot use the speech muscles to produce understandable speech. The person understands speech and knows what to say. However, the brain cannot coordinate the speech muscles to make the words. Apraxia is caused by damage to the motor speech area in the brain.
- *Dysarthria* means "difficult or poor *(dys)* speech *(arthria)*." It is caused by damage to the nervous system. Mouth and face muscles are affected. Slurred speech, speaking slowly or softly, hoarseness, and drooling are other problems that can occur.

To communicate with the speech-impaired person, practice the measures in Box 33.2.

See *Focus on Rehabilitation: Speech Disorders.*

🍃 FOCUS ON REHABILITATION

Speech Disorders
Some persons need speech rehabilitation. The goal is to improve the person's ability to communicate. A speech-language pathologist and other health team members help the person to:
- Improve affected language skills.
- Use remaining abilities.
- Restore language abilities to the extent possible.
- Learn other methods of communicating.
- Strengthen the muscles of speech.

The amount of improvement possible depends on many factors. They include the cause, amount, and area of brain damage and the person's age and health. The person's willingness and ability to learn are other factors.

Aphasia

Aphasia is the total or partial loss *(a)* of the ability to use or understand language *(phasia)*. Aphasia is a language disorder. It results from damage to parts of the brain responsible for language. Stroke, head injury, brain infections, and cancer are common causes. Most people who have aphasia are middle-aged or older adults.

Expressive aphasia (motor aphasia, Broca aphasia) relates to difficulty expressing or sending out thoughts. Thinking is clear. The person knows what to say but has difficulty or cannot speak the words. There are problems with speaking, spelling, counting, gesturing, or writing. The person may:
- Omit small words such as "is," "and," "of," and "the."
- Speak in single words or short sentences. For example, "Walk dog" can mean "I will take the dog for a walk" or "You take the dog for a walk."
- Put words in the wrong order. Instead of "bathroom," the person may say "room bath."
- Think one thing but say another. The person may want food but asks for a book.
- Call people by the wrong names.
- Make up words.
- Produce sounds and no words.
- Cry or swear for no reason.

BOX 33.2 **Measures to Communicate with the Speech-Impaired Person**

The Person
- Ask the person to repeat or rephrase statements if necessary.
- Repeat what the person has said. Ask if your understanding is correct.
- Ask the person to write down key words or the message.
- Ask the person to point, gesture, or draw to communicate key words.

You
- Follow the care plan. A consistent approach is needed.
- Provide a calm, quiet setting. Turn off the TV, radio, music, and other distractions.
- Include the person in conversations.
- Listen and give the person your full attention.
- Use short, simple sentences.

- Repeat what you are saying as needed.
- Write down key words as needed.
- Speak to the person in a normal, adult tone. Do not treat or talk to the person in a babyish or childlike way.
- Ask the person questions to which you know the answers. This helps you learn how the person speaks.
- Allow the person plenty of time to talk.
- Determine the topic being discussed. This helps you understand main points. Watch the person's lip movements.
- Watch facial expressions, gestures, and body language. They give clues about what is being said.
- Do not correct the person's speech.

Receptive aphasia (Wernicke aphasia) is difficulty understanding language. The person has trouble understanding what is said or read. The person may speak in long sentences that have no meaning. Because of difficulty understanding speech, the person may not be aware of the mistakes. People and common objects are not recognized. The person may not know how to use a fork, toilet, cup, TV, phone, or other items.

With *expressive aphasia*, the person has difficulty expressing or sending out thoughts. With *receptive aphasia*, the person has difficulty understanding language. Some people have both types. This is called *expressive-receptive aphasia (global aphasia, mixed aphasia)*. The person has problems speaking and understanding language.

The person has many emotional needs. Frustration, depression, and anger are common. Communication is needed to function and relate to others. The person wants to communicate but cannot. Be patient and kind.

EYE DISORDERS

Vision loss occurs at all ages. Problems range from mild loss to complete blindness. *Blindness* is the absence of sight. Vision loss is sudden or gradual. One or both eyes are affected.

Glaucoma

Glaucoma causes damage to the optic nerve. The eye produces a fluid that nourishes certain eye structures. The fluid normally drains from the eye. When the fluid cannot drain properly, it builds up in the eye, causing pressure on the optic nerve. The optic nerve is damaged. Vision loss with eventual blindness occurs.

Glaucoma can develop in one or both eyes. Onset is sudden or gradual. Peripheral vision (side vision) is lost. The person sees through a tunnel (Fig. 33.7), has blurred vision, and sees halos around lights. Severe eye pain, nausea, and vomiting occur with sudden onset.

Risk Factors

Glaucoma is a leading cause of vision loss in the United States. Persons at risk include the following:

- Blacks over 40 years of age
- Everyone over 60 years of age
- Those with a family history of the disease
- Those who have diabetes, high blood pressure, or heart disease
- Those who have eye diseases or eye injuries
- Those who have had eye surgery

Treatment

The damage caused by glaucoma cannot be reversed. Medications, surgery, and laser procedures can control glaucoma and prevent further damage to the optic nerve. Glaucoma is treated by lowering the pressure within the eye.

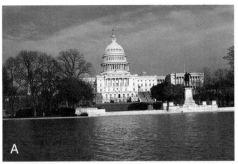
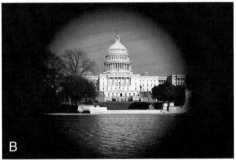
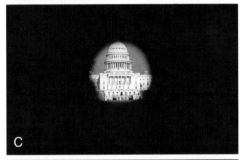
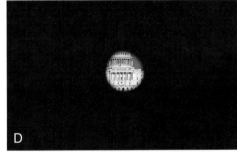

Fig. 33.7 Vision loss from glaucoma. (A) Normal vision. (B) Loss of peripheral vision begins. (C–E) Vision loss continues, with eventual blindness.

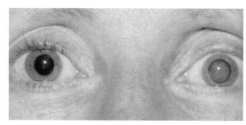

Fig. 33.8 One eye is normal. The other has a cataract. (From Swartz MH: *Textbook of physical diagnosis*, ed. 7, Philadelphia, 2014, Saunders.)

Cataracts

Cataract is a clouding of the lens (Fig. 33.8). The normal lens is clear. *Cataract* comes from the Greek word that means "waterfall." Trying to see is like looking through a waterfall. A cataract can occur in one or both eyes. Signs and symptoms include the following:

- Cloudy, blurry, or dimmed vision (Fig. 33.9)
- Colors seem faded; blues and purples are hard to see
- Sensitivity to light and glares
- Poor vision at night
- Halos around lights
- Double vision in the affected eye

Risk Factors

Most cataracts are caused by aging. By age 80, more than 50% of all Americans have a cataract or have had cataract surgery. Diabetes, smoking, alcohol use, and prolonged exposure to sunlight are risk factors. So is a family history of cataracts.

Treatment

Surgery is the only treatment. The lens is removed and a plastic lens is implanted. Surgery is done when the cataract starts to interfere with daily activities. Driving, reading, and watching TV are examples. Vision improves after surgery.

Postoperative care includes the following:

- Keep the eye shield in place as directed. The shield is worn for sleep, including naps.
- Follow measures for persons who are visually impaired or blind (p. ··) when an eye shield is worn. The person may have vision loss in the other eye.
- Remind the person not to rub or press the affected eye.
- Do not bump the eye.
- Place the overbed table and the bedside stand on the unoperative side.
- Place the call light within reach.
- Report eye drainage or complaints of pain at once.

Age-Related Macular Degeneration

Age-related macular degeneration (AMD) blurs central vision. *Central vision* is what you see "straight-ahead." AMD causes a blind spot in the center of vision (Fig. 33.10). Central vision is needed for reading, sewing, driving, and seeing faces and fine detail.

The disease damages the macula in the center of the retina. The retina receives light and sends messages to the brain through the optic nerve. Normal signals are not sent to the brain. Onset is gradual and painless. AMD is the leading cause of blindness in persons 60 years of age and older.

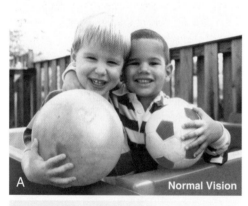

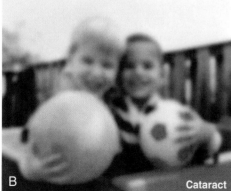

Fig. 33.9 Vision loss from a cataract. (A) Normal vision. (B) Scene viewed with a cataract. (From National Eye Institute: Cataract: what you should know, Bethesda, MD, National Institutes of Health.)

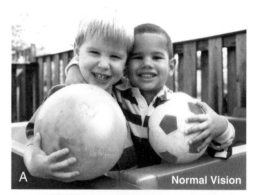

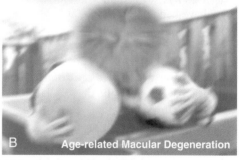

Fig. 33.10 Vision loss from macular degeneration. (A) Normal vision. (B) Central vision is blurred. (From National Eye Institute: Age-related macular degeneration: what you should know, Bethesda, MD, National Institutes of Health.)

The two types of AMD are:
- *Wet AMD*—Blood vessels behind the retina start to grow under the macula. The blood vessels leak blood and fluid. Loss of central vision occurs quickly. An early symptom is that straight lines appear wavy. Wet AMD is considered advanced. It is more severe than dry AMD.
- *Dry AMD*—Light-sensitive cells in the macula slowly break down. Central vision gradually blurs. As dry AMD gets worse, a blurred spot is seen in the center of the eye. Usually, both eyes are affected.

Dry AMD is more common than wet AMD. People who have wet AMD had dry AMD first. Dry AMD can suddenly turn into wet AMD.

Risk Factors

AMD can occur during middle age. However, the risk increases with aging. Besides age, risk factors include the following:
- Smoking
- Obesity
- Race; Whites are at greater risk than any other group
- Family history
- Gender; women are at greater risk than men
- Light-colored eyes
- Exposure to sunlight
- Cardiovascular disease; this includes high blood pressure, coronary artery disease, and stroke

Treatment

For advanced dry AMD, no treatment can prevent vision loss. For wet AMD, some treatments may stop or slow the disease progress. They may save what is left of central vision. Laser surgery is an example.

The following can reduce the risk of AMD:
- Eating a healthy diet high in green leafy vegetables and fish
- Not smoking
- Maintaining a normal blood pressure
- Managing cardiovascular diseases
- Maintaining a normal weight
- Exercising
- Wearing sunglasses
- Having regular eye exams

Diabetic Retinopathy

In diabetic retinopathy, the tiny blood vessels in the retina are damaged. A complication of diabetes, it is a leading cause of blindness. Usually, both eyes are affected.

Vision blurs (Fig. 33.11). The person may see spots "floating." Often, there are no early warning signs.

Risk Factors

Everyone with diabetes (Chapter 37) is at risk for diabetic retinopathy.

Treatment

The person needs to control diabetes, blood pressure, and blood cholesterol. Laser surgery may help. In another surgery, blood is removed from the center of the eye. The person may need low vision services.

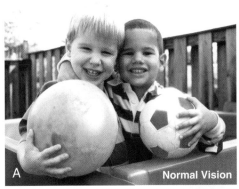
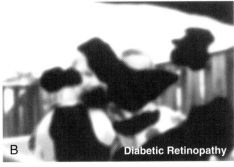

Fig. 33.11 Vision loss from diabetic retinopathy. (A) Normal vision. (B) Vision with diabetic retinopathy. (From National Eye Institute: Diabetic retinopathy: what you should know, Bethesda, MD, National Institutes of Health.)

Low Vision

Low vision is eyesight that cannot be corrected with eyeglasses, contact lenses, medications, or surgery. Reading, shopping, cooking, watching TV, writing, and other tasks are hard to do.

While wearing eyeglasses or contact lenses, the person has problems:
- Recognizing the faces of family and friends.
- Doing tasks that require close vision—reading, cooking, sewing, and so on.
- Picking out and matching the color of clothing.
- Reading signs.
- Doing things because lighting seems dimmer.

Risk Factors

Persons at risk for low vision have:
- Eye diseases.
- Glaucoma.
- Cataracts.
- Age-related macular degeneration.
- Diabetes.
- Eye injuries.
- Birth defects.

Treatment

The person learns to use one or more visual and adaptive devices. The devices used depend on the person's needs. Examples include the following:
- Prescription reading glasses
- Large-print reading materials

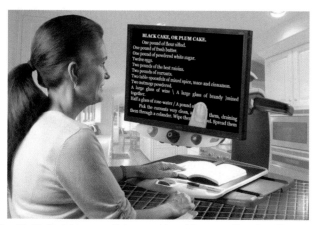

Fig. 33.12 A vision magnifying machine. (Courtesy Freedom Scientific, St. Petersburg, FL.)

- Magnifying aids for close vision
- Telescopic aids for far vision
- A black felt tip marker for writing
- Paper with bold lines for writing
- Audiotapes
- Electronic reading machines or vision magnifiers (Fig. 33.12)
- Computer systems using large print
- Computer systems that talk
- Smart speakers that can answer questions, play music, read books, etc.
- Smartphone applications that identify objects
- Closed-circuit TV
- Phones, clocks, and watches with large numbers
- Phones designed for people who have low vision, are visually impaired, or are blind
- Lighting that can be adjusted
- Dark-colored light switches and electrical outlets against light-colored walls
- Motion lights that turn on when the person enters a room

Impaired Vision and Blindness

Birth defects, accidents, and eye diseases are among the causes of impaired vision and blindness. They also are complications of some diseases. Some people are totally blind. Others sense some light but have no usable vision. Others have some usable vision but cannot read newsprint. The legally blind person sees at 20 feet what a person with normal vision sees at 200 feet. Box 33.3 lists signs and symptoms of vision problems.

According to the American Foundation for the Blind (AFB), about 1.3 million Americans are legally blind. According to AFB reports, about 6.2 million older persons (age 65 and older) are blind or visually impaired.

Loss of sight is serious. Adjustments can be hard and long. Special education and training are needed. Moving about, performing daily tasks, reading and writing, communicating with others, and using a guide dog are among the tasks the person needs to learn. All are needed for quality of life. The person may need some of the devices used for low vision. When caring for blind or visually impaired persons, follow the practices in Box 33.4.

See *Focus on Rehabilitation: Impaired Vision and Blindness.*

FOCUS ON REHABILITATION

Impaired Vision and Blindness

Rehabilitation programs help the person adjust to the vision loss and learn to be independent. The goal is for the person to be as active as possible and to have quality of life. The AFB describes these rehabilitation services:
- Counseling, to help with adjusting to the vision loss.
- Support groups. Members talk about their problems and how to cope.
- Training in home and personal skills. Preparing meals, personal care, managing money, and labeling medications are examples.
- Communication skills. This includes using large print, special computers, tape recorders, Braille, talking watches and clocks, and phones with large buttons.
- Movement and travel skills. How to orient oneself in new settings, asking for help, using a long cane, and using a guide dog are examples.

BOX 33.3   Signs and Symptoms of Vision Problems

The Person Complains of the Following:
- Halos or rings around lights
- Headaches with blurry vision
- Not being able to see at night
- Spots in front of the eyes
- Eyes hurting
- Seeing flashes of light
- Seeing double
- Things looking distorted
- Needing more light

You Observe the Person Doing the Following:
- Bumping into things
- Hesitating when moving
- Walking close to the wall

- Groping for objects
- Touching things in an uncertain way
- Squinting to see
- Tilting the head to see
- Asking for more or different lighting
- Holding books, newspapers, and so on close to the face
- Dropping food when eating
- Having trouble making out faces
- Having trouble reading signs
- Not seeing stains on clothing
- Wearing clothes that do not match
- Acting disoriented or confused in strange settings
- Tripping on rugs

Information from the American Foundation for the Blind: Understanding vision loss, 2010.

BOX 33.4 Caring for Blind and Visually Impaired Persons

The Environment

- Report worn carpeting and other flooring.
- Keep furniture, equipment, and electrical cords out of areas where the person will walk.
- Keep table and desk chairs pushed in under the table or desk.
- Keep doors fully open or fully closed. This includes room, closet, and cabinet doors.
- Keep drawers fully closed.
- Report burned-out lightbulbs in rooms, lounges, dining areas, hallways, stairways, and other areas.
- Provide lighting as the person prefers. Tell the person when the lights are on or off.
- Adjust window coverings to prevent glares. Sunny days and bright, snowy days cause glares.
- Provide a consistent mealtime setting.
  - Avoid plates, napkins, placemats, and tablecloths with patterns and designs. Use solid colors and provide contrast. For example, place a white plate on a dark placemat or tablecloth.
  - Have the person sit in good light above the table for mealtime.
  - Keep place settings the same. The knife and spoon are to the right of the plate. The fork and napkin are to the left of the plate. The glass or cup is to the right of the plate if the person is right-handed. It is to the left of the plate if the person is left-handed.
  - Arrange main dishes, side dishes, seasonings, and condiments in a straight line or in a semicircle just beyond the person's place setting. Arrange things in the same way for each meal.
  - Explain the location of food and beverages. Use the face of a clock (Chapter 20) or guide the person's hand to each item on the tray or place setting.
  - Cut meat, open containers, butter bread, and perform other tasks as needed.
- Keep the call light and TV, light, and other controls within the person's reach.
- Turn on nightlights in the person's room and bathroom and in hallways.
- Practice safety measures to prevent falls (Chapter 12).
- Orient the person to the room. Describe the layout. Also describe the location and purpose of furniture and equipment.
- Let the person move about. Let the person touch and find furniture and equipment.
- Do not rearrange furniture and equipment.
- Complete a safety check before leaving the room. (See the inside of the front cover.)

The Person

- Have the person use railings when climbing stairs.
- Make sure the person wears comfortable shoes that fit correctly.
- Assist with walking as needed. Offer to guide the person. Ask if the person would like help. Respect the person's answers. If your help is accepted:
  - Offer your arm. Tell the person which arm is offered. Tap the back of your hand against the person's hand.
  - Have the person hold on to your arm just above the elbow (Fig. 33.13). Do not grab the person's arm.
  - Walk at a normal pace. Walk one step ahead of the person. Stand next to the person at the top and bottom of stairs and when crossing streets.
  - Never push, pull, or guide the person in front of you.
  - Pause when changing direction, stepping up, and stepping down.
  - Tell the person about stairs, elevators, escalators, doors, turns, furniture, and other obstructions. State if steps are up or down.
  - Have the person hold on to a railing, the wall, or other strong surface if you need to leave the person's side. Tell the person that you are leaving and what to hold on to.
- Guide the person to a seat by placing your guiding arm on the seat. The person will move a hand down your arm to the seat.
- Let the person do as much for oneself as possible. Do not do things that the person can do. Cutting meat, seasoning food, getting dressed, and putting on shoes are examples.
- Assist the person to arrange clothes in the closet. Some suggest pinning a safety pin to distinguish colors. "The black pants have a safety pin, and the blue ones do not."
- Provide visual and adaptive devices. Follow the care plan.

You

- Identify yourself when you enter the room. Give your name, title, and reason for being there. Do not touch the person until you have indicated your presence.
- Ask how much the person can see. Do not assume the person is totally blind or that the person has some vision.
- Identify others. Explain where each person is located and what the person is doing.
- Offer to help. Simply say, "May I help you?" Respect the person's answer.
- Leave the person's belongings in the same place you found them. Do not move or rearrange things. If you have to move things, tell the person what you moved and where.

Communication

- Face the person when speaking. Speak slowly and clearly.
- Use a normal tone of voice. Do not shout or speak loudly. Vision loss does not mean the person has hearing loss.
- Address the person by name. This tells you are directing a comment or question to the person.
- Speak directly to the person. Do not just talk to family and friends who are present.
- Feel free to use words such as "see," "look," "read," or "watch TV." You also can use "blind" and "visually impaired."
- Feel free to refer to colors, sizes, shapes, patterns, designs, and so on.
- Describe people, places, and things thoroughly. Do not leave out a detail because you do not think it is important.
- Warn the person of dangers. Provide a calm and clear warning. You can say "wait" first. Then describe the danger. For example: "Wait, there is ice on the walk."
- Greet the person by name when the person enters a room. This alerts the person to your presence in the room. Tell the person who you are. Also identify others in the room.
- Listen to the person. Give the person verbal cues that you are listening. Say "Yes," "Okay," "I see," "Tell me more," "I don't understand," and so on.
- Answer the person's questions. Provide specific and descriptive responses.
- Give step-by-step explanations of procedures as you perform them. Say when the procedure is over.
- Give specific directions.
  - Say "right behind you," "on your left," or "in front of you." Avoid phrases such as "over here" or "over there."
  - Tell the distance. For example: "Three steps in front of you" or "At the end of the hallway by the nurses' station."
  - Give landmarks if possible. Sounds and scents can serve as "landmarks." "By the kitchen" is an example.
- Tell the person when you are leaving the room or the area. If appropriate, tell the person where you are going. For example: "I'm going to go into your bathroom now."
- Tell the person when you are ending a conversation. For example: "I enjoyed hearing about your children. Thank you for sharing stories with me."

Information from the American Foundation for the Blind: Understanding vision loss, 2010.

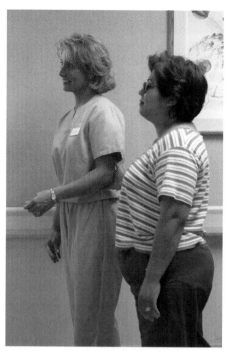

Fig. 33.13 The blind person walks slightly behind the nursing assistant. She touches the nursing assistant's arm lightly.

Braille

Braille is a touch reading and writing system that uses raised dots for each letter of the alphabet (Fig. 33.14). The first 10 letters also represent the numbers 0 through 9. Braille is read by moving the hands from left to right along each line of the "text" (Fig. 33.15).

Special devices allow computer access. A "Braille display" sits on a desk. Using Braille, the person reads information on the computer display. Certain printers allow computer information to be printed in Braille. Braille keyboards also are available.

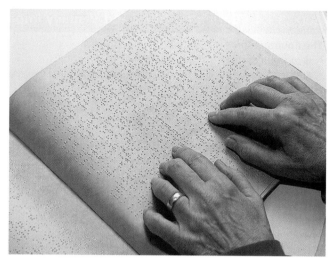

Fig. 33.15 Braille is read by moving the fingers from left to right across the lines.

Mobility

Blind and visually impaired persons learn to move about using a long cane with a red tip or using a guide dog. Both are used worldwide. The AFB describes them and measures to help as follows:

- Long canes are white or silver-gray. Some are one piece. Others fold or collapse for storage. To assist a person, announce your presence first. Ask if you can assist before trying to help. Do not interfere with the arm holding the cane. The person stores the cane. If you store it, tell the person where to find the cane.
- The guide dog sees for the person. The dog moves in response to the master's commands. Commands are disobeyed to avoid danger. For example, the master wants to cross the street. The guide dog disobeys the command if a car is approaching. Do not pet, feed, or distract a guide dog. Such actions can place the person in danger.

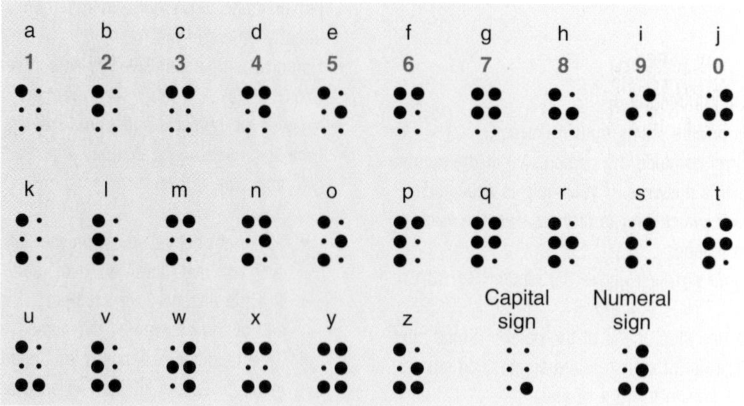

Fig. 33.14 Braille.

Corrective Lenses

Eyeglasses and contact lenses can correct many vision problems. Some people wear eyeglasses for reading or seeing at a distance. Others wear them for all activities. Contact lenses are usually worn while awake. Some contacts can be worn day and night for up to 30 days.

✴ Eyeglasses

Lenses are made of hardened glass or plastic. Clean them daily and as needed. Wash glass lenses with warm water. Dry them with a lens cloth or cotton cloth. Plastic lenses scratch easily. Use special cleaning solutions and cloths.

　See *Delegation Guidelines: Eyeglasses.*
　See *Promoting Safety and Comfort: Eyeglasses.*

📄 DELEGATION GUIDELINES

Eyeglasses

Cleaning eyeglasses is a routine care measure. Do not wait until the nurse tells you to clean them. Clean them daily and as needed.

　To clean eyeglasses, find out if you need a special cleaning solution. Then follow the manufacturer instructions.

👤 PROMOTING SAFETY AND COMFORT

Eyeglasses
Safety
Eyeglasses are costly. Protect them from loss or damage. When not worn, put them in their case. Place the case in the top drawer of the bedside stand.

✴ CARING FOR EYEGLASSES

Quality of Life
Remember to:
* Knock before entering the person's room.
* Address the person by name.
* Introduce yourself by name and title.
* Explain the procedure to the person before beginning and during the procedure.
* Protect the person's rights during the procedure.
* Handle the person gently during the procedure.

Preprocedure
1. Follow Delegation Guidelines: Eyeglasses. See *Promoting Safety and Comfort: Eyeglasses.*
2. Practice hand hygiene.
3. Collect the following:
   * Eyeglass case
   * Cleaning solution or warm water
   * Disposable lens cloth or cotton cloth

Procedure
4. Remove the eyeglasses.
   a. Hold the frames in front of the ears (Fig. 33.16A).

b. Lift the frames from the ears. Bring the eyeglasses down away from the face (see Fig. 33.16B).
5. Clean the lenses with cleaning solution or warm water. Clean in a circular motion. Dry the lenses with the cloth.
6. *If the person will not wear the eyeglasses:*
   a. Open the eyeglass case.
   b. Fold the glasses. Put them in the case. Do not touch the clean lenses.
   c. Place the case in the top drawer of the bedside stand.
7. *If the person wears the eyeglasses:*
   a. Unfold the eyeglasses.
   b. Hold the frames at each side. Place them over the ears.
   c. Adjust the eyeglasses so the nosepiece rests on the nose.
   d. Return the case to the top drawer in the bedside stand.

Postprocedure
8. Provide for comfort. (See the inside of the front cover.)
9. Place the call light within reach.
10. Return the cleaning solution to its proper place.
11. Discard the disposable cloth.
12. Complete a safety check of the room. (See the inside of the front cover.)
13. Decontaminate your hands.
14. Report and record your observations.

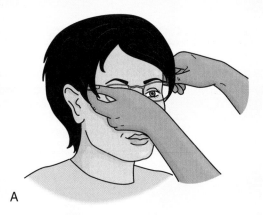 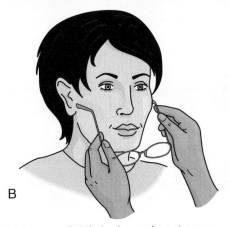

Fig. 33.16 Removing eyeglasses. (A) Hold the frames in front of the ears. (B) Lift the frames from the ears. Bring the glasses down away from the face.

Contact Lenses

Contact lenses fit on the eye. There are hard and soft contacts. Disposable ones are discarded daily, weekly, or monthly. Contacts are cleaned, removed, and stored according to the manufacturer instructions.

Report and record the following:

- Eye redness or irritation
- Eye drainage
- Complaints of eye pain, blurred or fuzzy vision, or uncomfortable lenses

See *Promoting Safety and Comfort: Contact Lenses.*

👤 PROMOTING SAFETY AND COMFORT

Contact Lenses
Safety

Some centers let nursing assistants remove and insert contact lenses. Others do not. Know your center's policy. If allowed to insert and remove contacts, follow the center's procedures.

Ocular Prosthesis

Removal of an eyeball is sometimes done because of injury or disease. The person is fitted with an ocular (eye) prosthesis (Fig. 33.17). This artificial eye does not provide vision. It matches the other eye in color and shape. The other eye may have normal, some, or no vision.

Some prostheses are permanent implants. Others are removable. If removable, the person is taught to remove, clean, and insert it.

Follow these measures if the prosthesis is not inserted after removal:

- Wash it with mild soap and warm water. Rinse well.
- Line a container with a soft cloth or 4 × 4 gauze. This prevents scratches and damage.

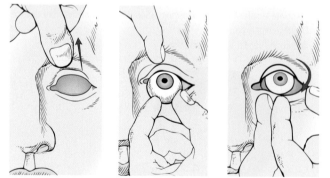

Fig. 33.17 An ocular prosthesis is inserted. (From Lewis SM, Heitkemper MM, Dirksen SR: *Medical-surgical nursing: assessment and management of clinical problems,* ed. 5, St. Louis, 2000, Mosby.)

- Fill the container with sterile water or saline (salt) solution.
- Place the eye in the container. Close the container.
- Label the container with the person's name and room and bed number.
- Place the labeled container in the top drawer of the bedside stand.
- Wash the eye socket with warm water or saline. Use a washcloth or gauze square. Remove excess moisture with a gauze square.
- Wash the eyelid and eyelashes with warm water. Clean from the inner to the outer aspect of the eye (Chapter 18). Dry the eyelid.
- Rinse the prosthesis with sterile water before the person inserts the eye.

See *Promoting Safety and Comfort: Ocular Prosthesis.*

👤 PROMOTING SAFETY AND COMFORT

Ocular Prosthesis
Safety

When an ocular prosthesis is removed, you must prevent chips and scratches. It must not fall on the floor or other hard surface. Always hold the eye over a towel or other soft surface.

The prosthesis is the person's property. Protect it from loss or damage.

👫 QUALITY OF LIFE

Hearing, speech, and vision problems can interfere with quality of life. Adjustment is often long and hard. The focus is on the person's abilities. The health team promotes independence to improve quality of life. The person is allowed to control own life to the extent possible. The person is encouraged to take part in the care planning process.

Provide a safe and secure setting (see Boxes 33.1, 33.2, and 33.4). Follow the person's care plan for specific safety measures. Always protect communication, hearing, and vision devices from loss or damage. This includes hearing aids, eyeglasses, and contact lenses.

Always treat the person with dignity and respect. Refer to the person first, then to the disability. Say "The person who is blind" rather than "the blind person." Do not pity the person. Treat the person like an adult, not like a child. Be patient, understanding, and sensitive to the person's needs and feelings.

❓ TIME TO REFLECT

Mr. Thomas has a severe hearing loss. He has been fitted for hearing aids in both ears. However, they do not seem to help him much. His son has brought a small white board and marker to his room for the staff to write messages on. This method of communication has worked until recently. Now Mr. Thomas's macular degeneration does not allow him to read the words on the white board. What are some methods of communication that you might try with Mr. Thomas?

REVIEW QUESTIONS

Circle the BEST answer.

1. A person with Meniere disease has
   a. A middle ear infection
   b. Vertigo
   c. A hearing aid to correct the problem
   d. A speech problem

2. Care of the person with Meniere disease includes preventing
   a. Infection
   b. Falls
   c. Pain
   d. Deafness

3. Which is *not* an obvious sign of hearing loss?
   a. Loneliness and boredom
   b. Speaking too loudly
   c. Asking to repeat things
   d. Answering questions poorly

4. You are talking to a person with hearing loss. You should do the following *except*
   a. Speak clearly, distinctly, and slowly
   b. Sit or stand in good light
   c. Shout
   d. Stand or sit on the side of the better ear

5. You are talking to a person with hearing loss. You can do the following *except*
   a. State the topic
   b. Change the subject if the person does not seem to understand
   c. Use short sentences and simple words
   d. Write out key words and names

6. A hearing aid
   a. Corrects a hearing problem
   b. Makes sounds louder
   c. Makes speech clearer
   d. Lowers background noise

7. A hearing aid does not seem to be working. Your *first* action is to
   a. See if it is turned on
   b. Wash it with soap and water
   c. Have it repaired
   d. Remove the batteries

8. A person has aphasia. You know that
   a. The person cannot use the muscles of speech
   b. Mouth and face muscles are affected
   c. The person has a language disorder
   d. The person cannot speak

9. A person with receptive aphasia has trouble
   a. Talking
   b. Writing
   c. Understanding messages
   d. Using gestures

10. A person has a speech disorder. You should do the following *except*
    a. Correct the person's speech
    b. Have the person write key words
    c. Ask the person to repeat or rephrase when necessary
    d. Watch lip movements

11. A person has a cataract. Which is *false*?
    a. Vision is cloudy, blurry, or dimmed
    b. Colors seem faded
    c. Central vision is lost
    d. The person is sensitive to light and glares

12. A person had cataract surgery. You should do the following *except*
    a. Follow measures for blind or visually impaired persons if an eye shield is worn
    b. Let the person rub the eye
    c. Place the overbed table on the unoperative side
    d. Have the person wear an eye shield during naps

13. A person has age-related macular degeneration. Which is *true*?
    a. There is a blind spot in the center of the eye
    b. Lost vision can be restored with surgery
    c. Peripheral (side) vision is lost
    d. Vision is blurry with spots

14. These statements are about low vision. Which is *false*?
    a. The person has usable vision
    b. Eyesight can be corrected
    c. The person needs visual or adaptive devices
    d. The person has problems doing things that require close vision

15. Who is at risk for low vision?
    a. The person with diabetic retinopathy
    b. The person with global aphasia
    c. The person with Meniere disease
    d. The person who is blind

16. Braille involves
    a. A long cane for walking
    b. Raised dots arranged for letters of the alphabet
    c. A guide dog
    d. Special computers and printers

17. Which are dangers to persons who are blind or visually impaired?
    a. Drawers that are fully closed
    b. Doors that are fully open
    c. Burnt-out bulbs
    d. Nightlights

18. A person is blind. The mealtime setting should
    a. Be the same for every meal
    b. Provide variety for mental stimulation
    c. Include plates, napkins, and placemats with designs
    d. Be arranged like the face of a clock

19. A person is blind. You should do the following *except*
    a. Identify yourself
    b. Move furniture to provide variety
    c. Explain procedures step-by-step
    d. Have the person walk behind you
20. You are talking to a person who is visually impaired. You should
    a. Face the person when talking
    b. Avoid words such as "see" and "look"
    c. Avoid using colors when describing things
    d. Assume that the person has no sight

21. A person is blind. To give directions you can say
    a. "Over there"
    b. "Right here"
    c. "Across the room"
    d. "On your left"
22. When eyeglasses are not worn they should be
    a. Soaked in a cleansing solution
    b. Kept within the person's reach
    c. Put in the eyeglass case
    d. Placed on the overbed table

See Appendix A for answers to these questions.

34

Cancer, Immune System, and Skin Disorders

OBJECTIVES

- Define the key terms and key abbreviations listed in this chapter.
- Explain the difference between benign tumors and cancer.
- Identify cancer risk factors.
- Identify the signs and symptoms of cancer.
- Explain the common cancer treatments.
- Describe the needs of a person with cancer.
- Explain how immune system disorders occur.
- Describe the common immune system disorders.

- Explain how the human immunodeficiency virus (HIV) is spread.
- Identify the signs and symptoms of acquired immunodeficiency syndrome (AIDS).
- Explain how to assist in the care of persons with AIDS.
- Describe the causes, signs and symptoms, and treatment of shingles.
- Explain how to promote quality of life.

KEY TERMS

autoimmune disorder A condition where the body attacks itself

benign tumor A tumor that does not spread to other body parts; it can grow to a large size

cancer See "malignant tumor"

malignant tumor A tumor that invades and destroys nearby tissue; it can spread to other body parts; cancer

metastasis The spread of cancer to other body parts

port An implanted device in the body that allows medications or fluids to be given into a vein; blood can also be withdrawn if needed

stem cells Cells with the potential to develop into many different types of cells in the body

stomatitis Inflammation (*-itis*) of the mouth (*stomat-*)

tumor A new growth of abnormal cells; tumors are benign or malignant

KEY ABBREVIATIONS

AIDS Acquired immunodeficiency syndrome
HIV Human immunodeficiency virus

IV Intravenous

Understanding cancer, the immune system, and skin disorders gives meaning to the required care. Refer to Chapter 8 while you study this chapter.

CANCER

Cells reproduce for tissue growth and repair. Cells divide in an orderly way. Sometimes cell division and growth are out of control. A mass or clump of cells develops. This new growth of abnormal cells is called a tumor. Tumors are benign or malignant (Fig. 34.1).

- Benign tumors do not spread to other body parts. They can grow to a large size but rarely threaten life. They usually do not grow back when removed.
- Malignant tumors (cancer) invade and destroy nearby tissue (Fig. 34.2). They can spread to other body parts. They may be life threatening. Sometimes they grow back after removal. Metastasis is the spread of cancer to other body parts (Fig. 34.3). Cancer cells break off the tumor and travel to other

body parts. New tumors grow in other body parts. This occurs if cancer is not treated and controlled.

Cancer can occur almost anywhere. Common sites are the skin, lung and bronchus, colon and rectum, breast, prostate, uterus, ovary, urinary bladder, kidney, mouth and pharynx, pancreas, and thyroid gland. Cancer is the second leading cause of death in the United States.

Risk Factors

Certain factors increase the risk of cancer. The National Cancer Institute describes these risk factors:

- *Growing older.* Cancer occurs in all age groups. However, most cancers occur in persons over 65 years of age.
- *Tobacco.* This includes using tobacco (smoking, snuff, and chewing tobacco) and being around tobacco (secondhand smoke). This risk can be avoided.
- *Sunlight.* Sun, sunlamps, and tanning booths cause early aging of the skin and skin damage. These can lead to skin cancer. Limit time in the sun. Avoid sunlamps and tanning booths.

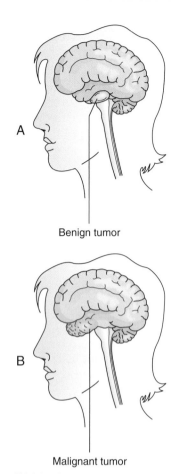

Benign tumor

Malignant tumor

Fig. 34.1 Tumors. (A) A benign tumor grows within a local area. (B) A malignant tumor invades other tissues.

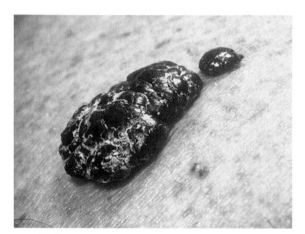

Fig. 34.2 Malignant tumor on the skin. (From Belcher AE: *Cancer nursing*, St. Louis, 1992, Mosby.)

- *Ionizing radiation.* This can cause cell damage that leads to cancer. Sources are x-rays and radon gas that forms in the soil and some rocks. Miners are at risk for radon exposure. Radon is found in some homes. Radioactive fallout is another source. It can come from nuclear power plant accidents and from the production, testing, or use of atomic weapons.

- *Certain chemicals and other substances.* Painters, construction workers, and those in the chemical industry are at risk. Household substances also carry risks—paint, pesticides, used engine oil, and other chemicals.
- *Some viruses and bacteria.* Certain viruses increase the risk of these cancers—cervical, liver, lymphoma, leukemia, Kaposi sarcoma (a cancer associated with acquired immunodeficiency syndrome [AIDS], p. ··), stomach.
- *Certain hormones.* Hormone replacement therapy for menopause may increase the risk of breast cancer. Some pregnant women received diethylstilbestrol (DES), a form of estrogen, between the early 1940s and 1971. They are at risk for breast cancer. Their daughters are at risk for a certain type of cervical cancer.
- *Family history of cancer.* Certain cancers tend to occur in families. They include melanoma and cancers of the breast, ovary, prostate, and colon.
- *Alcohol.* More than two drinks a day increases the risk of certain cancers. Such cancers are of the mouth, throat, esophagus, larynx, liver, and breast. Women should have only one drink a day. Men should have only two drinks a day.
- *Poor diet, lack of physical activity, and being overweight.* A high-fat diet increases the risk of cancers of the colon, uterus, and prostate. Lack of physical activity and being overweight increase the risk for cancers of the breast, colon, esophagus, kidney, and uterus.

Treatment

If detected early, cancer may be treated or controlled (Box 34.1). Treatment depends on the tumor type, its site and size, and if it has spread. The treatment goal may be to:
- Cure the cancer.
- Control the disease.
- Reduce symptoms for as long as possible.

Some cancers respond to one type of treatment. Others respond best to two or more types. Cancer treatments also damage healthy cells and tissues. Side effects depend on the type and extent of the treatment.

Surgery

Surgery removes tumors. It is done to cure or control cancer or to relieve pain from advanced cancer.

Postoperative pain is controlled with pain-relief medications. The person may feel weak or tired for a while.

Radiation Therapy

Radiation therapy *(radiotherapy)* kills cells. X-ray beams are aimed at the tumor. Sometimes radioactive material is implanted in or near the tumor.

Cancer cells and normal cells receive radiation. Both are destroyed. Radiation therapy:
- Destroys certain tumors.
- Shrinks a tumor before surgery.
- Destroys cancer cells that remain after surgery.
- Controls tumor growth to prevent or relieve pain.

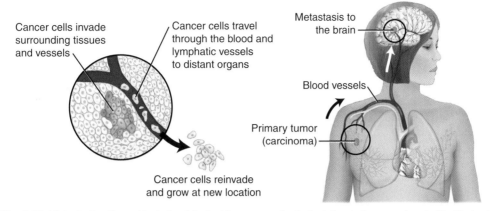

Cancer cells invade surrounding tissues and vessels

Cancer cells travel through the blood and lymphatic vessels to distant organs

Metastasis to the brain

Blood vessels

Primary tumor (carcinoma)

Cancer cells reinvade and grow at new location

Fig. 34.3 Metastasis. (From *Exploring Medical Language: A student-directed approach*, ed. 11, St. Louis, 2022, Elsevier.)

BOX 34.1 Possible Warning Signs of Cancer

- Changes in bowel or bladder habits
- Chronic coughing; trouble breathing
- Chronic headache
- Difficulty swallowing
- Frequent fevers or infections
- Hoarseness
- Lump or area of thickening that can be felt under the skin
- Pain that lasts
- Persistent fatigue
- Persistent indigestion or discomfort after eating
- Skin changes, such as yellowing, darkening or redness of the skin, sores that won't heal, or changes to existing moles
- Unexplained bleeding; excessive bruising
- Unexplained weight loss or gain

Data from Mayo Clinic, Patient Care & Health Information: Cancer, 2023, https://www.mayoclinic.org/diseases-conditions/cancer/symptoms-causes/syc-20370588; and University of California San Francisco Health, 17 Cancer Symptoms You Shouldn't Ignore, 2021. The Regents of The University of California, https://www.ucsfhealth.org/en/covid/17-cancer-symptoms-you-shouldnt-ignore.

Burns, skin breakdown, and hair loss can occur at the treatment site. The doctor may order special skin care measures. Extra rest is needed for fatigue. Discomfort, nausea, vomiting, diarrhea, and loss of appetite *(anorexia)* are other side effects.

Chemotherapy

Chemotherapy involves medications that kill cells. The medications may be taken orally or given intravenously. Sometimes the doctor creates a port, an implanted device in the body that allows medications or fluids to be given into a vein (Fig. 34.4). Blood may also be drawn from the port for testing. The port may be covered with a dressing while it is healing and needs to be kept dry. After it has healed, the person is allowed to get the port wet and to shower. The port should always be kept clean. Any signs of redness or swelling should be reported to the nurse immediately. If the person complains of pain or burning at the

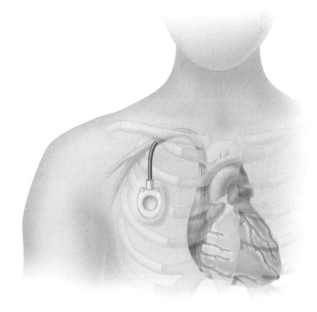

Fig. 34.4 An implanted port. (From Ignatavicius DD, Workman ML: *Medical-surgical nursing, patient-centered collaborative care*, ed. 7, St. Louis, 2013, Elsevier.)

site of the port, also report this to the nurse. When chemotherapy is completed, the port is removed.

Chemotherapy is used to:
- Shrink a tumor before surgery.
- Kill cells that break off the tumor; the goal is to prevent metastasis.
- Relieve symptoms caused by the cancer.

Cancer cells and normal cells are affected. Side effects depend on the medication used:
- Hair loss *(alopecia)*.
- Gastrointestinal irritation. Poor appetite, nausea, vomiting, and diarrhea can occur. Stomatitis, an inflammation *(itis)* of the mouth *(stomat)*, may occur.
- Decreased blood cell production. Bleeding and infection are risks. The person may feel weak and tired.

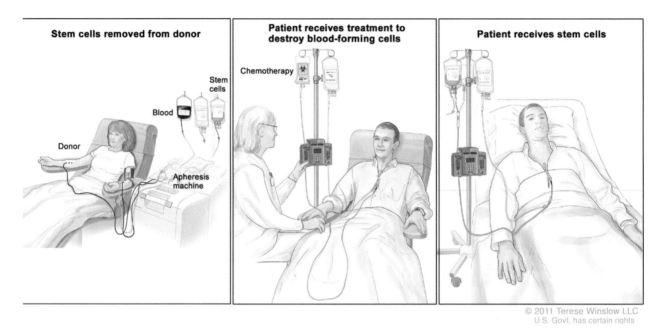

Stem cells removed from donor

Stem cells

Blood

Donor

Apheresis machine

Patient receives treatment to destroy blood-forming cells

Chemotherapy

Patient receives stem cells

© 2011 Terese Winslow LLC
U.S. Govt. has certain rights

Fig. 34.5 Stem cell transplant. (From National Cancer Institute.)

Stem Cell Transplants

When some cancer patients have high doses of chemotherapy or radiation, their blood cells may be destroyed. Stem cell transplants are procedures that restore blood-forming stem cells. Stem cells are cells with the potential to develop into many different types of cells in the body. The stem cells can come from the patient or a donor. Stem cells that are used in transplants may come from the bloodstream, bone marrow, or umbilical cord blood (Fig. 34.5).

Stem cell transplants may be most beneficial for these types of cancer:

- Leukemia
- Lymphoma
- Neuroblastoma
- Multiple myeloma

There can be side effects to stem cell transplants. The person must be protected from infections and abnormal bleeding. Rejection can also be a complication. It can be a long process and the person's immune system needs to recover and become restored.

Hormone Therapy

Hormone therapy prevents cancer cells from getting or using hormones needed for their growth. Medications are given that prevent the production of certain hormones. Organs or glands that produce a certain hormone are removed. For example, the ovaries are removed if a breast cancer needs estrogen for growth. A prostate cancer may need testosterone for growth. The testicles may be removed.

Side effects include fatigue, fluid retention, weight gain, hot flashes, nausea, vomiting, appetite changes, and blood clots. Fertility is affected in men and women. Men may experience impotence (Chapter 10) and loss of sexual desire.

Immunotherapy or Biologic Therapy

Biologic therapy (*immunotherapy*) helps the immune system fight the cancer. It also protects the body from the side effects of cancer treatments.

Side effects include flulike symptoms—chills, fever, muscle aches, weakness, loss of appetite, nausea, vomiting, and diarrhea. Bleeding, bruising, swelling, and skin rashes may occur.

The Person's Needs

Persons with cancer have many needs. These include the following:

- Pain relief or control
- Rest and exercise
- Fluids and nutrition
- Preventing skin breakdown
- Preventing bowel problems (constipation from pain-relief medications; diarrhea from some cancer treatments)
- Dealing with treatment side effects
- Psychologic and social needs
- Spiritual needs
- Sexual needs

Psychologic and social needs are great. Anger, fear, and depression are common. Some surgeries are disfiguring. The person may feel unwhole, unattractive, or unclean. The person and family need support.

Talk to the person. Do not avoid the person because you are uncomfortable. Cancer is not contagious. Listen and use touch to show that you care. Often, the person needs to talk and have someone listen. Being there when needed is important. You may not have to say anything. Just listen.

Spiritual needs are important. A spiritual leader may provide comfort. To many people, spiritual needs are just as important as physical needs.

Persons dying of cancer often receive hospice care (Chapters 1 and 45). Support is given to the person and family.

IMMUNE SYSTEM DISORDERS

The immune system protects the body from microbes, cancer cells, and other harmful substances. It defends against threats both inside and outside the body.

Immune system disorders occur from problems with the immune response. The response may be inappropriate, too strong, or lacking. Autoimmune disorders can occur. The immune system can attack the body's own *(auto)* normal cells, tissues, or organs. One of the following may occur:

- One or more types of body tissues are destroyed
- An organ grows abnormally
- There is a change in how an organ functions
The organs and tissues commonly affected are:
- Red blood cells.
- Blood vessels.
- Connective tissue.
- The endocrine glands (thyroid gland, pancreas).
- Muscles.
- Joints.
- Skin.

Signs and symptoms depend on the type of disease. Fatigue, dizziness, not feeling well, and fever are common.

There are over 80 known types of autoimmune disorders. Some common autoimmune disorders include the following:

- Celiac disease—a disease in which the body cannot tolerate gluten (found in wheat, rye, and barley) (Chapter 20)
- Graves disease—the most common form of hyperthyroidism. The immune system attacks the thyroid gland. The thyroid gland produces excess *(hyper)* amounts of the hormone thyroxine. Signs and symptoms include anxiety, problems sleeping, rapid heart rate, weight loss, and bulging of the eyeballs (Fig. 34.6).
- Lupus—an inflammatory disease affecting the blood cells, joints, skin, kidneys, lungs, heart, or brain. Lupus comes from the Latin word for "wolf." It was thought that the lupus rash looked like a wolf bite (Fig. 34.7).

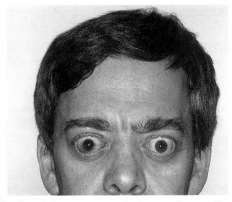

Fig. 34.6 Bulging of the eyes occurs in Graves disease. (From Belchetz PE, Hammond P: *Diabetes and endocrinology*, London, 2003, Mosby.)

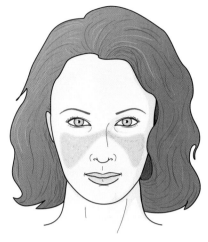

Fig. 34.7 The rash from lupus is across the nose and cheeks. (Redrawn from National Institute of Arthritis and Musculoskeletal and Skin Diseases: *Do I have lupus?* Bethesda, MD, 2009, National Institutes of Health.)

- Multiple sclerosis (Chapter 35)
- Rheumatoid arthritis (Chapter 35)
- Scleroderma—a disease causing abnormal growth of connective tissue in the skin and blood vessels
- Type 1 diabetes (Chapter 37)
- Vitiligo—a condition where the immune system destroys the cells that give skin its color

Most autoimmune disorders are chronic. Treatment depends on the disorder and the tissues and organs affected. Treatment is aimed at:

- Reducing symptoms.
- Controlling the autoimmune response.
- Maintaining the body's ability to fight disease.

Acquired Immunodeficiency Syndrome

Acquired immunodeficiency syndrome (AIDS) is caused by a virus. The virus is called *the human immunodeficiency virus (HIV)*. It attacks the immune system. Therefore, it destroys the body's ability to fight infections and certain cancers. Some infections are life threatening.

The virus is spread through body fluids—blood, semen, vaginal secretions, and breast milk. HIV is not spread by saliva, tears, sweat, sneezing, coughing, insects, or casual contact. The virus is transmitted mainly by:

- Unprotected anal, vaginal, or oral sex with an infected person; "unprotected" means without a new latex or polyurethane condom.
- Needle and syringe sharing among intravenous (IV) drug users.
- HIV-infected mothers before or during childbirth.
- HIV-infected mothers through breastfeeding.

The virus enters the bloodstream through the rectum, vagina, penis, mouth, or skin breaks. Small breaks in the vagina or rectum may occur when the penis, finger, or other objects are inserted. Gum disease can cause breaks in the gums. The virus can enter the bloodstream through these mucous

---

BOX 34.2 Signs and Symptoms of AIDS

- Appetite: loss of
- Cough
- Depression
- Diarrhea lasting more than 1 week
- Energy: lack of
- Fever
- Headache
- Memory loss, confusion, and forgetfulness
- Mouth or tongue:
  - Brown, red, pink, or purple spots or blotches
  - Sores or white patches
- Night sweats
- Pneumonia
- Shortness of breath
- Skin:
  - Rashes or flaky skin
  - Brown, red, pink, or purple spots or blotches on the skin, eyelids, or nose
- Swallowing: painful or difficult
- Swollen glands: neck, underarms, and groin
- Tiredness: may be extreme
- Vision loss
- Weight loss

BOX 34.3 Caring for the Person with AIDS

- Practice Standard Precautions.
- Follow the Bloodborne Pathogen Standard.
- Provide daily hygiene. Avoid irritating soaps.
- Provide oral hygiene according to the care plan. A toothbrush with soft bristles is best.
- Provide oral fluids as ordered.
- Measure and record intake and output.
- Measure weight daily.
- Encourage deep-breathing and coughing exercises as ordered.
- Prevent pressure ulcers.
- Assist with range-of-motion exercises and ambulation as ordered.
- Encourage self-care as able. The person may need assist devices (walker, commode, eating devices).
- Encourage the person to be as active as possible.
- Change linens and garments as often as needed when fever or night sweats are present.
- Be a good listener. Provide emotional support.

---

membrane breaks (mouth, vagina, rectum). Breaks in the skin pose a risk. The virus can enter the bloodstream when infected body fluids come in contact with open skin areas. Babies can become infected during pregnancy, shortly after birth, or from breastfeeding.

The virus is carried in contaminated blood left in needles or syringes. When the devices are shared, contaminated blood enters the bloodstream. Needlesticks are a threat to the health team.

The virus is very fragile. It cannot live outside the body. HIV is not spread by casual, everyday contact. Such contact includes using public telephones, restrooms, swimming pools, hot tubs, or water fountains. Other forms of casual contact include talking to, hugging, or dancing with an infected person. HIV is not transmitted through food prepared by the infected person.

Box 34.2 lists the signs and symptoms of AIDS. Some HIV-infected persons have symptoms within a few months. Others are symptom-free for more than 10 years. However, they carry the virus. They can spread it to others.

The person with AIDS can develop other health problems. The immune system is damaged. Pneumonia, tuberculosis, Kaposi sarcoma (a cancer), and nervous system damage are risks. Memory loss, loss of coordination, paralysis, mental health disorders, and dementia signal nervous system damage.

Many new medications help slow the spread of HIV in the body. They also reduce complications and prolong life. AIDS has no vaccine at present. Bone marrow (stem cell) transplants are showing some success for persons with AIDS. It is a life-threatening disease.

You may care for persons with AIDS or persons who are HIV carriers (Box 34.3). You may have contact with the person's blood or body fluids. Protect yourself and others from the virus. Follow Standard Precautions and the Bloodborne Pathogen Standard. A person may have HIV but no symptoms. In some persons, HIV or AIDS is not yet diagnosed.

Persons age 45 years and older are at risk. When people think of HIV or AIDS, older persons are often the last to come to mind. However, older people are at increasing risk for HIV and AIDS. People age 50 years and older represent almost one-fourth of all people with HIV or AIDS in the United States. Many factors contribute to the increasing risk of infection in older people. Older persons get and spread HIV through sexual contact and IV drug use. Many do not consider themselves to be at risk. Older persons tend to be less informed about the disease. They tend not to practice safe sex. Older persons are less likely than younger people to talk about their sex lives or drug use with their doctors. Aging and some diseases can mask the signs and symptoms of AIDS. Older persons are less likely to be tested for HIV and AIDS. Often, the person dies without the disease being diagnosed. A blood transfusion between 1978 and 1985 increases the HIV risk. You must follow Standard Precautions and the Bloodborne Pathogen Standard.

SKIN DISORDERS

There are many types of skin disorders. Alopecia, hirsutism, dandruff, lice, and scabies are discussed in Chapter 19. Skin tears and pressure injuries are discussed in Chapters 31 and 32. Burns are discussed in Chapter 44. Shingles, psoriasis, and eczema are discussed here.

Shingles

Shingles (herpes zoster) is caused by the same virus that causes chickenpox. The virus lies *dormant (inactive)* in nerve tissue. The virus can become active years later.

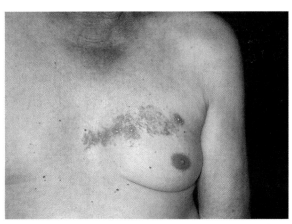

Fig. 34.8 Shingles. (Courtesy Department of Dermatology, School of Medicine, University of Utah, Salt Lake City, UT. From McCance KL, Huether SE: *Pathophysiology: the biologic basis for disease in adults and children*, ed. 6, St. Louis, 2010, Mosby.)

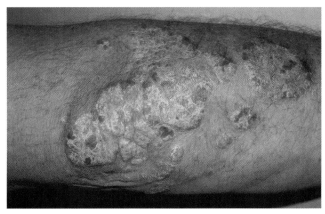

Fig. 34.9 Psoriasis. (From Lookingbill D, Marks J: *Principles of dermatology*, ed. 4, Philadelphia, 2006, Saunders.)

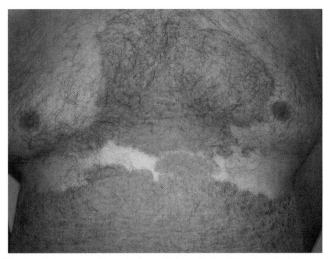

Fig. 34.10 Eczema. (From Ralston SH et al.: *Davidson's principles and practice of medicine*, ed. 23, Oxford, UK, 2018, Elsevier Ltd.)

A rash or blisters occur on the skin. At first there is burning or tingling pain, numbness, or itching. This occurs in an area on one side of the body or one side of the face. After a few days or a week, a rash with fluid-filled blisters appears (Fig. 34.8). Pain is mild to intense. Itching is a common complaint.

Shingles is most common in persons over 50 years of age. Persons who have had chickenpox are at risk. So are persons with weakened immune systems from HIV infection, cancer treatments, transplant surgeries, and stress. Persons who have shingles cannot transmit shingles to another person. Persons who have not had chickenpox, however, can be at risk if they come in contact with someone who currently has shingles.

The doctor orders antiviral and pain-relief medications. For some people, cool moist cloths offer relief. For many healthy people, blisters heal and pain is gone in 3 to 5 weeks. A vaccine is now available to help prevent shingles or lessen the complications that come with shingles.

Psoriasis

The American Academy of Dermatology defines psoriasis as a chronic disease that develops when a person's immune system sends faulty signals that tell skin cells to grow too quickly. New skin cells form in days rather than weeks. The body does not shed the excess skin cells. The cells pile up on the skin causing patches to appear (Fig. 34.9). The condition is not contagious. The person who has the patches, however, can be very self-conscious and want to cover the area. Treatment for psoriasis consists of creams, oral medication, and sometimes phototherapy (light therapy).

Eczema

Eczema (also called *contact dermatitis*) is a condition that consists of itchy, rough, inflamed patches on the skin (Fig. 34.10). The intense itching sensation often causes the person to scratch. This makes the areas bleed and ooze drainage. There is no known cause for eczema. Certain foods may trigger symptoms. Environmental factors such as smoke and pollen can also be triggers for eczema. Like psoriasis, eczema is not contagious. It is often present in persons who have asthma. Treatment includes keeping the skin moisturized, prescription creams, avoiding harsh fabrics, taking lukewarm baths, using mild soaps, and keeping fingernails cut short.

QUALITY OF LIFE

Any illness changes affect the family. This is especially true of cancer. Unlike a cold or the flu, the person with cancer may have health problems for a long time. Cancer treatments require hospital stays and medical and clinical appointments. The same is true for AIDS and some immune system disorders. Short-term or long-term nursing center care may be needed. Persons with skin conditions are often very self-conscience of their image. They are afraid people will feel they can "catch" a skin disease from them.

The person and family have many reactions. Fear, anger, worry, and guilt are common. Good communication skills are important. Sometimes all you have to do is listen.

Remember to protect the person's rights. Privacy, confidentiality, and personal choice are very important. Also meet the person's basic needs to the best of your ability.

TIME TO REFLECT

Mr. Logan is an 85-year-old male who lives at the nursing center where you work. He has been having chemotherapy treatments for lung cancer at the outpatient clinic. Three days a week, Mr. Logan's daughter arrives at the center to take him for his chemotherapy sessions. This morning, as you come to his room to help him get ready for his appointment, he tells you he feels an intense itching and pain on his side. He lifts up his pajama shirt to show you a reddened rash in a line on the right side of his chest. What may have caused this rash? How do you proceed from here? What are some likely measures that will be taken to help Mr. Logan? Do other residents and staff need to be protected?

REVIEW QUESTIONS

Circle the BEST answer.

1. A person has cancer. You know that
   a. The tumor will not threaten life
   b. The tumor can spread to other body parts
   c. The tumor is benign
   d. The person's mouth is inflamed

2. Who has the greatest risk for cancer?
   a. The person who smokes
   b. The person who is physically active
   c. The person who limits time in the sun
   d. The person who is 40 years old

3. Which is *not* a warning sign of cancer?
   a. Painful, swollen joints
   b. A sore that does not heal
   c. Unusual bleeding or discharge
   d. Discomfort after eating

4. A person had surgery for cancer. The person's care will likely include
   a. Pain-relief measures
   b. Mouth care for stomatitis
   c. Skin care for burns at the treatment site
   d. Measures to prevent hair loss

5. Which of the following side effects might a person receiving chemotherapy experience?
   a. Skin breakdown
   b. Burns
   c. Diarrhea
   d. Weight gain

6. Mrs. Jones has cancer. She is telling you about her treatments and how she feels. What should you do?
   a. Listen
   b. Change the subject
   c. Call for the nurse
   d. Ask about her feelings

7. HIV is spread through
   a. Coughing and sneezing
   b. Body fluids
   c. Using public telephones and restrooms
   d. Hugging or dancing with an infected person

8. HIV can enter the bloodstream in the following ways *except*
   a. Through gum disease
   b. Through the rectum, vagina, penis, mouth, or skin breaks
   c. Through needle-sharing
   d. Through swimming pools and hot tubs used by infected persons

9. Which of the following is used to prevent the spread of HIV and AIDS?
   a. Isolation precautions
   b. Radiation therapy
   c. Chemotherapy
   d. Standard Precautions

10. A person has shingles. You will likely assist the nurse with measures to
    a. Prevent diarrhea
    b. Relieve pain
    c. Prevent skin breakdown
    d. Prevent weight loss

11. A person has psoriasis. Which is *false*?
    a. It can be very painful
    b. The person is contagious
    c. Creams may be applied by the nurse
    d. Light therapy may be used to treat it

12. Which is *not* an example of an autoimmune disorder?
    a. Celiac disease
    b. Graves disease
    c. Osteoporosis
    d. Scleroderma

See Appendix A for answers to these questions.

35

Nervous System and Musculoskeletal Disorders

OBJECTIVES

- Define the key terms and key abbreviations listed in this chapter.
- Describe stroke and the care required.
- Describe Parkinson disease and the care required.
- Describe multiple sclerosis and the care required.
- Describe amyotrophic lateral sclerosis and the care required.
- Describe traumatic brain injury and spinal cord injury and the care required.
- Describe autonomic dysreflexia and the care required.

- Describe arthritis and the care required.
- Explain how to assist in the care of persons after total joint replacement surgery.
- Describe the care required for osteoporosis.
- Explain how to assist in the care of persons in casts, in traction, and with hip pinnings.
- Describe the effects of amputation.
- Explain how to promote quality of life.

KEY TERMS

amputation The removal of all or part of an extremity
arthritis Joint (*arthr-*) inflammation (*-itis*)
arthroplasty The surgical replacement (*-plasty*) of a joint (*arthr-*)
closed fracture The bone is broken but the skin is intact; simple fracture
compound fracture See "open fracture"
fracture A broken bone
gangrene A condition in which there is death of tissue

hemiplegia Paralysis (*-plegia*) on one side (*hemi-*) of the body
open fracture The broken bone has come through the skin; compound fracture
paralysis Loss of motor function, loss of sensation, or both
paraplegia Paralysis in the legs and trunk
quadriplegia Paralysis in the arms, legs, and trunk; tetraplegia
simple fracture See "closed fracture"
tetraplegia See "quadriplegia"

KEY ABBREVIATIONS

ADL   Activities of daily living
AKA   Above-the-knee amputation
ALS   Amyotrophic lateral sclerosis
BKA   Below-the-knee amputation
CVA   Cerebrovascular accident
EMS   Emergency Medical Services

FAST   Facial drooping, Arm weakness, Speech difficulty, Time to call EMS
MS   Multiple sclerosis
RA   Rheumatoid arthritis
ROM   Range of motion
TBI   Traumatic brain injury
TIA   Transient ischemic attack

Understanding disorders of the nervous and musculoskeletal systems gives meaning to the required care. Refer to Chapter 8 while you study this chapter.

NERVOUS SYSTEM DISORDERS

Nervous system disorders can affect mental and physical function. They can affect the ability to speak, understand, feel, see, hear, touch, think, control bowels and bladder, and move.

Stroke

Stroke is a disease affecting the arteries that supply blood to the brain. It also is called a *brain attack* or *cerebrovascular accident (CVA)*. It occurs when one of the following happens:

- A blood vessel in the brain bursts. Bleeding occurs in the brain (cerebral hemorrhage).
- A blood clot blocks blood flow to the brain.

Brain cells in the affected area do not get enough oxygen and nutrients. Brain cells die. Brain damage occurs. Functions controlled by that part of the brain are lost (Fig. 35.1).

Stroke is the third leading cause of death in the United States. It is a leading cause of disability in adults. Box 35.1 provides warning signs. The person needs emergency care. Blood flow to the brain must be restored as soon as possible.

Sometimes warning signs last a few minutes. This is called a *transient ischemic attack (TIA)*. (*Transient* means "temporary or short term." *Ischemic* means "to hold back [*ischein*] blood [*hemic*]."") Blood supply to the brain is interrupted for a short

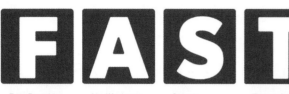

Face Drooping   Arm Weakness   Speech   Time to Call 9-1-1

DOES ONE SIDE OF THE FACE DROOP OR IS IT NUMB?
Ask the person to smile. Is the person's smile uneven?

IS ONE ARM WEAK OR NUMB?
Ask the person to raise both arms. Does one arm drift downward?

IS SPEECH SLURRED? Is the person unable to speak or hard to understand? Ask the person to repeat a simple sentence, like "The sky is blue."

Check the time so you'll know when the first symptoms appeared.

Fig. 35.1 *FAST:* Facial drooping, *Arm* weakness, *Speech* difficulty, *Time* to call EMS. (From the National Stroke Association. Copyright 2020 National Stroke Association, All Rights Reserved.)

BOX 35.1   Warning Signs of Stroke

- Sudden numbness or weakness of the face, arm, or leg, especially on one side of the body
- Sudden confusion, trouble speaking, or understanding speech
- Sudden trouble seeing in one or both eyes
- Sudden trouble walking, dizziness, loss of balance or coordination
- Sudden severe headache with no known cause

From National Institute for Neurological Disorders and Stroke: *What you need to know about stroke,* NIH Publication No. 04-5517, Bethesda, MD, updated May 16, 2017, National Institutes of Health.

---

time. Sometimes a TIA occurs before a stroke. All strokelike symptoms signal the need for emergency care.

Risk Factors

There are several risk factors for stroke. Some can be controlled, others cannot.

- *Age.* Older persons are at greater risk than younger persons.
- *Family history.* The risk increases if a parent, sister, or brother had a stroke.
- *Gender.* Both men and women are affected.
- *Race.* Blacks are at greater risk than other groups because they have high rates of hypertension and diabetes.
- *Hypertension (high blood pressure).* This damages and weakens blood vessels. Clots can form or arteries can burst.
- *Heart disease.* Heart diseases can increase the risk of stroke. They include heart failure, heart attack, valve diseases, abnormal heart rhythm, and atherosclerosis (Chapter 36).
- *Smoking.* Blood vessels are damaged. The nicotine in cigarettes makes the heart work harder, increases the heart rate, and raises blood pressure. The amount of oxygen in the blood decreases.
- *Diabetes.* Blood vessels are damaged. The person is at risk for high blood pressure and blood clots.
- *High blood cholesterol.* Fatty materials build up on the walls of the artery and block blood flow.

- *Obesity.* The overweight person is at risk for high blood pressure, heart disease, diabetes, and high blood cholesterol.
- *Previous stroke or TIA.* Persons who had a stroke or a TIA are at great risk.

Signs and Symptoms

Stroke can occur suddenly. The person may have warning signs (see Box 35.1). The person also may have nausea, vomiting, and memory loss. Unconsciousness, noisy breathing, high blood pressure, slow pulse, redness of the face, and seizures may occur. So can hemiplegia—paralysis (*plegia*) on one side (*hemi*) of the body. The person may lose bowel and bladder control and the ability to speak. (See "Aphasia" in Chapter 33.) The acronym *FAST* is helpful in recognizing a possible stroke. It stands for *facial* drooping, *arm* weakness, *speech* difficulties, *time* to call emergency medical services (EMS) (see Fig. 35.1).

Effects on the Person

If the person survives, some brain damage is likely. Functions lost depend on the area of the brain damaged (Fig. 35.2). The effects of stroke include the following:

- Loss of face, hand, arm, leg, or body control
- Hemiplegia
- Changing emotions (crying easily or mood swings, sometimes for no reason)
- Difficulty swallowing (dysphagia)
- Aphasia or slowed or slurred speech (Chapter 33)
- Changes in sight, touch, movement, and thought
- Impaired memory
- Urinary frequency, urgency, or incontinence
- Loss of bowel control or constipation
- Depression and frustration

Behavior changes occur. The person may forget about or ignore the weaker side. This is called *neglect.* It is from the loss of vision or movement and feeling on that side. Sometimes thinking is affected. The person may not recognize or know how to use common items. Activities of daily living (ADL) and other tasks are hard to do. The person may forget what to do and how to do it. If the person does know, the body may not respond.

Rehabilitation starts at once. The person may depend in part or totally on others for care. The health team helps the person regain the highest possible level of function (Box 35.2).

Parkinson Disease

Parkinson disease is a slow, progressive disorder with no cure. The area of the brain controlling muscle movement is affected. Persons over the age of 50 are at risk. Signs and symptoms become worse over time (Fig. 35.3). These include the following:

- *Tremors*—often start in one finger and spread to the whole arm. Pill-rolling movements—rubbing the thumb and index finger—may occur. The person may have trembling in the hands, arms, legs, jaw, and face.

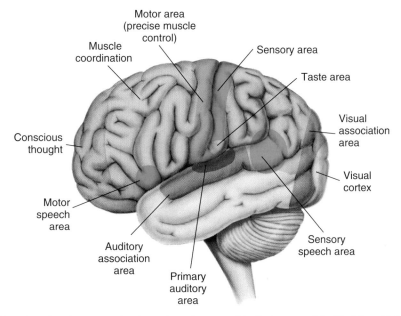

Fig. 35.2 Functions lost from a stroke depend on the area of brain damage. (Modified from Thibodeau GA, Patton KT: *Structure and function of the body,* ed 14, St Louis, 2012, Mosby.)

BOX 35.2   Care of the Person With a Stroke

- Position the person in the lateral (side-lying) position to prevent aspiration.
- Keep the bed in semi-Fowler position.
- Approach the person from the strong (unaffected) side. Place objects on the strong (unaffected) side. The person may have loss of vision on the affected side.
- Turn and reposition the person at least every 2 hours.
- Use assist devices to move, turn, reposition, and transfer the person.
- Encourage incentive spirometry and deep breathing and coughing.
- Prevent contractures.
- Meet food and fluid needs. The person may need a dysphagia diet (Chapter 20).
- Apply compression stockings to prevent thrombi (blood clots) in the legs.
- Assist with range-of-motion (ROM) exercises to prevent contractures. They also strengthen affected extremities.
- Meet elimination needs.
  - The person has a catheter or bladder training program.
  - A bowel training program is started if needed.
- Practice safety precautions.
  - Keep the call light within reach. It is on the person's strong (unaffected) side.
  - Check the person often if he or she cannot use the call light. Follow the care plan.
  - Use bed rails according to the care plan.
  - Prevent falls.
- Have the person do as much self-care as possible. This includes turning, positioning, and transferring. The person uses assist, self-help, and ambulation aids as needed.
- Follow established communication methods (Chapters 4 and 33).
- Give support, encouragement, and praise.
- Complete a safety check before leaving the room. (See the inside of the front cover.)

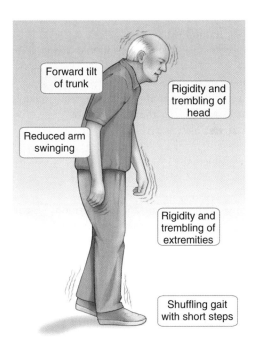

Fig. 35.3 Signs of Parkinson disease. (From Patton KT, Thibodeau GA: *The human body in health & disease,* ed 6, St Louis, 2014, Mosby.)

- *Rigid, stiff muscles*—in the arms, legs, neck, and trunk.
- *Slow movements*—the person has a slow, shuffling gait.
- *Stooped posture and impaired balance*—it is hard to walk. Falls are a risk.
- *Masklike expression*—the person cannot blink and smile. A fixed stare is common.

Other signs and symptoms develop over time. They include swallowing and chewing problems, constipation, and bladder problems. Sleep problems, depression, and emotional changes (fear, insecurity) can occur, as can memory loss and slow thinking. The person may have slurred, monotone, and soft speech. Some people talk too fast or repeat what they say.

Medications are ordered to treat and control the disease. Exercise and physical therapy are ordered to improve strength, posture, balance, and mobility. Therapy is needed for speech and swallowing problems. The person may need help with eating and self-care. Normal elimination is a goal. Safety measures are needed to prevent falls and injury.

Multiple Sclerosis

Multiple sclerosis (MS) is a chronic disease. (*Multiple* means "many"; *sclerosis* means "hardening or scarring.") The myelin (which covers nerve fibers) in the brain and spinal cord is destroyed. Nerve impulses are not sent to and from the brain in the normal way. Functions are impaired or lost. There is no cure.

Symptoms often start between the ages of 20 and 40. More women are affected than men. Whites are at greater risk than other groups. A person's risk increases if a family member has MS.

Signs and symptoms depend on the damaged area. These may include the following:

- Vision problems—blurred or double vision, blindness in one eye
- Numbness or weakness in the arms and legs
- Balance problems that affect standing and walking
- Tingling, prickling, or numb sensations
- Partial or complete paralysis
- Pain
- Speech problems
- Tremors
- Dizziness
- Problems with concentration, attention, memory, and judgment
- Depression
- Bowel and bladder problems
- Problems with sexual function
- Hearing loss
- Fatigue
- Coordination problems and clumsiness
  MS can present as follows:
- *Relapsing-remitting.* Symptoms last for a few weeks or a few months. They gradually disappear with partial or total recovery. That is, symptoms *remit* or the person is in *remission*. Later, symptoms flare up again *(relapse).*
- *Primary-progressive.* The person's condition gradually declines with more and more symptoms. There are no remissions.
- *Secondary-progressive.* Symptoms relapse and remit. More symptoms occur with each flare-up. The person's condition declines.

- *Progressive relapsing.* The person's condition gradually declines. Flare-ups occur, leaving new symptoms and more damage.

The person is kept active and independent for as long as possible. The care plan reflects the person's changing needs. Skin care, hygiene, and range-of-motion (ROM) exercises are important. So are turning, positioning, and deep breathing and coughing. Bowel and bladder elimination are promoted. Injuries and complications from bedrest are prevented.

Amyotrophic Lateral Sclerosis

Amyotrophic lateral sclerosis (ALS) attacks the nerve cells that control voluntary muscles. Commonly called *Lou Gehrig disease,* it is rapidly progressive and fatal. (Lou Gehrig was a New York Yankees baseball player. He died of the disease in 1941.)

ALS usually strikes between 40 and 60 years of age. The person usually dies 3 to 5 years after onset. Some survive for 10 or more years.

Motor nerve cells in the brain, brainstem, and spinal cord degenerate or die. They stop sending messages to the muscles. Muscles weaken, waste away (atrophy), and twitch. Over time, the brain cannot start voluntary movements or control them. The person cannot move the arms, legs, and body. Muscles for speaking, chewing, swallowing, and breathing also are affected. Eventually muscles in the chest wall fail. The person needs a ventilator for breathing (Chapter 26). The disease usually does not affect the mind or memory. Sight, smell, taste, hearing, and touch are not affected. Usually bowel and bladder functions remain intact.

ALS has no cure. Medications may slow disease progression. Damage cannot be reversed. The person is kept active and independent for as long as possible. The care plan reflects the person's changing needs. The care plan may include:

- Physical, occupational, and speech-language therapies.
- ROM exercises.
- Braces, a walker, or a wheelchair for mobility.
- Measures to relieve pain and promote comfort.
- Communication methods.
- Dysphagia diet or feeding tube.
- Suctioning to remove excess fluids and saliva.
- Mechanical ventilation.
- Safety measures to prevent falls and injuries.
- Psychologic and social support.
- Hospice care.

Traumatic Brain Injury

Head injuries result from trauma to the scalp, skull, or brain. Some injuries are minor and do not need health care. Or the person only needs emergency care.

Traumatic brain injury (TBI) occurs when a sudden trauma damages the brain. Brain tissue is bruised or torn. Bleeding is in the brain or in nearby tissues. Spinal cord injuries are likely. Motor vehicle crashes, falls, and firearms are common causes. So are assaults and sports and recreation injuries.

Death can occur at the time of injury or later. If the person survives TBI, some permanent damage is likely. Disabilities depend on the severity and site of the injury. They include:

- Cognitive problems—thinking, memory, reasoning.
- Sensory problems—sight, hearing, touch, taste, smell.
- Communication problems—expressing or understanding language.
- Behavior or mental health problems—depression, anxiety, personality changes, aggressive behavior, socially inappropriate behavior.
- Stupor—an unresponsive state; the person can be briefly aroused.
- Coma—the person is unconscious, does not respond, is unaware, and cannot be aroused.
- Vegetative state—the person is unconscious and unaware of surroundings; the person has sleep-wake cycles and alert periods.
- Persistent vegetative state (PVS)—being in a vegetative state for more than 1 month.

Rehabilitation is required. Physical, occupational, speech-language, and mental health therapies are ordered depending on the person's needs. Nursing care depends on the person's needs and remaining abilities.

Spinal Cord Injury

Spinal cord injuries can permanently damage the nervous system. Paralysis (loss of motor function, loss of sensation, or both) can result. Young adult men have the highest risk. Common causes are stab or gunshot wounds, motor vehicle crashes, falls, and sports injuries.

Problems depend on the amount of damage to the spinal cord and the level of injury. Damage may be:

- *Incomplete*—the spinal cord can send messages to and from the brain. The person has some sensory (feeling) and motor (movement) function below the level of the injury.
- *Complete*—the spinal cord cannot send messages to and from the brain. The person has no sensory or motor function below the level of the injury.

The higher the level of injury, the more functions lost (Fig. 35.4).

- *Lumbar injuries*—sensory and muscle functions in the legs are lost. Paraplegia is paralysis in the legs and trunk. (*Para* means "beside or beyond"; *plegia* means "paralysis.")
- *Thoracic injuries*—sensory and muscle function below the chest is lost. The person has paraplegia.
- *Cervical injuries*—sensory and muscle functions of the arms, legs, and trunk are lost. Paralysis in the arms, legs, and trunk is called quadriplegia or tetraplegia. (*Quad* and *tetra* mean "four.")

Cervical traction may be needed (p. 543). Cervical traction requires a special bed to keep the spine straight at all times. Box 35.3 provides care measures. Emotional needs require attention. Reactions to paralysis and loss of function are often severe.

If the person survives, rehabilitation is necessary. See *Focus on Rehabilitation: Spinal Cord Injury.*

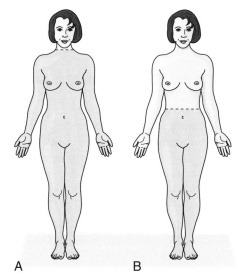

Fig. 35.4 The shaded areas show the area of paralysis. (A) Quadriplegia (tetraplegia). (B) Paraplegia.

BOX 35.3 Care of Persons With Paralysis

- Prevent falls. Follow the care plan for safety measures and bed rail use.
- Keep the bed in the low position.
- Keep the call light within reach. If unable to use the call light, check the person often.
- Prevent burns. Check bath water, heat applications, and food for proper temperature.
- Turn and reposition the person at least every 2 hours. Follow the care plan.
- Prevent pressure injuries. Follow the care plan.
- Maintain good alignment at all times. Use supportive devices according to the care plan.
- Follow bowel and bladder training programs.
- Keep intake and output records.
- Maintain muscle function and prevent contractures. Assist with ROM exercises.
- Assist with food and fluids as needed. Provide self-help devices as ordered.
- Give emotional and psychologic support.
- Follow the person's rehabilitation plan.
- Complete a safety check of the room. (See the inside of the front cover.)

FOCUS ON REHABILITATION

Spinal Cord Injury

Some rehabilitation centers focus on spinal cord injuries. The person learns to function at the highest possible level. The person learns to use self-help, assist, and other devices.

Some persons return home and live independently. Others need nursing center care, home care, or assisted-living settings.

Autonomic Dysreflexia

This syndrome affects persons with spinal cord injuries above the midthoracic level. There is uncontrolled stimulation of the sympathetic nervous system (Chapter 8). If untreated, stroke, heart attack, and death are risks. Report any of these signs and symptoms to the nurse at once:

- High blood pressure
- Throbbing or pounding headache
- Bradycardia—heart rate less than 60 beats per minute
- Blurred vision
- Sweating above the level of injury
- Flushing, reddening of the skin above the level of injury
- Cold, clammy skin below the level of injury
- "Goose bumps" *(piloerection)* below the level of injury
- Nasal congestion or stuffiness
- Nausea
- Anxiety

PROMOTING SAFETY AND COMFORT

Autonomic Dysreflexia
Safety
Constipation and fecal impaction can cause autonomic dysreflexia, as can checking for an impaction and enemas. Do not perform these procedures if the person is at risk for autonomic dysreflexia. Such procedures are best done by a nurse.

The head of the bed is raised 45 degrees or the person sits upright if allowed. The identified cause is removed.

The most common causes are a full bladder, constipation or fecal impaction, and skin disorders. The measures in Box 35.4 are part of the person's care plan.

See *Promoting Safety and Comfort: Autonomic Dysreflexia.*

MUSCULOSKELETAL DISORDERS

Musculoskeletal disorders affect movement. ADL, social activities, and quality of life are affected. Injury and age-related changes are common causes.

Arthritis

Arthritis means joint *(arthr)* inflammation *(itis)*. It is the most common joint disease. Pain, swelling, and stiffness occur in the affected joints. Joints are hard to move.

BOX 35.4 Preventing Autonomic Dysreflexia

- Monitor urinary output.
- Follow measures for the person with an indwelling catheter. See Box 22.3 (Chapter 22). Do not let the drainage bag get too full.
- Prevent urinary tract infections.
- Promote bowel elimination. Prevent constipation and fecal impaction.
- Prevent pressure injuries.
- Prevent skin injuries—skin tears, cuts, bruises, blisters, and so on.
- Check the person's feet for ingrown toenails, blisters, pressure injuries, and so on. Report any problems to the nurse.
- Prevent burns. This includes burns from hot water.
- Have the person wear clothing that is loose and comfortable. Avoid tight clothing.
- Make sure the person does not sit or lie on wrinkled clothing or linens.
- Reposition the person at least every 2 hours. Avoid prolonged pressure from the bed or chair.
- Report menstrual cramps to the nurse.

Osteoarthritis (Degenerative Joint Disease)

This is the most common type of arthritis. Aging, being overweight, and joint injury are causes. Stress, muscle weakness, and heredity are other causes. The fingers, spine (neck and lower back), and weight-bearing joints (hips, knees, and feet) are often affected (Fig. 35.5).

Signs and symptoms include joint stiffness, pain, swelling, and tenderness. Joint stiffness occurs with rest and lack of motion. Pain occurs with weight-bearing and joint motion. Or pain can be constant or occur from lack of motion. Pain can affect rest, sleep, and mobility. Swelling is common after using the joint. Cold weather and dampness seem to increase symptoms.

There is no cure. Treatment involves:

- *Pain relief.* Medications help to decrease swelling and inflammation and relieve pain.
- *Heat and cold applications.* Heat relieves pain, increases blood flow to the part, and reduces swelling. Heat applications and warm baths or showers are helpful. So is water therapy in a heated pool. Sometimes cold applications are used after joint use.
- *Exercise.* Exercise decreases pain, increases flexibility, and improves blood flow. It helps with weight control and promotes fitness. Mental well-being improves. The person is taught what exercises to do.
- *Rest and joint care.* Good body mechanics, posture, and regular rest protect the joints. Relaxation methods are helpful. Canes and walkers provide support. Splints support weak joints and keep them in alignment. Adaptive and self-help devices for hands and wrists are useful for ADL. See Chapters 20 and 42.
- *Weight control.* Weight loss reduces stress and injury on weight-bearing joints.
- *Healthy lifestyle.* Arthritis support programs can help the person develop a healthy outlook. Abilities and strengths are stressed. The focus is on fitness, exercise, rest, managing stress, and good nutrition.

Falls are prevented. Help is given with ADL as needed. Toilet seat risers are helpful when hips and knees are affected. So are

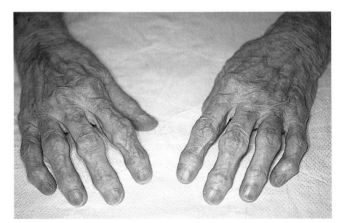

Fig. 35.5 Bony growths called Heberden nodes occur in the finger joints. (From Swartz MH: *Textbook of physical diagnosis*, ed 7, Philadelphia, 2014, Saunders.)

chairs with higher seats and armrests. Some people need joint replacement surgery.

Rheumatoid Arthritis

Rheumatoid arthritis (RA) is a chronic inflammatory disease. It causes joint pain, swelling, stiffness, and loss of function. More common in women than in men, it generally develops between the ages of 20 and 50.

RA occurs on both sides of the body. For example, if the right wrist is involved, so is the left wrist. The wrist and finger joints closest to the hand are often affected (Fig. 35.6). Other joints affected are the neck, shoulders, elbows, hips, knees, ankles, and feet. Joints are tender, warm, and swollen. Fatigue and fever are common. The person does not feel well. Symptoms may last for several years.

Other body parts may be affected. Decreased red blood cell production and dry eyes and mouth are common. Inflammation of the linings of the heart, blood vessels, and lungs can occur but is rare.

RA varies from person to person. Some people have flare-ups and then feel better. In others, the disease is active most of the time.

Treatment goals are to:
- Relieve pain.
- Reduce inflammation.
- Slow down or stop joint damage.
- Improve well-being and function.
The person's care plan may include:
- *Rest balanced with exercise.* More rest is needed when RA is active. More exercise is needed when it is not. Short rest periods during the day are better than long times in bed. The doctor and physical therapist prescribe an exercise program. ROM exercises are included. Exercise helps maintain healthy and strong muscles, joint mobility, and flexibility. Exercise also promotes sleep, reduces pain, and helps weight control.
- *Proper positioning.* Prevent contractures and deformities. Bed-boards, a bed cradle, trochanter rolls, and pillows are used.
- *Joint care.* Good body mechanics and body alignment, wrist and hand splints, and self-help devices for ADL reduce stress on the joints. Walking aids may be needed.

- *Weight control.* Excess weight places stress on the weight-bearing joints. Exercise and a healthy diet help control weight.
- *Measures to reduce stress.* Relaxation, distraction, and regular rest help reduce stress, as does exercise.
- *Measures to prevent falls.* See Chapter 12.

Medications are given for pain relief and to reduce inflammation. Heat and cold applications may be ordered. Some persons need joint replacement surgery.

Emotional support is needed. A good outlook is important. Persons with RA need to stay as active as possible. The more they can do for themselves, the better off they are. Give encouragement and praise. Listen when the person needs to talk.

Total Joint Replacement Surgery

Arthroplasty is the surgical replacement *(plasty)* of a joint *(arthro)*. The damaged joint is removed and replaced with an artificial joint—a prosthesis (Fig. 35.7).

Hip and knee replacements are the most common (Box 35.5). Ankle, foot, shoulder, elbow, and finger joints also can be replaced. The surgery can relieve pain, restore, or preserve joint function, or correct a deformed joint.

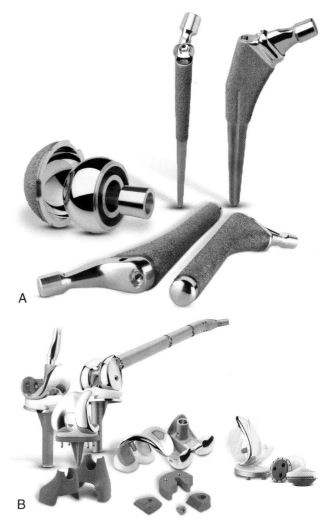

A

B

Fig. 35.7 (A) Hip replacement prosthesis and hip replacement prosthesis stems. (B) Knee replacement prosthesis. (Courtesy Zimmer, Inc., a Bristol-Meyers Squibb Co., Warsaw, IN.)

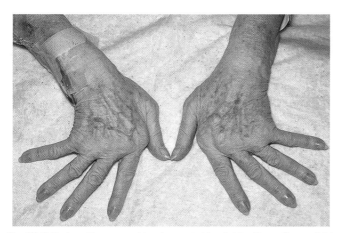

Fig. 35.6 Deformities caused by rheumatoid arthritis. (From Swartz MH: *Textbook of physical diagnosis,* ed 7, Philadelphia, 2014, Saunders.)

BOX 35.5 Care of the Person After Total Joint Replacement Surgery—Hip and Knee

- Incentive spirometry and deep-breathing and coughing exercises to prevent respiratory complications.
- Compression stockings to prevent thrombi (blood clots) in the legs.
- Exercises to strengthen the hip or knee. These are taught by a physical therapist.
- Measures to protect the hip as shown in Fig. 35.8.
- Food and fluids for tissue healing and to restore strength.

- Safety measures to prevent falls.
- Measures to prevent infection. Wound, urinary tract, and skin infections must be prevented.
- Measures to prevent pressure injuries.
- Assist devices for moving, turning, repositioning, and transfers.
- Assistance with walking and a walking aid. The person may need a cane, walker, or crutches.

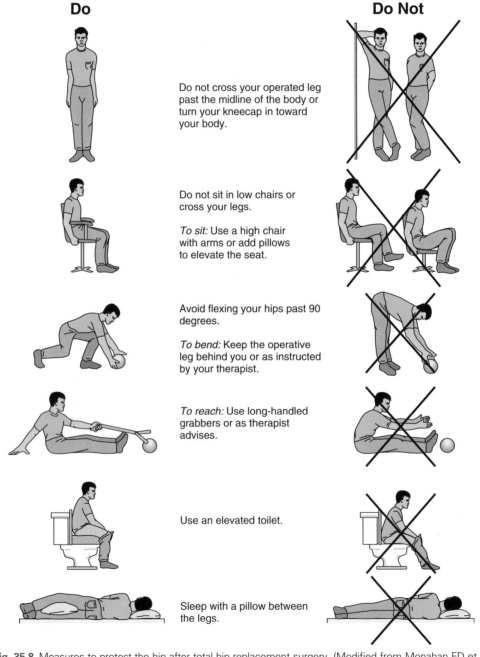

Do   **Do Not**

Do not cross your operated leg past the midline of the body or turn your kneecap in toward your body.

Do not sit in low chairs or cross your legs.

To sit: Use a high chair with arms or add pillows to elevate the seat.

Avoid flexing your hips past 90 degrees.

To bend: Keep the operative leg behind you or as instructed by your therapist.

To reach: Use long-handled grabbers or as therapist advises.

Use an elevated toilet.

Sleep with a pillow between the legs.

Fig. 35.8 Measures to protect the hip after total hip replacement surgery. (Modified from Monahan FD et al: *Phipps' medical-surgical nursing: health and illness perspectives,* ed 8, St Louis, 2007, Mosby.)

Osteoporosis

With osteoporosis, the bone *(osteo)* becomes porous and brittle *(porosis)*. Bones are fragile and break easily. Spine, hip, wrist, and rib fractures are common. Older men and women are at risk. The risk for women increases after menopause. The ovaries do not produce estrogen after menopause. The lack of estrogen causes bone changes, as do low levels of dietary calcium.

All ethnic groups are at risk. A family history of the disease, being thin or having a small frame, eating disorders, tobacco use, alcoholism, lack of exercise, bedrest, and immobility are risk factors. Exercise and activity are needed for bone strength. To form properly, bone must bear weight. If not, calcium leaves the bone. The bone becomes porous and brittle.

Back pain, gradual loss of height, and stooped posture occur. Fractures are a major threat. Even slight activity can cause fractures. They can occur from turning in bed, getting up from a chair, or coughing. Fractures are great risks from falls and accidents.

Prevention is important. Doctors often order calcium and vitamin supplements. Estrogen is ordered for some women. Other preventive measures include the following:

- Exercising weight-bearing joints—walking, jogging, stair climbing
- Strength-training (lifting weights)
- No smoking
- Limiting alcohol and caffeine
- Back supports or corsets if needed for good posture
- Walking aids if needed
- Safety measures to prevent falls and accidents
- Good body mechanics
- Safe handling, moving, transfer, and turning and positioning procedures

Fractures

A fracture is a broken bone. Tissues around the fracture—muscles, blood vessels, nerves, and tendons—are injured. Fractures are open or closed (Fig. 35.9).

- Closed fracture (simple fracture). The bone is broken but the skin is intact.
- Open fracture (compound fracture). The broken bone has come through the skin.
- Falls and accidents are causes. Bone tumors, metastatic cancer, and osteoporosis are other causes. Signs and symptoms of a fracture are the following:

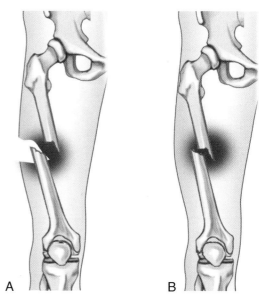

Fig. 35.9 (A) Open fracture. (B) Closed fracture. (From Patton KT, Thibodeau GA: *The human body in health & disease*, ed 6, St Louis, 2014, Mosby.)

- Pain
- Swelling
- Loss of function
- Limited or no movement of the part
- Movement where motion should not occur
- Deformity (the part is in an abnormal position)
- Bruising and skin color changes at the fracture site
- Bleeding (internal or external)

For healing, bone ends are brought into and held in normal position. This is called *reduction* and *fixation*.

- *Closed reduction and external fixation.* The bone is moved back into place. The bone is not exposed.
- *Open reduction and internal fixation.* This requires surgery. The bone is exposed and moved into alignment. Nails, rods, pins, screws, plates, or wires keep the bone in place (Fig. 35.10).

After reduction, movement of the bone ends is prevented. This is done with a cast or traction. Other devices—splints, walking boots, external fixators—also are used (Fig. 35.11).

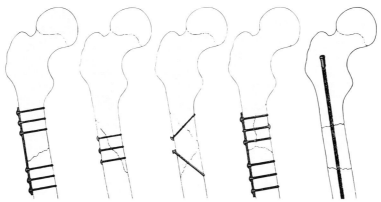

Fig. 35.10 Devices used for open reduction of a fracture. (From Beare PG, Meyers JL: *Adult health nursing*, ed 3, St Louis, 1998, Mosby.)

Casts

Casts are made of plaster of Paris, plastic, or fiberglass (Fig. 35.12). Before casting, the skin is protected with stockinette or cotton padding. Moistened cast rolls are wrapped around the part. Plastic and fiberglass casts dry quickly. A plaster of Paris cast dries in 24 to 48 hours. It is odorless, white, and shiny when dry. A wet cast is gray and cool and has a musty smell. Assist with care as directed (Box 35.6).

Traction

Traction reduces and immobilizes fractures. A steady pull from two directions keeps the bone in place. Traction also is used for muscle spasms and to correct deformities or contractures. Weights, ropes, and pulleys are used (Fig. 35.15). Traction is applied to the neck, arms, legs, or pelvis.

Skin traction is applied to the skin. Boots, wraps, tape, or splints are used. Weights are attached to the device (Fig. 35.15). *Skeletal traction* is applied to the bone. Wires or pins are inserted through the bone (Fig. 35.16). For cervical traction,

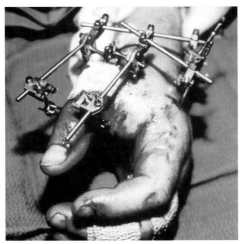

Fig. 35.11 External fixator. (From Lewis SM et al: *Medical-surgical nursing: assessment and management of clinical problems,* ed 9, St Louis, 2014, Mosby.)

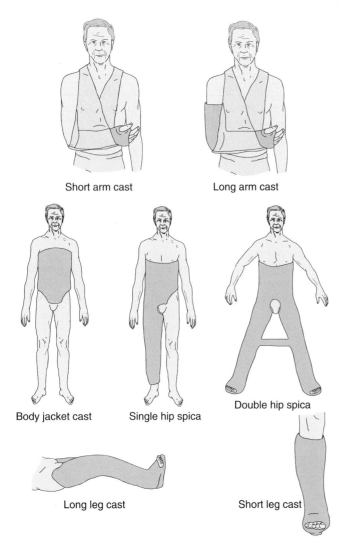

Short arm cast   Long arm cast

Body jacket cast   Single hip spica   Double hip spica

Long leg cast   Short leg cast

Fig. 35.12 Common casts.

BOX 35.6 Rules for Cast Care

- Do not cover the cast with blankets, plastic, or other material. A cast gives off heat as it dries. Covers prevent the escape of heat. Burns can occur if heat cannot escape.
- Turn the person every 2 hours or as directed by the nurse and the care plan. All cast surfaces need exposure to air. Turning promotes even drying.
- Do not place a wet cast on a hard surface. It flattens the cast. The cast must keep its shape. Use pillows to support the entire length of the cast (Fig. 35.13).
- Support the wet cast with your palms when turning and positioning the person (Fig. 35.14). Fingertips can dent the cast. The dents can cause pressure areas that lead to skin breakdown.
- Report rough cast edges. The nurse needs to cover the cast edges with tape.
- Keep the cast dry. A wet cast loses its shape. Some casts are near the perineal area. The nurse may apply a waterproof material around the perineal area after the cast dries.
- Do not let the person insert anything into the cast. Itching under the cast causes an intense desire to scratch. Items used for scratching (pencils, coat hangers, knitting needles, back scratchers, and so on) can open the skin. Infection is a risk. Scratching items can wrinkle the stockinette or cotton padding, or they can be lost into the cast. Both can cause pressure and lead to skin breakdown.
- Elevate a casted arm or leg on pillows to reduce swelling.
- Have enough help to turn and reposition the person. Plaster casts are heavy and awkward. Balance is lost easily.
- Position the person as directed.
- Follow the care plan for elimination needs. Some persons use a fracture pan.
- Report these signs and symptoms at once:
  - *Pain*—pressure injury, poor circulation, nerve damage
  - *Swelling and a tight cast*—reduced blood flow to the part
  - *Pale skin*—reduced blood flow to the part
  - *Cyanosis (bluish skin color)*—reduced blood flow to the part
  - *Odor*—infection
  - *Inability to move the fingers or toes*—pressure on a nerve
  - *Numbness*—pressure on a nerve, reduced blood flow to the part
  - *Temperature changes*—cool skin means poor circulation; hot skin means inflammation
  - *Drainage on or under the cast*—infection or bleeding
  - *Chills, fever, nausea, and vomiting*—infection
- Complete a safety check before leaving the room. (See the inside of the front cover.)

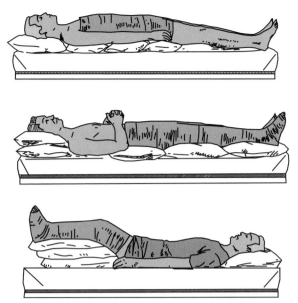

Fig. 35.13 Pillows support the entire length of the wet cast. (From Harkness GA, Dincher JR: *Medical-surgical nursing: total patient care,* ed 10, St Louis, 1999, Mosby.)

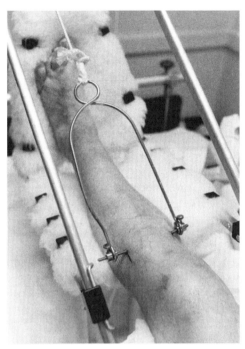

Fig. 35.16 Skeletal traction is attached to the bone. (From Christensen BL, Kockrow EO: *Adult health nursing,* ed 6, St Louis, 2011, Mosby.)

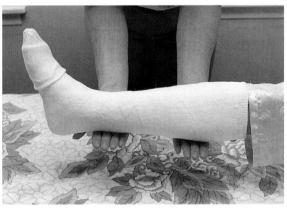

Fig. 35.14 The cast is supported with the palms.

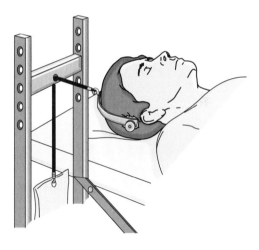

Fig. 35.17 Tongs are inserted into the skull for cervical spine traction. (From Monahan FD et al: *Phipps' medical-surgical nursing: health and illness perspectives,* ed 8, St Louis, 2007, Mosby.)

tongs are applied to the skull (Fig. 35.17). Weights are attached to the device.

Assist with the person's care as directed (Box 35.7).

Hip Fractures

Fractured hips are common in older persons (Fig. 35.18). Older women are at risk. Slow healing and other health problems affect the older person's condition and care.

Postoperative problems present life-threatening risks. They include pneumonia, atelectasis (collapse of a part of a lung), urinary tract infections, and thrombi (blood clots) in the leg veins. Pressure injuries, constipation, and confusion are other risks.

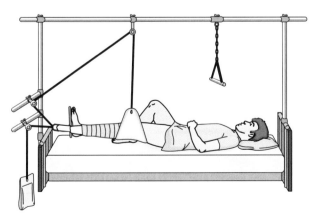

Fig. 35.15 Traction setup. Note the weights, pulleys, and ropes. (From Monahan FD et al: *Phipps' medical-surgical nursing: health and illness perspectives,* ed 8, St Louis, 2007, Mosby.)

BOX 35.7 Caring for Persons in Traction

- Keep the person in good alignment.
- Do not remove the traction.
- Keep the weights off the floor. Weights must hang freely from the traction setup (see Fig. 35.15).
- Do not add or remove weights from the traction setup.
- Check for frayed ropes. Report fraying at once.
- Perform ROM exercises for the uninvolved joints as directed.
- Position the person as directed. Usually only the back-lying position is allowed. Sometimes slight turning is allowed.
- Provide the fracture pan for elimination.
- Give skin care as directed.
- Put bottom linens on the bed from the top down. The person uses a trapeze to raise the body off the bed.
- Check pin, nail, wire, or tong sites for redness, drainage, and odors. Report observations at once.
- Observe for the signs and symptoms listed under cast care (see Box 35.6). Report them at once.
- Complete a safety check before leaving the room. (See the inside of the front cover.)

BOX 35.8 Care of the Person With a Hip Fracture

- Give good skin care. Skin breakdown can occur rapidly.
- Follow the care plan to prevent pressure injuries.
- Follow the care plan to prevent wound, skin, and urinary tract infections.
- Encourage incentive spirometry and deep-breathing and coughing exercises as directed.
- Turn and position the person as directed. Turning and positioning depend on the type of fracture and the surgery. Usually the person is not positioned on the operative side.
- Prevent external rotation of the hip. Use trochanter rolls, pillows, and sandbags as directed.
- Keep the leg abducted at all times. The leg is abducted when the person is supine, being turned, or in a side-lying position. Use pillows (Fig. 35.19A) or a hip abduction wedge (abductor splint) (Fig. 35.19B) as directed. Do not exercise the affected leg.
- Provide a straight-back chair with armrests. The person needs a high, firm seat. A low, soft chair is not used.
- Place the chair on the unaffected side.
- Use assist devices to move, turn, reposition, and transfer the person.
- Do not let the person stand on the operated leg unless allowed by the doctor.
- Elevate the leg according to the care plan. With an internal fixation device, the leg is not elevated when the person sits in a chair. Elevating the leg puts strain on the device.
- Apply compression stockings to prevent thrombi (blood clots) in the legs.
- Remind the person not to cross the legs.
- Assist with ambulation according to the care plan. The person uses a walker or crutches.
- Follow measures to protect the hip. See Box 35.5 and Fig. 35.8.
- Practice safety measures to prevent falls.
- Complete a safety check before leaving the room. (See the inside of the front cover.)

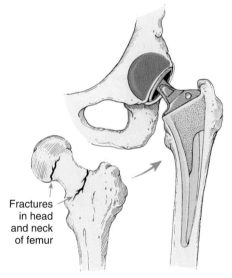

Fractures in head and neck of femur

Fig. 35.18 Hip fracture repaired with a prosthesis. (Modified from Christensen BL, Kockrow EO: *Adult health nursing,* ed 6, St Louis, 2011, Mosby.)

The fracture requires internal fixation (p. 541). Some hip fractures require partial or total hip replacement. Adduction, internal rotation, external rotation, and severe hip flexion are avoided after surgery. Rehabilitation is usually needed. If home care is not possible, the person needs subacute or long-term care. Recovery can take 6 months. Some persons return home after successful rehabilitation. Others stay in nursing centers. Box 35.8 lists the care required after surgery for a hip fracture.

Loss of Limb

An amputation is the removal of all or part of an extremity. Most amputations involve a lower extremity. Severe injuries, tumors, severe infection, gangrene, and vascular disorders are common causes. Diabetes is a common cause of vascular changes leading to amputation.

Gangrene is a condition in which there is death of tissue. It can cause death. Causes include infection, injuries, and vascular disorders. Blood flow is affected. Tissues do not get enough oxygen and nutrients. Poisonous substances and wastes build up in the tissues. Tissues die and become black, cold, and shriveled (Fig. 35.20). Surgery is needed to remove dead tissue. If untreated, gangrene spreads throughout the body. For example, in diabetes the toes are usually affected first. If affected toes are not removed, gangrene spreads up the foot and to the knee.

The amputation affects the person's life (Box 35.9). Body image, appearance, daily activities, movement, and work are

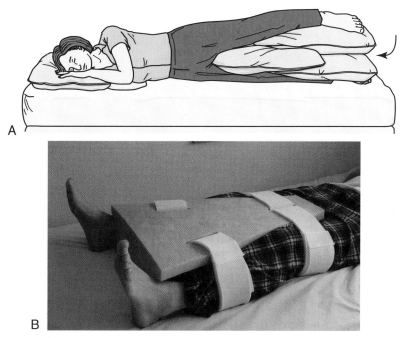

Fig. 35.19 (A) Pillows are used to keep the hip in abduction. (B) A hip abductor wedge. (A, From Monahan FD et al: *Phipps' medical-surgical nursing: health and illness perspectives,* ed 8, St Louis, 2007, Mosby.)

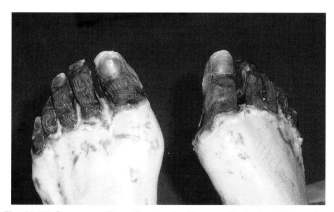

Fig. 35.20 Gangrene. (From Centers for Disease Control and Prevention/ Christina Nelson, MD, MPH, 2012.)

some areas affected. It may be better to refer to the remaining portion of the limb as the *residual limb* rather than use the term *stump.* Some persons report negative feelings associated with *stump,* as though being compared to a tree. Follow the care plan and use the term the person prefers. Fear, shock, anger, denial, and depression are also common emotions. Much support is needed. It may help to have a rehabilitated amputee visit with the person.

The person may be fitted with a prosthesis—an artificial replacement for a missing body part (Fig. 35.23). First the residual limb is conditioned so the prosthesis fits. This involves shrinking and shaping the limb into a cone shape with bandages (see Fig. 35.21) or a shrinker sock (see Fig. 35.22). The person learns exercises to strengthen other limbs. Occupational and physical therapists help the person use the prosthesis.

BOX 35.9 Care of the Person With a Limb Amputation

- Follow the care plan for specific instructions for ADL.
- Refer to the affected limb as the *residual limb* rather than the *stump.*
- Position the person and the residual limb according to the care plan.
- Reposition at least every 2 hours.
- Some persons may use a trapeze to position themselves while in bed.
- Transfer the person according to the care plan. If using a mechanical lift, a special sling may be needed.
- Observe the residual limb for signs of swelling, redness, or skin breakdown.

- Give good skin care and make close observations of the residual limb while bathing the person.
- Apply any elastic wraps (Fig. 35.21) or shrinker socks (Fig. 35.22) according to the care plan.
- Follow the care plan when assisting the person with applying the prosthesis.
- Report complaints of pain promptly to the nurse.
- Care for the person with dignity and respect. Be patient and aware that this is a change in the person's body image. Listen to the person's concerns and report signs of depression to the nurse.

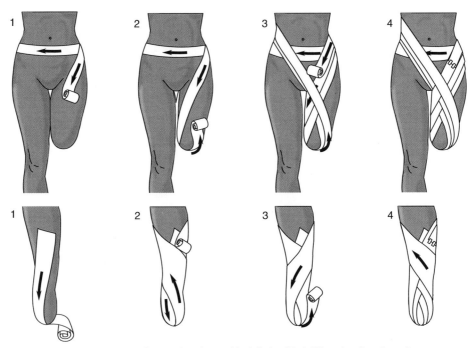

Fig. 35.21 A common method of wrapping the residual limb. (*Top*) Wrapping for above-knee amputation. (*Bottom*) Wrapping for below-knee amputation. (From Ignatavicius DD, Workman ML: *Medical-surgical nursing: patient-centered collaborative care,* ed 8, St Louis, 2013 Mosby.)

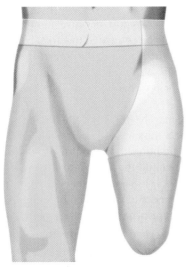

Fig. 35.22 Prosthetic shrinker sock. (Courtesy Knit-Rite, Inc., Kansas City, KS.)

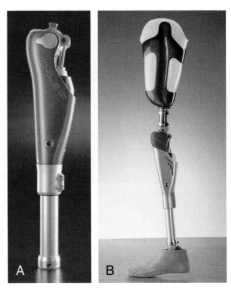

Fig. 35.23 Leg prostheses. (A) Above-the-knee prosthesis. (B) Below-the-knee prosthesis. (Courtesy Otto Bock Health Care, Minneapolis, MN.)

The person may feel that the limb is still there. Aching, tingling, and itching are common sensations. The person may also complain of pain in the amputated part. Called *phantom limb pain,* this is a normal reaction. It may occur for a short time or for many years.

Lower limb amputations are common in older persons. The amputation may occur above the knee (AKA) or below the knee (BKA). Because of other health problems, many persons cannot use a prosthesis. They need to use wheelchairs. After amputation, most older persons need temporary or permanent nursing center care.

QUALITY OF LIFE

A person may have one or many problems affecting the nervous and musculoskeletal systems. For example, a person with a stroke may fall and fracture a hip. The person may also have arthritis and osteoporosis. The care plan depends on the person's problems and needs.

The care you give affects the person's quality of life. Safety, good alignment, and turning and repositioning are important. So is skin care. Quality-of-life issues discussed for such care apply.

Always protect the person's rights. Privacy, confidentiality, and personal choice are examples. Also guard against abuse, mistreatment, and neglect.

TIME TO REFLECT

Mr. Ross is a kind, quiet gentleman who has Parkinson disease. One evening, as you are assisting him into bed, he begins to tell you how frustrated he is. He confides: "I feel so helpless lately. I can't even button my own shirt. Today in the dining room, my hands were shaking so hard that I spilled soup all over myself. Tonight I wanted to write a letter to my grandson, telling him how proud I am that he graduated from college. Instead, I ripped it up because my handwriting looked so messy. I guess I'm just not the man I used to be." How would you respond to Mr. Ross? What measures might be tried to help him regain some independence and confidence?

REVIEW QUESTIONS

Circle the BEST answer.

1. A stroke also is called
   a. A cerebrovascular accident
   b. Aphasia
   c. Hemiplegia
   d. A transient ischemic attack
2. Warning signs of stroke occur
   a. With exertion
   b. Suddenly
   c. Between the ages of 20 and 40
   d. At rest
3. A person had a stroke. Which measure should you question?
   a. Semi-Fowler position
   b. Range-of-motion exercises every 2 hours
   c. Turn, reposition, and give skin care every 2 hours
   d. Bed in the highest horizontal position
4. A person has Parkinson disease. Which is *false*?
   a. The part of the brain controlling muscle movements is affected
   b. Mental function is affected first
   c. Tremors, slow movements, and a shuffling gait occur
   d. The person needs protection from injury
5. Parkinson disease
   a. Can be cured with medications
   b. Can be cured with surgery
   c. Is a slow, progressive disorder
   d. Progresses rapidly
6. A person has multiple sclerosis. Which is *false*?
   a. There is no cure
   b. Only voluntary muscles are affected
   c. Symptoms begin in young adulthood
   d. Over time, the person depends on others for care

7. Amyotrophic lateral sclerosis affects nerve cells that control
   a. Involuntary muscles
   b. Voluntary muscles
   c. The brain
   d. The lungs
8. A person has amyotrophic lateral sclerosis. Which measure should you question?
   a. ROM exercises
   b. Dysphagia diet
   c. Walker for mobility
   d. Measures to prevent confusion
9. Persons with brain or spinal cord injuries require
   a. Rehabilitation
   b. Speech therapy
   c. Long-term care
   d. Chemotherapy
10. A person has quadriplegia from a spinal cord injury. Which measure should you question?
    a. Keep the bed in the low position
    b. Assist with active ROM exercises
    c. Follow the bowel training program
    d. Turn and reposition every hour
11. Autonomic dysreflexia occurs
    a. After spinal cord injuries
    b. In Parkinson disease
    c. With Lou Gehrig disease
    d. Following stroke
12. Autonomic dysreflexia is usually triggered by
    a. High blood sugar
    b. High blood pressure
    c. A full bladder
    d. A virus

13. Arthritis affects
    a. The joints
    b. The bones
    c. The muscles
    d. The hips and knees
14. A person has arthritis. Care includes the following *except*
    a. Preventing contractures
    b. ROM exercises
    c. A cast or traction
    d. Assisting with ADL
15. A person had hip replacement surgery. Which measure should you question?
    a. Provide a chair with a low seat
    b. Do not cross the legs
    c. Keep a hip abduction wedge between the legs
    d. Provide a long-handled brush for bathing
16. A person with osteoporosis is at risk for
    a. Fractures
    b. An amputation
    c. Phantom limb pain
    d. Paralysis
17. A cast needs to dry. Which is *false?*
    a. The cast is covered with blankets and plastic
    b. The person is turned so the cast dries evenly
    c. The entire cast is supported with pillows
    d. The cast is supported by the palm when lifted

18. A person has a cast. You report the following at once *except*
    a. Pain, numbness, or inability to move the fingers
    b. Chills, fever, nausea, or vomiting
    c. Odor, cyanosis, or temperature changes of the skin
    d. Pulse rate of 75 beats per minute
19. A person is in traction. Care includes the following *except*
    a. Performing ROM exercises as directed
    b. Keeping weights off the floor
    c. Removing weights if the person is uncomfortable
    d. Giving skin care at frequent intervals
20. After a hip pinning, the operated leg is
    a. Abducted at all times
    b. Adducted at all times
    c. Externally rotated at all times
    d. Flexed at all times
21. After an amputation, the person
    a. May be fitted with a prosthesis
    b. Needs a wheelchair
    c. Has quadriplegia
    d. Needs arthroplasty
22. Which is false concerning amputation?
    a. The person may feel phantom limb pain
    b. Refer to the portion of the limb that remains as the stump
    c. Diabetes is a common reason for amputation
    d. The person's body image is affected

See Appendix A for answers to these questions.

36

Cardiovascular and Respiratory Disorders

OBJECTIVES

- Define the key terms and key abbreviations listed in this chapter.
- Describe hypertension, its risk factors, signs and symptoms, complications, and treatment.
- Describe coronary artery disease, its risk factors, and complications.
- Describe cardiac rehabilitation.
- Describe angina, its signs and symptoms, and treatment.
- Describe myocardial infarction, its signs and symptoms, and treatment.
- Describe heart failure, its signs and symptoms, and treatment.
- Describe chronic obstructive pulmonary disease, its signs and symptoms, and treatment.
- Describe asthma, its signs and symptoms, and treatment.
- Explain the difference between a cold and influenza.
- Explain how influenza is treated.
- Describe pneumonia, its signs and symptoms, and treatment.
- Describe tuberculosis, its signs and symptoms, and treatment.
- Explain how to promote quality of life.

KEY TERMS

elevated blood pressure The systolic pressure is 120 to 129 mm Hg and the diastolic pressure is less than 80 mm Hg

hypertension (high blood pressure) The resting blood pressure is too high

hypertension stage 1 The systolic pressure is 130 to 139 mm Hg or the diastolic pressure is 80 to 89 mm Hg

hypertension stage 2 The systolic pressure is 140 mm Hg or higher or the diastolic pressure is 90 mm Hg or higher

hypertensive crisis The systolic pressure is higher than 180 mm Hg and/or the diastolic pressure is higher than 120 mm Hg

KEY ABBREVIATIONS

AHA American Heart Association
CAD coronary artery disease
CDC Centers for Disease Control and Prevention
CO₂ Carbon dioxide
COPD Chronic obstructive pulmonary disease

COVID-19 Coronavirus disease 2019
MI Myocardial infarction
mm Hg Millimeters of mercury
O₂ Oxygen
TB Tuberculosis

Cardiovascular and respiratory system disorders are leading causes of death in the United States. Many people have these disorders. Refer to Chapter 8 while you study this chapter.

CARDIOVASCULAR DISORDERS

Problems occur in the heart or blood vessels. See Chapter 31 for circulatory ulcers. Risk factors for cardiovascular disorders are listed in Box 36.1.

Hypertension

With hypertension (high blood pressure), the resting blood pressure is too high. In 2017, the American College of Cardiology and the American Heart Association (AHA) revised the guidelines for the detection and treatment of hypertension. With early detection of hypertension and lifestyle changes it is hoped that heart disease and stroke can be prevented. The new definition of hypertension will result in nearly half of the US adult population having high blood pressure. Doctors will decide what treatment is best for the person with hypertension (Box 36.1 lists risk factors).

Normal blood pressure for an adult is less than 120 mm Hg (millimeters of mercury) systolic and less than 80 mm Hg diastolic. Elevated blood pressure is 120 to 129 mm Hg systolic and less than 80 mm Hg diastolic. Hypertension stage 1 is 130 to 139 mm Hg systolic or 80 to 89 mm Hg diastolic. Hypertension stage 2 is systolic 140 mm Hg or higher or diastolic 90 mm Hg or higher. Hypertensive crisis is defined as systolic higher that 180 mm Hg and/or diastolic higher than 120 mm Hg. Always report elevated blood pressure readings to the nurse immediately.

Narrowed blood vessels are a common cause of hypertension. The heart pumps with more force to move blood through narrowed vessels. Kidney disorders, head injuries, some pregnancy problems, and adrenal gland tumors are causes.

BOX 36.1 Risk Factors for Cardiovascular Disorders

Hypertension
Factors You Cannot Change
- Age—45 years or older for men; 55 years or older for women
- Gender—younger men are at greater risk than younger women; the risk increases for women after menopause
- Race—Blacks are at greater risk than Whites
- Family history—tends to run in families

Factors You Can Change
- Being overweight
- Stress
- Tobacco use
- High-salt diet
- Excessive alcohol
- Lack of exercise
- Atherosclerosis
- Prehypertension

Coronary Artery Disease
Factors You Cannot Change
- Gender—men are at greater risk than women
- Age—in men, the risk increases after age 45; in women, the risk increases after age 55
- Family history
- Race—Blacks are at greater risk than other groups

Factors You Can Change
- Being overweight
- Lack of exercise
- High blood cholesterol
- Hypertension
- Smoking
- Diabetes

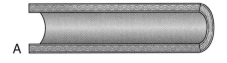

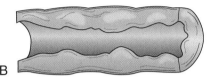

Fig. 36.1 (A) Normal artery. (B) Plaque on the artery wall in atherosclerosis.

collects on artery walls. The narrowed arteries block blood flow. Blockage may be total or partial. Blood clots can form along the plaque and block blood flow.

The major complications of CAD are angina, myocardial infarction (heart attack), irregular heartbeats, and sudden death. The more risk factors, the greater the chance of CAD and its complications (see Box 36.1 for risk factors).

CAD can be treated. Treatment goals are to:
- Relieve symptoms (see "Angina").
- Slow or stop atherosclerosis.
- Lower the risk of blood clots.
- Widen or bypass clogged arteries.
- Reduce cardiac events (see "Angina" and "Myocardial Infarction").

Persons with CAD need to make lifestyle changes. The person must quit smoking, exercise, and reduce stress. A healthy diet is needed to reduce high blood pressure, lower blood cholesterol, and maintain a healthy weight. If overweight, the person must lose weight.

Some persons need medications to decrease the heart's workload and relieve symptoms. Other medications are given to prevent a heart attack or sudden death. Medications can delay the need for medical and surgical procedures that open or bypass diseased arteries (Fig. 36.2).

A person can be unaware of hypertension for many years. That is why hypertension is called "the silent killer." Hypertension is found when blood pressure is measured (Chapter 27). Signs and symptoms develop over time. Headache, blurred vision, dizziness, and nose bleeds occur. Hypertension can lead to stroke, hardening of the arteries, heart attack, heart failure, kidney failure, and blindness.

Lifestyle changes can lower blood pressure. A diet low in fat and salt, a healthy weight, and regular exercise are needed. No smoking is allowed. Alcohol and caffeine are limited. Managing stress and sleeping well also lower blood pressure. Certain medications lower blood pressure.

Coronary Artery Disease

The coronary arteries are on the heart. They supply the heart with blood. In coronary artery disease (CAD), the coronary arteries become hardened and narrow. One or all are affected. The heart muscle gets less blood and oxygen (O₂). CAD also is called *coronary heart disease* and *heart disease*.

The most common cause is *atherosclerosis* (Fig. 36.1). Plaque—made up of cholesterol, fat, and other substances—

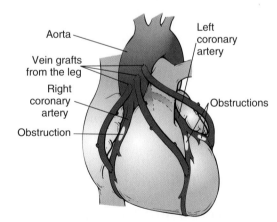

Fig. 36.2 Triple coronary artery bypass surgery. (Modified from Patton KT, Thibodeau GA: *The human body in health & disease*, ed 6, St Louis, 2014, Mosby.)

See *Focus on Rehabilitation: Coronary Artery Disease.*

🍃 FOCUS ON REHABILITATION

Coronary Artery Disease

Persons with complications from CAD may need cardiac rehabilitation (cardiac rehab). The cardiac rehab team includes doctors (the person's doctor, a heart specialist, a heart surgeon), nurses, exercise specialists, physical and occupational therapists, dietitians, and mental health professionals.

Cardiac rehab has two parts:

- *Exercise training.* The person learns to exercise safely. Exercises are done to strengthen muscles and improve stamina (staying power, endurance). The exercise plan is based on the person's abilities, needs, and interests.
- *Education, counseling, and training.* The person learns about:
  - The heart condition.
  - How to reduce the risk of future problems.
  - How to adjust to a new lifestyle.
  - How to deal with fears about the future.

Angina

Angina *(pain)* is chest pain from reduced blood flow to part of the heart muscle (myocardium). It occurs when the heart needs more O_2. Normally blood flow to the heart increases when O_2 needs increase. Exertion, a heavy meal, stress, and excitement increase the heart's need for O_2, as does smoking and very hot or cold temperatures. In CAD, narrowed vessels prevent increased blood flow.

Chest pain is described as tightness, pressure, squeezing, or burning in the chest (Fig. 36.3). Pain can occur in the shoulders, arms, neck, jaw, or back. Pain in the jaw, neck, and down one or both arms is common. The person may be pale, feel faint, and perspire. Dyspnea is common. Nausea, fatigue, and weakness may occur. Some persons complain of "gas" or indigestion. Rest often relieves symptoms in 3 to 15 minutes.

Rest reduces the heart's need for O_2. Therefore normal blood flow is achieved. Heart damage is prevented.

Besides rest, a medication called nitroglycerin is taken when angina occurs. The tablet is placed under the tongue. There it dissolves and is rapidly absorbed into the bloodstream. Some persons use nitroglycerin in a spray form. The person sprays the nitroglycerin into the mouth. Either way, the medications are kept within the person's reach at all times. The person takes a tablet or uses the spray and then tells the nurse. Some persons have nitroglycerin patches. The nurse applies and removes them.

Things that cause angina are avoided. These include overexertion, heavy meals and overeating, and emotional stress. The person needs to stay indoors during cold weather or during hot, humid weather. Doctor-supervised programs are helpful.

See "Coronary Artery Disease" for the treatment of angina. The goal is to increase blood flow to the heart. Doing so may prevent or lower the risk of heart attack and death. Chest pain lasting longer than a few minutes and not relieved by rest and nitroglycerin may signal heart attack. The person needs emergency care.

Myocardial Infarction

Myocardial refers to the heart muscle. *Infarction* means "tissue death." With myocardial infarction (MI), part of the heart muscle dies. Sudden cardiac death *(sudden cardiac arrest)* can occur (Chapter 44).

MI has other names as well:

- Heart attack
- Acute myocardial infarction (AMI)
- Acute coronary syndrome (ACS)
- Coronary
- Coronary thrombosis
- Coronary occlusion

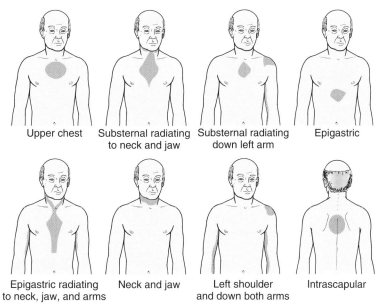

| Upper chest | Substernal radiating to neck and jaw | Substernal radiating down left arm | Epigastric |

| Epigastric radiating to neck, jaw, and arms | Neck and jaw | Left shoulder and down both arms | Intrascapular |

Fig. 36.3 Shaded areas show where the pain of angina is located. (From Lewis SM, Heitkemper MM, Dirksen SR: *Medical-surgical nursing: assessment and management of clinical problems,* ed 7, St Louis, 2007, Mosby.)

In MI, blood flow to the heart muscle is suddenly blocked. A thrombus (blood clot) blocks blood flow in an artery with atherosclerosis. The damaged area may be small or large (Fig. 36.4).

CAD, angina, and previous MI are risk factors. Box 36.2 provides signs and symptoms. MI is an emergency. Efforts are made to:

- Relieve pain.
- Restore blood flow to the heart.
- Stabilize vital signs.
- Give oxygen.
- Calm the person.
- Prevent death and life-threatening problems.

The person may need medical or surgical procedures to open or bypass the diseased artery. Cardiac rehabilitation is needed. The goals are to:

- Recover and resume normal activities.
- Prevent another MI.

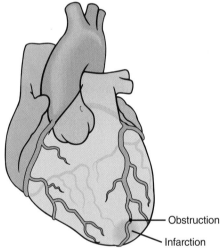

Fig. 36.4 Myocardial infarction. (Modified from Lewis SM, Heitkemper MM, Dirksen SR: *Medical-surgical nursing: assessment and management of clinical problems*, ed 7, St Louis, 2007, Mosby.)

BOX 36.2 Signs and Symptoms of Myocardial Infarction

- Chest pain
  - Sudden, severe; usually on the left side
  - Described as crushing, stabbing, or squeezing; some describe it as someone sitting on the chest
  - More severe and lasts longer than angina
  - Not relieved by rest and nitroglycerin
- Pain or numbness in one or both arms, the back, neck, jaw, or stomach
- Indigestion or "heartburn"
- Dyspnea
- Nausea
- Dizziness
- Perspiration and cold, clammy skin
- Pallor or cyanosis
- Blood pressure: low
- Pulse: weak and irregular
- Fear, apprehension, and a feeling of doom

- Prevent complications such as heart failure or sudden cardiac arrest.

Heart Failure

Heart failure or congestive heart failure (CHF) occurs when the weakened heart cannot pump normally. Blood backs up. Tissue congestion occurs.

When the left side of the heart cannot pump blood normally, blood backs up into the lungs. Respiratory congestion occurs. The person has dyspnea, increased sputum, cough, and gurgling sounds in the lungs. The body does not get enough blood. Signs and symptoms occur from the effects on other organs. Poor blood flow to the brain causes confusion, dizziness, and fainting. The kidneys produce less urine. The skin is pale. Blood pressure falls.

When the right side of the heart cannot pump blood normally, blood backs up into the venous system. Feet and ankles swell. Neck veins bulge. Liver congestion affects liver function. The abdomen is congested with fluid. Less blood is pumped to the lungs. The left side of the heart receives less blood from the lungs. The left side has less blood to pump to the body. As with right-sided heart failure, organs receive less blood. The signs and symptoms of left-sided failure occur.

Pulmonary edema (fluid in the lungs) is a very severe form of heart failure. It is an emergency. The person can die.

A damaged or weak heart usually causes heart failure. CAD, MI, hypertension, diabetes, age, and irregular heart rhythms are common causes. So are damaged heart valves and kidney disease.

Medications strengthen the heart. They also reduce the amount of fluid in the body. A sodium-controlled diet is ordered. Oxygen is given. A semi-Fowler position is preferred for breathing. The person must reduce CAD risk factors. If acutely ill, the person needs hospital care.

You assist with these aspects of the person's care:

- Promoting rest and activity as ordered
- Measuring intake and output
- Measuring weight daily
- Assisting with pulse oximetry
- Restricting fluids as ordered
- Promoting a diet that is low in sodium, fat, and cholesterol
- Preventing skin breakdown and pressure ulcers injuries
- Assisting with range-of-motion and other exercises
- Assisting with transfers and ambulation
- Assisting with self-care activities
- Maintaining good alignment
- Applying compression stockings

Many older persons have heart failure. Skin breakdown is a risk. Tissue swelling, poor circulation, and fragile skin combine to increase the risk of pressure ulcers injuries. Good skin care and regular position changes are needed.

RESPIRATORY DISORDERS

The respiratory system brings oxygen (O_2) into the lungs and removes carbon dioxide (CO_2) from the body. Respiratory disorders interfere with this function and threaten life.

Chronic Obstructive Pulmonary Disease

Chronic obstructive pulmonary disease (COPD) involves two disorders: chronic bronchitis and emphysema. These disorders interfere with O_2 and CO_2 exchange in the lungs. They obstruct airflow. Lung function is gradually lost.

Cigarette smoking is the most important risk. Pipe, cigar, and other smoking tobaccos are also risk factors, as is exposure to secondhand smoke. Not smoking is the best way to prevent COPD. COPD has no cure.

COPD affects the airways and alveoli (Chapter 8). Less air gets into the lungs; less air leaves the lungs. These changes occur:

- The airways and alveoli (air sacs) become less elastic. They are like old rubber bands.
- The walls between many alveoli are destroyed.
- Airway walls become thick, inflamed, and swollen.
- The airways secrete more mucus than usual. Excess mucus clogs the airways.

Chronic Bronchitis

Chronic bronchitis occurs after repeated episodes of bronchitis. *Bronchitis* means "inflammation *(itis)* of the bronchi *(bronch)*." Smoking is the major cause. Infection, air pollution, and industrial dusts are risk factors.

Smoker's cough in the morning is often the first symptom. At first the cough is dry. Over time, the person coughs up mucus. Mucus may contain pus. The cough becomes more frequent. The person has difficulty breathing and tires easily. Mucus and inflamed breathing passages obstruct airflow into the lungs. The body cannot get normal amounts of O_2.

The person must stop smoking. Oxygen therapy and breathing exercises are often ordered. Respiratory tract infections are prevented. If one occurs, the person needs prompt treatment.

Emphysema

In emphysema, the alveoli enlarge. They become less elastic. They do not expand and shrink normally with breathing in and out. As a result, some air is trapped in the alveoli when exhaling. Trapped air is not exhaled. Over time, more alveoli are involved. O_2 and CO_2 exchange cannot occur in affected alveoli. As more air is trapped in the lungs, the person develops a *barrel chest* (Fig. 36.5).

Smoking is the most common cause. Air pollution and industrial dusts are risk factors.

The person has shortness of breath and a cough. At first, shortness of breath occurs with exertion. Over time, it occurs at rest. Sputum may contain pus. Fatigue is common. The person works hard to breathe in and out, and the body does not get enough O_2. Breathing is easier when the person sits upright and slightly forward (Chapter 26).

The person must stop smoking. Respiratory therapy, breathing exercises, oxygen, and medications are ordered.

Airborne Allergies

Airborne allergies are the allergies that occur when the immune system has an overreaction to an airborne allergen (usually

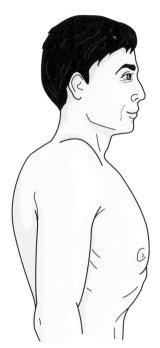

Fig. 36.5 Barrel chest from emphysema.

pollen or spores). Pet dander and dust mites can be other sources of allergens. The environment can greatly affect the person's response. Some people are more sensitive to allergens than others.

Asthma

Asthma comes from the Greek word that means "panting." With asthma, the airway becomes inflamed and narrow. Extra mucus is produced. Dyspnea results. Wheezing and coughing are common, as are pain and tightening in the chest. Symptoms are mild to severe.

Asthma usually is triggered by allergies. Other triggers include air pollutants and irritants, smoking and secondhand smoke, respiratory infections, exertion, and cold air.

Sudden attacks *(asthma attacks)* can occur. There is shortness of breath, wheezing, coughing, rapid pulse, sweating, and cyanosis. The person gasps for air and is very frightened. Fear makes the attack worse. Asthma is treated with medications. For some persons, the doctor orders an inhaler (Chapter 26). The person needs to use the inhaler quickly to help with breathing. Some persons are allowed to keep their inhaler with them. For others, the nurse brings it to them when needed. Severe attacks may require emergency care. The person and family learn how to prevent asthma attacks. Repeated attacks can damage the respiratory system. Always tell the nurse immediately if you observe someone having trouble breathing.

Influenza

Influenza *(flu)* is a respiratory infection. Table 36.1 contrasts *cold, flu, allergies, and COVID-19.* Caused by viruses, November through March is the usual flu season. According to the Centers for Disease Control and Prevention (CDC), about 12,000 to

TABLE 36.1 Comparing Cold, Flu, Allergies, and COVID-19

Symptoms	Cold	Flu	Airborne Allergy	COVID-19
Fever	Rare	Usually high (100—102°F); lasts 3—4 days	Never	Common
Headache	Uncommon	Common	Uncommon	Common
General aches and pains	Slight	Usual; often severe	Never	Common
Fatigue; weakness	Sometimes	Usual; can last 2—3 weeks	Sometimes	Common
Extreme exhaustion	Never	Usual; at the beginning of the illness	Never	Common
Stuffy nose	Common	Sometimes	Common	Common
Sneezing	Usual	Sometimes	Usual	Rarely
Sore throat	Common	Sometimes	Sometimes	Common
Cough	Common	Common; can be severe	Sometimes	Common, dry cough
Chest discomfort	Mild to moderate	Common	Rare	Common; can cause trouble breathing that calls for emergency care
Loss of taste or smell	Rarely	Rarely	Rarely	Common

Modified from National Institute of Allergy and Infectious Disease: *Is it flu, COVID-19, allergies, or a cold?* Bethesda, MD, 2022, National Institutes of Health.

52,000 people die every year from flu-related causes. Older persons are at great risk.

Older persons may not have the signs and symptoms listed in Table 36.1. The following may signal flu in older persons:
- Changes in mental status
- Worsening of other health problems
- A body temperature below the normal range
- Fatigue
- Decreased appetite and fluid intake

Treatment involves fluids and rest. The doctor orders medications for symptom relief and to shorten the flu episode. Most people are better in about 1 week.

Coughing and sneezing spread flu viruses. Some centers restrict visitors if many residents are suffering from the flu. Health care workers should stay home if they are having flu symptoms. Thorough and frequent hand hygiene is stressed. Masks may be made available to visitors who have a cough. Follow Standard Precautions. The flu vaccine is the best way to prevent the disease. Many health care facilities require an annual flu vaccine for their employees. Some centers may give their employees the vaccine free of charge. The CDC recommends the flu vaccine for all persons over the age of 6 months but especially for those who:
- Are 50 years of age and older.
- Have chronic heart, lung, liver, or kidney diseases.
- Have diabetes.
- Have immune system problems.
- Have nervous system disorders.
- Have a severe form of anemia (a decrease in hemoglobin in the blood).

- Are pregnant.
- Are residents of nursing centers or other long-term care centers.
- Are in close contact with children under 5 years of age.
- Are health care workers.
- Have contact with persons at high risk for flu-related complications.

Pneumonia is a common complication.

Pneumonia

Pneumonia is an inflammation and infection of lung tissue. (*Pneumo* means "lungs.") Affected tissues fill with fluid. O_2 and CO_2 exchange is affected.

Bacteria, viruses, and other microbes are causes. Microbes reach the lungs by being inhaled, aspirated, or carried in the blood to the lungs from an infection elsewhere in the body. Children under 2 years of age and adults over 65 years of age are at risk and are often vaccinated to prevent pneumonia. Smoking, aging, stroke, bedrest, immobility, chronic diseases, and tube feedings are some factors that increase the pneumonia risk.

Onset may be sudden. The person is very ill. Signs and symptoms are listed in Box 36.3.

Older adults are at great risk of dying from the disease. Changes from aging, diseases, and decreased mobility increase the risk of pneumonia in older persons. Decreased mobility after surgery also is a risk factor. Aspiration pneumonia is common in older persons. Dysphagia, decreased cough and gag reflexes, and nervous system disorders are risk factors. So are substances that depress the brain—narcotics, sedatives, alcohol, and medications for anesthesia.

BOX 36.3 Signs and Symptoms of Pneumonia

- High fever
- Chills
- Painful cough
- Chest pain on breathing
- Pulse: rapid
- Shortness of breath
- Breathing: rapid
- Cyanosis
- Sputum: thick and white, green, yellow, or rust-colored.
- Nausea
- Vomiting
- Headache
- Tiredness
- Muscle aches

Older persons may not have the signs and symptoms listed in Box 36.3. Medications and other diseases can mask signs and symptoms. Older persons may show signs of confusion, dehydration, and rapid respirations.

Medications are ordered for infection and pain. Fluid intake is increased because of fever and to thin secretions. Thin secretions are easier to cough up. Intravenous therapy and oxygen may be needed. A semi-Fowler position eases breathing. Rest is important. Standard Precautions are followed. Isolation precautions are used depending on the cause. Mouth care is important. Frequent linen changes are needed because of fever.

COVID-19

According to the CDC, COVID-19 (Chapter 14) is caused by a virus called SARS-CoV-2. It is part of the coronavirus family. This group includes common viruses that cause a variety of diseases from head or chest colds to more severe (but rarer) diseases like severe acute respiratory syndrome (SARS) and Middle East respiratory syndrome (MERS). Like many other respiratory viruses, coronaviruses spread quickly through droplets that project from the mouth or nose when you breathe, cough, sneeze, or speak. COVID-19 infection control principles are explained in Chapter 14. Viruses often mutate to form new variants. Long-term care facilities receive directions from the CDC to help protect residents in the best way possible.

Tuberculosis

Tuberculosis (TB) is a bacterial infection in the lungs. It also can occur in the kidneys, bones, joints, nervous system (including the spine), muscles, and other parts of the body. If TB is not treated, the person can die.

TB is spread by airborne droplets with coughing, sneezing, speaking, singing, or laughing (Chapter 14). Nearby persons can inhale the bacteria. Those who have close, frequent contact with an infected person are at risk. TB is more likely to occur in close, crowded areas. Age, poor nutrition, and human immunodeficiency virus (HIV) infection are other risk factors.

TB can be present in the body but not cause signs and symptoms. An active infection may not occur for many years. Only persons with an active infection can spread the disease to others. Increased numbers of nursing center residents have active TB. Infected long ago, the TB becomes active because general health declines with aging. Other older people become newly infected from lengthy, extended contact with those already infected.

Chest x-rays and TB testing can detect the disease. Most health care workers are required to have a TB test prior to employment and every year thereafter. Signs and symptoms of TB are tiredness, loss of appetite, weight loss, fever, and night sweats. Cough and sputum increase over time. Sputum may contain blood. Chest pain occurs.

Medications for TB are given. Standard Precautions and isolation precautions are needed (Chapter 14). The person must cover the mouth and nose with tissues when sneezing, coughing, or producing sputum. Tissues are flushed down the toilet, placed in a BIOHAZARD bag, or placed in a paper bag and burned. Hand washing after contact with sputum is essential.

QUALITY OF LIFE

A person's condition can change very quickly. A person with angina may have an MI. A person with hypertension may have a stroke. Sudden changes in a person's condition require the nurse's attention. Assist the nurse as directed. You may need to help other residents while the nurse readies the person for transport to a hospital. Always help willingly. The entire nursing team may need to make that "extra effort" to meet resident needs.

To promote quality of life, follow the care plan to meet the person's basic needs. This includes the person's emotional needs. Heart and lung function are essential for life. Fears of death are common.

Also protect the person's rights. Privacy, confidentiality, and personal choice are important to the person. So is the right to be free of abuse, mistreatment, or neglect. This is very important for persons with TB, a cold, or the flu. Do not avoid the person out of fear of getting the disease. Treat the person with dignity and respect. Follow Standard Precautions and the Bloodborne Pathogen Standard. They protect you and others from contamination.

TIME TO REFLECT

Mr. Byers has a history of angina. Today he wanted to take a walk outdoors in the courtyard. It was warmer and more humid than he anticipated. As he reenters the center through the door, you notice he is pale, perspiring, and having trouble catching his breath. He tells you he has discomfort in his chest. What should you do first in this situation? What are some actions the nurse may take? Do you think Mr. Byers's condition is serious?

REVIEW QUESTIONS

Circle the BEST answer.

1. In hypertension, the systolic blood pressure is over
   a. 120 mm Hg
   b. 100 mm Hg
   c. 90 mm Hg
   d. 80 mm Hg

2. Which is *not* a complication of hypertension?
   a. Stroke
   b. Heart attack
   c. Renal failure
   d. Diabetes

3. Treatment of hypertension may include the following *except*
   a. No smoking and regular exercise
   b. A high-sodium diet
   c. A low-calorie diet if the person is obese
   d. Medications to lower blood pressure

4. A person has angina. Which is *true*?
   a. There is heart muscle damage
   b. Pain is described as crushing, stabbing, or squeezing
   c. Pain is relieved with rest and nitroglycerin
   d. Pain is always on the left side of the chest

5. Cardiac rehabilitation involves
   a. Exercise
   b. Surgery
   c. Catheter procedures
   d. Receiving a vaccine

6. A person is having an MI. Which is *false*?
   a. The person is having a heart attack
   b. This is an emergency
   c. The person may have a cardiac arrest
   d. The person does not have enough blood

7. The pain of MI is usually
   a. On the left side of the chest
   b. On the right side of the chest
   c. In the upper abdomen
   d. In the midback region

8. A person has heart failure. Which should you question?
   a. Encourage fluids
   b. Measure intake and output
   c. Measure weight daily
   d. Perform range-of-motion exercises

9. The most common cause of COPD is
   a. Smoking
   b. Allergies
   c. Being overweight
   d. A high-sodium diet

10. A person has emphysema. Which is *false*?
    a. The person has dyspnea
    b. The person has an infection
    c. Breathing is usually easier sitting upright
    d. The person tires easily

11. The flu virus is spread by
    a. Coughing and sneezing
    b. The fecal-oral route
    c. Blood
    d. Needle sharing

12. A person has pneumonia. You know that this is
    a. An inflammation of the airway
    b. A narrowing of the airway
    c. An inflammation and infection of lung tissue
    d. A bacterial infection in the lungs

13. Which position eases breathing in the person with pneumonia?
    a. Supine
    b. Prone
    c. Semi-Fowler
    d. Trendelenburg

14. Tuberculosis is spread by
    a. Coughing and sneezing
    b. Contaminated drinking water
    c. Contact with wound drainage
    d. The fecal-oral route

15. A person has TB. You had contact with the person's sputum. What should you do?
    a. Wash your hands
    b. Put on gloves
    c. Use an alcohol-based hand rub
    d. Tell the nurse

See Appendix A for answers to these questions.

Digestive and Endocrine Disorders

OBJECTIVES

- Define the key terms and key abbreviations listed in this chapter.
- Describe gastroesophageal reflux disease and the care required.
- Describe the care required for vomiting.
- Describe diverticular disease and the care required.
- Describe gallstones and the care required.
- Describe hepatitis and the care required.
- Describe cirrhosis and the care required.
- Describe diabetes and the care required.
- Explain how to promote quality of life.

KEY TERMS

emesis See "vomitus"

heartburn A burning sensation in the chest and sometimes the throat

hyperglycemia High *(hyper-)* sugar *(glyc-)* in the blood *(-emia)*

hypoglycemia Low *(hypo-)* sugar *(glyc-)* in the blood *(-emia)*

jaundice Yellowish color of the skin or whites of the eyes

vomitus Food and fluids expelled from the stomach through the mouth; emesis

KEY ABBREVIATIONS

GERD Gastroesophageal reflux disease
HBV Hepatitis B virus
IBD Inflammatory bowel disease

I&O Intake and output
IV Intravenous

Problems can develop in any part of the digestive system. This includes the liver, gallbladder, and pancreas—the accessory organs of digestion. The pancreas also is part of the endocrine system. Refer to Chapter 8 while you study this chapter.

DIGESTIVE DISORDERS

The digestive system breaks down food for the body to absorb. Solid wastes are eliminated. Diarrhea, constipation, flatulence, and fecal incontinence are discussed in Chapter 23, as is ostomy care.

Gastroesophageal Reflux Disease

In gastroesophageal reflux disease (GERD), stomach contents flow back *(reflux)* from the stomach *(gastro)* into the esophagus *(esophageal)*. Stomach contents contain acid. The acid can irritate and inflame the esophagus lining. This is called *esophagitis*—inflammation *(itis)* of the esophagus.

Heartburn is the most common symptom of GERD. Heartburn is a burning sensation in the chest and sometimes the throat. The person may have a sour taste in the back of the mouth. Occasional heartburn is not a problem. If it occurs more than twice a week, the person may have GERD. Besides heartburn, other signs and symptoms of GERD include the following:

- Chest pain, often when lying down
- Hoarseness in the morning
- Dysphagia
- Choking sensation
- Feeling like food is stuck in the throat
- Feeling like the throat is tight
- Dry cough
- Sore throat
- Bad breath

GERD risk factors include being overweight, alcohol use, pregnancy, and smoking. Hiatal hernia is a risk. With hiatal hernia, the upper part of the stomach is above the diaphragm. Large meals and lying down after eating can cause gastric reflux, as can certain foods—citrus fruits, chocolate, caffeine drinks, fried and fatty foods, garlic, onions, spicy foods, and tomato-based foods (pasta sauce, chili, pizza).

The doctor may order medications to prevent stomach acid production or to promote stomach emptying. Surgery may be needed if medications and lifestyle changes do not work. Lifestyle changes include the following:

- Not smoking
- Not drinking alcohol
- Losing weight
- Eating small meals
- Avoiding spicy foods

- Wearing loose belts and loose-fitting clothes
- Not lying down for 3 hours after meals
- Raising the head of the bed 6 to 8 inches; see "Reverse Trendelenburg Position" in Chapter 16

Vomiting

Vomiting means expelling stomach contents through the mouth. It signals illness or injury. Vomitus (emesis) is the food and fluids expelled from the stomach through the mouth. Aspirated vomitus can obstruct the airway. Vomiting large amounts of blood can lead to shock. These measures are needed:

- Follow Standard Precautions and the Bloodborne Pathogen Standard.
- Turn the person's head well to one side to prevent aspiration.
- Place a kidney basin under the person's chin.
- Move vomitus away from the person.
- Provide oral hygiene. This helps remove the bitter taste of vomitus.
- Observe vomitus for color, odor, and undigested food. If it looks like coffee grounds, it contains undigested blood, which signals bleeding. Report your observations.
- Measure, report, and record the amount of vomitus. Also record the amount on the intake and output (I&O) record.
- Save a specimen for laboratory study.
- Dispose of vomitus after the nurse observes it.
- Eliminate odors.
- Provide for comfort. (See the inside of the front cover.)

Inflammatory Bowel Disease

Inflammatory bowel disease (IBD) occurs when there is inflammation of the digestive tract. The two main types of IBD are Crohn disease and ulcerative colitis. Crohn disease can affect any part of the GI tract, but most commonly affects the end of the small bowel and the beginning of the colon. It can affect the entire thickness of the bowel wall.

Ulcerative colitis is only found in the large intestine. It usually affects only the inner lining of the colon. The signs and symptoms of IBD may include the following:

- Diarrhea
- Fever
- Fatigue
- Abdominal pain
- Bloody stools
- Mouth sores
- Reduced appetite
- Weight loss

Diverticular Disease

Small pouches can develop in the colon. The pouches bulge outward through weak spots in the colon (Fig. 37.1). Each pouch is called a *diverticulum*. (*Diverticulare* means "to turn inside out.") *Diverticulosis* is the condition of having these pouches. (*Osis* means "condition of.") The pouches can become infected or inflamed—*diverticulitis*. (*Itis* means "inflammation.")

About half of all people over 60 years of age have diverticulosis. Age, a low-fiber diet, and constipation are risk factors.

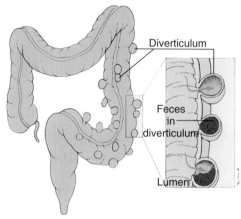

Fig. 37.1 Diverticulosis. (From Christensen BL, Kockrow EO: *Adult health nursing*, ed. 6, St. Louis, 2011, Mosby.)

When feces enter the pouches, they can become inflamed and infected. The person has abdominal pain and tenderness in the lower left abdomen. Fever, nausea and vomiting, chills, cramping, and constipation are likely. Bloating, rectal bleeding, frequent urination, and pain while voiding can occur.

A ruptured pouch is a rare complication. Feces spill out into the abdomen. This leads to a severe, life-threatening infection. A pouch also can cause a blockage in the intestine (intestinal obstruction). Feces and gas cannot move past the blocked part.

Dietary changes are ordered. The person may need a fiber and residue-restricted diet (Chapter 20). Sometimes antibiotics are ordered. Surgery is needed for severe disease, obstruction, and ruptured pouches. The diseased part of the bowel is removed. Sometimes a colostomy is necessary (Chapter 23).

PROMOTING SAFETY AND COMFORT

Assisting the Person Having GI Disturbances

Safety

Always practice Standard Precautions when assisting the person who is vomiting or has diarrhea. Wear gloves when handling body fluids. Wear the necessary personal protective equipment when assisting with personal care or changing clothing. You must practice hand hygiene before and after giving care.

Comfort

A person experiencing vomiting or diarrhea is very uncomfortable. You must act quickly to assist. The person may need an emesis basin or bedpan immediately. If the person puts on the call light, respond as quickly as possible. The person may need assistance to get to the bathroom quickly. Reassure the person and help with hygiene needs. Try to be understanding in difficult situations.

Gallstones

Bile is a greenish liquid made in the liver. It is stored in the gallbladder until needed to digest fat. Gallstones form when the bile hardens into stonelike pieces (Fig. 37.2).

Bile is carried from the liver to the gallbladder through ducts (tubes). The gallbladder contracts and pushes bile through the common bile duct to the small intestine. Gallstones can lodge in any of the ducts (Fig. 37.3). Bile flow is blocked. The trapped bile can cause inflammation of the gallbladder and the ducts. Liver and pancreas involvement are possible. Death can result from severe infections or damage.

Gallstones vary in size. They can be as small as a grain of sand or as large as a golf ball. A person may have one large stone. Some people have large and small stones. Risk factors include the following:

- *Gender.* Women are at greater risk than men.
- *Family history.* A genetic link is possible.
- *Diet.* A diet high in fat and cholesterol increases the risk, as does a low-fiber diet.
- *Age.* People over age 60 are at greater risk than younger people.
- *Native Americans.* These individuals have genetic factors that increase the risk of gallstones. High levels of cholesterol are secreted into the bile.

- *Latinos.* Men and women of all ages are at risk.
- *Being overweight.* Increased cholesterol reduces gallbladder emptying.
- *Rapid weight loss and fasting.* To burn fat, the liver secretes more cholesterol into the bile. Cholesterol can cause gallstones. The gallbladder does not empty properly.
- *Cholesterol-lowering medications.* They increase the amount of cholesterol secreted into bile.
- *Diabetes.* Persons with diabetes have high levels of fatty acids. The fatty acids may increase the risk of gallstones.

Signs and symptoms of a "gallbladder attack" or "gallstone attack" occur suddenly (Box 37.1). They often follow a fatty meal. The most common treatment is surgical removal of the gallbladder.

Hepatitis

Hepatitis is an inflammation *(itis)* of the liver *(hepat)*. It can be mild or cause death. Signs and symptoms are listed in Box 37.2. Some people do not have symptoms.

Protect yourself and others. Follow Standard Precautions and the Bloodborne Pathogen Standard. Isolation precautions are ordered as necessary (Chapter 14). Assist the person with hygiene and hand washing as needed.

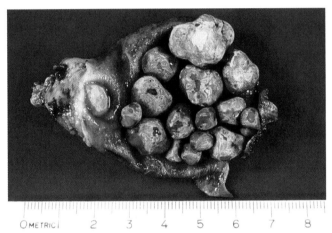

Fig. 37.2 Inflamed gallbladder filled with gallstones. (From Thompson JM, Wilson SF: *Health assessments for nursing practice*, St. Louis, 1996, Mosby.)

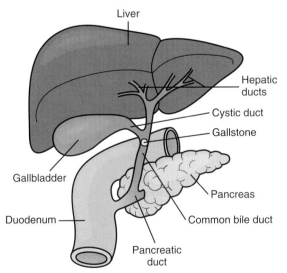

Fig. 37.3 The gallbladder and ducts that carry bile from the liver, gallbladder, and pancreas to the small intestine. (Modified from National Digestive Diseases Information Clearinghouse [NDDIC]: *Gallstones*, NIH Publication No. 07-2897, Bethesda, MD, 2007, National Institutes of Health.)

BOX 37.1 Signs and Symptoms of Gallstones

- Steady pain in the upper abdomen
  - Increases rapidly
  - Lasts 30 minutes to several hours
- Pain
  - In the back between the shoulder blades
  - Under the right shoulder
- Prolonged pain—lasting more than 5 hours
- Nausea and vomiting
- Chills
- Fever
- Jaundice—yellowish color of the skin or whites of the eyes (Fig. 37.4). (Jaundice comes from the French word *jaune* meaning "yellow.")
- Clay-colored stools

Modified from National Digestive Diseases Information Clearinghouse (NDDIC): *Gallstones*, NIH Publication No. 07-2897, Bethesda, MD, 2007, National Institutes of Health.

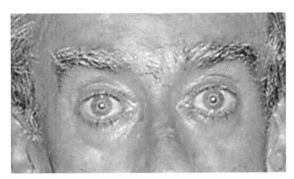

Fig. 37.4 Jaundice. (From Butcher GP: *Gastroenterology: an illustrated colour text*, London, 2004, Churchill Livingstone.)

BOX 37.2 Signs and Symptoms of Hepatitis

- Jaundice (yellowish color of the skin or whites of the eyes)
- Fatigue, weakness
- Pain and discomfort: abdominal, joint, muscles
- Appetite: loss of
- Nausea and vomiting
- Diarrhea
- Bowel movements: light, clay colored
- Urine: dark
- Fever
- Chills
- Headache
- Itching
- Weight loss
- Skin rash

There are five major types of hepatitis. See Box 37.3 for persons at risk.

Hepatitis A

This type is spread by food or water contaminated with feces from an infected person. Spread through the fecal-oral route, the hepatitis A virus is ingested when:

- Eating or drinking food or water contaminated with feces.
- Eating or drinking from a contaminated vessel.

Treatment involves rest, a healthy diet, fluids, and no alcohol. Recovery takes 1 to 2 months.

Persons with fecal incontinence, confusion, and dementia can cause contamination. Look carefully for contaminated items and areas.

Handle bedpans, feces, and rectal thermometers carefully. Good hand washing is needed by everyone, including the person. Assist with hand washing after bowel movements. The hepatitis A vaccine provides protection against the disease.

Hepatitis B

This type is caused by the hepatitis B virus (HBV). It is spread through infected blood or blood products and body fluids (saliva, semen, vaginal secretions) of infected persons. It is spread by:

- Intravenous (IV) drug use and sharing needles and syringes.
- Accidental needlesticks.
- Sex without a condom, especially anal sex.
- Contaminated tools used for tattoos or body piercings.
- Sharing a toothbrush, razor, or nail clippers with an infected person.

For the HBV vaccine, see Chapter 14. Medications are ordered to treat chronic hepatitis B.

Hepatitis C

This type is spread by blood contaminated with the hepatitis C virus. A person may have the virus but no symptoms. Serious liver disease and damage may show up years later. Even without symptoms, the person can transmit the disease. Hepatitis C is treated with medications. The virus is spread by:

- Blood contaminated with the virus.
- IV drug use and sharing needles.

BOX 37.3 Persons at Risk for Hepatitis

Hepatitis A
- International travelers (especially to developing countries)
- People who live with an infected person
- People who have sex with an infected person
- People living in areas where children are not routinely vaccinated against hepatitis A
- Children in day care (during outbreaks)
- Day care workers (during outbreaks)
- Men who have sex with men
- Users of illegal drugs

Hepatitis B
- People who live with an infected person
- People who have sex with an infected person
- People who have multiple sex partners
- Injection drug users
- Immigrants from areas with high rates of hepatitis B
- Children of immigrants from areas with high rates of hepatitis B
- Infants born to infected mothers
- Health care workers
- Hemodialysis patients (Chapter 38)

- People who received blood or blood products before 1987
- International travelers (especially to developing countries)

Hepatitis C
- Injection drug users
- People who have sex with an infected person
- People who have multiple sex partners
- Health care workers
- Infants born to infected mothers
- Hemodialysis patients
- People who received blood or blood products before 1992
- People who received blood clotting factors made before 1987

Hepatitis D
- People who have sex with an infected person
- People who received blood or blood products before 1987

Hepatitis E
- International travelers (especially to developing countries)
- People living in areas where hepatitis E outbreaks are common
- People who live with an infected person
- People who have sex with an infected person

Modified from National Digestive Diseases Information Clearinghouse (NDDIC): *Viral hepatitis: A through E and beyond*, NIH Publication No. 08-4762, Bethesda, MD, 2008, National Institutes of Health.

- Inhaling cocaine through contaminated straws.
- Contaminated tools used for tattoos or body piercings.
- High-risk sexual activity—sex with an infected person, multiple sex partners.
- Sharing a toothbrush, razor, or nail clippers with an infected person.

Hepatitis D and Hepatitis E

Hepatitis D occurs only in people infected with hepatitis B. It is spread the same way as HBV.

Hepatitis E is spread through food or water contaminated by feces from an infected person. It is spread by the fecal-oral route. This disease is not common in the United States.

Cirrhosis

Cirrhosis is a liver condition caused by chronic damage to the liver (Fig. 37.5). (*Cirrho* comes from the Greek word meaning "yellow-orange"; *osis* means "condition.") Healthy tissue is replaced by scar tissue. Blood flow through the liver is blocked. Normal liver functions are affected:

- Controlling infection
- Removing bacteria and toxins from the blood
- Processing nutrients, hormones, and medications
- Making proteins for blood clotting
- Producing bile for fat digestion

Cirrhosis has many causes. Chronic alcohol abuse and chronic hepatitis B and C are common causes. Obesity is becoming a common cause.

Signs and symptoms do not appear early in the disease. The following may occur as the disease progresses:

- Weakness
- Fatigue
- Loss of appetite
- Nausea
- Vomiting
- Weight loss
- Abdominal pain and bloating when fluid collects in the membrane lining the abdominal cavity (Fig. 37.6)

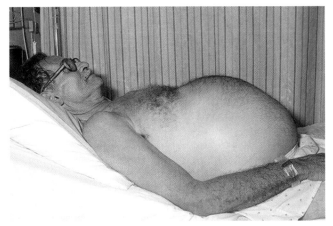

Fig. 37.6 Fluid in the membrane lining the abdominal cavity (ascites). (From Swartz MH: *Textbook of physical diagnosis*, ed. 7, Philadelphia, 2014, Saunders.)

- Itching
- Spiderlike blood vessels on the skin

Cirrhosis has many serious complications. Fluid collects in the legs *(edema)* and abdomen *(ascites)*. Infection, jaundice, and bruising and bleeding occur. Blood vessels in the esophagus and stomach may enlarge and can burst. Gallstones may develop. Toxins build up in the brain causing confusion, personality changes, and memory loss. The person is at risk for diabetes and liver cancer.

Treatment is aimed at preventing the progress of scar tissue. Complications also are treated. The person must have a healthy diet limited in protein. A low-sodium diet is needed for edema and ascites. Diuretic medications (water pills) are ordered to remove fluid from the body. Antibiotics are ordered for infection. Medications and enemas are ordered to remove toxins. The person must avoid alcohol. The person may need a liver transplant.

Assist with the person's care as directed. The measures listed in Box 37.4 may be part of the person's care plan.

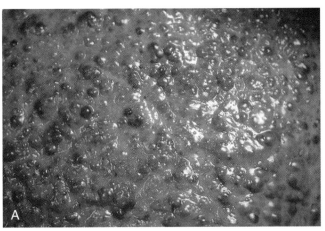
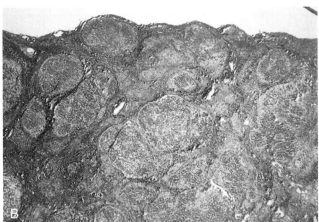

Fig. 37.5 A & B Liver damage from alcohol. (A, From Patton KT, Thibodeau GA: *The human body in health & disease*, ed. 6, St. Louis, 2014, Mosby; B, from Kumar V et al.: *Robbins basic pathology*, ed. 9, Philadelphia, 2013, Saunders.)

BOX 37.4 Care of the Person with Cirrhosis

- Use bed rails according to the care plan.
- Keep the call light within reach.
- Observe vomitus and stools for blood.
- Observe for signs of decreased mental function—confusion, memory loss, behavior changes, and so on.
- Measure vital signs every 2 to 4 hours. Follow the care plan.
- Measure I&O.
- Follow fluid restriction orders.
- Weigh the person daily.
- Provide good skin care.
- Apply lotion to the skin.
- Turn the person at least every 2 hours or as noted in the care plan.
- Provide mouth care every 2 hours.
- Use warm water with baking soda for bathing to decrease itching.
- Assist with activities of daily living (ADL) as needed.
- Complete a safety check before leaving the room. (See the inside of the front cover.)

ENDOCRINE DISORDERS

The endocrine system is made up of glands. The endocrine glands secrete hormones that affect other organs and glands. Diabetes is the most common endocrine disorder.

Diabetes

In this disorder, the body cannot produce or use insulin properly. Insulin is needed for glucose to move from the blood into the cells. The cells need glucose for energy. The pancreas secretes insulin. Without enough insulin, sugar builds up in the blood. Blood glucose (sugar) is high. Cells do not have enough sugar for energy and cannot function.

Types of Diabetes

A family history of the disease is a common risk factor for the three types of diabetes:

- *Type 1 diabetes.* Occurs most often in children, teens, and young adults. It is more common in Whites than in non-Whites. The pancreas produces little or no insulin. Onset is rapid.
- *Type 2 diabetes.* This type is more common after age 45. However, it is becoming more common in children, teens, and young adults. Being overweight, lack of exercise, and hypertension are risk factors. The pancreas secretes insulin. However, the body cannot use it well. Onset is slow. Infections are frequent. Wounds heal slowly. Gum disease (Chapter 18) is common. These ethnic groups are at risk:
  - Alaskan Natives
  - Native Americans
  - Blacks
  - Hispanics and Latinos
  - Asians
  - Pacific Islanders
- *Gestational diabetes.* This type develops during pregnancy. (Gestation comes from *gestare*, meaning "to bear.") The condition usually goes away after the baby is born. However, the mother is at risk for type 2 diabetes later in life.

Signs and Symptoms

Signs and symptoms of diabetes are the following:

- Being very thirsty
- Urinating often
- Feeling very hungry or tired
- Losing weight without trying
- Having sores that heal slowly
- Having dry, itchy skin
- Tingling or loss of feeling in the feet
- Blurred vision

Complications

Diabetes must be controlled to prevent complications. They include blindness, renal failure, nerve damage, and damage to the gums and teeth. Heart and blood vessel diseases are very serious problems. They can lead to stroke, heart attack, and slow healing. Foot and leg wounds and ulcers are very serious (Chapter 31). Infection and gangrene can occur. Sometimes amputation is necessary.

Treatment

Type 1 diabetes is treated with daily insulin therapy, healthy eating (Chapter 20), and exercise. Type 2 diabetes is treated with healthy eating and exercise. Many persons with type 2 take oral medications. Some need insulin. Overweight persons need to lose weight. Types 1 and 2 involve controlling blood pressure, cholesterol, and the risk factors for coronary artery disease.

Good foot care is needed. Corns, blisters, calluses, and other foot problems can lead to an infection and possibly the need for amputation (see Chapters 19 and 31).

The person's blood sugar level can fall too low or go too high. Blood glucose (Chapter 29) is monitored daily or three to four times a day for:

- Hypoglycemia—low *(hypo)* sugar *(glyc)* in the blood *(emia)*.
- Hyperglycemia—high *(hyper)* sugar *(glyc)* in the blood *(emia)*.

Table 37.1 lists causes, signs, and symptoms of hypoglycemia and hyperglycemia. Both can lead to death if not corrected. You must call for the nurse at once.

Assist with the person's care as directed by the nurse. Also follow the person's care plan.

TABLE 37.1 Hypoglycemia and Hyperglycemia

Condition	Causes	Signs and Symptoms
Hypoglycemia (low blood sugar)	Too much insulin or diabetic medications Omitting or missing a meal Delayed meal Eating too little food Increased exercise	Vomiting Drinking alcohol Hunger Fatigue; weakness Trembling; shakiness Sweating Headache Dizziness Faintness Pulse: rapid Blood pressure: low Respirations: rapid and shallow Motions: clumsy and jerky Tingling around the mouth Confusion Vision: changes in Skin: cold and clammy Convulsions Unconsciousness
Hyperglycemia (high blood sugar)	Undiagnosed diabetes Not enough insulin or diabetic medications Eating too much food Too little exercise Emotional stress Infection or sickness	Weakness Drowsiness Thirst Dry mouth (very) Hunger Urination: frequent Leg cramps Face: flushed Breath odor: sweet Respirations: rapid, deep, and labored Pulse: rapid, weak Blood pressure: low Skin: dry Vision: blurred Headache Nausea and vomiting Convulsions Coma

Hyperthyroidism

Hyperthyroidism occurs when the thyroid gland produces too many hormones. Graves disease (Chapter 34) is defined as inflammation of the thyroid. Signs and symptoms include the following:

- A rapid or irregular heartbeat
- Difficulty sleeping
- Irritability and nervousness
- Tiredness
- Poor temperature regulation

- Frequent bowel movements
- Weight loss with an increased appetite
- A goiter (a growth in the neck)

Surgery, medication, and radioiodine therapy are forms of treatment.

Hypothyroidism

Hypothyroidism occurs when the thyroid does not produce enough hormones. It is the most common thyroid disorder. It causes body processes to slow down. Signs and symptoms may include the following:

- Fatigue
- Sensitivity to cold
- Slow speech
- Droopy eyelids and facial swelling
- A slow heartbeat
- Muscle cramps
- Confusion
- Weight gain
- Tingling of the hands
- Constipation
- Dry skin

The condition is usually treated with medication. Hashimoto disease is a type of hypothyroidism. It is also an autoimmune condition.

QUALITY OF LIFE

For some health problems, family history is a risk factor. Others result from lifestyle choices. Poor diet, drug abuse, and alcohol abuse are examples, as is lack of exercise. Do not judge the person or the person's actions. Always treat the person with dignity and respect.

Also protect the person's rights. Privacy, confidentiality, and personal choice are important to the person. So is the right to be free of abuse, mistreatment, or neglect. Always provide a safe setting to protect the person from harm and injury. Be attentive to the person's discomfort and offer reassurance.

TIME TO REFLECT

Mrs. Dober has type 1 diabetes. She needs insulin to control her blood sugar. The nurses test her blood sugar before each meal and at bedtime. Today, Mrs. Dober received her insulin injection and then walked to the dining room for the noon meal. She drank a cup of black coffee and told her tablemates that she was not very hungry. She excused herself and went back to her room to take a nap. The nursing assistants were busy helping other residents with their meals. They did not notice when Mrs. Dober left. Upon returning to her room, Mrs. Dober vomited in her bathroom. She did not turn on her call light but lay down on her bed to rest. What are the potential problems in this situation? What actions, if any, should take place?

REVIEW QUESTIONS

Circle the BEST answer.

1. A person has gastroesophageal reflux disease. Which nursing measure should you question?
   a. Person will wear loose clothing
   b. Supine position after meals
   c. Person will have small meals
   d. No smoking or alcohol

2. A person with gastroesophageal reflux disease has the following food choices. Which is *best* for the person?
   a. Baked chicken
   b. Pasta with tomato sauce
   c. Pizza
   d. Salad with orange slices

3. A person is vomiting. How should you position the person?
   a. Supine
   b. Prone
   c. Semi-Fowler
   d. With the head turned to the side

4. Vomiting is dangerous because of
   a. Aspiration
   b. Diverticular disease
   c. Fluid loss
   d. Jaundice

5. Vomitus looks like coffee grounds. You need to report this at once because it signals
   a. Bleeding
   b. Gastroesophageal reflux disease
   c. Gallstones
   d. A ruptured pouch

6. A person has diverticular disease. You will likely assist the nurse with
   a. Preventing diarrhea
   b. Giving antibiotics
   c. Giving enemas
   d. Preventing constipation

7. Gallbladder attacks usually occur
   a. On awakening
   b. During a fast
   c. After a fatty meal
   d. When the person is lying down

8. Which is *not* a sign of gallstones?
   a. Jaundice
   b. Pain under the right shoulder
   c. Clay-colored stools
   d. Hoarseness and choking sensation

9. Hepatitis is an inflammation of the
   a. Gallbladder
   b. Liver
   c. Pancreas
   d. Stomach

10. Hepatitis A is spread by
    a. Needle sharing
    b. IV drug use
    c. Contaminated blood
    d. The fecal-oral route

11. Hepatitis requires
    a. Sterile gloves
    b. Double-bagging
    c. Standard Precautions
    d. Masks, gowns, and goggles

12. Which is a common cause of cirrhosis?
    a. Alcohol abuse
    b. Diabetes
    c. Gallstones
    d. GERD

13. A person has cirrhosis. Which measure should you question?
    a. Measure I&O
    b. Weigh the person daily
    c. Use warm water with baking soda for bathing
    d. Encourage fluids

14. A person has hypothyroidism. Which is *false*?
    a. It is an autoimmune disease
    b. The thyroid gland does not produce enough hormones
    c. The person likely has a rapid, irregular heartbeat
    d. Tiredness and fatigue are common

15. Which is *not* a sign of diabetes?
    a. Increased urine production
    b. Weight gain
    c. Hunger
    d. Increased thirst

16. A person with diabetes needs the following *except*
    a. Exercise
    b. Good foot care
    c. A sodium-controlled diet
    d. Healthy eating

17. A person with diabetes is vomiting after a meal. The person is at risk for
    a. Hypoglycemia
    b. Hyperglycemia
    c. Jaundice
    d. Bleeding

18. A person has diabetes. Blood glucose is monitored daily or
    a. 2 or 3 times a day
    b. 3 or 4 times a day
    c. 4 or 5 times a day
    d. 5 or 6 times a day

See Appendix A for answers to these questions.

38

Urinary and Reproductive Disorders

OBJECTIVES

- Define the key terms and key abbreviations listed in this chapter.
- Describe urinary tract infections and the care required.
- Describe prostate enlargement and the care required.
- Describe urinary diversions and the care required.
- Describe renal calculi and the care required.
- Describe acute and chronic kidney failure and the care required.
- Describe sexually transmitted diseases and the care required.
- Explain how to promote quality of life.

KEY TERMS

cystocele Occurs when the bladder drops down

dialysis The process of removing waste products from the blood

diuresis The process (*-esis*) of passing (*di*) urine (*ur*); large amounts of urine are produced—1000 to 5000 milliliters (mL) a day

dysuria Difficult or painful (*dys-*) urination (*-uria*)

hematuria Blood (*hemat-*) in the urine (*-uria*)

oliguria Scant (*olig-*) urine (*-uria*)

pyuria Pus (*py-*) in the urine (*-uria*)

rectocele Occurs when the rectum shifts downward

suprapubic Above (*supra-*) the pubic bone (*pubic*)

urinary diversion A new pathway for urine to exit the body

urostomy A surgically created opening (*-stomy*) between a ureter (*uro-*) and the abdomen

uterine prolapse Occurs when the uterus shifts downward into the vaginal canal

KEY ABBREVIATIONS

AIDS Acquired immunodeficiency syndrome
BPH Benign prostatic hyperplasia
HIV Human immunodeficiency virus
mL Milliliter

STI Sexually transmitted infection
TURP Transurethral resection of the prostate
UTI Urinary tract infection

Understanding urinary and reproductive disorders gives meaning to the required care. Refer to Chapter 8 while you study this chapter.

URINARY SYSTEM DISORDERS

The kidneys, ureters, bladder, and urethra are the major urinary system structures. Disorders can occur in these structures. Men can develop prostate problems.

Urinary Tract Infections

Urinary tract infections (UTIs) are common. Infection in one area can progress through the entire system. Microbes can enter the system through the urethra. Catheterization, urologic exams, intercourse, poor perineal hygiene, immobility, and poor fluid intake are common causes. UTI is a common healthcare-associated infection (Chapter 14).

Women are at high risk. Microbes can easily enter the short female urethra. Prostate gland secretions help protect men from UTIs. However, an enlarged prostate increases the risk of UTI.

Older persons are at high risk for UTIs. Incomplete bladder emptying, perineal soiling from fecal incontinence, poor fluid intake, urinary catheters, and poor nutrition increase the risk of UTI in older men and women.

Cystitis

Cystitis is a bladder *(cyst)* infection *(itis)* caused by bacteria. These signs and symptoms are common:

- Urinary frequency
- Oliguria—scant *(olig)* urine *(uria)*
- Urgency
- Dysuria—difficult or painful *(dys)* urination *(uria)*
- Pain or burning on urination
- Foul-smelling urine
- Hematuria—blood *(hemat)* in the urine *(uria)*
- Pyuria—pus *(py)* in the urine *(uria)*
- Fever

Antibiotics are ordered. Fluids are encouraged—usually 2000 milliliters (mL) per day. If untreated, cystitis can lead to pyelonephritis.

Pyelonephritis

Pyelonephritis is inflammation *(itis)* of the kidney *(nephr)* pelvis *(pyelo)*. Infection is the most common cause. Cloudy urine may contain pus, mucus, and blood. Chills, fever, back pain, and nausea and vomiting occur. So do the signs and symptoms of cystitis. Treatment involves antibiotics and fluids.

Prostate Enlargement

The prostate is a gland in men. It lies in front of the rectum and just below the bladder (Chapter 8). The prostate also surrounds the urethra. In young men, the prostate is about the size of a walnut. The prostate grows larger (enlarges) as the man grows older. This is called benign prostatic hyperplasia (BPH) (Fig. 38.1). (*Benign* means "nonmalignant"; *hyper* means "excessive"; *plasia* means "formation or development.") Benign prostatic hypertrophy is another name for enlarged prostate. (*Trophy* means "growth.")

Most men age 60 and older have some symptoms of BPH. The enlarged prostate presses against the urethra, obstructing urine flow. Bladder function is gradually lost. These problems are common:

- A weak urine stream
- Frequent voidings of small amounts of urine
- Urgency and leaking or dribbling of urine
- Frequent voiding at night
- Urinary retention (The man cannot void. Urine remains in the bladder.)

Treatment depends on the extent of the problem. For mild BPH, medications can shrink the prostate or stop its growth. Some microwave and laser treatments destroy excess prostate tissue.

Transurethral resection of the prostate (TURP) is a common surgical procedure. The doctor inserts a lighted scope through the penis. The scope has a wire loop. The loop is used to cut tissue and seal blood vessels. The removed tissue is flushed out of the bladder. A special catheter is inserted and left in place for a few days. Flushing fluid enters the bladder through the catheter. Urine and the flushing fluid flow out of the bladder through the same catheter. Some bleeding and blood clots are normal. After surgery, the person's care plan may include the following:

- No straining or sudden movements
- Drinking at least 8 cups of water daily to flush the bladder
- No straining to have a bowel movement
- A balanced diet to prevent constipation
- No heavy lifting

Prostate Cancer

Prostate cancer is one of the most common types of cancer in men. Some types of prostate cancer grow slowly and may not need any treatment. Other types can grow and spread quickly. Early detection is important for successful treatment. Report any unusual urinary symptoms to the nurse.

Urinary Diversions

Sometimes the urinary bladder is surgically removed. Cancer and bladder injuries are common reasons. When the bladder is removed, urine must still leave the body. A new pathway—urinary diversion—is needed for urine to exit the body.

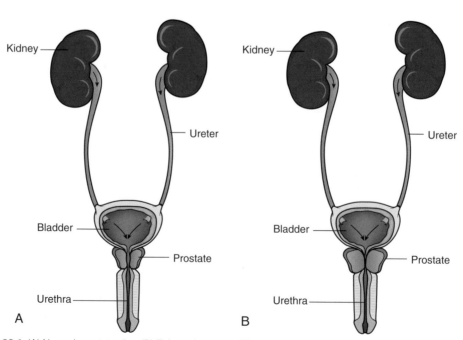

Fig. 38.1 (A) Normal prostate size. (B) Enlarged prostate. The prostate presses against the urethra. Urine flow is obstructed. (Redrawn from National Kidney and Urologic Diseases Information Clearinghouse: *Prostate enlargement: benign prostatic hyperplasia,* NIH Publication No. 07-3012, Bethesda, MD, 2006, National Institutes of Health.)

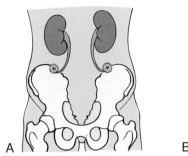
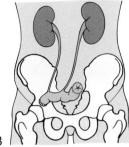

Fig. 38.2 Urostomies. (A) Both ureters are brought through the skin onto the abdomen. The person has two stomas. (B) The ileal conduit. A small section of the small intestine is removed. One end is sutured closed. The other end is brought through the skin onto the abdomen to form a stoma. The ureters are attached to this part of the small intestine. (From Beare PA, Myers JL: *Principles and practices of adult health nursing,* ed 3, St Louis, 1998, Mosby.)

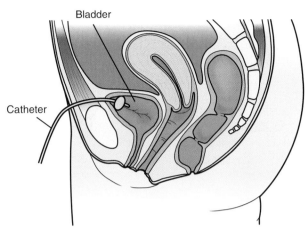

Fig. 38.4 Suprapubic catheter.

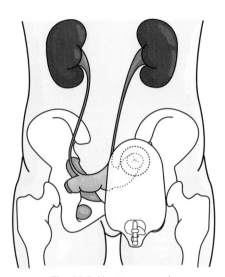

Fig. 38.3 Urostomy pouch.

Often an ostomy is involved. A urostomy is a surgically created opening *(stomy)* between a ureter *(uro)* and the abdomen (Fig. 38.2). The nurse provides care after surgery. You may care for persons with longstanding urostomies. The person assists with care as able.

A pouch is applied over the stoma (Fig. 38.3). Urine drains through the stoma into the pouch. Pouches are changed every 5 to 7 days. A pouch is replaced any time it leaks. Skin irritation, breakdown, and infection can occur if urine leaks onto the skin.

Urine drains constantly into the pouch. Empty pouches every 3 to 4 hours, or empty them when they are becoming one-third (1/3) full. Pouches become heavy as they fill with urine. A heavy pouch can loosen the seal between the pouch and the skin. Urine can leak onto the skin.

The person needs good skin care. You must help prevent skin breakdown. Observe the skin for changes around the stoma. Report changes to the nurse. See "The Person with an Ostomy" in Chapter 23.

Another type of urinary diversion is a suprapubic catheter (Fig. 38.4). This type of catheter is placed directly into the

bladder through the abdomen. It is inserted above *(supra)* the pubic bone *(pubic)*. The catheter is often attached to a urinary drainage bag (Chapter 22). Suprapubic catheters may be used for persons who have injury or blockage to the urethra. They also may be used for persons who require long-term catheterization.

See *Promoting Safety and Comfort: Urinary Diversions.*

> ### PROMOTING SAFETY AND COMFORT
>
> **Urinary Diversions**
> *Safety*
> Microbes can grow in urine, and urine may contain blood. Also, you have contact with mucous membranes. Follow Standard Precautions and the Bloodborne Pathogen Standard.
>
> *Comfort*
> The best time to change a pouch is after sleep and before eating or drinking fluids. Urine flow is less when the person has not had anything to eat or drink for 2 to 3 hours.
> The stoma does not have sensation. Touching the stoma does not cause pain or discomfort.

Kidney Stones

Kidney stones (calculi) are most common in White men between the ages of 20 and 40 years. Bedrest, immobility, and poor fluid intake are risk factors. Stones vary in size from as small as grains of sand to as big as golf balls (Fig. 38.5). Signs and symptoms include the following:

- Severe, cramping pain in the back and side just below the ribs (Fig. 38.6)
- Pain in the abdomen, thigh, and urethra
- Nausea and vomiting
- Fever and chills
- Dysuria
- Urinary frequency
- Urinary urgency
- Burning on urination
- Oliguria

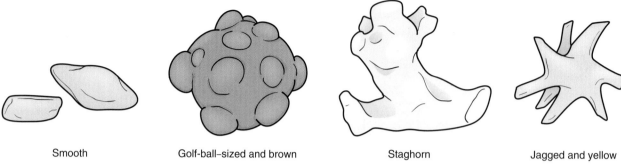

Smooth   Golf-ball–sized and brown   Staghorn   Jagged and yellow

Fig. 38.5 Kidney stones.

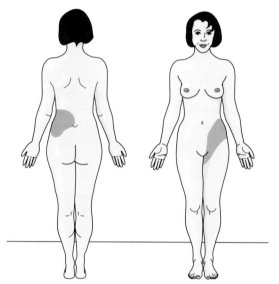

Fig. 38.6 Shaded areas show where the pain from kidney stones is located.

- Hematuria
- Cloudy urine
- Foul-smelling urine

Medications are given for pain relief. The person needs to drink 2000 to 3000 mL of fluid a day. The fluids help stones pass from the body through the urine. All urine is strained (Chapter 29). Surgical removal of the stone may be necessary. Some dietary changes can prevent stones.

Kidney Failure

In kidney failure (renal failure), the kidneys do not function or are severely impaired. Waste products are not removed from the blood. Fluid is retained. Heart failure and hypertension easily result. Kidney failure may be acute or chronic. The person is very ill.

Acute Kidney Failure

Acute kidney failure is sudden. Blood flow to the kidneys is severely decreased. Causes include severe injury or bleeding, heart attack, heart failure, burns, infection, and severe allergic reactions. Hospital care is needed.

At first, *oliguria* (scant amount of urine) occurs. Urine output is less than 500 mL in 24 hours. This phase lasts a few days to 2 weeks. Then diuresis occurs—the process *(esis)* of passing *(di)* urine *(ur)*. Large amounts of urine are produced—1000 to 5000 mL a day. Kidney function improves and returns to normal during the recovery phase. This can take 1 month to 1 year. Some persons develop chronic kidney failure.

Every system is affected when waste products build up in the blood. Death can occur.

Treatment involves medications, restricted fluids, and diet therapy. The diet is high in carbohydrates and low in protein and potassium. The care plan may include:

- Measuring and recording urine output every hour. Report an output of less than 30 mL per hour to the nurse at once.
- Measuring and recording intake and output.
- Restricting fluid intake.
- Measuring weight daily.
- Turning and repositioning at least every 2 hours.
- Measures to prevent pressure injuries.
- Frequent oral hygiene.
- Measures to prevent infection.
- Deep-breathing and coughing exercises.
- Measures to meet emotional needs.

Chronic Kidney Failure

The kidneys cannot meet the body's needs. Nephrons in the kidney are destroyed over many years. Hypertension and diabetes are common causes. Infections, urinary tract obstructions, and tumors are other causes.

Signs and symptoms appear when 75% of kidney function is lost (Box 38.1). Every system is affected as waste products build up in the blood.

Treatment includes fluid restriction, diet therapy, medications, and dialysis. Dialysis is the process of removing waste products from the blood. Persons receiving dialysis often feel fatigued. They need periods of rest.

- *Hemodialysis* removes waste and fluid by filtering the blood *(hemo)* through an artificial kidney (Fig. 38.7). The doctor creates a site where the blood can flow in and out of the body. This is the dialysis access. The most common type of access is a *fistula*. The doctor connects one of the arteries

BOX 38.1 Signs and Symptoms of Chronic Kidney Failure

- Skin
  - Color: yellow, tan, or dusky
  - Dry, itchy
  - Thin, brittle
- Bruises
- Breath: bad breath *(halitosis)*
- Mouth: inflammation of *(stomatitis)*
- Nausea
- Vomiting
- Appetite: loss of
- Weight loss
- Diarrhea or constipation
- Urine output: decreased
- Bleeding tendencies
- Infection: susceptible to
- Hypertension
- Heart failure
- Gastric ulcers
- Gastrointestinal bleeding
- Pulse: irregular
- Breathing: abnormal patterns
- Legs and ankles: swelling
- Legs and feet: burning sensation in
- Muscles: twitching and cramps
- Fatigue
- Sleep disorders
- Headache
- Convulsions
- Confusion
- Coma

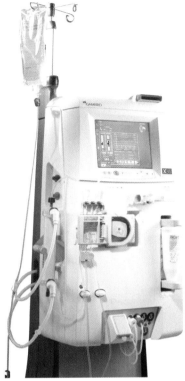

Fig. 38.7 Dialysis machine. (Courtesy Baxter Healthcare Corp., Deerfield, IL.)

to one of the veins in the lower arm. It is important not to take the person's blood pressure in this arm. Persons receiving hemodialysis usually go to a center or hospital three times a week for this treatment. Some are taught how to do it at home.

- *Peritoneal dialysis* uses the lining of the abdominal cavity *(peritoneal membrane)* to remove waste and fluid from the blood (Fig. 38.8). The fluid goes into the body through a catheter and remains for a certain amount of time (dwell time). When the dwell time is over, the solution, waste products, and excess fluid are drained into a collection bag. Peritoneal dialysis is often done at home. For some persons it may take place at night while they are sleeping.

You will assist the nurse in the care of persons with chronic kidney failure (Box 38.2).

REPRODUCTIVE DISORDERS

Sexual activities involve the structures and functions of the reproductive system. The male reproductive system:

- Produces and transports sperm.
- Deposits sperm in the female reproductive tract
- Secretes hormones.

The female reproductive system:

- Produces eggs (ova).
- Secretes hormones.
- Protects and nourishes the fetus during pregnancy.

Aging affects the reproductive system (Chapter 10). Many injuries, diseases, and surgeries can affect reproductive structures and functions.

Pelvic Organ Prolapse

The female reproductive organs are held in place in the pelvic cavity by muscles and connective tissue. As a woman ages, these muscles may weaken. Pelvic organs may drop down (prolapse) into the vaginal canal. Childbirth, loss of estrogen, surgery, or obesity can contribute to weakening of pelvic muscles.

When the bladder drops down, this is called a cystocele (Fig. 38.9A). When the rectum shifts downward, it is called a rectocele (see Fig. 38.9B). Uterine prolapse (see Fig. 38.9C) can occur when the uterus shifts downward into the vaginal canal. Any of these conditions can range from mild to severe.

The woman might have some improvement by practicing Kegel exercises. These are performed by tightening the pelvic muscles as if stopping the flow of urine. The doctor may prescribe a pessary for some women (Fig. 38.10). This device is placed in the vagina to support the prolapsed organ. In severe cases of prolapse, surgery may be necessary. For some women in long-term care settings, surgery may not be an option. The doctor may order bedrest instead. In certain cases, it may be possible for the nurse to reinsert the prolapsed organ. This should never be performed by the nursing assistant. When

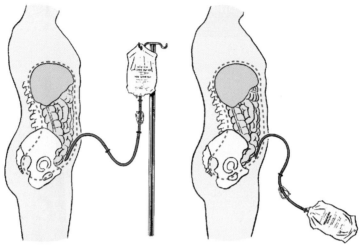

Fig. 38.8 Peritoneal dialysis system. (From Tucker S et al: *Patient care standards: collaborative practice planning guides,* ed 6, St Louis, 1996, Mosby.)

BOX 38.2 **Care of the Person With Chronic Kidney Failure**

- A diet low in protein, potassium, phosphorus, and sodium
- Fluid restriction
- Measuring blood pressure in the supine, sitting, and standing positions
- Measuring daily weight
- Measuring and recording intake and output
- Turning and repositioning
- Measures to prevent pressure injuries
- Range-of-motion exercises
- Measures to prevent itching (bath oils, lotions, creams)
- Measures to prevent injury and bleeding
- Frequent oral hygiene
- Measures to prevent infection
- Measures to prevent diarrhea or constipation
- Measures to meet emotional needs
- Measures to promote rest

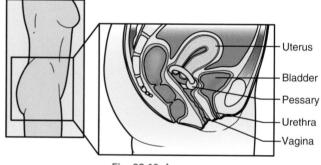

Fig. 38.10 A pessary.

helping women with perineal care, always report observations of anything unusual.

Sexually Transmitted Infection

A sexually transmitted infection (STI) is spread by oral, vaginal, or anal sex (Table 38.1). Some people do not have signs and symptoms or are not aware of an infection. Others know but do not seek treatment because of embarrassment.

STIs often occur in the genital and rectal areas. They also occur in the ears, mouth, nipples, throat, tongue, eyes, and nose. Condom use helps prevent the spread of STIs, especially the human immunodeficiency virus (HIV) and acquired immunodeficiency syndrome (AIDS). (HIV and AIDS are discussed in Chapter 34.) Some STIs are also spread through skin breaks, by contact with infected body fluids (blood, semen, saliva), or by contaminated blood or needles.

Standard Precautions and the Bloodborne Pathogen Standard are followed.

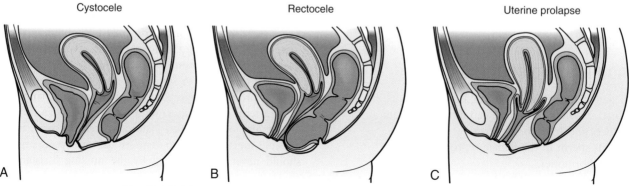

Fig. 38.9 Pelvic organ prolapse. (A) Cystocele. (B) Rectocele. (C) Uterine prolapse.

TABLE 38.1 Sexually Transmitted Infections

Disease	Signs and Symptoms	Treatment
Herpes	Painful, blisterlike sores on or near the genitals, mouth, or anus (Fig. 38.11) Pain, itching, burning, and tingling in the affected area Vaginal discharge Pain during urination or intercourse Fever Swollen glands	No known cure Antiviral medications
Genital warts	*Male*—Warts in or on the penis, anus, genitalia, mouth, or throat *Female*—Warts in or on the vagina, cervix, labia, anus, mouth, or throat	Application of special ointment that causes the warts to dry up and fall off Surgical removal may be necessary if the ointment is not effective
HIV/AIDS	See Chapter 34	See Chapter 34
Gonorrhea	Burning and pain on urination Urinary frequency and urgency Genital discharge (vagina, urethra, rectum)	Antibiotic medications
Chlamydia	May not show symptoms Discharge from the penis or vagina Burning or pain on urination Testicular pain or swelling Vaginal bleeding Rectal inflammation and/or discharge Pain during intercourse Diarrhea Nausea Abdominal pain Fever	Antibiotic medications
Pubic lice (Chapter 19)	Intense itching	Over-the-counter or prescription lice treatment Washing or dry-cleaning all exposed clothing, bedding, and towels
Trichomoniasis (occurs in women; men are carriers)	No symptoms in men Frothy, thick, foul-smelling, yellow vaginal discharge Genital itching and irritation Burning and pain on urination Genital swelling	Metronidazole
Syphilis	*Stage 1*—10 to 90 days after exposure • Painless sores (chancres) on the penis, in the vagina, or on the genitalia; the chancre may also be on the lips or inside the mouth, or anywhere on the body *Stage 2*—About 3 to 6 weeks after the sores • General fatigue, loss of appetite, nausea, fever, headache, rash, swollen glands, sore throat, bone and joint pain, hair loss, lesions on the lips and genitalia • Symptoms may come and go for many years *Stage 3*—3 to 15 years after infection • Central nervous system damage (including paralysis), heart damage, blindness, liver damage, mental health disorders, death	Penicillin and other antibiotic medications

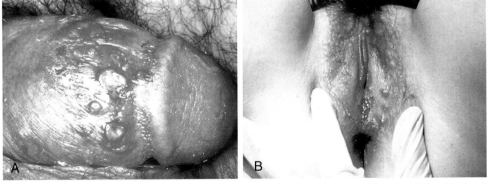

Fig. 38.11 Herpes. (A) Sores on the penis. (B) Sores on the female perineum. (Courtesy US Public Health Service, Washington, DC.)

QUALITY OF LIFE

Urinary and reproductive disorders can vary from mild to severely uncomfortable to life threatening. Follow the care plan and the nurse's directions carefully. Report your observations promptly. They can make a difference in the person's life.

Many older people are sexually active. They get and can spread STIs in the same ways as younger persons do. However, many do not think they are at risk. Always practice Standard Precautions and the Bloodborne Pathogen Standard. Do not assume that older people are too old to have sex.

TIME TO REFLECT

Mrs. Lightfoot has chronic kidney failure. She travels to a dialysis center three times a week for hemodialysis. The van will be arriving at your nursing center in 1 hour to pick her up. Mrs. Lightfoot has a fistula in her right forearm. The nurse asks you to provide AM care for Mrs. Lightfoot, obtain her weight, and measure her vital signs. What factors must you consider while offering this care? Does it matter which arm you use for her blood pressure? When Mrs. Lightfoot returns from her dialysis session, she is usually very tired. How would you care for her upon her return?

REVIEW QUESTIONS

Circle the BEST answer.

1. A person has cystitis. This is a
   a. Kidney infection
   b. Kidney stone
   c. Urinary diversion
   d. Bladder infection

2. The person with cystitis needs to drink about
   a. 500 mL daily
   b. 1000 mL daily
   c. 1500 mL daily
   d. 2000 mL daily

3. BPH causes urinary problems because
   a. The person has a weak urine stream
   b. The person voids frequently at night
   c. The enlarged prostate presses against the urethra
   d. Voidings are in small amounts

4. Mr. Jones had a TURP. Which measure should you question?
   a. No sudden movements
   b. No heavy lifting
   c. No straining to have a bowel movement
   d. No oral fluids

5. A person with a urostomy
   a. Has a new pathway for urine to exit the body
   b. Needs dialysis
   c. Had surgery for an enlarged prostate
   d. Has pyuria

6. A person has kidney stones. You need to
   a. Empty the pouch
   b. Strain all urine
   c. Collect a urine specimen
   d. Change the urinary drainage bag

7. A person has kidney failure. Which statement is *false?*
   a. The kidneys remove waste products from the blood in a normal manner
   b. The body retains fluid
   c. Every body system is affected
   d. Diuresis follows oliguria

8. For chronic kidney failure, care includes the following *except*
   a. A diet low in protein, potassium, and sodium
   b. Measuring urine output every hour
   c. Measures to prevent pressure injuries
   d. Measuring weight daily

9. These statements are about STIs. Which is *false?*
   a. They are usually spread by sexual contact
   b. They can affect the genital area and other body parts
   c. Signs and symptoms are obvious
   d. Some result in death

10. STIs require
    a. Masks and protective eyewear
    b. Gowns
    c. Double-bagging
    d. Standard Precautions

11. Mr. Sanchez has a suprapubic catheter. Which is *false?*
    a. The catheter drains his bladder
    b. He needs good skin care
    c. His catheter is connected to a drainage bag
    d. He voids in a urinal

12. Which does *not* contribute to pelvic organ prolapse?
    a. Loss of estrogen
    b. Kegel exercises
    c. Childbirth
    d. Weakened pelvic floor muscles

See Appendix A for answers to these questions.

39

Mental Health Disorders

OBJECTIVES

- Define the key terms and key abbreviations listed in this chapter.
- Explain the difference between mental health and mental illness.
- List the causes of mental illness.
- Describe four anxiety disorders.
- Explain the defense mechanisms used to relieve anxiety.
- Describe common phobias.
- Describe schizophrenia.

- Describe bipolar disorder and depression.
- Describe personality disorders.
- Describe substance abuse and addiction.
- Describe suicide and the persons at risk.
- Describe the care required by persons with mental health disorders.
- Explain how to promote quality of life.

KEY TERMS

affect Feelings and emotions

anxiety A vague, uneasy feeling in response to stress

compulsion Repeating an act over and over again

defense mechanism An unconscious reaction that blocks unpleasant or threatening feelings

delusion A false belief

delusion of grandeur An exaggerated belief about one's importance, wealth, power, or talents

delusion of persecution A false belief that one is being mistreated, abused, or harassed

emotional illness See "mental disorder"

flashback Reliving a trauma in thoughts during the day and in nightmares during sleep

hallucination Seeing, hearing, smelling, or feeling something that is not real

mental Relating to the mind; something that exists in the mind or is done by the mind

mental disorder A disturbance in the ability to cope with or adjust to stress; behavior and function are impaired; mental illness, emotional illness, psychiatric disorder

mental health The person copes with and adjusts to everyday stresses in ways accepted by society

mental illness See "mental disorder"

obsession A recurrent, unwanted thought, idea, or image

panic An intense and sudden feeling of fear, anxiety, terror, or dread

paranoia A disorder (para-) of the mind (-noia); false beliefs (delusions) and suspicion about a person or situation

phobia An intense fear

psychiatric disorder See "mental disorder"

psychosis A state of severe mental impairment

stigma A feeling of shame or judgment from someone else

stress The response or change in the body caused by any emotional, physical, social, or economic factor

stressor The event or factor that causes stress

substance use disorder A mental disorder that affects a person's brain and behavior

suicide To kill oneself

suicide contagion Exposure to suicide or suicidal behaviors within one's family, one's peer group, or media reports of suicide

withdrawal syndrome The person's physical and mental response after stopping or severely reducing the use of a substance that was used regularly

KEY ABBREVIATIONS

BPD Borderline personality disorder
GI Gastrointestinal
NAMI National Alliance on Mental Illness
NIAAA National Institute on Alcohol Abuse and Alcoholism

NIMH National Institute of Mental Health
OCD Obsessive-compulsive disorder
PTSD Posttraumatic stress disorder
SUD Substance use disorder

The whole person has physical, social, psychologic, and spiritual parts. Each part affects the other.
- A physical problem has social, mental, and spiritual effects.
- A mental health disorder can affect the person physically, socially, and spiritually.
- A social problem can have physical, mental health, and spiritual effects.

BASIC CONCEPTS

Mental relates to the mind. It is something that exists in the mind or is done by the mind. Therefore, mental health involves the mind. Mental disorders are the leading cause of disability in the United States. According to the National Alliance for Mental Illness (NAMI), people experiencing mental health conditions often deal with the stigma of mental illness. They often face rejection, bullying, and discrimination. This can make their recovery longer and more difficult. NAMI encourages health care workers to see the person, not the condition. Health care workers are encouraged to get to know the person and always treat the person with kindness and empathy.

Mental health and mental disorders may involve stress:
- Stress—is the response or change in the body caused by any emotional, physical, social, or economic factor.
- Mental health—means that the person copes with and adjusts to everyday stresses in ways accepted by society.
- Mental disorder—is a disturbance in the ability to cope with or adjust to stress. Behavior and function are impaired. Mental illness, emotional illness, and psychiatric disorder are other names.

Causes of mental health disorders include the following:
- Not being able to cope or adjust to stress
- Chemical imbalances
- Genetics
- Physical or biologic factors
- Psychologic factors
- Drug or substance abuse
- Social and cultural factors

ANXIETY DISORDERS

Anxiety is a vague, uneasy feeling in response to stress. The person may not know why or the cause. Danger or harm—real or imagined—is sensed. The person acts to relieve the unpleasant feeling. Often, anxiety occurs when needs are not met.

Some anxiety is normal. Persons with mental health disorders have higher levels of anxiety. Signs and symptoms depend on the degree of anxiety (Box 39.1).

Anxiety level depends on the stressor. A stressor is the event or factor that causes stress. It can be physical, emotional, social, or economic. Past experiences affect how a person reacts, as does the number of stressors. A stressor may produce mild anxiety. The same stressor can cause higher anxiety at another time.

Coping and defense mechanisms are used to relieve anxiety. Some are healthy. Others are not—eating, drinking, smoking, and fighting are examples. Healthy ways to cope include

---

BOX 39.1 Signs and Symptoms of Anxiety

- "Lump" in the throat
- "Butterflies" in the stomach
- Pulse: rapid
- Respirations: rapid
- Blood pressure: increased
- Speech: rapid, voice changes
- Mouth: dry
- Sweating
- Nausea
- Diarrhea
- Urinary frequency and urgency
- Attention span: poor
- Directions: difficulty following
- Sleep: difficulty
- Appetite: loss of

---

discussing the problem, exercising, playing music, taking a hot bath, and wanting to be alone.

Defense mechanisms are unconscious reactions that block unpleasant or threatening feelings (Box 39.2). Some use of defense mechanisms is normal. In mental disorders, they are used poorly.

Panic Disorder

Panic is the highest level of anxiety. Panic is an intense and sudden feeling of fear, anxiety, terror, or dread. Onset is sudden with no obvious reason. The person cannot function. Signs and symptoms of anxiety are severe (see Box 39.1). The person may also have:
- Chest pain.
- Shortness of breath.
- Rapid heart rate ("heart pounding").
- Numbness and tingling in the hands.
- Dizziness.
- A smothering sensation.
- Feeling of impending doom or loss of control.

These persons may feel that they are having a heart attack, losing their mind, or on the verge of death. Attacks can occur at any time, even during sleep.

Panic attacks can last for 10 minutes or longer. They can occur often. Panic disorder can last for a few months or for many years.

Many people avoid places where panic attacks occurred. For example, a person had a panic attack in a shopping mall so she now avoids malls.

Phobias

Phobia means an intense fear. The person has an intense fear of an object, situation, or activity that has little or no actual danger. Common phobias are fear of the following:
- Being in an open, crowded, or public place (agoraphobia—*agora* means "marketplace")
- Being in pain or seeing others in pain (algophobia—*algo* means "pain")

BOX 39.2 Defense Mechanisms

Compensation. *Compensate* means "to make up for, replace, or substitute." The person makes up for or substitutes a strength for a weakness.

EXAMPLE: Not good in sports, a child develops another talent.

Conversion. *Convert* means "to change." An emotion is shown as a physical symptom or changed into a physical symptom.

EXAMPLE: Not wanting to read aloud in school, a child complains of a headache.

Denial. *Deny* means "refusing to accept or believe something that is true." The person refuses to face or accept unpleasant or threatening things.

EXAMPLE: After a heart attack, a person continues to smoke.

Displacement. *Displace* means "to move or take the place of." An individual moves behaviors or emotions from one person, place, or thing to a safe person, place, or thing.

EXAMPLE: Angry at your boss, you yell at a friend.

Identification. *Identify* means "to relate or recognize." A person assumes the ideas, behaviors, and traits of another person.

EXAMPLE: A neighbor is a high school cheerleader. A little girl practices cheerleading in her backyard.

Projection. *Project* means "to blame another." An individual blames another person or object for unacceptable behaviors, emotions, ideas, or wishes.

EXAMPLE: Sleeping too long, a worker blames the traffic when late for work.

Rationalization. *Rational* means "sensible, reasonable, or logical." An acceptable reason or excuse is given for behaviors or actions. The real reason is not given.

EXAMPLE: Often late for work, an employee does not get a raise. The employee thinks: "My boss doesn't like me."

Reaction formation. A person acts in a way opposite to own true feelings.

EXAMPLE: A worker does not like his boss. He buys the boss an expensive gift.

Regression. *Regress* means "to move back or to retreat." The person retreats or moves back to an earlier time or condition.

EXAMPLE: A 3-year-old wants a baby bottle when a new baby comes into the family.

Repression. *Repress* means "to hold down or keep back." The person keeps unpleasant or painful thoughts or experiences from the conscious mind. The person cannot recall or remember such things.

EXAMPLE: A child was sexually abused. Now 33 years old, there is no memory of the event.

- Water (aquaphobia—*aqua* means "water")
- Being in or being trapped in an enclosed or narrow space (claustrophobia—*claustro* means "closing")
- The slightest uncleanliness (mysophobia—*myso* means "anything that is disgusting")
- Night or darkness (nyctophobia—*nycto* means "night or darkness")
- Fire (pyrophobia—*pyro* means "fire")
- Strangers (xenophobia—*xeno* means "strange")

The person avoids what is feared. When faced with the fear, the person has high anxiety and cannot function.

Obsessive-Compulsive Disorder

The person with obsessive-compulsive disorder (OCD) has obsessions and compulsions. An obsession is a recurrent, unwanted thought, idea, or image. Some people are obsessed with microbes, dirt, violent thoughts, or things forbidden by religious beliefs. Compulsion is repeating an act over and over again (a ritual). The act may not make sense. However, the person has much anxiety if the act is not done.

Common rituals are hand washing, constant checking to make sure the stove is off, cleaning, counting things to a certain number, or touching things in a certain order. Such rituals can take over an hour every day. They are very distressing and affect daily life. Some persons with OCD also have depression, eating disorders, substance abuse, and other anxiety disorders.

Posttraumatic Stress Disorder

Posttraumatic stress disorder (PTSD) occurs after a terrifying ordeal. The ordeal involved physical harm or the threat of physical harm. Signs and symptoms of PTSD are listed in Box 39.3. PTSD can develop after these events:
- Being harmed
- A loved one being harmed
- Seeing a harmful event happen to loved ones or strangers
  PTSD can result from many traumatic events. They include the following:
- War
- A terrorist attack
- Mugging
- Rape
- Torture
- Kidnapping
- Being held captive
- Child abuse
- A crash—vehicle, train, plane

BOX 39.3 Signs and Symptoms of Posttraumatic Stress Disorder

- Startles easily
- Emotionally numb—especially to those with whom the person used to be close
- Difficulty trusting people
- Difficulty feeling close to people
- Loss of interest in things the person used to enjoy
- Problems being affectionate
- Feelings of intense guilt
- Irritability
- Avoiding situations that remind the person of the harmful event
- Difficulty around the anniversary of the harmful event
- Gets mad easily
- Outbursts of anger
- Problems sleeping
- Increasingly aggressive
- Becoming more violent
- Physical symptoms:
  - Headache
  - Gastrointestinal (GI) distress
  - Immune system problems
  - Dizziness
  - Chest pain
  - Discomfort in other body parts

- Bombing
- A natural disaster—flood, tornado, hurricane

Most people with PTSD have flashbacks. A flashback is reliving the trauma in thoughts during the day and in nightmares during sleep. Flashbacks may involve images, sounds, smells, or feelings. Everyday things can trigger them. A door slamming is an example. During a flashback, the person may lose touch with reality. The person may believe that the trauma is happening all over again. For example, Mr. Butler served in the Army during World War II. When he hears a loud noise, he grabs his electric shaver and holds it as though it is a gun. The loud noise makes him relive the trauma of war.

Signs and symptoms usually develop about 3 months after the harmful event. However, they may not emerge until years later. Some people recover within 6 months. PTSD lasts longer in other people. The condition may become chronic.

PTSD can develop at any age, including during childhood. The person may also suffer from depression, substance abuse, and other anxiety disorders.

SCHIZOPHRENIA

Schizophrenia means split *(schizo)* mind *(phrenia)*. It is a severe, chronic, disabling brain disorder. It involves:

- Psychosis—a state of severe mental impairment. The person does not view the real or unreal correctly.
- Delusion—a false belief. For example, the person believes that a radio station is broadcasting the person's thoughts.
- Hallucination—seeing, hearing, smelling, or feeling something that is not real. A person may see animals, insects, or people that are not real. "Voices" are the most common type of hallucination in schizophrenia. These may comment on behavior, order the person to do things, warn of danger, or talk to other voices.
- Paranoia—a disorder *(para)* of the mind *(noia)*. The person has false beliefs (delusions). The person is suspicious about other individuals or situations, such as believing that others are cheating, harassing, poisoning, spying on, or plotting against the person.
- Delusion of grandeur—an exaggerated belief about one's importance, wealth, power, or talents. For example, a man believes he is Superman, or a woman believes she is the Queen of England.
- Delusion of persecution—a false belief that one is being mistreated, abused, or harassed. For example, such persons believe that someone is "out to get" them.

The person with schizophrenia has severe mental impairment *(psychosis)*. Thinking and behavior are disturbed. The person has false beliefs *(delusions)*. The person also has *hallucinations*. That is, the person sees, hears, smells, or feels things that are not real. The person has problems relating to others. The person may be *paranoid*, meaning being suspicious about a person or situation. The person may have difficulty organizing thoughts. Responses are not appropriate. Communication is disturbed. The person may ramble or repeat what another says. Sometimes speech cannot be understood. The person may make up words. The person may withdraw. That is, the person lacks interest in others and is not involved with people or society.

Disorders of movement occur. These include the following:

- Being clumsy and uncoordinated
- Involuntary movements
- Grimacing
- Unusual mannerisms
- Sitting for hours without moving, speaking, or responding

Some persons regress. To *regress* means "to retreat or move back to an earlier time or condition." For example, a 5-year-old wets the bed when there is a new baby. This is normal. Healthy adults do not act like infants or children.

In men, the symptoms usually begin in the late teens or early 20s. In women, symptoms usually begin in the 20s and 30s. In rare cases, it can appear in childhood. People with schizophrenia do not tend to be violent. However, if a person with paranoid schizophrenia becomes violent, it is often directed at family members. The violence usually occurs at home. Some persons with schizophrenia attempt suicide (p. ··).

See *Focus on Communication: Schizophrenia.*

FOCUS ON COMMUNICATION

Schizophrenia

Delusions, hallucinations, and paranoia can frighten a person. Good communication is important.

- Speak slowly and calmly.
- Do not pretend you experience what the person does. Help the person focus on reality.
- Do not try to convince the person that the experience is not real. To the person, it is real.

For example, a person is hearing voices. You can say: "I don't hear the voices, but I believe that you do. Try to listen to my voice and not the other voices."

MOOD DISORDERS

Mood or affect relates to feelings and emotions. Mood (or affective) disorders involve feelings, emotions, and moods.

Bipolar Disorder

Bipolar means two *(bi)* poles or ends *(polar)*. The person with bipolar disorder has severe extremes in mood, energy, and ability to function. There are emotional lows *(depression)* and emotional highs *(mania)*. The disorder also is called manic-depressive illness. The person may:

- Be more depressed than manic.
- Be more manic than depressed.
- Alternate between depression and mania.

The disorder tends to run in families. It usually develops in the late teens or in early adulthood. Lifelong management is required.

Signs and symptoms can range from mild to severe (Box 39.4). Mood changes are called "episodes." Bipolar disorder can damage relationships and affect school or work performance. Some people are suicidal.

BOX 39.4 Signs and Symptoms of Bipolar Disorder

Mania (Manic Episode)
- Increased energy, activity, and restlessness
- Excessively "high," overly good mood
- Extreme irritability
- Racing thoughts and talking very fast
- Jumping from one idea to another
- Easily distracted; problems concentrating
- Little sleep needed
- Unrealistic beliefs in one's abilities and powers
- Poor judgment
- Spending sprees
- A lasting period of behavior that is different from usual
- Increased sexual drive
- Drug abuse (particularly cocaine, alcohol, and sleeping pills)
- Aggressive behavior
- Denial that anything is wrong

Depression (Depressive Episode)
- Lasting sad, anxious, or empty mood
- Feelings of hopelessness
- Feelings of guilt, worthlessness, or helplessness
- Loss of interest or pleasure in activities once enjoyed
- Loss of interest in sex
- Decreased energy; a feeling of fatigue or being "slowed down"
- Problems concentrating, remembering, or making decisions
- Restlessness or irritability
- Sleeping too much or unable to sleep
- Change in appetite
- Unintended weight loss or gain
- Chronic pain or other symptoms not caused by physical illness or injury
- Thoughts of death or suicide
- Suicide attempts

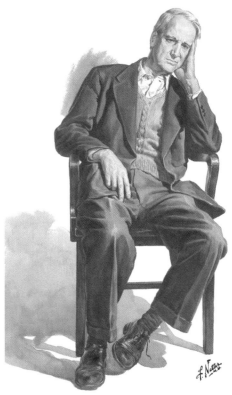

Fig. 39.1 The person feels sad and depressed. (From Solomon PR, Budson AE: *Memory loss, Alzheimer's disease, and dementia: a practical guide for clinicians*, ed. 3, St. Louis, 2022, Elsevier.)

Major Depression

Depression involves the body, mood, and thoughts. Symptoms (see Box 39.4) affect work, study, sleep, eating, and other activities. The person is very sad (Fig 39.1) and loses interest in daily activities. Table 39.1 lists types of depression.

Depression may occur because of a stressful event such as the death of a partner, parent, or child. Divorce and job loss are other stressful events. Some physical disorders can cause depression. Stroke, heart attack, cancer, and Parkinson disease are examples. Hormonal factors may cause depression in women—menstrual cycle changes, pregnancy, miscarriage, after childbirth (postpartum depression), and before and during menopause.

Depression in Older Persons

Depression is common in older persons. They have many losses—death of family and friends, loss of health, loss of body functions, loss of independence. Loneliness and the side effects of some medications also are causes. Elderly persons in long-term care settings may be afraid to admit that they are suffering from depression. Many older persons feel that depression is a character flaw. They may be ashamed and blame themselves. They may think treatment would cost too much. Report your observations to the nurse. Box 39.5 lists signs and symptoms of depression in older persons.

Depression in older persons is often overlooked or a wrong diagnosis is made. Often, the person is thought to have a cognitive disorder (Chapter 40). Therefore, the depression may not be treated.

Treatment for Depression

Medication is effective in treating depression in a majority of older persons. Other forms of treatment are psychotherapy (counseling) or electroconvulsive (shock) therapy. Psychosocial treatment also may play a role. For some individuals, being isolated and having few social contacts can promote depression. For this reason, nursing assistants should encourage activities that include socialization. Sharing meals at a table instead of eating alone in a room is one way to promote socialization. Some older persons benefit greatly from the camaraderie of playing cards regularly with friends. Others meet with members of their church or faith-based group to help improve their mood and reduce feelings of sadness. Getting to know the person's likes and dislikes will help you to offer suggestions for activities. The health care providers, nursing staff, social worker, activity director, and chaplain (religious advisor) assist persons dealing with depression.

TABLE 39.1 Types of Depression

Types of Depression

There are different types of depressive disorders, and while there are many similarities, each depressive disorder has its own unique set of symptoms.

Persistent Depressive Disorder (Dysthymia)	Major Depressive Disorder	Adjustment Disorder with Depressed Mood
The essential feature of this mood disorder is a low, dark, or sad mood that is persistently present for most of the day and on most days, for at least 2 years	Major depression is characterized by having at least five of nine common symptoms. One of the symptoms must be either an overwhelming feeling of sadness or a loss of interest and pleasure in most usual activities. The symptoms must persist for 2 weeks or longer and represent a significant change from previous functioning. Social, occupational, educational, or other important functioning are impacted by major depressive disorder.	This is diagnosed when symptoms of depression are triggered within 3 months of onset of a stressor. The stressor usually involves a change of some kind in the life of the individual who finds it stressful. Sometimes the stressor can even be a positive event such as a new job, marriage, or baby, which is nevertheless stressful for the individual.

From Anxiety and Depression Association of America, Understanding depression, 2021, https://understandingdepression.adaa.org.

BOX 39.5 Signs and Symptoms of Depression in Older Persons

- Fatigue and lack of interest
- Inability to experience pleasure
- Feelings of uselessness, hopelessness, and helplessness
- Decreased sexual interest
- Increased dependency
- Anxiety
- Slow or unreliable memory
- Paranoia
- Agitation
- Focus on the past
- Thoughts of death and suicide
- Difficulty completing activities of daily living
- Changes in sleep patterns
- Poor grooming
- Withdrawal from people and interests
- Muscle aches, abdominal pain, and headaches
- Nausea and vomiting
- Dry mouth
- Loss of appetite
- Weight loss

PERSONALITY DISORDERS

Personality disorders involve rigid and maladaptive behaviors. (To *adapt* means "to change or adjust"; *mal* means "bad, wrong, or ill"; *maladaptive* means "to change or adjust in the wrong way.") Because of their behaviors, those with personality disorders cannot function well in society.

Antisocial Personality Disorder

This is a chronic disorder in which the person's thinking and behaviors show no regard for right and wrong. The person has poor judgment, lacks responsibility, and is hostile. The person is not loyal to any person or group. Morals and ethics are lacking. The rights of others do not matter. The person lies, charms, or cons others for personal gain or pleasure. The person has no guilt and does not learn from experiences or punishment. The person is often in trouble with the police.

Signs and symptoms may include the following:
- Lying or cheating
- Child abuse or neglect
- Aggressive or violent behaviors
- Poor or abusive relationships
- Blaming others for actions and behaviors
- Problems functioning in work or school

Symptoms tend to peak during the 20s and then decrease.

Risk factors include the following:
- A conduct disorder in childhood
- A family history of antisocial personality disorder
- A family history of mental disorders
- Childhood abuse—verbal, physical, sexual
- Unstable family life during childhood
- Loss of parents during childhood—death, divorce

Borderline Personality Disorder

The person with borderline personality disorder (BPD) has problems with moods, relationships, self-image, and behavior. The person has problems controlling emotions and may have intense bouts of anger, depression, and anxiety that last hours or most of the day. Aggression, self-injury, and drug or alcohol abuse may occur. The person may engage in risky behaviors—unsafe driving, unsafe sex, gambling sprees. The person may greatly admire and love family and friends and then suddenly shift to intense anger and dislike. The person may have thoughts of suicide and other mental health disorders.

BPD is more common in women than in men. Risk factors may include the following:
- A family history of BPD
- Childhood abuse—sexual, physical
- Childhood neglect or being abandoned
- Changes in the brain
- Brain chemicals that do not function properly

SUBSTANCE USE DISORDER AND ADDICTION

According to the National Institute of Mental Health (NIMH), a substance use disorder (SUD) is a mental disorder that affects a person's brain and behavior. This leads to a person's inability to control the use of substances such as legal or illegal drugs, alcohol, or medications. Symptoms can range from moderate to severe, with addiction being the most severe form of SUDs. Addiction is the inability to stop using a substance even though it has harmful effects. Physical and mental health are affected, as is the welfare of others.

Substances involved in abuse and addiction affect the nervous system. Some depress the nervous system. Others stimulate it. All affect the mind and thinking.

Alcoholism and Alcohol Abuse

Alcohol slows brain activity. It affects alertness, judgment, coordination, and reaction time. Over time, heavy drinking damages the brain, central nervous system, liver, heart, kidneys, blood vessels, and stomach. It also can cause forgetfulness and confusion.

According to the National Institute on Alcohol Abuse and Alcoholism (NIAAA), *alcoholism* (alcohol dependence) includes these symptoms:

- *Craving.* The person has a strong need or urge to drink.
- *Loss of control.* The person cannot stop drinking once drinking has begun.
- *Physical dependence.* The person has withdrawal symptoms when stopping drinking. They include nausea, sweating, shakiness, and anxiety.
- *Tolerance.* The person needs to drink greater amounts of alcohol to get "high."

Alcoholism is a chronic disease. It lasts throughout life. Lifestyle and genetics are risk factors. Some people drink alcohol for relief from life stresses—retirement, lowered income, job loss, failing health, loneliness, or the deaths of loved ones or friends. The alcohol craving can be as strong as the need for food or water. An alcoholic will continue to drink despite serious family, health, or legal problems.

Alcoholism can be treated but not cured. Counseling and medications are used to help the person stop drinking. The person must avoid all alcohol to avoid a relapse.

Alcohol abuse is just as harmful as alcoholism. A person who abuses alcohol drinks too much but is not dependent on alcohol.

Problems linked to alcoholism and alcohol abuse include the following:

- Not being able to meet work, school, or family responsibilities
- Motor vehicle crashes
- Drunk-driving arrests
- Drinking-related medical conditions

Drinking occasionally or regularly does not mean a drinking problem. According to the NIAAA, a person needs help when the following occur:

- Drinks to calm nerves, forget worries, or reduce depression

- Has lost interest in food
- Gulps drinks down quickly
- Lies or tries to hide drinking habits
- Drinks alone more often
- Has hurt oneself or someone else while drinking
- Was drunk more than three or four times in 1 year
- Needs more alcohol to get "high"
- Feels irritable, resentful, or unreasonable when not drinking
- Has medical, social, or money problems caused by drinking

Alcohol and Older Persons

Alcohol effects vary with age. Even small amounts can make older persons feel "high." Older persons are at risk for falls, motor vehicle crashes, and other injuries from drinking. They have:

- Slower reaction times.
- Hearing and vision problems.
- A lower tolerance for alcohol.

Older people tend to take more medications than younger persons. Mixing alcohol with some medications can be harmful, even fatal. Alcohol also makes some health problems worse. High blood pressure is an example.

Drug Abuse and Addiction

Drugs interfere with normal brain function. While they create powerful feelings of pleasure, they have long-term effects on the brain. At some point, changes in the brain can turn drug abuse into addiction.

- *Drug abuse*—is the overuse of a drug for nonmedical or nontherapy effects.
- *Drug addiction*—is a chronic, relapsing brain disease. The person has an overwhelming desire to take a drug. The person repeatedly takes the drug because of its effect. Usually, the effect is altered mental awareness. The person has to have the drug. Often, higher doses are needed. The person cannot stop taking the drug without treatment.

A diagnosis of drug abuse or addiction is based on three or more of the following. They must have occurred at any time during a 12-month period.

- The substance is often taken in larger amounts, or it is taken longer than intended.
- There is a constant desire for the substance, or the person cannot cut down or control substance use.
- A lot of time is spent using the substance or recovering from its effects, or a great deal of time is spent trying to obtain the substance. For example, the person visits many doctors to obtain the substance or drives long distances to get the substance.
- The person gave up or reduced important social, occupational, or recreational activities because of substance abuse.
- The person continues to use the substance. The person does so despite knowing that a constant or recurring problem is caused by or made worse by using the substance. The problem may be physical or psychologic.
- The person has tolerance to the substance.

- Increased amounts are needed to achieve intoxication or the desired effect.
- Continued use of the same amount has a greatly reduced effect on the person.
- The person has withdrawal from the substance (*withdraw* means "to stop, remove, or take away").
  - The withdrawal syndrome is that expected for the drug. Withdrawal syndrome is the person's physical and mental response after stopping or severely reducing the use of a substance that was used regularly. The body responds with anxiety, restlessness, insomnia, irritability, impaired attention, and physical illness.
  - The same (or similar) substance is taken to relieve or avoid withdrawal symptoms.

Drug abuse and addiction affect social and mental function. Drug abuse and addiction are linked to crimes, violence, and motor vehicle crashes. Physical effects can occur from one use, high doses, or prolonged use:

- Human immunodeficiency virus (HIV) and acquired immunodeficiency syndrome (AIDS) (Chapter 34)
- Cardiovascular disease
- Stroke
- Sudden death
- Hepatitis
- Lung disease
- Cancer

Both legal and illegal drugs may be abused. Legal drugs are approved for use in the United States. Doctors prescribe them. Illegal drugs are not approved for use. They are obtained through illegal means. Often, legal drugs also are obtained through illegal means. Currently in the United States we are facing an enormous problem of addiction to opioid drugs. In the beginning people may take them as prescribed by a doctor, but then they cannot stop taking them. They become addicted and find other ways to get the drugs. Prescription pain relievers can possibly lead to addiction. Some people use stronger and stronger drugs. Overdose due to heroin and other opioids is a serious health crisis in the United States.

Treatment depends on the drug and the person. A drug treatment program combines various therapies and services to meet the person's needs. The person's age, race, culture, sexual orientation, and gender are considered. So are issues such as pregnancy, parenting, housing, employment, and physical and sexual abuse.

Drug abuse and addiction are chronic problems. Relapses can occur. A short-term, one-time treatment is often not enough. Treatment is a long-term process. Drug and alcohol addiction are often symptoms of underlying mental disorders that are not treated.

SUICIDE

Suicide means "to kill oneself." According to a 2019 NIMH report and a 2019 report from the Centers for Disease Control and Prevention (CDC):

- Suicide was the 10th leading cause of death in the United States. In 2019, there were more than 47,500 deaths from suicide.

- Risk factors for attempted suicide include the following:
  - Depression and other mental health disorders
  - Alcohol or other substance abuse
  - Separation or divorce
- Firearms, suffocation, and poison are the most common methods of suicide. Firearms are the most common method for men. Poison is the most common method for women.
- More men than women die by suicide.
- Native Americans and Alaskan Natives have high rates of suicide.
- Youth, the elderly, and veterans are at risk for suicide.
- The highest rate of suicide was among White men aged 75 years and older.
- Suicide was the third leading cause of death among persons aged 15 to 24. More males than females in this age group died by suicide. Risk factors for attempted suicide are the following:
  - Depression
  - Alcohol or other substance abuse
  - Physical or sexual abuse
  - Disruptive behavior

Risk factors for suicide are listed in Box 39.6. If a person mentions or talks about suicide, take the person seriously. Call for the nurse at once. Do not leave the person alone.

Centers that treat persons with mental health disorders must identify persons at risk for suicide. They must:

- Identify specific factors or features that increase or decrease the risk for suicide.
- Meet the person's immediate safety needs.
- Provide the most appropriate setting for treating the person.
- Provide crisis information to the person and family. A crisis "hotline" phone number is an example. The US National Suicide Prevention Lifeline is 1-800-273-TALK (8255). It is a free, 24/7 service that provides suicidal persons or those around them with support, information, and local resources. Fig. 39.2 gives additional information to help someone in emotional pain.

See *Focus on Communication: Suicide.*

BOX 39.6 Risk Factors for Suicide

- A history of suicide attempts
- Depression and other mental disorders
- History of alcohol or drug abuse
- Chronic pain
- Stressful life event or loss (example: divorce)
- Family history of a mental disorder or substance abuse
- Family history of suicide
- Family violence (including physical or sexual abuse)
- Having guns or other firearms in the home
- Having recently been released from prison or jail
- Being exposed to others' suicidal behavior, such as that of family, peers, or celebrities

Modified from National Institute of Mental Health: *Suicide in the US: statistics and prevention*, NIH Publication No. 06-4594, Bethesda, MD, 2021, National Institutes of Health.

5 Action Steps for Helping Someone in Emotional Pain

Suicide is a major public health concern and a leading cause of death in the United States. Suicide affects people of all ages, genders, races, and ethnicities.

Suicide is complicated and tragic, but it can be preventable. **Knowing the warning signs for suicide and how to get help can help save lives.**

Here are 5 steps you can take to #BeThe1To help someone in emotional pain:

1. ASK:
"Are you thinking about killing yourself?" It's not an easy question but studies show that asking at-risk individuals if they are suicidal does not increase suicides or suicidal thoughts.

2. KEEP THEM SAFE:
Reducing a suicidal person's access to highly lethal items or places is an important part of suicide prevention. While this is not always easy, asking if the at-risk person has a plan and removing or disabling the lethal means can make a difference.

3. BE THERE:
Listen carefully and learn what the individual is thinking and feeling. Research suggests acknowledging and talking about suicide may in fact reduce rather than increase suicidal thoughts.

4. HELP THEM CONNECT:
Save the National Suicide Prevention Lifeline number **(1-800-273-TALK)** and the Crisis Text Line **(741741)** in your phone so they're there if you need them. You can also help make a connection with a trusted individual like a family member, friend, spiritual advisor, or mental health professional.

5. STAY CONNECTED:
Staying in touch after a crisis or after being discharged from care can make a difference. Studies have shown the number of suicide deaths goes down when someone follows up with the at-risk person.

For more information on suicide prevention:
www.nimh.nih.gov/suicideprevention
www.bethe1to.com

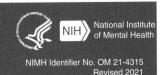

NIMH Identifier No. OM 21-4315
Revised 2021

Fig. 39.2 Action steps for helping someone in emotional pain. (**From National Institute of Mental Health, 5 action steps for helping someone in emotional pain, 2021;** www.nimh.nih.gov/suicideprevention)

FOCUS ON COMMUNICATION

Suicide

Persons thinking of suicide may talk about their thoughts. A person may say:
- "I just don't want to live anymore."
- "I wish I were dead."
- "I wish I had never been born."
- "Everyone would be better off without me."

Call for the nurse at once if a person mentions thoughts of suicide.

A person may ask you not to tell anyone about the suicidal thoughts. Protecting personal information is important, but the person's safety is the priority. Never promise the person that you will not tell anyone. Report the statements to the nurse at once. It is the right thing to do.

Suicide and Older Persons

According to NIMH, older persons have higher suicide rates than younger persons. Older White males have the highest rates. Among White males 65 years and older, the risk goes up with age. White men 75 years and older have the highest suicide rates. Some older persons are less likely to recover from a suicide attempt.

Many older persons suffer from depression (p. ··). Depression often occurs with other serious illnesses. Heart disease, stroke, diabetes, cancer, and Parkinson disease are examples. The person also may have social and financial problems.

Most older suicide victims did not report depression to their health care providers, or depression was not detected by the health care providers.

Suicide Contagion

NIMH defines suicide contagion as exposure to suicide or suicidal behaviors within one's family, peer group, or media reports of suicide. The exposure has led to an increase in suicide and suicidal behaviors in persons at risk for suicide. Adolescents and young adults are at risk for suicide contagion.

Following suicide exposure, those close to the victim should be evaluated by a mental health professional. They include family, friends, peers, and coworkers. Persons at risk for suicide need mental health services.

CARE AND TREATMENT

Treatment of mental health disorders involves having persons explore their thoughts and feelings. This is done through psychotherapy and behavior, group, occupational, art, and family therapies. Often, medications are ordered.

The care plan reflects each person's needs. The needs of the total person must be met. This includes physical, safety and security, and emotional needs.

Communication is important. Be alert to nonverbal communication. This includes the person's nonverbal communication and your own.

Persons with mental health disorders may respond to stress with anxiety, panic, or anger. Some may become violent. You must take responsibility for your safety. Your first priority is to protect yourself. Once you are safe, the health team can work together to protect the person and others. To protect yourself:

- Call for help. Do not try to handle the situation on your own.
- Keep a safe distance between you and the person.
- Be aware of your surroundings. Do not let the violent person get between you and the exit. (See "Workplace Violence" in Chapter 11.)

See *Focus on Communication: Care and Treatment.*

FOCUS ON COMMUNICATION

Care and Treatment

Nonverbal communication involves eye contact, tone of voice, facial expressions, body movements, and posture. Persons with major depression often have little eye contact, poor posture, and speak softly. Some do not speak much at all. Facial expressions may not change. Some persons cry.

Persons with anxiety feel uneasy. They may be restless and unable to sit still. Anxious persons often speak quickly. Eye contact may be prolonged and intense. Others have poor eye contact. The eyes may move quickly from one place to another. Be alert to nonverbal cues. Tell the nurse what you observe.

Your nonverbal communication also is important. When interacting with persons with mental disorders:

- Face the person.
- Maintain eye contact.
- Position yourself near the person but not too close. Do not invade the person's space.
- Crouch, sit, or stand at the person's level if it is safe to do so.
- Show interest and concern through your posture and facial expressions.
- Speak calmly.

QUALITY OF LIFE

Persons with mental health disorders have the right to quality of life. They have the same rights as other residents. Some are very ill. They cannot exercise their rights. Legal representatives do so for them.

People do not choose to have physical or mental health disorders. Just as a person does not choose to have diabetes, a person does not choose to have anxiety or depression. How you view the person's illness affects the way you treat the person. Persons with mental health disorders deserve the same dignity and respect given to persons with physical illnesses. Always treat them with kindness and empathy. See the person, not the illness.

Persons with mental health disorders may respond to stress in different ways. They may say or do things that seem strange or odd to you. Do not laugh at or insult the person. Do not joke with others about the person. Treat the person with kindness and respect. Also protect the person's right to privacy and confidentiality. Share what the person said or did only with the nurse. The nurse shares it with the health team as needed. No one else needs to know what the person said or did.

Protect the right to personal choice. The person may have problems making choices. Follow the care plan. Sometimes choices are limited. This helps the person make simple choices. It helps the person feel in control.

Protect the person from abuse, mistreatment, and neglect. Some persons cannot protect themselves. They do not know that they are being mistreated. Report signs of abuse, mistreatment, or neglect to the nurse.

Provide a safe setting. Some persons with mental disorders are dangerous to themselves or others. The care plan includes safety measures. If suicide is a threat, all harmful items are removed from the person's setting. The nurse tells you what to do.

TIME TO REFLECT

Mrs. Westfield is an 87-year-old resident who was admitted to your care center 3 weeks ago. She needs assistance with her personal hygiene. She is incontinent and wears a brief. She becomes very agitated and uncooperative when you assist her with perineal care. She is particularly uncooperative when male staff members assist with her personal care. Mrs. Westfield's daughter attended the care conference this week. She shared with the staff that her mother was raped when she was 20 years old. Why is this information important? How could something that happened more than 60 years ago be significant today? Should this information be passed on to the caregivers? What measures can be put in place to help Mrs. Westfield as care is offered?

REVIEW QUESTIONS

Circle the BEST answer.

1. Stress is
   a. The way a person copes with and adjusts to everyday living
   b. A response or change in the body caused by some factor
   c. A mental disorder
   d. A thought or idea
2. Defense mechanisms are used to
   a. Blame others
   b. Make excuses for behavior
   c. Return to an earlier time
   d. Block unpleasant feelings
3. These statements are about defense mechanisms. Which is *false*?
   a. Mentally healthy persons use them
   b. They relieve anxiety
   c. They prevent mental disorders
   d. Persons with mental disorders use them
4. A phobia is
   a. The event that causes stress
   b. A false belief
   c. An intense fear of something
   d. Feelings and emotions
5. A person cleans and cleans. This behavior is a(n)
   a. Delusion
   b. Hallucination
   c. Compulsion
   d. Obsession
6. A person has nightmares about a trauma. The person is having
   a. Phobias
   b. Panic attacks
   c. Flashbacks
   d. Anxiety
7. A woman believes she is married to a rock singer. This is called a
   a. Fantasy
   b. Delusion of grandeur
   c. Delusion of persecution
   d. Hallucination

8. A man believes that someone is trying to kill him. This belief is called a
   a. Fantasy
   b. Delusion of grandeur
   c. Delusion of persecution
   d. Hallucination
9. These statements are about schizophrenia. Which is *false*?
   a. It is a brain disorder
   b. It can be cured with medications and therapy
   c. Thinking and behavior are disturbed
   d. Suicide is a risk
10. Bipolar disorder means that the person
    a. Is very suspicious
    b. Has anxiety
    c. Is very unhappy and feels unwanted
    d. Has severe mood swings
11. In bipolar disorder, an "emotional high" is called
    a. Depression
    b. Psychosis
    c. An obsession
    d. Mania
12. These statements are about antisocial personality disorder. Which is *false*?
    a. The person has regard for right and wrong
    b. The person blames others
    c. The person lies or cons others for pleasure
    d. The person is hostile and lacks morals
13. Substances involved in abuse and addiction affect the
    a. Circulatory system
    b. Respiratory system
    c. Nervous system
    d. Immune system
14. These statements are about alcoholism. Which is *false*?
    a. The person has a strong craving for alcohol
    b. The disease lasts throughout life
    c. After treatment, the person can have a social drink
    d. The person physically depends on alcohol

15. These statements are about drug addiction. Which is *false*?
    a. It is a chronic brain disease
    b. Higher doses of the drug may be needed
    c. The person has to have the drug
    d. The person can stop taking the drug without treatment
16. A person has withdrawal syndrome. This means that
    a. The person has a physical and mental response when the drug is not taken
    b. The person needs higher doses of the drug
    c. The effect is reduced with the same amount of drug
    d. The person has a relapse after treatment
17. Which group has the highest suicide rate?
    a. White men over 75 years of age
    b. Persons between the ages of 15 and 24
    c. Men
    d. Women
18. For men, the most common method of suicide involves
    a. Firearms
    b. Suffocation
    c. Self-poisoning
    d. Drug overdose
19. Most persons who commit suicide have
    a. A mental disorder
    b. Schizophrenia
    c. A phobia
    d. Suicide contagion
20. A person talks about suicide. What should you do?
    a. Restrain the person
    b. Identify factors that increase the risk of suicide
    c. Ask what method the person intends to use
    d. Call for the nurse

See Appendix A for answers to these questions.

40

Confusion and Dementia

OBJECTIVES

- Define the key terms and key abbreviations listed in this chapter.
- Describe confusion and its causes.
- List the measures that help confused persons.
- Explain the differences between delirium, depression, and dementia.
- Describe Alzheimer disease (AD).
- Describe the signs, symptoms, and behaviors of AD.
- Explain the care required by persons with AD and other dementias.
- Describe the effects of AD on the family.
- Explain validation therapy.
- Explain how to promote quality of life.

KEY TERMS

cognitive function Involves memory, thinking, reasoning, ability to understand, judgment, and behavior
delirium A state of sudden, severe confusion and rapid brain changes
delusion A false belief
dementia The loss of cognitive function that interferes with routine personal, social, and occupational activities
elopement When a person leaves the center without staff knowledge

hallucination Seeing, hearing, smelling, or feeling something that is not real
paranoia A disorder *(para-)* of the mind *(-noia)*; the person has false beliefs (delusions) and suspicion about a person or situation
pseudodementia False (pseudo) dementia
sundowning Signs, symptoms, and behaviors of AD increase during hours of darkness

KEY ABBREVIATIONS

AD Alzheimer disease
ADL Activities of daily living
GDS Global deterioration scale

MCI Mild cognitive impairment
NIA National Institute on Aging
OBRA Omnibus Budget Reconciliation Act of 1987

Changes in the brain and nervous system occur with aging (Box 40.1). Certain diseases affect the brain. Changes in the brain can affect cognitive function. (*Cognitive* relates to knowledge.) Quality of life is affected. Cognitive function involves the following:

- Memory
- Thinking
- Reasoning
- Ability to understand
- Judgment
- Behavior

CONFUSION

Confusion has many causes. Diseases, infections, hearing and vision loss, and medication side effects are some causes. So is brain injury. With aging, blood supply to the brain is reduced. Personality and mental changes can result. Memory and the ability to make good judgments are lost. A person may not know people, the time, or the place. Some people gradually lose the ability to perform daily activities. Behavior changes are common. The person may be angry, restless, depressed, and irritable.

Acute confusion (delirium) occurs suddenly. It is usually temporary. Causes include infection, illness, injury, medications, and surgery. Treatment is aimed at the cause.

Confusion caused by physical changes cannot be cured. Some measures help to improve function (Box 40.2). You must meet the person's basic needs.

DEMENTIA

Dementia is the loss of cognitive function that interferes with routine personal, social, and occupational activities. (*De* means "from"; *mentia* means "mind.") The person may have changes in personality, mood, or behavior. Dementia is a group of symptoms that may occur with certain diseases or conditions.

Dementia is not a normal part of aging. Most older people do not have dementia. Early warning signs include the following:

- Recent memory loss that affects job skills

BOX 40.1 Changes in the Nervous System from Aging

- Nerve cells are lost.
- Nerve conduction slows.
- Responses and reaction times are slower.
- Reflexes are slower.
- Vision and hearing decrease.
- Taste and smell decrease.
- Touch and sensitivity to pain decrease.
- Blood flow to the brain is reduced.
- Sleep patterns change.
- Memory is shorter.
- Forgetfulness occurs.
- Dizziness can occur.

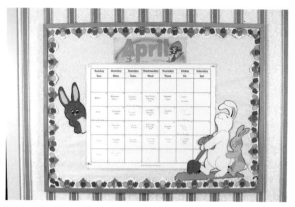

Fig. 40.1 A large calendar can help persons who are confused.

BOX 40.2 Caring for the Person with Confusion

- Follow the person's care plan.
- Provide for safety.
- Face the person. Speak clearly.
- Call the person by name every time you meet.
- State your name. Show your name tag.
- Give the date and time each morning. Repeat as needed during the day or evening.
- Explain what you are going to do and why.
- Give clear, simple directions and answers to questions.
- Ask clear and simple questions. Give the person time to respond.
- Redirect the person's attention.
- Keep calendars and clocks with large numbers in the person's room and in nursing areas (Fig. 40.1). Remind the person of holidays, birthdays, and special events.
- Have the person wear eyeglasses and hearing aids as needed.
- Use touch to communicate (Chapter 6).
- Place familiar objects and pictures within the person's view.
- Provide security item if needed such as a doll, blanket, or stuffed animal (see Fig. 40.12).
- Provide newspapers, magazines, TV, and radio. Read to the person if appropriate.
- Discuss current events with the person.
- Maintain the day-night cycle.
  - Open window coverings during the day. Close them at night.
  - Use nightlights at night. Use them in rooms, bathrooms, hallways, and other areas.
  - Have the person wear regular clothes during the day—not sleepwear.
- Provide a calm, relaxed, and peaceful setting. Prevent loud noises, rushing, and congested hallways and dining rooms. Turn off television if needed.
- Follow the person's routine. Meals, bathing, exercise, TV, bedtime, and other activities have a schedule. This promotes a sense of order and what to expect.
- Break tasks into small steps when helping the person.
- Do not rearrange furniture or the person's belongings.
- Encourage the person to take part in self-care.
- Look for reasons behind the behavior.
- Be consistent. Avoid being confrontational.

- Problems with common tasks (for example, dressing, cooking, driving)
- Problems with language; forgetting simple words
- Getting lost in familiar places
- Misplacing things and putting things in odd places (for example, putting a watch in the oven)
- Personality changes
- Poor or decreased judgment (for example, going outdoors in the snow without shoes)
- Loss of interest in life

If changes in the brain have not occurred, some dementias can be reversed. When the cause is removed, so are the signs and symptoms. Treatable causes include the following:

- Medications and alcohol
- Delirium and depression
- Tumors
- Heart, lung, and blood vessel problems
- Head injuries
- Infection
- Vision and hearing problems

Permanent dementias result from changes in the brain. They have no cure. Function declines over time. Causes of permanent dementia are listed in Box 40.3. Alzheimer disease is the most common type of permanent dementia.

Pseudodementia means false *(pseudo)* dementia. The person has signs and symptoms of dementia. However, there are no changes in the brain. This can occur with delirium and depression. Both can be mistaken for dementia.

Delirium

Delirium is a state of sudden, severe confusion and rapid brain changes. It occurs with physical or mental illness. Usually temporary and reversible, it is common in older persons with acute or chronic illnesses. Infections, heart and lung diseases, and poor nutrition are common causes. So are hormone disorders. Hypoglycemia is also a cause (Chapter 37). Alcohol and many drugs (including prescription medications) can cause delirium. Delirium often lasts for about 1 week. However, it may take several weeks for normal mental function to return.

BOX 40.3 Causes of Permanent Dementia

- AIDS-related dementia
- Alcohol-related dementia and Korsakoff syndrome
- Alzheimer disease
- Dementia with Lewy bodies
- Frontotemporal dementia
- Mixed dementia
- Creutzfeldt-Jakob disease
- Brain tumors
- Cerebrovascular disease
- Huntington disease (a nervous system disease)
- Multiinfarct dementia (MID) (many *[multi]* strokes leave areas of damage *[infarct]*)
- Multiple sclerosis
- Parkinson disease
- Stroke
- Syphilis
- Trauma and head injury

BOX 40.4 Signs and Symptoms of Delirium

- Alertness: changes in (The person is usually more alert in the morning and less alert at night.)
- Changing levels of consciousness
- Awareness: changes in
- Hallucinations and delusions
- Disorganized thinking, talking in a way that doesn't make sense
- Confusion about time or place
- Memory problems, especially with short-term memory
- Problems concentrating
- Disrupted sleep patterns, sleepiness
- Emotional changes:
  - Anger
  - Anxiety
  - Apathy
  - Depression
  - Agitation
  - Irritability
- Incontinence
- Restlessness

Modified from Medline Plus: *Delirium*, Bethesda, MD, 2021, US National Library of Medicine, National Institutes of Health.

Delirium signals physical illness in older persons and in persons with dementia. It is an emergency. The cause must be found and treated. Signs and symptoms are listed in Box 40.4.

Depression

Depression is the most common mental health disorder in older persons. It is often overlooked. Depression, aging, and some medication side effects have similar signs and symptoms. See Chapter 39 for signs and symptoms of depression in older persons.

Mild Cognitive Impairment

Mild cognitive impairment (MCI) is a type of memory change. The person has problems with memory, language, and other mental functions (attention, judgment, reading, writing). The person or others may notice the problems. However, the problems do not interfere with daily life. The person is at risk for Alzheimer disease.

ALZHEIMER DISEASE

Alzheimer disease (AD) is the fifth-leading cause of death among those 65 and older in the United States. According to the Alzheimer's Association, more than 6 million Americans are living with AD. By the year 2050, this number is predicted to rise as high as 12.7 million. In 2022 Alzheimer disease and other dementias cost the nation $321 billion. By 2050, this figure may rise to nearly $1 trillion. Alzheimer disease is a brain disease. Many nerve cells that control intellectual and social function are damaged and die (Fig. 40.2). These functions are affected:

- Memory
- Thinking
- Reasoning
- Judgment
- Language
- Behavior
- Mood
- Personality

The person has problems with work and everyday functions. Problems with family and social relationships occur. There is a steady decline in memory and mental function.

The disease is gradual in onset. It gets worse and worse over time. Persons with AD usually live 8 to 10 years after diagnosis. Some persons live as few as 3 years. Others live as long as 20 years. Some people in their 40s and 50s have AD. However, usually symptoms first appear after the age of 60. The risk increases with age. It is often diagnosed around the age of 80. Nearly half of the persons age 85 and older have AD.

The cause is unknown. A family history of AD increases a person's risk of developing the disease. More women than men have AD. Women live longer than men.

Signs of AD

The classic sign of AD is *gradual loss of short-term memory*. At first, the only symptom may be forgetfulness. Box 40.5 lists the warning signs and other signs of AD. Box 40.6 lists the differences between AD and normal age-related changes.

Stages of AD

Signs and symptoms become more severe as the disease progresses. The disease ends in death. AD is often described in terms of three stages (Box 40.7; Fig. 40.3). The Alzheimer's Association describes seven stages:

- *No impairment.* The person shows no signs of memory problems.
- *Very mild cognitive decline.* The person is aware of a memory loss or lapse. Familiar words or names are forgotten. The person does not know where to find keys, eyeglasses, or other objects. These problems are not apparent to family, friends, or the health team.

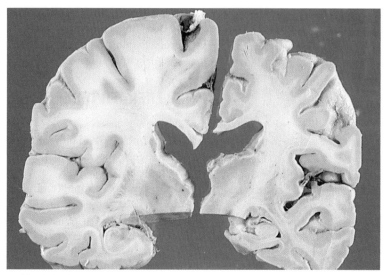

Fig. 40.2 Normal brain is shown on the left. Brain of a person with Alzheimer disease is shown on the right. (From Lewis SL et al.: *Medical-surgical nursing: assessment and management of clinical problems*, ed. 9, St. Louis, 2014, Mosby.)

BOX 40.5 Signs of Alzheimer Disease

Warning Signs
- Gradual loss of short-term memory.
- Asking the same question over and over again.
- Repeating the same story—word for word, again and again.
- Forgetting how to cook, how to make repairs, or how to play cards. The person forgets activities that were once done regularly and with ease.
- Losing the ability to pay bills or balance a checkbook.
- Getting lost in familiar places.
- Misplacing household items.
- Neglecting to bathe. Or wearing the same clothes over and over again. Meanwhile, the person insists that a bath was taken or that clothes are clean.
- Relying on someone else to make decisions or answer questions that the person normally would have handled.

Other Signs
- Forgets recent events, conversations, and appointments.
- Forgets simple directions.
- Forgets names (including family members).
- Forgets the names of everyday things (clock, radio, TV, and so on).
- Forgets words. Loses train of thought.
- Substitutes unusual words and names for what is forgotten.
- Speaks in a native language.
- Curses or swears.

- Misplaces things. Puts things in odd places.
- Has problems writing checks.
- Gives away large amounts of money.
- Does not recognize or understand numbers.
- Has problems following conversations.
- Has problems reading and writing.
- Becomes lost in familiar settings.
- Forgets where own self is.
- Does not know how to get back home.
- Wanders from home.
- Cannot tell or understand time or dates.
- Cannot solve everyday problems (iron left on, stove burners left on, food burning on the stove, and so on).
- Cannot perform everyday tasks (dressing, bathing, brushing teeth, and so on).
- Distrusts others.
- Is stubborn.
- Withdraws socially.
- Is restless.
- Becomes suspicious.
- Becomes fearful.
- Does not want to do things.
- Sleeps more than usual.

Warning signs written by Eric Pfeiffer, MD, Director of the University of South Florida Suncoast Alzheimer's and Gerontology Center. Reprinted with permission.

- *Mild cognitive decline.* Family, friends, and others notice problems. The person has problems with memory or concentration and with words or names. The person loses or misplaces something valuable. Functioning in social or work settings declines.
- *Moderate cognitive decline (mild or early stage).* Memory of recent or current events declines. There are problems with shopping, paying bills, and managing money. The person may withdraw or be quiet in social situations.

- *Moderately severe cognitive decline (moderate or midstage).* The person has major memory problems. There may be confusion about the date or day of the week. The person may need help choosing the correct clothing to wear. The person knows own name, a partner's name, and children's names. Usually, help is not needed with eating or elimination.
- *Severe cognitive decline (moderately severe or midstage).* Memory problems are worse. Personality and behavior changes

develop—delusions, hallucinations, repetitive behavior. The person needs much help with daily activities, including dressing and elimination. Names may be forgotten but faces may be recognized. Sleep problems, incontinence (urinary and fecal), and wandering are common.

- *Very severe cognitive decline (severe or late stage).* The person cannot respond to own setting, speak, or control movement. The person cannot walk without help. Over time, the person cannot sit up without support or hold the head up. Muscles become rigid. Swallowing is impaired.

Another tool that is often used to assess the stage of dementia is the Global Deterioration Scale (GDS).

Behaviors and Problems

AD changes how a person behaves and acts. These changes are common:

- Getting upset, worried, or angry more easily
- Acting depressed
- Losing interest in things
- Hiding things (p. 594)
- Believing other people are hiding things
- Pacing a lot of the time
- Wandering
- Sundowning (p. 591)
- Hallucinations (p. 591)
- Delusions (p. 591)
- Catastrophic reactions (p. 591)
- Agitation and restlessness (p. 591)
- Aggression and combativeness (p. 592)
- Screaming (p. 593)
- Problems with intimacy and sexuality (p. 592)
- Repetitive behaviors (p. 592)
- Communication problems (p. 593)

BOX 40.6 Alzheimer Disease and Normal Age-Related Changes

Signs of AD	Normal Age-Related Changes
Poor judgment and decision-making.	Makes a bad decision once in a while.
Cannot manage a budget.	Misses a monthly payment.
Loses track of the date or season.	Forgets which day it is but remembers later.
Problems having a conversation.	Sometimes forgets which word to use.
Misplaces things. Cannot retrace steps to find them.	Loses things from time to time.

Modified from Alzheimer's Association: *10 signs of Alzheimer's*, Chicago, 2022, Author.

👤 PROMOTING SAFETY AND COMFORT

Behaviors and Problems
Safety
Some behaviors and problems are not caused by AD. They may be caused by an illness, injury, or medication. If the cause is not treated, it may threaten the person's life. Always report changes in behaviors to the nurse.

BOX 40.7 Stages of Alzheimer Disease

Stage 1: Mild AD
- Memory loss—forgetfulness; forgets recent events
- Problems finding words, finishing thoughts, following directions, and remembering names
- Poor judgment; bad decisions (including when driving)
- Disoriented to time and place
- Lack of spontaneity—less outgoing or interested in things
- Blames others for mistakes, forgetfulness, and other problems
- Moodiness
- Problems performing everyday tasks

Stage 2: Moderate AD
- Restlessness—increases during the evening hours
- Sleep problems
- Memory loss increases:
  - May not know family and friends
  - May not know where own self is
  - May not know the day or year
- May wander
- Dulled senses—cannot tell the difference between hot and cold; cannot recognize dangers
- Fecal and urinary incontinence
- Needs help with activities of daily living (ADL)—bathing, feeding, and dressing self; afraid of bathing; will not change clothes

- Loses impulse control—foul language, poor table manners, sexual aggression, rudeness
- Movement and gait problems—walks slowly, has a shuffling gait
- Communication problems—cannot follow directions; problems with reading, writing, and math; speaks in short sentences or single words; statements may not make sense
- Repeats motions and statements—moves things back and forth constantly; says the same thing over and over again
- Agitation—behavior may be violent
- May make threats, accuse others of stealing, curse, kick, hit, bite, scream, or grab things

Stage 3: Severe AD
- Seizures (Chapter 44)
- Cannot speak—may groan, grunt, or scream
- Does not recognize self or family members
- Depends totally on others for all ADL
- Disoriented to person, time, and place
- Totally incontinent of urine and feces
- Cannot swallow—choking and aspiration are risks
- Sleep problems increase
- Becomes bed bound—cannot sit or walk
- Coma
- Death

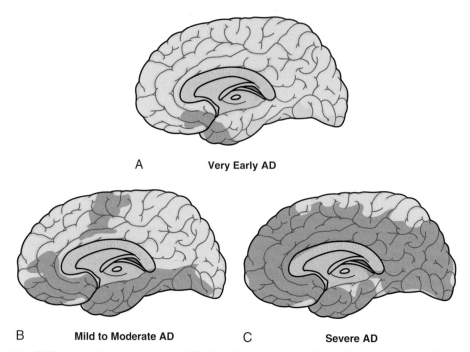

Fig. 40.3 (A) Very early Alzheimer disease (AD). (B) Mild to moderate AD. (C) Severe AD. (From Alzheimer's Disease Education & Referral [ADEAR] Center: *Alzheimer's disease fact sheet*, NIH Publication No. 08-6423, Bethesda, MD, 2010, National Institutes of Health.)

Health-related issues can make the problems worse. Examples include illness, infection, medications, lack of sleep, constipation, hunger, thirst, poor vision or hearing, alcohol, and caffeine. So can problems in the person's setting. According to the National Institute on Aging (NIA), they include the following:

- A strange setting. The person does not know the setting well.
- Too much noise. TV, radio, people talking at once, and other noises can cause confusion and frustration.
- Stepping from one type of flooring to another. With changes in floor color or texture, the person may want to step down.
- Not understanding signs. The person may think that a WET FLOOR sign means to urinate on the floor.
- Mirrors. The person may think that a mirror image is another person in the room.

See *Promoting Safety and Comfort: Behaviors and Problems.*

TEAMWORK AND TIME MANAGEMENT

Wandering

Every staff member must be alert to persons who wander. Such persons are allowed to wander in safe areas (Fig. 40.4). However, the person may wander into an unsafe area. Kitchens, shower rooms, and utility rooms are examples.

Tell your team members when you are caring for a person who wanders. You cannot be with the person all the time. The team can assist and monitor the person. Help your team members in the same way. If you see a person wandering into an unsafe area, gently guide the person to a safe place (Fig 40.5). Report the problem to the nurse.

Wandering

Persons with AD are not oriented to person, time, and place. They may wander away and not find their way back. Wandering may be by foot, car, bike, or other means. They may be with you one moment and gone the next.

Judgment is poor. They cannot tell what is safe or dangerous. Life-threatening accidents are great risks. They can walk into traffic or into a nearby river, lake, ocean, or forest. If not properly dressed, heat or cold exposure is a risk.

Residents may try to wander to another nursing unit or out of the center. Leaving the center without staff knowledge is called elopement. Serious injury and death have resulted from elopement. Centers must follow state and federal guidelines to prevent elopement.

Wandering may have no cause. Or the person may be looking for something or someone—the bathroom, the bedroom, a child, or a partner. Pain, medication side effects, stress, restlessness, and anxiety are possible causes. Sometimes finding the cause prevents wandering.

See *Teamwork and Time Management: Wandering.*

MedicAlert + Safe Return

MedicAlert + Safe Return is a 24-hour emergency service for persons who wander or have a medical emergency. It was formed by the MedicAlert Foundation and the Alzheimer's Association. The program is nationwide.

The purpose is to identify and safely return persons who wander and become lost. A small fee is charged. A family member completes a form and provides a photo. These are entered into a national database. The person receives identification (ID) information—wallet card, bracelet, or necklace.

When reported missing, the person's information is sent to the police. When the person is found, someone calls the

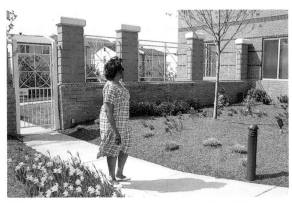

Fig. 40.4 An enclosed garden allows persons with AD to wander in a safe setting.

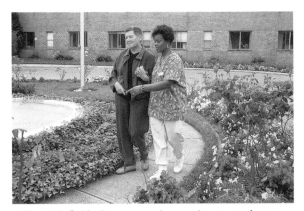

Fig. 40.5 Guide the person who wanders to a safe area.

toll-free number on the ID. *MedicAlert + Safe Return* then calls the family member or caregiver. The person is returned home safely.

Sundowning

With sundowning, signs, symptoms, and behaviors of AD increase during hours of darkness. It occurs in the late afternoon and evening hours. As daylight ends and darkness starts, confusion and restlessness increase, as do anxiety, agitation, and other symptoms. Behavior is worse after the sun goes down. It may continue throughout the night.

Sundowning may relate to being tired or hungry. Poor light and shadows may cause the person to see things that are not there. Persons with AD may be afraid of the dark.

Hallucinations and Delusions

A hallucination is seeing, hearing, smelling, or feeling something that is not real. Senses are dulled. Affected persons see animals, insects, or people that are not present. Some hear voices. They may feel bugs crawling or feel that they are being touched.

Sometimes the problem is caused by poor vision or hearing. The person needs to wear eyeglasses and hearing aids as prescribed.

Delusions are false beliefs. People with AD may think they are some other person. Some believe they are in jail, are being killed, or are being attacked. A person may believe that the caregiver is someone else. Many other false beliefs can occur.

Paranoia

Paranoia is a disorder *(para)* of the mind *(noia)*. The person has false beliefs (delusions) and suspicion about a person or situation. Paranoia is a type of delusion. Such persons believe that others are mean, lying, not fair, or "out to get" them. They may be suspicious, fearful, or jealous.

According to the NIA, paranoia may worsen as memory loss gets worse. The NIA uses these examples:

- The person forgets where he put something. He may believe that someone is taking his things.
- The person forgets that you are a caregiver. She may think that you are a stranger and not trust you.
- The person forgets people to whom he was introduced. The person may believe that strangers are harmful.
- The person forgets directions that you gave. The person may think that you are trying to trick her.

The person may express loss through paranoia. Reasons for the loss do not make sense. Therefore, the person blames or accuses others. The NIA offers these helpful measures:

- Do not react if the person blames you for something.
- Do not argue with the person.
- Assure the person of own safety.
- Use touch or gently hug the person. This shows that you care.
- Search for missing things. This helps distract the person. Talk about what you found. For example, you find a photo, so talk about the photo.

See *Promoting Safety and Comfort: Paranoia.*

Catastrophic Reactions

These are extreme responses. The person reacts as if there is a disaster or tragedy. The person may scream, cry, or be agitated or combative. These reactions are common from too many stimuli. Eating, music or TV playing, and being asked questions all at once can overwhelm the person.

Agitation and Restlessness

The person may pace, hit, or yell. Common causes are pain or discomfort, anxiety, lack of sleep, and too many or too few stimuli. Hunger, the need to eliminate, and incontinence also are causes. A calm, quiet setting helps calm the person, as does meeting basic needs.

Caregivers can cause these behaviors. A caregiver may rush the person or be impatient. Or mixed verbal and nonverbal messages are sent. For example, a caregiver may talk too fast or too loud. Caregivers always need to consider how their behaviors affect other persons.

PROMOTING SAFETY AND COMFORT

Paranoia

Safety

The person's behaviors may not mean paranoia. Fears of harm, strangers, stealing, mistreatment, and so on may be real. Some people do take advantage of vulnerable adults (Chapter 2). This includes sexual abuse and financial abuse.

The abuse may be by phone, mail, email, or in person. The abuser may be a friend or family member. The NIA describes financial abuse as including:

- "Scams" such as identity theft, phony prizes, and threats.
- Borrowing money and not paying it back.
- Giving away or selling the person's property without permission.
- Signing or cashing the person's check without permission.
- Misusing bank cards or credit cards.
- Forcing the person to sign over property.
- Stealing prescription medications.

You must protect the person from harm, abuse, and mistreatment. Report the following at once:

- What the person is saying
- The person seems afraid or worried about money
- Some of the person's items are missing
- The person's behaviors
- Signs and symptoms of problems
- Visitors or family members acting strangely

The NIA suggests these measures to help with agitation and restlessness:

- Observe for early signs of agitation and restlessness. Such signs may help you remove the cause before the behaviors worsen.
- Do not ignore the problem. Try to find the cause.
- Allow personal choice. Let the person decide things to the extent possible.
- Try to distract the person. A snack, safe object, or activity may help.
- Reassure the person.
  - Speak calmly.
  - Listen to the person's concerns.
  - Try to show that you understand the person's anger or fears.
- Keep personal items within the person's sight. Photos and treasures are examples.
- Reduce noise and clutter.
- Limit the number of people in the room.
- Use gentle touch.
- Provide soothing music.
- Read to the person using a gentle voice.
- Provide quiet times.
- Follow a set routine for bathing, dressing, eating, and so on.

Aggression and Combativeness

These behaviors include hitting, pinching, grabbing, biting, or swearing. They may result from agitation and restlessness. They frighten others.

Sometimes these behaviors are personality traits. Or pain, fatigue, too much stimulation, caregiver stress, and feeling lost or abandoned are causes. The behaviors can occur during care measures (bathing, dressing) that upset or frighten the person. See Chapter 6 for dealing with the angry person. See Chapter 11 for workplace violence. Also follow the person's care plan. The measures listed for agitation and restlessness may be helpful.

Intimacy and Sexuality

Intimacy is a special bond between people who love and respect each other. It involves the way people talk and act toward each other. *Sexuality* is a type of intimacy. It is the way partners physically express their feelings for each other. AD can affect intimacy and sexuality. The person with AD may:

- Depend on and cling to a partner.
- Not remember life with a partner.
- Not remember feelings for a partner.
- Fall in love with another person.
- Have side effects from medications that affect sexual interest.
- Have memory loss, changes in the brain, or depression that affect sexual interest.
- Have abnormal sexual behaviors.

Sexual behaviors are labeled abnormal because of how and when they occur. Persons with AD are not oriented to person, time, and place. Sexual behaviors may involve the wrong person, the wrong place, and the wrong time. Also, persons with AD cannot control their behavior.

Healthy persons do not undress or expose themselves in front of others. They do not masturbate or engage in sexual pleasures in public. They know their sexual partners. Persons with AD often mistake someone else for a sexual partner. The person kisses and hugs the other person.

Being overly *(hyper)* interested in sex is called *hypersexuality*. The person may try to seduce others. Or the person may masturbate often. These behaviors are symptoms of AD. They may not mean that the person wants to have sex. When such persons masturbate in public, lead the person to their room. Provide for privacy and safety.

Some behaviors are not sexual. Touching, scratching, and rubbing the genitals can signal infection, pain, or discomfort in the urinary or reproductive systems. Poor hygiene is another cause. So is being wet or soiled from urine or feces. Good hygiene prevents itching. Clean the person quickly and thoroughly after elimination. Do not let the person stay wet or soiled. The nurse assesses the person for urinary or reproductive system problems. The doctor is contacted as necessary.

The nurse encourages the person's partner to show affection. Their normal practices are encouraged. Examples include hand holding, hugging, kissing, touching, and dancing.

Repetitive Behaviors

Repetitive means "to repeat over and over again." Persons with AD repeat the same motions over and over again. For example, the person folds the same napkin over and over, or the person says the same words over and over, or the person asks the same question repeatedly. Such behaviors do not harm the person. However, they can annoy caregivers and the family.

Harmless acts are allowed. Music, picture books, exercise, and movies are distracting. Taking the person for a walk can help. Such measures help when words or questions are repeated.

CARING ABOUT CULTURE

Communication Problems

Some persons with AD learned English as a second language. For example, the first language learned may be Spanish, Italian, French, Russian, Chinese, Japanese, and so on. With AD the person may forget or no longer understand English. The person may use and understand only the first language learned.

FOCUS ON COMMUNICATION

Communication Problems

Impaired communication is a common problem among persons with AD and other dementias. Communication abilities decline over time. Some persons can have brief conversations. To promote communication, practice the measures in Box 40.8. Avoid the following:

- *Giving orders.* For example: "Sit down and eat." The statement is bossy. It does not show respect for the person. Instead you can say: "Let me help you sit down."
- *Wanting the truth.* For example, do not say: "Don't you remember?" "What's my name?" "What day is it?" Instead you can say: "Today is Friday."
- *Correcting the person's errors.* For example, do not say: "No, that is your daughter Rose. That's not Mary." Or: "I just told you that it's time to get dressed. You already had breakfast." Instead you can say: "Let me help you get dressed."
- *Pointing out errors.* Instead of saying: "You missed a button," say: "Let's try it this way."
- *Giving many choices.* For example: "What would you like for dinner?" involves many choices. Instead, limit choices. You can say: "Do you want potatoes or rice?"
- *Asking open-ended questions.* For example, do not say: "How did you sleep last night?" Instead, ask "yes" or "no" questions. You can say: "Did you sleep okay last night?"

Communication Problems

People with AD have trouble remembering things. Communication problems include the following:

- Struggling to find the right word
- Forgetting what one wants to say
- Problems understanding the meaning of words
- Attention problems during conversations
- Losing one's train of thought when talking
- Problems blocking out background noises—radio, TV, phones, and so on
- Frustration with problems communicating
- Being sensitive to touch, tone, and voice volume
  See *Caring About Culture: Communication Problems.*
  See *Focus on Communication: Communication Problems.*

Screaming

Persons with AD have communication problems. At first, it is hard to find the right words. As AD progresses, the person

---

BOX 40.8 Communicating with Persons with AD and Other Dementias

- Approach the person in a calm, quiet manner.
- Approach the person from the front, not from the side or the back. This avoids startling the person.
- Make eye contact to get the person's attention.
- Have the person's attention before you start speaking.
- Call the person by name.
- Identify other people by their names. Avoid pronouns (*he, she, them,* and so on).
- Follow the rules of communication (Chapters 4 and 6).
- Practice measures to promote communication (Chapter 6).
- Use gestures or cues. Point to objects.
- Speak in a calm, gentle voice.
- Hold the person's hand while you talk.
- Speak slowly. Use simple words and short sentences.
- Ask or say one thing at a time. Present one idea, question, or instruction at a time.
- Do not "baby talk" or use a "baby voice."
- Let the person speak. Do not interrupt or rush the person.
- Give the person time to respond.
- Try different words if the person does not seem to understand.
- Do not criticize, correct, interrupt, argue, or try to reason with the person.
- Give simple, step-by-step instructions.
- Repeat instructions as needed. Give the person time to respond or react.
- Ask simple questions having simple answers. Do not ask complex questions.
- Do not present the person with many questions.
- Provide simple explanations of all procedures and activities.
- Give consistent responses.
- Practice measures to promote hearing (Chapter 33).
- Practice measures to communicate with speech-impaired persons (Chapter 33).
- Practice measures for blind and visually impaired persons (Chapter 33).

---

speaks in short sentences or just in words. Often, speech is not understandable.

The person screams to communicate. This is common in persons who are very confused and have poor communication skills. The person may scream a word or a name, or the person just makes screaming sounds.

Possible causes include hearing and vision problems, pain or discomfort, fear, and fatigue. Too much or not enough stimulation is another cause. The person may react to a caregiver or family member by screaming.

Sometimes these measures are helpful:

- Providing a calm, quiet setting
- Playing soft music
- Having the person wear hearing aids and eyeglasses
- Having a family member or favorite caregiver comfort and calm the person
- Using touch to calm the person

Rummaging and Hiding Things

To *rummage* means "to search for things by moving things around, turning things over, or looking through something such as a drawer or closet." The behavior may not have meaning. Or the person may be looking for a certain item but cannot tell you what or why.

The person may hide things, throw things away, or lose something. Some things need to stay with the person or in a safe storage area. Eyeglasses, hearing aids, and dentures are examples. Always make sure these items are safe. Look for them before discarding linens, returning food trays, or emptying wastebaskets. Money, jewelry, and other important items usually are sent home with the family.

These measures may help with rummaging and hiding behaviors:

- Keep harmful items and products out of the person's sight and reach.
- Remove spoiled items from refrigerators and cabinets. The person may go into a kitchen looking for food and snacks. The person may not know or be able to taste spoiled food.
- Do not let the person go into another resident's room.
- Keep wastebaskets covered or out of sight. The person may rummage through a wastebasket or throw things away.
- Check wastebaskets before you empty them. Look for items thrown away or hidden.
- Keep bathroom doors closed and toilet seats down. This helps prevent the person from flushing things down the toilet.
- Allow the person to rummage in a safe place. The center may have a drawer, closet, bag, box, basket, or chest with safe items.

CARE OF PERSONS WITH AD AND OTHER DEMENTIAS

Usually, the person is cared for at home until symptoms are severe. Adult day care may help. Often, assisted living or nursing center care is required. Some nursing centers have separate memory care units. These are built with special features that allow the person to live in a safe environment. Sometimes hospital care is needed for other illnesses. You may care for persons with AD or other dementias in such settings. Nursing assistants play a vital role in caring for dementia residents. At times, the tasks may seem overwhelming. Talk to the nurse if you are becoming stressed. Sometimes a change in assignment can reduce the burden. Patience and empathy must always be practiced. The person and family need your support and understanding.

People with AD do not choose to be forgetful, incontinent, agitated, or rude. Nor do they choose to have other behaviors, signs, and symptoms of the disease. They cannot control what is happening to them. The disease causes the behaviors. *The disease is responsible, not the person.*

Currently AD has no cure. Symptoms worsen over many years. The rate varies from person to person. Over time, persons with AD depend on others for care. Safety, hygiene, nutrition and fluids, elimination, and activity needs must be met. So must comfort and sleep needs. The person's care plan will include many of the measures listed in Box 40.9.

TEAMWORK AND TIME MANAGEMENT

Care of Persons with AD and Other Dementias
The entire staff must protect the person from harm. Always look for dangers in the person's room and in hallways, lounges, dining areas, and other areas on the nursing unit. Remove the danger if you can and tell the nurse at once. If you cannot remove the danger, also tell the nurse at once.

Comfort and safety are important. Check for pain, hunger, thirst, constipation, full bladder, fatigue, and infections. Good skin care and alignment prevent skin breakdown and contractures. Maintain a comfortable room temperature. You must treat these persons with dignity and respect. They have the same rights as persons who are alert and active. Talk to them in a calm voice. Always explain what you are going to do. Massage, soothing touch, music, and aromatherapy are comforting and relaxing. Avoid noise, glare, and too much background distraction. Allow adequate rest. Some persons are comforted by a security object. This may be a doll, stuffed animal (Fig. 40.11), or special blanket. The person may need hospice care as death nears (Chapter 45).

The person can have other health problems and injuries. However, the person may not be aware of pain, fever, constipation, incontinence, or other signs and symptoms. Carefully observe the person. Report any change in the person's usual behavior to the nurse.

Infection is a risk. The person cannot fully tend to self-care. Infection can occur from poor hygiene. This includes poor skin care, oral hygiene, and perineal care after bowel and bladder elimination. Inactivity and immobility can cause pneumonia and pressure injuries.

The person needs to feel useful, worthwhile, and active. This promotes self-esteem. Therapists work with one person, a small group, or a large group. Therapies and activities focus on the person's strengths and past successes. For example:

- A woman used to cook. She helps clean fruit.
- A man was a good dancer. Activities are planned so he can dance.
- A man likes to clean. He helps with dusting.

Supervised activities meet the person's needs and cognitive abilities. The person's interests are considered. Activities are based on what the person enjoys and can do. Some people like crafts, exercise, gardening, and listening and moving to music. Others like sing-alongs, reminiscing, and board games. Some like to string beads, fold towels, or roll dough. Some enjoy animals. Some centers have resident dogs or cats. An aviary (bird cage) may offer interest to some persons with AD. Therapy dogs and cats are brought to the center for visits. There are even robotic pets that can be used to calm an agitated person (see Fig. 40.11). An agitated person may calm down when a robotic cat begins to purr on their lap. This might be an alternative to medication that would otherwise be given for agitation.

BOX 40.9 Care of Persons with AD and Other Dementias

Environment
- Follow set routines.
- Avoid changing rooms or roommates.
- Place picture signs by room doors, bathrooms, dining rooms, and other areas (Fig. 40.6).
- Keep personal items where the person can see them.
- Stay within the person's sight to the extent possible.
- Place memory aids (large clocks and calendars) where the person can see them.
- Place familiar items and pictures near the person's room in the hallway. Some centers have built-in memory cabinets next to each person's doorway. This helps them find their room (see Fig. 40.13).
- Keep noise levels low.
- Play music and show movies from the person's past.
- Select tasks and activities that fit the person's abilities and interests.

Safety
- Reassure the person that you are there to help.
- Remove harmful, sharp, and breakable items from the area. This includes knives, scissors, glass, dishes, razors, and tools. Do not use thumb tacks on bulletin boards.
- Provide plastic eating and drinking utensils. This helps prevent breakage and cuts.
- Place safety plugs in electrical outlets or cover outlets with safety plates.
- Keep cords and electrical items out of reach.
- Remove electrical appliances from the bathroom. Hair dryers, curling irons, makeup mirrors, and electric shavers are examples.
- Store personal care items (shampoo, deodorant, lotion, and so on) in a safe place.
- Keep childproof caps on medication containers and household cleaners.
- Store household cleaners and medications in locked storage areas.
- Store dangerous equipment and tools in a safe place.
- Remove knobs from stoves or place safety covers on the knobs (Fig. 40.8).
- Remove dangerous appliances and power tools from the home.
- Remove firearms from the home.
- Store car keys in a safe place.
- Supervise the person who smokes.
- Store cigarettes, cigars, pipes, matches, and other smoking materials in a safe place.
- Practice safety measures to prevent falls (Chapter 12).
- Practice safety measures to prevent fires (Chapter 11).
- Practice safety measures to prevent burns (Chapter 11).
- Practice safety measures to prevent poisoning (Chapter 11).
- Keep locked all doors to kitchens, utility rooms, and housekeeping closets.

Wandering
- Follow center policy for locking doors and windows. Locks are often placed at the top and bottom of doors (Fig. 40.8). The person is not likely to look for a lock there.
- Keep door alarms and electronic doors turned on. The alarm goes off when the door is opened. Respond to door alarms at once.
- Follow center policy for fire exits. Everyone must be able to leave the building if there is a fire.
- Make sure the person wears an ID bracelet or *MedicAlert + Safe Return* at all times.
- Exercise the person as ordered. Adequate exercise may reduce wandering.
- Involve the person in activities—folding napkins, dusting a table, sorting socks, rolling yarn, sweeping, sanding blocks of wood, or watering plants.

- Do not use restraints. Restraints require a doctor's order. They also tend to increase confusion and disorientation.
- Do not argue with the person who wants to leave. The person does not understand what you are saying. Instead, try to redirect the person.
- Go with the person who insists on going outside. Make sure the person is properly dressed. Guide the person inside after a few minutes.
- Let the person wander in enclosed areas. The center may have enclosed areas for walking about. They provide a safe place for the person to wander.

Sundowning
- Complete treatments and activities early in the day.
- Provide a calm, quiet setting late in the day.
- Do not restrain the person.
- Encourage exercise and activity early in the day.
- Meet nutrition needs. Hunger can increase restlessness.
- Promote elimination. The need to eliminate can increase restlessness.
- Do not try to reason with the person. The person cannot understand what you are saying.
- Do not ask the person to tell you what is the problem. Communication is impaired. The person does not understand what you are asking and cannot think or speak clearly.

Hallucinations and Delusions
- Have the person wear eyeglasses and hearing aids as needed. Follow the care plan.
- Do not argue with the person. The person does not understand what you are saying.
- Reassure the person. State that you will provide protection from harm.
- Try to comfort if the person is afraid.
- Distract the person with some item or activity. Go to another room. Taking the person for a walk may be helpful.
- Turn off TV or movies when violent and disturbing programs are on. The person may believe that the story is real.
- Use touch to calm and reassure the person (Fig. 40.9).
- Eliminate noises that the person could misinterpret. TV, radio, stereos, furnaces, air conditioners, and other things could affect the person.
- Check lighting. Make sure there are no glares, shadows, or reflections.
- Cover or remove mirrors. The person could misinterpret the reflection.
- Make sure the person cannot reach anything that could be used to hurt self or others.

Sleep
- Develop a regular bedtime. Keep the bedtime at the same time each evening.
- Provide a quiet, peaceful mood in the evening—dim lights, low noise level, and soothing music.
- Follow bedtime rituals.
- Use nightlights so the person can see. Use them in rooms, hallways, bathrooms, and other areas. They help prevent accidents and disorientation.
- Limit caffeine during the day.
- Discourage naps during the day.
- Follow the person's exercise plan. Play music to the exercise.
- Reduce noises.

Basic Needs
- Follow a daily routine. This helps the person know when certain things will happen.
- Meet food and fluid needs (Chapter 20). Provide finger foods. Cut food and pour liquids as needed.

Continued

BOX 40.9 Care of Persons with AD and Other Dementias—cont'd

- Provide good skin care (Chapters 18, 31, and 32). Keep the person's skin free of urine and feces.
- Promote urinary and bowel elimination (Chapters 22 and 23).
- Provide incontinence care as needed (Chapters 22 and 23).
- Promote exercise and activity during the day (Chapter 24). This helps reduce wandering and sundowning behaviors. The person also may sleep better.
- Reduce intake of coffee, tea, and cola drinks. These contain caffeine. Caffeine is a stimulant. It can increase restlessness, confusion, and agitation.
- Provide a quiet, restful setting. Soft music is better than loud TV programs.
- Play music during care activities such as bathing and during meals.
- Promote personal hygiene (Chapter 18). Do not force the person into a shower or tub. People with AD are often afraid of bathing. Try bathing when the person is calm. Use the person's preferred bathing method (tub bath, shower). Provide privacy and keep the person warm. Do not rush the person.
- Provide oral hygiene (Chapter 18).

- Choose clothing that is comfortable and simple to put on. Front-opening garments are easy to put on. Pullover tops are harder to put on. The person may become frightened when the head is inside the pullover top.
- Select clothing that closes with Velcro. Such items are easy to put on and take off. Buttons, zippers, snaps, and other closures can frustrate the person.
- Offer simple clothing choices (Fig. 40.10). Let the person choose between two shirts or two blouses, two pants or two slacks, and so on.
- Lay clothing out in the order it will be put on. Hand the person one clothing item at a time. Tell or show the person what to do. Do not rush the process.
- Have equipment ready for any procedure. This reduces the amount of time the person is involved in care measures.
- Protect hearing aids, eyeglasses, and dentures from being misplaced or discarded accidently.
- Observe for signs and symptoms of health problems (Chapter 5).
- Prevent infection (Chapter 14).

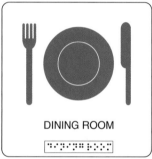

TOILET   DINING ROOM

Fig. 40.6 Signs give cues to persons with dementia.

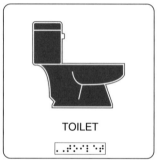

Fig. 40.7 Safety covers are on stove knobs.

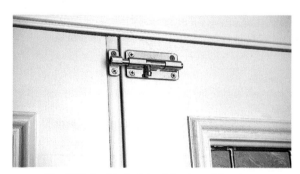

Fig. 40.8 A slide lock is at the top of the door.

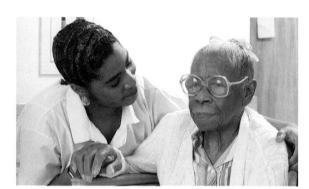

Fig. 40.9 Use touch to calm the person.

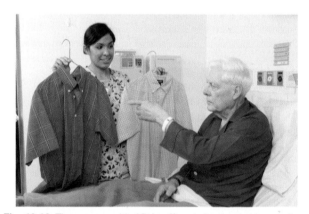

Fig. 40.10 The person with AD is offered simple clothing choices.

See *Teamwork and Time Management: Care of Persons with AD and Other Dementias.*

Special Care Units

Many nursing centers have special memory care units for persons with AD and other dementias. Some units are secured. This means that entrances and exits are locked. Persons in these

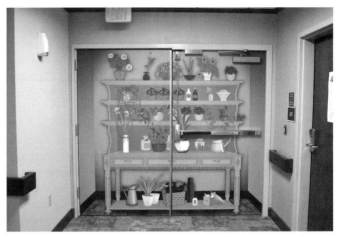

Fig. 40.12 Exit door of memory care unit disguised to reduce the tendency of AD residents to elope. (Courtesy Roxanne Strike, Green Hills Retirement Community, Ames, IA.)

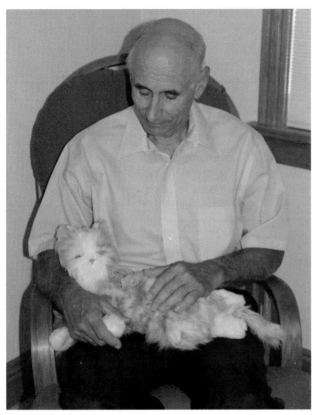

Fig. 40.11 A robotic therapy cat offers comfort to the person with AD.

units have a safe setting for moving about. They cannot wander away. Some units disguise the exit doors so that the person with AD is not inclined to try to leave through the door (Fig. 40.12). Some persons have aggressive behaviors that disrupt or threaten others. They may need a secured unit. Bathrooms may be modified to meet the needs of the person with AD. For example, a bathroom door may be replaced with a curtain for safety. The mirror may be replaced with a picture if the person's reflection upsets them.

❖ According to the Omnibus Budget Reconciliation Act of 1987 (OBRA), secured units are physical restraints. The center must follow OBRA rules. They must use the least restrictive approach. A dementia diagnosis and a doctor's order are needed to place a person on a secured unit. At least every 90 days, the health team reviews the person's need for a secured ◆ unit. The person's rights are always protected.

At some point, the secured unit is no longer needed for safe care. For example, the person's condition progresses from stage 2 to stage 3. The person cannot sit or walk. Wandering is not a concern. The person may be transferred to another unit.

Licensing and accrediting agencies have standards of care for special care units. Staff must have special training in the care of persons with dementia. The unit must have programs that promote dignity, personal freedom, and safety.

The Family

The person may live at home or with a partner, children, or other family members. The family gives care or someone stays with the person. Health care is sought when the family cannot deal with the situation or meet the person's needs. Home health care may help for a while. Adult day care is an option. Long-term care is needed when:

- Family members cannot meet the person's needs.
- The person no longer knows the caregiver.
- Family members have health problems.
- Money problems occur.
- The person's behavior presents dangers to self and others.

Diagnostic tests, doctor's visits, medications, and home care are costly. So is long-term care. The person's medical care can drain family finances.

The family has special needs. Home care and nursing center care are stressful. There are physical, emotional, social, and financial stresses. Adult children are in the *sandwich generation.* They are caught between their own children needing attention and an ill parent needing care. Caring for two families is stressful. Often, adult children have jobs too.

Caregivers can suffer from anger, anxiety, guilt, depression, and sleeplessness. Some cannot concentrate or are irritable. Health problems can develop. They need to focus on their own health. They need a healthy diet, exercise, and plenty of rest. Asking family and friends for help is important. However, asking for help is hard for some people. According to the NIA, they may feel that:

- They should do everything themselves.
- It is wrong to leave the person with someone else.
- No one will help if they ask.
- They do not have money to pay someone to help or watch the person for 1 or 2 hours.

Caregivers need much support and encouragement. AD support groups are helpful. They are sponsored by hospitals, nursing centers, and the Alzheimer's Association. The Alzheimer's Association has chapters in cities across the country. Support groups offer encouragement and advice. Members share their feelings, anger, frustration, guilt, and other emotions. They also share coping and caregiving ideas.

The family often feels hopeless. No matter what is done, the person gets worse. Much time, money, energy, and emotion are needed to care for the person. Anger and resentment may result. Guilt feelings are common. The family knows that the person did not choose the disease. They know that the person does not choose to have its signs, symptoms, and behaviors. Sometimes behaviors are embarrassing. The family may be upset and angry that the loved one cannot show love or affection.

The family is an important part of the health team. They help plan care whenever possible. They need to learn how to bathe, feed, dress, and give oral hygiene to the person. They also need to learn how to provide a safe setting. The nurse and support group help the family learn how to give necessary care.

Some family members take part in unit activities. Some nursing centers have memory curio cabinets next to the resident's room (Fig. 40.13). Family members may enjoy placing special photos and memorabilia in these cabinets. Seeing familiar objects and photos might help the person find own room. For many persons, family members provide comfort. They also need support and understanding from the health team. Many families benefit from support groups that meet regularly. Therapists and volunteers help them understand dementia and provide understanding and support.

The NIA suggests ways that family members can take care of themselves (Box 40.10).

Validation Therapy

Validation therapy may be part of the person's care plan. The therapy is based on these principles:

- All behavior has meaning.

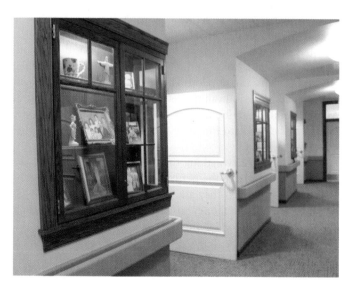

Fig. 40.13 Memory curio cabinet near person's room entry.

- Development occurs in a sequence, order, and pattern (Chapter 9). Certain tasks must be completed during a stage of development. A stage cannot be skipped. Each stage is the basis of the next stage.
- If a person does not successfully complete a stage of development, unresolved issues and emotions may surface later in life.
- A person may return to the past to resolve such issues and emotions.
- Caregivers need to listen and provide empathy.
- Attempts are not made to correct the person's thoughts or bring the person back to reality. For example:
  - While going from room to room, Mrs. Bell calls for her mother. In reality, her mother died 20 years ago. The caregiver does not tell Mrs. Bell that her mother has died. Instead, the caregiver says: "Tell me about your mother."

BOX 40.10 Family Caregivers—Taking Care of Yourself

- Ask for help when you need it. Asking for something specific may be useful. For example:
  - "Can you make Mom's dinner on Sunday night?"
  - "Can you stay with Dad from 2 to 4 on Monday afternoon?"
  - "Can Mom stay at your house on Saturday afternoon?"
- Join a caregiver's support group.
- Take breaks every day.
- Spend time with friends.
- Maintain hobbies and interests.
- Eat healthy foods.
- Exercise often.
- See a doctor regularly.
- Keep health, legal, and financial information current.
- Remember that these feelings are normal—being sad, lonely, frustrated, confused, angry. Say the following to yourself:
  - "I'm doing the best I can."
  - "What I'm doing would be hard for anyone."
  - "I'm not perfect and that's okay."
  - "I can't control some things."
  - "I need to do what works for me right now."
  - "Even when I do everything that I can, the person with AD will still have problem behaviors. They are caused by the illness, not what I do."
  - "I will enjoy the times when we can be together in peace."
  - "I will get counseling if caregiving becomes too much for me."
- Meet spiritual needs—attending religious services, believing that larger forces or a higher power is at work.
  - Understand that you may feel powerless and hopeless about what is happening.
  - Understand that you feel a sense of loss and sadness.
  - Understand why you are caring for a person with AD. Was the choice made out of love, loyalty, duty, religious obligation, money concerns, fear, habit, or self-punishment?
  - Let yourself feel day-to-day "uplifts." Examples include good feelings about the person, support from caring people, and time for your own interests.

Modified from National Institute on Aging: *Alzheimer's caregiving: caring for yourself*, 2017, Author, https://www.nia.nih.gov/health/alzheimers-caregiving-caring-yourself.

- Mrs. Brown sits all day on a bench by the window. She says that she is at the train station waiting to meet her husband. In reality, her husband was killed during World War II. Buried in England, he never returned home. The caregiver does not remind Mrs. Brown of what happened. Instead, the caregiver encourages Mrs. Brown to talk about her husband.
- Mr. Garcia was 3 years old when his father died. He holds a ball constantly. He is very upset when anyone tries to remove it from his hand. He calls for his father and repeats "play ball, play ball." The caregiver does not remind Mr. Garcia that he is 80 years old and that his father died many years ago. Instead, the caregiver says: "Tell me about playing ball."

The health team decides if validation therapy might help a person. If so, it will be part of the person's care plan. Proper use of validation therapy requires special training. If the therapy is used in your center, you will receive the training needed to use it correctly.

QUALITY OF LIFE

Quality of life is important for all persons with confusion and dementia. Nursing center residents have rights under OBRA. They may not know or be able to exercise their rights. However, the family knows the person's rights. They want those rights protected. They want respect and dignity for the loved one.

The person has the right to privacy and confidentiality. Protect the person from exposure. Only those involved in the person's care are present for care and procedures. The person is allowed to visit in private. Protect confidentiality. Do not share information about the person's care and condition with others.

Personal choice is important. Encourage simple choices. For example, a person chooses to wear a shirt or sweater. Watching or not watching TV may be a simple choice. The family makes choices if the person cannot. They choose bath times, menus, clothing, activities, and other care.

The person has the right to keep and use personal items. Some items provide comfort. A pillow, blanket, afghan, or sweater may have meaning to the person. The person may not know why or even recognize the item. Still, it is important. Keep personal items safe. Protect the person's property from loss or damage.

These persons must be kept free from abuse, mistreatment, and neglect. Caring for persons with confusion and dementia is often very frustrating. Some behaviors are hard to deal with. Family and staff can become short tempered and angry. Protect the person from abuse. Report any signs and symptoms of abuse to the nurse at once. Be patient and calm when caring for these persons. Talk with the nurse if you are becoming upset. Sometimes an assignment change is needed for a while.

All persons have the right to be free from restraints. Restraints require a doctor's order. They are used only if it is the best way to protect the person. They are not used for staff convenience. Restraints can make confusion and demented behaviors worse. The nurse tells you when to use restraints.

Activity and a safe setting promote quality of life. Safe, calm, and quiet activities are needed. The recreational therapist and other health team members will find activities that are best for each person. These are part of the person's care plan.

TIME TO REFLECT

You are working in the memory care unit of your long-term care facility. Mr. Conway is 86 years old and has AD. He is confused most of the time. He no longer recognizes family members. His wife visits nearly every afternoon. Recently, Mr. Conway has been spending time with a female resident who also lives in the memory care unit. Today when his wife arrives, she finds her husband sitting in the lounge holding the hand of this female resident. As you enter the lounge area you see that Mrs. Conway is visibly upset and has tears in her eyes. How would you respond from here?

▌ REVIEW QUESTIONS

Circle the BEST answer.

1. Cognitive function relates to the following *except*
   a. Memory loss and personality
   b. Thinking and reasoning
   c. Ability to understand
   d. Judgment and behavior
2. A person is confused after surgery. The confusion is likely to be
   a. Permanent
   b. Temporary
   c. Caused by an infection
   d. Caused by a brain injury
3. A person is confused. The care plan includes the following. Which should you question?
   a. Restrain in bed at night
   b. Give clear, simple directions
   c. Use touch to communicate
   d. Open drapes during the day
4. A person has delusions. A delusion is
   a. A false belief
   b. An illness caused by changes in the brain
   c. Seeing, hearing, or feeling something that is not real
   d. Alzheimer disease
5. A person has AD. Which is *true*?
   a. AD occurs only in older persons
   b. Diet and medications can cure the disease
   c. AD and delirium are the same
   d. AD ends in death
6. The following are common in persons with AD *except*
   a. Memory loss, poor judgment, and sleep disturbances
   b. Loss of impulse control and loss of the ability to communicate
   c. Wandering, delusions, and hallucinations
   d. Paralysis, dyspnea, and pain

7. A person leaves the center without staff knowledge. This is called
   a. Elopement
   b. Wandering
   c. Bad behavior
   d. Poor judgment

8. Sundowning means that
   a. The person becomes sleepy when the sun sets
   b. Behaviors become worse in the late afternoon and evening hours
   c. Behavior improves at night
   d. The person goes to bed when the sun sets

9. A person with AD keeps telling you that someone is stealing things. What should you do?
   a. Nothing. You know that the person suffers from paranoia.
   b. Tell the nurse. Someone could be abusing the person.
   c. Replace missing items.
   d. Send other items home with the family.

10. A person has AD. To communicate with this person, you should
    a. Give orders
    b. Correct the person's mistakes
    c. Ask open-ended questions
    d. Limit the person's choices

11. A person with AD is screaming. You know that this is
    a. An agitated reaction
    b. A way to communicate
    c. Caused by a delusion
    d. A repetitive behavior

12. A person with AD is rummaging through a drawer. Which is *false*?
    a. The person may be looking for something
    b. The behavior may have no meaning
    c. The behavior is allowed if items in the drawer are safe
    d. You must distract the person with another activity

13. Which is the best way to approach a person with AD?
    a. From the front
    b. From the back
    c. From the right side
    d. From the left side

14. A person with AD tends to wander. You should do the following *except*
    a. Make sure door alarms are turned on
    b. Make sure an ID bracelet is worn
    c. Assist with exercise as ordered
    d. Tell the person where to wander safely

15. Safety is important for the person with AD. Which is *false*?
    a. Safety plugs are placed in electrical outlets
    b. Cleaners and medications are kept locked up
    c. The person can keep smoking materials
    d. Sharp and breakable objects are removed from the person's setting

16. Which of these can cause delusions in persons with AD?
    a. Eyeglasses
    b. Hearing aids
    c. Mirrors
    d. Nightlights

17. You are caring for a person with AD. Which is *false*?
    a. You can reason with the person
    b. Touch can calm and reassure the person
    c. A calm, quiet setting is important
    d. Help is needed with ADL

18. Which helps prevent many of the behaviors and problems of AD?
    a. Soothing music
    b. Support groups
    c. Caffeine
    d. Validation therapy

19. AD support groups do the following *except*
    a. Provide care
    b. Offer encouragement and care ideas
    c. Provide support for the family
    d. Promote the sharing of feelings and frustrations

20. A woman with AD tells you her husband is coming soon to pick her up. You know that her husband is no longer living. Which approach is best?
    a. Tell her that her husband died years ago
    b. Help her get ready to wait for her husband
    c. Sit with her and ask her to tell you about her husband
    d. Call her daughter and report the confusion

See Appendix A for answers to these questions.

41

Intellectual and Developmental Disabilities

OBJECTIVES

- Define the key terms and key abbreviations listed in this chapter.
- Identify the areas of function limited by intellectual and developmental disabilities.
- Explain how intellectual and developmental disabilities affect the person and family across the lifespan.
- Explain when intellectual and developmental disabilities occur.
- Describe the causes of intellectual and developmental disabilities.
- Explain how various intellectual and developmental disabilities affect a person's function.
- Explain how to promote quality of life.

KEY TERMS

birth defect An abnormality present at birth that can involve a body structure or function

developmental disability A disability occurring before 22 years of age

diplegia Similar body parts are affected on both sides of the body

disability Any lost, absent, or impaired physical or mental function

inherited That which is passed down from parents to children

intellectual disability Involves severe limits in intellectual function and adaptive behavior occurring before age 18

spastic Uncontrolled contractions of skeletal muscles

KEY ABBREVIATIONS

ADA Americans with Disabilities Act of 1990
ASD Autism spectrum disorder
CP Cerebral palsy
DS Down syndrome
FXS Fragile X syndrome

IDD Intellectual and developmental disability
IQ Intelligence quotient
OBRA Omnibus Budget Reconciliation Act of 1987
SB Spina bifida

A disability is any lost, absent, or impaired physical or mental function. Many diseases, illnesses, and injuries cause disabilities in adulthood. Intellectual and developmental disabilities (IDDs) can be intellectual, physical, or both. IDDs occur before, during, or after birth. They can also be caused by childhood illnesses and injuries.

Developmental disability is a severe and chronic mental or physical impairment occurring before the age of 22. Function is limited in three or more life skills:

- Self-care
- Understanding and expressing language
- Learning
- Mobility
- Self-direction
- Capacity for independent living
- Economic self-sufficiency (supporting oneself financially)

Some disabilities involve birth defects. A birth defect is an abnormality present at birth that can involve a body structure or function. It can be inherited (p. ··), occur during pregnancy, or occur during birth. The defect causes disabilities or death. Causes of birth defects include the following:

- Genetic problems
- Problems with the number or structure of chromosomes
- Problems during pregnancy:
  - Rubella (German measles)
  - Cytomegalovirus
  - Untreated or uncontrolled diabetes
  - Contact with dangerous chemicals
  - Using drugs or alcohol
  - Smoking

Developmentally disabled children become adults. Not children forever, they need lifelong help, support, and special services in these areas:

- Housing
- Employment
- Education
- Civil and human rights protection
- Health care

An IDD affects the family throughout life. The infant or child becomes a teenager, young adult, middle-aged adult, and older adult. Both the child and the parents grow older. Often, it is hard to care for an older child or adult. It may be hard to handle or move the person. A parent may become ill, injured, or disabled or may die. Still, the disabled person needs care.

Some severely disabled children need long-term care in centers for the developmentally disabled. Some adults with IDDs need nursing center care. *They are further protected by the Omnibus Budget Reconciliation Act of 1987 (OBRA). OBRA requires that centers provide age-appropriate activities. Staff must have special training to meet their care needs.*

INTELLECTUAL DISABILITIES

An intellectual disability involves severe limits in intellectual function and adaptive behavior. It occurs before age 18. *Intellectual function* relates to learning, thinking, reasoning, and solving problems. *Adapt* means "to change or adjust." The person has low intellectual function. Adaptive behavior is impaired.

See *Focus on Communication: Intellectual Disabilities.*

The Arc describes an intellectual disability as:

- An IQ score of about 70 or below. (IQ means intelligence quotient.) The person learns at a slower rate than normal. Learning ability is less than normal.
- A significant limit in at least one adaptive behavior. Adaptive behaviors are skills needed to function in everyday life—to live, work, and play. They involve communication, reading and writing, and money concepts.
  - Social skills involve interpersonal skills, responsibility, not being tricked by others, following rules, and obeying laws.
  - Practical skills involve personal activities of daily living: eating, dressing, mobility, and elimination.
  - Other personal skills include preparing meals, taking medications, using the phone, managing money, using transportation, housekeeping, job skills, and maintaining a safe setting.

BOX 41.1   Causes of Intellectual Disabilities

Genetic Conditions
- Abnormal genes from parents
- Errors when genes combine
- Gene disorders during pregnancy caused by infections, overexposure to x-rays, and other factors
- Down syndrome (p. XX)
- Fragile X syndrome (p. XX)

Problems During Pregnancy
- Alcohol use (fetal alcohol syndrome)
- Drug use
- Smoking
- Malnutrition (*mal* means "bad")
- Infections

Problems at Birth
- Prematurity
- Low birth weight
- Head injury
- Lack of oxygen to the brain

Problems After Birth
- Childhood diseases (whooping cough, chickenpox, measles, meningitis, encephalitis)
- Head injuries
- Near drowning
- Exposure to poisons (lead, mercury, etc.)
- Shaken baby syndrome
- Malnutrition
- Dehydration
- Poor health care

Data from *What causes intellectual and developmental disabilities (IDDs)?*, 2021, National Institutes of Health, US Department of Health and Human Services, Author. https://www.nichd.nih.gov/health/topics/idds/conditioninfo/causes; and Intellectual Disabilities: *What is intellectual disability?*, 2023, Special Olympics, Author. https://www.specialolympics.org/about/intellectual-disabilities/what-is-intellectual-disability

---

FOCUS ON COMMUNICATION

Intellectual Disabilities

Mental retardation is a common term for intellectual disabilities. However, the term is offensive and outdated. *Intellectual disabilities* is the newer term preferred by The Arc of the United States. The Arc is a national organization focused on people with intellectual and related developmental disabilities.

In June 2003, the President's Committee on Mental Retardation was changed to the President's Committee for People with Intellectual Disabilities. The name was changed to:
- Update and improve the image of people with mental retardation.
- Help reduce discrimination against such persons.
- Reduce confusion between "mental illness" and "mental retardation."

Avoid using *mental retardation* and *mentally retarded.* Instead use the terms *intellectual disabilities* and *intellectually disabled.*

Brain development is impaired. It can occur before birth, during birth, or before age 18. Causes are listed in Box 41.1.

According to The Arc, alcohol use during pregnancy is the leading preventable cause of intellectual disabilities.

Intellectual disabilities range from mild to severe. Persons mildly affected are slow to learn in school. As adults, they can function in society with some support. For example, they need help finding a job. Support is not needed every day. Some people need much support every day at home and at work. Still others need constant support in all areas.

The Arc believes that persons with intellectual disabilities must be able to enjoy and maintain a good quality of life. A good quality of life involves friendships, health and safety, and the right to make choices and take risks.

The Arc believes that children should live in a family. They should learn and play with children without disabilities. As adults, they should control their lives to the greatest extent possible. They should speak, make choices, and act for themselves. They should live in a home and have friends. They should do meaningful work and enjoy adult activities.

Sexuality

Persons with intellectual and developmental disabilities have physical, emotional, and social needs and desires. Reproductive organs develop. Some have life partners. Others marry and have children. Some persons can control their sexual urges. Others cannot. The type and location of sexual responses may be inappropriate. Also, sometimes persons with intellectual disabilities are sexually abused.

The Arc's beliefs about sexuality include the right to:

- Develop friendships and emotional and sexual relationships. This involves the right to:
  - Love and be loved.
  - End a relationship as the person chooses.
- Dignity and respect.
- Privacy and confidentiality.
- Freely choose associations.
- Sexual expression.
- Learn about sex, marriage and family, abstinence, safe sex, sexual orientation, sexual abuse, and emotional abuse.
- Be protected from sexual harassment and abuse—physical, sexual, emotional.
- Decide about having and raising children.
- Make birth control decisions.
- Have control over one's own body.
- Protection from sterilization because of the disability. *Sterilization* means "to remove or block sex organs so the person cannot have children."

DOWN SYNDROME

Down syndrome (DS) is named for the doctor who identified the syndrome. DS is a common genetic cause of mild to moderate intellectual disabilities. It is caused by an error in cell division. At fertilization, a male sex cell (sperm) unites with a female sex cell (ovum). Each cell has 23 chromosomes. When they unite, the cell has 46 chromosomes. In DS, an extra 21st chromosome is present. The fertilized cell has 47 chromosomes. Thus DS occurs at fertilization. There are three types of DS. Trisomy 21 accounts for 95% of cases.

According to the National Down Syndrome Society (NDSS), persons with DS are living longer than ever before. In 1910 a child born with DS was expected to survive to 9 years. Today, with improved care and heart surgeries, as many as 80% of adults reach the age of 60 or beyond.

The child with DS has certain features caused by the extra chromosome (Fig. 41.1):

- Small head
- Eyes that slant upward
- Flat face
- Short, wide neck
- Large tongue
- Wide, flat nose
- Abnormally shaped ears
- Short stature
- Short, wide hands with stubby fingers
- Poor muscle tone

Many children with DS have heart defects and thyroid gland problems. They tend to have hearing and vision problems and to be overweight. They are at risk for ear and respiratory infections. Leukemia is a risk. (*Leukemia* is a malignant disease in which there is an abnormal increase in the number of white blood cells.) Dementia may appear in adults with DS.

Persons with DS need speech, language, physical, and occupational therapies. Most learn self-care skills. They also need health and sex education. Weight gain and constipation are problems. They need a healthy diet and regular exercise.

FRAGILE X SYNDROME

Fragile X syndrome (FXS) is inherited from one's parents. Inherited means "to be passed down from parents to children." FXS is the most common form of inherited intellectual

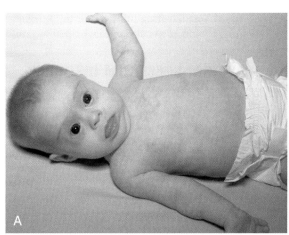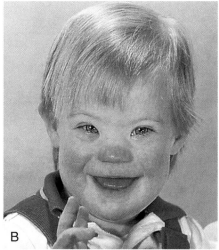

Fig. 41.1 (A) An infant with Down syndrome. (B) A child with Down syndrome. (A, From Hockenberry MJ, Wilson D: *Wong's nursing care of infants and children*, ed. 9, St. Louis, 2011, Mosby; B, from Zitelli BJ, Davis HW: *Atlas of pediatric physical diagnosis*, ed. 5, Philadelphia, 2007, Mosby.)

disability. With FXS there is a change in the gene that makes a protein needed for brain development. The body makes only a little or none of the protein.

Signs and symptoms vary from person to person. Girls often have milder symptoms than boys. FXS has no cure. The person needs help to reduce or eliminate these common signs and symptoms:

- *Learning.* The person may have mild learning disabilities or severe intellectual disabilities.
- *Physical.* Teenagers and adults may have long ears, faces, and jaws. Joints may be loose and flexible. They may be able to extend the elbow, thumb, and knee further than normal.
- *Social and emotional.* Behavior problems are common.
  - Fear and anxiety in new situations
  - Boys: attention problems, aggression
  - Girls: shy around new people
- *Speech and language.* Girls usually do not have severe problems. Most boys may have these problems:
  - Speaking clearly
  - Stuttering
  - Leaving out parts of words
  - Understanding "clues" when talking to people (voice tone, body language)
- *Sensory.* Bright lights, loud noises, and how something feels may bother many children. Some do not like being touched. They may have trouble making eye contact with others.

CEREBRAL PALSY

Cerebral palsy (CP) is a term applied to a group of disorders involving muscle weakness or poor muscle control *(palsy)*. The defect is in the motor region of the brain *(cerebral)*. CP permanently affects the ability to move and to maintain balance and posture. Abnormal movements, posture, and coordination result. Problems walking are likely.

The defects result from brain damage. It occurs before, during, or within a few years after birth. Lack of oxygen to the brain is the usual cause. Brain defects (from faulty brain development) are other causes. There is no cure.

Infants at risk include those who:
- Are premature.
- Have low birthweight.
- Do not cry within the first 5 minutes after birth.
- Need mechanical ventilation.
- Have bleeding in the brain.
- Have heart, kidney, or spinal cord defects.
- Have blood problems.
- Have seizures.
- Have fetal alcohol syndrome.

Brain damage in infancy and early childhood also can result in CP. Lack of oxygen to the brain can occur from:
- Poisoning.
- Traumatic brain injuries from accidents, falls, or child abuse (including shaken baby syndrome).
- Encephalitis and meningitis.
- Rubella (German measles).

Body movements and body parts are affected. These types are the most common:

- *Spastic.* Spastic comes from *spastikos*, "to draw in," which means uncontrolled contractions of skeletal muscles. Muscles contract or shorten. They are stiff and cannot relax. One or both sides of the body may be involved. Posture, balance, and movement are affected. The arms may be affected. If so, there are problems with eating, writing, dressing, and other activities of daily living.
- *Athetoid.* The person cannot control movements. *Athetoid* comes from *athetos*, meaning "not fixed." The person has constant, slow, weaving, or writhing motions. These occur in the trunk, arms, hands, legs, and feet. Sometimes the tongue, face, and neck muscles are involved. Drooling and grimacing result.

Certain terms describe the body parts involved:
- *Hemiplegia.* The arm and leg on one side are paralyzed.
- *Diplegia. Di* means "twice." Diplegia means that similar body parts are affected on both sides of the body. Both arms or both legs are paralyzed. The legs are commonly involved.
- *Quadriplegia.* Both arms and both legs are paralyzed, as are the trunk and neck muscles.

The person with CP can have many other impairments:
- Intellectual disabilities
- Learning disabilities
- Hearing, vision, and speech impairments
- Drooling
- Bladder and bowel control problems
- Seizures
- Difficulty swallowing
- Attention deficit hyperactivity disorder (short attention span, poor concentration, increased activity)
- Breathing problems from poor posture
- Pressure ulcers from immobility

Care needs depend on the degree of brain damage. Disabilities range from mild to severe. Some persons are very smart. Others have severe intellectual disabilities. The goal is independence to the extent possible. Physical, occupational, and speech therapies can help. Some persons need braces and use walkers or crutches. Others need wheelchairs. Some need vision and hearing aids. Medications can control seizures. Surgery and medications can help some muscle problems.

AUTISM SPECTRUM DISORDER

Autism spectrum disorder (ASD) is an umbrella term that covers these five different types of autism:
- Asperger syndrome
- Rett syndrome
- Childhood disintegrative disorder
- Kanner syndrome (classic autistic disorder)
- Pervasive developmental disorder

ASD is a complex neurologic condition that affects the development of the brain. Some signs of delayed development are seen at about 18 months of age. The child has:
- Problems with social skills.

- Verbal and nonverbal communication problems.
- Repetitive behaviors and routines and narrow interests. (*Repetitive* means "to repeat or be repeated.")

There are early signs of ASD:

- No babbling or pointing by the age of 1
- No single words by 16 months
- No two-word phrases by age 2
- No response to own name
- Loss of language or social skills
- Poor eye contact
- Excessive lining up of toys or objects
- No smiling or social responses

ASD is more common in boys than in girls. The Centers for Disease Control and Prevention (CDC) reports that 1 in every 59 children in the United States meets the criteria for ASD. The cause is unknown. Genetics and environmental factors may be involved.

The disorder can range from mild to severe. Signs of ASD are listed in Box 41.2. With therapy, the person can learn to change or control behaviors. Some persons with ASD can be high functioning and lead productive lives. The therapies used include the following:

- Behavior modification
- Speech and language therapy
- Music therapy
- Auditory therapy
- Sensory therapies
- Physical and occupational therapies
- Medication therapy
- Diet therapy
- Communication therapy
- Recreation therapy
- Family therapy

The person needs to develop social and work skills. Children with ASD become adults. Some adults work and live independently. Others need support from family and community services. Some live in group homes or residential facilities.

Persons with ASD may have other disorders. They include FXS and seizure disorders.

SPINA BIFIDA

Spina bifida (SB) is a defect of the spinal column. (*Spina* means "backbone"; *bifid* means "split in two parts.") The defect occurs during the first month of pregnancy. Hydrocephalus (p. ··) often occurs with SB.

Spinal column bones (*vertebrae*) protect the spinal cord. In SB, vertebrae do not form properly. This leaves a split in the vertebrae. The split leaves the spinal cord unprotected. Only a membrane covers the spinal cord, which contains nerves. The nerves send messages to and from the brain. If the spinal cord is not protected, nerve damage occurs. Affected body parts do not function properly. Paralysis may occur. Bowel and bladder problems are common. Infection is a threat.

SB can occur anywhere in the spine. The lower back is the most common site. Types of SB include the following:

- *Spina bifida occulta.* (*Occult* means "hidden.") Vertebrae are closed. A defect occurs in the vertebrae closure. In other words, the defect is hidden. The spinal cord and nerves are normal. The person has a dimple or tuft of hair on the back (Fig. 41.2). Often, there are no symptoms. Foot weakness and bowel and bladder problems can occur.
- *Spina bifida cystica.* (*Cystica* means "pouch or sac.") Part of the spinal column is in the pouch or sac. A membrane or a thin layer of skin covers the sac. It looks like a large blister.

BOX 41.2 Signs of Autism Spectrum Disorder

- Shows no interest in other people
- Poor eye contact
- Wants to be alone
- Has trouble understanding the feelings of others
- Has trouble talking about own feelings
- Does not like to be held or cuddled; screams to be put down
- Overreacts to touch
- Shows little reaction to pain
- Has frequent tantrums for no apparent reason
- Does not notice when others try to engage in a conversation
- May not know how to talk, play, or relate to others
- May not talk
- Has slow language development
- Talks later than other children
- Repeats what others say at the moment or later
- Repeats words or phrases
- May not understand gestures (such as waving good-bye)
- Has a voice that sounds flat
- Cannot control voice volume (loudness or softness)
- Does not start or maintain conversations
- Stands too close to people when talking to them
- Stays with one topic of conversation for too long
- Has problems listening to what others say
- May act deaf
- Does not respond to own name
- Repeats actions over and over again
- Has routines where things stay the same
- Does not like change
- Repeats body movements (hand flapping, hand twisting, rocking)
- Has strong attachment to one item, idea, activity, or person
- Is very active or very quiet

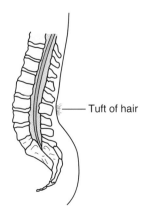

Fig. 41.2 Spina bifida occulta.

Tuft of hair

The pouch is easily injured. Infection is a threat. There are two types of spina bifida cystica (Fig. 41.3):

- *Meningocele.* (*Meningo* comes from *meninx*, meaning "membrane"; *cele* means "hernia or swelling.") Meninges are the connective tissue that covers and protects the brain and spinal cord. Cerebrospinal fluid also protects the brain and spinal cord. The sac contains meninges and cerebrospinal fluid (Fig. 41.4; also see Fig. 41.3A). The sac does not contain nerve tissue. The spinal cord and nerves are usually normal. Nerve damage usually does not occur. Surgery corrects the defect.
- *Myelomeningocele* (or *meningomyelocele*). (*Myelo* means "spinal cord.") The pouch contains nerves, spinal cord, meninges, and cerebrospinal fluid (see Fig. 41.3B). Nerve damage occurs. Loss of function occurs below the level of damage. Leg paralysis and lack of sensation are common problems. So is lack of bowel and bladder control. The defect is closed with surgery. Some children walk with braces or crutches. Others use wheelchairs.

Some children have learning problems. They may have problems with attention, language, reading, and math. They are at high risk for gastrointestinal disorders and mobility problems. Skin breakdown, depression, and social and sexual issues are other risks.

HYDROCEPHALUS

With hydrocephalus, cerebrospinal fluid collects in and around the brain. (*Hydro* means "water"; *cephalo* means "head.") The head enlarges (Fig. 41.5). Pressure inside the head increases. Intellectual disabilities and neurologic damage occur without treatment.

A shunt is placed in the brain. It allows cerebrospinal fluid to drain from the brain. The shunt is a long, flexible tube. It goes from the brain into a body cavity (Fig. 41.6). Usually, it drains into the abdomen or a heart chamber. The shunt must remain open (*patent*). If blocked, the cerebrospinal fluid cannot drain from the brain.

The person can have many problems. Vision problems, seizures, and learning disabilities can occur.

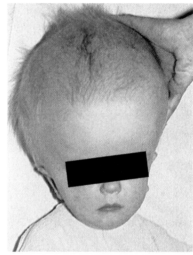

Fig. 41.5 Hydrocephalus. (From Hart CA, Broadhead RL: *Color atlas of pediatric infectious diseases*, London, 1992, Mosby-Wolfe.)

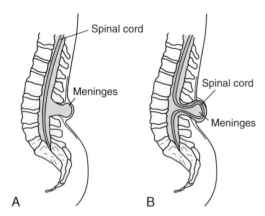

Fig. 41.3 (A) Meningocele. (B) Meningomyelocele.

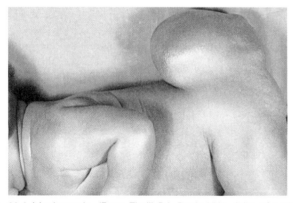

Fig. 41.4 Meningocele. (From Zitelli BJ, Davis HW: *Atlas of pediatric physical diagnosis*, St. Louis, 1987, Gower Medical Publishing.)

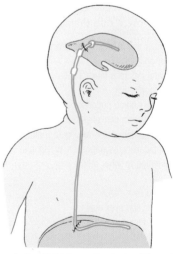

Fig. 41.6 A shunt drains fluid from the brain. (From Hockenberry MJ, Wilson D: *Wong's nursing care of infants and children*, ed. 9, St. Louis, 2011, Mosby.)

QUALITY OF LIFE

Persons with IDDs have the same rights as every citizen. They have the right to live, learn, work, and enjoy life. The Americans with Disabilities Act of 1990 (ADA) further protects their rights. So does the Developmental Disabilities Assistance and Bill of Rights Act of 2000. Some persons with IDDs need nursing center care. They are further protected by OBRA.

Independence to the extent possible is the goal for these persons. This includes having a job and living in the community. The many resources to assist the person and family include the following:

- Assist and self-help devices
- Education
- Job training
- Personal assistive services
- Home and vehicle changes
- Financial help
- Physical and occupational therapies
- Speech and language therapy
- Respiratory therapy
- Recreation therapy
- Assistance with hearing and vision

TIME TO REFLECT

Mr. Murphy is a 40-year-old resident who has an intellectual disability. He used to live in a group home with six other men until he needed more assistance with his activities of daily living and monitoring of his diabetes. Lately he has been spending most of the day in his room watching television. You are caring for him today and ask if he would like to come to the activity room to hear a visiting musical group. He replies: "No, I don't think so. All the programs here are for *old* people. There's nobody here who I can relate to. This place is pretty boring." Can you think of some ideas that could be tried to make Mr. Murphy happier at the nursing center? Can you understand how it might be difficult for a younger resident to live in a care center where most persons are much older?

REVIEW QUESTIONS

Circle the BEST answer.

1. All developmental disabilities occur
   a. At birth
   b. From trauma
   c. During pregnancy
   d. Before 22 years of age
2. These statements are about IDDs. Which is *true*?
   a. Self-care, learning, and mobility are always affected
   b. The disability is permanent
   c. The person can never live independently
   d. The person cannot hold a job
3. The person with intellectual disabilities
   a. Has delayed development of sexual organs
   b. Does not have the skills to live, work, and play
   c. Needs care in a special setting
   d. Learns at a slower rate than normal
4. Intellectual disabilities
   a. Are always severe
   b. Can occur before, during, or after birth
   c. Are caused by an extra chromosome
   d. Affect the motor region of the brain
5. Down syndrome occurs
   a. At fertilization
   b. During the first month of pregnancy
   c. Any time before, during, or after birth
   d. From trauma
6. The person with Down syndrome always has some degree of
   a. Cerebral palsy
   b. Autism
   c. Impaired mobility
   d. Intellectual disability

7. Fragile X syndrome is
   a. The result of brain injury
   b. Inherited from parents
   c. Caused by drug and alcohol use
   d. Caused by an infection
8. Cerebral palsy is usually caused by
   a. An extra chromosome
   b. High fever
   c. Lack of oxygen to the brain
   d. Infection during pregnancy
9. The person with the spastic type of cerebral palsy has problems with
   a. Learning
   b. Drooling
   c. Posture, balance, and movement
   d. Weaving motions of the trunk, arms, and legs
10. Autism spectrum disorder begins
    a. At fertilization
    b. During pregnancy
    c. At birth
    d. In early childhood
11. The person with autism spectrum disorder has
    a. Impaired movement
    b. Social and communication problems
    c. Diplegia and brain damage
    d. Intellectual disabilities
12. Spina bifida involves
    a. Nerve damage
    b. A defect in the spinal column
    c. Seizures
    d. Intellectual disabilities

13. Which is common in spina bifida?
    a. Short attention span
    b. Hearing and vision problems
    c. Seizures
    d. Bowel and bladder problems
14. Hydrocephalus often occurs with
    a. Down syndrome
    b. Cerebral palsy
    c. Spina bifida
    d. Autism

15. Hydrocephalus is treated with
    a. Braces and crutches
    b. A shunt
    c. Medications
    d. Social services

See Appendix A for answers to these questions.

42

Rehabilitation and Restorative Nursing Care

OBJECTIVES

- Define the key terms and key abbreviations listed in this chapter.
- Describe how rehabilitation and restorative care involve the whole person.
- Identify the complications to prevent.
- Identify the common reactions to rehabilitation.
- List the common rehabilitation programs and services.
- Explain your role in rehabilitation and restorative care.
- Explain how to promote quality of life.

KEY TERMS

activities of daily living (ADL) The activities usually done during a normal day in a person's life

disability Any lost, absent, or impaired physical or mental function

prosthesis An artificial replacement for a missing body part

rehabilitation The process of restoring the person to the highest possible level of physical, psychological, social, and economic function

restorative aide A nursing assistant with special training in restorative nursing and rehabilitation skills

restorative nursing care Care that helps persons regain health, strength, and independence

KEY ABBREVIATIONS

ADL Activities of daily living
OBRA Omnibus Budget Reconciliation Act of 1987
OT Occupational therapy

PT Physical therapy
ROM Range of motion
SNF Skilled nursing facility

Disease, injury, and surgery can affect body function. So can birth injuries and birth defects (Chapter 41). Often, more than one function is lost. Losses are temporary or permanent. Eating, bathing, dressing, and walking are hard or seem impossible. Some persons cannot work. Others cannot care for children or family.

A *disability* is any lost, absent, or impaired physical or mental function. Causes are acute or chronic (Box 42.1).

- An *acute problem* has a short course. Recovery is complete. A fracture is an acute problem.
- A *chronic problem* has a long course. The problem is controlled—not cured—with treatment. Diabetes and arthritis are chronic health problems.

Disabilities are short term or long term. A leg fracture is short term. The person has a cast. Crutches are used until the bone heals. A spinal cord injury is long term if paralysis results.

The person may depend totally or in part on others for basic needs. The degree of disability affects how much function is possible.

A goal of health care is to prevent and reduce the degree of disability. Helping the person adjust is another goal. *Rehabilitation* is the process of restoring the person to the highest possible level of physical, psychological, social, and economic function. The focus is on improving abilities. This promotes function at the highest level of independence. For some persons, the goal is to return to a job. For others, self-care is the goal. Sometimes improved function is not possible. Then the goal is to prevent further loss of function. This helps the person maintain the best possible quality of life.

Some nursing center residents have physical disabilities. Causes include strokes, fractures, amputations, and injuries. They need to regain function or adjust to a long-term disability. Often, these residents return home. The rehabilitation may continue in home or community settings.

RESTORATIVE NURSING

Some persons are weak. Many cannot perform daily functions. They need *restorative nursing care*, which helps persons regain health, strength, and independence. With progressive illnesses, the person becomes more and more disabled. Restorative nursing programs:

- Help maintain the highest level of function.
- Prevent unnecessary decline in function.

Restorative nursing may involve measures that promote the following:

- Self-care
- Elimination

BOX 42.1 Common Health Problems Requiring Rehabilitation

- Amputation
- Birth defects
- Brain tumor
- Burns
- Cerebral palsy
- Chronic obstructive pulmonary disease
- Fractures
- Head injury
- Myocardial infarction (heart attack)
- Spinal cord injury
- Spinal cord tumor
- Stroke
- Substance abuse—drug, alcohol

- Positioning
- Mobility
- Communication
- Cognitive function

Many persons need restorative nursing and rehabilitation. Often, it is hard to separate them. In many centers, they mean the same thing. Both focus on the whole person. Skilled nursing facilities (SNFs) provide health care and nursing care for those who need rehabilitation. The care may include physical therapy (PT) and occupational therapy (OT). These therapists may give you direction about how to care for the resident.

Restorative Aides

Some centers have restorative aides. A restorative aide is a nursing assistant with special training in restorative nursing and rehabilitation skills. These aides assist the nursing and health teams as needed.

Usually, nursing assistants are promoted to restorative aide positions. Professional behaviors are highly valued when considering staff to promote. Restorative aides need patience, kindness, and good communication skills. Those chosen have a positive attitude and excellent work ethics, job performance, and skills. Required training varies among states. If there are no state requirements, the center provides the needed training.

REHABILITATION AND THE WHOLE PERSON

A health problem has physical, psychological, and social effects. So does a disability. Suppose an illness left you paralyzed from the waist down.

- Would you be angry, afraid, or depressed?
- How would you move about?
- How would you care for yourself?
- How would you care for your family?
- How would you worship, shop, or visit friends?
- What job could you do?
- How would you support yourself?

The person must learn to adjust physically, psychologically, socially, and economically. Abilities—what the person can

do—are stressed. Complications are prevented. They can cause further disability.

Rehabilitation takes longer in older persons than in other age groups. Changes from aging affect healing, mobility, vision, hearing, and other functions. Chronic health problems can slow recovery. Older persons also are at risk for injuries. Fast-paced rehabilitation programs are hard for them. Their programs usually are slower paced.

Physical Aspects

Rehabilitation starts when the person first seeks health care. Complications are prevented. They can occur from bedrest, a long illness, or recovery from surgery or injury. Bowel and bladder problems are prevented, as are contractures and pressure injuries. Good alignment, turning and repositioning, range-of-motion (ROM) exercises, and supportive devices are needed (Chapters 15 and 24). Good skin care also prevents pressure injuries (Chapters 18 and 32).

Elimination

Some persons need bladder training (Chapter 22). The method depends on the person's problems, abilities, and needs. Some need bowel training (Chapter 23). Control of bowel movements and regular elimination are goals. Fecal impaction, constipation, and fecal incontinence are prevented. Follow the care plan and the nurse's instructions.

Self-Care

Self-care is a major goal. Activities of daily living (ADL) are the activities usually done during a normal day in a person's life. ADL include bathing, oral hygiene, dressing, eating, elimination, and moving about. The health team evaluates the person's ability to perform ADL. The need for self-help devices is considered.

Sometimes the hands, wrists, and arms are affected. Self-help devices are often needed. Equipment is changed, made, or bought to meet the person's needs.

- Eating devices include glass holders, plate guards, and silverware with curved handles or cuffs (Chapter 20). Some devices attach to splints (Fig. 42.1).
- Electric toothbrushes are helpful. They have back-and-forth brushing motions for oral hygiene.
- Longer handles attach to combs, brushes, and sponges; or the devices have long handles (Chapters 18 and 19).
- Self-help devices are useful for cooking, dressing, writing, phone calls, and other tasks (Fig. 42.2).

Mobility

The person may need crutches or a walker, cane, or brace. Physical and occupational therapies are common for musculoskeletal and nervous system problems (Fig. 42.3). Some people need wheelchairs. If possible, they learn wheelchair transfers. Such transfers include to and from the bed, toilet, bathtub, sofa, and chair and in and out of vehicles (Figs. 42.4, 42.5, and 42.6).

A prosthesis is an artificial replacement for a missing body part. The person learns how to use the artificial arm or leg (Chapter 35). The goal is for the device to be like the missing body part in function and appearance.

Nutrition

Difficulty swallowing *(dysphagia)* may occur after a stroke. The person may need a dysphagia diet (Chapter 20). When possible, the person learns exercises to improve swallowing. Some persons cannot swallow. They need enteral nutrition (Chapter 21).

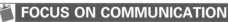

FOCUS ON COMMUNICATION

Communication

Speaking is difficult or impossible for some persons. Persons with speech disorders may need the services of a speech therapist. They may be introduced to other communication methods. Pictures, reading, writing, facial expressions, and gestures are examples. The person and health team decide on the best method. All health team members and the family use the same method with the person. Changing methods can cause confusion and delay progress.

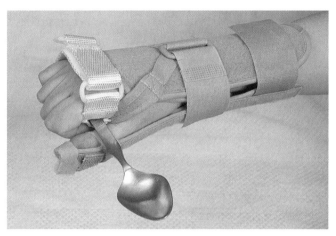

Fig. 42.1 Eating device attached to a splint.

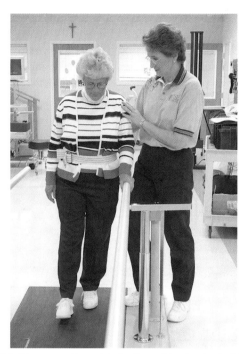

Fig. 42.3 The person is assisted with walking in physical therapy.

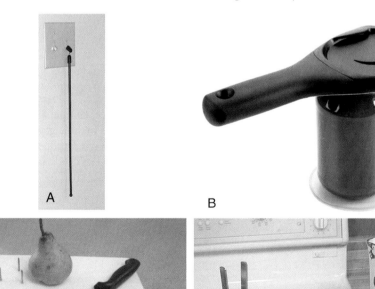

Fig. 42.2 (A) Light switch extender. (B) Power gripper. (C) cutting board. (D) Pot stabilizer. (A, C, D, courtesy Parsons ADL, Inc., Tottenham, Ontario; B, courtesy OXO International, Inc., New York, NY.)

Communication

Aphasia may occur from a stroke (Chapter 33). Aphasia is the total or partial loss *(a)* of the ability to use or understand language *(phasia)*. It is a language disorder resulting from damage to parts of the brain responsible for language. The person does not have normal speech. Speech therapy and communication devices are helpful (Chapter 6).

See *Focus on Communication: Communication.*

Mechanical Ventilation

Some persons need mechanical ventilation (Chapter 26). Some are weaned from the ventilator. That is, the person learns to breathe without the machine. The process may take many weeks. Other persons must learn to live with lifelong mechanical ventilation.

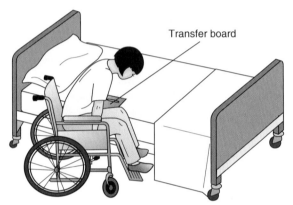

Fig. 42.4 The person uses a transfer board to transfer from the wheelchair to bed.

Psychological and Social Aspects

A disability can affect function and appearance. Self-esteem and relationships may suffer. Some persons may feel unwhole, useless, unattractive, unclean, or undesirable. They may deny

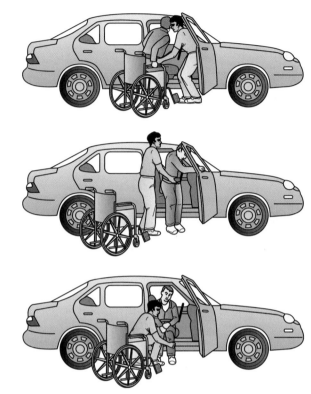

Fig. 42.6 The person transfers from the wheelchair to the car.

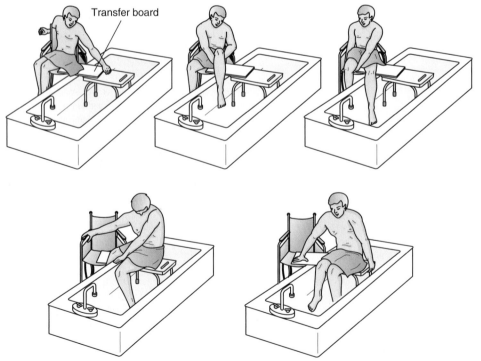

Fig. 42.5 The person transfers from the wheelchair to the bathtub. A transfer board is used.

the disability and expect therapy to correct the problem. Some persons are depressed, angry, and hostile.

FOCUS ON COMMUNICATION

Psychological and Social Aspects

Denial, anger, depression, fear, and frustration are common during rehabilitation. Good communication and support provide encouragement. To deal with such emotions:
- Listen to the person.
- Show concern, not pity.
- Focus on what the person can do. Point out even slight progress.
- Be polite but firm. Do not let the person control you.
- Do not shout at or insult the person. Such behaviors are abuse and mistreatment.
- Do not argue with the person.
- Tell the nurse. The person may need other support measures.

Successful rehabilitation depends on the person's attitude. The person must be helped to accept the limits and be motivated. The focus is on abilities and strengths. Despair and frustration are common. Progress may be slow. Learning a new task is a reminder of the disability. Old fears and emotions may recur.

Remind persons of their *progress.* They need help accepting disabilities and limits. Give support, reassurance, and encouragement. Psychologic and social needs are part of the care plan. The activity department can often play an important role in rehabilitation. Understanding the person's interests helps to motivate the person to work harder. Music therapy and pet therapy (Fig. 42.7) may inspire the person. Spiritual support helps some persons.

See *Focus on Communication: Psychological and Social Aspects.*

Economic Aspects

Some persons return to their jobs. Others cannot do so. They are assessed for work skills, work history, interests, and talents. A job skill may be restored or a new one learned. The goal is for the person to become gainfully employed. Help is given finding a job.

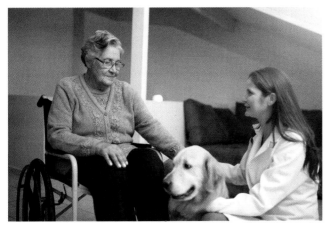

Fig. 42.7 Pet therapy can be helpful in rehabilitation settings. (From iStock/Capuski.)

THE REHABILITATION TEAM

Rehabilitation is a team effort. The person is the key team member. The family, doctor, nursing team, and other health team members help the person set goals and plan care. The focus is on regaining function and independence.

The team meets often to discuss the person's progress. The rehabilitation plan is changed as needed. The person and family attend the meetings when possible. Families are important. They provide support and encouragement. Often, they help with care when the person returns home.

Your Role

Every part of your job focuses on promoting the person's independence. Preventing decline in function also is a goal. The many procedures, care measures, and rules in this book apply. Safety, communication, legal, and ethical aspects apply, as do the measures in Box 42.2.

See *Focus on Communication: Your Role.*

See *Teamwork and Time Management: Your Role.*

BOX 42.2 Assisting with Rehabilitation and Restorative Care

- Follow the nurse's instructions carefully.
- Follow the person's care plan.
- Follow the person's daily routine.
- Provide for safety.
- Protect the person's rights. Privacy and personal choice are very important.
- Report early signs and symptoms of complications. They include pressure injuries, contractures, and bowel and bladder problems.
- Keep the person in good alignment at all times.
- Turn and reposition the person as directed.
- Use safe transfer methods.
- Practice measures to prevent pressure injuries.
- Perform ROM exercises as instructed.
- Apply assist devices as ordered.
- Do not pity the person or give sympathy.
- Encourage the person to perform ADL to the extent possible.
- Give the person time to complete tasks. Do not rush the person.
- Give praise when even a little progress is made.
- Provide emotional support and reassurance.
- Try to understand and appreciate the person's situation, feelings, and concerns.
- Provide for spiritual needs.
- Practice the methods developed by the rehabilitation team. This helps you better assist the person.
- Practice the task the person must do. This helps you guide and direct the person.
- Know how to apply the person's self-help devices.
- Know how to use the person's equipment.
- Stress what the person can do. Focus on abilities and strengths. Do not focus on disabilities and weaknesses.
- Remember that muscles will atrophy if not used, and contractures can develop.
- Have a hopeful outlook.

FOCUS ON COMMUNICATION

Your Role

You may need to guide and direct the person during care measures. First, listen to how the nurse or therapist guides and directs the person. Use those words. Hearing the same thing helps the person learn and remember what to do.

TEAMWORK AND TIME MANAGEMENT

Your Role

Rehabilitation can frustrate the person, you, and other team members. Teamwork is about helping with care. But it is also about giving each other emotional support. Talking about your feelings may help. The team can help you control or express your feelings. You may need to assist with other residents for a while.

REHABILITATION PROGRAMS AND SERVICES

Rehabilitation begins when the person first needs health care. Often, this is in the hospital. Common rehabilitation programs include the following:

- *Cardiac rehabilitation*—for heart disorders (Chapter 36)
- *Brain injury rehabilitation*—for nervous system disorders, including traumatic brain injury (Chapter 35)
- *Spinal cord rehabilitation*—for spinal cord injuries (Chapter 35)
- *Stroke rehabilitation*—after a stroke (Chapter 35)
- *Respiratory rehabilitation*—for respiratory system disorders such as chronic obstructive pulmonary disease, after lung surgery, for respiratory complications from other health problems (Chapter 36), and for mechanical ventilation (Chapter 26)
- *Musculoskeletal rehabilitation*—for fractures, joint replacement surgery, and so on (Chapter 35)
- *Rehabilitation for complex medical and surgical conditions*—for wound care (Chapters 31 and 32), diabetes (Chapter 37), burns (Chapter 44), and so on

Depending on the person's needs and problems, the process may continue after the person leaves the hospital. The person may need nursing center care. Some persons transfer to rehabilitation agencies. There are agencies for persons who are blind or deaf, have intellectual disabilities (formerly called mental retardation), are physically disabled, or have speech problems. Some agencies are for persons who are mentally ill. Many substance abuse programs are available.

Home care agencies also provide rehabilitation services, as do some assisted living residences (Chapter 43) and adult day care centers.

❖ OBRA Requirements

The Omnibus Budget Reconciliation Act of 1987 (OBRA) requires that nursing centers provide rehabilitation services. If not provided by center staff, service is obtained from another source. For example, a center does not have a speech-language pathologist. Instead, the service is obtained from a hospital or other agency.

The center must provide services required by a person's comprehensive care plan. If a person requires physical therapy, it must be provided. If a person requires occupational therapy, it must be provided. If a person requires speech therapy, it must be provided. Such services require a doctor's order.
◆

QUALITY OF LIFE

Successful rehabilitation and restorative care improve the person's quality of life. The goal is independence to the greatest extent possible. A hopeful and winning outlook is needed. The more the person can do alone, the better that person's quality of life. To promote independence:

- Focus on what the person can do.
- Offer support and encouragement.
- Remain patient. Do not rush the person.
- Resist the urge to do things for the person that the person is able to do. This hinders the person's ability to regain function. Remind the family to resist as well.
- Use self-help devices as needed.

Promoting quality of life helps the person's attitude. To promote quality of life:

- *Protect the right to privacy.* The person relearns old skills or practices new skills in private. No one needs to watch. Others do not need to see mistakes, falls, spills, or clumsiness. Nor do they need to see anger or tears. Privacy protects dignity and promotes self-respect.
- *Encourage personal choice.* This gives the person control. Not being able to control body movements or functions is very frustrating. Allow and encourage persons to control their lives to the extent possible. Persons who are sad and depressed may not want to make choices. Encourage them to do so. It can help them feel in control of things that affect them. Personal choice is important in planning care.
- *Protect the right to be free from abuse and mistreatment.* Sometimes improvement is not seen for weeks. Learning to use a self-help device takes time. Learning to speak again can take a long time. So can learning how to dress when there is paralysis. What seems simple is often very hard to do. Repeated explanations and demonstrations may have no or little results. You may become upset and short tempered. Other staff or the family may have such behaviors. Protect the person from abuse and mistreatment. No one can shout at, scream at, yell at, or call the person names. They cannot hit or strike the person. Unkind remarks are not allowed. Report signs of abuse or mistreatment to the nurse.
- *Learn to deal with your anger and frustration.* The person does not choose loss of function. If the process upsets you, think how the person must feel. Share your feelings with the nurse. The nurse can suggest ways to help you control or express your feelings. Perhaps you can assist other persons for a while.
- *Encourage activities.* Often, a person worries about how others view the disability. Provide support and reassurance. Remind the person that others have disabilities. They can give support and understanding. Allow personal choice. Let the person do what is of interest. The person usually chooses activities that provide meaning and success.
- *Provide a safe setting.* It must meet the person's needs. Needed changes are made. The overbed table, bedside stand, call light, and other needed items are moved to the person's strong side. If unable to use the call light, another way is used to communicate with the staff. The person may need a special chair. The rehabilitation team suggests these and other changes. They explain the need and purpose to the person and family.
- *Show patience, understanding, and sensitivity.* Disability affects the whole person. Many emotions are felt. Anger and frustration are common. Some persons have trouble controlling such feelings. They may have outbursts. Progress may be slow and hard to see. The person may be upset and discouraged. You may feel short tempered. You still must show respect. Control your words and actions. Give support, encouragement, and praise. Stress the person's abilities and strengths. Do not give pity or sympathy.

TIME TO REFLECT

Mrs. Lee is a 77-year-old woman who suffered a stroke 3 weeks ago. She has right-sided weakness of both her upper and her lower extremities. Her speech is slurred, and she needs help with most ADL. She has been admitted to the care center and has begun physical, occupational, and speech therapy as part of her rehabilitation program. You are assisting her in the dining room during the evening meal. She uses a special spoon attached to a splint. You open her milk carton and make sure her food is cut into small pieces. Then you move on to help another resident. Suddenly you hear dishes, food, and drink crashing to the floor. You see Mrs. Lee crying in frustration and knocking dishes off her table. She has become angry and upset about her inability to feed herself as she used to. What is your first reaction? How will you help Mrs. Lee? How can the rehabilitation team work together to help Mrs. Lee? Do you understand how easy it is for a stroke victim to become discouraged with the lack of progress?

REVIEW QUESTIONS

Circle the BEST answer.

1. Rehabilitation and restorative nursing care focus on
   a. What the person cannot do
   b. Self-care
   c. The whole person
   d. The person's rights

2. Rehabilitation begins with preventing
   a. Angry feelings
   b. Contractures and pressure injuries
   c. Illness and injury
   d. Loss of self-esteem

3. A person has weakness on the right side. ADL are
   a. Done by the person to the extent possible
   b. Done by you
   c. Postponed until the right side can be used
   d. Supervised by a therapist

4. Persons with disabilities are likely to feel the following *except*
   a. Undesirable
   b. Angry and hostile
   c. Depressed
   d. Relief

5. During a therapy, a person asks to have music played. You should
   a. Explain that music is not allowed
   b. Choose some music
   c. Ask the person to choose some music
   d. Ask a therapist to choose some music

6. A person's right side is weak. You move the call light to the left side. You have promoted quality of life by
   a. Protecting the person from abuse and mistreatment
   b. Allowing personal choice
   c. Providing for safety
   d. Taking part in activities

7. Good communication and support are important during rehabilitation. Which of the following is incorrect?
   a. Be polite but firm
   b. Show concern
   c. Listen to the person
   d. Show pity

8. The total or partial loss of the ability to use or understand language is
   a. Dysphagia
   b. Aphasia
   c. Dyspnea
   d. Apnea

9. Which would not likely be part of the rehabilitation team?
   a. Speech therapist
   b. Occupational therapist
   c. Physical therapist
   d. Dental hygienist

10. Which of the following actions does not promote independence for the person?
    a. Focus on what the person can do
    b. Use self-help devices
    c. Rush the person
    d. Resist the urge to do things for the person that he or she can do alone

11. An artificial replacement for a missing body part is
    a. A prosthesis
    b. Quadriplegia
    c. Hemiplegia
    d. Aphasia

12. Mr. Hanson has the goal of returning to the job he had before suffering a stroke. Which of the following is *not* helpful?
    a. Remind him of the progress he has made
    b. Be understanding when he seems depressed
    c. Apply assist devices as ordered
    d. Encourage him to work faster

See Appendix A for answers to these questions.

43

Assisted Living

OBJECTIVES

- Define the key terms and key abbreviations listed in this chapter.
- Identify the purpose of assisted living.
- Identify the person's rights.
- Identify the types of assisted living residences and the living areas offered.
- Describe the physical and environmental requirements for assisted living.
- Describe the requirements for assisted living staff.

- Describe the requirements for persons who want to live in an assisted living residence.
- Explain the purpose of a service plan.
- Explain how to assist with housekeeping and laundry.
- Identify food safety measures.
- Explain how to assist with medications.
- Identify the reasons for transferring, discharging, or evicting a person.
- Explain how to promote quality of life.

KEY TERMS

assisted living A housing option for older persons who need help with activities of daily living yet wish to remain independent for as long as possible

medication reminder Reminding the person to take medications, observing them being taken as prescribed, and charting that they were taken

service plan A written plan listing the services needed by the person, how much help is needed, and who provides the services

KEY ABBREVIATIONS

AD Alzheimer disease
ADL Activities of daily living

ALR Assisted living residence
F Fahrenheit

Many older persons cannot or do not want to live alone. Some need help with self-care. Some have physical or cognitive problems and disabilities (Chapter 40). Still others need help taking medications. Yet these people do not need constant care.

Assisted living offers quality of life with independence, companionship, and social involvement. Assisted living is a housing option for older persons who need help with activities of daily living (ADL) yet wish to remain independent for as long as possible. Little or no medical care is provided. Housing, personal care, support services, health care, and social activities are provided in a homelike setting. Assisted living usually offers these services:

- Two to three meals a day
- Help with ADL—bathing, dressing, grooming, toileting, eating, walking
- Housekeeping and maintenance
- Linens and personal laundry
- 24-hour emergency communication system for use in an emergency or to call for help
- 24-hour security

- 24-hour supervision
- Transportation arrangements
- Social, educational, recreational, and spiritual services
- Help with shopping, banking, and money management
- Some health services
- Exercise and wellness programs
- Medication management or help taking medications
- Supervision for persons with Alzheimer disease (AD), dementia, and other disabilities

Living areas vary. A small apartment has a bedroom, bathroom, living area, and kitchen (Figs. 43.1 and 43.2). Some people want only a bedroom and bathroom. Box 43.1 lists the requirements and features of assisted living units. Box 43.2 lists environment requirements.

Assisted living residences (ALRs) also are called *assisted living facilities (ALFs)*. Some are part of retirement communities. Others are separate facilities. State laws and licensing requirements for ALRs vary. Resident rights are part of such laws.

See *Promoting Safety and Comfort: Assisted Living.*

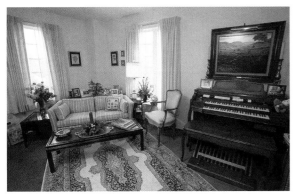

Fig. 43.1 A living area in an assisted living apartment.

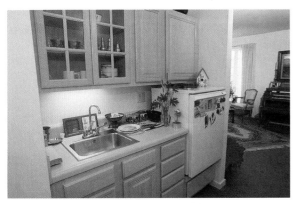

Fig. 43.2 A kitchen in an assisted living apartment.

BOX 43.1 Requirements and Features of Assisted Living Units

- A door that locks; the person keeps a key
- A telephone jack
- A 24-hour emergency communication system
- A window or door that provides natural light
- Wheelchair access
- Lighted common areas
- A window or door that allows safe exit in an emergency
- A mailbox for each person
- A bathroom that provides privacy:
  - A sink in the bathroom or the next room (sink is not used for food preparation)
  - A bathtub or shower with a shower curtain and nonslip surfaces
  - Ventilation or a window that opens
  - Grab bars for the toilet and bathtub or shower
  - Other assist devices needed for safety and identified in the service plan (p. ··)
- Smoke detectors
- A fire sprinkler system
- A bed (frame and mattress) that is clean and in good repair
- Adequate general and task lighting
- An easy chair
- A table and chair for meals
- Adjustable window covers that provide privacy
- A dresser or storage space for clothing and personal items
- Appliances for food—sink, refrigerator with freezer, and storage for food and cooking items

👤 PROMOTING SAFETY AND COMFORT

Assisted Living
Safety
Residents have the same diseases and illnesses as persons at home, in hospitals, and in nursing centers. They are at risk for infections. This includes sexually transmitted and other communicable diseases. Follow Standard Precautions and the Bloodborne Pathogen Standard when contact with blood, body fluids, secretions, excretions, or potentially contaminated items and surfaces is likely.

BOX 43.2 Environment Requirements

- The assisted living residence (ALR) is clean, safe, orderly, odor free, and in good repair.
- The ALR is free of insects and rodents.
- Garbage is stored in covered containers lined with plastic bags. Bags are removed from the ALR at least once a week.
- Hot water temperatures are between 95°F (Fahrenheit) and 120°F in areas used by residents.
- The hot/cold water supply meets hygiene needs.
- Common bathrooms have toilet paper, soap, and cloth towels, paper towels, or a hand dryer.
- Clean linens are handled, transported, and stored to prevent contamination.
- Soiled linen and clothing are stored in closed containers away from food, kitchen, and dining areas.
- Oxygen containers are stored according to the manufacturer instructions.
- Cleaning solutions, insecticides, and other hazardous substances are stored in their original containers. They are in locked cabinets in rooms separate from food, dining areas, and medications.
- Pets or animals are controlled to protect residents and maintain sanitation.
- Employees have access to a first aid kit.

PURPOSE

People choose assisted living for many reasons. People are living longer, and there are more older persons than before. Men and women lose life partners through death or divorce. Some remarry. Others do not. Some persons have never married. Some older persons enjoy being independent but do not want the burdens that come with maintaining a home. Children grow up and move away from their families. For these reasons, many older persons live alone. Often, there is no family nearby to help them.

ALR RESIDENTS

ALR residents usually need some help with one or more ADL:
- Personal care—bathing, dressing, grooming, elimination
- Meals—cooking, eating
- Taking medications
- Housekeeping
- Laundry
- Personal safety
- Transportation

ALR residents do not need 24-hour nursing care. And they are not bedridden. Some persons have chronic illnesses or are cognitively impaired.

Mobility is often a requirement. The person walks or uses a wheelchair or motor scooter. The person must be able to leave the building in an emergency. Stable health is another requirement. Only limited health care or treatment is needed.

RESIDENT RIGHTS

ALR residents have rights and liberties as US citizens. They also gain special rights under state laws and rules (Box 43.3). If a person is unable to exercise one's own rights, then family members, legal representatives, or ombudsmen act on the person's behalf.

BOX 43.3 Assisted Living Residents' Rights

Quality of Life—Residents have the right to:
- Receive a list of current resident rights when accepted into an ALR. Language barriers or disabilities will not interfere with becoming aware of one's rights.
- Receive current phone numbers of state and local agencies that protect the rights of older persons. Adult Protective Services and a long-term care ombudsman are examples.
- Be treated with dignity and respect.
- Make choices about how to live one's everyday life.
- Make choices about how to receive care.
- Receive the care and services needed to attain or maintain the highest level of physical, mental, and social well-being.
- Take part in deciding what services he or she will receive.

Self-Determination—Residents have the right to:
- Live in a setting that promotes and supports dignity, individuality, independence, self-determination, privacy, and choice.
- Exercise free choice in selecting a primary care provider, pharmacy, or other service provider and assume costs resulting from such choices.
- Submit grievances to employees and outside agencies.
- Take part in developing a written service plan (p. ··).
- Receive a copy of service plans.
- Receive services specified in the service plan.
- Review and revise the service plan at any time.
- Refuse services, unless:
  - Such services are court ordered.
  - Refusing services endangers the health, safety, or welfare of others.
- Free choice in selecting activities, schedules, and daily routines.
- Have the same civil and human rights as other persons.
- Terminate living at an ALR without notice if a government agency has proven:
  - Neglect.
  - Exploitation.
  - Conditions that are an immediate threat to life, health, or safety.
- Terminate living at an ALR after giving 14 days' written notice if documentation shows that the ALR failed to comply with the service plan or residency agreement.
- Receive written notice from the ALR when it terminates the person's residency. The notice shall include:
  - The effective date.
  - The right to submit a grievance.
  - The grievance procedure.
  - The ALR's refund policy.

Transfer and Discharge—Residents have the right to:
- Request to relocate or refuse to relocate within the ALR.
- Understand the reasons why the ALR may terminate residency.
  Without notice:

- If behavior is an immediate threat to the health and safety of others in the ALR
- For urgent medical or health needs that require immediate transfer to another health care agency
- If care and service needs exceed the level of care provided by the ALR
  Within 14 days of written notice for:
- Failure to pay fees or charges
- Not complying with the residency agreement or ALR requirements

Personal and Privacy Rights—Residents have the right to:
- Take part in or refuse to take part in social, recreational, rehabilitative, religious, political, or community activities.
- Perform or refuse to perform work for the ALR.
- Privacy in correspondence, communication, visits, and financial and personal matters.
- Privacy in hygiene and health-related services.
- Receive visitors.
- Make private phone calls.
- Maintain and use personal items, unless the health, safety, or welfare of others is affected.
- Have financial and other records kept in confidence. Release of such records requires written consent except when required by law.
- Be treated with consideration and respect.
- Have access to common areas in the ALR.

Rights Against Restraints and Abuse—Residents have the right to:
- Be free from physical, mental, and sexual abuse and sexual assault.
- Be free from involuntary seclusion.
- Not be deprived of the care and services needed to maintain physical or mental health.
- Not have one's resources used for another's profit or advantage.
- Be free from the use of physical restraints used for discipline or staff convenience.
- Be free from chemical restraints used to control behavior.
- Be free from discrimination in regard to race, color, national origin, sex, sexual orientation, and religion.

Right to Information—Residents have the right to:
- Review the ALR's most recent survey conducted by the state. This includes any plan of correction in effect.
- Review a copy of the state's administrative code for ALRs.
- Be informed, in writing, of any change to a fee or charge at least 30 days before the change. The exception is a change in one's service plan.
- Review one's records during normal business hours or at an agreed-upon time.

Modified from Assisted Living Residents' Rights, Arizona Administrative Code R9, Chapter 10, Article 7.

STAFF REQUIREMENTS

Staff requirements vary among states. Some require that the staff complete a nursing assistant training and competency evaluation program. In some assisted living residences, the staff may be required to perform many duties. For example, a worker might serve meals, clean apartments, and assist with the personal care of the residents. Some workers are provided with additional training that allows them to help with the administration of medications. Most staff are provided training in these areas:

- The needs and goals of ALR residents
- Promoting dignity, independence, and resident rights
- Using service plans
- Ethics, privacy, and confidentiality of records and information
- Hygiene and infection control
- Nutrition and menu planning
- Food preparation, service, and storage
- Housekeeping and sanitation
- Preventing and reporting abuse and neglect
- Incident reports
- Fire, emergency, and disaster plans
- Assisting with medications
- Early signs of illness and the need for health care
- Safety measures
- Communication skills
- Special needs of persons with AD and other dementias
- Cardiopulmonary resuscitation and first aid (Chapter 44)

Criminal background and fingerprint checks are common requirements. The ALR cannot employ a person with a criminal record.

SERVICE PLAN

A service plan is a written plan listing the following:
- The services needed by the person
- How much help is needed
- Who provides the services

The plan relates to ADL, activities and social services, dietary needs, taking medications, and special needs. Health services are included.

For example, a person needs help getting dressed. The service plan states that you will assist the person. The service plan also states that a nurse will replace the person's catheter. The person needs physical therapy after a hip fracture. The service plan states that a physical therapist will visit. And the person needs help taking medications. A family member will assist the person with this.

The plan is reviewed when the person's condition, wants, or service needs change. Services are added or reduced as the person's needs change.

Meals

Three meals a day and snacks are often provided. Usually, there are no more than 14 hours between the evening meal and breakfast. It can be longer if there is a nutritious evening snack. Special dietary needs are met. Menus are posted for residents to see.

Residents are encouraged to eat in the dining room with others. If they are not feeling well, meals may be delivered to their apartment. Assist devices are provided as needed. So is help with eating, opening cartons, buttering bread, cutting meat, and so on (Chapter 20).

Housekeeping

The following housekeeping measures help prevent infection and keep assisted living units neat and clean.
- Dust furniture at least weekly.
- Vacuum floors at least weekly and as needed.
- Wipe up spills right away.
- Use a dust mop or broom to sweep. Use a dustpan to collect dust and crumbs.
- Sweep daily or more often as needed.
- Make sure toilets are flushed after each use.
- Rinse the sink after washing, shaving, or oral hygiene.
- Clean the tub or shower after each use.
- Remove and dispose of hair from the sink, tub, or shower.
- Hang towels to dry, or place them in a hamper.
- Clean bathroom surfaces every day. Use a disinfectant or water and detergent to clean all surfaces. They include the following:
  - Toilet bowl, seat, and outside areas of the toilet
  - The floor
  - Sides, walls, and curtain or door of the tub or shower
  - Towel racks and toilet tissue, toothbrush, and soap holders
  - The sink and mirror
  - Windowsills
- Mop or vacuum the bathroom floor every day.
- Empty bathroom wastebaskets every day.
- Put out clean towels and washcloths every day.
- Wash bathmats, the wastebasket, and the laundry hamper every week.
- Replace toilet and facial tissue as needed.
- Open bathroom windows for a short time. Also use air fresheners.

Food Safety

Certain measures are needed when handling, preparing, and storing food. They protect against infection (Chapter 20). Also practice these measures:
- Handle meat and poultry safely. Follow the safe handling instructions on food labels.
- Check and record the food temperature according to ALR policy (Fig. 43.3).
- Protect leftover food. Place leftover food in small containers. Cover containers with lids, foil, or plastic wrap. Date and refrigerate containers as soon as possible.
- Use leftover food within 2 or 3 days.
- Use liquid detergent and hot water to wash eating and cooking items. Wash glasses and cups first. Follow with

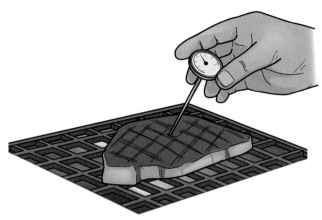

Fig. 43.3 Thermometer checking the correct temperature of food.

silverware, plates, bowls, and then pots and pans. Rinse well with hot water.

- Place washed eating and cooking items in a drainer to dry. Air-drying is more aseptic than towel drying.
- Rinse dishes before loading them into a dishwasher. Use dishwasher soap.
- Do not wash pots and pans and cast iron, wood, and some plastic items in a dishwasher.
- Clean appliances, counters, tables, and other surfaces after each meal. Use hot, soapy water and paper towels or clean cloths.
- Remove grease spills and splashes. Use a liquid surface cleaner.
- Clean sinks with a sink cleaner.

TEAMWORK AND TIME MANAGEMENT

Laundry

Residents may share washers and dryers. If assisting with laundry, remove clothes from washers and dryers promptly. Other residents and staff may want to use them. Some facilities establish a schedule where people sign up for a time to use the washers and dryers. You may find someone's laundry left in a washer or dryer when you are ready to use the machine. First, try to find the person who left the laundry. Politely tell the person that the washer or dryer is done and that you are ready to use the machine. Offer to remove laundry if the other person is busy. If you cannot find that person, do the following:

- *If left in a washer*—place the wet laundry on a clean surface. Do not put it in the dryer. Some items may need to dry flat or hang to dry. Some fabrics may need certain dryer settings. Or the resident may have drying preferences.
- *If left in a dryer*—fold the laundry. Then place it on a clean surface.

While laundry is in the washer or dryer, use the time for other tasks. Assist with ADL, do housekeeping tasks, prepare meals, and so on.

- Dispose of garbage, leftovers, and other soiled supplies after each meal. A garbage disposal is best for food and liquid garbage. Do not put bones in the garbage disposal.
- Recycle paper, boxes, cans, and plastic containers according to ALR policy.
- Empty garbage at least once a day.

Laundry

Laundry services include providing clean linens. Residents can use a washing machine, dryer, iron, and ironing board for personal laundry. When assisting with laundry:

- Wear gloves when handling soiled laundry (see *Promoting Safety and Comfort: Assisted Living,* p. ··).
- Follow the person's preferences.
- Follow care label directions.
- Sort items by color and fabric. Separate white, colored, and dark items. Separate sturdy and delicate fabrics.
- Empty pockets.
- Fasten buttons, zippers, snaps, hooks, and other closures.
- Wash heavily soiled items separately.
- Follow detergent directions.
- Select the correct wash cycle and water temperature. Follow care label directions and the person's preferences.
- Select the correct drying temperature and cycle. Follow care label directions and the person's preferences.
- Fold, hang, or iron clothes as the person prefers. See *Teamwork and Time Management: Laundry.*

Nursing Services

Some ALRs provide limited nursing services. The nurse assesses each person and monitors health. The nurse supervises tasks delegated to you. If a person cannot manage own medications, the nurse gives them.

Medication Assistance

Medications must be taken as prescribed. The six rights of medication administration are:

- The right medication.
- The right dose (amount).
- The right route (by mouth, injection, applied to the skin, inhalation, vaginally, or rectally).
- The right time.
- The right person.
- The right documentation.

Your role in assisting with medications depends on your state's laws, ALR policy, and your training and education. It may involve one or more of the following. *Remember, you do not give medications* (Chapter 1). *Also remember that the person has the right to refuse to take prescribed medications.*

- Reminding the person it is time to take a medication
- Reading the medication label to the person
- Opening containers for a person who cannot do so
- Checking the dosage against the medication label
- Providing water, juice, milk, crackers, applesauce, or other food and fluids as needed
- Making sure the person takes the right medication, in the right amount, at the right time, and in the right way
- Charting that the person took or refused to take the medication (right documentation)
- Storing medications

Residents manage and take their own medications if able. This is called *self-directed medication management.* The person knows medications by name, color, or shape. The person knows

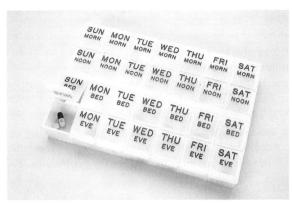

Fig. 43.4 Pill organizer.

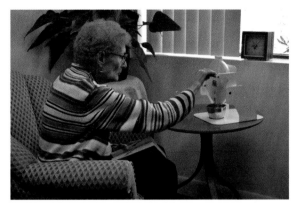

Fig. 43.5 Automatic pill-dispensing machine. (Courtesy e-pill Medication Reminders, www.epill.com, 1-800-549-0095.)

what medications to take, the correct doses, and when and how to take them. The person is able to question changes in the usual medication routine. For example, the person comments that a pill is not broken in half. Or the person says that a pill looks different. Report comments or questions to the nurse.

Pill organizers (Fig. 43.4) have sections for days and times. Some are for a week. Others are for a month. The person, a family member or legal representative, a nurse, or a pharmacist prepares the pill organizer. The person then takes the medications on the right day and at the right time. Automatic pill dispensing machines are sometimes used (Fig. 43.5). This machine is filled and programmed by a nurse or pharmacist. A voice recording tells the person that it is time to take the medication. The pill is released into a small cup. If the person fails to pick up the cup, the machine will dial a phone number that has been programmed in its memory. The responsible party will then go to the person's unit to see why the person has not taken the medication.

📋 FOCUS ON COMMUNICATION

Medication Assistance

Your role may include assisting the person with medications. To remind a person to take medications, you can say:

- "Ms. Parks, it's time to take your 8-o'clock pills."
- "Mr. Ladd, you'll need to take your pills in about 10 minutes."
- "Mrs. Young, are you ready to take your medicine?"

To read a medication label to a person, read the following:

- The name of the person on the label
- The name of the medication
- How to take the medication (by mouth, with food, with a full glass of water, apply to the skin, rectally, and so on)
- The dosage
- When to take the medication (before meals, with meals, after meals, and so on)
- How often to take the medication
- Warnings and other information on the medication label

You may need to remind some people. A medication reminder means reminding the person to take medications, observing them being taken as prescribed, and charting that they were taken.

See *Focus on Communication: Medication Assistance.*

Medication Record

A medication record is kept for each person who needs help with medications. The record includes the following:

- The person's name
- Medication name, dose, directions, and route of administration
- Date and time to take the medication
- Date and time help was given
- Signature or initials of the person assisting

Medication Errors

Report any medication error to the nurse. Also complete an incident report. An error means one or more of the following:

- Taking another person's medications
- Taking the wrong medication
- Taking the wrong dose
- Taking an extra dose
- Missing or skipping a dose
- Taking a medication at the wrong time
- Taking a medication by the wrong route
- Not taking a medication when ordered
- Not recording that a medication was taken

Storing Medications

Medications are kept in a secure place. This prevents others from taking them. If the ALR stores the medications, they are kept in a locked container, cabinet, or area.

Some persons store their own medications. This is on the service plan. If sharing a room, each person's ability to safely have medications is assessed. Medications are kept in a locked container or locked drawer if safety is a factor.

Medications must have the original pharmacy label. They are stored as directed on the label. For example, some medications are refrigerated. Others are kept away from light. The label also has an expiration date. The ALR has procedures for disposing of expired or discontinued medications.

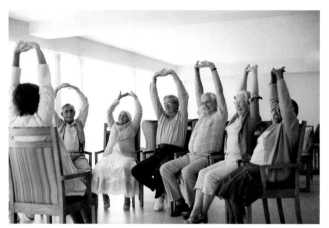

Fig. 43.6 Assisted living facilities offer recreational activities to promote and maintain health. (From iStock/Squaredpixels.)

Activities and Recreation

Residents are urged to take part in activity and recreational programs (Fig. 43.6). Social, physical, and community activities promote well-being and independence. An activities director plans, organizes, and conducts the ALR's activity program. These activities are on a weekly or monthly calendar. The calendar also tells about community events and activities.

Special Services and Safety Needs

Sometimes emergencies occur. Some people need help getting out of bed or transferring to a wheelchair. Then they can leave the building with little or no help.

Other people cannot walk or they may use a wheelchair or motor scooter. They need attendants. If an attendant is needed, the ALR and the person agree on who will meet the person's needs and how they will be met. An attendant is needed 24 hours a day. The ALR must follow state fire safety regulations. It must have documentation of emergency procedures, evacuation plans, and fire drills.

TRANSFER, DISCHARGE, AND EVICTION

Residents can be transferred, discharged, or evicted. State laws require that the ALR tell the person about the action. Reasons for such action are:

- The ALR can no longer meet the person's health needs. The person is a threat to the health and safety of self or others. Or the ALR cannot provide needed care.
- The person fails to pay for services as agreed upon.
- The person fails to comply with ALR policies or rules.
- The person wants to transfer.
- The ALR closes.

QUALITY OF LIFE

ALR residents have rights. Federal and state laws protect their rights as citizens. State laws usually protect the rights listed in Box 43.3. You need to protect those rights.

People choose assisted living for many reasons. Most residents need some help, but they want to live independently with dignity and respect. You can help them by following their service plans. Assist them as needed while allowing as much privacy and personal choice as possible.

TIME TO REFLECT

Mr. Ladd moved into the assisted living residence 3 years ago, shortly after his wife died. He was able to care for himself independently when he first arrived. He enjoyed sharing meals with other residents in the dining room and always participated in planned activities. Gradually, he has become forgetful and even confused at times. He has no family members who live close by. This month he has fallen on three separate occasions. He refuses to use his walker. Today, in the dining room, you notice he has not changed his clothing for 3 days and has a body odor. Should these observations be reported? Do you think Mr. Ladd is safe to continue living in his assisted living unit? Can you understand how it might be difficult for some persons to give up their independence when they are told they must transfer to an area that offers a higher level of care?

REVIEW QUESTIONS

Circle the BEST answer.
1. ALRs provide the following *except*
   a. 24-hour nursing care
   b. Housing
   c. Help with ADL
   d. Support services
2. These statements are about ALRs. Which is *false*?
   a. Each person must have medications given by a nurse
   b. Some residents may have Alzheimer disease
   c. If requested, cleaning and laundry services may be provided
   d. Meals are provided

3. Which statement is *false*?
   a. Residents can refuse care
   b. Residents must plan and organize their own activities
   c. Residents are able to lock their doors
   d. An emergency communication system is provided
4. Which of these violates an ALR resident's rights?
   a. Covering the person during personal care
   b. Giving the person unopened mail
   c. Keeping information confidential
   d. Choosing activities for the person

5. A person wants to attend a concert. Which statement is true?
   a. The ALR must approve the concert
   b. The person must return by 10 PM
   c. An attendant must go with the person
   d. The ALR must respect the person's choice

6. Assisted living staff must
   a. Complete a nursing assistant training and competency evaluation program
   b. Meet state requirements
   c. Assist with medications
   d. Provide transportation

7. ALRs often require the following *except that persons*
   a. Be mobile
   b. Have stable health
   c. Require only limited care
   d. Speak English

8. A service plan
   a. Describes nursing care needs
   b. Describes the services needed and who provides them
   c. Lists the medications the person needs to take
   d. Lists service fees and charges

9. ALR residents are encouraged to eat
   a. In their rooms
   b. In the dining room
   c. At home
   d. At community events

10. You assist with housekeeping. Which is *false*?
    a. Dusting and vacuuming are done at least weekly
    b. Spills are wiped up right away
    c. Bathroom surfaces are cleaned regularly
    d. Laundry is done for all residents

11. You assist with food. Which is *false*?
    a. Safe handling instructions are followed
    b. Leftover food is used in 5 to 7 days
    c. Garbage is emptied at least once a day
    d. Pots and pans are washed by hand

12. You assist with laundry. Which is *true*?
    a. Care label directions are followed
    b. Clothes are always washed in hot water
    c. Clothes are ironed
    d. White fabrics are washed with dark fabrics

13. Usually, assisted living staff are allowed to
    a. Give medications
    b. Give medication reminders
    c. Refill medications
    d. Prepare pill organizers

14. Medications are kept
    a. In the person's closet
    b. In the person's bathroom
    c. In a locked container, cabinet, or drawer
    d. By the family

15. The ALR cannot provide a person with all needed services. Which is *true*?
    a. The ALR must hire more staff
    b. The family must provide the needed care
    c. The ALR can ask the person to transfer
    d. The person's service plan needs to change

See Appendix A for answers to these questions.

44

Basic Emergency Care

OBJECTIVES

- Define the key terms and key abbreviations listed in this chapter.
- Describe the rules of emergency care.
- Identify the signs of sudden cardiac arrest and the emergency care required.
- Identify the signs of choking and the emergency care required to remove a foreign-body airway obstruction.
- Describe the signs, symptoms, and emergency care for hemorrhage.

- Identify the common causes and emergency care for fainting.
- Identify the signs, symptoms, and emergency care for shock.
- Describe the signs, symptoms, and emergency care for stroke.
- Explain the causes and types of seizures and how to care for a person during a seizure.
- Identify the causes, types, and emergency care for burns.
- Perform the procedures described in this chapter.
- Explain how to promote quality of life.

KEY TERMS

anaphylaxis A life-threatening sensitivity to an antigen

cardiac arrest See "sudden cardiac arrest"

convulsion See "seizure"

fainting The sudden loss of consciousness from an inadequate blood supply to the brain

first aid Emergency care given to an ill or injured person before medical help arrives

hemorrhage The excessive loss of blood in a short time

respiratory arrest Breathing stops but heart action continues for several minutes

seizure Violent and sudden contractions or tremors of muscle groups; convulsion

shock Results when organs and tissues do not get enough blood

sudden cardiac arrest (SCA) The heart stops suddenly and without warning; cardiac arrest

KEY ABBREVIATIONS

ACS American College of Surgeons
AED Automated external defibrillator
AHA American Heart Association
BLS Basic Life Support
CPR Cardiopulmonary resuscitation
DNR Do Not Resuscitate

EMS Emergency Medical Services
FAST Facial drooping, Arm drifting downward, Speech slurred, Time to call 911
FBAO Foreign-body airway obstruction
SCA Sudden cardiac arrest
VF (or **V-fib**) Ventricular fibrillation

Emergencies can occur anywhere. Sometimes you can save a life if you know what to do. You are encouraged to take a first-aid course, a Stop the Bleed® course, and a Basic Life Support (BLS) course. These courses prepare you to give emergency care.

The BLS procedures in this chapter are given as basic information. They do not replace certification training. You need a BLS course for health care providers.

EMERGENCY CARE

First aid is the emergency care given to an ill or injured person before medical help arrives. The goals of first aid are to prevent the following:
- Death
- Injuries from becoming worse

In an emergency, the Emergency Medical Services (EMS) system is activated. Emergency personnel (paramedics, emergency medical technicians) rush to the scene. They treat, stabilize, and transport persons with life-threatening problems. Their ambulances have emergency medications, equipment, and supplies. They have guidelines for care and communicate with doctors in hospital emergency departments. The doctors can tell them what to do. To activate the EMS system, do one of the following:
- Dial 911
- Call the local fire or police department
- Call the phone operator

In nursing centers, a nurse decides when to activate the EMS system. The nurse tells you how to help. Some centers have emergency carts (Chapter 11) that are brought to the scene of the emergency. Know where this emergency cart is located. It may be your job to bring this cart or an automated external defibrillator (AED). If a person has stopped breathing or is in sudden cardiac arrest, the nurse may start cardiopulmonary resuscitation (CPR) (p. 626). Some centers train nursing assistants in CPR. They allow nursing assistants to start CPR if cardiac arrest occurs. Others do not. Allow nursing assistants to do this. Know your center's policy about CPR.

Death is expected in persons with terminal illnesses. Usually, these persons are not resuscitated (Chapter 45). The person may have advance directives (Chapter 45) in place. The doctor may have written a Do Not Resuscitate (DNR) order on the person's chart. This information is on the care plan. In some centers the person may wear a special DNR wristband. It is important for the nursing assistant to know this information and the center's policy about who may start CPR.

Each emergency is different. The rules in Box 44.1 apply to any emergency.

See *Focus on Communication: Emergency Care.*
See *Promoting Safety and Comfort: Emergency Care.*
See *Teamwork and Time Management: Emergency Care.*

📋 FOCUS ON COMMUNICATION

Emergency Care
Some illnesses and injuries are life threatening. To find out what happened and the person's condition, you can say:
- "Tell me what happened."
- "Where does it hurt?"
- "If you can, please point to where it hurts."
- "Is the pain constant or does it come and go?"
- "Tell me what's wrong."
- "Can you move your arms and legs?"

👤 PROMOTING SAFETY AND COMFORT

Emergency Care
Safety
During emergencies, contact with blood, body fluids, secretions, and excretions is likely. Follow Standard Precautions and the Bloodborne Pathogen Standard to the extent possible.

When an emergency occurs in a long-term care center, call for the nurse at once. You may need to activate the EMS system or take the person's vital signs (Chapter 27). Assist as instructed by the nurse.

Comfort
Mental comfort is important during emergencies. Help the person feel safe and secure. Provide reassurance and explanations about care. Use a calm approach.

👥 TEAMWORK AND TIME MANAGEMENT

Emergency Care
Onlookers can threaten privacy and confidentiality. During an emergency, your main concern is the person's illness or injuries. You cannot give care and manage onlookers at the same time. Ask someone to deal with onlookers. If someone else is giving care, keep onlookers away from the person.

BASIC LIFE SUPPORT FOR ADULTS

When the heart and breathing stop, the person is clinically dead. Blood is not circulated through the body. Heart, brain, and other organ damage occur within minutes. The American Heart Association's (AHA) BLS procedures support circulation and breathing.

BOX 44.1 Rules of Emergency Care

- Know your limits. Do not do more than you are able. Do not perform an unfamiliar procedure. Do what you can under the circumstances.
- Verify that the scene is safe for you and the victim. You do not want to become a victim yourself.
- Stay calm. This helps the person feel more secure.
- Know where to find emergency supplies.
- Follow Standard Precautions and the Bloodborne Pathogen Standard to the extent possible.
- Check for life-threatening problems. Check to see if the person responds. Check for breathing, a pulse, and bleeding.
- Keep the person lying down or as you found the person. Moving the person could make an injury worse.
- Move the person only if the setting is unsafe. Examples include the following:
  - A burning building or car
  - A building that might collapse
  - Stormy conditions with lightning
  - In water
  - Near electrical wires
- Wait for help to arrive if the scene is not safe enough for you to approach.
- Perform necessary emergency measures.

- Call for help. Or have someone activate the EMS system. *Do not hang up until the operator has hung up.* Give the operator the following information:
  - Your location: street address and city, cross streets or roads, and landmarks
  - Phone number you are calling from
  - What seems to have happened (for example: heart attack, crash, fire)—police, fire equipment, and ambulances may be needed
  - How many people need help
  - Conditions of victims, obvious injuries, and life-threatening situations
  - What aid is being given
- Do not remove the person's clothes unless necessary. If you must remove clothing, tear or cut garments along the seams.
- Do not remove motorcycle or sports helmets unless necessary to provide CPR.
- Keep the person warm. Cover the person with a blanket, coats, or sweaters.
- Reassure the person. Explain what is happening and that help was called.
- Do not give the person food or fluids.
- Keep onlookers away. They invade privacy and tend to stare, give advice, and comment about the person's condition. The person may think the situation is worse than it really is.
- Keep the person's information confidential. Only share information with EMS personnel that would help with the care of the victim.

Chain of Survival for Adults

The AHA's BLS courses teach the adult *Chain of Survival.* These actions are taken for heart attack (Chapter 36), sudden cardiac arrest, respiratory arrest, stroke (Chapter 35 and p. ··), and choking (p. ··). They also apply to other life-threatening problems. They are done as soon as possible. Any delay reduces the person's chance of surviving.

Chain of Survival actions for the adult are:

*   *Recognizing cardiac arrest and activating the EMS system at once.*
*   *Early CPR.*
*   *Early defibrillation* (see p. ··).
*   *Early advanced care.* This is given by EMS staff, doctors, and nurses. They give medications and perform life-saving measures.
*   *Organized postcardiac arrest care.* This care is given to improve survival following cardiac arrest.

You will learn the Chain of Survival for children in the AHA's *BLS for Healthcare Providers* course.

See *Focus on Communication: Chain of Survival for Adults.*

Sudden Cardiac Arrest

Sudden cardiac arrest (SCA) or cardiac arrest is when the heart stops suddenly and without warning. Within moments, breathing stops as well. Permanent brain and other organ damage occur unless circulation and breathing are restored. There are three major signs of SCA:

*   No response
*   No breathing or no normal breathing (The person may have *agonal gasps* or *agonal respirations* early during SCA. [*Agonal* comes from the Greek word that means "to struggle." Agonal is used in relation to death and dying.] Agonal gasps do not bring enough oxygen into the lungs. Gasps are not normal breathing.)
*   No pulse

📋 **FOCUS ON COMMUNICATION**

Chain of Survival for Adults

Calling for help is a critical step in the Chain of Survival. If others are around, tell a certain person to activate the EMS system. You may not know the person's name. Point at the person. Make eye contact. You can say, "Call 911 and get an AED." (AED stands for *automated external defibrillator.*) Begin care. Follow up soon. Make sure the person was able to contact help.

The person's skin is cool, pale, and gray. The person is not coughing or moving.

SCA is a sudden, unexpected, and dramatic event. It can occur anywhere and at any time—while driving, shoveling snow, playing golf or tennis, watching TV, eating, or sleeping. Common causes include heart disease, drowning, electric shock, severe injury, choking, and drug overdose. These causes lead to an abnormal heart rhythm called ventricular fibrillation (p. 629). The heart cannot pump blood. A normal rhythm must be restored or the person will die.

Respiratory Arrest

Respiratory arrest is when breathing stops but heart action continues for several minutes. If breathing is not restored, cardiac arrest occurs. Causes of respiratory arrest include the following:

*   Drowning
*   Stroke
*   Choking
*   Drug overdose
*   Electric shock (including lightning strikes)
*   Smoke inhalation
*   Suffocation
*   Heart attack
*   Coma
*   Other injuries

Rescue Breathing

Rescue breaths are given when there is a pulse but no breathing or only gasping. To give rescue breaths:

*   Open the airway (p. 627).
*   Give 1 breath every 5 to 6 seconds for adults.
*   Give each breath over 1 second. The chest should rise when breaths are given.
*   Check the pulse every 2 minutes. If there is no pulse, begin CPR.

Cardiopulmonary Resuscitation for Adults

When the heart and breathing stop, blood and oxygen are not supplied to the body. Brain and other organ damage occur within minutes.

CPR must be started at once when a person has SCA. CPR supports circulation and breathing. It provides blood and oxygen to the heart, brain, and other organs until advanced emergency care is given. CPR involves the following:

*   Chest compressions
*   Airway
*   Breathing
*   Defibrillation

CPR procedures require speed, skill, and efficiency. Chest compressions and airway and breathing procedures are done until a defibrillator arrives. The defibrillator is used as soon as possible.

See *Promoting Safety and Comfort: Cardiopulmonary Resuscitation for Adults.*

👤 **PROMOTING SAFETY AND COMFORT**

Cardiopulmonary Resuscitation for Adults
Safety

The discussion and procedures that follow assume that the person does not have injuries from trauma (Chapter 31). If injuries are present, special measures are needed to position the person and open the airway. Such measures are learned during a BLS certification course.

You will learn CPR for infants and children in the AHA's *BLS for Healthcare Providers* course.

Chest Compressions

The heart, brain, and other organs must receive blood. Otherwise, permanent damage results. In cardiac arrest, the heart has stopped beating. Blood must be pumped through the body in some other way. Chest compressions force blood through the circulatory system.

Before starting chest compressions, check for a pulse. Use the carotid artery on the side near you. To find the carotid pulse, place two or three fingertips on the trachea (windpipe). Then slide your fingertips down to the groove of the neck (Fig. 44.1). While checking for a pulse, look for signs of circulation. See if the person has started breathing or is coughing or moving.

The heart lies between the sternum (breastbone) and the spinal column. When pressure is applied to the sternum, the sternum is depressed. This compresses the heart between the sternum and spinal column (Fig. 44.2). For

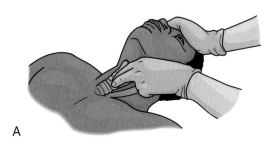

A

B

Fig. 44.1 Locating the carotid pulse. (A) Two fingers are placed on the trachea. (B) The fingertips are moved down into the groove of the neck to the carotid artery.

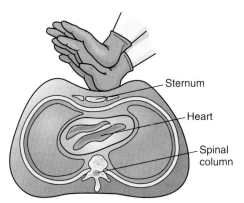

Fig. 44.2 The heart lies between the sternum and the spinal column. The heart is compressed when pressure is applied to the sternum.

effective chest compressions, the person must be supine on a hard, flat surface—floor or backboard. You are positioned at the person's side.

Hand position is important for effective chest compressions (Fig. 44.3). You use the heels of your hands—one on top of the other—for chest compressions. For proper placement:

- Expose the person's chest. Remove clothing or move it out of the way. You need to be able to see the person's bare skin for proper hand position.
- Place the heel of one hand (usually your dominant hand) in the center of the bare chest. The heel of this hand is placed on the sternum between the nipples.
- Place the heel of your other hand on top of the heel of the first hand.

To give chest compressions, your arms are straight. Your shoulders are directly over your hands and your fingers are interlocked (Fig. 44.4). Exert firm downward pressure to depress the adult sternum at least 2 inches. Release pressure without removing your hands from the chest. Releasing pressure allows the chest to recoil—to return to its normal position. Recoil lets the heart fill with blood.

The AHA recommends that you:

- Give compressions at a rate of 100 to 120 per minute.
- Push hard and push fast.
- Push deeply into the chest (at least 2 inches).
- Interrupt chest compressions only when necessary. Interruptions should be less than 10 seconds. When there are no chest compressions, blood does not flow to the heart, brain, and other organs.

Airway

The respiratory passages (airway) must be open to restore breathing. The airway is often obstructed (blocked) during SCA. The person's tongue falls toward the back of the throat and blocks the airway. The head tilt-chin lift method opens the airway (Fig. 44.5).

- Place the palm of one hand on the forehead.
- Tilt the head back by pushing down on the forehead with your palm.
- Place the fingers of your other hand under the lower jaw. Use your index and middle fingers. Do not use your thumb.
- Lift the jaw. This brings the chin forward.
- Do not close the person's mouth. The mouth should be slightly open.

Breathing

Air is not inhaled when breathing stops. The person must get oxygen. If not, permanent heart, brain, and other organ damage occur. The person is given *breaths*. That is, a rescuer inflates the person's lungs.

Each breath should take 1 second. *You should see the chest rise with each breath.* Then 2 breaths are given after every 30 chest compressions.

Mouth-to-mouth breathing. Mouth-to-mouth breathing (Fig. 44.6) is one way to give breaths. You place your mouth

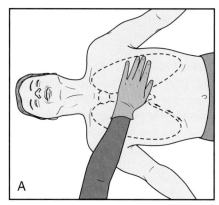
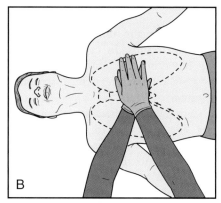

Fig. 44.3 Proper hand position for cardiopulmonary resuscitation (CPR). (A) The heel of the dominant hand is placed in the center of the chest between the nipples. (B) The heel of the nondominant hand is placed on top of the dominant hand.

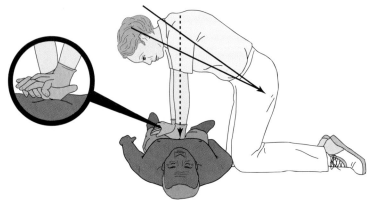

Fig. 44.4 Giving chest compressions. The arms are straight. The shoulders are over the hands. The fingers are interlocked.

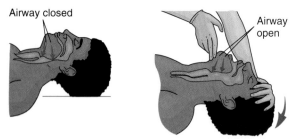

Fig. 44.5 The head tilt-chin lift method opens the airway. One hand is on the person's forehead. Pressure is applied to tilt the head back. The chin is lifted with the fingers of the other hand.

over the person's mouth. Contact with the person's blood, body fluids, secretions, or excretions is likely. To give mouth-to-mouth breathing:

- Keep the airway open with the head tilt-chin lift method.
- Pinch the person's nostrils shut. Use your thumb and index finger. Use the hand on the forehead. Shutting the nostrils prevents air from escaping through the nose.
- Take a breath. A regular breath is needed, not a deep breath.
- Place your mouth tightly over the person's mouth. Seal the person's mouth with your lips.
- Blow air into the person's mouth. You should see the chest rise as the lungs fill with air. You should also hear air escape when the person exhales.

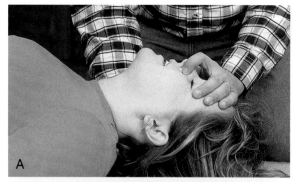
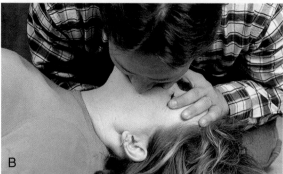

Fig. 44.6 Mouth-to-mouth breathing. (A) The person's airway is opened. The nostrils are pinched shut. (B) The person's mouth is sealed by the rescuer's mouth.

- Repeat the head tilt-chin lift method if the person's chest did not rise.
- Remove your mouth from the person's mouth. Then take in a quick breath.
- Give another breath. You should see the chest rise.

Barrier device breathing. A barrier device is used for giving breaths when possible. The device prevents contact with the person's mouth and blood, body fluids, secretions, or excretions. A face shield may be used (Figs. 44.7 and 44.8). A face shield is replaced with a face mask as soon as possible (Fig. 44.9A). The mask is placed over the person's mouth and nose (see Fig. 44.9B). When using a barrier device, seal the device against the person's face. The seal must be tight. Then open the airway with the head tilt-chin lift method.

A bag valve mask (Fig. 44.10) is another device used to give rescue breaths. The device consists of a handheld bag attached to a mask. It is used when there are two rescuers. The mask is held securely to the person's face, and the bag is squeezed to give breaths. The bag can be connected to an oxygen source.

Defibrillation

Ventricular fibrillation (VF or V-fib) is an abnormal heart rhythm (Fig. 44.11). It causes SCA. Rather than beating in a regular rhythm, the heart shakes and quivers like a bowl of gelatin. The heart does not pump blood. The heart, brain, and other organs do not receive blood and oxygen. If VF (V-fib) is not reversed, the person will die.

A *defibrillator* is used to deliver a shock to the heart. The shock stops the VF (V-fib). This allows the return of a regular heart rhythm. Defibrillation as soon as possible after the onset of VF (V-fib) increases the person's chance of survival.

For adults, the AHA recommends that rescuers:

- Attach and use the AED as soon as it is available.
- Minimize interruptions in chest compressions before and after a shock is delivered.
- Give one shock. Then resume CPR at once. Begin with compressions. Do five cycles of 30 compressions and two breaths.
- Check for a heart rhythm.

AEDs are found in hospitals, nursing centers, dental offices, and other health care agencies (Fig. 44.12). They are on airplanes and in airports, health clubs, malls, schools, churches, and many other public places. Some people with heart conditions have them in their homes.

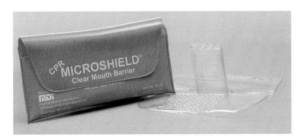

Fig. 44.7 Face shield.

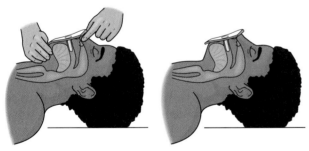

Fig. 44.8 The face shield is in place.

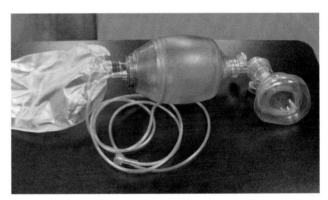

Fig. 44.10 A bag valve mask.

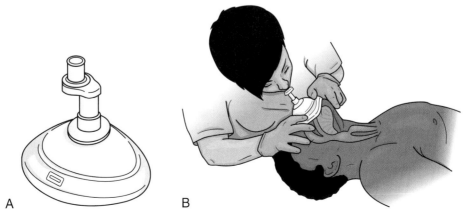

Fig. 44.9 (A) Mask for giving breaths. (B) The mask is in place.

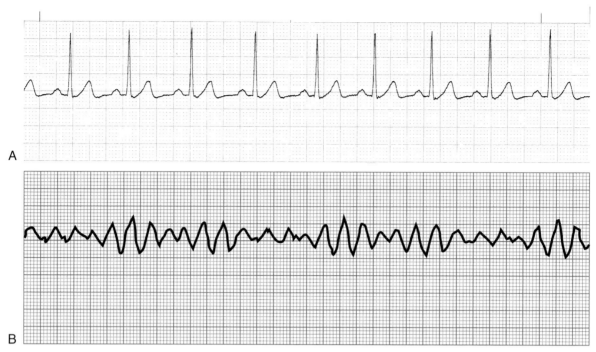

A

B

Fig. 44.11 (A) Normal rhythm. (B) Ventricular fibrillation. (From Ignatavicius DD, Workman ML, Rebar CR, et al.: *Medical-surgical nursing: concepts for interprofessional collaborative care*, ed. 10, St. Louis, 2021, Elsevier.)

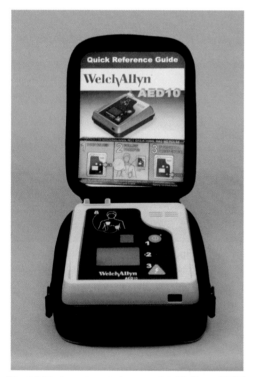

Fig. 44.12 An automated external defibrillator (AED).

You will learn more about using an AED in the AHA's *BLS for Healthcare Providers* course.

Performing Adult CPR

CPR is done only for cardiac arrest. You must determine if cardiac arrest or fainting (p. 635) has occurred. *CPR is done if*

the person does not respond, is not breathing (or has no normal breathing), and has no pulse.

FOCUS ON COMMUNICATION

Performing Adult CPR

Good communication is needed when two rescuers perform CPR. The rescuer giving compressions must count aloud so the other rescuer is ready to give breaths. Clear communication prevents delays and minimizes interruptions in chest compressions.

PROMOTING SAFETY AND COMFORT

Performing Adult CPR

Safety

Never practice CPR on another person. Serious damage can be done. Mannequins are used to learn and practice CPR.

Make sure you have a safe setting for CPR. Move the person only if the setting is unsafe (see Box 44.1). Do not approach the person if the scene is unsafe for you.

The person must be on a hard, flat surface for CPR. If the person is in bed, place a board under the person. Or move the person to the floor.

CPR is done alone or with another person. When done alone, chest compressions and rescue breathing are done by the one rescuer. With two rescuers, one person gives chest compressions and the other person does rescue breathing. Rescuers switch tasks about every 2 minutes to avoid fatigue and inadequate compressions. The second rescuer uses the AED if one is available.

See *Focus on Communication: Performing Adult CPR.*

See *Promoting Safety and Comfort: Performing Adult CPR.*

Hands-only CPR. When an adult has SCA, the person's survival depends on others nearby. Outside of the health care setting, persons trained in BLS are often not available. Bystanders may worry that they will not do CPR correctly or they may injure the person.

The AHA developed "Hands-Only CPR" to improve the response of bystanders who witness an adult collapse suddenly in an out-of-hospital setting. In "Hands-Only CPR," CPR is simplified to two steps.
1. Call 911.
2. Push hard and fast in the center of the chest.

"Hands-Only CPR" is used to educate persons not trained in BLS. As a health care provider, use the CPR method presented in this chapter and in a BLS course.

✴ ADULT CPR—ONE RESCUER

Procedure
1. Make sure the scene is safe.
2. Take 5 to 10 seconds to check for a response and breathing.
   a. Check if the person is responding. Tap or gently shake the person. Call the person by name, if known. Shout: "Are you okay?"
   b. Check for no breathing or no normal breathing (gasping).
3. Call for help. Activate the EMS system or the center's emergency response system if the person is not responding and not breathing or not breathing normally (gasping).
4. Tell someone to bring an AED, if available.
5. Position the person supine on a hard, flat surface. Logroll the person so there is no twisting of the spine. Place the arms alongside the body.
6. Check for a carotid pulse. This should take 5 to 10 seconds. Start chest compressions if you do not feel a pulse.
7. Expose the person's chest.
8. Give chest compressions at a rate of 100 to 120 per minute. Push hard and fast. Establish a regular rhythm. Count aloud. Press down at least 2 inches. Allow the chest to recoil between compressions. Give 30 chest compressions.
9. Open the airway. Use the head tilt-chin lift method.
10. Give two breaths. Each breath should take only 1 second. Each breath must make the chest rise. (If the first breath does not make the chest rise, try opening the airway again. Use the head tilt-chin lift method.)
11. Continue the cycle of 30 compressions followed by two breaths. Limit interruptions in compressions to less than 10 seconds. Continue cycles until the AED arrives. See Procedure: *Adult CPR with AED—Two Rescuers*. Or continue until help arrives or the person begins to move. If movement occurs, place the person in the recovery position.

✴ ADULT CPR—TWO RESCUERS

Procedure
1. Make sure the scene is safe.
2. *Rescuer 1:* Take 5 to 10 seconds to check for a response and breathing.
   a. Check if the person is responding. Tap or gently shake the person. Call the person by name, if known. Shout: "Are you okay?"
   b. Check for no breathing or no normal breathing (gasping).
3. *Rescuer 2:*
   a. Activate the EMS system or the center's emergency response system if the person is not responding and not breathing or not breathing normally (gasping).
   b. Get a defibrillator (AED) if one is available. (See Procedure: *Adult CPR with AED—Two Rescuers*.)
4. *Rescuer 1:* Position the person supine on a hard, flat surface. Logroll the person so there is no twisting of the spine. Place the arms alongside the body. Begin one-rescuer CPR until the second rescuer returns. (See Procedure: *Adult CPR—One Rescuer*, steps 6–11.)
5. When the second rescuer returns, perform two-person CPR (Fig. 44.13).
   a. *Rescuer 1:* Give chest compressions at a rate of 100 to 120 per minute. Push hard and fast. Establish a regular rhythm. Count aloud. Press down at least 2 inches. Allow the chest to recoil between compressions. Give 30 chest compressions. Pause to allow the other rescuer to give two breaths.
   b. *Rescuer 2:*
      (1) Open the airway. Use the head tilt-chin lift method.
      (2) Give two breaths after every 30 compressions. Each breath should take only 1 second and make the chest rise. (If the first breath does not make the chest rise, try opening the airway again. Use the head tilt-chin lift method.)
   c. Continue cycles of 30 compressions and two breaths.
   d. Change positions every 2 minutes (after about five cycles of 30 compressions and two breaths). The switch should take no more than 5 seconds.
   e. Continue until the AED arrives. See Procedure: *Adult CPR with AED—Two Rescuers*. Or continue until help takes over or the person begins to move. If movement occurs, place the person in the recovery position (p. 633).

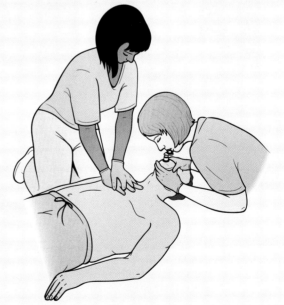

Fig. 44.13 Two people perform cardiopulmonary resuscitation (CPR).

✦ ADULT CPR WITH AED—TWO RESCUERS

Procedure

1. Make sure the scene is safe.
2. *Rescuer 1:* Take 5 to 10 seconds to check for a response and breathing.
   a. Check if the person is responding. Tap or gently shake the person. Call the person by name, if known. Shout: "Are you okay?"
3. *Rescuer 2:*
   a. Activate the EMS system or the center's emergency response system if the person is not responding and not breathing or not breathing normally (gasping).
   b. Get a defibrillator (AED) if one is available.
4. *Rescuer 1:*
   a. Position the person supine on a hard, flat surface. Logroll the person so there is no twisting of the spine. Place the arms alongside the body.
   b. Check for a carotid pulse. This should take 5 to 10 seconds. Start chest compressions if you do not feel a pulse.
   c. Expose the person's chest.
   d. Give chest compressions at a rate of 100 to 120 per minute. Push hard and fast. Establish a regular rhythm. Count aloud. Press down at least 2 inches. Allow the chest to recoil between compressions. Give 30 chest compressions.
   e. Open the airway. Use the head tilt-chin lift method.
   f. Give two breaths. Each breath should take only 1 second. Each breath must make the chest rise. (If the first breath does not make the chest rise, try opening the airway again. Use the head tilt-chin lift method.)
   g. Continue the cycle of 30 chest compressions followed by two breaths. Limit interruptions in compressions to less than 10 seconds.

5. *Rescuer 2:*
   a. Open the case with the AED.
   b. Turn on the AED (Fig. 44.14A).
   c. Apply adult electrode pads to the person's chest (see Fig. 44.14B). Follow the instructions and diagram provided with the AED.
   d. Attach the connecting cables to the AED (see Fig. 44.14C).
   e. Clear away from the person. Make sure no one is touching the person (see Fig. 44.14D).
   f. Let the AED check the person's heart rhythm.
   g. Make sure everyone is clear of the person if the AED advises a "shock" (see Fig. 44.14D). Loudly instruct others not to touch the person. Say: "I am clear, you are clear, everyone is clear!" Look to make sure no one is touching the person.
   h. Press the "SHOCK" button if the AED advises a "shock" (see Fig. 44.14E).
6. *Rescuers 1 and 2:*
   a. Perform two-person CPR.
      (1) Begin with compressions. One rescuer gives chest compressions at a rate of 100 to 120 per minute. Push hard and fast. Establish a regular rhythm. Count aloud. Allow the chest to recoil between compressions. Give 30 chest compressions. Pause to allow the other rescuer to give two breaths.
      (2) The other rescuer gives two breaths after every 30 chest compressions.
7. Repeat steps 5e–h after 2 minutes of CPR (five cycles of 30 compressions and two breaths). Change positions and continue CPR beginning with compressions.
8. Continue until help takes over or the person begins to move. If movement occurs, place the person in the recovery position.

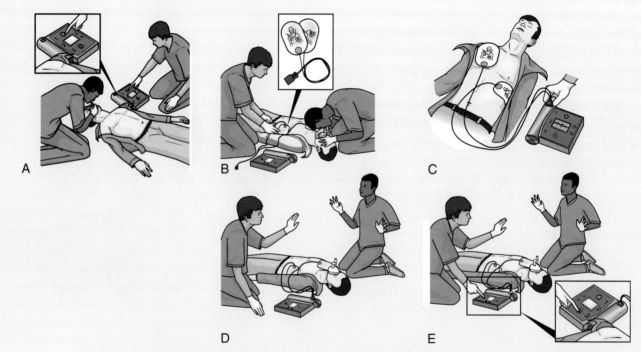

Fig. 44.14 (A) The rescuer turns on the automated external defibrillator (AED). (B) Electrode pads are placed on the person's chest. (C) The cables are connected to the AED. (D) The rescuer "clears" the person. The rescuer makes sure no one is touching the person. (E) The "SHOCK" button is pressed to deliver a shock.

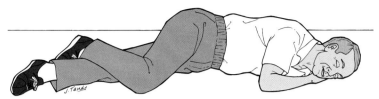

Fig. 44.15 Recovery position.

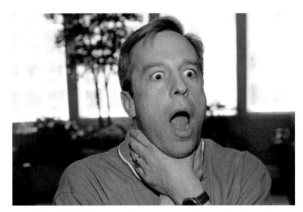

Fig. 44.16 The choking person clutches the throat.

Recovery Position

The recovery position is used when the person is breathing and has a pulse but is not responding (Fig. 44.15). The position helps keep the airway open and prevents aspiration.

Logroll the person into the recovery position. Keep the head, neck, and spine straight. A hand supports the head. *Do not use this position if the person might have neck injuries or other trauma.*

Choking

Choking may occur for a variety of causes. Foreign-body airway obstruction (FBAO) may be caused by a piece of meat lodged in the airway. Persons with dysphagia (Chapter 20) may be at risk. The conscious person clutches at the throat (Fig. 44.16). Clutching at the throat is often called the "universal sign of choking." The conscious person is very frightened. If the obstruction is not removed, the person will die. Severe airway obstruction is an emergency.

✳ Relieving Choking

Abdominal thrusts are used to relieve severe airway obstruction. Abdominal thrusts are quick, upward thrusts to the abdomen. They force air out of the lungs and create an artificial cough. They are done to try to expel the foreign body from the airway.

Abdominal thrusts are not used for very obese persons or pregnant women. Chest thrusts are used (p. 634).

You may observe a person choking; and you may perform emergency measures to relieve choking. Report and record what happened, what you did, and the person's response.

Relief of choking occurs when the foreign body is removed. Or it occurs when you feel air move and see the chest rise and fall when giving rescue breaths. The person may still be unresponsive.

Self-Administered Abdominal Thrusts. You may choke when by yourself. Perform abdominal thrusts to relieve the obstructed airway.

1. Make a fist with one hand.
2. Place the thumb side of the fist above your navel and below the lower end of the sternum.
3. Grasp your fist with your other hand.
4. Press inward and upward quickly.
5. Press the upper abdomen against a hard surface if the thrust did not relieve the obstruction. Use the back of a chair, a table, or railing.
6. Use as many thrusts as needed.

The Unresponsive Adult. You may find an adult who is unresponsive. You did not see the person lose consciousness, and you do not know the cause. Do not assume the cause is choking. Check to see if the person is responding. If not, start CPR (p. ··).

✳ RELIEVING CHOKING—ADULT OR CHILD (OVER 1 YEAR OF AGE)

Procedure

1. Ask the person, "Are you choking?" Help if the person nods "yes" and cannot talk.
2. Have someone call for help.
   a. *In a public area,* have someone activate the EMS system by calling 911. Send someone to get an AED.
   b. *In a center,* call the emergency response system. This team quickly responds to give care in life-threatening situations. Send someone to get the AED and emergency cart.
3. *If the person is sitting or standing,* give abdominal thrusts.
   a. Stand or kneel behind the person.
   b. Wrap your arms around the person's waist.
   c. Make a fist with one hand.

   d. Place the thumb side of the fist against the abdomen. The fist is slightly above the navel in the middle of the abdomen and well below the end of the sternum (breastbone) (Fig. 44.17A).
   e. Grasp the fist with your other hand (see Fig. 44.17B).
   f. Press your fist into the person's abdomen with a quick, upward thrust (Fig. 44.18).
   g. Repeat thrusts until the object is expelled or the person becomes unresponsive.
4. *If the person is obese or pregnant,* give chest thrusts (Fig. 44.19).
   a. Stand behind the person.
   b. Place your arms under the person's underarms. Wrap your arms around the person's chest.
   c. Make a fist. Place the thumb side of the fist on the middle of the sternum (breastbone).

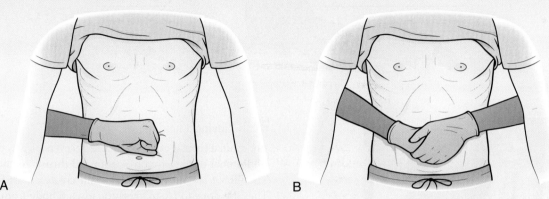

Fig. 44.17 Hand positioning for abdominal thrusts. (A) The fist is slightly above the navel in the midline of the abdomen. (B) The other hand clasps the fist.

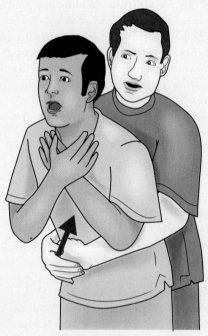

Fig. 44.18 Abdominal thrusts for choking victim. (From Harding M, et al.: *Lewis's medical-surgical nursing: assessment and management of clinical problems*, ed. 11, St. Louis, 2020, Elsevier.)

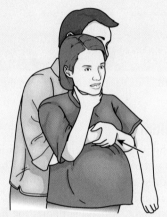

Fig. 44.19 Chest thrusts to relieve choking in pregnant woman. (From Remmert LN, Sorrentino SA: *Mosby's essentials for nursing assistants*, ed. 7, St. Louis, 2023, Elsevier.)

  d. Grasp the fist with your other hand.
  e. Give thrusts to the chest until the object is expelled or the person becomes unresponsive.
5. *If the object is dislodged,* encourage the person to go to the hospital. Injuries can occur from abdominal or chest thrusts.
6. *If the person becomes unresponsive,* gently lower the person to the floor or ground. Position the person supine (lying flat on the back). Make sure EMS or the emergency response system was called (step 2). If alone, provide five cycles (2 minutes) of CPR first. Then call EMS or the emergency response system.
7. Start CPR (p. 630).
  a. Do not check for a pulse. Begin with compressions. Give 30 compressions. Chest compressions help dislodge an obstruction.

  b. Use the head tilt-chin lift method to open the airway (see Fig. 44.5). Open the person's mouth. The mouth should be wide open. Look for an object. Remove the object if you see it and can remove it easily. Use your fingers.
  c. Give two breaths.
  d. Continue cycles of 30 compressions and two breaths. Look for an object every time you open the airway for rescue breaths.
8. *If you relieve choking in an unresponsive person:*
  a. Check for a response, breathing, and a pulse.
    1. *If no response, normal breathing, or pulse*—continue CPR. Attach an AED (p. 629).
    2. *If no response and no normal breathing but there is a pulse*—give rescue breaths. For an adult, give one breath every 5 to 6 seconds (10–12 breaths per minute). For a child, give one breath every 3 to 5 seconds (12–20 breaths per minute). Check for a pulse every 2 minutes. If no pulse, begin CPR.
    3. *If the person has normal breathing and a pulse*—place the person in the recovery position (p. 633). Continue to check the person until help arrives. Encourage the person to go to the hospital if the person responds.

HEMORRHAGE

Life and body functions require an adequate blood supply. If a blood vessel is cut or torn, bleeding occurs. The larger the blood vessel, the greater the bleeding and blood loss. Hemorrhage is the excessive loss of blood in a short time. If bleeding is not stopped, the person will die. Someone who is severely bleeding can bleed to death in as little as 5 minutes.

Internal bleeding

Bleeding can be internal or external. You cannot see internal hemorrhage. The bleeding is inside body tissues and body cavities. Pain, shock, vomiting blood, coughing up blood, and loss of consciousness signal internal hemorrhage.

Follow the rules in Box 44.1. This includes activating the EMS system.

- Keep the person warm, flat, and quiet until help arrives.
- Do not give fluids.

External bleeding

If not hidden by clothing, external bleeding is usually seen. Bleeding can come from capillaries, veins, or arteries that have been cut (Fig. 44.20). Blood loss from capillaries is usually minor. There is a steady flow of blood from a vein. Bleeding from an artery occurs in spurts and can be life threatening.

The American College of Surgeons (ACS) and the ACS Committee on Trauma (ACS COT) have recommendations to control bleeding. A recent national public campaign called Stop the Bleed® (Fig. 44.21) is promoted across the United States. Unexpected violence and injuries—on the highway, in the workplace, at schools, and in other public places has prompted the need for such a program. Just as people are trained in CPR, they may also be trained to save lives by stopping severe bleeding. There is a free online course that can be taken at www.stopthebleed.org/training. Further instruction can be taken with hands-on applications.

Wall-mounted Stop the Bleed® cabinets can be found in many public places (Fig. 44.22A). These cabinets contain supplies, including tourniquets (Fig. 44.22B) and dressings and bandages (Fig. 44.22C) to stop severe bleeding. The cabinets are often mounted next to where an AED is located.

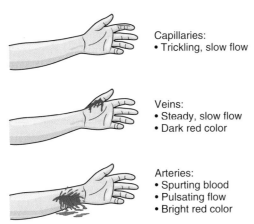

Fig. 44.20 Bleeding from a capillary, vein, and artery.

Capillaries:
- Trickling, slow flow

Veins:
- Steady, slow flow
- Dark red color

Arteries:
- Spurting blood
- Pulsating flow
- Bright red color

To control external bleeding:
- Follow the rules in Box 44.1. This includes activating the EMS system.
- Do not remove any objects that have pierced or stabbed the person.
- Place a sterile dressing directly over the wound. Or use any clean material (handkerchief, towel, cloth, or sanitary napkin).
- Apply pressure with your hand directly over the bleeding site. Do not release pressure until bleeding stops.
- If direct pressure does not control bleeding, pack the wound with clean material (dressings).
- If available, correctly apply tourniquet. Write the time that the tourniquet was applied.

See *Promoting Safety and Comfort: Hemorrhage.*

> **PROMOTING SAFETY AND COMFORT**
>
> **Hemorrhage**
> *Safety*
> Contact with blood is likely with hemorrhage. Follow Standard Precautions and the Bloodborne Pathogen Standard to the extent possible. Wear gloves if possible. Practice hand hygiene as soon as you can.

FAINTING

Fainting is the sudden loss of consciousness from an inadequate blood supply to the brain. Hunger, fatigue, fear, and pain are common causes. Some people faint at the sight of blood or injury. Standing in one position for a long time and being in a warm, crowded room are other causes. Dizziness, perspiration, and blackness before the eyes are warning signals. The person looks pale. The pulse is weak. Respirations are shallow if consciousness is lost. Emergency care for fainting includes the following:

- Have the person sit or lie down before fainting occurs.
- If sitting, the person bends forward and places the head between the knees (Fig. 44.23).
- If the person is lying down, raise the legs.
- Loosen tight clothing (belts, ties, scarves, collars, and so on).
- Keep the person lying down if fainting has occurred. Raise the legs.
- Do not let the person get up until symptoms have subsided for about 5 minutes.
- Help the person to a sitting position after recovery from fainting. Observe for fainting.

SHOCK

Shock results when organs and tissues do not get enough blood. Blood loss, heart attack (myocardial infarction), burns, and severe infection are causes. Signs and symptoms include the following:

- Low or falling blood pressure
- Rapid and weak pulse

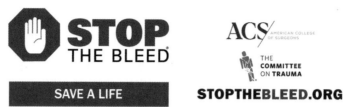

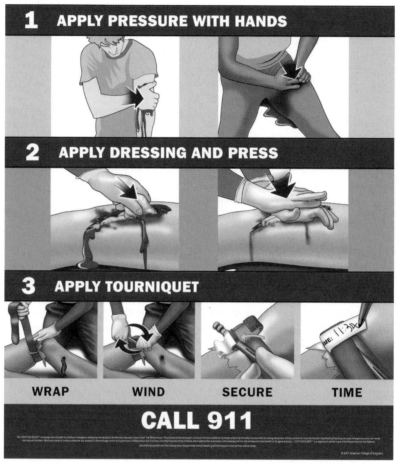

Fig. 44.21 Stop the Bleed poster. (©2021 American College of Surgeons.)

- Rapid respirations
- Cold, moist, and pale skin
- Thirst
- Restlessness
- Confusion and loss of consciousness as shock worsens

Shock is possible in any person who is acutely ill or severely injured. Follow the rules in Box 44.1. Keep the person lying down, maintain an open airway, and control bleeding. Begin CPR if cardiac arrest occurs.

Anaphylactic Shock

Some people are allergic or sensitive to foods, insects, chemicals, and medications. For example, many people are allergic to *penicillin*—an antibiotic medication. An *antigen* is a substance that the body reacts to. The body releases chemicals to fight or attack the antigen. The person may react with an area of redness, swelling, or itching. Or the reaction can involve the entire body.

Anaphylaxis is a life-threatening sensitivity to an antigen. (*Ana* means "without"; *phylaxis* means "protection.") The reaction can occur within seconds. Signs and symptoms include the following:

- Sweating
- Shortness of breath
- Low blood pressure
- Irregular pulse
- Respiratory congestion
- Swelling of the larynx (laryngeal edema)
- Hoarseness
- Dyspnea

Anaphylactic shock is an emergency. The EMS system must be activated. The person needs special medications to reverse

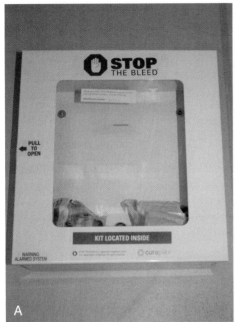

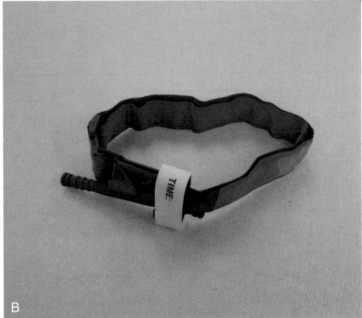

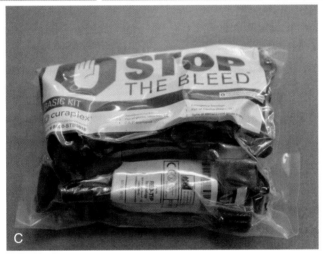

Fig. 44.22 (A) Stop the Bleed cabinet mounted on a wall. (B) Item (tourniquet) contained in cabinet. (C) Package of bandages and dressings.

the allergic reaction. Some residents may have an order for an epinephrine pen. The nurse is aware of these residents and follows the care plan and health care provider orders. In some cases, the person is allowed to keep it and self-administer epinephrine. Keep the person calm and the airway open. Start CPR if cardiac arrest occurs.

STROKE

Stroke (cerebrovascular accident) occurs when the brain is suddenly deprived of its blood supply (Chapter 35). Usually, only part of the brain is affected. A stroke may be caused by a thrombus, an embolus, or hemorrhage if a blood vessel in the brain ruptures.

Signs of stroke vary (Chapter 35). They depend on the size and location of brain injury. Loss of consciousness or semi-consciousness, rapid pulse, labored respirations, high blood pressure, facial drooping, and hemiplegia (paralysis on one side of the body) are signs of a stroke. The person may have slurred speech or aphasia (the inability to have normal speech). Remember the acronym **FAST** (**f**acial drooping, **a**rm drifting downward, **s**peech slurred, **t**ime to call 911). Loss of vision in one eye, unsteadiness, and falling also are signs. Seizures may occur.

Emergency care includes the following:
- Follow the rules in Box 44.1. This includes activating the EMS system.
- Position the person in the recovery position on the affected side (see Fig. 44.17). The affected side is limp, and the cheek appears puffy.
- Raise the head without flexing the neck.
- Loosen tight clothing (belts, ties, scarves, collars, and so on).
- Keep the person quiet and warm.
- Reassure the person.

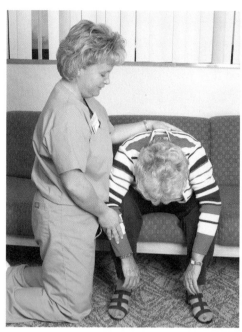

Fig. 44.23 The person bends forward and lowers the head between the knees to prevent fainting.

- Provide CPR if necessary.
- Provide emergency care for seizures if necessary.

SEIZURES

Seizures (convulsions) are violent and sudden contractions or tremors of muscle groups. Movements are uncontrolled. The person may lose consciousness. Seizures are caused by an abnormality in the brain. Causes include head injury during birth or from trauma, high fever, brain tumors, poisoning, and nervous system disorders or infections. Lack of blood flow to the brain, seizure disorders, and epilepsy are other causes. About 1 in 10 people may have a seizure during their lifetime. Seizures are common, so it is good to know how to help.

Epilepsy

Epilepsy is a brain disorder in which clusters of nerve cells sometimes signal abnormally. There are brief changes in the brain's electrical function. The person can have strange sensations, emotions, and behavior. Sometimes there are seizures, muscle spasms, and loss of consciousness.

A single seizure does not mean epilepsy. In epilepsy, seizures recur. The person has a permanent brain injury or defect.

Children and young adults are commonly affected. However, epilepsy can develop at any time in a person's life. It can occur with any problem affecting the brain. Such causes include the following:

- Brain injury before, during, or after birth (Chapter 41)
- Problems with brain development before birth
- The mother having an injury or infection during pregnancy
- Head injury (accidents, gunshot wounds, sports injuries, falls, blows to the head)
- Poor nutrition

- Brain tumor
- Childhood fevers
- Poisoning—such as lead and alcohol
- Infection—such as meningitis and encephalitis
- Stroke

There is no cure at this time. Doctors order medications to prevent seizures. The medications control seizures in many people. In others, medications may not work.

When controlled, epilepsy usually does not affect learning and activities of daily living. Activity and job limits occur in severe cases. For example, a person has seizures at any time. The person may not be allowed to drive a car or operate machinery. This may limit job choices. Also, the person is at risk for accidents and injuries. Safety measures are needed. They are needed for the home, workplace, transportation, and recreation.

Types of Seizures

The major types of seizures are:

- *Partial seizure.* Only one part of the brain is involved. A body part may jerk. Or the person has a hearing or vision problem or stomach discomfort. The person does not lose consciousness.
- *Generalized tonic-clonic seizure (grand mal seizure).* This type has two phases. In the *tonic phase*, the person loses consciousness. If standing or sitting, the person falls to the floor. The body is rigid because all muscles contract at once. The *clonic phase* follows. Muscle groups contract and relax. This causes jerking and twitching movements. Urinary and fecal incontinence may occur. A deep sleep is common after the seizure. Confusion and headache may occur on awakening.
- *Generalized absence (petit mal) seizure.* This type usually lasts a few seconds. There is loss of consciousness, twitching of the eyelids, and staring. No first aid is necessary. However, you should guide the person away from dangers—stairs, streets, a hot stove, fireplaces, and so on.

Emergency Care for Seizures

You cannot stop a seizure. However, you can protect the person from injury.

- Follow the rules in Box 44.1. This includes activating the EMS system.
- Do not leave the person alone.
- Lower the person to the floor. This protects the person from falling.
- Turn the person gently onto one side. This will help the person breathe.
- Clear the area around the person of any hard or sharp objects. This can prevent injury.
- Note the time the seizure started.
- Place something soft and flat under the person's head (Fig. 44.24). It prevents the person's head from striking the floor. You can use a pillow, a cushion, or a folded blanket, towel, or jacket.
- Remove eyeglasses.
- Loosen tight jewelry and clothing around the person's neck. Ties, scarves, collars, and necklaces are examples.

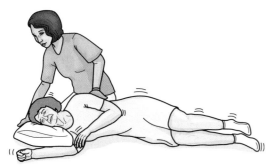

Fig. 44.24 A pillow protects the person's head during a seizure.

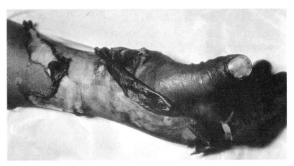

Fig. 44.25 Full-thickness burn. (From Ignatavicius DD, Workman ML, Rebar CR, et al.: *Medical-surgical nursing: concepts for interprofessional collaborative care*, ed. 10, St. Louis, 2021, Elsevier.)

BOX 44.2 Seizures—When to Call 911 (EMS)

- The person has never had a seizure before.
- The person has difficulty breathing or walking after the seizure.
- The seizure lasts longer than 5 minutes.
- The person has another seizure soon after the first one.
- The person is hurt during the seizure.
- The seizure happens in water.
- The person has a health condition such as diabetes, heart disease, or is pregnant.

Centers for Disease Control and Prevention: Seizure first aid, https://www.cdc.gov/epilepsy/about/first-aid.htm, 2022.

- Time the seizure. Call 911 if the seizure lasts longer than 5 minutes (Box 44.2).
- Do not put any object or your fingers between the person's teeth. The person can bite down on your fingers during the seizure.
- Do not try to stop the seizure or control the person's movements.
- Make sure the mouth is clear of food, fluids, and saliva after the seizure.
- Stay with the person until the seizure ends and the person is fully awake. Help the person sit in a safe place. Comfort the person and speak calmly.

PROMOTING SAFETY AND COMFORT

Seizures

Safety

Precautions may be taken for persons who may be prone to having seizures. The bed siderails may be padded to prevent injury. The bed should always be in the lowest position. Fall precautions are in place. If the person is standing or sitting, gently ease the person to the floor. Place a soft, flat object under the person's head. Showers are generally safer than bathing in a tub.

BURNS

Burns can severely disable a person (Fig. 44.25). They can also cause death. Most burns occur in the home. Infants, children, and older persons are at risk. Common causes of burns and fires are the following:

- Scalds from hot liquids
- Playing with matches and lighters
- Electrical injuries
- Cooking accidents (barbecues, microwaves, stoves, ovens)
- Falling asleep while smoking
- Fireplaces
- Space heaters
- No smoke detectors or nonfunctioning smoke detectors
- Sunburn
- Chemicals

The skin has two layers: the dermis and epidermis. Burns are described as superficial, partial thickness, and full thickness.

- *Superficial (first-degree) burns*—involve the epidermis only. They are painful but the burn is not severe.
- *Partial-thickness (second-degree) burns*—involve the epidermis and part of the dermis. They are very painful. Nerve endings are exposed.
- *Full-thickness (third-degree) burns*—involve the entire epidermis and dermis. Fat, muscle, and bone may be injured or destroyed. These burns are not painful. Nerve endings are destroyed.

Some burns are minor; others are severe. Severity depends on burn size and depth, the body part involved, and the person's age. Burns to the face, eyes, ears, hands, and feet are more serious than burns to an arm or leg. Infants, young children, and older persons are at high risk for death.

Emergency care for severe burns includes the following:

- Follow the rules in Box 44.1. This includes activating the EMS system.
- Do not touch the person if in contact with an electrical source. Have the power source turned off or remove the electrical source. Use an object that does not conduct electricity (rope or wood) to remove the electrical source.
- Remove the person from the fire or burn source.
- Stop the burning process. Put out flames with water or roll the person in a blanket. Or smother flames with a coat, sheet, or towel.
- Do not remove burned clothing.
- Remove hot clothing that is not sticking to the skin. If you cannot remove hot clothing, cool the clothing with water.
- Remove jewelry and any tight clothing that is not sticking to the skin.

- Provide rescue breathing and CPR as needed.
- Cover burns with sterile, cool, moist coverings. Or use towels, sheets, or any other clean cloth. Keep the covering wet.

- Do not put oil, butter, salve, or ointments on the burns.
- Cover the person with a blanket or coat to prevent heat loss.

QUALITY OF LIFE

During emergencies, promoting quality of life is important. Remember the person's rights. And treat the person with dignity and respect.

Protect the right to privacy. Do not expose the person unnecessarily. You may be in a place where you cannot close doors or window coverings. The person may be in a lounge, dining area, or public place. Do what you can to provide privacy.

Protect the person from onlookers. (See *Teamwork and Time Management: Emergency Care*, p. 625.) People are curious. They want to know what happened, the extent of injuries or illness, and if the person will be okay. Do not discuss the situation or offer ideas of what is wrong with the person. Information about the person's care, treatment, and condition is confidential.

Protect the right to personal choice. Choices are few in emergencies. They are given when possible. Hospital care may be required. The person has the right to

choose a hospital. Sometimes the person may choose to refuse care. The EMS has guidelines to follow for persons who refuse care. For example, the person must be competent and able to legally make one's own medical decisions. The person must also be informed of the risks, benefits, and alternatives to the care recommended.

Protect personal items from loss and damage. Dentures, eyeglasses, and hearing aids are often lost or broken in emergencies. Watches and jewelry are easily lost. Clothing may be torn or cut. Be very careful to protect the person's property. In public places, personal items are given to police or EMS personnel.

Physical and psychologic safety is important. Protect the person from further injury. For example, protect the person from falls after a stroke. Protect the person's head during a seizure. The person needs to feel safe and secure. Reassurance, explanations about care, and a calm approach are helpful.

TIME TO REFLECT

The nursing center where you work provides CPR training for its entire nursing staff. You have received this training. One day, you witness a man collapse in the parking lot of the nursing center. What action would you take first? You

notice two visitors sitting near the main entrance. If you determine that the man has suffered a sudden cardiac arrest, what would you do from here?

REVIEW QUESTIONS

Circle the BEST answer.

1. The goals of first aid are to
   a. Call for help and keep the person warm
   b. Prevent death and prevent injuries from becoming worse
   c. Stay calm and give emergency care
   d. Calm the person and keep bystanders away

2. When giving first aid, you should
   a. Be aware of your own limits
   b. Move the person
   c. Give the person fluids
   d. Remove clothing

3. Sudden cardiac arrest is
   a. The same as stroke
   b. The sudden stopping of heart action
   c. The sudden loss of consciousness
   d. When organs and tissues do not get enough blood

4. The signs of sudden cardiac arrest are
   a. Confusion, hemiplegia, and slurred speech
   b. Restlessness, rapid breathing, and a weak pulse
   c. No response, no normal breathing, and no pulse
   d. Dizziness, pale skin, and rapid breathing

5. Rescue breathing for an adult involves
   a. Giving each breath over 2 seconds
   b. Watching the abdomen rise with each breath
   c. Giving a breath every 3 to 5 seconds
   d. Giving a breath every 5 to 6 seconds

6. In adult CPR, the chest is compressed
   a. ½ inch with the index and middle fingers
   b. 2 inches with the heel of one hand
   c. At least 2 inches with two hands
   d. At least 1 inch with two hands

7. When checking for breathing
   a. Use the head tilt-chin lift method to open the airway
   b. Look for no breathing or for gasping
   c. Look, listen, and feel for air moving in and out of the lungs
   d. Take 10 to 15 seconds to listen for breathing

8. Which pulse is used during adult CPR?
   a. Apical pulse
   b. Brachial pulse
   c. Carotid pulse
   d. Femoral pulse

9. Which compression rate is used for CPR?
   a. 150 compressions per minute
   b. 100 to 120 compressions per minute
   c. At least 30 compressions per minute
   d. At least 15 compressions per minute

10. When doing adult CPR alone, give
    a. Two breaths after every 15 compressions
    b. Two breaths after every 30 compressions
    c. One breath after every 5 compressions
    d. Two breaths when you are tired from giving compressions

11. After delivering a shock with an AED, you should
    a. Deliver another shock
    b. Place the person in the recovery position
    c. Look, listen, and feel for breathing
    d. Perform CPR beginning with compressions
12. Arterial bleeding
    a. Cannot be seen
    b. Occurs in spurts
    c. Is dark red
    d. Oozes from the wound
13. A person is hemorrhaging from the left forearm. Your first action is to
    a. Lower the arm
    b. Apply pressure to the brachial artery
    c. Apply direct pressure to the wound
    d. Tape a dressing in place
14. A person is about to faint. Which is *false*?
    a. Take the person outside for fresh air
    b. Have the person sit or lie down
    c. Loosen tight clothing
    d. Raise the legs if the person is lying down
15. Which is *not* a sign of shock?
    a. High blood pressure
    b. Rapid pulse
    c. Rapid respirations
    d. Cold, moist, and pale skin
16. A person in shock needs
    a. Rescue breathing
    b. To be kept lying down
    c. Clothes removed
    d. The recovery position
17. A person is having a stroke. Emergency care involves the following *except*
    a. Positioning the person on the affected side
    b. Giving the person sips of water
    c. Loosening tight clothing
    d. Keeping the person quiet and warm

18. These statements relate to tonic-clonic seizures. Which is *false*?
    a. There is contraction of all muscles at once
    b. Incontinence may occur
    c. The seizure lasts 5 seconds
    d. There is loss of consciousness
19. A person is having a seizure. Which is *not* emergency treatment?
    a. Ease the person to the floor
    b. Gently turn the person on their side
    c. Place something soft under the person's head
    d. Insert a spoon in the person's mouth to hold the tongue in place
20. A pregnant woman is choking. What should you do?
    a. Perform abdominal thrusts
    b. Perform chest thrusts
    c. Start chest compressions on the floor
    d. Give two rescue breaths
21. A person was burned. There are no complaints or signs of pain. You know that
    a. The burn is minor
    b. The burn is partial thickness
    c. The burn is full thickness
    d. The dermis was destroyed
22. Burns are covered with
    a. A clean, moist cloth or dressing
    b. Butter, oil, or salve
    c. Water
    d. Nothing

See Appendix A for answers to these questions.

45

End-of-Life Care

OBJECTIVES

- Define the key terms and key abbreviations listed in this chapter.
- Describe terminal illness.
- Describe the factors that affect attitudes about death.
- Describe how different age groups view death.
- Describe the five stages of dying.
- Explain how to meet the needs of the dying person and family.
- Describe palliative care and hospice care.

- Explain the purpose of the Patient Self-Determination Act.
- Explain what is meant by a Do Not Resuscitate order.
- Identify the signs of approaching death and the signs of death.
- Explain how to assist with postmortem care.
- Perform the procedure described in this chapter.
- Explain how to promote quality of life.

KEY TERMS

advance directive A document stating a person's wishes about health care when that person cannot make one's own decisions

autopsy The examination of the body after death

end-of-life care The support and care given during the time surrounding death

hospice care Care that focuses on comfort and quality of life of a person with a serious illness who is approaching the end of life

palliative care Care that involves relieving or reducing the intensity of uncomfortable symptoms without producing a cure

postmortem care Care of the body after (*post*) death (*mortem*)

reincarnation The belief that the spirit or soul is reborn in another human body or in another form of life

rigor mortis The stiffness or rigidity (*rigor*) of skeletal muscles that occurs after death (*mortis*)

terminal illness An illness or injury from which the person will not likely recover

KEY ABBREVIATIONS

AD Alzheimer disease
CPR Cardiopulmonary resuscitation
DNR Do Not Resuscitate
EMS Emergency Medical Services

ID Identification
OBRA Omnibus Budget Reconciliation Act of 1987
POLST Portable (or Physician) Orders for Life-Sustaining Treatment

---

End-of-life care describes the support and care given during the time surrounding death. Sometimes death is sudden. Often, it is expected. Some people gradually fail. End-of-life care may involve days, weeks, or months.

According to the National Institute on Aging, most people die in hospitals or nursing centers. Hospice care is becoming a common option; therefore, the health team sees death often. Many team members are not sure of their feelings about death. Dying persons and the subject of death cause discomfort. Death and dying mean helplessness and failure to cure. They also remind us that we and our loved ones will die.

Your feelings about death affect the care you give. You will help meet the dying person's physical, psychologic, social, and spiritual needs. Therefore, you must understand the dying process. Then you can approach the dying person with caring, kindness, and respect.

See *Teamwork and Time Management: End-of-Life Care.*

> ### TEAMWORK AND TIME MANAGEMENT
> **End-of-Life Care**
> The nurse may need to spend a lot of time with the dying person. Often, it is a busy time before and after someone dies. Offer to take equipment and supplies to and from the room. Also offer to help with other residents.

TERMINAL ILLNESS

Many illnesses and diseases have no cure. Some injuries are so serious that the body cannot function. Recovery is not expected. The disease or injury ends in death. An illness or injury from which the person will not likely recover is a terminal illness.

Doctors cannot predict the time of death. A person may have days, months, weeks, or years to live. People expected to live for a short time have lived for years. Others have died sooner than expected.

Modern medicine has found cures or has prolonged life in many cases. Research will bring new cures. However, hope and the will to live strongly influence living and dying. Many people have died for no apparent reason when they have lost hope or the will to live.

Types of Care

Persons with terminal illnesses can choose palliative care or hospice care. The person may opt for palliative care and then change to hospice care.

- *Palliative care. Palliate* comes from the Latin word meaning "to cloak." It means to soothe or relieve. Palliative care involves relieving or reducing the intensity of uncomfortable symptoms without producing a cure. The person receives care to relieve symptoms. The person's illness also is treated. The intent is to improve the person's quality of life and provide support for the family. This type of care is for anyone with a long-term illness that will cause death. Settings include hospitals, nursing centers, and the person's home.
- *Hospice care.* Hospice care focuses on the physical, emotional, social, and spiritual needs of dying persons and their families. Often, the person has less than 6 months to live. No attempts are made to cure the person. It is not concerned with cure or life-saving measures. Pain relief and comfort are stressed. The goal is to improve the dying person's quality of life. Hospitals, nursing centers, and home care agencies offer hospice care. Or a hospice may be a separate agency. Follow-up care and support groups for survivors are hospice services. Hospice also provides support for the health team to help deal with a person's death.

Attitudes about Death

Experiences, culture, religion, and age influence attitudes about death. Many people fear death. Others do not believe they will die. Some look forward to and accept death. Attitudes about death often change as a person grows older and with changing circumstances.

Dying people often need hospital, nursing center, hospice, or home care. The family is often involved in the person's care. They usually gather at the bedside to comfort the person and each other. When death occurs, the funeral director is called. The funeral director takes the body to the funeral home to prepare it for funeral practices.

Many adults and children have never had contact with a dying person. Nor have they been present at the time of death. Some have not attended a visitation (wake) or funeral. They have not seen the process of dying and death. Therefore, it may be frightening, morbid, or mysterious.

Culture and Spiritual Needs

Practices and attitudes about death differ among cultures (Chapter 7). In some cultures, dying people are cared for at home by the family. Some families prepare the body for burial.

Spiritual needs relate to the human spirit and to religion and religious beliefs. They do not involve material or physical things. Rather, they involve finding meaning in one's life. Some people need to resolve issues with family and friends. Many people strengthen their religious beliefs when dying. Religion provides comfort for the dying person and the family.

Attitudes about death are closely related to religion. Some believe that life after death is free of suffering and hardship. They also believe in reunion with loved ones. Many believe that sins and misdeeds are punished in the afterlife. Some feel it is necessary to confess sins. Others do not believe in the afterlife. To them, death is the end of life.

There also are religious beliefs about the body's form after death. Some believe that the body keeps its physical form. Others believe that only the spirit or soul is present in the afterlife. Reincarnation is the belief that the spirit or soul is reborn in another human body or in another form of life.

Many religions practice rites and rituals during the dying process and at the time of death (Chapter 7). Prayers, blessings, scripture readings, and religious music are common sources of comfort. So are visits from a spiritual leader—minister, priest, rabbi, or other cleric (Fig. 45.1).

📋 FOCUS ON COMMUNICATION

Culture and Spiritual Needs

You may have different cultural or religious practices and beliefs about death. You must not judge the person by your standards. Do not make negative comments or insult the person's beliefs. Respect the person as a whole. This includes the person's beliefs and customs. If the dying person or a family member requests to talk to a spiritual leader, convey this information to the nurse at once.

Age

Infants and toddlers do not understand the nature or meaning of death. They know or sense that something is different. They sense that a caregiver is absent or that there is a different

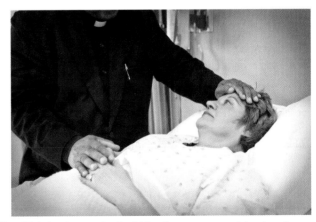

Fig. 45.1 A priest at the bedside of a person receiving hospice care. (From Yoost LC: *Conceptual care mapping: case studies for improving communication, collaboration, and care,* ed. 1, St. Louis, 2018, Elsevier.)

caregiver. They also sense changes in when and how their needs are met. They may feel a sense of loss.

Between 2 and 6 years old, children think death is temporary. It can be reversed. The dead person continues to live and function in some ways and can come back to life. These ideas come from fairy tales, cartoons, movies, video games, and television. For example, a cartoon character is injured and dies. Later the character comes back to life, whole and intact. Children this age often blame themselves when someone or something dies. To them, death is punishment for being bad. They know when family members or pets die. They notice dead birds or bugs. Answers to questions about death often cause fear and confusion. Children who are told "He is sleeping" may be afraid to go to sleep.

Between 6 and 11 years old, children learn that death is final. They do not think they will die. Death happens to others, especially adults. It can be avoided. Children relate death to punishment and body mutilation. It also involves witches, ghosts, goblins, and monsters.

By age 11, death is more fully understood. Death is still viewed as something that happens to other people. One's own death is an event in the distant future. Without correct information, children may have some wrong ideas. However, understanding increases as they grow older and have more experiences with death.

Adults fear pain and suffering, dying alone, and the invasion of privacy. They also fear loneliness and separation from loved ones. Some may fear an undignified death. They may worry about the care and support of those left behind. Adults often resent death because it affects plans, hopes, dreams, and ambitions.

Older persons usually have fewer fears than younger adults. They know death will occur. They have had more experiences with dying and death. Many have lost family and friends. Some welcome death as freedom from pain, suffering, and disability. Death also means reunion with those who have died. Like younger adults, many fear dying alone.

THE STAGES OF DYING

Dr. Elisabeth Kübler-Ross described five stages of dying. They also are known as the "stages of grief." *Grief* is the person's response to loss.

- *Stage 1: Denial.* The person refuses to believe that death is coming. "No, not me" is a common response. The person believes a mistake was made. Information about the illness or injury is not heard. The person cannot deal with any problem or decision about the matter. This stage can last for a few hours, days, or much longer. Some people are still in denial when they die.
- *Stage 2: Anger.* The person thinks "Why me?" There is anger and rage. Dying persons envy and resent those with life and health. Family, friends, and the health team are often targets of anger. The person blames others and finds fault with

those who are loved and needed the most. It is hard to deal with the person during this stage. Anger is normal and healthy. Do not take the person's anger personally. Control any urge to be angry back or avoid the person.

- *Stage 3: Bargaining.* Anger has passed. The person now says, "Yes, me, but. . . ." Often, the person bargains with God or a higher power for more time. Promises are made in exchange for more time. The person may want to see a child marry, see a grandchild born, have one more Christmas, or live for some other event. Usually, more promises are made as the person makes "just one more" request. You may not see this stage. Bargaining is usually private and spiritual.
- *Stage 4: Depression.* The person thinks "Yes, me" and is very sad. The person mourns things that were lost and the future loss of life. The person may cry or say little. Sometimes the person talks about people and things that will be left behind.
- *Stage 5: Acceptance.* The person is calm and at peace. The person has said what needs to be said. Unfinished business is completed. The person accepts death. This stage may last for many months or years. Reaching the acceptance stage does not mean death is near.

Dying persons do not always pass through all five stages. A person may never get beyond a certain stage. Some move back and forth between stages. For example, Mr. Jones reached acceptance but moves back to bargaining. Then he moves forward to acceptance. Some people stay in one stage.

COMFORT NEEDS

Comfort is a basic part of end-of-life care. It involves physical, mental, emotional, and spiritual needs. For spiritual needs, see Chapter 7. Comfort goals are to:

- Prevent or relieve suffering to the extent possible.
- Respect and follow end-of-life wishes.

Persons may want family and friends present. They may want to talk about their fears, worries, and anxieties. Some want to be alone. Often, they need to talk during the night. Things are quiet, distractions are few, and there is more time to think. You need to listen and use touch.

- *Listening.* Persons need to talk and share worries and concerns. Let them express feelings and emotions in their own way. Do not worry about saying the wrong thing or finding comforting words. You do not need to say anything. Being there for each person is what counts.
- *Touch.* Touch shows caring and concern when words cannot. Sometimes persons do not want to talk but need you nearby. Do not feel that you need to talk. Silence, along with touch, is a powerful and meaningful way to communicate.

Some people may want to see a spiritual leader or take part in religious practices. Provide privacy during prayer and spiritual moments. Be courteous to the spiritual leader. The person has the right to have religious objects nearby—medals, rosaries, pictures, statues, writings, prayer books, and so on. Handle these valuables with care and respect.

See *Focus on Communication: The Person's Needs*
See *Residents With Dementia: The Person's Needs.*

 FOCUS ON COMMUNICATION

The Person's Needs

You may not know what to say to the dying person. That is hard for many experienced health team members. Unless you have been near death yourself, do not say "I understand what you are going through." The statement is a communication barrier. Instead you can say:

- "Would you like to talk? I have time to listen."
- "You seem sad. How can I help?"
- "Is it okay if I sit quietly with you for a while?"

RESIDENTS WITH DEMENTIA

The Person's Needs

Persons with Alzheimer disease (AD) become more and more disabled. Those with advanced AD cannot share their concerns, discomforts, or problems. It is hard to provide emotional and spiritual comfort.

Focusing on the person's senses—hearing, touch, sight—can promote comfort. Comforting touch or massage can be soothing. So can soft music or sounds from nature—birds chirping, gentle breezes, ocean waves, and so on.

Mental, Emotional, and Spiritual Needs

Mental, emotional, and spiritual needs are very personal. There may be times when dying persons seem to see or talk to someone who is not there. If this occurs when you are present, do not correct them or tell them that this is their imagination. For some, this is very real. They may describe in detail meeting a deceased friend or relative. The person may describe seeing religious figures or angels. Let them share their experience by listening and being present.

Some persons are anxious or depressed. Others have specific fears and concerns. Examples include the following:

- Severe pain
- When and how death will occur
- What will happen to loved ones
- Dying alone

The doctor may order medications for anxiety or depression. Simple measures may soothe the person—touch, holding a hand, back massage, soft lighting, music at a low volume.

Physical Needs

Dying may take a few minutes, hours, days, or weeks. Body processes slow. The person is weak. Changes occur in levels of consciousness. To the extent possible, independence is allowed. As the person weakens, basic needs are met. The person may depend on others for basic needs and activities of daily living. Every effort is made to promote physical and psychologic comfort. The person is allowed to die in peace and with dignity.

Pain

Some dying persons do not have pain. Others do and it may be severe. Always report signs and symptoms of pain at once (Chapter 25). Pain management is important. The nurse can give pain-relief medications ordered by the doctor. Preventing and controlling pain is easier than relieving pain.

Skin care, personal and oral hygiene, back massages, and good alignment promote comfort. Frequent position changes and supportive devices promote comfort. Turn the person slowly and gently. The person's care plan will include other measures to prevent and control pain.

Breathing Problems

Shortness of breath and difficulty breathing (dyspnea) are common end-of-life problems. Semi-Fowler position is usually best for breathing problems. The doctor may order oxygen (Chapter 26). Opening a window for fresh air may help some people. For others, a fan circulating air is helpful.

Noisy breathing—called the *death rattle*—is common as death nears. This is due to mucus collecting in the airway. The following may help:

- The side-lying position
- Suctioning by the nurse
- Medications ordered by the doctor to reduce the amount of mucus

Vision, Hearing, and Speech

Vision blurs and gradually fails. The person naturally turns toward light. A darkened room may frighten the person. The eyes may be half-open. Secretions may collect in the eye corners.

Because of failing vision, explain who you are and what you are doing to the person or in the room. The room should be well lit. However, avoid bright lights and glares.

Good eye care is essential (Chapter 18). If the eyes stay open, a nurse may apply a protective ointment. Then the eyes are covered with moist pads to prevent injury.

Hearing is one of the last functions lost. Many people hear until the moment of death. Even unconscious persons may hear. Always assume that the person can hear. Speak in a normal voice. Provide reassurance and explanations about care. Offer words of comfort. Avoid topics that could upset the person. Do not talk about the person.

Speech becomes harder. It may be hard to understand the person. Sometimes the person cannot speak. Anticipate the person's needs. Do not ask questions that need long answers. Ask "yes" or "no" questions. These should be few in number. Despite speech problems, you must talk to the person.

Mouth, Nose, and Skin

Oral hygiene promotes comfort. Give routine mouth care if the person can eat and drink. Give frequent oral hygiene as death nears and when taking oral fluids is difficult. Oral hygiene is needed if mucus collects in the mouth and the person cannot swallow. A lip balm may help dry lips.

Crusting and irritation of the nostrils can occur. Nasal secretions, an oxygen cannula, and a nasogastric tube are common causes. Carefully clean the nose. Apply lubricant as directed by the nurse and the care plan.

Circulation fails and body temperature rises as death nears. The skin feels cool, pale, and mottled (blotchy). Perspiration increases. Skin care, bathing, and preventing pressure injuries are necessary. Linens and gowns are changed when needed. Although the skin feels cool, only light bed coverings are needed. Blankets may make the person feel warm and cause restlessness. However, observe for signs of cold. Shivering, hunching the shoulders, and pulling covers up may signal that the person is cold. Prevent drafts and provide more blankets.

Nutrition

Nausea, vomiting, and loss of appetite are common at the end of life. The doctor can order medications for nausea and vomiting.

Some persons are too tired or too weak to eat. You may need to feed them. Providing the person's favorite foods may help with loss of appetite. Small, frequent meals may be preferred.

As death nears, loss of appetite is common. The person may choose not to eat or drink. Do not force the person to eat or drink. Doing so may add to the person's discomfort. Report refusal to eat or drink to the nurse.

Elimination

Urinary and fecal incontinence may occur. Use incontinence products or bed protectors as directed. Give perineal care as needed. Constipation and urinary retention are common. Enemas and catheters may be needed. Provide catheter care according to the care plan.

The Person's Room

Provide a comfortable and pleasant room. It should be well lit and well ventilated. Remove unnecessary equipment. Some equipment is upsetting to look at (suction machines, drainage containers). If possible, keep these items out of the person's sight.

Mementos, pictures, cards, flowers, and religious items provide comfort. Arrange them within the person's view. The person and family arrange the room as they wish. This helps meet love, belonging, and esteem needs. The room should reflect the person's choices.

THE FAMILY

This is a difficult time for the family. It may be hard to find comforting words. To show you care, be available, courteous, and considerate. Use touch to show your concern (Fig. 45.2).

The family usually can stay as long as they wish. Sometimes family members keep a *vigil*. That is, someone is with the person at all times, including during the night. They watch over or pray for the person. The health team makes them as comfortable as possible. Never make them feel like they are a burden or "in the way."

Respect the right to privacy. The person and family need time together. However, do not neglect care because the family

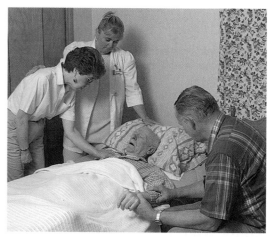

Fig. 45.2 A hospice nurse helps the family say goodbye. (From Williams P: *DeWit's fundamental concepts and skills for nursing*, ed. 5, St. Louis, 2018, Elsevier.)

is present. Most centers let family members help give care. Or you can suggest that they take a break for a beverage or meal.

The family may be very tired, sad, and tearful. Watching a loved one die is very painful. So is dealing with the eventual loss of that person. The family goes through stages like the dying person. They need support, understanding, courtesy, and respect. A spiritual leader may provide comfort. Communicate a request for a spiritual leader to the nurse at once.

LEGAL ISSUES

Much attention is given to the right to die. Many people do not want machines or other measures keeping them alive. Consent is needed for any treatment. When able, the person makes care decisions. Some people make end-of-life wishes known.

The Patient Self-Determination Act

The Patient Self-Determination Act and the Omnibus Budget Reconciliation Act of 1987 (OBRA) give persons the right to accept or refuse treatment. They also give the right to make advance directives.

An advance directive is a document stating a person's wishes about health care when that person cannot make one's own decisions. It lets others know the type of care desired if seriously ill or dying. Advance directives usually forbid certain care if there is no hope of recovery. Living wills and a durable power of attorney for health care are common advance directives.

These laws protect quality of care. Quality of care cannot be less because of the person's advance directives. Some elderly people may think they will not be cared for the same if they sign an advance directive. They need to be reassured that this is not the case.

Nursing centers must inform all persons of the right to advance directives on admission. This information is in writing. The medical record must document whether the person has made them.

If a person expresses a desire to complete or change an advance directive, tell the nurse as soon as possible. Most centers have procedures for completing these forms. If a resident asks you to sign as a witness on one of these documents, it is best to refer that request to the nurse. Know your facility's policy for witnessing legal documents.

Living Wills

A living will is a document about measures that support or maintain life when death is likely. Tube feedings, ventilators, and resuscitation are examples. A living will may instruct doctors:

- Not to start measures that prolong dying.
- To remove measures that prolong dying.

Durable Power of Attorney for Health Care

This advance directive gives the power to make health care decisions to another person. That person is often called a *health care proxy*. Usually, this is a family member, friend, or lawyer. When a person cannot make health care decisions, the health care proxy can do so. This advance directive does not cover property or financial matters.

Portable Orders for Life-Sustaining Treatment (POLST)

The National POLST program is an independent nonprofit organization that promotes advance care planning. It encourages all states to create a POLST program that meets national standards yet is specific to each state. POLST programs are run by the state, not by National POLST. The POLST form is a physician order sheet based on the person's current medical condition and wishes. POLST has different names in different states. It is a standardized form usually printed on brightly colored paper (Fig. 45.3). It specifically identifies which life-sustaining treatments will be performed or withheld. The form becomes a part of the person's medical record. It follows whenever the person is transferred to another care setting. For example, it goes with the person when a resident leaves the care center for the hospital. In some states, the information on the form can be retrieved from a computerized database. For example, Emergency Medical Services (EMS) might need this important information. The program helps health team members to communicate the person's wishes. The person can change or cancel a POLST form at any time.

Do Not Resuscitate Orders

When death is sudden and unexpected, efforts are made to save the person's life (Chapter 44).

For terminally ill persons, doctors often write Do Not Resuscitate (DNR) or No Code orders. The person will not be resuscitated. The person is allowed to die with peace and dignity. The orders are written after consulting with the person and family. The family and doctor make the decision if the person is not mentally able to do so. Some advance directives address resuscitation. Each nursing center may have its own method of denoting which residents have DNR orders. To promote dignity and privacy there should not be a DNR sign posted by the person's doorway. The resident may wear a special wristband (Chapter 11). The order is noted in the care plan. Know your center's method of communicating DNR status of residents.

You may not agree with care and resuscitation decisions. However, you must follow the person's or family's wishes and the doctor's orders. These may be against your personal, religious, and cultural values. If so, discuss the matter with the nurse. You may need an assignment change.

SIGNS OF DEATH

In the weeks before death, the following may occur:

- Restlessness and agitation
- Shortness of breath (dyspnea)
- Depression
- Anxiety
- Drowsiness
- Confusion
- Constipation or incontinence
- Nausea
- Loss of appetite
- Healing problems
- Swelling in the hands, feet, or other body areas
- Pauses in breathing
  As death nears, these signs may occur fast or slowly:
- Movement, muscle tone, and sensation are lost. This usually starts in the feet and legs. When mouth muscles relax, the jaw drops. The mouth may stay open. The facial expression is often peaceful.
- Peristalsis and other gastrointestinal functions slow down. Abdominal distention, fecal incontinence, nausea, and vomiting are common.
- Body temperature rises. The person feels cool or cold, looks pale, and perspires heavily.
- Circulation fails. The pulse is fast or slow, weak, and irregular. Blood pressure starts to fall.
- The respiratory system fails. Slow or rapid and shallow respirations are observed. Mucus collects in the airway. Breathing sounds are noisy and gurgling—commonly called the *death rattle*.
- Pain decreases as the person loses consciousness. However, some people are conscious until the moment of death.

The signs of death include no pulse, no respirations, and no blood pressure. The pupils are fixed and dilated. A doctor determines that death has occurred. The doctor pronounces the person dead. The cause, time, and place are noted for the death certificate.

✳ CARE OF THE BODY AFTER DEATH

Care of the body after (*post*) death (*mortem*) is called postmortem care. A nurse gives postmortem care. You may be asked to assist. Postmortem care begins when the doctor pronounces the person dead.

HIPAA PERMITS DISCLOSURE OF POLST TO OTHER HEALTH CARE PROVIDERS AS NECESSARY

Physician Orders for Life-Sustaining Treatment (POLST)

EMSA #111 B
(Effective 4/1/2011)

First follow these orders, then contact physician. This is a Physician Order Sheet based on the person's current medical condition and wishes. Any section not completed implies full treatment for that section. A copy of the signed POLST form is legal and valid. POLST complements an Advance Directive and is not intended to replace that document. Everyone shall be treated with dignity and respect.

Patient Last Name:	Date Form Prepared:
Patient First Name:	Patient Date of Birth:
Patient Middle Name:	Medical Record #: *(optional)*

A
Check
One

CARDIOPULMONARY RESUSCITATION (CPR):　*If person has no pulse and is not breathing.*
When NOT in cardiopulmonary arrest, follow orders in Sections B and C.

☐ **Attempt Resuscitation/CPR** (Selecting CPR in Section A **requires** selecting Full Treatment in Section B)
☐ **Do Not Attempt Resuscitation/DNR**　(<u>A</u>llow <u>N</u>atural <u>D</u>eath)

B
Check
One

MEDICAL INTERVENTIONS:　*If patient is found with a pulse and/or is breathing.*

☐ <u>**Full Treatment**</u> – primary goal of prolonging life by all medically effective means.
In addition to treatment described in Selective Treatment and Comfort-Focused Treatment, use intubation, advanced airway interventions, mechanical ventilation, and cardioversion as indicated.
　　☐ *Trial Period of Full Treatment.*

☐ <u>**Selective Treatment**</u> – goal of treating medical conditions while avoiding burdensome measures.
In addition to treatment described in Comfort-Focused Treatment. use medical treatment, IV antibiotics, and IV fluids as indicated. Do not intubate. May use non-invasive positive airway pressure. Generally avoid intensive care.
　　☐ *Request transfer to hospital <u>only</u> if comfort needs cannot be met in current location.*

☐ <u>**Comfort-Focused Treatment**</u> – primary goal of maximizing comfort.
Relieve pain and suffering with medication by any route as needed; use oxygen, suctioning, and manual treatment of airway obstruction. Do not use treatments listed in Full and Selective Treatment unless consistent with comfort goal. *Request transfer to hospital <u>only</u> If comfort needs cannot be met in current location.*

Additional Orders: _____
_____

C
Check
One

ARTIFICIALLY ADMINISTERED NUTRITION:　*Offer food by mouth if feasible and desired.*

☐ Long-term artificial nutrition, including feeding tubes.　　**Additional Orders:** _____
☐ Trial period of artificial nutrition, including feeding tubes.　_____
☐ No artificial means of nutrition, including feeding tubes.　_____

D

INFORMATION AND SIGNATURES:

Discussed with:　　☐ Patient (Patient Has Capacity)　　☐ Legally Recognized Decisionmaker

☐ Advance Directive dated _____ available and reviewed →　Health Care Agent if named in Advance Directive:
☐ Advance Directive not available　　　　　　　　　　　　　Name: _____
☐ No Advance Directive　　　　　　　　　　　　　　　　　Phone: _____

Signature of Physician
My signature below indicates to the best of my knowledge that these orders are consistent with the person's medical condition and preferences.

| Print Physician Name: | Physician Phone Number: | Physician License Number: |
| Physician Signature: *(required)* | | Date: |

Signature of Patient or Legally Recognized Decisionmaker
By signing this form, the legally recognized decisionmaker acknowledges that this request regarding resuscitative measures is consistent with the known desires of, and with the best interest of, the individual who is the subject of the form.

Print Name:	Relationship: *(write self if patient)*
Signature: *(required)*	Date:
Address:	Daytime Phone Number:	Evening Phone Number:

SEND FORM WITH PERSON WHENEVER TRANSFERRED OR DISCHARGED

Fig. 45.3 Physician Orders for Life-Sustaining Treatment (POLST). (From Coalition for Compassionate Care, Sacramento, CA.)

HIPAA PERMITS DISCLOSURE OF POLST TO OTHER HEALTH CARE PROVIDERS AS NECESSARY

Patient Information

Name (last, first, middle):	Date of Birth:	Gender: M F

Health Care Provider Assisting with Form Preparation

Name:	Title:	Phone Number:

Additional Contact

Name:	Relationship to Patient:	Phone Number:

Directions for Health Care Provider

Completing POLST

- Completing a POLST form is voluntary. California law requires that a POLST form be followed by health care providers, and provides immunity to those who comply in good faith. In the hospital setting, a patient will be assessed by a physician who will issue appropriate orders.
- POLST does not replace the Advance Directive. When available, review the Advance Directive and POLST form to ensure consistency, and update forms appropriately to resolve any conflicts.
- POLST must be completed by a health care provider based on patient preferences and medical indications.
- A legally recognized decisionmaker may include a court-appointed conservator or guardian, agent designated in an Advance Directive, orally designated surrogate, spouse, registered domestic partner, parent of a minor, closest available relative, or person whom the patient's physician believes best knows what is in the patient's best interest and will make decisions in accordance with the patient's expressed wishes and values to the extent known.
- POLST must be signed by a physician and the patient or decisionmaker to be valid. Verbal orders are acceptable with follow-up signature by physician in accordance with facility/community policy.
- Certain medical conditions or treatments may prohibit a person from residing in a residential care facility for the elderly.
- If a translated form is used with patient or decisionmaker, attach it to the signed English POLST form.
- Use of original form is strongly encouraged. Photocopies and FAXes of signed POLST forms are legal and valid. A copy should be retained in patient's medical record, on Ultra Pink paper when possible.

Using POLST

- Any incomplete section of POLST implies full treatment for that section.

Section A:
- If found pulseless and not breathing, no defibrillator (including automated external defibrillators) or chest compressions should be used on a person who has chosen "Do Not Attempt Resuscitation."

Section B:
- When comfort cannot be achieved in the current setting, the person, including someone with "Comfort-Focused Treatment" should be transferred to a setting able to provide comfort (e.g., treatment of a hip fracture).
- Non-invasive positive airway pressure includes continuous positive airway pressure (CPAP), bi-level positive airway pressure (BiPAP), and bag valve mask (BVM) assisted respirations.
- IV antibiotics and hydration generally are not "Comfort Measures."
- Treatment of dehydration prolongs life. If person desires IV fluids, indicate "Limited Interventions" or "Full Treatment."
- Depending on local EMS protocol, "Additional Orders" written in Section B may not be implemented by EMS personnel.

Reviewing POLST

It is recommended that POLST be reviewed periodically. Review is recommended when:
- The person is transferred from one care setting or care level to another, or
- There is a substantial change in the person's health status, or
- The person's treatment preferences change.

Modifying and Voiding POLST

- A patient with capacity can, at any time, request alternative treatment.
- A patient with capacity can, at any time, revoke a POLST by any means that indicates intent to revoke. It is recommended that revocation be documented by drawing a line through Sections A through D, writing "VOID" in large letters, and signing and dating this line.
- A legally recognized decisionmaker may request to modify the orders, in collaboration with the physician, based on the known desires of the individual or, if unknown, the individual's best interests.

This form is approved by the California Emergency Medical Services Authority in cooperation with the statewide POLST Task Force. For more information or a copy of the form, visit **www.caPOLST.org**.

SEND FORM WITH PERSON WHENEVER TRANSFERRED OR DISCHARGED

Fig. 45.3, cont'd

Postmortem care is done to maintain a good appearance of the body. Discoloration and skin damage are prevented. Valuables and personal items are gathered for the family. The right to privacy and the right to be treated with dignity and respect apply after death.

Within 2 to 4 hours after death, rigor mortis develops. Rigor mortis is the stiffness or rigidity (*rigor*) of skeletal muscles that occurs after death (*mortis*). The body is positioned in normal alignment before rigor mortis sets in. The family may want to see the body. The body should appear in a comfortable and natural position for this viewing.

In some centers, the body is prepared only for viewing by the family. The funeral director completes postmortem care.

Sometimes an autopsy is done. An autopsy is the examination of the body after death. (*Autos* means "self"; *opsis* means "view.") Its purpose is to determine the cause of death. The coroner or medical examiner can order an autopsy, or the family may request one. Follow center procedures when an autopsy is to be done. Postmortem care is not done. Doing so could remove or destroy evidence.

Postmortem care involves moving the body. For example, soiled areas are bathed and the body is placed in good alignment. Moving the body can cause remaining air in the lungs, stomach, and intestines to be expelled. When air is expelled, sounds are produced. Do not let these sounds alarm or frighten you. They are normal and expected.

See *Delegation Guidelines: Care of the Body After Death.*

See *Promoting Safety and Comfort: Care of the Body After Death.*

📄 DELEGATION GUIDELINES

Care of the Body After Death

When assisting with postmortem care, you need this information from the nurse:

- If dentures are inserted or placed in a denture cup
- If tubes and dressings are removed or left in place
- If rings are removed or left in place
- If the family wants to view the body
- Special center policies and procedures

👤 PROMOTING SAFETY AND COMFORT

Care of the Body After Death

Safety

Standard Precautions and the Bloodborne Pathogen Standard are followed. You may have contact with blood, body fluids, secretions, or excretions.

✳ ASSISTING WITH POSTMORTEM CARE

Preprocedure

1. Follow *Delegation Guidelines: Care of the Body After Death.* See *Promoting Safety and Comfort: Care of the Body After Death.*
2. Practice hand hygiene.
3. Collect the following:
   - Postmortem kit (shroud or body bag, gown, identification [ID] tags, gauze squares, safety pins)
   - Bed protectors
   - Wash basin
   - Bath towel and washcloths
   - Denture cup
   - Tape
   - Dressings
   - Gloves
   - Cotton balls
   - Valuables envelope
4. Provide for privacy.
5. Raise the bed for body mechanics.
6. Make sure the bed is flat.

Procedure

7. Put on the gloves.
8. Position the body supine. Arms and legs are straight. A pillow is under the head and shoulders. Or raise the head of the bed 15 to 20 degrees if this is center policy.
9. Close the eyes. Gently pull the eyelids over the eyes. Apply moist cotton balls gently over the eyelids if the eyes will not stay closed.
10. Insert dentures if it is center policy to do so. If not, put them in a labeled denture cup.
11. Close the mouth. If necessary, place a rolled towel under the chin to keep the mouth closed.
12. Follow center policy for jewelry. Remove all jewelry, except for wedding rings if this is center policy. List the jewelry that you removed. Place the jewelry and the list in a "valuables" envelope.
13. Place a cotton ball over the rings. Tape them in place.
14. Remove drainage containers.
15. Remove tubes and catheters. Use the gauze squares as needed. (Omit this step if autopsy will be performed.)
16. Bathe soiled areas with plain water. Dry thoroughly.
17. Place a bed protector under the buttocks.
18. Remove soiled dressings. Replace them with clean ones.
19. Put a clean gown on the body. Position the body as in step 8.
20. Brush and comb the hair if necessary.
21. Cover the body to the shoulders with a sheet if the family will view the body.
22. Gather the person's belongings. Put them in a bag labeled with the person's name. Make sure you include eyeglasses, hearing aids, and other valuables.
23. Remove supplies, equipment, and linens. Straighten the room. Provide soft lighting.
24. Remove the gloves. Decontaminate your hands.
25. Let the family view the body. Provide for privacy. Return to the room after they leave.
26. Decontaminate your hands. Put on gloves.
27. Fill out the ID tags. Tie one to the ankle or to the right big toe.
28. Place the body in the body bag or cover it with a sheet. Or apply the shroud (Fig. 45.4).
    a. Position the shroud under the body.
    b. Bring the top down over the head.
    c. Fold the bottom up over the feet.
    d. Fold the sides over the body.
    e. Pin or tape the shroud in place.

Continued

✳ ASSISTING WITH POSTMORTEM CARE—cont'd

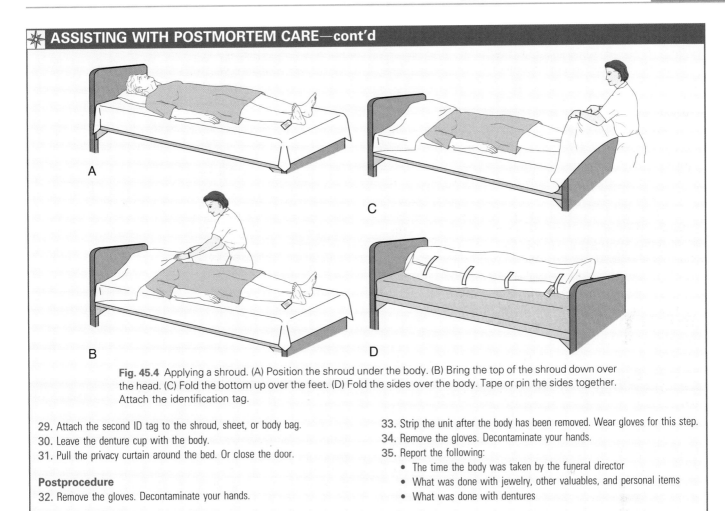

Fig. 45.4 Applying a shroud. (A) Position the shroud under the body. (B) Bring the top of the shroud down over the head. (C) Fold the bottom up over the feet. (D) Fold the sides over the body. Tape or pin the sides together. Attach the identification tag.

29. Attach the second ID tag to the shroud, sheet, or body bag.
30. Leave the denture cup with the body.
31. Pull the privacy curtain around the bed. Or close the door.

Postprocedure
32. Remove the gloves. Decontaminate your hands.

33. Strip the unit after the body has been removed. Wear gloves for this step.
34. Remove the gloves. Decontaminate your hands.
35. Report the following:
    - The time the body was taken by the funeral director
    - What was done with jewelry, other valuables, and personal items
    - What was done with dentures

CARE FOR THE CAREGIVER

It is natural for nursing assistants and other staff members to grow close to the people they care for. In some cases, long-term relationships have grown over a period of years. When death takes a person you are close to, it can be a very sad time. Often, the caregivers experience grief as well. Nursing assistants who experience these losses for the first time may find it somewhat frightening. If this happens to you, confide in a nurse or other staff member. Others may not realize the sadness you are experiencing. For some caregivers it may be helpful to discuss feelings with their spiritual adviser or other member of their faith. Sometimes, just talking can be helpful. Do not be hard on yourself for feeling sad. Healing comes with time. Remembering the good times and positive characteristics of the person helps to ease the pain. With more exposure, caregivers come to understand how important their role is to support the dying person and the family.

It is also important to consider the feelings of other residents. They too may be sad over the loss of their friend. They may want to express their feelings of grief. Some nursing centers may have a chapel where a memorial service takes place. This might offer an opportunity for residents and caregivers to socialize and share memories with each other and the person's family. Some funerals, memorial services, or visitations are held at funeral homes or churches. Caregivers sometimes attend these. They may find comfort and peace by remembering the person in this manner. For some persons, a private service for family members only is held. If you have questions about whether it is appropriate for you to attend a service, discuss this with the nurse.

QUALITY OF LIFE

A person has the right to die in peace and with dignity. Box 45.1 contains the dying person's bill of rights. The dying person also has these rights under OBRA:

- *The right to privacy before and after death.* Do not expose the person unnecessarily. The person has the right not to have the body seen by others. Properly drape and screen the person.
- *The right to visit others in private.* If the person is too weak to leave the room, the roommate may have to do so. The nurse and social worker develop a plan that satisfies everyone. Moving the dying person to a private room provides privacy. The family can stay as long as they like.
- *The right to confidentiality before and after death.* Only those involved in care need to know the person's diagnosis and condition. The final moments and cause of death also are kept confidential. So are statements, conversations, and family reactions.
- *The right to be free from abuse, mistreatment, and neglect.* Some health team members avoid dying persons. They are uncomfortable with death and dying. Others have religious or cultural beliefs about being near dying people. Neglect is possible. So is abuse or mistreatment. Family, friends, or staff may be sources of such actions. The dying person may be too weak to report the abuse or mistreatment. Or the person may feel that the punishment is deserved for needing so much care. The person has the right to receive kind and respectful care before and after death. Always report signs of abuse, mistreatment, or neglect to the nurse at once.
- *Freedom from restraint.* Restraints are used only if ordered by the doctor. Dying persons are often too weak to pose dangers to themselves or others.
- *The right to have personal possessions.* You must protect the person's property. The person may want photos and religious items nearby. Protect the person's property from loss or damage before and after death. They may be family treasures or mementos.
- *The right to a safe and homelike setting.* Dying persons depend on others for safety. Everyone must keep the setting safe and homelike. The center is the person's home. Try to keep equipment and supplies out of view. The room also should be free from unpleasant odors and noises. Do your best to keep the room neat and clean.
- *The right to personal choice.* The person has the right to be involved in treatment and care. The dying person may refuse treatment. Advance directives are common. Some persons cannot make treatment decisions. The family or health care proxy does so. The decision may be to allow the person to die with peace and dignity. The health team must respect choices to refuse treatment or not prolong life.

TIME TO REFLECT

Mr. Nieman lives in the assisted living residence where you work. He is 86 years old but still active for his age. His wife died 2 years ago. He has a passion for golf and plays several times a week. He is a retired biology professor and loves being outdoors. When he arrived at the assisted living residence, he completed some advance directives that were placed in his medical record. He signed a living will. He once told you: "When the Good Lord takes me, I sure don't want anyone pounding on my chest to bring me back!" This afternoon, he collapsed at the golf course. Another player called 911 from his cell phone. EMS arrived and began cardiopulmonary resuscitation (CPR). Mr. Nieman was transported to the hospital. Before his family could be reached, he was placed on life-support machines. The assisted living residence was not notified until later in the day. Do you think that Mr. Nieman's wishes were followed? Is there anything that could have defined his wishes more clearly? What do you think should happen from here?

BOX 45.1 A Dying Patient's Bill of Last Rights

- *The Right to BE IN CONTROL.* Grant me the right to make as many decisions as possible regarding my care. Please do not take choices from me. Let me make my own decisions.
- *The Right to HAVE A SENSE OF PURPOSE.* I have lost my job. I can no longer fulfill my role in my family. Please help me find some sense of purpose in my last days.
- *The Right to REMINISCE.* There has been pleasure in my life, moments of pride, moments of love. Please give some time to recollect those moments. And please listen to my recollections.
- *The Right to TOUCH AND BE TOUCHED.* Sometimes I need distance. Yet sometimes I have a strong need to be close. When I want to reach out, please come to me and hold me as I hold you.
- *The Right to LAUGH.* People often—far too often—come to me wearing masks of seriousness. Although I am dying, I still need to laugh. Please laugh with me and help others to laugh as well.
- *The Right to BE ANGRY AND SAD.* It is difficult to leave behind all of my attachments and all that I love. Please allow me the opportunity to be angry and sad.
- *The Right to HAVE A RESPECTED SPIRITUALITY.* Whether I am questioning or affirming, doubting or praising, I sometimes need your ear, a nonjudging ear. Please let my spirit travel its own journey, without judging its direction.
- *The Right to HEAR THE TRUTH.* If you withhold the truth from me, you will treat me as if I am no longer living. I am still living and I need to know the truth about my life. Please help me find that truth.
- *The Right to BE IN DENIAL.* If I hear the truth and choose not to accept it, that is my right.

Honor these rights. One day you, too, will want the same rights.

Modified from *The hospice RN: patient's bill of rights: a dying patient's bill of last rights.*

REVIEW QUESTIONS

Circle the BEST answer.

1. Which is *true*?
   a. Death from terminal illness is sudden and unexpected
   b. Doctors know when death will occur
   c. An illness is terminal when recovery is not likely
   d. All severe injuries end in death

2. These statements relate to attitudes about death. Which is *false*?
   a. Dying people are often cared for in health care agencies
   b. Religion influences attitudes about death
   c. Infants and toddlers understand death
   d. Young children often blame themselves when someone dies

3. Reincarnation is the belief that
   a. There is no afterlife
   b. The spirit or soul is reborn into another human body or another form of life
   c. The body keeps its physical form in the afterlife
   d. Only the spirit or soul is present in the afterlife

4. A 6-year-old views death as
   a. Temporary
   b. Final
   c. Adults do
   d. Going to sleep

5. Adults and older persons usually fear
   a. Dying alone
   b. Reincarnation
   c. The five stages of dying
   d. Advance directives

6. Persons in the stage of denial
   a. Are angry
   b. Are calm and at peace
   c. Are sad and quiet
   d. Refuse to believe they are dying

7. A dying person tries to gain more time during the stage of
   a. Anger
   b. Bargaining
   c. Depression
   d. Acceptance

8. When caring for the dying person, you should
   a. Use touch and listen
   b. Do most of the talking
   c. Keep the room darkened
   d. Speak in a loud voice

9. As death nears, the last sense lost is
   a. Sight
   b. Taste
   c. Smell
   d. Hearing

10. The dying person's care includes the following *except*
    a. Eye care
    b. Mouth care
    c. Active range-of-motion exercises
    d. Position changes

11. The dying person is positioned in
    a. The supine position
    b. Fowler position
    c. Good body alignment
    d. The dorsal recumbent position

12. A DNR order was written. This means that
    a. CPR will not be done
    b. The person has a living will
    c. Life-prolonging measures will be carried out
    d. The person is kept alive as long as possible

13. Which are *not* signs of approaching death?
    a. Increased body temperature and rapid pulse
    b. Loss of movement and muscle tone
    c. Increased pain and blood pressure
    d. Slow or rapid and shallow respirations

14. The signs of death are
    a. Convulsions and incontinence
    b. No pulse, respirations, or blood pressure
    c. Loss of consciousness and convulsions
    d. The eyes stay open, no muscle movements, and the body is rigid

15. Postmortem care is done
    a. After rigor mortis sets in
    b. With respect and dignity
    c. Before an autopsy
    d. Without wearing gloves

See Appendix A for answers to these questions.

46

Getting a Job

OBJECTIVES

- Define the key terms and key abbreviations listed in this chapter.
- Understand different methods to search for a job.
- Know the common forms required for employment.
- Know what a résumé is and methods of creating one.
- Understand the purpose of a cover letter.
- Understand how to accurately complete a job application.
- Prepare for a job interview.

- Be aware of possible interview questions.
- How to follow up after an interview.
- Understand a job description.
- Understand a dress code policy.
- Explain how to resign from a job.
- Identify the common reasons for losing a job.
- Explain how to promote quality of life.

KEY TERMS

application A form used by an employer to collect information from a potential employee

cover letter A letter written with the purpose of obtaining an interview

preceptor A staff member who guides another staff member; a mentor

résumé A summary of personal information

KEY ABBREVIATIONS

CNA Certified nursing assistant
CPR Cardiopulmonary resuscitation
DON Director of nursing

NATCEP Nursing Assistant Training and Competency Evaluation Program
OBRA Omnibus Reconciliation Act of 1987
RN Registered nurse

BEGINNING A JOB SEARCH

Many students are eager to begin the search for a nursing assistant job. This is an exciting time to begin a career helping people. It is good to make this a thoughtful process. If a job is accepted hastily, it may not turn out to be a good fit. Be prepared and do some research before applying for a position.

There are easy ways to find out about jobs and places to work.
- Websites of places where you would like to work
- Job search websites
- People you know—your instructor, family, and friends
- Newspaper ads
- Local state employment services
- Social media
- Your school's or college's job placement counselors
- Your clinical experience site

Your clinical experience site is an important source. The staff always looks at students as future employees. They look for good work ethics (Chapter 3). They watch how students treat residents and coworkers. If that center is not hiring, the staff may suggest other places to apply.

What Employers Look For

If you owned a business, who would you want to hire? Your answer helps you better understand the employer's point of view. Employers want people who:
- Are dependable.
- Are well-groomed.
- Have needed job skills and training.
- Have values and attitudes that fit with the center.
- Treat others with kindness and respect.

Applicants who look good communicate many things to the employer. You have one chance to make a good first impression. A well-groomed person will likely get the job. A sloppy person with wrinkled or dirty clothes may not get the job, nor will someone with body or breath odors. See p. ·· for how to dress for an interview.

Job Skills and Training

Employers need to know that you have the required job skills. To work in long-term care, you must complete a state-approved Nursing Assistant Training and Competency Evaluation Program (NATCEP).

This is a requirement of the Omnibus Budget Reconciliation Act of 1987 (OBRA). The employer checks the nursing assistant registry and requests proof of training.

- A certificate of course completion
- A high school, college, or technical school transcript
- An official grade report (report card)

Give the employer only a *copy* of your certificate, transcript, or grade report. Never give the original to the employer. Keep it for future use. The employer may want a transcript sent directly from the school or college.

Job Applications

You get a job application from the personnel office or human resources office (Fig. 46.1). An application is a form used by an employer to collect information from a potential employee. You may be asked to complete the application there. Other centers

EMPLOYMENT APPLICATION

APPLICANT INSTRUCTIONS

If you need help filling out this application form or for any phase of the employment process, please notify the person that gave you this form and every effort will be made to accommodate your needs in a reasonable amount of time.

1. Please read "APPLICANT NOTE" below.
2. Complete both sides of this page.
3. If more space is needed to complete any question, use comments section at the bottom of this page.
4. Print clearly: incomplete or illegible applications will not be processed. PLEASE NOTE "NOT APPLICABLE" IF NOT ANSWERING A QUESTION.
5. Provide only requested information. Failure to do so may result in disqualification of your application.
6. Some packets may include an AFFIRMATIVE ACTION QUESTIONNAIRE. This information is being gathered for affirmative action under Section 503 of the Rehabilitation Act of 1973. The information requested is voluntary and will be kept confidential. An applicant will not be subject to any adverse treatment for refusing to complete the questionnaire.
7. DO NOT FILL OUT ANY OTHER ATTACHED FORMS OR PAGES UNTIL INSTRUCTED.

TODAY'S DATE: _____

NAME: _____
LAST   FIRST   MI

SOCIAL SECURITY NUMBER: _____

HOME PHONE: _____ WORK PHONE: _____

CURRENT ADDRESS: _____
STREET

CITY   STATE   ZIP

PRIOR ADDRESS: _____
STREET

CITY   STATE   ZIP

APPLICANT NOTE

This application form is intended for use in evaluating your qualifications for employment. This is not an employment contract. Please answer all appropriate questions completely and accurately. False or misleading statements during the interview and on this form are grounds for terminating the application process or, if discovered after employment, terminating employment. All qualified applicants will receive consideration without discrimination based on sex, marital status, race, color, age, creed, national origin, sexual orientation, military reserve membership, ancestry, religion, height, weight, use of a guide or support animal because of blindness, deafness or physical handicap, or the presence of disabilities. A conviction will not necessarily bar an applicant from employment. Additional testing of job-related skills and for the presence of drugs in your body may be required prior to employment. After an offer of employment, and prior to reporting to work, you may be required to submit to a medical review. Depending on company policy and the needs of the job, you will be required to complete a medical history form and may be required to be examined by a medical professional designated by the company.

AVAILABILITY

For which position are you applying? _____

What date can you start?_____ What category would you prefer? ❑ Full time ❑ Part time ❑ Temporary ❑ Labor pool

For which schedules are you available?* ❑ Weekdays ❑ Weekends ❑ Evenings ❑ Nights ❑ Overtime ❑ Shift ❑ Other_____
*reasonable efforts will be made to accommodate sincerely held moral and ethical beliefs, (WI) religious beliefs and practices (All other States)

JOB-RELATED SKILLS

NOTE: Do not fill out any part of this section you believe to be non-job related.

❑ Yes ❑ No   If the job requires, do you have the appropriate valid drivers license?
Name on license _____DL#_____Type _____State of Issue_____

❑ Yes ❑ No   Have you had any moving violations within the last seven years? Please describe._____
Please list any other skills, licenses or certificates that may be job-related or that you feel would be of value to this job or company. _____

❑ Yes ❑ No   Have you been given a job description or had the essential functions of the job explained to you?

❑ Yes ❑ No   Do you understand these essential functions?

❑ Yes ❑ No   Can you perform the essential functions of this job with or without reasonable accommodation?

SECURITY

List states and counties of residence for the past seven years: _____

❑ Yes ❑ No   Have you used any names or Social Security Numbers other than given above? If so, please list in comments, below.

❑ Yes ❑ No   Have you been convicted of a crime in the past seven years? If so, please describe in the boxes below. (Conviction will not necessarily be a bar to employment. In accordance with company policy and applicable state and federal laws, factors such as age at time of the offense, remoteness of the offense, time since last conviction, nature of the job sought and rehabilitation effort will be reviewed.)

INCIDENT	CITY/STATE	CHARGE
1.		
2.		

COMMENTS
(ASK FOR AN ADDITIONAL PAGE IF NECESSARY)

_____
_____
_____
_____

© ADP SCREENING & SELECTION SERVICES 2002

Fig. 46.1 A sample job application. (Courtesy ADP Screening and Selection Services, Fort Collins, CO.)

PREVIOUS EMPLOYERS

PLEASE NOTE: Your application will <u>not</u> be considered unless every question in this section is answered. Since we will make every effort to contact previous employers, the **correct telephone numbers of past employers are critical.** Ask for a phone book or call information if necessary. FOR EMPLOYERS OUTSIDE THE U.S., A CURRENT FAX NUMBER IS MANDATORY.

MOST RECENT EMPLOYER   ☐ Yes ☐ No   Are you currently working for this employer?

☐ Yes ☐ No   If yes, may we contact?

PHONE (   )
FAX   (   )

COMPANY NAME _____   CITY _____   STATE _____

FROM _____ TO _____
DATES EMPLOYED   JOB TITLE _____   SUPERVISOR NAME _____

DUTIES _____

SALARY _____ PER _____ (HOUR, WEEK, MONTH)   REASON FOR LEAVING _____

SECOND MOST RECENT EMPLOYER

PHONE (   )
FAX   (   )

COMPANY NAME _____   CITY _____   STATE _____

FROM _____ TO _____
DATES EMPLOYED   JOB TITLE _____   SUPERVISOR NAME _____

DUTIES _____

SALARY _____ PER _____ (HOUR, WEEK, MONTH)   REASON FOR LEAVING _____

THIRD MOST RECENT EMPLOYER

PHONE (   )
FAX   (   )

COMPANY NAME _____   CITY _____   STATE _____

FROM _____ TO _____
DATES EMPLOYED   JOB TITLE _____   SUPERVISOR NAME _____

DUTIES _____

SALARY _____ PER _____ (HOUR, WEEK, MONTH)   REASON FOR LEAVING _____

REFERENCES

Include only individuals familiar with your work ability. Do not include relatives.

NAME	ADDRESS/PHONE	YEARS KNOWN/RELATIONSHIP
1.		
2.		

EDUCATION

NOTE: Do not fill out any part of this section you believe to be non-job related.
Please circle highest grade completed.   7   8   9   10   11   12   13   14   15   16   16+

If your school records are under a different name than listed on page 1, please enter that name _____

NAME	CITY/STATE	GRADUATED	DEGREE?
HIGH SCHOOL			
COLLEGE			
OTHER			

CERTIFICATION AND RELEASE

I certify that I have read and understand the applicant note on page one of this form and that the answers given by me to the foregoing questions and the statements made by me are complete and true to the best of my knowledge and belief. I understand that any false information, omissions or misrepresentations of facts called for in this application, whether on this document or not, may result in rejection of my application or discharge at any time during my employment. I authorize the company and/or its agents, including consumer reporting bureaus, to verify any of this information. I authorize all former employers, persons, schools, companies and law enforcement authorities from any liability for any damage whatsoever for issuing this information. I also understand that the use of illegal drugs is prohibited during employment. If company policy requires, I am willing to submit to drug testing to detect the use of illegal drugs prior to and during employment.

SIGNATURE _____   DATE _____

© ADP SCREENING & SELECTION SERVICES 2002

Fig. 46.1 con'd

allow you to take it home and return it by mail or in person. When completing an application at the site, come prepared. The application may ask for dates of former employment, dates of graduation, and references. Have this information written down on a card so you can complete the application easily. Many nursing centers require references. They will call these references to see if you would be a good employee. It is courteous to ask people in advance if you may list them as references. Then they will not be surprised if an employer contacts them. Also bring copies of any certifications you have received. Nurse aide certification, cardiopulmonary resuscitation (CPR), first aid, and abuse reporting training are examples. Some facilities might want to copy your social security card or driver's license. You must be well groomed and behave pleasantly when seeking or returning a job application. It may be your first chance to make a good impression.

To complete a job application, follow the guidelines in Box 46.1. How you fill out the application may mean getting or not getting the job. Often, the application is your first chance to impress the employer. A neat, readable, and complete application gives a good image. A sloppy or incomplete one does not. Use black or dark blue ink when completing the application.

Some centers provide job applications online. Follow the center's instructions for completing and sending an online

BOX 46.1   Guidelines for Completing a Job Application

- Read and follow the directions. They may ask you to print using black ink. You need to follow directions on the job. Employers look at job applications to see if you can follow directions.
- Write neatly. Your writing must be readable. A messy application gives a bad image. Readable writing gives the correct information. The center cannot contact you if unable to read your phone number. You may miss getting the job.
- Complete the entire form. Something may not apply to you. If so, write "nonapplicable" or "N/A." Or draw a line through the space. This tells the employer that you read the section. It also shows that you did not skip the item on purpose.
- When completing an online application, proofread it carefully and make sure any necessary attachments are added before clicking the "submit" button.
- Report any felony arrests or convictions as directed. Write "no" or "none" as appropriate. Criminal background and fingerprint checks are common requirements.
- Give information about employment gaps. If you did not work for a time, the employer wonders why. Provide this information to give a good impression about your honesty. Some reasons are an illness, going to school, raising your children, or caring for an ill or older family member.
- Tell why you left a job, if asked. Be brief but honest. People leave jobs for one that pays better. Some leave for career advancement. Other reasons include those given for employment gaps. If you were fired from a job, give an honest but positive response. Do not talk badly about a former employer.
- Provide references. Be prepared to give names, titles, addresses, and phone numbers of at least four references who are not relatives. You should have this information written down before completing an application. (Always ask references if an employer can contact them.) You may get the job faster or over another applicant if the employer can check references quickly. If they are missing or not complete, the employer waits for all the information. This wastes your time and the employer's time. Also, the employer wonders if you are hiding something with incomplete reference information.
- Be prepared to provide the following:
  - Social security number
  - Proof of citizenship or legal residency
  - Proof of required training and competency evaluation
  - Identification—driver's license or government-issued ID card
- Give honest responses. Lying on an application is fraud. It is grounds for being fired.
- Keep a file of your education, certifications, work history, and copies of performance evaluations.

application. Make sure it is complete and truthful. Proofread it carefully before clicking the "submit" button.

Résumé

A résumé is a summary of your personal information. It includes contact information such as your address, phone number, and email address. It also includes information about your education and work experience. A sample résumé is shown in Fig. 46.2. Your résumé should be neatly typed in a Word document. Always be truthful about the information that is included. It is a good idea to save your résumé as a Word document so you can update it frequently as you gain new skills, education, or work experience. If completing an online application, the employer may request that you include your résumé as an attachment. Print the résumé on quality paper. There are many templates available to help write a résumé. There are also services and professionals that can help with this. Make sure all information is accurate and truthful.

Cover Letter

A cover letter often accompanies a résumé. The purpose of a cover letter is to help you obtain an interview. A sample cover letter is shown in Fig. 46.3. If mailing a cover letter and résumé to an employer, place it in an envelope large enough so the pages do not have to be folded.

The Job Interview

A job interview is the employer's chance to get to know and evaluate you. You also find out more about the center.

The interview may be when you complete the job application. Some centers schedule interviews after reviewing applications. Write down the interviewer's name and the interview date and time. If you need directions to the center, ask for them at this time.

Box 46.2 lists common interview questions. It may be helpful to have a friend or relative ask you some practice interview questions. This puts you more at ease for the real interview. Prepare your answers before the interview. Also prepare a list of your skills. Give the list to the interviewer. A neat and current job résumé is also helpful to bring to the interview.

Preparing for the Interview

You must present a good image. You need to be neat, clean, and well groomed. How you dress is important. Follow the guidelines in Box 46.3. If possible, do a little research on the facility. Look at the center's website to get a feel for the organization and the different levels of care that are offered. This may also give you information that could be used during the interview. For example, you may ask, "I notice there is construction taking place. Could you tell me what is planned for that area?"

Be on time. It shows you are dependable. Arriving late for a job interview creates a very negative first impression. Go to the center some day before your interview. Note how long it takes to get there and where to park. Also find the personnel office.

Suzanne M. Browning
1525 Hazelnut Drive, Upper Peninsula, MI 49930
(201) 344-1234, Suzanneb@gmail.com

Job Objective
To work as a nursing assistant in a long-term care center.

Education
A.S., Adult Services, Grand Valley Community College (expected 2023).
East Valley High School (2020).

Certifications
Nurse Aide (February, 2021).
Health Care Provider CPR (January, 2021).

Nursing Home Experience
Nurse Aide, Riverbend Care Center, Oakton, MI (March 2021–present).
- Provided personal care for residents (bathing, grooming, transfers, etc).
- Served on safety committee.

Volunteer, Meadow View Care Center, Sterling, MI (2019–20).
- Read to residents, assisted with activities.
- Trained new volunteers.

Other Experience

Clerk, Main Street Health Foods, Appleton, MI (2019–20).
- Stocked shelves, checked out customers, balanced cash register.
- Answered customer inquiries about health products.

Activities

Captain, Volleyball Team, East Valley High School (2020).
Chair, Homecoming Planning Committee (2019).

References available upon request.

Fig. 46.2 A sample résumé.

A *dry run* (practice run) gives an idea of how long it takes to get from your home to the personnel office. It is best to arrive about 10 minutes before the scheduled appointment.

When you arrive for the interview, turn off your cell phone or pager. Tell the receptionist your name and why you are there. Also give the interviewer's name. Then sit quietly in the waiting area. Do not smoke, chew gum, or use your phone. While you wait, review your answers to the common interview questions. Waiting may be part of the interview. The interviewer may ask the receptionist about how you acted while waiting. Smile and be polite and friendly.

During the Interview
Politely greet the interviewer. A firm handshake is correct for men and women. Address the interviewer appropriately (for example, Miss, Mrs., Ms., Mr., Dr.). Stand until asked to take a seat. When sitting, use good posture. Sit in a professional manner. If offered a beverage, you may accept. Be sure to thank the person.

Good eye contact is needed. Look directly at the interviewer when you answer or ask questions. Poor eye contact sends negative information—being shy, insecure, dishonest, or lacking interest.

Watch your body language (Chapter 6). Body language involves facial expressions, gestures, posture, and body movements. What you say is important. However, how you use and move your body also tells a great deal. Avoid distracting habits—biting nails; playing with jewelry, clothing, or your hair; crossing your arms; and swinging legs back and forth. Keep your mind on the interview. Do not touch or read things on the person's desk.

The interview usually lasts between 15 and 45 minutes. Give complete and honest answers. If the interviewer asks you a question that takes you off guard, pause, reflect, and then

1525 Hazelnut Drive
Upper Peninsula, MI 49930
July 24, 2022

Mr. Dennis Davis
Deerfield Retirement Center
1322 Shorewood Drive
Green Bay, WI 54302

Dear Mr. Davis:

I wish to apply for your position of Nurse Aide advertised recently in the *Green Bay Press Gazette*. With my experience as a Nurse Aide and my expected A.A. degree in Adult Services from Grand Valley Community College, I believe that I have the qualifications that you are seeking for this position.

My experience as a Nurse Aide at Riverbend Care Center in Oakton, Michigan, included a range of personal care services for residents, including bathing, transfers, grooming, and assisting with meals. I performed all of these activities competently and enthusiastically, with my supervisor, Ann Smith, rating my overall performance as "excellent" for my six-month evaluation. I was also pleased to serve on the Safety Committee at Riverbend, which entailed devising a new plan for responding effectively to emergency conditions.

The degree program at Grand Valley Community College has prepared me well for a career in Adult Services. My coursework included Adult Recreation, Adult Nutrition, Anatomy and Physiology, and Geriatric Psychology, as well as courses in Interpersonal Communication, Speech, and Business Writing.

My activities have helped me develop skills in teamwork, communication, and leadership. In high school I served as captain of the volleyball team and served on the Homecoming Planning Committee. I also volunteered at a local care center, where I read to residents and trained new volunteers.

Enclosed is my resume that includes additional details about my qualifications. If you would like to arrange an interview, you can reach me on my cell phone at 201-344-1234 or by email at Suzanneb@gmail.com. I look forward to hearing from you.

Sincerely,

Suzanne Browning

Fig. 46.3 A sample cover letter.

answer to the best of your ability. Always be truthful. Do not lie or exaggerate an answer in an attempt to impress the interviewer. Speak clearly and with confidence. Avoid short and long answers. "Yes" and "no" answers give little information. Briefly explain "yes" and "no" responses.

The interviewer will ask about your skills. Share your skills list or résumé. The interviewer may ask about a skill not on your list. Explain that you are willing to learn the skill if your state of residence allows nursing assistants to perform the task.

Find the right job for you. An employer wants to hire someone who will be happy in the job and the center. Box 46.2 lists some questions for you to ask at the end of the interview. The person's answers will help you decide if the job is right for you.

BOX 46.2   Common Interview Questions

What the Interviewer May Ask You
- Tell me about yourself.
- Tell me about your career goals.
- What are you doing to reach these goals?
- Describe your idea of *professional* behavior.
- Tell me about your last job. Why did you leave?
- What did you like the most about your last job? What did you like the least?
- What would your supervisor and coworkers tell me about you? Your dependability? Your skills? Your flexibility?
- Which functions are the hardest for you? How do you handle this difficulty?
- How do you set your priorities?
- How have your experiences prepared you for this job?
- What would you like to change about your last job?
- How do you handle problems with residents and coworkers?
- Why do you want to work here?
- Why should this center hire you?

Questions to Ask the Interviewer
- Which job functions do you think are the most important?
- What employee qualities and traits are the most important to you?
- Who will I work with?
- When are performance evaluations done? Who does them? How are they done?
- What performance factors are evaluated?

- How does the supervisor handle problems?
- What are the most common reasons that nursing assistants lose their jobs here?
- What are the most common reasons that nursing assistants resign from their jobs here?
- How do you see this job in the next year? In the next 5 years?
- What is the greatest reward from this job?
- What is the greatest challenge from this job?
- What do you like the most about nursing assistants who work here? What do you like the least?
- Why should I work here rather than in another center?
- Why are you interested in hiring me?
- How much will I make an hour?
- What hours will I work?
- What uniforms are required?
- What benefits do you offer?
  - Health and disability insurance
  - Continuing education
  - Vacation time
- Does the center have a new employee orientation program?
- May I have a tour of the center and the unit I will work on? Will you introduce me to the nurse manager and unit staff?
- Can I have a few minutes to talk to the nurse manager?

BOX 46.3   Grooming and Dressing for an Interview

- Bathe and brush your teeth. Wash your hair.
- Use deodorant or antiperspirant.
- Make sure your hands and fingernails are clean.
- Apply makeup in a simple, attractive manner.
- Style your hair in a neat and attractive way. Wear it as you would for work.
- Do not wear jeans, shorts, tank tops, halter tops, or other casual clothing.
- Iron clothing. Sew on loose buttons and mend garments as needed.
- Wear clothing that covers tattoos (body art).
- Wear a simple dress, skirt and blouse, suit, or slacks with a coordinating top (women). Men wear a suit or dark slacks and a shirt and tie. A jacket is optional. A long-sleeved white or light blue shirt is best (Fig. 46.4).

- Wear socks (men and women) or hose (women). Hose should be free of runs and snags.
- Make sure shoes are clean and in good repair.
- Avoid heavy perfumes, colognes, and aftershave lotions. A lightly scented fragrance is okay.
- Wear only simple jewelry that complements your clothes. Avoid adornments in body piercings. If you have multiple ear piercings, wear only one set of earrings.
- Stop in the restroom when you arrive for the interview. Check your hair, makeup, and clothes.

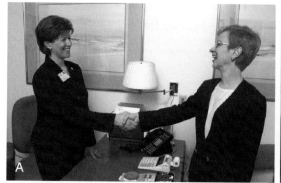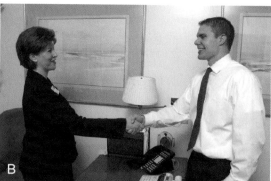

Fig. 46.4 (A) A simple suit is worn for a job interview. (B) This man wears slacks and a shirt and tie for his interview.

Review the job description with the interviewer. If you have questions about it, ask them at this time. Advise the interviewer of functions you cannot perform because of training, legal, ethical, or religious reasons. Also tell the person who is conducting the interview about any shifts or dates that you may not be able to work. Honesty now prevents problems later.

The interviewer signals when the interview is over. You may be offered a job at this time. Or you are told when to expect a call or letter. Follow-up is acceptable. Ask when you can check on your application. Before leaving, thank the interviewer. Say that you look forward to hearing from the interviewer. Shake the person's hand before you leave.

After the Interview

A thank-you letter or note is advised (Fig. 46.5). This note may be the difference of getting the job over other applicants. Write this within 24 hours after the interview. Write neatly and clearly. Use a computer or typewriter if your writing is hard to read. It is also acceptable to send a thank-you letter by email. The thank-you note should include the following:

- The date
- The interviewer's formal name using Miss, Mrs., Ms., Mr., or Dr.
- A statement thanking the person for the interview
- Comments about the interview, the center, and your eagerness to hear about the job
- Your signature using your first and last names

Accepting a Job

Accept the job that is best for you. You can apply many places and have many interviews. Think about all offers before accepting one. You might have more questions about a center. Ask them before accepting the job. To help decide what to do, discuss the offer with a family member, friend, coworker, or your instructor.

When you accept a job, agree on a starting date, pay rate, and work hours. Find out where to report on your first day. Ask for such information in writing. That way you and the center

---

December 12

Dear Ms. O'Neal,

Thank you for the interview yesterday. I enjoyed meeting you and learning more about the nursing center. I was impressed by the friendliness of the staff and would enjoy working in that environment.

Again, thank you. I look forward to hearing from you soon.

Sincerely,
Alison M. Teal

Fig. 46.5 Sample thank-you note written after a job interview.

---

have the same understanding of the job offer. Use the written offer later if questions arise. Also ask for the employee handbook and other center information. Make sure you understand what the dress code requirements are. Read everything before you start working.

New Employee Orientation

Centers have orientation programs for new employees. The center's policy and procedure manual is reviewed. Your skills are checked. That is, the center has you perform the procedures in your job description. This is to make sure that you do them safely and correctly. Also, you are shown how to use the center's supplies and equipment.

Many centers have preceptor programs. A preceptor (mentor) is a staff member who guides another staff member. A nurse or nursing assistant:

- Helps you learn the center's layout so you can find what you need.
- Introduces you to residents and staff.
- Helps you organize your work.
- Helps you feel comfortable as a part of the nursing team.
- Answers questions about the policy and procedure manual.

A nursing assistant preceptor is not your supervisor. Only nurses can supervise. A preceptor program usually lasts 2 to 4 weeks. Its purpose is to help you succeed in your role. It also helps ensure quality care. After the preceptor program, you should feel comfortable with the setting and your role. If not, ask for more orientation time.

PREPARING FOR WORK

You successfully completed a NATCEP. You had a successful job interview. To keep your job, you must function well and work well with others. You must:

- Work when scheduled.
- Get to work on time.
- Stay the entire shift.

Absences and tardiness (being late) are common reasons for losing a job. Child care and transportation issues often interfere with getting to work. Plan for them in advance by having a backup plan to cover unexpected circumstances.

Child Care

Someone needs to care for your children when you leave for work, while you are at work, and before you get home from work. Also plan for emergencies:

- Your child care provider is ill or cannot care for your children that day.
- A child becomes ill while you are at work.
- You will be late getting home from work.

Transportation

Plan for how you get to and from work. If you drive, keep your car in good working order. Keep enough gas in the car. Or leave early to get gas.

BOX 46.4 Common Reasons for Losing a Job

- Poor attendance—not going to work or excessive tardiness (being late)
- Abandonment—leaving the job during your shift
- Falsifying a record—job application or a person's medical record
- Violent behavior in the workplace
- Having weapons in the work setting—guns, knives, explosives, or other dangerous items
- Having, using, or distributing alcohol in the work setting
- Having, using, or distributing drugs in the work setting (This excludes taking drugs ordered by a doctor.)
- Taking a person's drugs for your own use or giving them to others
- Harassment
- Using offensive speech and language
- Stealing the center's or a person's property
- Destroying the center's or a person's property
- Showing disrespect to residents, families, visitors, coworkers, or supervisors
- Abusing or neglecting a person
- Invading a person's privacy
- Failing to maintain resident, family, center, or coworker confidentiality (This includes access to computer and other electronic information.)
- Using the center's supplies and equipment for your own use
- Defamation (Chapter 2) and gossip (Chapter 3)
- Abusing meal breaks and break periods
- Sleeping on the job
- Violating the center's dress code
- Violating any center policy
- Failing to follow center care procedures
- Tending to personal matters while on duty

Carpooling is an option. Carpool members depend on each other. If the driver is late leaving, everyone is late for work. If one person is not ready when the driver arrives, everyone is late for work. Carpool with persons you trust to be ready and on time. When you drive, leave and pick up others on time. As a passenger, be ready to be picked up on time.

Know your bus or train schedule. Know what other bus or train to take if delays occur. Always carry enough money for fares to and from work.

Always have a backup plan for getting to work. Your car may not start, the carpool driver may not go to work, or public transportation may not operate.

RESIGNING FROM A JOB

A job closer to home, better pay, returning to school, or new opportunities may prompt you to leave your job. Child care and illness are other reasons. Whatever the reason, tell your employer. Do one of the following:

- Give a written notice
- Write a resignation letter
- Complete a form in the human resources office

Giving a 2-week notice is good practice. Do not leave a job without notice. Doing so can affect resident care. Include the following in your notice:

- Reason for leaving
- The last date you will work
- Comments thanking the employer for the opportunity to work in the center

An exit interview is common practice. You and the employer talk before you leave the center. The employer asks what you liked about the center and your job. Often, employees are asked how the center can improve.

LOSING A JOB

A job is a privilege. You must perform your job well and protect residents from harm. No pay raise or losing your job results from poor performance. Failure to follow center policy is often grounds for termination. So is failure to get along with others. Box 46.4 lists the many reasons why you can lose your job. To protect your job, function at your best. Always practice good work ethics.

QUALITY OF LIFE

Getting a job as a nursing assistant is an important step. You have studied and prepared for this position. The work can be very enjoyable and rewarding. You want to put forth your best effort to obtain the job that fits you best. By being honest in an interview and when completing an application, you give the employer information to make a decision. If you must resign from a position, always give adequate notice so that the residents are provided the necessary care that promotes their quality of life and safety. Through your work you will contribute to the quality of life of the residents by offering them compassionate care.

TIME TO REFLECT

Kathy O'Brien has completed her nursing assistant training and is now certified in her state. She is eager to get her first job. She also has plans to take a cruise with her family members in 6 weeks. She completes the interview, and the Director of Nursing (DON) offers her a position. The DON would like her to start orientation immediately. During the interview Kathy did not mention her vacation plans. What do you think should happen at this point?

REVIEW QUESTIONS

Circle the BEST answer.

1. You are completing a job application. You should do the following *except*
   a. Write neatly and clearly
   b. Provide references
   c. Give information about employment gaps
   d. Leave spaces blank that do not apply to you

2. Which of the following do employers look for the *most*?
   a. Cooperation
   b. Courtesy
   c. Dependability
   d. Empathy

3. What should you wear to a job interview?
   a. A uniform
   b. Party clothes
   c. A simple dress or suit
   d. Whatever is most comfortable

4. Which is a poor behavior during a job interview?
   a. Good eye contact with the interviewer
   b. Shaking hands with the interviewer
   c. Asking the interviewer questions
   d. Crossing your arms and legs

5. Which is the best response to an interview question?
   a. "Yes" or "no"
   b. Long answers
   c. Brief explanations
   d. A written response

6. A resignation letter should *not* include
   a. Your reasons for leaving
   b. The last day you will work
   c. A thank-you to the employer
   d. Problems you had during your work

7. Which is *not* a reason for losing your job?
   a. Leaving the job during your shift
   b. Using alcohol in the work setting
   c. Sleeping on the job
   d. Taking a meal break

8. When should you ask questions about your job description?
   a. After completing the job application
   b. Before completing the job application
   c. When your interview is scheduled
   d. During the interview

9. Lying on a job application is
   a. Negligence
   b. Fraud
   c. Libel
   d. Defamation

10. A thank-you letter after an interview
    a. Is not necessary
    b. May make the difference in getting the job
    c. Should never be sent electronically
    d. Can be mailed weeks later

11. How much notice should be given when resigning from a position?
    a. 1 week
    b. 2 weeks
    c. 1 month
    d. It does not matter

12. When completing a job application
    a. Use black ink
    b. Blacken out any errors
    c. Use pencil
    d. Use red ink

See Appendix A for answers to these questions.

APPENDIX A

Chapter 1

1 d
2 c
3 b
4 a
5 a
6 c
7 a
8 b
9 a
10 d
11 c
12 c
13 d
14 c
15 b
16 c
17 c
18 a
19 c
20 b

Chapter 2

1 b
2 b
3 c
4 d
5 a
6 a
7 a
8 a
9 d
10 b
11 a
12 b
13 d
14 b
15 c
16 a
17 c
18 a
19 d
20 c
21 b
22 a
23 a
24 c
25 c

Chapter 3

1 c
2 d
3 a
4 b
5 b
6 a
7 a
8 b
9 c
10 d
11 c
12 b
13 a
14 c
15 b
16 b
17 c
18 a
19 c
20 b

Chapter 4

1 a
2 c
3 a
4 c
5 a
6 c
7 d
8 c
9 c
10 c
11 d
12 d
13 b
14 b
15 c
16 a
17 d
18 b

Chapter 5

1 a
2 d
3 b
4 c

5 d
6 b
7 a
8 c
9 c
10 b
11 c
12 d

Chapter 6

1 d
2 c
3 b
4 a
5 a
6 c
7 b
8 c
9 b
10 d
11 c
12 a
13 c
14 a
15 d
16 a
17 d
18 c
19 d
20 b

Chapter 7

1 d
2 d
3 b
4 c
5 d
6 c
7 b
8 b
9 c
10 a
11 c
12 a
13 b
14 b

15 c
16 d

Chapter 8

1 a
2 b
3 d
4 c
5 a
6 b
7 c
8 d
9 d
10 b
11 a
12 b
13 b
14 b
15 c
16 d
17 a
18 d
19 a
20 b

Chapter 9

1 c
2 c
3 a
4 d
5 c
6 b
7 c
8 a
9 b
10 a
11 b
12 d
13 c
14 d
15 c
16 a
17 d
18 b
19 a
20 b
21 d

22 c
23 c
24 a

Chapter 10

1 a
2 d
3 c
4 d
5 b
6 c
7 d
8 b
9 b
10 b

Chapter 11

1 a
2 d
3 c
4 a
5 a
6 b
7 c
8 d
9 a
10 d
11 b
12 a
13 b
14 b
15 c
16 b
17 d
18 b
19 b
20 a
21 b
22 c
23 c
24 c
25 b
26 d

Chapter 12

1 b

2 d
3 c
4 a
5 a
6 c
7 d
8 c
9 a
10 b
11 a
12 c
13 c
14 a
15 b

Chapter 13

1 a
2 c
3 b
4 c
5 a
6 d
7 c
8 c
9 d
10 b
11 a
12 d

Chapter 14

1 b
2 d
3 d
4 b
5 a
6 b
7 a
8 d
9 a
10 a
11 d
12 c
13 a
14 d
15 b
16 d
17 c

18 b
19 a
20 c

Chapter 15

1 d
2 b
3 a
4 b
5 c
6 b
7 a
8 c
9 b
10 a
11 a
12 a
13 a
14 d
15 a
16 d
17 b
18 c

Chapter 16

1 c
2 d
3 a
4 b
5 d
6 a
7 b
8 d
9 c
10 b
11 c
12 c
13 b
14 b
15 d
16 b

Chapter 17

1 b
2 d
3 b
4 a
5 b
6 a
7 d
8 c
9 c
10 a

11 b
12 a

Chapter 18

1 d
2 d
3 b
4 c
5 d
6 b
7 b
8 c
9 c
10 d
11 b
12 c
13 a
14 c
15 a

Chapter 19

1 d
2 b
3 c
4 a
5 d
6 d
7 b
8 a
9 b
10 c
11 c
12 b

Chapter 20

1. b
2. a
3. a
4. d
5. d
6. c
7. a
8. c
9. a
10. c
11. d
12. a
13. b
14. c
15. c
16. b
17. b
18. c

19. d
20. b
21. c
22. d
23. d
24. b

Chapter 21

1 c
2 a
3 a
4 b
5 d
6 a
7 c
8 a
9 a
10 c
11 a
12 b
13 a
14 d
15 b
16 b
17 a
18 a

Chapter 22

1 b
2 d
3 a
4 b
5 a
6 b
7 d
8 a
9 a
10 c
11 a
12 d
13 d
14 a
15 c

Chapter 23

1 a
2 b
3 d
4 a
5 b
6 c
7 a
8 a

9 d
10 d
11 d
12 c

Chapter 24

1 a
2 b
3 d
4 d
5 b
6 b
7 c
8 b
9 c
10 b
11 c
12 a
13 a
14 c
15 b

Chapter 25

1 d
2 a
3 b
4 a
5 c
6 d
7 c
8 a
9 b
10 c
11 d
12 b
13 c
14 d
15 a
16 b

Chapter 26

1 a
2 c
3 c
4 b
5 b
6 d
7 c
8 d
9 a
10 a
11 a
12 d

13 d
14 b
15 b
16 a
17 c
18 d
19 b
20 c

Chapter 27

1 c
2 b
3 a
4 c
5 c
6 c
7 a
8 a
9 b
10 b
11 c
12 b
13 d
14 a
15 b
16 b
17 d
18 b
19 a
20 c

Chapter 28

1 b
2 d
3 c
4 b
5 c
6 d
7 b
8 a
9 b
10 d
11 c
12 b
13 a
14 d

Chapter 29

1 d
2 b
3 a
4 c
5 b

6 a
7 d
8 a
9 b
10 c
11 a
12 a

Chapter 30

1 d
2 c
3 c
4 b
5 d
6 a
7 b
8 d

Chapter 31

1 a
2 c
3 a
4 c
5 a
6 b
7 a
8 a
9 d
10 b
11 d
12 c
13 b
14 d
15 d
16 a
17 c
18 d
19 b
20 b
21 b
22 d
23 a
24 d

Chapter 32

1 b
2 a
3 a
4 a
5 d
6 c
7 b
8 b

9 d
10 a
11 b
12 a
13 d
14 c
15 d
16 d
17 b
18 b
19 c
20 d

Chapter 33

1 b
2 b
3 a
4 c
5 b
6 b
7 a
8 c
9 c
10 a
11 c
12 b
13 a
14 b
15 a
16 b
17 c
18 a
19 b
20 a
21 d
22 c

Chapter 34

1 b
2 a
3 a
4 a
5 c
6 a
7 b
8 d

9 d
10 b
11 b
12 c

Chapter 35

1 a
2 b
3 d
4 b
5 c
6 b
7 b
8 d
9 a
10 b
11 a
12 c
13 a
14 c
15 a
16 a
17 a
18 d
19 c
20 a
21 a
22 b

Chapter 36

1 a
2 d
3 b
4 c
5 a
6 d
7 a
8 a
9 a
10 b
11 a
12 c
13 c
14 a
15 a

Chapter 37

1 b
2 a
3 d
4 a
5 a
6 d
7 c
8 d
9 b
10 d
11 c
12 a
13 d
14 c
15 b
16 c
17 a
18 b

Chapter 38

1 d
2 d
3 c
4 d
5 a
6 b
7 a
8 b
9 c
10 d
11 d
12 b

Chapter 39

1 b
2 d
3 c
4 c
5 c
6 c
7 b
8 c
9 b
10 d
11 d

12 a
13 c
14 c
15 d
16 a
17 a
18 a
19 a
20 d

Chapter 40

1 a
2 b
3 a
4 a
5 d
6 d
7 a
8 b
9 b
10 d
11 b
12 b
13 a
14 d
15 c
16 c
17 a
18 a
19 a
20 c

Chapter 41

1 d
2 b
3 d
4 b
5 a
6 d
7 b
8 c
9 c
10 d
11 b
12 b
13 d

14 c
15 b

Chapter 42

1 c
2 b
3 a
4 d
5 c
6 c
7 d
8 b
9 d
10 c
11 a
12 d

Chapter 43

1 a
2 a
3 b
4 d
5 d
6 b
7 d
8 b
9 b
10 d
11 b
12 a
13 b
14 c
15 c

Chapter 44

1 b
2 a
3 b
4 c
5 d
6 c
7 b
8 c
9 b
10 b

11 d
12 b
13 c
14 a
15 a
16 b
17 b
18 c
19 d
20 b
21 c
22 a

Chapter 45

1 c
2 c
3 b
4 a
5 a
6 d
7 b
8 a
9 d
10 c
11 c
12 a
13 c
14 b
15 b

Chapter 46

1 d
2 c
3 c
4 d
5 c
6 d
7 d
8 d
9 b
10 b
11 b
12 a

NATIONAL NURSE AIDE ASSESSMENT PROGRAM (NNAAP®) WRITTEN EXAMINATION CONTENT OUTLINE

The NNAAP® Written Examination is comprised of 70 multiple-choice questions. Ten of these questions are pretest (nonscored) questions on which statistical information will be collected.

I Physical Care Skills

A. Activities of Daily Living — 14% of exam
  1 Hygiene
  2 Dressing and Grooming
  3 Nutrition and Hydration
  4 Elimination
  5 Rest/Sleep/Comfort
B. Basic Nursing Skills — 39% of exam
  1 Infection Control
  2 Safety/Emergency
  3 Therapeutic/Technical Procedures
  4 Data Collection and Reporting
C. Restorative Skills — 8% of exam
  1 Prevention
  2 Self-Care/Independence

II Psychosocial Care Skills

A. Emotional and Mental Health Needs — 11% of exam
B. Spiritual and Cultural Needs — 2% of exam

III Role of the Nurse Aide

A. Communication — 8% of exam
B. Client Rights — 7% of exam
C. Legal and Ethical Behavior — 3% of exam
D. Member of the Health Care Team — 8% of exam

NATIONAL NURSE AIDE ASSESSMENT PROGRAM (NNAAP®) SKILLS EVALUATION

List of Skills

1 Performs hand hygiene (hand washing)
2 Applies one knee-high elastic stocking
3 Assists to ambulate using transfer belt
4 Assists with use of bedpan
5 Cleans upper or lower denture
6 Counts and records radial pulse
7 Counts and records respirations
8 Donning and removing PPE (gown and gloves)
9 Dresses client with affected (weak) right arm
10 Feeds client who cannot feed self
11 Gives modified bed bath (face and one arm, hand and underarm)
12 Measures and records electronic blood pressure
13 Measures and records urinary output
14 Measures and records weight of ambulatory client
15 Performs modified passive range of motion (PROM) for one knee and one ankle
16 Performs modified passive range of motion (PROM) for one shoulder
17 Positions on side
18 Provides catheter care for female
19 Provides foot care on one foot
20 Provides mouth care
21 Provides perineal care for female
22 Transfers from bed to wheelchair using transfer belt
23 Measures and records manual blood pressure

Reproduced and used with permission from the National Council of State Boards of Nursing (NCSBN), Chicago, Ill, ©2016.
Note: Not all states participate in the program. Such states have other arrangements for nurse aide competency and evaluation programs.

GLOSSARY

abbreviation A shortened form of a word or phrase

abduction Moving a body part away from the midline of the body

abrasion A partial-thickness wound caused by the scraping away or rubbing of the skin

abuse The willful infliction of injury, unreasonable confinement, intimidation, or punishment that results in physical harm, pain, or mental anguish; depriving the person (or the person's caretaker) of the goods or services needed to attain or maintain well-being

accountable Being responsible for one's actions and the actions of others who performed delegated tasks; answering questions about and explaining one's actions and the actions of others

acetone See *ketone*

activities of daily living (ADL) The activities usually done during a normal day in a person's life

acute illness A sudden illness from which a person is expected to recover

acute pain Pain that is felt suddenly from injury, disease, trauma, or surgery

adduction Moving a body part toward the midline of the body

admission Official entry of a person into a nursing center

advance directive A document stating a person's wishes about health care when that person cannot make his or her own decisions

affect Feelings and emotions

agnostic A person who believes it is impossible to know if a god exists

allergy A sensitivity to a substance that causes the body to react with signs and symptoms

alopecia Hair loss

Alzheimer disease (AD) A disease that affects brain tissue; memory loss and confusion increase until the person cannot tend to simple personal needs

ambulation The act of walking

amputation The removal of all or part of an extremity

AM care See *early morning care*

anaphylaxis A life-threatening sensitivity to an antigen

anorexia The loss of appetite

anticoagulant A medication that prevents or slows down *(anti)* blood clotting *(coagulate)*

anxiety A vague, uneasy feeling in response to stress

aphasia The total or partial loss *(a)* of the ability to use or understand language *(phasia)*; a language disorder resulting from damage to parts of the brain responsible for language

apical-radial pulse Taking the apical and radial pulses at the same time

apnea The lack or absence *(a)* of breathing *(pnea)*

application A form used by an employer to collect information from a potential employee

arterial ulcer An open wound on the lower legs or feet caused by poor arterial blood flow

artery A blood vessel that carries blood away from the heart

arthritis Joint *(arthr)* inflammation *(itis)*

arthroplasty The surgical replacement *(plasty)* of a joint *(arthr)*

asepsis Being free of disease-producing microbes

aspiration Breathing fluid, food, vomitus, or an object into the lungs

assault Intentionally attempting or threatening to touch a person's body without the person's consent

assessment Collecting information about the person; a step in the nursing process

assisted living A housing option for older persons who need help with activities of daily living yet wish to remain independent for as long as possible

assisted living residence (ALR) Provides housing, personal care, support services, health care, and activities in a homelike setting

asymptomatic Without symptoms

atheist A person who denies the existence of a god or deity

atrophy The decrease in size or the wasting away of tissue

autoimmune disorder A condition where the body attacks itself

autopsy The examination of the body after death

avoidable pressure injury A pressure injury that develops from the improper use of the nursing process

base of support The area on which an object rests

battery Touching a person's body without his or her consent

bed bugs Small, flat insects that feed on the blood of sleeping people and animals

bed rail A device that serves as a guard or barrier along the side of the bed; side rail

bedfast Confined to bed

benign tumor A tumor that does not spread to other body parts; it can grow to a large size

bias To prefer something or someone, often without sound judgment

biohazardous waste Items contaminated with blood, body fluids, secretions, or excretions; *bio* means "life" and *hazardous* means "dangerous or harmful"

Biot respirations Rapid and deep respirations followed by 10 to 30 seconds of apnea

birth defect An abnormality present at birth that can involve a body structure or function

bisexual A person who is attracted to both sexes

blanchable To become white

blindness The absence of sight

blood pressure (BP) The amount of force exerted against the walls of an artery by the blood

board and care home Provides rooms, meals, laundry, and supervision to independent residents in a homelike setting; group home

body alignment The way the head, trunk, arms, and legs are aligned with one another; posture

body language Messages sent through facial expressions, gestures, posture, hand and body movements, gait, eye contact, and appearance

body mechanics Using the body in an efficient and careful way

body temperature The amount of heat in the body that is a balance between the amount of heat produced and the amount lost by the body

bony prominence An area where the bone sticks out or projects from the flat surface of the body

boundary crossing A brief act or behavior outside the helpful zone

boundary sign An act, behavior, or thought that warns of a boundary crossing or violation

boundary violation An act or behavior that meets your needs, not the person's needs

bradycardia A slow *(brady)* heart rate *(cardia)*; less than 60 beats per minute

bradypnea Slow *(brady)* breathing *(pnea)*; respirations are fewer than 12 per minute

braille A touch reading and writing system that uses raised dots for each letter of the alphabet; the first 10 letters also represent the numbers 0 through 9

Broca aphasia See "expressive aphasia"

calorie The fuel or energy value of food

cancer See *malignant tumor*

capillary A tiny blood vessel; food, oxygen, and other substances pass from the capillaries into the cells

cardiac arrest See *sudden cardiac arrest*

care plan A record of the measures to be offered to best care for the resident

carrier A human or animal that is a reservoir for microbes but does not have the signs and symptoms of infection

case management A nursing care pattern; a case manager (a registered nurse) coordinates a person's care from admission through discharge and into the home setting

catheter A tube used to drain or inject fluid through a body opening

catheterization The process of inserting a catheter

cell The basic unit of body structure

cerumen Earwax

chairfast Confined to a chair

chart See *medical record*

chemical restraint Any medication that is used for discipline or convenience and not required to treat medical symptoms

Cheyne-Stokes respirations Respirations gradually increase in rate and depth and then become shallow and slow; breathing may stop (apnea) for 10 to 20 seconds

chronic illness An ongoing illness, slow or gradual in onset; it has no cure; the illness can be controlled and complications prevented with proper treatment

chronic pain Pain that continues for a long time (months or years) or occurs off and on; persistent pain

chronic wound A wound that does not heal easily

circadian rhythm Daily rhythm based on a 24-hour cycle; the day-night cycle or body rhythm

civil law Laws concerned with relationships between people

clean-contaminated wound A wound that occurs from the surgical entry of the reproductive, urinary, respiratory, or gastrointestinal system

clean technique See *medical asepsis*

clean wound A wound that is not infected

cleric A leader or representative from an organized religion (a pastor, priest, or rabbi)

closed fracture The bone is broken but the skin is intact; simple fracture

closed wound Tissues are injured but the skin is not broken

cognitive function Involves memory, thinking, reasoning, ability to understand, judgment, and behavior

colonized The presence of bacteria on the wound surface or in wound tissue; the person does not have signs and symptoms of an infection

colostomy A surgically created opening (*stomy*) between the colon (*colo*) and abdominal wall

coma A state of being unaware of one's surroundings and being unable to react or respond to people, places, or things

comatose Being unable to respond to stimuli

comfort A state of well-being; the person has no physical or emotional pain and is calm and at peace

communicable disease A disease caused by pathogens that spreads easily; contagious disease

communication The exchange of information—a message sent is received and correctly interpreted by the intended person

compound fracture See *open fracture*

comprehensive care plan A written guide about the care a person should receive; developed by the interdisciplinary team (IDT); care plan

compress A soft pad applied over a body area

compulsion Repeating an act over and over again

confidentiality Trusting others with personal and private information

conflict A clash between opposing interests or ideas

constipation The passage of a hard, dry stool

constrict To narrow

contagious disease See *communicable disease*

contaminated wound A wound with a high risk of infection

contamination The process of becoming unclean

contracture The lack of joint mobility caused by abnormal shortening of a muscle

contusion A closed wound caused by a blow to the body; a bruise

convulsion See *seizure*

cotton drawsheet A drawsheet made of cotton; it helps keep the mattress and bottom linens clean

courtesy A polite, considerate, or helpful comment or act

cover letter A letter written with the purpose of obtaining an interview

crime An act that violates a criminal law

criminal law Laws concerned with offenses against the public and society in general

culture The characteristics of a group of people—language, values, beliefs, habits, likes, dislikes, customs—passed from one generation to the next

cyanosis Bluish color to the skin, lips, mucous membranes, and nail beds

cystocele Occurs when the bladder drops down

Daily Value (DV) How a serving fits into the daily diet; expressed in a percentage (%) based on a daily diet of 2000 calories

dandruff Excessive amounts of dry, white flakes from the scalp

deafness Hearing loss in which it is impossible for the person to understand speech through hearing alone

deconditioning The loss of muscle strength from inactivity

deep tissue injury Trauma to the skin and subcutaneous tissue causing rupture of blood vessels; also called bruising

defamation Injuring a person's name and reputation by making false statements to a third person

defecation The process of excreting feces from the rectum through the anus; a bowel movement

defense mechanism An unconscious reaction that blocks unpleasant or threatening feelings

dehiscence The separation of wound layers

dehydration A decrease in the amount of water in body tissues

delegate To authorize another person to perform a nursing task in a certain situation

delirium A state of sudden, severe confusion and rapid brain changes

delusion A false belief

delusion of grandeur An exaggerated belief about one's importance, wealth, power, or talents

delusion of persecution A false belief that one is being mistreated, abused, or harassed

dementia The loss of cognitive and social function caused by changes in the brain

denture An artificial tooth or a set of artificial teeth

development Changes in mental, emotional, and social function

developmental disability (DD) A disability occurring before 22 years of age

developmental task A skill that must be completed during a stage of development

diabetic foot ulcer An open wound on the foot caused by complications from diabetes

diagnosis The term used when symptoms, signs, or reasons for a problem are identified

dialysis The process of removing waste products from the blood

diarrhea The frequent passage of liquid stools

diastole The period of heart muscle relaxation; the heart is at rest

diastolic pressure The pressure in the arteries when the heart is at rest

digestion The process of physically and chemically breaking down food so it can be absorbed for use by the cells

dilate To expand or open wider

diplegia Similar body parts are affected on both sides of the body

dirty wound See *infected wound*

disability Any lost, absent, or impaired physical or mental function

disaster A sudden catastrophic event in which people are injured and killed and property is destroyed

discharge Official departure of a person from a nursing center

discomfort See *pain*

disinfection The process of destroying pathogens

distraction To change the person's center of attention

diuresis The process (*esis*) of passing (*di*) urine (*ur*); large amounts of urine are produced—1000 to 5000 milliliters (mL) a day

dorsal recumbent position See *supine position*

dorsiflexion Bending the toes and foot up at the ankle

drawsheet A small sheet placed over the middle of the bottom sheet

dysphagia Difficulty (*dys*) swallowing (*phagia*)

dyspnea Difficult, labored, or painful (*dys*) breathing (*pnea*)

dysuria Painful or difficult (*dys*) urination (*uria*)

early morning care Care given before breakfast; AM care

edema The swelling of body tissues with water

electric shock When electrical current passes through the body

elevated blood pressure The systolic pressure is 120 to 129 mm Hg and the diastolic pressure is less than 80 mm Hg.

elopement When a person leaves the center without staff knowledge

embolus A blood clot (or other foreign matter) that travels through the vascular system until it lodges in a vessel

emesis See *vomitus*

emotional illness See *mental disorder*

end-of-life care The support and care given during the time surrounding death

enema The introduction of fluid into the rectum and lower colon

enteral nutrition Giving nutrients into the gastrointestinal (GI) tract (*enteral*) through a feeding tube

enuresis Urinary incontinence in bed at night

epidemic A sudden outbreak of disease in a certain geographical area

erectile dysfunction (ED) See *impotence*

ergonomics The science of designing a job to fit the worker

erythema Redness of the skin

eschar Thick, leathery dead tissue that may be loose or adhered to the skin; it is often black or brown

esteem The worth, value, or opinion one has of a person

ethics Knowledge of what is right conduct and wrong conduct

ethnicity A classification of people based on national origin or culture

evaluation To determine if goals in the planning step were met; a step in the nursing process

evening care Care given in the evening at bedtime; PM care

evisceration The separation of the wound along with the protrusion of abdominal organs

expressive aphasia Difficulty expressing or sending out thoughts; motor aphasia, Broca aphasia

expressive-receptive aphasia Difficulty expressing or sending out thoughts and difficulty understanding language; global aphasia, mixed aphasia

extended family A family composed of parents, their children, grandparents, aunts, uncles, and cousins

extension Straightening a body part

external catheter A catheter placed on the outside of the body (male or female) and drains urine to a collection container

external rotation Turning the joint outward

fainting The sudden loss of consciousness from an inadequate blood supply to the brain

false imprisonment Unlawful restraint or restriction of a person's freedom of movement

fast To refrain from consuming food (sometimes food and drink)

fecal impaction The prolonged retention and buildup of feces in the rectum

fecal incontinence The inability to control the passage of feces and gas through the anus

feces The semisolid mass of waste products in the colon that is expelled through the anus

fever Elevated body temperature

first aid Emergency care given to an ill or injured person before medical help arrives

flashback Reliving the trauma in thoughts during the day and in nightmares during sleep

flatulence The excessive formation of gas or air in the stomach and intestines

flatus Gas or air passed through the anus

flexion Bending a body part

flow rate The number of drops per minute (gtt/min)

Foley catheter See *indwelling catheter*

footdrop The foot falls down at the ankle; permanent plantar flexion

Fowler position A semisitting position; the head of the bed is raised between 45 and 60 degrees

fracture A broken bone

fraud Saying or doing something to trick, fool, or deceive a person

freedom of movement Any change in place or position of the body or any part of the body that the person is physically able to control

friction The rubbing of one surface against another

full-thickness wound The dermis, epidermis, and subcutaneous tissue are penetrated; muscle and bone may be involved

full visual privacy Having the means to be completely free from public view while in bed

functional incontinence The person has bladder control but cannot use the toilet in time

gait belt See *transfer belt*

gangrene A condition in which there is death of tissue

gastrostomy tube A tube inserted through a surgically created opening *(stomy)* in the stomach *(gastro)*; stomach tube

gavage The process of giving a tube feeding

genupectoral position See *knee-chest position*

geriatrics The care of aging people

germicide A disinfectant applied to the skin, tissues, or nonliving objects

gerontology The study of the aging process

global aphasia See *expressive-receptive aphasia*

glucosuria Sugar *(glucos)* in the urine *(uria)*; glycosuria

glycosuria Sugar *(glycos)* in the urine *(uria)*; glucosuria

goal That which is desired for or by a person as a result of nursing care

gossip To spread rumors or talk about the private matters of others

graduate A measuring container for fluid

ground That which carries leaking electricity to the earth and away from an electrical item

group home See *board and care home*

growth The physical changes that are measured and that occur in a steady, orderly manner

guided imagery Creating and focusing on an image

hallucination Seeing, hearing, smelling, or feeling something that is not real

harassment To trouble, torment, offend, or worry a person by one's behavior or comments

hazard Anything in the person's setting that may cause injury or illness

hazardous substance Any chemical in the workplace that can cause harm

healthcare-associated infection (HAI) An infection that develops in a person cared for in any setting where health care is given; the infection is related to receiving health care

healthcare provider A medical doctor, doctor of osteopathy, nurse practitioner, or physician assistant

hearing loss Not being able to hear the normal range of sounds associated with normal hearing

heartburn A burning sensation in the chest and sometimes the throat

hematoma A swelling *(oma)* that contains blood *(hemat)*

hematuria Blood *(hemat)* in the urine *(uria)*

hemiplegia Paralysis *(plegia)* on one side *(hemi)* of the body

hemoglobin The substance in red blood cells that carries oxygen and gives blood its color

hemoptysis Bloody *(hemo)* sputum *(ptysis* means "to spit")

hemorrhage The excessive loss of blood in a short time

hemothorax Blood *(hemo)* in the pleural space *(thorax)*

heterosexual A person who is attracted to members of the other sex

high blood pressure See *hypertension*

high-Fowler position A semisitting position; the head of the bed is raised 60 to 90 degrees

hirsutism Excessive body hair

holism A concept that considers the whole person; the whole person has physical, social, psychologic, and spiritual parts that are woven together and cannot be separated

homosexual A person who is attracted to members of the same sex

horizontal recumbent position See *supine position*

hormone A chemical substance secreted by the endocrine glands into the bloodstream

hospice A healthcare agency or program for persons who are terminally ill

hospice care Care that focuses on comfort, and quality of life of a person with a serious illness who is approaching the end of life

HS care See *evening care*

hyperextension Excessive straightening of a body part

hyperglycemia High *(hyper)* sugar *(glyc)* in the blood *(emia)*

hypertension Blood pressure measurements remaining above *(hyper)* a systolic pressure of 140 mm Hg or a diastolic pressure of 90 mm Hg; high blood pressure

hypertension stage 1 The systolic pressure is 130 to 139 mm Hg or the diastolic pressure is 80 to 89 mm Hg.

hypertension stage 2 The systolic pressure is 140 mm Hg or higher or the diastolic pressure is 90 mm Hg or higher.

hypertensive crisis The systolic pressure is higher than 180 mm Hg and/or the diastolic pressure is higher than 120 mm Hg.

hyperthermia A body temperature *(thermia)* that is much higher *(hyper)* than the person's normal range

hyperventilation Respirations *(ventilation)* are rapid *(hyper)* and deeper than normal

hypoglycemia Low *(hypo)* sugar *(glyc)* in the blood *(emia)*

hypotension When the systolic blood pressure is below *(hypo)* 90 mm Hg and the diastolic pressure is below 60 mm Hg

hypothermia A very low *(hypo)* body temperature *(thermia)*

hypoventilation Respirations *(ventilation)* are slow *(hypo)*, shallow, and sometimes irregular

hypoxemia A reduced amount *(hypo)* of oxygen *(ox)* in the blood *(emia)*

hypoxia Cells do not have enough *(hypo)* oxygen *(oxia)*

ileostomy A surgically created opening *(stomy)* between the ileum (small intestine [*ileo*]) and the abdominal wall

immunity Protection against a disease or condition; the person will not get or be affected by the disease

implementation To perform or carry out nursing measures in the care plan; a step in the nursing process

impotence The inability of the male to have an erection; erectile dysfunction

incident Any event that has harmed or could harm a resident, visitor, or staff member

incision A cut produced surgically by a sharp instrument; it creates an opening into an organ or body space

incontinence The inability to control urination or defecation

independence Not relying on or requiring care from others

indwelling catheter A catheter left in the bladder, so urine drains constantly into a drainage bag; retention catheter, Foley catheter

infected wound A wound containing large amounts of microbes that shows signs of infection; dirty wound

infection A disease state resulting from the invasion and growth of microbes in the body

infection control Practices and procedures that prevent the spread of infection

inherited That which is passed down from parents to children

insomnia A chronic condition in which the person cannot sleep or stay asleep all night

intact skin Normal skin without openings or damage

intake The amount of fluid taken in

intellectual disability Involves severe limits in intellectual function and adaptive behavior occurring before age 18

intentional wound A wound created for therapy

interdisciplinary team (IDT) The many health care workers whose skills and knowledge focus on the person's total care; health team

internal rotation Turning the joint inward

intravenous (IV) therapy Giving fluids through a needle or catheter inserted into a vein; IV and IV infusion

intubation Inserting an artificial airway

invasion of privacy Violating a person's right not to have his or her name, photo, or private affairs exposed or made public without giving consent

involuntary seclusion Separating a person from others against his or her will, keeping the person confined to a certain area, or keeping the person away from his or her room without consent

jaundice Yellowish color of the skin or whites of the eyes

jejunostomy tube A feeding tube inserted into a surgically created opening (*stomy*) in the jejunum of the small intestine

job description A document that describes what the center expects an employee to do

Kardex A type of card file that summarizes information found in the medical record—medications, treatments, diagnoses, routine care measures, equipment, and special needs

ketone A substance that appears in urine from the rapid breakdown of fat for energy; acetone, ketone body

ketone body See *ketone*

knee-chest position The person kneels and rests the body on the knees and chest; the head is turned to one side, the arms are above the head or flexed at the elbows, the back is straight, and the body is flexed about 90 degrees at the hips; genupectoral position

Kussmaul respirations Very deep and rapid respirations

laceration An open wound with torn tissues and jagged edges

laryngeal mirror An instrument used to examine the mouth, teeth, and throat

lateral position The person lies on one side or the other; side-lying position

law A rule of conduct made by a government body

left semiprone position A lateral position in which the upper leg (right leg) is sharply flexed so it is not on the lower leg (left leg) and the lower arm (left arm) is behind the person. Used for rectal procedures.

libel Making false statements in print, writing, or through pictures or drawings

lice See *pediculosis*

licensed practical nurse (LPN) A nurse who has completed a 1-year nursing program and has passed a licensing test; called licensed vocational nurse (LVN) in some states

licensed vocational nurse (LVN) See *licensed practical nurse*

lithotomy position The woman lies on her back with her hips at the edge of the exam table; her knees are flexed, her hips are externally rotated, and her feet are in stirrups

logrolling Turning the person as a unit, in alignment, with one motion

low vision Eyesight that cannot be corrected with eyeglasses, contact lenses, medications, or surgery

malignant tumor A tumor that invades and destroys nearby tissue and can spread to other body parts; cancer

malpractice Negligence by a professional person

mastectomy The surgical removal of a breast

mechanical ventilation Using a machine to move air into and out of the lungs

Medicaid A healthcare payment program sponsored by the federal government and operated by the states

medical asepsis Practices used to remove or destroy pathogens and to prevent their spread from one person or place to another person or place; clean technique

medical diagnosis The identification of a disease or condition by a doctor

medical record A written or electronic document of a person's condition and response to treatment and care; often referred to as a chart or clinical record

medical symptom An indication or characteristic of a physical or psychologic condition

Medicare A federal health insurance program for persons 65 years of age or older and younger people with certain disabilities

medication reminder Reminding the person to take medications, observing them being taken as prescribed, and charting that they were taken

melena A black, tarry stool

menopause When menstruation stops and there has been at least 1 year without a menstrual period

menstruation The process in which the lining of the uterus breaks up and is discharged from the body through the vagina

mental Relating to the mind; something that exists in the mind or is done by the mind

mental disorder A disturbance in the ability to cope with or adjust to stress; behavior and function are impaired; mental illness, emotional illness, psychiatric disorder

mental health The person copes with and adjusts to everyday stresses in ways accepted by society

mental illness See *mental disorder*

metabolism The burning of food for heat and energy by the cells

metastasis The spread of cancer to other body parts

microbe See *microorganism*

microorganism A small (*micro*) living plant or animal (*organism*) seen only with a microscope; microbe

micturition See *urination*

mite A very small, spiderlike organism

mixed aphasia See *expressive-receptive aphasia*

mixed incontinence The combination of stress incontinence and urge incontinence

morning care Care given after breakfast; hygiene measures are more thorough at this time

motor aphasia See *expressive aphasia*

nasal speculum An instrument used to examine the inside of the nose

nasoenteral tube A feeding tube inserted through the nose (*naso*) into the small bowel (*enteral*)

nasogastric (NG) tube A feeding tube inserted through the nose (*naso*) into the stomach (*gastro*)

natal sex A person's genital anatomy that is present at birth

need Something necessary or desired for maintaining life and mental well-being

neglect Failure to provide the person with the goods or services needed to avoid physical harm, mental anguish, or mental illness

negligence An unintentional wrong in which a person did not act in a reasonable and careful manner and a person or the person's property was harmed

nocturia Frequent urination (*uria*) at night (*noct*)

nonpathogen A microbe that does not usually cause an infection

nonverbal communication Communication that does not use words

normal flora Microbes that live and grow in a certain area

norovirus A very contagious virus that causes vomiting and diarrhea

NREM sleep The phase of sleep when there is no rapid eye movement; non-REM sleep

nuclear family   A family consisting of parents and their children

nurse practitioner (NP)   a registered nurse (RN) who has completed graduate education at the master's or doctoral level and has obtained national board certification

nursing assistant   A person who gives basic nursing care under the supervision of a licensed nurse; nurse aide, nursing attendant, and health care assistant are some other titles

nursing center   Provides health care and nursing care to persons who need regular or continuous care; licensed nurses are required; nursing facility, nursing home

nursing diagnosis   Describes a health problem that can be treated by nursing measures; a step in the nursing process

nursing facility (NF)   See *nursing center*

nursing home   See *nursing center*

nursing intervention   An action or measure taken by the nursing team to help the person reach a goal

nursing process   The method nurses use to plan and deliver nursing care; its five steps are assessment, nursing diagnosis, planning, implementation, and evaluation

nursing task   Nursing care or a nursing function, procedure, activity, or work that can be delegated to nursing assistants when it does not require an RN's professional knowledge or judgment

nursing team   Those who provide nursing care—registered nurses (RNs), licensed practical nurses/licensed vocational nurses (LPNs/LVNs), and nursing assistants

nutrient   A substance that is ingested, digested, absorbed, and used by the body

nutrition   The processes involved in the ingestion, digestion, absorption, and use of foods and fluids by the body

objective data   Information that is seen, heard, felt, or smelled by an observer; signs

observation   Using the senses of sight, hearing, touch, and smell to collect information

obsession   A recurrent, unwanted thought, idea, or image

oliguria   Scant amount (*olig*) of urine (*uria*); less than 500 mL in 24 hours

ombudsman   Someone who supports or promotes the needs and interests of another person

open fracture   The broken bone has come through the skin; compound fracture

open wound   The skin or mucous membrane is broken

ophthalmoscope   A lighted instrument used to examine the internal eye structures

optimal level of function   A person's highest potential for mental and physical performance

oral hygiene   Mouth care

organ   Groups of tissues with the same function

orthopnea   Breathing (*pnea*) deeply and comfortably only when sitting (*ortho*)

orthopneic position   Sitting up (*ortho*) and leaning over a table to breathe (*pneic*)

orthostatic hypotension   Abnormally low (*hypo*) blood pressure when the person suddenly stands up (*ortho* and *static*); postural hypotension

ostomy   A surgically created opening for the elimination of body wastes; see *colostomy* and *ileostomy*

otoscope   A lighted instrument used to examine the external ear and the eardrum (tympanic membrane)

output   The amount of fluid lost

overflow incontinence   Small amounts of urine leak from a full bladder

oxygen concentration   The amount (percentage) of hemoglobin containing oxygen

pack   Wrapping a body part with a wet or dry application

pain   To ache, hurt, or be sore; discomfort

palliative care   Care that involves relieving or reducing the intensity of uncomfortable symptoms without producing a cure

pandemic   An outbreak of disease that spreads easily and extends across several countries or continents

panic   An intense and sudden feeling of fear, anxiety, terror, or dread

paralysis   Loss of muscle function, loss of sensation, or loss of both muscle function and sensation

paranoia   A disorder (*para*) of the mind (*noia*); false beliefs (delusions) and suspicion about a person or situation

paraphrasing   Restating the person's message in your own words

paraplegia   Paralysis in the legs and lower trunk

parenteral nutrition   Giving nutrients through a catheter inserted into a vein; *para* means "beyond"; *enteral* relates to the bowel

partial-thickness wound   The dermis and epidermis of the skin are broken

patent   Open and unblocked

pathogen   A microbe that is harmful and can cause an infection

pediculosis   Infestation with wingless insects; lice

pediculosis capitis   Infestation of the scalp (*capitis*) with lice; head lice

pediculosis corporis   Infestation of the body (*corporis*) with lice

pediculosis pubis   Infestation of the pubic (*pubis*) hair with lice

penetrating wound   An open wound that breaks the skin and enters a body area, organ, or cavity

percussion hammer   An instrument used to tap body parts to test reflexes; reflex hammer

percutaneous endoscopic gastrostomy (PEG) tube   A feeding tube inserted into the stomach (*gastro*) through a small incision (*stomy*) made through (*per*) the skin (*cutaneous*); a lighted instrument (*scope*) is used to see inside a body cavity or organ (*endo*)

pericare   See *perineal care*

perineal care   Cleaning the genital and anal areas; pericare

peristalsis   Involuntary muscle contractions in the digestive system that move food down the esophagus through the alimentary canal

persistent pain   See *chronic pain*

personal space   The distance that people require to comfortably communicate

phantom pain   Pain felt in a body part that is no longer there

phlebitis   Inflammation (*itis*) of a vein (*phleb*)

phobia   An intense fear

physical restraint   Any manual method or physical or mechanical device, material, or equipment attached to or near the person's body that he or she cannot remove easily and that restricts freedom of movement or normal access to one's body

physician assistant (PA)   A medical professional who may diagnose, treat, and prescribe medication for patients. They often work together with other healthcare providers

planning   Setting priorities and goals; a step in the nursing process

plantar flexion   The foot (*plantar*) is bent (*flexion*); bending the foot down at the ankle

plaque   A thin film that sticks to the teeth; it contains saliva, microbes, and other substances

pleural effusion   The escape and collection of fluid (*effusion*) in the pleural space

PM care   See *evening care*

pneumothorax   Air (*pneumo*) in the pleural space (*thorax*)

podiatrist   A medical professional who treats disorders of the foot, ankle, and related structures of the leg

pollutant   A harmful chemical or substance in the air or water

polyuria   Abnormally large amounts (*poly*) of urine (*uria*)

port   An implanted device in the body that allows medications or fluids to be given into a vein; blood can also be withdrawn if needed

postmortem care   Care of the body after (*post*) death (*mortem*)

postural hypotension   See *orthostatic hypotension*

posture   See *body alignment*

preceptor   A staff member who guides another staff member; mentor

prefix   A word element placed before a root; it changes the meaning of the word

prehypertension   When the systolic pressure is between 120 and 139 mm Hg or the diastolic pressure is between 80 and 89 mm Hg

prejudice   Forming an opinion without having facts or information

presbyopia   Age-related (*presby*) farsightedness (*opia* means "eye")

pressure injury   Localized damage to the skin and/or underlying soft tissue, usually over a bony prominence or related to a medical or other device. The injury can present as intact skin or an open ulcer and may be painful. Injury occurs as a result of intense and/or prolonged pressure or pressure in combination with shear

priority   The most important thing at the time

professional boundary   That which separates helpful behaviors from behaviors that are not helpful

professional sexual misconduct   An act, behavior, or comment that is sexual in nature

professionalism   Following laws, being ethical, having good work ethics, and having the skills to do the work

progress note A written description of the care given and the person's response and progress

pronation Turning the joint downward

prone position Lying on the abdomen with the head turned to one side

prosthesis An artificial replacement for a missing body part

protected health information Identifying information and information about the person's health care that is maintained or sent in any form (paper, electronic, oral)

pseudodementia False (*pseudo*) dementia

psychiatric disorder See *mental disorder*

psychosis A state of severe mental impairment

pulse The beat of the heart felt at an artery as a wave of blood passes through the artery

pulse deficit The difference between the apical and radial pulse rates

pulse rate The number of heartbeats or pulses felt in 1 minute

puncture wound An open wound made by a sharp object

purulent drainage Thick green, yellow, or brown drainage

pyuria Pus (*py*) in the urine (*uria*)

quadriplegia Paralysis in the arms, legs, and trunk; tetraplegia

race A classification of persons based on physical and biologic characteristics

radiating pain Pain felt at the site of tissue damage and in nearby areas

range of motion (ROM) The movement of a joint to the extent possible without causing pain

receptive aphasia Difficulty understanding language; Wernicke aphasia

recording The written account of care and observations; charting

rectocele Occurs when the rectum shifts downward

reflex incontinence Urine is lost at predictable intervals when the bladder is full

registered nurse (RN) A nurse who has completed a 2-, 3-, or 4-year nursing program and has passed a licensing test

regurgitation The backward flow of stomach contents into the mouth

rehabilitation The process of restoring the person to his or her highest possible level of physical, psychologic, social, and economic function

reincarnation The belief that the spirit or soul is reborn in another human body or in another form of life

relaxation To be free from mental and physical stress

religion Spiritual beliefs, needs, and practices

REM sleep The phase of sleep when there is rapid eye movement

remove easily The manual method, device, material, or equipment used to restrain the person that can be removed intentionally by the person in the same manner it was applied by the staff

reporting The oral account of care and observations

representative Any person who has the legal right to act on the resident's behalf when he or she cannot do so for oneself

reservoir The environment in which a microbe lives and grows; host

Resident Assessment Instrument (RAI) Helps staff to gather information on a resident's strengths and needs, which must be addressed in an individualized care plan

Resident Assessment Protocols (RAP) identify social, medical, and psychological problems and form the basis for individualized care planning

resident unit The personal space, furniture, and equipment provided for the person by the nursing center

respiration The process of supplying the cells with oxygen and removing carbon dioxide from them

respiratory arrest When breathing stops but heart action continues for several minutes

respiratory depression Slow, weak respirations at a rate of fewer than 12 per minute

responsibility The duty or obligation to perform some act or function

rest To be calm, at ease, and relaxed; no anxiety or stress

restorative aide A nursing assistant with special training in restorative nursing and rehabilitation skills

restorative nursing care Care that helps persons regain health, strength, and independence

résumé A summary of personal information

retention catheter See *indwelling catheter*

reverse Trendelenburg position The head of the bed is raised and the foot of the bed is lowered

rigor mortis The stiffness or rigidity (*rigor*) of skeletal muscles that occurs after death (*mortis*)

root A word element that contains the basic meaning of the word

rotation Turning the joint

sanguineous drainage Bloody (*sanguis*) drainage

seizure Violent and sudden contractions or tremors of muscle groups; convulsion

self-actualization Experiencing one's potential

self-esteem Thinking well of oneself and seeing oneself as useful and having value

self-neglect A person's behaviors that threaten his or her health and safety

semi-Fowler position The head of the bed is raised 30 degrees; or the head of the bed is raised 30 degrees and the knee portion is raised 15 degrees

semiprone side position See *Sims position*

sensitivity The ability to appreciate the personal characteristics of others

serosanguineous drainage Thin, watery drainage (*sero*) that is blood tinged (*sanguineous*)

serous drainage Clear, watery fluid (*serum*)

service plan A written plan listing the services needed by the person, how much help is needed, and who provides the services

sex Physical activities involving the reproductive organs; done for pleasure or to have children

sexuality The physical, emotional, social, cultural, and spiritual factors that affect a person's feelings and attitudes about his or her sex

shear When layers of the skin rub against each other; when the skin remains in place and underlying tissues move and stretch and tear underlying capillaries and blood vessels, causing tissue damage

shearing When skin sticks to a surface while muscles slide in the direction the body is moving

shock Results when organs and tissues do not get enough blood

side-lying position See *lateral position*

signs See *objective data*

simple fracture See *closed fracture*

skilled care Daily services provided by a registered nurse (RN) and/or therapist for rehabilitation or other complex services; provided in nursing centers for short periods of time

skilled nursing facility (SNF) Provides health care and nursing care for residents who have many or severe health problems or who need rehabilitation; may be part of a nursing center or a hospital

skin tear A break or rip in the outer layers of the skin; the epidermis (top skin layer) separates from the underlying tissues

slander Making false statements orally

sleep A state of unconsciousness, reduced voluntary muscle activity, and lowered metabolism

slough Dead tissue that is soft, often moist, and appears white, yellow, green, or tan; it may be firmly attached or loose and stringy

spastic Uncontrolled contractions of skeletal muscles

sphygmomanometer A cuff and measuring device used to measure blood pressure

spirituality A person's need to find meaning and purpose in life

spore A bacterium protected by a hard shell

sputum Mucus from the respiratory system that is expectorated (expelled) through the mouth

standard of care The skills, care, and judgments required by a health team member under similar conditions

stasis ulcer See *venous ulcer*

stem cells Cells with the potential to develop into many different types of cells in the body

stereotyping Believing that everyone in a group is the same

sterile The absence of all microbes

sterile field A work area free of all pathogens and nonpathogens (including spores)

sterile technique See *surgical asepsis*

sterilization The process of destroying all microbes

stethoscope An instrument used to listen to sounds produced by the heart, lungs, and other body organs

stigma A feeling of shame or judgment from someone else

stoma An opening that can be seen through the abdominal wall; see *colostomy* and *ileostomy*

stomatitis Inflammation (*itis*) of the mouth (*stomat*)

stool Excreted feces

straight catheter A catheter that drains the bladder and then is removed

stress The response or change in the body caused by any emotional, physical, social, or economic factor

stress incontinence When urine leaks during exercise and certain movements that cause pressure on the bladder

stressor The event or factor that causes stress

subjective data Things a person tells you about that you cannot observe through your senses; symptoms

suction The process of withdrawing or sucking up fluid (secretions)

sudden cardiac arrest (SCA) The heart stops suddenly and without warning; cardiac arrest

suffix A word element placed after a root; it changes the meaning of the word

suffocation When breathing stops from the lack of oxygen

suicide To kill oneself

suicide contagion Exposure to suicide or suicidal behaviors within one's family, one's peer group, or media reports of suicide

sundowning Signs, symptoms, and behaviors of Alzheimer disease (AD) increase during hours of darkness

supination Turning the joint upward

supine position The back-lying position; dorsal recumbent position, horizontal recumbent position

suppository A cone-shaped, solid medication that is inserted into a body opening; it melts at body temperature

suprapubic Above (supra) the pubic bone (pubic)

surgical asepsis The practices that keep items free of all microbes; sterile technique

symptoms See subjective data

syncope A brief loss of consciousness; fainting

system Organs that work together to perform special functions

systole The period of heart muscle contraction; the heart is pumping blood

systolic pressure The pressure in the arteries when the heart contracts

tachycardia A rapid (tachy) heart rate (cardia); more than 100 beats per minute

tachypnea Rapid (tachy) breathing (pnea); respirations are more than 20 per minute

tartar Hardened plaque

terminal illness An illness or injury from which the person will not likely recover

tetraplegia See quadriplegia

thrombus A blood clot

tinnitus A ringing, roaring, hissing, or buzzing sound in the ears or head

tissue A group of cells with similar functions

tort A wrong committed against a person or the person's property

tracheostomy A surgically created opening (stomy) into the trachea (tracheo)

transfer Moving the person to another health care setting; moving the person to a new room within the center

transfer belt A device used to support a person who is unsteady or disabled; gait belt

transgender A broad term used to describe people who express their sexuality or gender in other than the expected ways; persons who are undergoing hormone therapy or surgery for sexual reassignment (female to male; male to female)

transient incontinence Temporary or occasional incontinence that is reversed when the cause is treated

trauma An accident or violent act that injures the skin, mucous membranes, bones, and organs

treatment The care provided to maintain or restore health, improve function, or relieve symptoms

Trendelenburg position The head of the bed is lowered and the foot of the bed is raised

triggers Information that is collected from the minimum data set (MDS) for the care area assessments (CAAs)

tumor A new growth of abnormal cells; tumors are benign or malignant

tuning fork An instrument vibrated to test hearing

ulcer A shallow or deep craterlike sore of the skin or a mucous membrane

unavoidable pressure injury A pressure injury that occurs despite efforts to prevent one through proper use of the nursing process

unintentional wound A wound resulting from trauma

urge incontinence The loss of urine in response to a sudden, urgent need to void; the person cannot get to a toilet in time

urinary diversion A new pathway for urine to exit the body

urinary frequency Voiding at frequent intervals

urinary incontinence The involuntary loss or leakage of urine

urinary urgency The need to void at once

urination The process of emptying urine from the bladder; micturition, voiding

urostomy A surgically created opening (stomy) between a ureter (uro) and the abdomen

uterine prolapse Occurs when the uterus shifts downward into the vaginal canal

utilization Putting planned care into action in an efficient manner

vaccination Giving a vaccine to produce immunity against an infectious disease

vaccine A preparation containing dead or weakened microbes

vaginal speculum An instrument used to open the vagina for examining it and the cervix

vascular ulcer An open sore on the lower legs or feet caused by decreased blood flow through the arteries or veins

vein A blood vessel that returns blood to the heart

venous ulcer An open sore on the lower legs or feet caused by poor venous blood flow; stasis ulcer

verbal communication Communication that uses written or spoken words

vertigo Dizziness

vital signs Temperature, pulse, respirations, and blood pressure

voiding See urination

vomitus Food and fluids expelled from the stomach through the mouth; emesis

vulnerable adult A person 18 years old or older who has a disability or condition that puts him or her at risk to be wounded, attacked, or damaged

waterproof drawsheet A drawsheet made of plastic, rubber, or absorbent material used to protect the mattress and bottom linens from dampness and soiling

Wernicke aphasia See receptive aphasia

will A legal document of how a person wants property distributed after death

withdrawal syndrome The person's physical and mental response after stopping or severely reducing the use of a substance that was used regularly

word element A part of a word

work ethics Behavior in the workplace

workplace violence Violent acts (including assault and threat of assault) directed toward persons at work or while on duty

wound A break in the skin or mucous membrane

ABHR:	Alcohol-based hand rub
ACS:	American College of Surgeons
AD:	Alzheimer disease
ADA:	Americans With Disabilities Act of 1990
ADL:	Activities of daily living
AED:	Automated external defibrillator
AFB:	American Foundation for the Blind
AHA:	American Heart Association
AIDS:	Acquired immunodeficiency syndrome
AIIR:	Airborne infection isolation room
AKA:	Above-the-knee amputation
ALR:	Assisted living residence
ALS:	Amyotrophic lateral sclerosis
AMD:	Age-related macular degeneration
ARNP:	Advanced registered nurse practitioner
ASD:	Autism spectrum disorder
ASL:	American Sign Language
BKA:	Below-the-knee amputation
BLS:	Basic Life Support
BM:	Bowel movement
BP:	Blood pressure
BPD:	Borderline personality disorder
BPH:	Benign prostatic hyperplasia
C:	Centigrade
CAA:	Care area assessment
CAD:	Coronary artery disease
CAUTI:	Catheter-associated urinary tract infection
CCRC:	Continuing care retirement community
CDC:	Centers for Disease Control and Prevention
C. diff:	Clostridium difficile
cm:	Centimeter
CMS:	Centers for Medicare & Medicaid Services
CNA:	Certified nursing assistant; certified nurse aide
CO2:	Carbon dioxide
COPD:	Chronic obstructive pulmonary disease
COVID-19:	Coronavirus disease 2019
CP:	Cerebral palsy
CPAP:	Continuous positive airway pressure
CPR:	Cardiopulmonary resuscitation
CVA:	Cerebrovascular accident
DD:	Developmental disability
DNR:	Do not resuscitate
DON:	Director of nursing
DS:	Down syndrome
DV:	Daily value
ED:	Erectile dysfunction
EHR:	Electronic health record
EMR:	Electronic medical record
EMS:	Emergency Medical Services
EPHI:	Electronic protected health information
ET:	Endotracheal
F:	Fahrenheit
FAST:	Facial drooping, Arm weakness, Speech difficulty, Time to call EMS
FBAO:	Foreign-body airway obstruction
FDA:	Food and Drug Administration
FXS:	Fragile X syndrome
GDS:	Global deterioration scale
GERD:	Gastroesophageal reflux disease
GI:	Gastrointestinal
gtt:	Drops
gtt/min:	Drops per minute
HAI:	Healthcare-associated infection
HBV:	Hepatitis B virus
Hg:	Mercury
HIPAA:	Health Insurance Portability and Accountability Act of 1996
HIV:	Human immunodeficiency virus
HMO:	Health maintenance organization
HOH:	Hard of hearing
HS:	Hour of sleep
IBD:	Inflammatory bowel disease
ID:	Identification
IDD:	Intellectual and developmental disability
IDDSI:	International Dysphagia Diet Standardisation Initiative
IDT:	Interdisciplinary team
I&O:	Intake and output
IQ:	Intelligence quotient
IV:	Intravenous
kg:	Kilogram
lb:	Pound
LGBTQ+:	Lesbian, gay, bisexual, transgender, queer, or questioning community
L/min:	Liters per minute
LNA:	Licensed nursing assistant
LPN:	Licensed practical nurse
LVN:	Licensed vocational nurse
MCI:	Mild cognitive impairment
MDRO:	Multidrug-resistant organism
MDRPI:	Medical device-related pressure injuries
MDS:	Minimum Data Set
mg:	Milligram
MI:	Myocardial infarction
mL:	Milliliter
mm:	Millimeter
mm Hg:	Millimeters of mercury
MRSA:	Methicillin-resistant Staphylococcus aureus
MS:	Multiple sclerosis

MSD: Musculoskeletal disorder
NAMI: National Alliance on Mental Illness
NATCEP: Nursing assistant training and
            competency evaluation program
NCSBN: National Council of State Boards of
            Nursing
NDD: National Dysphagia Diet
NG: Nasogastric
NIA: National Institute on Aging
NIAAA: National Institute on Alcohol Abuse
            and Alcoholism
NIMH: National Institute of Mental Health
NIOSH: National Institute for Occupational
            Safety and Health
NOAA   National Oceanic and Atmospheric
            Association
NP: Nurse practitioner
NPIAP: National Pressure Injury Advisory Panel
NPO: Non per os; nothing by mouth
NREM: Nonrapid eye movement
O2:   Oxygen
OBRA: Omnibus Budget Reconciliation Act of
            1987
OCD: Obsessive-compulsive disorder
OPIM: Other potentially infectious materials
OSHA: Occupational Safety and Health
            Administration
OT: Occupational therapy
oz: Ounce
PA: Physician assistant
PASS: Pull the safety pin, aim low, squeeze the
            lever, sweep back and forth
PEG: Percutaneous endoscopic gastrostomy
PHE: Public Health Emergency
PHI: Protected health information
PICC: Peripherally inserted central catheter
POC: Point of care
POLST: Physician Orders for Life-Sustaining
            Treatment
PPE: Personal protective equipment
PPO: Preferred provider organization
PT: Physical therapy

PTSD: Posttraumatic stress disorder
RA: Rheumatoid arthritis
RACE: Rescue, Alarm, Confine, Extinguish
RAI: Resident Assessment Instrument
RAP: Resident Assessment Protocols
RBC: Red blood cell
REM: Rapid eye movement
RN: Registered nurse
RNA: Registered nurse aide
ROM: Range of motion
SARS: Severe acute respiratory syndrome
SB: Spina bifida
SCA: Sudden cardiac arrest
SDS: Safety Data Sheet
SNF: Skilled nursing facility
SpO2:   Saturation of peripheral oxygen (pulse
            oximetry)
SSE: Soapsuds enema
STD: Sexually transmitted disease
STI: Sexually transmitted infection
STNA: State-tested nursing assistant
SUD: Substance use disorder
TB: Tuberculosis
TBI: Traumatic brain injury
TENS: Transcutaneous electrical nerve
            stimulation
TIA: Transient ischemic attack
TJC: The Joint Commission
TPN: Total parenteral nutrition
TPR: Temperature, pulse, and respiration
TURP: Transurethral resection of the prostate
TWE: Tapwater enema
UAP: Unlicensed assistive personnel
USDA: United States Department of
            Agriculture
UTI: Urinary tract infection
VF: Ventricular fibrillation
V-fib: Ventricular fibrillation
VRE: Vancomycin-resistant Enterococcus
WBC: White blood cell
WHO: World Health Organization

Note: Page numbers followed by *f* indicate figures and *t* indicate tables.